Guy's Hospital 1994 Nursing Drug Reference

Edited by Anne Joshua, BPharm, DipClinPharm, MRPharmS
and Theo King, RN
With a team of Pharmacists and Nurses
from Guy's Hospital

Second Edition

Published by
Mosby–Year Book Europe Ltd
Lynton House
7–12 Tavistock Square
London WC1H 9LB

ISBN 0 7234 1896 9
ISSN 1350-5246
First edition published in 1993 by Mosby Year–Book Ltd

For full details of all Mosby–Year Book Europe Ltd titles please write to Mosby–Year Book Europe Ltd, Lynton House, 7–12 Tavistock Square, London WC1H 9LB, England.

A CIP record for this book is available from the British Library.

This book is based on an original work by Linda Skidmore-Roth, RN, MSN, NP published in the USA on an annual basis by Mosby–Year Book as *Mosby's Nursing Drug Reference*.

Printed and bound in Great Britain by The Bath Press, Avon

A note to the reader:

This book is intended to help nurses and midwives understand drug protocols and the management of patients under given drug regimens. This book should not be used as a prime source for prescribing and dispensing drugs. Guy's Hospital, the Editors, Contributors and the Publisher have undertaken reasonable endeavours to check dosage and nursing content for accuracy. Because the science of clinical pharmacology is continually advancing, our knowledge base continues to expand. Therefore, we recommend that the reader should always check the manufacturer's product information for changes in dosage or administration before administering any medication. This is particularly important with new or rarely used drugs.

Contents

Foreword

There are a number of excellent reference books on drugs in use in the UK, but all have been produced primarily with the clinician and pharmacist in mind, and there has been a lack of information tailored to the needs of nurses and midwives.

With the development of the professional role of the nurse, this gap has become more apparent. We therefore welcome the opportunity to contribute to the preparation and publication of a UK version of *Mosby's Nursing Drug Reference*, which has been in use in the USA for some years.

The unique feature of this book is the inclusion of 'Nursing Considerations' in each monograph, giving practical information of value to nurses and midwives when administering drugs and observing their actions, and in the contact with patients, their families or carers. This second edition includes more than 90 new drug monographs, and new appendixes on wound care products and UKCC standards for administering medicines.

Roger W. Horne, *Director of Pharmacy*
Wilma MacPherson, *Director of Nursing*
Guy's Hospital
December 1993

Editors' preface

In 1983 the Lewisham and North Southwark District Formulary Committee for Guy's and Lewisham Hospitals issued its first *District Formulary*, following the introduction two years earlier of a new type of *British National Formulary (BNF)* by the Joint Formulary Committee of the British Medical Association and the Royal Pharmaceutical Society of Great Britain (formerly the Pharmaceutical Society of Great Britain).

Both publications were intended as pocket book references for those health professionals concerned with the prescribing, dispensing and administration of medicines. Guy's, Lewisham and St. Thomas' Hospitals also produce a joint prescribing guide for paediatric medicines.

The *1994 Nursing Drug Reference* from Guy's Hospital has been designed to provide advice and drug information for the nurse and midwife consistent with the nursing process, and as such is a unique development not addressed by these previous publications. The intention is to produce a new edition every year so that the most up-to-date information on new and existing drugs is available to nurses and midwives.

Anne Joshua, BPharm, DipClinPharm, MRPharmS
Theo King, RN

Introduction

Who should use this book?

This book has been produced to provide a quick reference to essential drug information. It is intended for use in the clinical situation by the practising nurse, midwife or student. The guiding principle is to give the reader easy access to drug information and to highlight the nursing considerations relating to medication which assist in the nursing process.

Why use this book?

This reference is an annual publication which gives nurses and midwives accessible, up-to-date drug information. Perhaps more importantly, this book equips nurses and midwives to plan and improve care for patients/clients by assisting them in evaluating the patients'/clients' response to medication and in communicating with patients/clients and their carers.

When nurse prescribing is introduced in the UK, the specially trained nurse should be able to prescribe from a nurse's formulary according to certain criteria. Therefore, nurses should be aware of, and have easy access to, current information on the dosage, use and administration of these drugs.

The *Nursing Drug Reference* has been prepared by a team of nurses, midwives and pharmacists from various clinical specialities within the hospital and community care settings. The information is based on their clinical and pharmacological knowledge, confirmed by reference to the *British National Formulary*, Manufacturer's Product Data Sheets, *Martindale*, 30th edition and other sources listed in the bibliography.

About the drugs included in this book

This reference includes the most current information on existing and new drugs. Although this book is a comprehensive reference, the medications included have been selected according to the following criteria:

- Drugs primarily used in adult medicine. Where appropriate, doses for children have been included.
- All the drugs are available in the UK. Currently, some preparations available in other European countries are not routinely available in the UK, and vice versa. Although the centralised control and licensing of drugs for Europe is still a few years away, this will eventually affect the choice of drugs available to be prescribed and the way in which they will be monitored.
- The uses stated in each monograph in this book are those for which the drug is licensed in the UK. Some drugs and preparations may be prescribed for use in circumstances outside the product licence. In

these cases, the principal responsibility rests with the prescriber, but in practice there is a duty of care on both the pharmacist and the nurse or midwife.
- The restrictions on prescribing do not apply to the supply and administration of certain medicinal products by a certified midwife in the course of professional practice. These products are specifically related to their use for procedures in childbirth. *See* Appendix 1.

The information contained in each monograph should not be used in isolation. Multiple drug therapies and disease states will affect the patient's drug handling capacity and response to treatment. Each patient should be evaluated according to his or her own individual needs. A team approach with prescriber, pharmacist, patient and nurse should ensure that the patient receives the optimum therapy for his or her condition.

Always check the manufacturer's product information for any changes in dosage or administration before administering any medication. The local treatment protocol and the local pharmacy are useful additional sources of information which should be consulted.

Every attempt has been made to present this information in a consistent format; however, some drugs within the same therapeutic group may differ in the presentation of the information.

How to read the drug monographs

A combination of pharmacological and nursing care information is provided in each drug monograph; however, not every monograph requires or includes all of the information listed in the sample monograph below. It is assumed that good basic nursing care is provided by nurses to all patients, but there is minimal reiteration of general nursing points. Reminders are given only where it is helpful to the reader. Readers are advised to study the **entire monograph** and not just the nursing section, because details of dosage are given in the pharmacological section and are not repeated in the nursing section.

The drugs are listed in alphabetical order by generic name. The prefix 'co' indicates that the medication is a compound preparation.

▼ beside the generic name of some newer drugs means the prescriber must report all suspected reactions to the Committee on Safety of Medicines (CSM), i.e., to report any adverse or unexpected event, however minor, which could conceivably be attributed to the drug. The nurse is often the first carer to be alerted to an adverse event.

~~NHS~~ means the drug is not available on NHS prescription. It may be possible for certain individuals to obtain these black-listed preparations on NHS prescription in special circumstances.

captopril

Capoten, Acepril, combination product
Func. class: Antihypertensive
Chem. class: Angiotensin converting enzyme inhibitor
Legal class: POM

Action: Selectively suppresses renin angiotensin-aldosterone system; inhibits angiotensin converting enzyme, prevents conversion of angiotensin I to angiotensin II, reducing vasoconstriction
Uses: Mild to moderate hypertension, first-line treatment alone or with thiazide; severe resistant hypertension, where standard therapy is ineffective; adjunctive treatment of congestive heart failure with diuretics and digitalis where appropriate

The most commonly used proprietary or trade name(s). These are the brand names of specific drugs. The statement 'combination product' or 'many combination products' is included where there are one or more combination products of the drugs available.

Functional and chemical classification includes all known broad functional and chemical classifications. The functional classes enable you to recognise similarities between drugs or other drugs in the same functional class, but which are different chemically.

Legal class symbols indicate restrictions which apply to the prescribing, dispensing and storage of such medicines:
GSL – General Sales List Medicine
P – Pharmacy Medicine
POM – Prescription Only Medicine
CD – Controlled Drug subject to the prescription requirements of the Misuse of Drugs Act 1971.*

Action describes the pharmacological action and mechanism of the drug.

Uses sets out the purpose for which the drug has been granted a UK product licence.

*Controlled drugs are listed under five schedules of the Misuse of Drugs Regulations (1985). There are mandatory requirements that cover ordering, storage, and recording of these drugs by the nurse or midwife. Of these, the most important are Schedule 2 drugs, CD(Sch2)POM, e.g. diamorphine injection. For further details see: Pearce, M.S. (1984) **Medicines and Poisons Guide,** 4th edn, Sect. 1.9: The Pharmaceutical Press, or **Medicines, Ethics and Practice,** (1993), No. 11, October: Royal Pharmaceutical Society of Great Britain.

Dosage and routes:
Diuretics should be stopped if possible for 2–3 days before starting treatment to minimise the risk of a rapid fall of blood pressure and hypotension
Hypertension
• *Adult:* Initial dose alone, 12.5 mg twice daily; with thiazide, in elderly or in renal impairment, initially 6.25 mg twice daily; maintenance 25–50 mg twice daily, maximum 50 mg twice daily (rarely 3 times daily in severe hypertension)
Congestive heart failure
• *Adult:* By mouth with thiazide, initially 6.25–12.5 mg 2–3 times daily under supervision in hospital, maintenance 25 mg 3 times daily (maximum 50 mg 3 times daily)
Available forms include: Tablets 12.5 mg, 25 mg, 50 mg
Side effects/adverse reactions:
CV: Tachycardia, hypotension
GU: Dysuria, nocturia, proteinuria, nephrotic syndrome, acute reversible renal failure, polyuria, oliguria, urinary frequency
HAEM: Neutropenia, anaemia, thrombocytopenia, hyperkalaemia
INTEG: Rash, pruritus, photosensitivity
RESP: Bronchospasm, cough
CNS: Paraesthesia of hands
MISC: Angioedema of face, lips, mucous membranes, tongue and extremeties
Contraindictations: Hypersensitivity, pregnancy, breast–feeding, aortic stenosis, outflow obstruction, or renovascular disease, porphyria
Precautions: Dialysis patients, hypovolaemia, leukaemia, blood dyscrasias, congestive cardiac failure, renal disease, diuretics with first dose may cause hypotension, hypotension with low sodium diet, dialysis or dehydration
Pharmacokinetics:
Period of Onset: Peak 1 hr duration 2-6 hr; half-life 6-7 hr, metabolised by liver, metabolites, excreted in urine; crosses placenta, excreted in breast milk.

Dosages and routes are given for adults and children according to the UK product licence. Some of the doses shown may differ from those in current medical practice. Where differences occur, the reader should seek specialist advice, including the Manufacturer's Product Data Sheet.

All available forms are included: tablets, capsules, modified-release formulations, lozenges, aerosols, sprays, injectables (IV, IM, SC), solutions, creams ointments, lotions, gels, shampoos, elixirs, suspensions and suppositories. Please note that not all proprietary brands are available in all forms.

Side effects/adverse reactions are grouped by body system, without emphasis given to the frequency or severity of the reaction. Some categories include broad descriptions, eg, myelosuppression or blood disorders, because the range and severity of effects can vary between individuals, depending on the dose.

Contraindications lists instances in which the specified drug, absolutely, should NOT be used.

Precautions warns of potential clinical problems associated with the drug. These may vary according to the brand of drug to be used, and the manufacturer's recommendations.

Pharmacokinetics provides metabolism, absorption, distribution and elimination data for all dosage forms, where known. Each patient handles a particular drug according to his or her own individual parameters. Disease states will affect the pharmacokinetics of a drug.

Interactions/incompatabilities:
- Increased hypotension diuretics, other antihypertensives, ganglionic blockers, ardrenergic blockers
- Increased toxicity: potassium-sparing diuretics, lithium, NSAIDs, cyclosporin
- Do not use with vasodilators, hydralazine, prazosin
- Allopurinol, procainamide: Stevens-Johnson syndrome reported
- Azathioprine, cyclophosphamide: blood dyscrasias in patients with renal failure
- Probenecid: reduced renal clearance

Clinical assessment:
- Blood studies: neutrophils, decreased platelets
- Renal studies: protein, blood urea nitrogen, creatinine; watch for increased levels that may indicate nephrotic syndrome
- Baselines in renal, liver function tests before therapy begins
- Potassium levels, although hyperkalaemia rarely occurs

Lab test interferences
False positive: Urine acetone

Treatment of overdose: Monitor BP and if hypotensive give volume expansion. Removed by dialysis

NURSING CONSIDERATIONS

Assess:
- BP, apex/radial baselines

Administer:
- With patient in supine position if hypotensive
- IV infustion of sodium chloride 0.9% (as prescribed) to expand fluid volume if severe hypotension occurs

Interactions/incompatibilities are clinical effects which result from giving more than one medication during a course of treatment. Interactions occur whether medication is given concurrently or sequentially. Incompatibilities include pharmaceutical interactions which occur in infusion solutions, syringes, tubing or injection vials on dilution of the drug, when more than one drug is given at the same time. This section also includes drug, food and smoking interactions.

Clinical assessment lists procedures which are likely to be initiated by the clinician. In high dependency units, such as intensive or coronary care, some of the tests and procedures may be undertaken by nurses.

Laboratory test interferences are dependent on the type of test used in the laboratory, the body fluid being analysed, and the drug salt/ester. Tests can vary between laboratories.

Treatment of overdose gives brief information about antidotes and other treatments for drug overdose, wherever appropriate. See Appendix 3 for details of national poisons information services.

NURSING CONSIDERATIONS provide information to help the nurse or midwife to plan care.

Assess identifies the minimum baseline assessment which should be made before administering the drug under consideration.

Administer gives points of particular importance that relate to care during the administration of the drug.

Perform/provide:
• Supine or Trendelenburg position for severe hypotension

Evaluate:
• BP ¼ hrly for 1½hr, starting 1 hr after 1st dose. Continue if BP drops
• Apex/radial first dose. Report any significant change
• Daily urinalysis for protein (first morning specimen) 24 hr urine collection if positive.
• Assess ankle oedema daily
• Therapeutic response: decrease in BP in hypertensives, decreased signs of cardiac failure
• *Observe for:* Allergic reaction (rash, fever, pruritus, urticaria); drug should be stopped if anti-histamines fail to help. Renal symptoms (polyuria, oliguria, frequency)

Teach patient/family:
• Not to discontinue drug abruptly
• Not to use non-prescribed (cough, cold, or allergy) products unless directed by clinician
• Prescribed doses should be continued even if the patient feels better. Rise to sitting/standing position slowly to reduce effect of postural hypotension
• Inform clinician if mouth ulcers, sore throat, fever, palpitations, chest pain, or ankle oedema occur
• May experience dizziness or fainting during first days of therapy

Perform/provide identifies action(s) to be taken when administering the drug. Storage of drugs and medicines should be in accordance with the Medicines Act 1968; only special storage requirements have been included in the monograph. It is essential that nurses and midwives understand the storage required for controlled drugs, as referred to in the Misuse of Drugs Act 1971 and the Misuse of Drugs Regulations 1985. Certain preparations should be stored under specific environmental conditions, e.g. refrigerated storage.

Evaluate highlights the reassessment of the patient's condition after, and sometimes during, the administration of the medication in question. It also acts as a prompt to the nurse when writing care notes on the patient.

Teach patient/family provides information a patient, family or carer need to know about the continued use of the drug, including general effects on the patient and side effects. This information is of increasing importance as self-care or care by relatives becomes more important. An assumption is made that all nurses and midwives will remind patients and their families of the need for proper use and safe storage of medicines.

Appendixes

For your general reference, appendixes include:

1: Exemption from the Controls on Retail Sale: Midwives
2: Guide to Therapeutic Drug Monitoring
3: Drug and Poisons Information Services
4: Immunisation Against Infectious Diseases
5: Wound Care Products Available on FP10
6: Standards for the Administration of Medicines, UKCC

Indexes

List of drugs in alphabetical order by generic name.

Generic drugs grouped into functional classes. This allows the reader to compare drugs which have similar properties.

Every attempt has been made to be consistent in terms of style. Some drugs within the same therapeutic group may differ in the presentation of the information.

Thanks are due to all the nurses, midwives and pharmacists who contributed to this book at all stages prior to publication. Their enthusiasm and determination made this second edition possible.

We would welcome comments from readers of this book, via the publishers, so that we may continue to provide current and useful information in future editions.

A note to the reader:

This book is intended to help nurses and midwives understand drug protocols and the management of patients under given drug regimens. This book should not be used as a prime source for prescribing and dispensing drugs. Guy's Hospital, the Editors, Contributors and the Publisher have undertaken reasonable endeavours to check dosage and nursing content for accuracy. Because the science of clinical pharmacology is continually advancing, our knowledge base continues to expand. Therefore, we recommend that the reader should always check the manufacturer's product information for changes in dosage or administration before administering any medication. This is particularly important with new or rarely used drugs.

Abbreviations used

ACE	angiotensin converting enzyme
ACTH	adrenocorticotrophic hormone
ADH	antidiuretic hormone
AIDS	auto-immune deficiency syndrome
APTT	activated partial thromboplastin time
ATP	adenosine triphosphate
BCG	Bacillus Calmette-Guerin vaccine
BMR	basal metabolism rate
BP	blood pressure
CCF	congestive cardiac failure
CD	controlled drug
CNS	central nervous system
CO_2	carbon dioxide
CSF	cerebrospinal fluid
CSM	Committee on Safety of Medicines
CTG	cardiotocograph
CV	cardiovascular
CVA	cerebrovascular accident
CVP	central venous pressure
D&C	dilatation and curettage
DNA	deoxyribonucleic acid
DOA	dead on arrival
DOB	date of birth
DTP	Diptheria, Tetanus, Pertussis vaccine
ECT	electroconvulsive therapy
ECG	electrocardiogram
EDTA	ethylenediaminetetracetic acid
EEG	electroencephalogram
EENT	eye, ear, nose and throat
ELECT	electrolytes
ENDO	endocrine
ESR	erythrocyte sedimentation rate
exam	examination
FSH	follicle-stimulating hormone
GABA	gamma-aminobutyric acid
GFR	glomerular filtration rate
GI	gastrointestinal
G6PD	glucose-6 phosphate dehydrogenase
GSL	general sales list medicine
GU	genitourinary
Gyn	gynaecology
HAEM	haematology
Hb	haemoglobin
HCG	human chorionic gonadotropin
H_2O	water
HDL	high density lipoprotein
HDU	high density unit
HIV	Human Immunodeficiency Virus

HPA hypothalamic-pituitary-adrenal

HRT hormone replacement therapy

5HT 5-hydroxytryptamine

ICU intensive care unit

ID identification/intradermally

IgG immunoglobulin G

IM intramuscular

INTEG integument

IPV inactivated polio vaccine

IUD intrauterine contraceptive device

IV intravenous

IVP intravenous pyelogram

K potassium

LDL low density lipoprotein

LH luteinizing hormone

LMP last menstrual period

MAOIs monoamine oxidase inhibitors

META metabolic

MI myocardial infarction

MICs minimum inhibitor concentrations

MISC miscellaneous

MS motor sensory

MU mega units

Na sodium

neg negative

~~NHS~~ not available on NHS prescription

NIDDM non-insulin-dependent diabetes mellitus

NSAIDs non-steroidal anti-inflammatory drugs

O_2 oxygen

OPV oral polio vaccine

P pharmacy medicine

PABA para-aminobenzoic acid

PAS para-aminosalicylic acid

PCV packed cell volume

pH hydrogen ion concentration

POM prescription only medicine

postop postoperatively

preop preoperatively

prep preparation

PVC polyvinyl chloride

RBC(s) red blood count or cell(s)

REC rectal

REM rapid eye movement

RESP respiratory

Rh factor Rhesus factor

RNA ribonucleic acid

SC subcutaneous

SGOT serum glutamic oxalo-acetic transaminase

SROM spontaneous rupture of membranes

SYST systemic

STD sexually transmitted disease

TB	tuberculosis
TPN	total parenteral nutrition
TSH	thyroid-stimulating hormone
TT	thrombin time
UV	ultraviolet
VLDL	very low density lipoprotein
VMA	vanillylmandelic acid
WBC	white blood count or cell(s)
°C	degrees celsius (centigrade)
hr/hrly	hour/hourly
IU	International Units
mEq	milliequivalent
min	minute
temp	temperature
°	degree
%	percent
=	equal
▼	'new drug': report all reactions to CSM

Individual drugs

acarbose ▼

Glucobay
Func. class.: Oral hypoglycaemic
Chem. class.: α-glucosidase inhibitor
Legal class.: POM

Action: Inhibits the breakdown of starch and sucrose into absorbable monosaccharides in the small intestine by α-glucosidase enzymes. This slows absorption and, in diabetics, results in a lowering of postprandial hyperglycaemia and a smoothing effect on the blood glucose profile
Uses: As an adjunctive treatment to diet and oral hypoglycaemic agents in non-insulin dependent diabetes mellitus
Dosage and routes:
• *Adult:* By mouth initially 50 mg 3 times a day, increased after 6–8 weeks treatment to 100 mg 3 times a day if response inadequate, further increased to a maximum 200 mg 3 times a day if needed
Available forms include: Tablets 50, 100 mg
Side effects/adverse reactions:
GI: Flatulence, borborygmi, abdominal distension, abdominal pain, diarrhoea, raised liver enzymes
Contraindications: Hypersensitivity; children under 12 yr; pregnancy; breast-feeding; inflammatory bowel disease; colonic ulceration; partial intestinal obstruction; predisposition to intestinal obstruction; chronic intestinal diseases associated with disorders of digestion or absorption; conditions aggravated by increased gas formation, e.g. large hernias; liver impairment; severe renal impairment
Precautions: May potentiate hypoglycaemic effects of insulin and oral hypoglycaemics; existing therapy may require modification
Pharmacokinetics: Only 1–2% absorbed after oral administration, extensively degraded in the GI tract
Interactions:
• Antagonised by: Intestinal adsorbents e.g. charcoal, amylase, pancreatin, other carbohydrate splitting enzymes
• Potentiated by: Neomycin, cholestyramine
Treatment of overdose: Symptomatic treatment, avoid carbohydrate-containing beverages for 4–6 hr after ingestion

NURSING CONSIDERATIONS

Assess:
• Diabetic status, understanding of condition
Administer:
• Tablet (whole) with small quantity of liquid immediately before meals OR
• Tablet to be chewed with first mouthful of food
Teach patient/family:
• Correct method of taking tablets
• About their diabetic state including management of diet
• To report any side effects to nurse or clinician
• Not to take other medicines such as charcoal without seeking advice first

acebutolol

Sectral combination preparation
Func. class.: Antihypertensive, anti-anginal, anti-arrhythmic
Chem. class.: Cardioselective β-blocker
Legal class.: POM

Action: Has anti-arrythmic and intrinsic sympathomimetic activity. Blocks effects of excessive catecholamine stimulation resulting from stress. Competitively blocks stimulation of cardiac β-adrenergic receptors, decreases heart rate, which decreases O_2 consumption in myocardium; inhibits β-2 receptors in bronchial system at high doses. Lowers blood pressure in hypertensive subjects

Uses: Hypertension, tachyarrhythmias, prophylaxis of angina pectoris

Dosage and routes:

Hypertension

• *Adult:* By mouth 400 mg once daily or in 2 divided doses, may be increased to desired response, maximum 800 mg daily

Arrhythmias

• *Adult:* By mouth 400–1200 mg daily as required in 2–3 divided doses

Angina

• *Adult:* Initially 400 mg daily, or 200 mg twice daily; in severe cases, 300 mg daily; maximum 1200 mg daily

Available forms include: Capsules 100 mg, 200 mg; tablets 400 mg all acebutolol as the hydrochloride

Side effects/adverse reactions:

CV: Profound hypotension, bradycardia, congestive heart failure, cold extremities, postural hypotension, 2nd or 3rd degree heart block

CNS: Insomnia, fatigue, dizziness, mental changes, memory loss, hallucinations, depression, lethargy, drowsiness, nightmares, catatonia

GI: Nausea, diarrhoea, vomiting

RESP: Bronchospasm, dyspnoea, wheezing

Contraindications: Bronchospasm, asthma, history of obstructive airways disease, metabolic acidosis, sinus bradycardia, partial heart block, uncontrolled congestive heart failure

Precautions: Pregnancy, lactation, renal impairment, chronic obstructive pulmonary disease, BP 100/60 or below

Pharmacokinetics:

By mouth: Peak 2–4 hr; drug and metabolites are excreted in urine, protein binding 5%–15%, combined plasma half-life of drug and metabolite is 7–10 hr

Interactions/incompatibilities:

• Verapamil: should not be used with nor within several days of acebutolol, risk of asystole, severe hypotension and heart failure

• Effect reduced by: non-steroidal anti-inflammatory agent

• Increased side effects: cardiac glycosides, antidiabetics, clonidine, anaesthetics, sympathomimetics

• Reduces effect of: orxanthine bronchodilates

Clinical assessment:

• Anaesthetist must be informed that patient is on acebutolol

• Baseline measurements in renal and liver function tests before therapy begins

• Reduce dosage in renal dysfunction

• Maximal anti-arrythmic effect may not be achieved until 3 hr after oral dose

Lab. test interferences: Some patients develop anti-nuclear factor titres

Treatment of overdose: 1 mg atropine sulphate IV without delay. If insufficient follow by slow IV injection of isoprenaline (5 mcg per min). Monitor constantly until response occurs. If no response, IV glucagon 10–20 mg may produce dramatic improvement. Cardiac pacing if bradycardia becomes severe. Consider use of vasopressors, diazepam, phenytoin, lignocaine, digoxin and bronchodilators. Acebutolol can be removed from blood by haemodialysis

NURSING CONSIDERATIONS

Assess:

- Baseline weight, pulse and BP

Administer:

- If single daily dose take at breakfast

Perform/provide:

- Weight daily (fluid balance if significant increase)
- 4 hrly BP and pulse – report significant changes in rhythm and rate

Evaluate:

- Observe for signs of dehydration
- Observe for ankle oedema daily
- Evaluate therapeutic response: decreased BP after 1–2 weeks

Teach patient/family:

- Not to take unprescribed cold remedies (may contain α-adrenergic stimulants)
- How to take pulse, and advise when to inform clinician if rate is low
- To report dizziness, confusion, fever, breathlessness, swollen ankles
- To avoid driving or operating machines if dizzy
- To avoid alcohol, smoking and excess salt in diet

acemetacin ▼

Emflex

Func. class.: Anti-inflammatory, analgesic

Chem. class.: Non-steroidal anti-inflammatory (indomethacin derivative)

Legal class.: POM

Action: Reduces pain and inflammation by inhibiting synthesis and release of prostaglandins and other inflammatory mediators

Uses: Pain and inflammation in rheumatoid arthritis, osteo-arthritis, and post-operatively

Dosage and routes:

- *Adult:* By mouth 120 mg daily in divided doses, increased if necessary to 180 mg daily

Available forms include: Capsules 60 mg

Side effects/adverse reactions:

CNS: Headache, dizziness, vertigo, insomnia, confusion, depressed mood, irritability

CV: Oedema, chest pain, palpitations

EENT: Tinnitus, blurred vision, eye pain

GI: Discomfort, anorexia, nausea, vomiting, indigestion, diarrhoea, constipation, peptic ulceration, gastrointestinal perforation/haemorrhage

GU: Renal impairment

HAEM: Thrombocytopenia, leucopenia, reduced haemoglobin levels, agranulocytosis

INTEG: Pruritis, urticaria, erythema, rash, alopecia, excessive sweating

SYST: Allergic reactions including angio-neurotic oedema

Contraindications: Active peptic ulceration or history of recurrent ulceration; hypersensitivity to this drug or indomethacin; asthmatics in whom asthma, urticaria or rhinitis are precipitated by NSAIDs; children; pregnancy; breast-feeding

Precautions: History of gastro-intestinal ulceration; psychiatric disorder; epilepsy; parkinsonism; renal/hepatic impairment; congestive heart failure, electrolyte or fluid imbalance; elderly

Interactions:

- Increased effect of: oral anticoagulants, lithium, methotrexate
- Reduced effects of: thiazide diuretics, frusemide, mifepristone
- Risk of toxicity: ACE inhibitors, 4-quindone antibiotics, cyclosporin
- Risk of hyperkalaemia: ami-

loride, triamterene, spironolactone

Treatment of overdose: Gastric lavage in the first few hours after ingestion, symptomatic and supportive treatment. Antacids may help with gastrointestinal ulceration

NURSING CONSIDERATIONS

Assess:

• Pain levels, joint mobility

Administer:

• With or after food or milk

Evaluate:

• Therapeutic effect, reduction in pain, increased joint mobility

Teach patient/family:

• To take drug with food or milk

• About all side effects and to report any, particularly black tarry stools, difficulty in breathing, rashes, urticaria or mood changes

---

acetazolamide/ acetazolamide sodium

Diamox

Func. class.: Diuretic; carbonic anhydrase inhibitor

Chem. class.: Sulphonamide derivative

Legal class.: POM

Action: Inhibits carbonic anhydrase activity in proximal renal tubules to decrease reabsorption of water, sodium, potassium and bicarbonate; decreases carbonic anhydrase in CNS, increasing seizure threshold; decreases aqueous humour in eye, which lowers intraocular pressure

Uses: Open-angle glaucoma, pre-operative management of closed-angle glaucoma, epilepsy (petit mal, grand mal, mixed), oedema associated with pre-menstrual tension or drug induced oedema, obesity, and congestive heart failure in each case where fluid retention a problem. Also Ménière's, hydrocephalus in the infant

Dosage and routes:

• By mouth, IV or IM (IM preferably avoided because of alkaline pH)

Glaucoma

• *Adult:* 250–1000 mg daily. Divided doses if greater than 250 mg daily

• *Child:* 125–750 mg daily in divided doses

• *Elderly:* See precautions

Sustet dose (adult only): 500 mg night and morning

Abnormal retention of fluid (adult only): 250–375 mg single morning dose. Acetazolamide is often given alternating with rest days

Menstrual diuresis (adult) 125–375 mg daily

Epilepsy

• *Adult:* 250–1000 mg daily in divided doses

• *Child:* 125–750 mg daily in divided doses

Change over from other medication should be gradual

Available forms include: Tablets (scored) 250 mg; capsules modified release 500 mg (sustet); injection IM/IV 500 mg (as sodium salt)

Side effects/adverse reactions:

GU: Hypokalaemia, polydipsia and polyuria

CNS: Drowsiness, paraesthesia of extremities and face, depression, headache, dizziness, stimulation, fatigue, irritability, ataxia

GI: Anorexia, GI upsets, thirst

EENT: Myopia, loss of hearing

INTEG: Flushing

RESP: Hyperpnoea

Contraindications: Hypersensitivity to sulphonamides, idiopathic renal hyperchloraemic acidosis, adrenal gland failure, precoma associated with hepatic cirrhosis, renal insufficiency, electrolyte imbalances (hyponatreamia, hypokalaemia), Addison's disease, long-term use in chronic congestive angle-closure glaucoma, marked kidney and liver disease

Precautions: Pregnancy, chronic obstructive pulmonary disease, emphysema, lactation, elderly, urinary tract obstruction, liver dysfunction, precarious electrolyte balance. Increased dose does not increase diuresis. Discontinue drug if loss of hearing

Pharmacokinetics:

By mouth: Onset ½–1 hr, peak 2–4 hr, duration 6–12 hr

By mouth – sustained release: Onset 2 hr, peak 8–12 hr, duration 18–24 hr

IV: Onset 2 min, peak 15 min, duration 4–5 hr

65% absorbed if fasting (oral), 75% absorbed if given with food; half-life 2½–5½ hr; excreted unchanged by kidneys (80% within 24 hr)

Interactions/incompatibilities:

• Potentiates effects of: folic acid antagonists, hypoglycaemics, oral anticoagulants

• Increased side effects: cardiac glycosides, hypotensives, aspirin, phenytoin

• Increased elimination of lithium

• If hypokalaemia occurs: amiodarone, disopyramide, cardiac glycosides, flecainide, quinidine toxicity is increased, action of lignocaine, mexiletine, tocainide is antagonised, increased risk of ventricular arrythmias with pimozide and sotalol

• Increased risk of hypokalaemia with other diuretics, corticosteroids, corticotrophin and carbenoxolone

Clinical assessment:

• Take blood for measurement of potassium, sodium, chloride, urea, blood glucose levels and creatinine.

• Prescribe morning dosage to avoid sleep disturbance as this drug is a diuretic

• Evaluate therapeutic response: intraocular pressure should decrease as excess aqueous humour is drained

• Give potassium supplement if potassium is less than 3 mmol/litre

• Monitor fluid and electrolyte state

• Periodic blood cell counts recommended

• May need dose adjustments of cardiac glycosides or hypotensive agents administered with acetazolamide

Lab. test interferences: Possibly interferes with theophylline assay

Treatment of overdose: No specific antidote. Supportive measures with correction of electrolyte and fluid balance. Force fluids

NURSING CONSIDERATIONS

Assess:

• Baseline BP lying acid standing; weight

• Electrolytes: potassium, sodium, chloride; also blood glucose levels, serum creatinine, blood pH

Administer:

• Orally or intravenously if possible; IM injections are painful

• Reconstitute injection with at least 5 ml water for injection when given by slow iv bolus.

• In the morning to avoid disrupting sleep, especially if given as a diuretic

• Potassium supplement if potassium levels fall below 3.0 mmol/litre

• With food if nausea occurs; absorption may be reduced

Evaluate:

• Weigh daily and maintain fluid balance chart to determine urinary output; effectiveness of drug may be reduced if used daily

• BP lying and standing: postural hypotension may occur

• Therapeutic response indicated

by: reduction in oedema and CVP daily if medication is given for congestive cardiac failure; or decrease in intraocular pressure if used to treat glaucoma
- Signs of metabolic acidosis indicated by drowsiness and restlessness
- Signs of hypokalaemia: postural hypotension, malaise, fatigue, tachycardia, leg cramps and weakness
- Confusion, especially in the elderly

Teach patient/family:
- To increase fluid intake to 2–3 litres daily unless contraindicated
- To rise slowly when standing to avoid postural hypotension
- To inform the clinician of sore throat, bleeding, bruising, paresthesiae, tremors, pain or rashes
- To avoid driving or operating machinery if drowsiness occurs
- To report skin rash or loss of hearing (stop medication)

---

acetylcholine chloride (ophthalmic)

Miochol
Func. class.: Miotic, cholinergic
Chem. class.: Quaternary ammonium compound
Legal class.: POM

Action: Intense, immediate miosis (pupil constriction) by causing contraction of sphincter muscle of iris
Uses: Anterior segment surgery; cataract removal, peripheral iridectomy, penetrating keratoplasty
Dosage and routes:
- *Adult and child:* Instil 0.5–2 ml of a 1% sol in anterior chamber of eye (instillation by physician)

Available forms include: Solution 1% (with Mannitol 3%)

Side effects/adverse reactions:
CV: Hypotension, bradycardia
EENT: Blurred vision, lens opacities, lachrimation
Contraindications: Hypersensitivity, when miosis is undesirable
Precautions: Acute cardiac failure, bronchial asthma
Pharmacokinetics:
Instil: Miosis occurs immediately, duration 10 min

NURSING CONSIDERATIONS

Administer:
- Mix solution with powder and shake vial well to dissolve
- Clean stopper with alcohol before administration
- Use reconstituted solution immediately; unused portion must be discarded

Evaluate:
- Pulse and blood pressure
- Patient safety: in view of artificial pupil constriction ensure patient is accompanied if mobile

Teach patient/family:
- To report visual disturbances such as blurring or loss of sight, difficulty breathing, sweating or flushing

---

acetylcysteine

Parvolex
Func. class.: Antidote
Chem. class.: Amino acid L-cysteine derivative
Legal class.: POM

Action: Increases hepatic-reduced glutathione, which is necessary to inactivate toxic metabolites in paracetamol overdose or by acting as an alternative substrate for the toxic paracetamol metabolite
Uses: Paracetamol toxicity
Dosage and routes:
- *Adult and child:* By IV infusion, in glucose 5%, initially 150 mg/kg

in 200 ml over 15 min, followed by 50 mg/kg in 500 ml over 4 hr, then 100 mg/kg in 1000 ml over 16 hr
Available forms include: Injection 200 mg/ml, 10 ml ampoule
Side effects/adverse reactions:
INTEG: Rash
SYST: Anaphylaxis 15–60 min after infusion commenced
Contraindications: Hypersensitivity
Precautions: Asthma, history of bronchospasm, pregnancy
Pharmacokinetics: Contact Poisons Centre for information about paracetamol overdose
Incompatibilities:
• Do not use with iron, copper, rubber, nickel
Treatment of overdose: There is a theoretical risk of hepatic encephalopathy. There is no specific treatment, and general supportive measures should be carried out
NURSING CONSIDERATIONS:
Assess:
• Baseline vital signs (all)
• Obtain arterial blood gas estimations for increased CO_2 retention in asthmatic patients
• Liver function tests must be performed and dose must be received within 15 hr of overdose
• Monitor plasma potassium concentration
Administer:
• By IV infusion in glucose 5%
Evaluate:
• Vital signs at regular intervals as anaphylaxis can occur up to 60 min after start of infusion
• Skin—observe for rash

acipimox

Olbetam
Func. class.: Hypolipidaemic agent
Chem. class.: Nicotinic acid group
Legal class.: POM

Action: Lowers both cholesterol and triglyceride concentrations by inhibiting synthesis; increases high-density lipoproteins, inhibits release of fatty acids from adipose tissue
Uses: Hyperlipidaemias of types IIa, IIb and IV in patients who have not responded adequately to diet and other measures
Dosage and routes:
• *Adult:* By mouth, 500–750 mg daily, in divided doses, maximum 1200 mg daily (with meals). Reduce dose in renal impairment
Available forms include: Capsules 250 mg
Side effects/adverse reactions:
CNS: Flushing
INTEG: Itching, rashes, erythema, sensation of heat
CV: Skin vasodilation
Contraindications: Peptic ulcer, hypersensitivity, pregnancy, breast-feeding
Precautions: Modification of diet is preferred before treatment of hyperlipidaemia. Reduce dose in renal impairment
Pharmacokinetics: Rapidly and completely absorbed orally. Peak plasma concentration within 2 hr; not bound to plasma protein; half-life 2 hr, excreted unchanged in the urine
Clinical assessment:
• Monitor plasma triglyceride and cholesterol levels
• Assess renal function
Treatment of overdose: If toxic effects observed, administer supportive and symptomatic treatment

NURSING CONSIDERATIONS

Assess:

• BP and weight

Administer:

• With or soon after food

Perform/provide:

• Measures to reduce effects of itching and vasodilation, e.g. cotton clothes

• Observe for side effects

Teach patient/family:

• To understand the importance of concurrent cholesterol lowering diet and maintenance of ideal weight

• To understand the importance of not smoking, avoiding alcohol, and of positive stress management

• That they may feel malaise, GI upsets, flushing and warmth

acitretin ▼

Neotigason

Func. class.: Antipsoriatic systemic

Chem. class.: Retinoid

Legal class.: POM

Action: Reverses hyperkeratotic skin changes

Uses: Severe extensive psoriasis resistant to other treatments; palmar-plantar pustular psoriasis; severe congenital ichthyosis; severe Darier's disease

Dosage and routes:

• *Adult:* By mouth, 25–30 mg daily (Darier's disease 10 mg daily) for 2–4 weeks, then adjusted according to response, usually within range 25–50 mg daily (in some cases up to max. 75 mg daily) for further 6–8 weeks (in Darier's disease and ichthyosis not more than 50 mg daily for up to 6 months)

• *Child:* By mouth, 0.5–1 mg/kg/day (max. 35 mg/day)

Available forms include: Capsules 10, 25 mg

Side effects/adverse reactions:

CNS: Headache, malaise, lethargy, benign intracranial hypertension

EENT: Drying and erosion of lips, mucosa of mouth and nose, conjunctivae; nose bleed; conjunctivitis; intolerance of contact lenses; alopecia; decreased right vision

ELECT: Elevated serum triglycerides

GI: Nausea, hepatotoxicity

INTEG: Dry skin, scaling, thinning of skin, pruritus, palmar-plantar exfoliation, epidermal fragility; paronychia

MS: Myalgia, arthralgia, hyperostosis

MISC: Sweating

Contraindications: Pregnancy; females of child-bearing potential not taking adequate contraceptive precautions; breast-feeding

Precautions: Diabetes mellitus

Interactions:

• Increased risk of intracranial hypertension with tetracycline

• Risk of toxicity with vitamin A supplements

• Increased risk of hepatitis with methotrexate

Treatment of overdose: Gastric lavage within the first few hours of ingestion; supportive treatment

NURSING CONSIDERATIONS

Administer:

• With or after food

Evaluate:

• Therapeutic effect: reduction in scaling and itching; resolution of psoriasis

• For side effects, particularly neurological status: headache, nausea, vomiting or visual disturbance; blurring of vision, poor nocturnal vision, decreased visual acuity. Ophthalmic opinion should be sought

Teach patient/family:

• To take capsules with or immediately after food
• To discontinue taking acitretin if any side effects occur and to seek medical advice promptly
• A reliable method of contraception must be used by women of child-bearing age for 2 yr after treatment is complete
• Not to take if pregnancy is suspected
• Not to donate blood either during, or for at least two years after, treatment is discontinued
• Wearing contact lenses may be difficult or uncomfortable
• Not to take vitamin A supplements or tetracycline (prescribed)

---

acrivastine

Semprex
Func. class.: Antihistamine
Chem. class.: Derivative of triprolidine
Legal class.: POM

Action: Competitive histamine H_1 antagonist, providing symptomatic relief of allergy
Uses: Allergic rhinitis including hayfever, urticaria
Dosage and routes:
• *Adults and children over 12 yr:* By mouth 8 mg 3 times daily
Available forms include: Capsules 8 mg
Side effects/adverse reactions:
CNS: Drowsiness, headache
GU: Urinary retention
Lacks significant anticholinergic effects. Low penetration of CNS
Contraindications: Renal impairment; hypersensitivity to acrivastine or triprolidine; elderly; children; porphyria
Precautions: Pregnancy, lactation, driving or operating machinery. Alcohol, other CNS depressants may produce reduced mental alertness
Pharmacokinetics: Peak plasma concentration 1.5 hr; onset of effect 1 hr, maximum 2 hr, duration 8 hr; half-life 1.5 hr; excreted in urine
Interactions/incompatibilities: Effects potentiated by alcohol, other CNS depressants, tricyclic antidepressants, antimuscarinics
Treatment of overdose: No experience of overdosage. Appropriate supportive therapy, including gastric lavage, should be initiated if indicated

NURSING CONSIDERATIONS

Administer:
• Orally
Perform/provide:
• Observe for side effects—drowsiness, headaches or urinary retention
• Observe for signs of hypersensitivity
Evaluate:
• Mental alertness/drowsiness
• Urinary output (may cause urinary retention)
• Alleviation of allergic symptoms
Teach patient/family:
• Warn patient drowsiness rare but can occur—may affect driving or operating machinery. Alcohol may enhance this effect
• To avoid alcohol with medication
• To avoid driving or operating machinery

acyclovir (ophthalmic)

Zovirax Ophthalmic Ointment
Func. class.: Antiviral
Chem. class.: Synthetic purine analogue
Legal class.: POM

Action: Interferes with viral DNA replication
Uses: Treatment of herpes simplex keratitis
Dosage and routes: *Adults, children*: Topical 1 cm ribbon of ointment inside lower conjunctival sac 5 times a day (approximately 4 hrly intervals) omitting night-time application. Continue for at least 3 days after healing is complete
Available forms include: Eye ointment 3%
Side effects/adverse reactions:
EENT: Transient mild stinging, superficial punctate keratopathy, local irritation and inflammation (blepharitis, conjunctivitis)
Contraindications: Hypersensitivity
Precautions: For ophthalmic use only, pregnancy, lactation
Pharmacokinetics: Rapidly absorbed into aqueous humour. Clinically insignificant levels found in urine
Interactions: None known for application to eye
Lab. test interferences: None reported
Treatment of overdose: No untoward effects expected if the entire contents of the tube containing 135 mg acyclovir were ingested orally

NURSING CONSIDERATIONS

Administer:
- After washing hands. Cleanse crust or discharge from eyes before application
- Ensure separate application for each eye and wash hands between applications to avoid cross infection

Evaluate:
- Therapeutic response; absence of redness; inflammation
- Allergy, itching, lacrimation, redness and swelling

Teach patient/family:
- To wear gloves and handle carefully
- To use exactly as prescribed
- Not to use make up
- That drug container should not touch eye
- To report adverse reaction
- That drug may cause blurred vision when ointment applied
- To avoid using flannels and towels which may cause reinfection
- Not to use other people's flannels and towels
- To wash hands carefully after application

acyclovir (oral)

Zovirax
Func. class.: Antiviral
Chem. class.: Synthetic purine analogue
Legal class.: POM

Action: Interferes with viral DNA replication
Uses: Herpes simplex and varicella-zoster
Dosage and routes
Herpes simplex
- *Adult:* By mouth 200 mg 5 times daily, usually for 5 days. (Use 400 mg for immunocompromised)
- *Child under 2 yr:* Half adult dose, over 2 yr adult dose

Prevention of recurrence
- *Adult:* By mouth 200 mg 4 times daily or 400 mg twice daily possibly reduced to 200 mg 2 or 3 times

daily and interrupted every 6–12 months

Prophylaxis for immunocompromised

• *Adult:* By mouth 200–400 mg 4 times daily

Varicella-zoster

• *Adult:* By mouth 800 mg 5 times daily for 7 days

Available forms include: Tablets 200 mg, 400 mg, 800 mg; suspension 200 mg in 5 ml

Side effects/adverse reactions:

GI: Nausea, vomiting, diarrhoea, abdominal pains

INTEG: Rashes

Contraindications: Hypersensitivity

Precautions: Pregnancy, lactation, elderly, renal impairment. Maintain adequate hydration

Pharmacokinetics: Only partially absorbed from the gut. Bioavailability is very low when given orally. In normal adults terminal plasma half-life is 2.9 hr. Excreted mainly unchanged by the kidney. In children, renal impairment and the elderly, the excretion pattern differs

Interactions: Probenecid reduces acyclovir excretion (increased plasma concentrations and risk of toxicity)

Clinical assessment: Check for renal impairment; dosage adjustment may be necessary for patients with herpes zoster

Treatment of overdose: Unlikely that serious toxic effects would occur if a dose of up to 5 g were taken on a single occasion. No data on higher doses—closely observe patient. Acyclovir is dialysable

NURSING CONSIDERATIONS

Assess:

• Fluid balance

• Ask patient about any allergies before treatment and record on care plan/nursing notes

• Adequate hydration in elderly patients receiving high doses for herpes zoster

Administer:

• Adjust dosage in severe renal impairment

Perform/provide:

• Urinic testing, particularly for protein before and during medication

Evaluate:

• Maintain fluid balance chart. Report haematuria, oligouria, fatigue, weakness, which may indicate nephrotoxicity. Test urine for protein during treatment

• Pay particular attention to patients with known renal disease and inform doctor immediately if side effects occur

• Evaluate therapeutic response indicated by absence of painful, itching lesions

• Observe bowel pattern before and during treatment. Report severe abdominal pain with bleeding to clinician: drug should then be discontinued

• Observe skin for rashes, urticaria, itching

Teach patient/family:

• That for maximal effectiveness drug should be taken at the first sign of infection e.g. pain, irritation

• That patient has herpes; they could become infected

• Acyclovir does not cure infection, just controls symptoms

• To report sore throat, fever, fatigue could indicate secondary infection

• That drug must be taken at regular intervals throughout the day to maintain therapeutic blood levels for about 10 days

• To report side effects, e.g. bruising, bleeding, fatigue, malaise to clinician; may indicate blood dyscrasias

acyclovir (topical)

Zovirax
Func. class.: Antiviral
Chem. class.: Synthetic purine analogue
Legal class.: POM

Action: Interferes with viral DNA replication
Uses: Treatment of herpes simplex virus infections of the skin including initial and recurrent genital herpes and herpes labialis. DO NOT USE IN THE EYES
Dosage and routes: Apply topically to lesions every 4 hr (5 times daily) for 5 days
Available forms include: Cream 5%
Side effects/adverse reactions:
INTEG: Transient burning or stinging on application. Erythema or mild drying of the skin
Contraindications: Hypersensitivity to acyclovir or propylene glycol
Precautions: Avoid contact with eyes and mucous membranes, pregnancy, lactation
Pharmacokinetics: Absorption of acyclovir is usually slight following topical application
Interactions: None reported for topical application
Incompatibilities: Should not be diluted
Treatment of overdose: No untoward effects expected if entire contents of 10 g tube were ingested orally; acyclovir is dialysable

NURSING CONSIDERATIONS

Assess:
- Fluid balance

Administer:
- Begin therapy as early as possible (prodromal period or when lesions first appear)
- Apply after cleansing the local area with soap and water. Dry thoroughly
- Repeat 4 hrly
- Avoid contact with mucous membranes and eyes
- Apply sufficient medication to completely cover lesions

Perform/Provide:
- Fluids, boiled sweets, mouthwashes for dry mouth
- Store preparation below 25°C

Evaluate:
- Observe patient for signs of allergic reaction e.g. burning, stinging, swelling, redness
- Observe for therapeutic response as indicated by decrease in size and number of lesions

Teach patient/family:
- To wear gloves when applying topical medication
- To wash hands before and after each application
- To avoid use of other topical creams, lotions and ointments unless ordered by clinician

acyclovir sodium

Zovirax IV for Intravenous Infusion
Func. class.: Antiviral
Chem. class.: Synthetic purine analogue
Legal class.: POM

Action: Interferes with viral DNA replication
Uses: Herpes simplex and varicella zoster
Dosage and routes:
- *Slow intravenous infusion: Adult:* 5 mg/kg over 1 hr, repeated every 8 hr; doubled in zoster in the immunocompromised, and in simplex encephalitis
- *Child up to 3 months:* 10 mg/kg every 8 hr
- *Child 3 months–12 yr:* 250 mg/m^2 every 8 hr, doubled in the immunocompromised and in simplex encephalitis

Dosage should be adjusted according to creatinine clearance in renal impairment

Available forms include: Powder acyclovir sodium 250 mg and 500 mg

Side effects/adverse reactions:

CNS: Confusion, hallucinations, agitation, tremors, somnolence psychosis, convulsions, coma, fever

HAEM: Decrease in haematological indices

GI: Nausea, vomiting, increase in liver related enzymes

GU: Renal impairment, increase in blood urea and creatinine levels

INTEG: Rashes

Contraindications: Hypersensitivity

Precautions: Abnormal renal function, dehydration, not to be given orally, pregnancy, lactation

Pharmacokinetics: In normal adults terminal plasma half-life is 2.9 hr. Most of the drug is excreted unchanged by the kidney. In children, renal impairment and the elderly, the excretion pattern differs

Interactions/incompatibilities:

- Zidovudine: extreme lethargy with IV acyclovir
- Probenecid reduces excretion (risk of toxic plasma concentrations)

Clinical assessment:

- Maintain adequate hydration
- Monitor renal function during treatment

Treatment of overdose: Single doses of up to 80 mg per kg have been accidentally administered with no adverse consequences. Acyclovir is dialysable

NURSING CONSIDERATIONS

Assess:

- Hydration and fluid balance
- Renal and hepatic function
- Check for hypersensitivity, abnormal renal function, pregnancy, lactation

Administer:

- Reconstitute powder with 10 ml sterile water for injections 250 mg drug; shake; use within 12 hr; infuse over at least 1 hr to prevent nephrotoxicity
- By slow intravenous infusion over 1 hr following reconstitution and dilution
- Dilute with water for injections or sodium chloride 0.9% to 25 mg/ml; this solution may be given directly iv or further diluted to not more than 5 mg/ml for infusion

Perform/provide:

- Maintain fluid balance chart. Report haematuria, oliguria, fatigue, weakness, which may indicate nephrotoxicity. Test urine for protein during treatment
- Pay particular attention to patients with known renal disease and inform clinician immediately if side effects occur
- Store at room temperature for no more than 12 hr after reconstitution
- Ensure adequate fluid intake (2 litres/24 hr) to prevent renal damage

Evaluate:

- IV site as phelebitis is likely to occur when given peripherally
- By assessment of clinical symptoms
- Hepatic and renal function

Teach patient/family:

- That for maximal effectiveness drug should be taken at the first sign of infection e.g. pain, irritation
- That patient has herpes; they could become infected
- Acyclovir does not cure infection, just controls symptoms
- To report sore throat, fever, fatigue, which could indicate secondary infection
- That drug must be taken at regular intervals throughout the day

to maintain therapeutic blood levels for about 10 days
• To report side effects e.g. bruising, bleeding, fatigue, malaise to clinician; may indicate blood dyscrasias

adenosine ▼

Adenocor
Func. class.: Antiarrhythmic
Chem. class.: Purine
Legal class.: POM

Action: Slows conduction through the AV node, interrupting re-entry circuits involving the AV node and restoring normal sinus rhythm in patients with paroxysmal supraventricular tachycardias.
Uses: Treatment of supraventricular tachycardias, including those associated with accessory by-pass tracts (Wolff-Parkinson-White syndrome) and as an aid to the diagnosis of broad or narrow complex supraventricular tachycardias and other abnormalities of cardiac conduction
Dosage and routes:
Therapeutic dose
• *Adult:* By rapid IV injection (over 2 sec) 3 mg; if this fails to restore sinus rhythm within 1–2 min give a further 6 mg by rapid IV injection; if this fails to work within 1–2 min give a final dose of 12 mg by rapid IV injection. Additional or higher doses are not recommended
• *Child:* No controlled paediatric study has been undertaken, but doses of 0.0375–0.25 mg/kg have been used in children with similar effects to those seen in adults
Diagnostic dose
The above ascending dosage schedule should be followed until sufficient diagnostic information has been obtained
Available forms include: Injection 6 mg
Side effects/adverse reactions:
CNS: Lightheadedness, head pressure, headache, dizziness, apprehension
CV: Facial flushing, palpitations, bradycardia sometimes requiring temporary pacing, transient abnormalities of cardiac rhythm at the time of conversion to sinus rhythm
EENT: Blurred vision, metallic taste
GI: Nausea
INTEG: Sweating
MISC: Feeling of discomfort, burning sensation, chest pain, heaviness in arms, pains in arms, neck and back
RESP: Dyspnoea, feeling of thoracic constriction
Contraindications: Second or third degree heart block or sick sinus syndrome (except in patients with a functioning artificial pacemaker)
Precautions: Atrial flutter/fibrillation and an accessory by-pass tract; asthma; pregnancy
Pharmacokinetics: Taken up rapidly into tissues following IV injection
Interactions:
• Potentiated by: Dipyridamole (reduce doses of adenosine if use considered essential)
• Antagonised by: Caffeine, theophylline, aminophylline, other xanthines
Treatment of overdose: There is no experience of overdose, as the half-life of adenosine is very short; supportive treatment after overdose should be sufficient

NURSING CONSIDERATIONS

Assess:
• Baseline vital signs
• Patient's normal baseline cardiac pattern
Administer:
• Undiluted. If given into an IV

line this should be as proximally as possible and followed by a rapid saline flush

Perform/provide:

• Constant cardiac monitoring/pacing

• Bed in cardiac unit or ICU (if possible)

Evaluate:

• Therapeutic effect (return to patient's normal cardiac sinus rhythm)

• For any side effects

Teach patient/family:

• Reason for giving the drug

• About the side effects

---

adrenaline

Min-I-Jet Adrenaline

Func. class.: Adrenergic agonist

Chem. class.: Sympathomimetic amine

Legal class.: POM

Action: Activates α- and β-adrenergic receptors producing increased contractility and heart rate, peripheral vasoconstriction or vasodilation

Uses: 1 in 1000: emergency treatment of acute anaphylaxis

1 in 10,000: cardiac arrest

Dosage and routes:

Cardiac arrest

• Adrenaline 1 in 10,000 (1 mg per 10 ml) – 10 ml by central intravenous injection

Acute anaphylaxis

• IM route, volume of 1 in 1000 (1 mg/ml) injection:

• *Adult:* 0.5–1 ml

• *Child:* Under 1 yr 0.05 ml, 1 yr 0.1 ml, 2 yr 0.2 ml, 3–4 yr 0.3 ml, 5 yr 0.4 ml, 6–12 yr 0.5 ml. May need to use half recommended dose in underweight children

Available forms include:

• Injection 1 in 1000 (adrenaline 1 mg/ml as acid tartrate), 0.5 ml, 1 ml

• Injection 1 in 10,000 (adrenaline 100 mcg/ml as acid tartrate) 10 ml

• Min-I-Jet 1 in 1000 (adrenaline 1 mg/ml as hydrochloride) 0.5 ml, 1 ml

• Min-I-Jet 1 in 10,000 (adrenaline 100 mcg/ml as hydrochloride) 3 ml, 10 ml

Side effects/adverse reactions:

CNS: Anxiety, tremor, headache

CV: Tachycardia, cold extremities, arrhythmias

EENT: Dry mouth

In overdose: Cerebral haemorrhage, pulmonary oedema

Precautions: Hyperthyroidism, diabetes mellitus, ischaemic heart disease, hypertension, elderly

Interactions: Risk of hypertension and/or arrhythmias: MAOIs (concomitant administration and up to 3 weeks after MAOIs), tricyclic antidepressants, cyclopropane, halothane, β-blockers, doxapram, dopexamine

Treatment of overdose: Supportive measures – prompt injection of rapidly-acting α-adrenergic blocking agent (e.g. phentolamine) followed by a β-blocker (e.g. propranolol). Rapidly acting vasodilators (e.g. glyceryl trinitrate) have been used

NURSING CONSIDERATIONS

Administer:

• Into central vein by pumped, continuous infusion in mcg/kg/min

• Correct hypovolaemia prior to and during administration

Perform/provide:

• CVP monitoring is advisable

• Continuous ECG monitoring during administration

• BP and pulse every 5 min; arterial pressure monitoring advised if adrenaline given by infusion

• Detailed patient observation;

preferably in HDU or ICU environment
• Ensure infusion reservoir is replaced before emptied to avoid hypotension
• Do not use discoloured solutions
• Emergency equipment
Evaluate:
• Fluid balance
• Drug should be titrated against response until prescribed blood pressure is achieved
• Paraesthesias and coldness of extremities, peripheral blood flow may decrease
• Monitor peripheral and central temperatures
• Injection site: extravasation—inform medical staff immediately; find alternative access—if necessary stop infusion and observe blood pressure
• Therapeutic response—increased BP with stabilisation
Teach patient/family:
• Reason for drug administration and careful monitoring

---

adrenaline (inhaler)

Medihaler-epi
Func. class.: Adrenergic agonist
Chem. class.: Sympathomimetic amine
Legal class.: POM

Action: Activates α- and β-adrenergic receptors producing vasoconstriction, bronchodilatation, relief of mucosal congestion and causes cardiac stimulation. By inhalation: relaxes bronchial smooth muscle, constricts bronchial mucosal vessels, relieves congestion and oedema
Uses: Adjunct to anaphylaxis treatment only
Dose and routes:
• *Adult:* minimum dose of 20 puffs inhaled
• *Child:* 10–15 puffs under supervision
Available forms include: Aerosol inhalation adrenaline acid tartrate 280 mcg/metered inhalation
Side effects/adverse reactions:
GI: Gastric pain
Precautions: Use with caution if cardiac disease, hypertension, hyperthyroidism. Tolerance develops after prolonged use. Pregnancy
Pharmacokinetics: By inhalation: onset 1 min
Interactions: Risk of hypertension and/or arrhythmias: MAOIs (concomitant administration and up to 3 weeks after MAOIs), tricyclic antidepressants, cyclopropane, halothane, β-blockers, doxapram, dopexamine
Clinical assessment:
• Check inhaler technique
• Monitor for tolerance after repeated use of inhaler
Treatment of overdose: Acute poisoning: immediate IV injections of quick-acting sympatholytics (e.g. phentolamine or piperoxan)
NURSING CONSIDERATIONS
Perform/provide:
• Monitor respiratory pattern
• Provide reassurance and comfortable patient environment to maximise respiratory function
Evaluate:
• Heart and respiratory rate, general appearance
• Response to administration by reduction in bronchospasm (and acuteness of asthma attack)
Teach patient/family:
• Correct inhalation technique

adrenaline HCl/ adrenaline borate complex

Epifrin, Eppy, Simplene
Func. class.: Mydriatic
Chem. class.: Sympathomimetic amine
Legal class.: P or POM

Action: Reduces production of aqueous humour and increases outflow
Uses, dosage and routes: Primary open angle glaucoma
• *Adult*: One or two drops in affected eye(s) once or twice daily. Less frequently if necessary
Available forms include: Eye drops 0.5%, 1%. Product specific salts
Side effects/adverse reactions:
CNS: Headache, browache
EENT: Severe smarting and redness of the eye; blurred vision, photophobia, eye pain. After prolonged use – pigmentary deposits
Contraindications: Closed angle glaucoma, patients with narrow angle prone to angle block with mydriatics, hypersensitivity to any component of preparation, soft contact lenses (some products only)
Precautions: Hypertension, heart disease, pregnancy, lactation, evaluate anterior chamber angle before initiating therapy, aneurysms, arrhythmia or tachycardia, hyperthyroidism, cerebral arteriosclerosis, diabetes mellitus. Discontinue if visual acuity deteriorates in aphakic patients. Soft contact lenses. Do not drive or operate machinery if have blurred vision
Pharmacokinetics:
INSTIL: Onset 1 hr, peak 4–8 hr, duration 12–24 hr
Interactions: Risk of hypertension and arrhythmias, MAOIs (concomitant administration and up to 3 weeks after MAOIs), tricyclic antidepressants (or within several days of their discontinuation) cyclopropane, halothane, β-blockers, doxapram, dopexamine
Incompatibilities: Soft contact lenses (some products)
Clinical assessment:
• Assess visual acuity in aphakic patients
• Tonometer readings during long-term treatment
• Evaluate anterior chamber angle prior to treatment
Treatment of overdose: Treatment of severe toxic reaction – immediate IV α-adrenoreceptor blocking agent (5–10 mg phentolamine) followed by β-adrenoreceptor blocking agent (2.5–5 mg propranolol)

NURSING CONSIDERATIONS

Assess:
• BP, pulse, respirations
• Visual acuity
Evaluate:
• Allergic reaction: itching, oedema of eyelids, eye discharge; drug should be discontinued
Teach patient/family:
• Report change in vision, blurring or loss of sight, trouble breathing, sweating, flushing
• Method of instillation: pressure on lacrimal sac for 1 min, do not touch dropper to eye
• That long-term therapy may be required if using for glaucoma
• Some smarting and redness of the eye may occur. Report to clinician if this occurs

albumin, human serum 4.5%/5%/20%/25%

Albuminar-5, -20, -25, Human Albumin solution 4.5%, 20% Immuno, Albutein 5%, 20%, 25% Buminate 5%, 20%, Zenalb 4.5%, 20%, Albumin solution 20% SNBTS

Func. class.: Blood derivative
Chem. class.: human plasma protein
Legal class.: POM

Action: Exerts osmotic pressure on tissue fluids, which expands volume of circulating blood

Uses: Isotonic solutions (4%–5% protein): acute or subacute loss of plasma volume (e.g. burns, pancreatitis, trauma, complications of surgery) plasma exchange

Concentrated solutions (15%–25% protein): severe hypoalbuminaemia associated with low plasma volume and generalised oedema where salt and water restriction with plasma volume expansion are required, adjunct in treatment of hyperbilirubinaemia by exchange transfusion in newborn, priming heart-lung machines

Dosage and routes:
For intravenous use. Seek clinician's advice for dosage and rate of administration

Available forms include: Varying size vials from 50 ml to 1 litre for isotonic; 5 ml to 100 ml for concentrated

Side effects/adverse reactions:
GI: Nausea, vomiting, increased salivation
CNS: Fever, chills
CV: Hypotension, tachycardia

Contraindications: Hypersensitivity, cardiac failure, severe anaemia, premature infants, dialysis patients, defects in clotting mechanism

Precautions: Lack of albumin deficiency, pregnancy, history of cardiac or circulatory (including hypertensive) disease, risk of further haemorrhage or shock due to rise in BP. Correct any dehydration if necessary; watch for circulatory overload; seek clinician's advice for use in renal and hepatic disease

Pharmacokinetics: In hyponutrition states metabolized as protein energy source

Interactions/incompatibilities:
Protein hydrolysates, amino acid mixtures, solutions containing alcohol

Clinical assessment:
• Check for hypersensitivity, defects in clotting, cardiac failure or disease, severe anaemia, circulatory disease (including hypertension)

Lab. test interferences: Blood samples taken during or shortly after infusion show lower lab. test results (e.g. haematocrit). No interference with rhesus factor determination, thrombocyte function, blood coagulation

Treatment of overdose: Interrupt infusion immediately and watch patient's haemodynamic parameters carefully: Give any specific treatment necessary. Administration of large quantities of albumin should be supplemented with red cell concentrates or replaced by whole blood.

NURSING CONSIDERATIONS

Assess:
• Haemodynamic stability and correction of hypovolaemia

Administer:
• Intravenous infusion–rate/volume according to clinician's advice, patient response and blood picture
• Within 4–8 hr of opening
• Use new infusion set

Perform/provide:

• Appropriate storage facilities
• Observation of CVP/pulmonary wedge pressure, BP, heart rate, respirations, and temp, as often as patient's condition dictates
• Accurate fluid balance—NB: watch for possible deterioration in urinary output

Evaluate:

• Monitor BP
• Monitor any dehydration, watch for circulatory overload, not dialysis patients, pregnancy
• Therapeutic response: increased CVP and BP, decreased oedema, increased serum albumin (within normal limits)
• Allergic response, rash, itching, chills, flushing, urticaria, nausea, vomiting, hypotension, requires discontinuation of infusion, use of new lot if therapy reinstituted
• Overdose: circulatory overload, haemodilution. Increased CVP and BP recordings, distended neck veins, cyanosis, abnormal respiratory pattern, frothy sputum and blood

Teach patient/family:

• If appropriate, explain reason for treatment and possible adverse reactions so that these may be identified early and treated

alcuronium chloride

Alloferin
Func. class.: Non-depolarising muscle relaxant
Chem. class.: Derivative of toxiferine, a curare alkaloid
Legal class.: POM

Action: Causes relaxation by competing with acetylcholine as the neurotransmitter

Uses: Medium duration muscle relaxation during surgery and anaesthesia

Dosage and routes:

• *Adult:* Intravenous injection 200–250 mcg/kg (higher dose used for longer procedures) when non-potentiating anaesthetic agents used, then incremental doses of one-sixth to one-quarter of initial dose as required
• *Child over 28 days:* 125–200 mcg/kg

Available forms include: Injection IV 5 mg/ml (2 ml amp)

Side effects/adverse reactions:

CV: Tachycardia, decreased BP

Contraindications: Myasthenia gravis, hypersensitivity, pregnancy, porphyria, myasthenic (Eaton-Lambert) syndrome

Precautions: Reduce dose in renal impairment, pregnancy, hepatic disease, poliomyelitis, Duchenne muscular dystrophy, neurofibromatosis, amyotrophic lateral sclerosis, hypothermia, carcinomatosis. Anaesthetist must be present to control patient's ventilation, disturbed serum protein levels, acidosis, correct electrolyte or acid-base disturbances before administration, and correct any lack of effect

Pharmacokinetics: Laryngeal relaxation achieved within 90–120 seconds, muscle relaxation persists for 20–40 min. Half-life 3.3 hours; excreted unchanged in urine

Interactions/incompatibilities:

• Effects increased by: antibiotics of the polymixin and aminoglycoside groups, lincomycin, azlocillin, mezlocillin, nifedipine, verapamil, lithium, parenteral magnesium, clindamycin, volatile anaesthetics, quinidine, β-blockers, phenytoin, penicillamine, narcotic analgesics, ganglion-blocking agents, diazepam, high concentrations of magnesium ions
• Effects decreased by: neostigmine, pyridostigmine, demecarium and ecothiopate eye drops, high concentrations of calcium,

potassium and sodium ions; do not mix with thiopentone
• Adverse effects produced by: IV dantrolene and IV verapamil (hypotension, myocardial depression, hyperkalaemia)

Treatment of overdose:
Continue artificial ventilation; reverse neuromuscular blockade with IV injection of prostigmine 1–5 mg (child 50–70 mcg/kg) plus atropine 400–1250 mcg (child 20–30 mcg/kg); observe patient until neuromuscular function is restored. Do not leave unattended until adequate spontaneous respiration is present

NURSING CONSIDERATIONS

Assess:
• Baseline pulse, blood pressure and vital signs
• Check history of sensitivity or myasthenia gravis, porphyria, pregnancy
• Test for urea and electrolytes, blood gases and pH if appropriate
• Ensure acid-base/electrolyte disturbances are corrected before administration
• Airway and respirations constantly; temperature

Administer:
• If required, dilute with water for injections immediately before administration

Perform/provide:
• In theatre or intensive care unit
• Perform IV administration in the presence of an experienced anaesthetist
• Provide equipment for intubation/resuscitation

Evaluate:
• Therapeutic response
• Observe for muscle spasms, rashes

Teach patient/family:
• The effects of the drug and communication strategies where drug is used to facilitate ventilation in intensive care

aldesleukin (interleukin-II)

Proleukin
Func. class.: Antineoplastic, immunostimulant
Chem. class.: Cytokine
Legal class.: POM

Action: Stimulates host's immune response to tumour
Uses: Metastatic renal cell carcinoma
Dosage and routes:
• By continuous IV infusion, 18 million IU (1 mg)/M^2/day for 5 days repeated after 2–6 days without drug. This constitutes one induction cycle; it should be repeated after 3 weeks without drug. Responding patients may receive up to four maintenance cycles (18 million IU/m^2/day for 5 days by continuous IV infusion) at 4-week intervals

Available forms include: Powder for IV injection, 18-million IU (1 mg) vials

Side effects/adverse reactions:
CNS: Irritability, confusion, depression, lethargy, somnolence, coma
CV: Capillary leak syndrome, hypotension, oedema
ELECT: Electrolyte imbalances
GI: Nausea, vomiting, diarrhoea, hepatotoxicity
GU: Renal impairment, oliguria
INTEG: Rash, pruritis
RESP: Dyspnoea, pulmonary oedema, respiratory failure
MISC: Fever, worsening of malignant effusions

Contraindications: Hypersensitivity; pregnancy; breast-feeding; CNS metastases; seizure disorders; serious major organ dysfunction; resting pO_2-less than 60 mmHg; patients in whom dopamine or other pressor agents are contraindicated; serious active infection, serious cardiac disease, performance status of ECOG 2 or greater; patients with simultaneous prescence of performance status of ECOG 1 or greater *and* metastatic disease in more than one organ *and* a period of less than 24 months between tumour diagnosis and evaluation for aldesleukin treatment

Precautions: Malignant effusions, bone marrow suppression, impaired hepatic/renal function, organ allografts, corticosteroid treatment

Interactions:

• Increased risk of renal impairment: aminoglycoside antibiotics, vancomycin, amphotericin, cisplatin, non-steroidal anti-inflammatory drugs, ACE inhibitors, other nephrotoxic drugs

Incompatibilities:

• In-line filters, plastics in the absence of albumin

Treatment of overdose: Stop infusion; symptomatic and supportive treatment

NURSING CONSIDERATIONS

Assess:

• Baseline vital signs (temperature, pulse, respiration, BP); also ECG, fluid balance, weight, food likes and dislikes

• Full blood count, differential, platelet count weekly; withhold drug if WBC is less than 4000 or platelet count is less than 75,000

Administer:

• HANDLING: take safety precautions appropriate to antineoplastic agents

• Following local antineoplastic (cytotoxic) policies

• After ensuring that clinician is aware of blood results

• IV: by continuous infusion. All syringes, infusion bags, giving sets should be made of glass, PVC, polypropylene, polyolefine or polyethyline. Reconstitute with 1.2 ml water for injection, added gently to prevent foaming. DO NOT SHAKE. Dilute for infusion by adding to 5% dextrose containing 0.1% human albumin which must be added before Aldesleukin

• Other medications by mouth if possible. Avoid IV, IM, SC routes to prevent infection and bruising

• Anti-emetic 30–60 min before treatment

• All other medication as prescribed including analgesics, antibiotics, anti-emetics, antispasmodics

Perform/provide:

• Good aseptic technique when administering and/or connecting IV line (see Administer)

• Protective isolation (WBC levels are likely to be low)

• Regular FBC, urea and electrolytes for bone marrow depression, recordings of TPR and BP

• Fluids: increase fluid intake to 2–3 l daily to prevent urate deposits, calculi formation

• Diet: as nutritious as patient will eat, but low in purines (offal, dried beans, peas) to maintain urine alkalinity

• Skincare: rashes and pruritus occur as side effects

• Mouthcare: mouth rinsing 3–4 times daily; brush teeth with soft brush or use cotton-tipped applicators for stomatitis; use unwaxed dental floss

• Warm compresses and other suitable treatment at injection site if indicated

• Storage: vials in refrigerator

Evaluate:

• Vital signs: toxicity is severe and likely to affect all patients receiving Aldesleukin

• Hypotension, signs of pulmonary and other oedema caused by capillary leak

• Fluid balance: report fall in urinary output if below 30–50 ml/hr
• Condition of skin and mouth (dryness, sores, ulceration, white patches, pain, dysphagia)
• All side effects, affecting all systems
• Nausea and vomiting (may be severe)
• Unexpected bleeding; haematuria; bruising; petechiae (skin, mucosa and orifices)
• Yellowing of skin; sclera; dark urine; clay-coloured stools; itchy skin; abdominal pain; fever; diarrhoea
• Signs and symptoms of chest infection
• Psychological effect of changes in body image, alopecia

Teach patient/family:
• About the effects of the drug
• About major side effects of the drug
• To notify any side effects promptly to nurse or clinician
• The necessity for protective isolation and precautions related to this
• That hair may be lost but that a wig or hairpiece may be obtained free from the NHS. Regrown hair may be different in colour and texture
• About sexual changes: impotence, loss of libido, amenorrhoea, gynomaestia, which are often reversible after treatment, and the need to practise contraception (cytotoxic drugs are teratogenic)

alfentanil

Rapifen, Rapifen concentrate, Rapifen Intensive Care
Func. class.: Opioid analgesic
Chem. class.: Opioid, synthetic
Legal class.: CD (Sch 2), POM

Action: Inhibits ascending pain pathways in limbic system, thalamus, midbrain, hypothalamus
Uses: Analgesia especially during short operative procedure and outpatient surgery; enhancement of anaesthesia; analgesic and respiratory depressant in assisted respiration
Dosage and routes:
Spontaneous respiration
• *Adult:* IV injection, initially up to 500 mcg over 30 seconds, supplement, with increments of 250 mcg
• *Child:* Not recommended
Assisted ventilation
• *Adult and child:* IV injection, initially 30–50 mcg/kg, supplement with increments of 15 mcg/kg. Discontinue dosage at least 10 min before end of surgery
IV infusion, initially 50–100 mcg/kg over 10 min or as a bolus then maintenance 0.5–1.0 mcg/kg/min. Discontinue infusion at least 30 min before end of surgery. (Supplement with IV bolus if necessary)
Available forms include: Injection 500 mcg per ml (2 ml, 10 ml amps) 5 mg per ml (1 ml amps with sodium chloride and water for injection) (as hydrochloride)
Side effects/adverse reactions:
CNS: Dizziness
GI: Nausea, vomiting
CV: Bradycardia, hypotension
RESP: Respiratory depression
MS: Rigidity
Contraindications: Obstructive airways disease or respiratory

depression if not ventilating. Intolerance to alfentanil. Concurrent administration of monoamine oxidase inhibitors or within 2 weeks of their discontinuation. Administration in labour or before clamping of the cord during Caesarean section due to the possibility of respiratory depression in the newborn infant

Precautions: Reduce dose in elderly, hypothyroidism and chronic liver disease. Respiratory depression may persist or recur during postoperative period. Adequate spontaneous breathing must be established before leaving recovery room. Hypovolaemic patients, concomitant β-blocker or sedative medication. Reduced dose and extended interval may be required with concomitant use of erythromycin or cimetidine. Following cessation of Rapifen Intensive Care patient should be closely observed for at least 6 hr. Respiratory depression occurs following doses in excess of 1 mg. Seek clinician's advice on taking measures to avoid muscle rigidity

Pharmacokinetics: Half-life 1–2 hr. Peak analgesic and respiratory depressant effects occur within 90 seconds. Analgesia lasts up to 10 min

Interactions/incompatibilities:
- Cimetidine and erythromycin can inhibit alfentanil clearance leading to increased plasma levels
- Increased effects: hypnotics, CNS depressants

Treatment of overdose: Anticholinergics (e.g. atropine or glycopyrrolate)
Oxygen administration (assisted or controlled ventilation may be required)
IV neuromuscular blocking agent
Maintain body temperature and adequate fluid intake. Observe patient for 24 hr
Specific narcotic antagonist (e.g. naloxone) should be available to treat respiratory depression. All the effects of alfentanil may be antagonised if necessary by a specific narcotic antagonist such as naloxone

NURSING CONSIDERATIONS

Assess:
- Respiratory function if unventilated. If ventilated, maintenance of adequate analgesia/anaesthesia
- CNS function: dizziness, drowsiness, hallucinations, euphoria, level of consciousness and pupil reactions
- Fluid balance: decreasing urine output may indicate urinary retention

Administer:
- By prescribed bolus injection with maintenance infusion as prescribed, with assisted ventilation
- IV infusion in glucose 5%, sodium chloride 0.9% compound sodium lactate

Perform/provide:
- Dilute before use and for infusion
- Resuscitation equipment and narcotic antagonist (e.g. Naloxone) in case of respiratory depression

Evaluate:
- Response to treatment: maintenance of anaesthesia
- Allergic reactions: rash, urticaria
- Respiratory function: respiratory depression, rate and depth. Notify clinician if rate falls below 12 respirations per minute

allopurinol

Aloral, Aluline, Caplenal, Rimapurinol, Xanthomax, Cosuric, Hamarin, Zyloric, also others with no proprietary name
Func. class.: Antigout
Chem. class.: Enzyme inhibitor
Legal class.: POM

Action: Decreases uric acid levels by inhibiting xanthine oxidase
Uses: Gout prophylaxis, hyperuricaemia, management of some renal stones
Dosage and routes:
• *Adult:* By mouth, initially 100 mg/day, gradually increased over 1–3 weeks to 300 mg/day then 200–600 mg/day maintenance depending on severity
• *Child:* 10–20 mg/kg/day
• For dose in elderly, renal impairment and dialysis—seek clinician's advice
Available forms include: Tablets 100, 300 mg
Side effects/adverse reactions:
SYST: Generalised hypersensitivity reactions, withdraw drug. Initial exacerbation of acute gouty attacks
GI: Nausea, vomiting
INTEG: Fever, rashes (sometimes with fever) withdraw drug
Contraindications: Hypersensitivity, acute gout
Precautions: Pregnancy, lactation, renal disease, hepatic disease. Maintain adequate fluid intake (2 litres per day)
Asymptomatic hyperuricaemia. Withdraw immediately and permanently at first sign of intolerance
Neoplastic conditions—allopurinol should be commenced before cytotoxics
Administer prophylactic colchicine or NSAID (not aspirin or salicylates) until at least 1 month after hyperuricaemia corrected. Do not start therapy during or immediately after a gout attack
Pharmacokinetics:
By mouth: Peak 2–4 hr; excreted in faeces, urine, half-life 1–3 hr, terminal half-life 18–30 hr
Interactions/incompatibilities:
• Increased effects of: 6-mercaptopurine, azathioprine, cyclophosphamide, chlorpropamide, coumarin anticoagulants
• Effectiveness decrease of: salicylates, and uricosuric agents
• Renal calculi with: vitamin C
Lab. test interferences: Liver function tests
Clinical assessment:
• Monitor uric acid levels twice weekly. Levels should be 6 mg/dl
• Perform full blood count, blood urea and creatinine and serum aspartate aminotransferase levels before treatment commences, then monthly
• Check for any hypersensitivity, pregnancy, lactation, renal and hepatic disease
• For initial treatment prophylactic colchicine or NSAID (not aspirin or salicylate) should be prescribed
• Commence treatment a few days before anti-neoplastic therapy
Treatment of overdose: Adequate hydration to facilitate excretion. Dialysis if considered necessary. If taken with mercaptopurine or azathioprine inform clinician

NURSING CONSIDERATIONS

Assess:
• Fluid balance; increase fluid intake to at least 2 litres per 24 hr to prevent formation of renal calculi on clinical advice
• Diet: discourage offal, sardines, salmon, pulses, gravies (high purine foods)
Administer:
• With a full glass of water
• With meals to prevent gastro-

intestinal symptoms

Perform/provide:

• Sieve urine to detect renal calculi if calculi suspected

Evaluate:

• Therapeutic effectiveness e.g. decreased joint pain.

Teach patient/family:

• To report skin rashes, stomatitis, malaise, fever; aching; drug may have to be discontinued

• To avoid driving or handling machinery if drowsiness occurs

• To avoid alcohol, caffeine as they increase uric acid levels

• To avoid vitamin C preparations as renal calculi may develop

---

allyloestrenol

Gestanin

Func. class.: Progestogen

Chem. class.: Synthetic progestogen

Legal class.: POM

Action: Suppresses uterine motility, maintains pregnancy. Orally active progestogen

Uses: Threatened or habitual abortion, threatened premature labour

Dosage and routes: By mouth

Threatened abortion

• 5 mg 3 times daily for 5–7 days, extended if necessary, followed by gradual reduction in dose unless symptoms return

Habitual abortion

• 5–10 mg daily as soon as pregnancy is diagnosed and continued for at least 1 month after critical period ends

Threatened premature labour

• Dosage determined individually; high doses (up to 40 mg daily) have been used

Available forms include: Tablets 5 mg

Side effects/adverse reactions:

GI: Nausea and vomiting

Contraindications: Abnormal liver function. Porphyria

Interactions: Cyclosporin plasma concentration increased due to inhibition of metabolism

Clinical assessment:

• Liver function tests: bilirubin, alkaline phosphatase during long-term treatment

NURSING CONSIDERATIONS

Assess:

• BP at start of therapy, fluid balance, weight

Administer:

• With food or milk

Perform/provide:

• Blood/urine glucose monitoring in diabetes mellitus

Observe:

• Oedema and weight gain, clay coloured stools/dark urine, etc.

Evaluate:

• Vaginal bleeding

Teach patient/family:

• To inform clinician about: weight gain, PV loss, jaundice, light coloured stools, nausea and vomiting, headaches and breast lumps

• To perform breast examination

• If diabetic, to monitor glucose carefully

• To avoid over-exposure to sunlight

---

alprazolam

Xanax

Func. class.: Anxiolytic

Chem. class.: Benzodiazepine

Legal class.: CD (Sch 4) POM

Action: Depresses subcortical levels of CNS, including limbic system, reticular formation

Uses: Short-term treatment of moderate or severe anxiety and anxiety associated with depression

Dosage and routes:
• *Adult:* By mouth, 250–500 mcg 3 times daily increasing if necessary to a total of 3 mg daily
• *Elderly, debilitated:* 250 mcg, 2 to 3 times daily to be gradually increased, if required
Available forms include: Tablets 250 mcg, 500 mcg
Side effects/adverse reactions:
CNS: Drowsiness, sedation, unsteadiness and ataxia, impaired alertness, confusion, amnesia, dependence
EENT: Blurred vision
Contraindications: CNS depression, coma, respiratory depression, sleep apnoea
Precautions: Elderly, debilitated, hepatic disease, renal disease, chronic respiratory disease, lactation, pregnancy, psychosis, depression, labour, alcoholism, other CNS depressants, not for use under 18 years of age, personality disorders, loss or bereavement
Pharmacokinetics:
By mouth: Onset 30 min, peak 1–2 hr, duration 4–6 hr, therapeutic response 2–3 days, metabolised by liver, excreted by kidneys, breast milk, half-life 12–15 hr; can get accumulation
Interactions/incompatibilities:
• Increased effects: alcohol, anaesthetics, opioid analgesics, antidepressants, clonazepam, antihistamines, antipsychotics, CNS depressants
Treatment of overdose: Induce vomiting and/or gastric lavage, vital sign, supportive care

NURSING CONSIDERATIONS

Assess:
• Dosage to be assessed regularly
• Baseline BP (lying, standing), pulse
Administer:
• Crushed if patient is unable to swallow medication whole
Perform/provide:
• Mouthwashes; frequent sips of water for dry mouth
• Assistance with ambulation during beginning therapy; drowsiness/dizziness occurs
• Safety measures, including siderails
• Check to see oral medication has been swallowed
Evaluate:
• Therapeutic response: decreased anxiety, restlessness, sleeplessness
• Mental status: mood, alertness, affect, sleeping pattern, drowsiness, dizziness
• Physical dependency, withdrawal symptoms: headache, nausea, vomiting, muscle pain, weakness after long-term use
• Fluid balance, may indicate renal dysfunction
• Suicidal tendencies
Teach patient/family:
• That drug may be taken with food
• That drug is not to be used for everyday stress or longer than 4 months, unless directed by clinician
• To avoid non-prescribed preparations unless approved by clinician
• To avoid driving, activities that require alertness, since drowsiness may occur
• To avoid alcohol or other psychotropic medications, unless prescribed by clinician
• Not to discontinue medication abruptly after long-term use
• That drowsiness might worsen at beginning of treatment
• To see general practitioner/clinician each time a new supply is required (repeat prescriptions are not recommended)

alteplase INN

Actilyse
Func. class.: Fibrinolytic
Chem. class.: Tissue-type plasminogen activator (rtPA)
Legal class.: POM

Action: Accelerates conversion of plasminogen to plasmin; binds to fibrin, converts plasminogen in thrombus to plasmin, which leads to local fibrinolysis of clot. Alteplase is relatively inactive until it binds to fibrin

Uses: Fibrinolytic therapy of acute thrombotic coronary artery occlusion

Dosage and routes:

• *Adult:* IV 100 mg over 3 hr as 10 mg over 1–2 min, 50 mg over 1 hr, 40 mg over 2 hr. Patients under 67 kg receive 1.5 mg/kg in same proportions (10%, 50% and 40% of the total dose respectively). Treatment should be initiated within 6 hr of acute myocardial infarction

Available forms include: Powder for reconstitution 50 mg (29 million IU) per vial and 20 mg (11.6 million IU per vial)

Side effects/adverse reactions:

SYST: GI and GU bleeding, bleeding at site of injection, intracerebral haemorrhage, retroperitoneal bleeding, surface bleeding, nausea, vomiting

CV: Accelerated idioventricular rhythm associated with repofusion of the coronary artery

Contraindications: History of cerebrovascular disease or uncontrolled hypertension, known bleeding diathesis. Within 10 days of major surgery, severe internal bleeding episodes, or trauma or puncture of major non-compressible blood vessels. Acute pancreatitis, bacterial endocarditis, severe liver disease including hepatic failure, cirrhosis, portal hypertension (oesophageal varices) and active hepatitis, prolonged or traumatic resuscitation, active peptic ulcer

Precautions: Pregnancy, pay special attention to potential bleeding sites. Avoid IM injections, venepuncture and arterial puncture if possible, children, diabetes mellitus, diabetic retinopathy, severe renal impairment, avoid non-essential manipulation of patient. Anti-arrhythmic therapy should be available

Pharmacokinetics: Cleared by liver, 80% cleared within 10 min of administration

Interactions/incompatibilities:

• Increased risk of bleeding with prior or concomitant administration of anticoagulant

Treatment of overdose: Terminate infusion. If serious bleeding occurs fresh frozen plasma or fresh whole blood should be infused. Administer synthetic antifibrinolytic agents if necessary

NURSING CONSIDERATIONS

Assess:

• ECG, baseline temperature and neurological assessment
• Electrolytes—particular potassium (precipitates ectopics, etc.)
• Contraindications in patient

Administer:

• Reconstitute with diluting agent provided, then add sodium chloride 0.9% and dilute up to 1:5 if required
• Infuse via controlled pump delivery system over 3 hr period.
• Heparin after thrombolytic treatment has been discontinued, thrombin time or activated partial thromboplastin time less than 2 times baseline (about 3–4 hr)
• Within 6 hr of coronary occlusion for best results
• As prescribed by clinician

Perform/provide:

• Continuous ECG monitoring for arrhythmias/reperfusion dysrhythmias
• Emergency resuscitation equipment if anaphylaxis or cardiac arrest occurs
• Close observation of all IV puncture sites; urine; stools for evidence of haemorrhage – inform medical staff immediately
• Analgesics for the control of central chest pain (diamorphine/GTN)
• Issue card to patient stating time and nature of fibrinolytic administration. 1 hr post-administration

Evaluate:
• Vital signs: ½–1 hrly pulse respiration and BP
• Bleeding/haemorrhage during and immediately post-infusion: haematuria, haematemesis, bleeding from mucous membranes, epistaxis, ecchymosis
• ECG

Teach patient/family:
• To report any signs of bleeding, chest pain or malaise to nursing staff immediately
• Information concerning immediate and longer term counselling as to myocardial infarction, throughout hospital stay

aluminum acetate (otic, topical)

Func. class.: Astringent
Chem. class.: Aluminum salt
Legal class.: P

Action: Precipitate protein, form superficial protective layer
Uses: Suppurating an exudative eczema or wounds, treats inflammation in otitis externa
Dosage and routes:
• *Topical lotion 0.65%:* Use undiluted as a wet dressing
• *Ear drops 13% and 8%:* Instil into meatus or apply on gauze wick kept saturated with ear drops
Available forms include: Topical lotion 0.65%; ear drops 13%, 8%
Side effects/adverse reactions:
INTEG: Irritation, increasing inflammation
Contraindications: Tight, occlusive dressing
Interactions/incompatibilities:
• Inhibits action of topical collagenase ointment
• Soap decreases action

NURSING CONSIDERATIONS

Administer:
• Apply as moist dressings to the affected area. Avoid tight packing
• Avoid areas near the eyes

Evaluate:
• Observe area to receive topical application carefully for irritation, rashes, dryness and breaks in the skin

Teach patient/family:
• To discontinue use if irritation occurs
• To avoid using near eyes
• To retain ear drops by lying with affected ear uppermost for 10 min after instillation

aluminium hydroxide

Alu-Cap, NHS Aludrox, combination products
Func. class.: Antacid, phosphate-binder
Chem. class.: Aluminum salt
Legal class.: GSL or P

Action: Neutralises gastric acidity, adsorbs phosphates in GI tract
Uses: Antacid, hyperphosphataemia in chronic renal failure
Dosage and routes: By mouth
Antacid
• *Adult:* Suspension 5–10 ml 4 times a day between meals and at night

• *Child 6–12 yr:* up to 5 ml 3 times daily
• *Adult:* Tablets 500–1000 mg chewed 4 times daily and at night
Alu-Cap
• *Adult:* 1 capsule 4 times daily and at night. Not suitable as antacid for children
Hyperphosphataemia in renal failure
• Mixture 20–100 ml according to requirement of patient
Alu-Cap
• *Children and adult:* 2–10 g/day according to requirement of patient
Available forms include: Capsules 475 mg; tablets 500 mg; mixture 4%
Side effects/adverse reactions:
GI: Constipation
Contraindications: Hypersensitivity to this drug or aluminium products; hypophosphataemia; porphyria
Precautions: Renal impairment can cause aluminium accumulation. Watch for phosphate depletion. Porphyria
Pharmacokinetics:
By mouth: Onset 20–40 min, excreted in faeces and some in urine
Interactions/incompatibilities:
• Increased excretion: aspirin
• Reduced absorption: ciprofloxacin, isoniazid, norfloxacin, ofloxacin, tetracyclines, rifampicin, phenytoin, diflunisal, pivampicillin, itraconazole, ketoconazole, fosinopril, chloroquine, hydroxychloroquine, penicillamine
• Absorption of biphosphonates reduced
Treatment of overdose: Gastric lavage, mild aperient if required

NURSING CONSIDERATIONS
Assess:
• Monitor phosphate levels if using doses for phosphate binding
Administer:
• Shake suspension before use
• In cases of hyperphosphataemia, administer with food
• For antacid relief, administer between meals and at bedtime
Perform/provide:
• Give stool softeners as prescribed if constipated
• Test urine for pH
Evaluate:
• Therapeutic response: relief of pain/dyspepsia (antacid), relief of pruritus (hyperphosphataemia)
• Observe for pain, symptoms of dyspepsia
• Symptoms of hyperphosphataemia, e.g. persistent pruritus
• Signs of constipation
Teach patient/family:
• To drink at least 2 litres/day unless contraindicated
• To avoid foods rich in phosphates, e.g. dairy products, eggs, fruits
• Inform prescribing clinician regarding current medication
• High fibre diet unless contraindicated
• Appropriate administration technique
• To observe for side effects or signs of possible sub-therapeutic dosage

amantadine HCl

Symmetrel
Func. class.: Anti-viral, anti-parkinsonian agent
Chem. class.: Tricyclic amine
Legal class.: POM

Action: Inhibits viral replication. Prevents uncoating of viral nucleic acid and penetration of virus into host; potentiates dopaminergic activity in CNS
Uses: Prophylaxis or treatment of influenza type A, herpes zoster,

Parkinson's disease
Dosage and routes:
Herpes zoster
• *Adult:* 100 mg twice daily for 14 days. Repeat course if necessary for post-herpetic neuralgia
Influenza type A
• *Adult:* 100 mg twice daily for 5–7 days. Prophylaxis 100 mg daily for as long as required (usually 7–10 days)
• *Child 10–15 yr:* 100 mg daily
Parkinson's disease
• *Adult:* By mouth 100 mg daily or twice daily, second dose not later than 4 pm, maximum 400 mg daily
Available forms include: Capsules 100 mg; syrup 50 mg/5 ml
Side effects/adverse reactions:
CNS: Dizziness, anxiety, hallucinations, convulsions, inability to concentrate, insomnia
CV: Peripheral oedema
INTEG: Skin discolouration
EENT: Blurred vision
GI: Nausea, vomiting, constipation, dry mouth
Contraindications: Hypersensitivity, epilepsy, gastric ulceration or history of ulceration, severe renal disease
Precautions: Confusion, hallucinatory states, recurrent eczema. Renal impairment, liver disease, psychosis, congestive heart failure. Pregnancy, lactation, elderly. Avoid abrupt withdrawal
Pharmacokinetics:
By mouth: Peak plasma levels 4 hr, half-life 24 hr, not metabolised, excreted in urine (90%) unchanged, excreted in breast milk
Interactions/incompatibilities:
• Increased antimuscarinic side effects with: antimuscarinics
• Reduced antiparkinsonian action with: methyldopa, meticosine, antipsychotics, metoclopramide, reserpine, tetrabenazine
Treatment of overdose: No specific antidote. Supportive measures aimed at symptoms of excessive central stimulation

NURSING CONSIDERATIONS
Assess:
• Weight and fluid balance
Administer:
• Preferably before exposure to influenza and for 10 days after contact
• At least 4 hr before retiring to avoid insomnia
• After meals for better absorption and to avoid gastric upset
Evaluate:
• Therapeutic response: apyrexia, failure to develop malaise, cough, dyspnoea in infection: tremors, shuffling gait in Parkinson's disease
• For aggravation of side effects of anti-parkinsonian drugs
• Fluid balance, report urinary frequency and hesitancy
• Weight daily
• Bowel pattern before and during treatment
• Rashes, photosensitivity after administration of drug
• Rate and depth of respirations, wheezing, tightness in chest, limb oedema
• Allergies before commencing treatments and reaction to each administration of the drug. Note allergies in patient records and care plan and notify all staff responsible for drug administration
Teach patient/family:
• To alter position slowly to avoid postural hypotension
• All aspects of drug therapy: need to report breathlessness, weight gain, dizziness, lack of concentration, dysuria, behavioural changes
• To avoid situations where alertness is essential if there are CNS effects or blurred vision
• To take the drug exactly as prescribed, since parkinsonian crisis may occur if it is discontinued abruptly

amikacin sulphate

Amikin
Func. class.: Antibiotic
Chem. class.: Aminoglycoside
Legal class.: POM

Action: Interferes with protein synthesis in bacterial cell by binding to ribosomal subunit, which causes misreading of genetic code; inaccurate peptide sequence forms in protein chain, causing bacterial death

Uses: Serious gram-negative infection due to gentamicin-resistant organisms, e.g. some strains of *P. aeruginosa, E. coli, Enterobacter, Acinetobacter, Providencia, Citrobacter, Serratia, Proteus*

Dosage and routes:
- *Adult and child:* IM, slow IV injection, IV infusion 15 mg/kg/day in 2 doses; in life-threatening or pseudomonal infection, may be increased up to 1.5 g/day (500 mg 8 hrly), maximum 15 g total dose
- *Neonate and premature infant:* initial loading dose 10 mg/kg then 15 mg/kg/day in 2 doses
- ***Severe urinary tract infection*** (not due to *Pseudomonas* spp.) *Adult:* 7.5 mg/kg/day in 2 doses
- Reduce dose and/or decrease frequency in renal impairment. Other routes of administration: seek clinician's advice

Available forms include: Injection 50, 250 mg/ml

Side effects/adverse reactions:
GU: Oliguria, nephrotoxicity, azotaemia, renal irritation
CNS: Headache, numbness, paraesthesia, fever
EENT: Ototoxicity, deafness, tinnitus, vertigo
GI: Nausea, vomiting
INTEG: Rash

Contraindications: Mild-to-moderate infections, myasthenia gravis, hypersensitivity to aminoglycosides, pregnancy

Precautions: Renal impairment, lactation, hearing deficits, elderly, poor hydration. Renal irritation, prior administration of nephrotoxic and/or ototoxic agents

Pharmacokinetics:
IM: Onset rapid, peak 1 hr
IV: Onset immediate, peak 30 min
Plasma half-life 2–3 hr; not metabolised, excreted unchanged in urine

Interactions/incompatibilities:
- Increased risk of nephrotoxicity: cephalosporins, colistin, polymyxin, capreomycin, vancomycin, amphotericin, cyclosporin, cisplatin, diuretics
- Enhanced effects of: non-depolarising muscle relaxants
- Severe hypocalcaemia: bisphosphonates
- Do not mix in solution or syringe with other drugs

Clinical assessment:
- Monitor plasma concentrations of drug 1 hr after IV or IM injection when levels should peak and just before next dose when levels should trough. Plasma levels should be 2–4 times greater than bacteriostatic level. 1 hr (peak) concentration should not exceed 30 mg/litre, pre-dose (trough) concentration should be less than 10 mg/litre
- Prescribe to be given at regular intervals to maintain plasma concentrations
- Assess for signs of renal impairment by creatinine clearance tests, blood urea and creatinine levels; lower dosage should be given for renal impairment

Treatment of overdose: Haemodialysis or peritoneal dialysis, monitor serum levels of drug

NURSING CONSIDERATIONS

Assess:
- Weight before treatment commences: dose is usually calculated

on ideal body weight, but may be calculated on actual body weight
• Fluid balance

Administer:
• Preferably IM, but if necessary IV bolus over 2 to 3 min or IV infusion as 0.25% solution over 30 min. Adjust dosage according to renal and auditory function; pre-dose (trough) concentrations should be less than 10 mg/l
• Administer IM injection into large muscle mass, rotate injection sites
• Ensure drug is given at regular intervals as prescribed to maintain blood levels
• Bicarbonate, to keep urine alkaline if drug prescribed for urinary tract infection, as drug is most effective in an alkaline environment. Bladder wash out may be used

Perform/provide:
• Monitor vital signs during infusion, observe for hypotension, change in pulse
• Obtain culture and sensitivity before treatment commences to identify causative organism
• Encourage patient to drink 2–3 litres fluid daily to prevent renal damage
• Flush line with normal saline after infusion
• Observe for vestibular dysfunction

Evaluate:
• Urinalysis daily for proteinuria casts. Report sudden change in urinary output
• Observe IV site for signs of thrombophlebitis, e.g. pain, redness, swelling. Inform clinician if thrombophlebitis occurs
• Therapeutic effectiveness
• Record temperature, wounds for signs of infection
• For signs of deafness e.g. tinnitus, vertigo. Audiometric testing may be necessary
• Observe for dehydration: concentrated urine, decrease in skin elasticity, dry mucous membranes
• Secondary infection, pyrexia, malaise, redness, pain, swelling, perineal itching, stomatitis, change in cough or sputum, diarrhoea
• Vestibular dysfunction: nausea, vomiting, dizziness, headache and report: drug may have to be discontinued if severe

Teach patient/family:
• To report headache, dizziness, symptoms of secondary infection, renal impairment
• To report hearing loss, tinnitus, feeling of 'fullness' in head

---

amiloride HCl

Midamor, Berkamil, Amilospare, many combination products

Func. class.: Potassium-sparing diuretic

Legal class.: POM

Action: Acts primarily on distal tubule, secondarily by inhibiting reabsorption of sodium. Reduces excretion of potassium

Uses: Oedema, potassium conservation with thiazide and loop diuretics in hypertension, congestive heart failure, hepatic cirrhosis with ascites

Dosage and routes:

Adult: By mouth initially 10 mg daily or 5 mg twice daily, maximum 20 mg daily. Cirrhosis with ascites, initially 5 mg daily. Contraindicated in children. Monitor dose carefully in elderly

Available forms include: Tablets 5 mg, sugar-free oral solution 5 mg in 5 ml

Side effects/adverse reactions:

ELECT: Hyponatraemia, hyperkalaemia

CNS: Confusion

GI: Nausea, dry mouth, anorexia, abdominal pain, flatulence

INTEG: Rash

CV: Orthostatic hypotension
Contraindications: Anuria, hyperkalaemia, diabetic nephropathy, hypersensitivity, acute renal failure, severe renal disease, pregnancy, lactation, potassium supplements, potassium-conserving agents, use in children
Precautions: Ascites, hepatic disease, renal impairment, acidosis, diabetes mellitus, elderly, cardiac oedema, potassium-rich diet
Pharmacokinetics:
By mouth: Onset 2 hr, peak 6–10 hr, duration 24 hr; excreted in urine, faeces, excreted in breast milk, half-life 6–9 hr
Interactions/incompatibilities:
• Reduced renal clearance of lithium
• Increased risk of hyponatraemia with chlorpropamide in combination with thiazide diuretic
• Increased risk of hypokalaemia in combination with angiotensin—converting enzyme inhibitor
Clinical assessment:
• Monitor electrolytes; blood potassium, sodium and chloride.
• Order medication to be given in the morning to avoid diuretic effect at night
• Assess therapeutic response, e.g. oedema of feet, legs, sacral area daily if drug is given for congestive cardiac failure
Lab. test interferences:
Interfere: Glucose tolerance test. Discontinue at least 3 days before test
Treatment of overdose: Discontinue therapy. No antidote. Induce emesis or gastric lavage. Symptomatic and supportive treatment for dehydration, electrolyte imbalance, hyperkalaemia
NURSING CONSIDERATIONS
Assess:
• Fluid balance, weight, BP
Administer:
• In early morning to avoid nocturia
• With food if nausea occurs; absorption may be decreased slightly
Perform/provide:
• Weigh daily; maintain fluid balance chart
• BP (standing and lying) 6-hrly
Evaluate:
• Drowsiness and restlessness (signs of metabolic acidosis) and confusion, especially in the elderly
• Relief of dyspnoea and oedema
• Rashes, pyrexia daily
Teach patient/family:
• To increase fluid intake 2–3 litre daily unless contraindicated
• To rise slowly from lying or sitting position
• About adverse reactions
• To take medication as prescribed
• To avoid potassium-rich foods, e.g. oranges, bananas
• To inform prescribing clinician about current medication

amino acid solution

Aminoplasmal, Aminoplex, Branched Chain Aminoacids, FreAmine III, Hepanutrin, Heplex Amine
Nephramine, Perifusin, Primene, Synthamin, Vamin
Func. class.: Nutrition, intravenous
Chem. class.: Amino acids
Legal class.: POM

Action: Required for anabolism to maintain structure, decrease catabolism, promote healing
Uses: Supplemental or total parenteral nutrition (TPN) when adequate feeding via alimentary tract is not possible
Dosage and routes:
• Intravenous infusion
• Seek advice from clinician, dietician and pharmacist; folic acid, vitamin, electrolyte and mineral supplements may be necessary

Available forms include: Vary in composition of amino acids, often contain energy source and/or electrolytes

Side effects/adverse reactions:

GI: Nausea, cholestasis, abnormal liver function tests, portal tract fibrosis

GU: Hypercalciuria

ENDO: Hyperglycaemia, osteomalacia

INTEG: Phlebitis at injection site

Contraindications: Hypersensitivity, severe electrolyte imbalances, anuria, severe liver disease, errors of amino acid metabolism, acidosis, advanced renal disease (no dialysis available), severe uraemia, hyperhydration, disturbed protein metabolism, cardiac insufficiency

Precautions: Renal disease, pregnancy, children, diabetes mellitus, congestive cardiac failure, liver disease, electrolyte retention, cardiac disease, drug therapy requiring electrolyte monitoring, energy supply necessary

Interactions/incompatibilities: Contact pharmacy department

Clinical assessment:

• Before therapy commences ensure adequate circulating volume, liver and renal function, absence of acidosis or hypoxaemia and check vitamin B_{12} status

• Monitor plasma electrolytes, circulating volume, blood glucose, acid-base, fluid balance and nutritional status throughout treatment

• Monitor ECG for potassium replacement needs

• Monitor blood urea nitrogen in addition in renal impairment

• Monitor plasma phenylalanine in infants

Treatment of overdose: Reduce rate of infusion or stop

NURSING CONSIDERATIONS

Assess:

• Fluid balance

Administer:

• Via dedicated, tunnelled central venous feeding line for long-term use, i.e. Hickman line. Central venous access preferable to avoid phlebitis and extravasation

• TPN in combination with dextrose to promote (protein synthesis) anabolism

• Immediately after the freshly prepared solution has been received from pharmacy, using strict aseptic technique

Perform/provide:

• Urinalysis for glucose 6 hrly

• Blood glucose estimations are more accurate

• Monitor drip rate/infusion rate carefully. The infusion must never be speeded up; pulmonary oedema and hyperglycaemia will result

• Store all solutions according to manufacturer's instructions; slight variations may be necessary according to exact nature of solution

• Change dressing over intravenous site as necessary. Using strict aseptic technique

Evaluate:

• Infusion site for extravasation: inflammation, local oedema, necrosis, pain, hardening or tenderness; the site will need to be changed immediately

• Monitor respiratory function 4 hrly, observing respiratory rate and depth

• Monitor temperature 4 hrly. If infection is suspected the infusion must be discontinued and swabs from the tubing and container sent to the bacteriology laboratory for culture

• Hyperammonaemia: nausea, vomiting, malaise, tremors, anorexia, convulsions

• Therapeutic response: weight gain, resolution of jaundice if patient has hepatic dysfunction, increased serum albumin levels

• Urinary creatinine clearance and

nitrogen excretion with 24 hr urine collection twice a week

Teach patient/family:

• Why intravenous nutrition is necessary

• If chills, sweating are experienced they should be reported at once

• If the patient is to be discharged with intravenous nutrition in the community *all* aspects of nutrition must be taught, preferably by a specialist nurse or dietitian

aminoglutethimide

Orimeten

Func. class.: Antineoplastic, adrenal steroid inhibitor

Chem. class.: Enzyme inhibitor, glutethimide analogue

Legal class.: POM

Action: Inhibits conversion of androgens to oestrogens in the peripheral tissues

Uses: Advanced breast cancer in postmenopausal or oophorectomised women, advanced prostate cancer (palliative). Cushing's syndrome due to malignant disease

Dosage and routes:

• Doses are highly variable, and dependent on local treatment protocols, concomitant therapy and tumour type; the following dose schedules have been used

Breast or prostate cancer:

• *Adult:* By mouth, initially 250 mg daily increasing at weekly intervals to maximum 250 mg 4 times daily (lower doses may be adequate), in conjunction with a glucocorticoid.

Cushing's syndrome due to malignant disease:

• *Adult:* By mouth, 250 mg daily increasing gradually to 1 g (occasionally 2 g) daily in divided doses

Available forms include: Tablets, scored 250 mg

Side effects/adverse reactions:

HAEM: Thombocytopenia, leucopenia, agranulocytosis, pancytopenia

GI: Nausea, vomiting, diarrhoea

INTEG: Rash

RESP: Allergic alveolitis

METAB: Altered thyroid function

CNS: Dizziness, somnolence, lethargy, unsteadiness; fever

Contraindications: Hypersensitivity, pregnancy, breast-feeding children, porphyria

Pharmacokinetics: Half-life (long term therapy), 7 hr, peak plasma concentration 1–2 hr, metabolised in liver, excreted in urine

Interactions/incompatibilities:

• Aminoglutethimide accelerates metabolism of certain drugs: nicoumalone, warfarin, digitoxin, dexamethasone, theophylline, oral antidiabetics

Clinical assessment:

• Full blood count, platelet count every 2–3 weeks initially

• Prescribe hydrocortisone to replace drug-induced adrenal steroid production

• Response to stress may be impaired

Treatment of overdose: Remove tablets from GI tract. Supportive treatment to maintain fluid and electrolyte balance, IV steroids if needed. Symptoms may recur

NURSING CONSIDERATIONS

Assess:

• Fluid balance if GI symptoms occur

• BP and temperature

Administer:

• Handling: take safety precautions appropriate to antineoplastic agents

• Following local antineoplastic (cytotoxic) policies

• After ensuring that clinician is aware of blood results

- By mouth
- Antacid immediately before drug and at bedtime
- Anti-emetic 30–60 min before treatment
- With hydrocortisone to replace drug-induced adrenal steroid suppression
- Other medications by mouth if possible. Avoid IV, IM, SC routes to prevent infection and bruising

Perform/provide:
- Medication by oral route if possible: avoid IM, IV and subcutaneous injections to prevent infection
- Antacid before drug and at bedtime as ordered
- Anti-emetic as prescribed before drug to prevent vomiting
- Skin care
- Nutritious diet with iron and vitamin supplements

Evaluate:
- Temperature 4 hrly; may indicate beginning of infection, but only in first few days as early toxicity then settles
- Food preferences
- For side effects; including early toxicity (dizziness, somnolence, lethargy), tumour flare (spinal cord compression, increased bone pain), nausea, vomiting

Teach patient/family:
- That drowsiness drug fever and morbilliform eruption often settle spontaneously
- To report side effects to nurse or clinician
- That masculinisation can occur but is reversible after discontinuing treatment

aminophylline (theophylline ethylenediamine)

Phyllocontin Continus, Pecram, Amnivent

Func. class.: Bronchodilator
Chem. class.: Xanthine
Legal class.: Injection POM; Tablets P

Action: Relaxes smooth muscle of respiratory system, may have anti-inflammatory action in respiratory system

Uses: Reversible airways obstruction, status asthmaticus. In adults, cardiac asthma and left ventricular or congestive cardiac failure

Dosages and routes:
- *Adult:* By mouth, 100–300 mg 3 to 4 times daily – modified-release preparations usually 225 mg twice daily; initially increasing up to 450 mg twice daily after one week as appropriate. IV injection 250–500 mg (5mg/kg) over 20 min (if already taking xanthines, maximum dose 2.5 mg/kg over 20 min – measure levels). Slow IV infusion in patients not already taking xanthines 500 micrograms/kg/hr
- *Child over 3 yr:* By mouth, modified-release preparations usually 6 mg/kg twice daily for one week increasing to 12 mg/kg twice a day as appropriate
- *Child:* Slow IV injection in patients not already taking xanthines, 5 mg/kg over 20 min. Maintenance IV infusion in patients not already taking xanthines 6 months–9 years 1 mg/kg/hr, 10–16 yr 800 mcg/kg/hr

Narrow margin between therapeutic and toxic dose. Plasma levels must be monitored. Optimum plasma levels of theophylline 10–20 mg/l

Available forms include: Tablets 100 mg, modified release 100 mg, 225 mg, 350 mg; Injection IV 25 mg/ml; 10 ml amp. Some modified release are hydrate salt

Side effects/adverse reactions:

CNS: Insomnia, convulsions, headache, stimulation

CV: Palpitations, tachycardia, arrythmias

GI: Nausea, vomiting, diarrhoea, dyspepsia

Contraindications: Hypersensitivity to xanthines and ethylenediamine; porphyria. Concomitant use of ephedrine in children; concurrent use of other xanthines

Precautions: Elderly, congestive heart failure, hepatic disease, cardiac disease, hypokalaemia, smoking, alcohol, viral infections, epilepsy, lactation, fever, keep to same brand of tablet, pregnancy

Pharmacokinetics:

IV: Peak 30 min. Bioavailability of different oral preparations varies greatly

Interactions/incompatibilities:

- Do not mix in syringe with other drugs
- Increased plasma theophylline levels: thiabendazole, ciprofloxacin, enoxacin, erythromycin, norfloxacin, isoniazid, viloxazine, diltiazem, verapamil, disulfiram, interferons, combined oral contraceptives, cimetidine, possibly influenza vaccine
- Reduced plasma theophylline levels: rifampicin, carbamazepine, barbiturates, phenytoin, primidone, aminoglutethimide, sulphinpyrazone, alcohol, smoking
- Increased risk of side effects: β-blockers, lithium, respiratory stimulants, fenoterol, pirbuterol, reproterol, rimiterol, ritodrine, salbutamol, salmeterol, terbutaline, tulobuterol, allopurinol, isoprenaline, halothane, lomustine, glucagon, other xanthines, ephedrine, steroids, diuretics, hypoxia

Clinical assessment:

- Monitor theophylline blood levels (therapeutic level is 10–20 mg/litre); toxicity may occur with small increase above 20 mg/litre
- Monitor serum potassium levels in severe asthma–potentially serious hypokalaemia may result from concomitant treatment with β_2-adrenoceptor stimulants, theophylline and derivatives, corticosteroids, and diuretics, and by hypoxia
- Check whether theophylline was given recently and if modified release preparation. Measure theophylline plasma concentrations before instituting aminophylline therapy if patient has been taking oral theophylline preparations
- Once patient is stabilised on one modified-release product, do not change to another preparation without retitration and clinical assessment

Treatment of overdose: *Oral*: empty stomach. Monitor ECG, maintain fluid balance. Administer oral activated charcoal. In severe poisoning use charcoal-column haemoperfusion. Symptomatic treatment. NB: modified-release preparations will release aminophylline for several hours. If hypokalaemia, give potassium chloride by mouth or slow IV infusion. Monitor plasma potassium. Control convulsions by IV diazepam or if necessary thiopentone sodium

NURSING CONSIDERATIONS

Administer:

- Respiratory function
- Do not mix in syringe with other drugs
- IV injection slowly over 20 min

• IV infusion in 250–500 ml glucose 5%, sodium chloride 0.9% or compound sodium lactate
• Oral preparations after meals to decrease gastrointestinal symptoms; absorption may be affected
• Modified-release tablets should be swallowed whole with water and not chewed
• Same brand unless retitrate dose

Evaluate:
• Cardiac rhythm and rate during IV infusion
• Fluid balance: if diuresis occurs, dehydration may result in elderly or children
• Response to treatment; decreased dyspnoea, respiratory rate, depth
• Allergic reactions, e.g. rash, urticaria and inform clinician, who may discontinue drug

Teach patient/family:
• To avoid medicines that have not been prescribed; those containing ephedrine will increase CNS stimulation
• To avoid driving and operating machinery; dizziness may occur
• To be aware of possible side effects and to know when to contact clinician
• If gastrointestinal upset occurs to take dose with about 200 ml of water, and avoid food since absorption may be decreased

---

amiodarone hydrochloride

Cordarone X

Func. class.: Anti-arrhythmic (Class III)
Chem. class.: Iodinated benzofuran derivative
Legal class.: POM

Action: Delays repolarisation by prolonging action potential and refractory period

Uses: Wolff-Parkinson-White syndrome. Atrial flutter and fibrillation, supraventicular and ventricular tachycardias and recurrent ventricular fibrillation when other drugs ineffective or contraindicated

Dosage and routes:
• *Adult:* By mouth, initially 200 mg 3 times daily for 1 week, then twice daily for 1 week, then 200 mg or less daily for maintenance; in some cases more than 200 mg daily maintenance may be needed
• *Adult:* IV infusion via central venous catheter up to 5 mg/kg over 20–120 min under ECG, may be repeated 2–3 times in 24 hr, up to maximum daily dose of 1.2 g
• *Adult:* Emergency treatment at discretion of clinician, slow IV injection, 150–300 mg in 10–20 ml dextrose 5% over not less than 3 min; should not be repeated for at least 15 min

Available forms include: Tablets scored 100 mg, 200 mg; injection 50 mg/ml, or dilution

Side effects/adverse reactions:
CNS: Headache, benign raised intracranial pressure, nightmares, vertigo, sleeplessness, peripheral neuropathy, myopathy
GI: Hepatotoxicity
CV: Bradycardia, sinus arrest, anaphylaxis on rapid injection
INTEG: Rash, photosensitivity
EENT: Microdeposits in cornea
ENDO: Hyperthyroidism or hypothyroidism
RESP: Pulmonary fibrosis, dyspnoea, pulmonary alveolitis

Contraindications: Thyroid dysfunction, sinus bradycardia, atrioventricular block (unless pacemaker fitted) sino-atrial heartblock; IV contraindicated in severe respiratory failure, circulatory collapse or severe arterial hypotension, congestive heart failure; iodine sensitivity, lactation, pregnancy, porphyria

Precautions: Sinus node dysfunction, severe conduction disturbances, heart failure, elderly, renal impairment

Too high a dose may produce severe bradycardia and conduction disturbances

Pharmacokinetics:

By mouth: Onset 1–3 weeks, peak 2–10 hr; half-life 53 days; much interpatient variation; metabolised by liver, strongly protein-bound

IV: onset 1–30 min, duration 1–3 hr

Interactions/incompatibilities:

• Increased effect of: disopyramide, flecainide, procainamide, quinidine and other anti-arrhythmics, nicoumalone, warfarin, phenytoin

• Increased risk of side effects: B-blockers, diltiazem, verapamil, digoxin, cimetidine, general anaesthesia

• Toxicity increased if hypokalaemia with acetazolamide, loop diuretics, thiazides

Clinical assessment:

• Obtain blood for potassium, sodium and chloride estimations.

• Perform liver function tests; aspartate aminotransferase, alanine aminotransferase, bilirubin and alkaline phosphatase

• Monitor for hypovolaemia

• Reduce dose slowly with ECG monitoring

• During long-term therapy—monitor eyes, thyroid function, liver function

• Inform anaesthetist about amiodarone therapy, when appropriate

Lab. test interferences: Some thyroid function tests

Treatment of overdose: Gastric lavage and general supportive measures. Monitor patient and give β-adrenoceptor stimulants or glucagon if bradycardia. Prolonged surveillance

NURSING CONSIDERATIONS

Administer:

Infusion should be diluted as directed in 5% glucose solution. Amiodarone infusion may reduce drop size and, if appropriate, make adjustments to rate of infusion. At the discretion of the clinician, slow IV injection can be administered in extreme clinical emergency

Perform/provide:

• Patient will require continuous cardiac monitoring during IV therapy to determine drug effectiveness, check for premature ventricular contraction, other dysrhythmias

Evaluate:

• For rebound hypertension after 1–2 hr

• Changes in BP, bradycardia

• Hypothyroidism, e.g. lethargy, dizziness, constipation, enlarged thyroid, oedema of extremities, cool, dry skin

• Hyperthyroidism: restlessness, tachycardia, eyelid puffiness, weight loss, frequency of urine, menstrual irregularities, dyspnoea, warm, moist skin

• For dyspnoea, fatigue, cough, fever, chest pain may indicate pneumonitis

Teach patient/family:

• All aspects of drug therapy, side effects and when to report to clinician

• To report side effects immediately

• To protect the skin against ultra violet and visible light by using total sunblock

• That skin discoloration is reversible

• That dark glasses may be needed for photophobia and that drivers may be dazzled by headlights at night (micro-deposits in eyes)

• That metallic taste may be noted

amitriptyline hydrochloride

Tryptizol, Lentizol, Domical, Elavil

Func. class.: Antidepressant, tricyclic

Chem. class.: Tertiary amine

Legal class.: POM

Action: Blocks reuptake of noradrenaline, serotonin into nerve endings, increasing action of noradrenaline, serotonin on nerve cells. Mode of action in depression not known

Uses: Depression, nocturnal enuresis in children

Dosage and routes:

Depression:

• *Adult:* By mouth initially 50–75 mg daily increasing as required to maximum 200 mg daily, IM/IV 10–20 mg 4 times daily

• *Adolescent/geriatric:* By mouth initially 25–50 mg daily

• Not recommended for treatment of *depression* in children under 16 yr

Nocturnal enuresis:

• *Child:* 7–10 yr: 10–20 mg at night, 11–16 yr: 25–50 mg at night. Maximum duration 3 months

Available forms include: Tablets 10, 25, 50 mg, capsules modified release 25, 50, 75 mg, mixture 10 mg (as embonate)/5 ml; injection 10 mg/ml (10 ml vial)

Side effects/adverse reactions:

HAEM: Agranulocytosis, thrombocytopenia, eosinophilia, leucopenia, purpura

CNS: Convulsions, confusion, sedation, tremors, hypomania, behavioural disturbances (especially children)

GI: Dry mouth, nausea, black tongue, paralytic ileus, increased appetite, jaundice, constipation, weight gain (occasionally loss)

GU: Difficulty with micturition, interference with sexual function

INTEG: Rash, sweating

CV: Orthostatic hypotension, tachycardia, arrythmias, syncope

EENT: Blurred vision

METAB: Blood sugar changes

Contraindications: Hypersensitivity to tricyclic antidepressants, breast-feeding, arrythmias, coronary artery insufficiency, recovery phase of myocardial infarction, heart block, severe liver disease, children less than 6 yr, co-administration with MAOIs, mania, porphyria

Precautions: Suicidal patients, convulsive disorders, prostatic hypertrophy, schizophrenia, elderly, diabetes mellitus, psychoses, severe depression, manic depression, anaesthesia, increased intraocular pressure, narrow-angle glaucoma, urinary retention, hepatic disease, hyperthyroidism, thyroid medication or anticholinergic agents, electroshock therapy, elective surgery, pregnancy, cardiovascular disorders. Avoid abrupt cessation

Pharmacokinetics:

By mouth/IM: Onset 45 min, peak 2–12 hr, therapeutic response 2–4 weeks; metabolised by liver, excreted in urine/faeces, excreted in breast milk, half-life 10–50 hr

Interactions/incompatibilities:

• Enhanced effect: Alcohol, anaesthetics, MAOIs (stop for at least 2 weeks before starting tricyclics), fluoxetine, antiepileptics, antihistamines

• Increased side effects: Antimuscarinics, phenothiazines, anxiolytics, hypnotics, diltiazem, verapamil, disulfiram, diuretics, oral contraceptives, adrenaline noradrenaline, ephedrine, isoprenaline, phenylephrine, phenylpropanolamine, methylphenidate

• Reduced effect of: sublingual nitrates
• Amitriptyline increases response to alcohol, barbiturates and other CNS depressants
• Reduced antidepressant effect: barbiturates

Clinical assessment:
• Perform full blood count, differential white blood count, cardiac enzymes if patient is receiving treatment long-term
• Liver function tests; aspartate aminotransferase, alanine aminotransferase, bilirubin, creatinine
• Perform ECG for flattening of T wave, bundle branch block, atrioventricular block, dysrhythmias in cardiac patients

Treatment of overdose:
Symptomatic and supportive treatment. Emesis, gastric lavage, activated charcoal. ECG, close cardiac monitoring for at least 5 days. Maintain open airway, fluid intake. Regulate body temperature. IV physostigmine salicylate if clinically indicated (not for routine use). Administer anticonvulsant (non-barbiturate). Dialysis of no value. Manage circulatory shock and metabolic acidosis

NURSING CONSIDERATIONS

Assess:
• Baseline BP (lying, standing) and pulse
• Weight

Administer:
• At bedtime if over-sedation occurs during day; entire dose may be taken at bedtime; elderly may not be able to tolerate dosage once daily
• Increase fluid and fibre in diet if constipated. Urinary retention may occur, especially in children
• Give with food or milk for GI symptoms

Perform/provide:
• Mouth care and frequent sips of water for dry mouth
• Help when patient takes exercise at beginning of therapy since drowsiness/dizziness occurs
• Checking to ensure that oral medication is swallowed

Evaluate:
• BP (lying, standing), pulse 4 hrly; if systolic BP falls 20 mmHg withhold drug and inform clinician; take vital signs in all patients with cardiovascular disease
• Weight weekly; appetite may increase with drug
• Extrapyramidal symptoms in elderly, e.g. rigidity, dystonia, akathisia
• Mental status: mood, clarity of thought/mental alertness, affect, increase in psychiatric symptoms, e.g. depression, panic
• Withdrawal symptoms: headache, nausea, vomiting, muscle pain, weakness; do not usually occur unless drug is discontinued abruptly
• Alcohol consumption: if alcohol is consumed inform clinician and withhold dose until morning

Teach patient/family:
• Therapeutic effects may take 2–3 weeks
• Caution when driving or operating machinery because of drowsiness, dizziness, blurred vision
• To avoid alcohol, other CNS depressants
• Not to discontinue medication suddenly after long term; may cause nausea, headache, vomiting
• To avoid strong sunshine
• Careful supervision for risk of suicide

amlodipine besylate

Istin
Func. class.: Antihypertensive, anti-anginal
Chem. class.: Dihydropyridine calcium-channel blocker
Legal class.: POM

Action: Calcium slow channel blocker; relaxes vascular smooth muscle; reduces total ischaemic burden
Uses: Hypertension, prophylaxis of angina
Dosage and routes:
• *Adult:* By mouth, initially 5 mg daily; maximum 10 mg daily
Available forms include: Tablets 5 mg, 10 mg (as besylate)
Side effects/adverse reactions:
GI: Nausea
CNS: Headache, fatigue, dizziness
INTEG: Flushing
CV: Oedema
Contraindications: Hypersensitivity to dihydropyridines, cardiogenic shock
Precautions: Hepatic insufficiency
Pharmacokinetics:
By mouth: Half-life 35–50 hr, peak 6–12 hr. Excreted mainly as inactive metabolites in urine. Highly plasma protein bound
Treatment of overdose: Gastric lavage. Treat symptomatically for excessive peripheral vasodilation, systemic hypotension. Monitor cardiac and respiratory function, elevate extremities, monitor circulating fluid volume and urine output. If no contraindication, vasoconstrictor may be useful. Not dialysable
NURSING CONSIDERATIONS
Assess:
• Baseline BP
Administer:
• With or without food
Evaluate:
• Therapeutic response: decreased anginal pain
• If used as antihypertensive, record BP regularly. Note: full effect may not be seen for 10–14 days
Teach patient/family:
• To report immediately if pregnancy is suspected
• To report headaches, dizziness, parasthesia
• To avoid hazardous activities until stabilised on drug or dizziness no longer a problem

amoxycillin

Amoxil, Almodan, Flemoxin
Func. class.: Broad spectrum antibiotic
Chem. class.: Aminohydroxy penicillin
Legal class.: POM

Action: Interferes with cell wall replication of susceptible organisms; the cell wall, rendered osmotically unstable, swells, and bursts from osmotic pressure. Bactericidal
Uses: Include: urinary-tract infections, otitis media, chronic bronchitis, invasive salmonellosis, gonorrhoea, typhoid fever, dental prophylaxis, septicaemia
Dosage and routes:
• *Adult:* By mouth, 250 mg every 8 hr, doubled in severe infections; IM 500 mg every 8 hr; IV injection/infusion 500 mg every 8 hr increased to 1 g every 6 hr
• *Child up to 10 yr:* 125 mg every 8 hr, doubled in severe infections; IM/IV 50–100 mg/kg daily in divided doses
Severe or recurrent purulent respiratory infection
• *Adult:* By mouth, 3 g every 12 hr
• *Child 2–5 yr:* By mouth, 750 mg every 12 hr, 5–10 yr 1.5 g every 12 hr

Dental abscess
• *Adult:* By mouth, 3 g repeated after 8 hr
Urinary-tract infection
• *Adult:* By mouth, 3 g repeated after 10–12 hr
Gonorrhoea
• *Adult:* single dose of 3 g with probenecid 1 g
Otitis media
• *Child 3–10 yr:* 750 mg twice daily for 2 days

Available forms include: Capsules 250, 500 mg; powder for oral suspension, 125, 250 mg/5 ml; injection 250, 500 mg, 1 g vial for reconstitution. Dispersible sugar-free tablets 500 mg. Powder for sugar-free syrup 125, 250 mg/5 ml. Powder for paediatric suspension 125 mg/1.25 ml. Sugar-free sachets 750 mg, 3 g. Injection is sodium salt, oral preparations as trihydrate

Side effects/adverse reactions:
GI: Nausea, diarrhoea, indigestion
INTEG: Rashes (discontinue treatment)
MISC: Angioedema, anaphylaxis

Contraindications: Hypersensitivity to penicillins

Precautions: Hypersensitivity to cephalosporins. History of allergy, glandular fever, lactation, renal impairment, chronic lymphatic leukaemia, HIV-infection

Interactions/incompatibilities:
• Do not mix with blood products, protein hydrolysates, IV lipid emulsions, or aminoglycosides in same syringe
• Enhances effect of: warfarin, phenindione, probenecid
• Risk of reduced contraceptive effect: combined oral contraceptives

Pharmacokinetics:
By mouth: Peak 1–2 hr, duration 6–8 hr; half-life 1–1⅓ hr, metabolised in liver, excreted in urine, enters breast milk

Clinical assessment:
• Injection contains sodium, which may restrict use if salt restricted or problems with fluid balance

Treatment of overdose: Maintain adequate fluid intake and urinary output–crystalluria possible. Removed by haemodialysis

NURSING CONSIDERATIONS

Assess:
• Obtain specimen for bacteriology laboratory for culture and sensitivity testing before treatment commences and after course is completed
• Ask patient about allergies before treatment commences and record on drug chart

Administer:
• Preferably by mouth. If IV, dissolved in 5 ml water for injections per 250 mg and injected over 3–4 min, or added to IV infusion and given over half to one hour. IM solutions may be dissolved in 1% lignocaine hydrochloride solution or water for injections.

Perform/provide:
• Adequate fluid intake (2 litres daily) if diarrhoea occurs

Evaluate:
• Therapeutic response
• Temperature 4 hrly; observe condition of discharging wounds
• Bowel pattern before and during treatment
• Skin rashes (often related to penicillin allergy)
• Respiratory rate, character, wheezing, tightness in chest
• Observe patient with known renal impairment carefully; toxicity may develop rapidly

Teach patient/family:
• To take oral amoxycillin with a full glass of water
• All aspects of drug therapy: the entire course must be completed unless advised otherwise by clinician
• That medication must be taken

regularly to maintain blood levels
• To wear Medic Alert Identity if allergic to penicillins
• To report any diarrhoea to nurse or clinician

amphotericin (oral)

Fungilin
Func. class.: Antifungal
Chem. class.: Amphoteric polyene macrolide
Legal class.: POM

Action: Increases cell membrane permeability in susceptible organisms by binding sterols; decreases potassium, sodium and nutrients in cell
Uses: Intestinal candidosis, oral and perioral fungal infections, suppression of intestinal reservoir of *C. albicans*
Dosage and routes:
Intestinal candidiasis
• *Adult:* By mouth, 100–200 mg every 6 hr
Oral and perioral infections
• *Adult:* Lozenges, dissolve one lozenge slowly in mouth 4 times daily. If infection is severe, increase to 8 daily. May require 10–15 days
• *Adult, infant, child*: Suspension, place 1 ml in mouth after food and retain near lesions 4 times daily for 14 days
For further child doses seek advice from clinician/pharmacist
Available forms include: Tablets 100 mg; suspension 100 mg/ml; lozenges 10 mg
Side effects/adverse reactions: Few reported side effects when given orally, gastrointestinal upsets after long courses at high dose
Contraindications: No known contraindications
Precautions: No special precautions apply
Pharmacokinetics: Negligible absorption from GI tract
Interactions/incompatibilities:
• Decreased effect of: miconazole
Treatment of overdose: No systemic toxicity from oral overdose
NURSING CONSIDERATIONS
Administer:
• Retain in the mouth (in contact with lesions) as long as possible when given for oral infection
Evaluate:
• Therapeutic response
• Decreasing urinary output, concentrated urine and inform clinician immediately
Teach patient/family:
• That drug may need to be taken for 2 weeks to 3 months to clear infection

amphotericin intravenous ▼

Fungizone, AmBisome
Func. class.: Antifungal
Chem. class.: Amphoteric polyene macrolide
Legal class.: POM

Action: Increases cell membrane permeability in susceptible organisms by binding sterols; decreases K, Na, and nutrients in cell
Uses: Progressive, potentially fatal systemic fungal infections
Dosage and routes:
• By slow intravenous infusion over at least 6 hr, 250 mcg/kg daily, gradually increased if tolerated to 1 mg/kg daily; maximum (severe infection) 1.5 mg/kg daily or on alternate days. *Note* Prolonged treatment usually necessary; if interrupted for longer than 7 days recommence at 250 mcg/kg daily and increase gradually
• Liposomal amphotericin by IV infusion over 30 to 60 min, initially

1 mg/kg daily as a single dose increased gradually if necessary to 3 mg/kg daily as a single dose

Available forms include:

Fungizone: Powder for reconstitution 50 mg as sodium deoxycholate complex

AmBisome: Powder for reconstitution 50 mg encapsulated in liposomes

Side effects/adverse reactions:

EENT: Tinnitus, deafness, diplopia, blurred vision, transient vertigo

INTEG: Flushing, phlebitis, skin rash

CNS: Headache, fever, chills, peripheral neuropathy, convulsions, malaise

CV: Cardiovascular toxicity

GU: Hypokalaemia, permanent renal impairment, anuria, oliguria, abnormal renal function

GI: Nausea, vomiting, anorexia, diarrhoea, cramps, abnormal liver function (discontinue), dyspepsia, weight loss, gastroenteritis, acute liver failure

MS: Arthralgia, myalgia, generalised pain, weakness

HAEM: Normochromic, normocytic anaemia, thrombophlebitis, blood disorders, coagulation problems

SYST: Anaphylaxis

Contraindications: Hypersensitivity

Precautions: Renal disease, pregnancy, abnormal liver function, other drug therapy, frequent change of injection site

Pharmacokinetics:

IV: Peak 1–2 hr, initial half-life 24 hr, excreted very slowly in urine, highly bound to plasma proteins

Interactions/incompatibilities:

• Increased nephrotoxicity: other nephrotoxic drugs e.g. aminoglycosides, cisplatin, vancomycin, cyclosporin, polymyxin B, cephalothin, cytotoxic drugs

• Increased hypokalaemia following amphotericin therapy potentiates toxicity and/or actions of: cardiac glycosides, skeletal muscle relaxants

• Amphotericin-induced potassium loss increased by corticosteroids

• Do not give other drugs in same infusion or same cannula

• Antagonism: miconazole

• Do not mix in sodium solutions or diluent with preservatives

• Dextrose of pH below 4.2

Clinical assessment:

• Perform full blood count, potassium, sodium, calcium and magnesium levels weekly

• Drug is nephrotoxic: monitor blood urea nitrogen, serum creatinine for renal toxicity

• Commence treatment only after culture and sensitivity tests are positive for the infection suspected; drug should be used only for life-threatening conditions

• Symptomatic treatment for adverse reactions

• Perform liver function tests; discontinue therapy if increasing bromsulphalein, alkaline phosphatase and bilirubin levels indicate hepatotoxicity

NURSING CONSIDERATIONS

Assess:

• Baseline vital signs, fluid balance and weight

Administer:

• Administer after diluting with 10 ml sterile water, then dilute with 500 ml of 0.5% glucose solution to concentration of 0.1 mg/ml

• Aseptic technique for handling – no preservative

• Do not reconstitute with sodium chloride solutions. Use only recommended diluent

• Do not use initial concentrate or infusion solution if there is any evidence of precipitation

• Check IV site 8 hrly for signs of inflammation
• By intravenous infusion, as a solution containing 0.1 mg per ml over 6 hr (as sodium deoxycholate complex) or a solution containing 0.5 mg per ml over 30 to 60 min (as liposomal amphotericin); to be given under close supervision

Perform/protect:
• Protect from light during infusion
• Store away from moisture and light; diluted solution is stable for 24 hr

Evaluate:
• Vital signs every 15–30 min during first infusion
• Fluid balance chart; be alert for decreasing urinary output, concentrated urine and inform clinician immediately
• Weight weekly. Inform clinician if weight increases by more than 1 kg in a week or if there is evidence of oedema
• Patient's condition; temperature, malaise, rash
• Allergic reaction and report to clinician, who may discontinue drug or order antihistamines (mild reaction) or adrenaline (severe reaction), pethidine for rigors
• Anorexia, drowsiness, weakness, decreased reflexes, increased urinary output, thirst, paraesthesiae (signs of hypokalaemia)
• Hearing impairment and vestibular dysfunction e.g. tinnitus, vertigo, hearing loss (rare)

Teach patient/family:
• That drug may need to be taken for 2 weeks to 3 months to clear infection
• To recognise side effects and report them to clinician immediately

ampicillin/ampicillin sodium/ampicillin trihydrate

Amfipen, Penbritin, Vidopen, Rimacillin

Func. class.: Broad spectrum antibiotic
Chem. class.: Aminopenicillin
Legal class.: POM

Action: Interferes with cell wall replication of susceptible organisms; the cell wall, rendered osmotically unstable, swells, bursts from osmotic pressure. Bactericidal

Uses: Include the following infections: ear, nose, throat, urinary tract, gastrointestinal, gynaecological, bronchitis, pneumonia, peritonitis, gonorrhoea, septicaemia, endocarditis, enteric fever, meningitis

Dosage and routes:

Systemic infections
• *Adult:* By mouth 250 mg–1 g 6 hrly 30 min before food, IM/IV 500 mg 4–6 hrly
• *Child:* under 10 yr: half adult dose
• Also used intraperitoneal, intrapleural, intra-articular, extraperitoneal in conjunction with systemic therapy. Consult specialist

Meningitis
• *Adult:* IV 2 g 6-hrly
• *Child:* IV 150 mg/kg/day in divided doses

Gonorrhoea
• *Adult:* By mouth 2–3.5 g given with 1 g probenecid as a single dose

Available forms include: Powder for preparing injection IV, IM 250, 500 mg; capsules 250, 500 mg; powder for oral syrup or suspension 125, 250 mg/5 ml; paediatric suspension 125 mg/1.25 ml. Contain ampicillin base, sodium or trihydrate salt depending on preparation

Side effects/adverse reactions:

GI: Nausea, diarrhoea

INTEG: Rashes (discontinue treatment)

Contraindications: Hypersensitivity to penicillins

Precautions: Lactation; hypersensitivity to cephalosporins; history of allergy, renal impairment, erythematous rashes common in glandular fever, chronic lymphatic leukaemia, HIV infection

Pharmacokinetic:

By mouth: Peak 1–2 hr

IV: Peak 5 min

IM: Peak 1 hr

Half-life 50–110 min; metabolised in liver, excreted in urine, bile, faeces, breast milk; food can interfere with absorption

Interactions/incompatibilities:

- Enhances effect of: phenindione, warfarin, oral contraceptives
- Allopurinol increases risk of skin reactions
- Increased penicillin concentrations when used with: aspirin, probenicid
- Do not mix with blood products, proteinaceous fluids or lipid emulsions
- Do not mix with aminoglycosides in syringe, IV fluid or giving set

Clinical Assessment:

- Obtain specimen for bacteriology laboratory for culture and sensitivity testing before treatment commences and after course is completed. Consider resistance
- Ask patient about allergies before treatment commences and record on drug chart
- Test for renal impairment if problem suspected

Treatment of overdose: Problems unlikely. Treat symptomatically

NURSING CONSIDERATIONS

Assess:

- Any known allergies and record on care plan/nursing notes

Administer:

- Before food (action decreased by the presence of food in the gut)
- Oral, at least 30 min before food. If IV, dissolved in 5 ml water for injections per 250 mg and injected over 3–4 min, or added to IV infusion
- With full glass of water

Perform/provide:

- Adequate fluid intake (2 litres daily) if diarrhoea occurs

Evaluate:

- Observe patients with known renal impairment carefully; toxicity may develop rapidly
- Temperature 4 hrly
- Therapeutic response
- Bowel pattern before and during treatment
- Skin rashes (drug may be discontinued)

Teach patient/family:

- To take oral ampicillin on empty stomach with a full glass of water
- All aspects of drug therapy: the entire course must be completed unless advised otherwise by clinician
- To report any side effects
- Drug must be taken regularly to maintain blood levels
- To wear Medic Alert Identity if allergic to penicillins
- To report any diarrhoea to nurse or clinician

amsacrine

Amsidine

Func. class.: Antineoplastic agent
Chem. class.: Acridine derivative
Legal class.: POM

Action: Inhibits DNA synthesis

and may modify cell membrane function; active throughout entire cell cycle

Uses: Second-line treatment in refractory acute myeloid leukaemia

Dosage and routes:

• Doses are highly variable, and dependent on local treatment protocols, concomitant therapy and tumour type

Available forms include: Injection 50 mg/ml plus diluent to prepare concentrated solution of 5 mg/ml (as lactate)

Side effects/adverse reactions:

HAEM: Leucopenia, pancytopenia, haemorrhage, infections, myelosuppression

GI: Nausea, vomiting, stomatitis, oesophagitis

CNS: Seizures

SYSTEM: Abnormal liver function tests, jaundice

GU: Haematuria, anuria

CARDIAC: Ventricular tachycardia, congestive heart failure, cardiac arrest

INTEG: Local tissue irritation, necrosis, phlebitis, alopecia

Contraindications: Pre-existing bone marrow suppression induced by chemotherapy or radiotherapy, children under 12 yr

Precautions: Pregnancy, wear polythene gloves while handling (irritant to skin), use glass syringes, renal or hepatic impairment

Pharmacokinetics:

Half-life 7 hr; metabolised in liver and excreted as metabolites in bile

Interactions/incompatibilities:

• Incompatible with sodium chloride solutions and plastic (use glass syringes) protect from sunlight

• Increased risk of cardiotoxicity: diuretics, aminoglycosides and other nephrotoxic drugs, previous anthracycline therapy

Clinical assessment:

• Monitor CNS, cardiac, liver, kidney, bone marrow functions

• Ensure that potassium serum is normal.

• Perform frequent full blood counts

• Perform ECG

• Monitor urea, electrolytes, creatinine clearance

• Evaluate effects on condition

Treatment of overdose: Supportive treatments; monitor blood picture closely. If necessary administer appropriate blood products

NURSING CONSIDERATIONS

Assess:

• Temperature 4 hrly for infection, vital signs 4 hrly for arrhythmias. Fluid balance – report less than 30–60 ml urine/hr

Administer:

• HANDLING: take safety precautions appropriate to antineoplastic agents

• Following local antineoplastic (cytotoxic) policies

• After ensuring that clinician is aware of blood results

• NB: Use glass syringes

• IV; by infusion in 500 ml dextrose 5% over 60–90 min

• Other medications by mouth if possible. Avoid IV, IM, SC routes to prevent infection and bruising

• Anti-emetic 30–60 min before treatment

• All other medication as prescribed, including analgesics, antibiotics, anti-emetics, antispasmodics

Evaluate:

• IV site for leakage, pain and phlebitis

• For infection/inflammation; neutropenia (temperature, pulse, respiration 4 hrly)

• Fluid balance, BP and daily weight

• Mouth 8 hrly for infection

• Bleeding/bruising 8 hrly for thrombocytopenia

• Fits

• Jaundice; itchy, dark urine; light stools
• Haematuria and anuria
• Oedema, pain and dysphagia
• Effects of alopecia

Perform/provide:
• Analgesia, antiemetics, antibiotics, sedatives, antiuric acid drugs and transfusions as prescribed
• Storage out of sunlight, stable for 8 hr at room temperature
• Asepsis/isolation as appropriate
• Mouth care—fizzy mouth wash, gentle teeth cleaning and oral toilet; observe for mucositis
• Warm compresses for injection (IV) site
• Support/counselling—changes in body image

Teach patient/family:
• Need for isolation and high standard of hygiene
• About side effects of drug
• Counselling, wig, etc. available for alopecia
• Importance of mouth examination and reporting any effects, e.g. bleeding, mouth ulcers
• Avoid food/drink that may irritate mouth

---

amylobarbitone

Amytal, Sodium Amytal, combination product
Func. class.: Sedative/hypnotic
Chem. class.: Barbiturate (intermediate acting)
Legal class.: CD (Sch 3) POM

Action: Depresses activity in brain cells primarily in reticular activating system in brainstem, also selectively depresses neurons in posterior hypothalamus, limbic structures; able to decrease seizure activity by inhibition of epileptic activity in CNS

Uses: Severe intractable insomnia in patients already taking barbiturates; parenteral, status epilepticus

Dosage and routes:
• *Adult:* By mouth, 60–200 mg at bedtime, depending on preparation

Available forms include: Amylobarbitone tablets 50 mg, Amylobarbitone sodium capsules 60, 200 mg

Sides effects/adverse reactions:
CNS: Lethargy, drowsiness, hangover, dizziness, paradoxical excitement confusion pain sedation memory defects vertigo headache, ataxia
GI: Nausea, vomiting
INTEG: Hypersensitivity skin reactions, skin eruptions
CV: Circulatory collapse
RESP: Depression, apnoea

Contraindications: Hypersensitivity to barbiturates, respiratory disease, uncontrolled pain, pregnancy, breast-feeding, liver impairment, porphyria, children, young adults, drug/alcohol abusers, elderly, debilitated

Precautions: Labour, depression, suicidal tendencies, hepatic disease, renal disease, shock, respiratory depression. Withdraw gradually after long use, addiction potential, cumulative effect, borderline hypoadrenal function

Pharmacokinetics:
By mouth: Onset 30–60 min, duration 6–8 hr
Metabolised by liver, excreted mainly in urine, some in faeces and breast milk highly protein bound, half-life 20–25 hr

Interactions/incompatibilities:
• Increased CNS depression: alcohol, monoamine oxidase inhibitors, sedatives, narcotics, CNS depressants, anti-epileptics, tranquillisers
• Increased metabolism of: tri-

cyclic antidepressants, clonazepam, disopyramide, quinidine
• Decreased effect of: oral anticoagulants, corticosteroids, griseofulvin, phenytoin, digitoxin, cyclosporin, theophylline, thyroxine, oral contraceptives, rifampicin, gestrinone, tibolone, chloramphenicol doxycycline, metronidazole, chlorpromazine, isradipine, nicardipine, nifedipine
• Antagonism of anticonvulsant effect: antidepressants, antipsychotics
• Enhanced effects, reductions in plasma concentrations possible—antiepileptics or enhanced toxicity

Clinical assessment:
• Measure amylobarbitone plasma levels if on repeated IV/IM doses

Treatment of overdose: Symptomatic and supportive. Gastric lavage, monitor-vital signs. IV fluids. Maintain BP, body temperature, adequate respiratory exchange. Haemodialysis.

NURSING CONSIDERATIONS

Assess:
• Vital signs every 30 minutes for 2 hours after intravenous injection
• Barbiturate or other dependency

Administer:
• Only after all other measures for insomnia have proven ineffective
• 30 minutes to an hour before bedtime if used to treat insomnia

Perform/provide:
• Supervision to mobile patients once the drug is given
• Necessary safety precautions, e.g. cotsides. Ensure that the patient has a nightlight and knows how to summon the nurse quickly
• With resuscitative equipment available

Evaluate:
• Therapeutic response; ability to sleep throughout the night without early morning wakening
• Mental status: mood, whether oriented in time and place, memory (long and short term)
• Habituation to dependency on drug: increasingly frequent requests for medication, shaking, anxiety
• Barbiturate toxicity hypotension, bronchospasm, cold clammy skin, cyanosis of the lips, insomnia, nausea, vomiting, hallucinations, delirium, weakness. Mild symptoms may occur/persist 10–12 hours after receiving the drug
• Respiratory: respiratory depression, rate, depth and rhythm. Withhold drug if respirations are less than 1 per minute or if pupils are dilated
• Blood dyscrasias: pyrexia, sore throat, bruising, rashes, jaundice, epistaxis

Teach patient/family:
All points for treatment of insomnia:
• Hangover is to be expected
• Use of the drug is permitted only for short-term treatment of insomnia; that it will probably become ineffective after 2 weeks
• Drug dependency may result if used for extended periods (45–90 days depending on dose)
• To avoid driving, handling machinery, etc.
• To avoid alcohol or other CNS depressants: severe depression of the CNS may otherwise occur
• Not to stop taking the drug abruptly after long term use; dose should be reduced gradually over a period of 1–2 weeks
• To inform G.P. that a barbiturate has been prescribed
• That insomnia may recur after short-term use, but further doses are not indicated, as this will improve within 1–3 nights
• Benefits may not be noted until 2 nights after commencing drug
• Other additional measures to combat insomnia (reading,

exercise, warm bath, hot milk, drinks, television, deep breathing exercises)
• Self hypnosis as a form of meditation
• That drug must be kept well out of children's reach

ancrod

Arvin

Func. class.: Anticoagulant
Chem. class.: Enzymatic principle, derived from the venom of the Malayan pit viper
Legal class.: POM ('named-patient' basis)

Action: Reduces plasma fibrinogen by cleavage of fibrin; reduces blood viscosity but has no effect on established thrombi
Uses: Deep-vein thrombosis, prevention of postoperative thrombosis ('named-patient' basis only)
Dosage and routes:
• *Adult:* IV infusion, 2–3 units/kg in 50–500 ml sodium chloride 0.9% over 4–12 hr (usually 6–8 hr) then by infusion or slow IV injection over 5 min, 2 units/kg every 12 hr; initial infusion *must* be given slowly
• *Adult:* SC injection, for prophylaxis of deep-vein thrombosis, 280 units immediately after surgery, then 70 units daily for 4 days (fractured femur) or 8 days (hip replacement)
Available forms include: Injection 70 units/ml
Sides effects/adverse reactions:
• Drugs for anaphylaxis and antidote should be available. Alternatively reconstituted freeze-dried fibrinogen or 1 litre fresh frozen plasma
HAEM/CV: Haemorrhage, thrombocytopenia (stop treatment if thrombocytopenia), massive intravascular formation of unstable fibrin if drug not given slowly
INTEG: Alopecia, hypersensitivity reactions
MS: Osteoporosis if use is prolonged
SYSTEM: Hypersensitivity reactions
Contraindications: Hypersensitivity, bleeding tendencies, e.g. haemophilia, gastric or duodenal ulcer, severe hypertension, cerebrovascular disorders, thrombocytopenia, bacterial endocarditis, oesophageal varices
Precautions: Renal colic, cardiovascular disease, uraemia, resistance may develop, stroke
Pharmacokinetics: Duration 12–24 hours. May be necessary to give antidote—see Treatment of overdose
Interactions/incompatibilities:
• Avoid administration with dextrans, aminocaproic acid
Tests:
Perform
• Clotting function, aim for 2–3 mm clot after 2 hr standing or directly measure plasma fibrinogen concentrations
• Plasma fibrinogen, full blood count, prior to therapy. Platelet count also if treatment longer than 5 days
Treatment of overdose: Antidote (ancrod antivenom), reconstituted freeze-dried fibrinogen or fresh frozen plasma. For anaphylaxis adrenaline, antihistamines, corticosteroids

NURSING CONSIDERATIONS

Assess:
• Vital signs, fluid balance
Administer:
• After diluting in 50–500 ml sodium chloride

• Slowly (induction dose over at least 4 hr) and maintenance 10–50 ml/5 min

Perform/provide:

• Refrigerated storage at 4–8°C; do not freeze

• Emergency equipment in case of anaphylaxis

Evaluate:

• Observe for bleeding

Teach patient/family:

• To report any signs of haemorrhage immediately

anistreplase (APSAC)

Eminase

Func. class.: Thrombolytic enzyme
Chem. class.: Enzyme complex
*Legal class.:*POM

Action: An anisoylated complex of streptokinase with human plasminogen, the precursor of the natural fibrinolytic enzyme plasmin. Acylation of the plasminogen molecule retards its conversion to plasmin, but it does not affect its binding to fibrin. After IV injection deacylation produces enzymatically active plasminogen-streptokinase activator complex. This converts plasminogen to plasmin within the thrombus

Uses: Treatment of acute myocardial infarction

Dosage and routes:

• *Adult:* Slow IV injection 30 units single dose over 4 to 5 min, administered as soon as possible after the onset of symptoms and preferably within 6 hours

Available forms include: IV injection 30 units/vial, powder for reconstitution

Side effects/adverse reactions:

HAEM: Bleeding
GI: Nausea, vomiting
INTEG: Flushing, allergic reactions
CV: Bradycardia, hypotension (transient), anaphylaxis (uncommon)
CNS: Fever

Contraindications: Hypersensitivity, surgery or major trauma within previous 10 days, recent (previous 2 months) neurosurgical procedures or recent traumatic cardiopulmonary resuscitation, active peptic ulcer or internal bleeding (previous 6 months), cerebrovascular accident, bleeding diathesis, severe hypertension, intracranial neoplasms or aneurysm, menorrhagia

Precautions: Risk of bleeding increased. Risk of emboli with intramural ventricular thrombi or thrombi within abdominal aneurysms or enlarged left atrium with atrial fibrillation. Arrhythmias may develop. Patients over 70 yr. Pregnancy, lactation, external chest compression, recent or concurrent anticoagulant therapy. Keep invasive procedures to a minimum, e.g. cardiac catheterization. Repeated therapy (or streptokinase) from 5 days–12 months previously

Lab. test interferences: For 24–48 hr after therapy
Decreased plasma fibrinogen and plasminogen concentrations
Increased fibrin degradation products

Treatment of overdose: Transfusion with packed cells or whole blood if necessary—or cryoprecipitate or purified clotting factor concentrates. Tranexamic acid or aprotinin competitively inhibit fibrinolytic action

NURSING CONSIDERATIONS

Assess:

• All baseline vital signs, ECG

Administer:

• Mix solution with water for in-

jections or sodium chloride 0.9% as recommended. Avoid shaking to prevent foaming
• Infuse via peripheral line over 5 min
• As soon as thrombi identified; value of treatment within first 12 hr is established
• Cryoprecipitate or fresh, frozen plasma if bleeding occurs. Control local bleeding with pressure
• Heparin therapy after thrombolytic therapy is discontinued, TT or APTT less than 2 times control (about 3–4 hr)
• Have available antiarrhythmic therapy for bradycardia and/or ventricular irritability
• About 10% patients have high streptococcal antibody titres requiring increased loading doses

Perform/provide:
• Bed rest during entire course of treatment
• Avoidance of any other invasive procedures: injection, rectal temperature
• Treatment of fever with paracetamol or aspirin
• Pressure for 30 seconds to minor bleeding sites; inform clinician if this does not attain haemostasis; apply pressure dressing
• Pain relief as required
• Emergency resuscitation equipment if cardiac arrest occurs
• Continuous ECG monitoring for reperfusion arrhythmias

Evaluate:
• 12 lead ECG before and after drug administration
• Vital signs, BP, pulse, respiration, neurological signs, at least 4 hrly; temperature or other indications of internal bleed, cardiac rhythm following intracoronary administration
• Electrolytes, particularly potassium and magnesium
• Allergy: fever, rash, itching, chills; mild reaction may be treated with antihistamines
• For bleeding during first hr of treatment: haematuria, haematemesis, bleeding from mucous membranes, epistaxis, ecchymosis

Teach patient/family:
• Issue advice card stating that malaise or signs of bleeding need to be reported to clinician
• Provide information concerning immediate and long-term counselling provisions for myocardial infarction problems

---

anti-D (Rh_o) immunoglobulin, human

Partobulin
Func. class.: Immunising agent
Chem. class.: IgG

Action: Suppresses immune response of non-sensitised Rh_o negative patients who are exposed to Rh_o positive blood

Uses: To prevent a rhesus-negative mother from forming antibodies to fetal rhesus-positive cells which may pass into maternal circulation during childbirth, abortion or miscarriage. Transfusion of rhesus-incompatible blood. Also given in threatened miscarriage when blood loss has occurred

Dosage and routes:
Rh exposure/post-abortion
• Ideally within 72 hr. Intramuscular injection
• *Adult:* 500 units following birth of rhesus-positive infant; 250 units if before 20 weeks gestation

After transfusion
Consult clinician

Available forms include: Injection IM single use vial or preloaded syringe

Side effects/adverse reactions:
Well tolerated generally without reactions

Contraindications: Intravenous administration. Rh_o(D) positive individuals or neonates
Precautions: Active immunisation with live virus vaccines should be postposed until 3 months after last anti-D dose. If administration is essential, seek clinician's advice. If anti-D needs to be given within 2–4 weeks of live virus vaccination, efficacy of vaccination may be impaired
Lab. test interference: Previous anti-D therapy (even months before) may affect Rh_o(D) antibody levels. Additional antibodies (e.g. rubella) in anti-D may give false positive tests for such antibodies
Treatment of overdose: No problems anticipated in rhesus-negative individuals

NURSING CONSIDERATIONS

Administer:
• After sending neonate's cord blood to lab after delivery for cross match and type. Infant must be rhesus-positive, with rhesus-negative mother
• IM only
• Rhesus-negative clients routinely given anti-D in termination of pregnancy and miscarriage (rhesus status of foetus is not available)
• Only equal lot numbers of drug, cross-match

Perform/provide:
• Storage in refrigerator

Evaluate:
• Allergic reaction: rash, urticaria, nausea, fever, wheezing
• Therapeutic response in threatened miscarriages

Teach patient/family:
• How the therapy works
• That after subsequent deliveries doses may be needed if the baby is rhesus-positive or foetal blood group is not known

ascorbic acid (vitamin C)

~~NHS~~ Redoxon
Func. class.: Water-soluble vitamin
Legal class.: GSL
POM (Injection)

Action: Needed for collagen synthesis, antioxidant, carbohydrate metabolism
Uses: Vitamin C deficiency, prevention and treatment of scurvy
Dosage and routes:
Scurvy
• *Adult:* By mouth, IM, IV or subcutaneous not less than 250 mg/day in divided doses
Deficiency prophylactic 25–75 mg daily
Available forms include: Tablets 25, 50, 100, 200, 500 mg; tablets effervescent 1000 mg; injection IM/IV/subcutaneous 100 mg/ml 5 ml amp
Side effects/adverse reactions:
Large doses only
GI: Nausea, vomiting, diarrhoea, anorexia, heartburn, cramps
GU: Oxalate renal stones
HAEM: Haemolytic anaemia in patients with G-6-PD
Contraindications:
None significant
Precautions: Hyperoxaluria
Pharmacokinetics:
Readily absorbed from GI tract. Metabolised in liver, metabolites and unused amounts excreted in urine (unchanged), excreted in breast milk. Removed by haemodialysis
Clinical assessment:
• Monitor blood ascorbic acid levels if severe deficiency is present, e.g. scurvy
Lab. test interferences:
• False positive, negatives in tests involving oxidation and reduction reactions
• Plasma, faeces and urine may be affected

Assess:
• Fluid balance
Perform/provide:
• Diet with high content of vitamin C, e.g. citrus fruit, vegetables
Evaluate:
• Continued signs of deficiency, e.g. anorexia, pallor, joint pain, hyperkeratosis, petechiae
• Injection sites for inflammation
Teach patient/family:
• That foods rich in vitamin C should be included in diet
• Extra vitamin C is needed if patient smokes or takes oral contraceptives

aspirin

Caprin, Platet, Solprin, Nuseals Aspirin, Angettes 75, many single-ingredient and combination products
Func. class.: Minor analgesic; antiplatelet agent
Chem. class.: Salicylate
Legal class.: Aspirin BP Tablets packsize more than 25 P; tablets packsize 25 GSL

Action: Inhibition of prostaglandin synthesis; antipyretic action results from inhibition of hypothalamic heat-regulating centre, inhibits platelet aggregation
Uses: Mild to moderate pain or fever; pain and inflammation in rheumatic disease and other musculoskeletal disorders; prophylaxis of cerebrovascular disease or myocardial infarction
Dosage and routes:
Analgesic/antipyretic
• *Adult:* By mouth, 300–900 mg every 3–6 hr according to response; maximum 4 g daily
Musculoskeletal disorders
• *Adult:* By mouth, acute disorders, 4–8 g daily in divided doses; chronic disorders, up to 5.4 g in divided doses may be sufficient; dose may need to be adjusted according to plasma concentrations
Antiplatelet
• *Adult:* By mouth, 75–100 mg daily; up to 130 mg daily may be needed
Juvenile rheumatoid arthritis
• *Child:* By mouth, 80–100 mg/kg in 5–6 divided doses; up to 130 mg/kg may be needed
Available forms include: Tablets 75, 100, 300, 600 mg in various formulations
Side effects/adverse reactions:
HAEM: Increased bleeding time
GU: Urate kidney stones
CNS: Confusion
GI: Nausea, vomiting, GI bleeding, ulceration, diarrhoea, heartburn, anorexia
INTEG: Rash, urticaria
EENT: Tinnitus, subconjunctival haemorrhage, vertigo
RESP: Wheezing, bronchospasm
Contraindications: Hypersensitivity to salicylates, GI bleeding and ulceration, bleeding disorders, children under 12 yr except for juvenile arthritis, breast-feeding, gout
Precautions: G6PD-deficiency, hepatic disease, renal disease, allergic disease, asthma, pregnancy, dehydration, elderly, history of GI ulceration, gout, hypertension
Pharmacokinetics: Onset 15–30 min, peak 1–2 hr, by mouth duration 4–6 hr but values depend on formulation
Metabolized by liver, excreted by kidneys, excreted in breast milk, half-life 1–3½ hr
Interactions/incompatibilities:
• Decreased effects of aspirin: antacids, adsorbents, urinary alkalinisers
• Increased effects and toxicity of: anticoagulants, insulin, metho-

trexate, phenytoin, sodium valproate, acetazolamide
• Decreased effects of: probenecid, spironolactone, sulphinpyrazone
• Increased effect of aspirin: metoclopramide
• Avoid aspirin until 8–12 days after mifepristone

Clinical assessment:
• Monitor patients with hypertension for bleeding
• Monitor blood clotting picture

Treatment of overdose: Gastric lavage, forced alkaline diuresis, monitor electrolytes, ventricular systole. Haemodialysis in severe cases. Restore acid-base balance. Observe patient for at least 24 hr

NURSING CONSIDERATIONS

Assess:
• Pre-existing conditions, omit if known gastric ulcer or bleeding
• Prior drug history: there are many drug interactions

Administer:
• With food or milk to decrease gastric symptoms

Perform/provide:
• Repositioning to decrease pain
• Cool cloth for fever

Evaluate:
• Relief of pain (if reason for prescription)
• Hepatotoxicity: dark urine, clay-colored stools, yellowing of skin, sclera, itching, abdominal pain, fever, diarrhoea if patient is on long-term therapy
• Allergic reactions: rash, urticaria; if these occur, drug may need to be discontinued
• Renal dysfunction: decreased urine output
• Ototoxicity: tinnitus, ringing, roaring in ears; audiometric testing needed before, after long-term therapy
• Visual changes: blurring, halos, corneal, retinal damage
• Oedema in feet, ankles, legs

Teach patient/family:
• To report any symptoms of hepatotoxicity, renal toxicity, visual changes, ototoxicity, allergic reactions (long-term therapy)
• Not to exceed recommended dosage; acute poisoning may result
• To read label on other non-prescribed drugs; many contain aspirin
• That the therapeutic response may take 2 weeks (arthritis)
• To avoid alcohol ingestion; GI bleeding may occur
• To store in child-proof container and out of reach of children

astemizole

Hismanal, Pollon-eze

Func. class.: Antihistamine, H_1-receptor antagonist

Chem. class.: Substituted benzimidazole

Legal class.: POM (Hismanal preparations)/P (Pollon-eze tablets)

Action: Decreases allergic response by antagonising the action of histamine at H_1-receptor sites in the eyes, respiratory tract, GI tract and skin

Uses: Symptomatic relief of allergic conditions such as hay fever, urticaria

Dosage and routes:
• *Adult and child over 12 yr:* By mouth, 10 mg once daily; this dose must *not* be exceeded
• *Child 6–12 yr:* By mouth, 5 mg once daily; this dose must *not* be exceeded

Available forms include: Tablets, 10 mg; suspension 5 mg/5 ml

Side effects/adverse reactions:

CNS: Benign paraesthesias, convulsions

CV: Ventricular arrhythmias (torsade de pointes)

GI: Hepatotoxicity
INTEG: Allergic reactions including rash, pruritus and photosensitivity
SYST: Weight gain, anaphylactic and other allergic reactions
Contraindications: Hypersensivity; breast-feeding; hypokalaemia; co-administration of drugs predisposing to cardiac arrhythmias or hypokalaemia, or which inhibit astemizole metabolism
Pharmacokinetics: Rapid absorption from GI tract; extensive first-pass metabolism; plasma concentrations of astemizole and metabolites take 4–8 weeks to reach steady state; extensively metabolised in liver, excreted in urine and faeces; elimination half-life about 19 days
Interactions:
• Increased risk of ventricular arrhythmias (avoid): ketoconazole, intraconazole, fluconazole, erythromycin, azithromycin, clarithromycin, anti-arrhythmics, antipsychotics, tricyclic antidepressants, diuretics, sotalol
Treatment of overdose: Induce emesis; perform gastric lavage; observe closely with ECG monitoring; provide symptomatic and supportive treatment
NURSING CONSIDERATIONS:
Assess:
• Ensure prescribing clinician is aware of all concurrent medication and/or previous adverse reactions to anti-histamines
• Advise prescribing clinician r.e. relevant illnesses, e.g. respiratory disease/urinary outflow obstruction
• Baseline observations of BP and pulse
Administer:
• On empty stomach 1 hr before or 2 hr after meals
• If GI symptoms occur, administer with food and be aware of possible decreased absorption
• Ensure awareness of concurrent medication to prevent interaction
Perform/provide:
• Sips of water, frequent mouthwashes to alleviate dry mouth
Evaluate:
• Fluid balance: be alert for urinary retention, frequency, dysuria, especially in the elderly; drug should be discontinued on occurence
• For side effects. Discontinue treatment if serious reactions occur
• For signs of cardiac CNS instability during treatment
• Therapeutic response: absence of running or congested nose, or rashes
• Respiratory status: rate, rhythm, increase in bronchial secretions, wheezing, chest tightness
• For signs of hypersensitivity/allergy, e.g. rash, pruritus, photosensitivity
Teach patient/family:
• Avoid in breast-feeding mothers/during pregnancy
• To avoid driving or other hazardous activity if drowsiness occurs
• To avoid alcohol or other CNS depressants

---

atenolol

Antipressan, Tenormin, Atenix, Totamol, Vasaten, combination preparations
Func. class.: Antihypertensive, anti-anginal; anti-arrhythmic
Chem. class.: Selective β-blocker
Legal class.: POM

Action: Competitively blocks stimulation of β-adrenergic receptors, produces negative chronotropic, inotropic activity (decreases rate of SA node discharge, increases recovery time), slows conduction of atrioventricular node decreases heart rate, decreases O_2 consumption in myocardium. Cardioselective, without intrinsic sympathomimetic and membrane stabilising activities

Uses: Hypertension, cardiac dysrhythmias, acute phase after myocardial infarction, angina pectoris

Dosage and routes:

Hypertension

• *Adult:* By mouth, 50 mg daily

Angina

• *Adult:* By mouth, 100 mg daily in 1–2 doses

Arrhythmias

• *Adult:* By mouth, 50–100 mg daily

• *Adult:* IV injection, 2.5 mg at rate of 1 mg/min; repeat at 5-min intervals; maximum 10 mg

• *Adult:* IV infusion, 150 mcg/kg over 20 min; repeat every 12 hr if required

Following acute phase of myocardial infarction (within 12 hr)

• *Adult:* Slow IV injection, 5–10 mg, then by mouth 50 mg after 15 min, 50 mg after 12 hr, and then 100 mg daily

Available forms include: Tablets 25 mg, 50 mg, 100 mg; syrup 25 mg/5 ml; injection 500 mcg/ml (hospital only)

Side effects/adverse reactions:

CV: Cold extremities

MS: Muscle fatigue

INTEG: Rash

EENT: Dry burning eyes

Contraindications: Bronchospasm, asthma, history of obstructive airways disease, metabolic acidosis, sinus bradycardia, partial heart block, uncontrolled congestive heart failure

Precautions: Myasthenia gravis, pregnancy, lactation, diabetes mellitus, renal disease. Reversible obstructive airways disease, asthma, well compensated heart failure, poor cardiac reserve, anaesthesia. Avoid abrupt withdrawal. NB: verapamil treatment, clonidine.

Pharmacokinetics dynamics:

By mouth. Peak 2–4 hr; half-life 6–7 hr, excreted unchanged in urine, protein binding 3%

Interactions/incompatibilities:

• Increased effect: alcohol, anaesthetics, antihypertensives (NB: clonidine), anxiolytics and hypnotics, diuretics

• Increased side effects: mefloquine, diltiazem, nifedipine, verapamil, cardiac glycosides, antiarrhythmics, anti-diabetics

• Reduced effects: oestrogens, combined oral contraceptives, sympathomimetics, carbenoxolone, xamoterol, NSAIDs

Clinical assessment:

• Obtain baseline data of renal function before treatment commences

• Assess time lapse since infarction

• Prescribe reduced dosage for patients with known renal disease

• Evaluate therapeutic response (fall in BP) after 1–2 weeks

• Monitor respiratory function if appropriate

Lab test interferences:

Interference: Glucose/insulin tolerance tests

Treatment of overdose: IV atropine, follow if necessary with IV glucagon. Follow by IV prenalterol or dobutamine if required

NURSING CONSIDERATIONS

Assess:

• Fluid balance and weight

• Apex and radial pulses before dose is given

• Monitor peak flow rate (PEFR) in patients with reversible airways obstruction

Administer:

• Crushed or whole tablets before meals and at bedtime

Evaluate:

• Weight and fluid balance daily
• Pulse and BP at least 4 hrly
• Legs and feet for oedema daily
• Signs of dehydration e.g. loss of skin elasticity, dry mucous membranes
• Respiratory rate, rhythm, depth

Teach patient/family:

• That drug must not be discontinued suddenly, but should be reduced gradually over a period of 2 weeks
• Not to take other non-prescribed medicines without the clinician's permission
• To report bradycardia, dizziness, confusion, depression, fever
• How to take pulse and explain that this must be done at home. Ensure patient knows when to contact clinician
• To avoid alcohol, smoking, salt
• To reduce weight if necessary and take sufficient exercise
• To carry Medic Alert Card. (Alerts that patient is taking drug and lists any known allergies)
• To avoid driving or operating machinery if dizzy

---

atracurium besylate

Tracrium
Func. class.: Non-depolarising muscle relaxant
Chem. class.: Biquaternary non-chlorine diester
Legal class.: POM

Action: Inhibits transmission of nerve impulses by binding with cholinergic receptor sites, antagonising action of acetylcholine

Uses: Facilitation of endotracheal intubation, skeletal muscle relaxation during mechanical ventilation, surgery, or general anaesthesia. Caesarean section

Dosage and routes:

• *Adult and child over 1 month:* IV initially 300–600 mcg/kg then 100–200 mcg/kg as required; IV infusion 300–600 mcg/kg/hr

Available forms include: Injection IV 10 mg/ml, 2.5 ml, 5 ml, 25 ml ampoules

Side effects/adverse reactions:

CV: Transient hypotension
RESP: Respiratory depression
INTEG: Flushing

Contraindications: Hypersensitivity

Precautions: Pregnancy, cardiovascular disease, lactation, electrolyte imbalances, myasthenia gravis, hypothermia, neuromuscular disease, only under anaesthetist supervision

Pharmacokinetics:

IV: Onset 2 min, duration 15–35 min; half-life 2 min, 29 min (terminal), excreted in urine, faeces (metabolites). Duration not affected by impaired renal, hepatic or circulatory function

Interactions/incompatibilities:

• Increased neuromuscular blockade: aminoglycosides, clindamycin, lincomycin, quinidine, azlocillin, mezlocillin, propranolol, nifedipine, verapamil, parenteral magnesium, polypeptide antibiotics, lithium, inhalation anaesthetics
• Do not mix with barbiturates or any alkaline agent in solution or syringe
• Do not administer depolarising muscle relaxant to prolong neuromuscular block
• Hypotension, myocardial depression, hyperkalaemia with: IV dantrolene and verapamil
• Decreased neuromuscular blockade: demecarium and ecothiopate eye drops, neostigmine, pyridostigmine

Clinical assessment:

Treatment of overdose: (or delayed recovery) Administer atropine and neostigmine. Maintain artificial ventilation as required

NURSING CONSIDERATIONS

Assess:

• BP, pulse, respirations, temperature, airway, strength of handgrip until fully recovered

• Fluid balance chart; check for urinary retention, frequency, hesitancy

• Previous anaesthetic history to ensure patient has not had myasthenia gravis

• Test for urea and electrolytes, blood gases and pH if appropriate

Administer:

• IV, slowly (onset 1–2 min)

• Only under medical supervision of an anaesthetist

• Allow 90 seconds after initial administration before endotracheal tube is inserted

Perform/provide:

• Flush cannula before and after use

• Do not mix with barbiturates

Evaluate:

• Airway status, strength of handgrip, ability to raise head from pillow, reduced facial movement

Teach patient/family:

• About effects of drug, weakness, loss of muscle tone

---

atropine sulphate

Min-I-Jet, Atropine sulphate

Func. class.: Antimuscarinic

Chem. class.: Belladonna alkaloid

Legal class.: POM or P depending on preparation

Action: Competes for acetylcholine receptors at parasympathetic neuroeffector sites; increases cardiac output, heart rate by blocking vagal stimulation in heart

Uses: Bradycardia, anticholinesterase insecticide poisoning, blocking cardiac vagal reflexes, decreasing secretions before surgery, antispasmodic, with neostigmine for reversal of competitive neuromuscular block

Dosage and routes:

• Seek advice from clinician or pharmacist

Available forms include: Injection 600 mcg/ml, 1 ml; injection 100 mcg/ml, 5 ml, 10 ml

Side effects/adverse reactions:

GU: Retention, hesitancy

GI: Dry mouth, constipation, difficulty in swallowing, thirst

CV: Bradycardia followed by tachycardia, palpitations, arrhythmias

INTEG: Dry skin, flushing

EENT: Blurred vision, photophobia, glaucoma, dilatation of pupils

Contraindications: Hypersensitivity to belladonna alkaloids, prostatic hypertrophy, urinary retention, pyloric stenosis, paralyticileus, closed-angle glaucoma

Precautions: Pregnancy, elderly, urinary retention, prostatic enlargement, tachycardia, cardiovascular disease, paralytic ileus, ulcerative colitis, pyloric stenosis, lactation

Pharmacokinetics:

IV: Peak 2–4 min

IM: Peak 30 min

Half-life 2–3 hr, incompletely metabolised in liver, excreted in breast milk, excreted in urine unchanged and as metabolites

Interactions/incompatibilities:

• Decreased effects of: phenothiazines, ketoconazole, sublingual nitrates

• Increased side effects: other drugs with antimuscarinic effects, nefopam, disopyramide, tricyclics, MAOIs, antihistamines, phenothiazines, amantadine

- Delayed absorption: mexiletine
- Decreased GI effects: cisapride, metoclopramide, domperidone

Treatment of overdose: If overdose by mouth: aspiration, lavage or induction of emesis. Activated charcoal to reduce absorption. Supportive therapy. Neostigmine or carbachol antagonises only peripheral effects

NURSING CONSIDERATIONS

Administer:

- Intravenously usually as a bolus injection, directly into vein, can be repeated 4–6 hr later
- Intramuscularly, subcutaneously, orally as prescribed

Perform/provide:

- Frequent drinks to prevent dry mouth when taking oral medication

Evaluate:

- Cardiac rate, rhythm, character; blood pressure, respirations
- Input and output of fluids, check for urinary retention
- For bowel sounds; check for constipation
- Pulse, respiration and blood pressure especially during intravenous infusion; monitor with electrocardiograph
- Dry mouth, dry skin, urinary retention dilation of pupils
- Therapeutic response, increase in cardiac output, decrease in secretions before surgery and parkinsonism
- Allergy to atropine sulphate—rash on face upper trunk, rapid respirations, tachycardiac, hyperpyrexia
- Effect of any other drug therapy

Teach patient family:

- To report blurred vision, chest pain, palpitations
- That long term medication may be required to improve cardiac output

atropine sulphate (ophthalmic)

Isopto Atropine, Minims

Func. class.: Mydriatic, cycloplegic

Chem. class.: Belladonna alkaloid

Legal class.: POM

Action: Blocks response of iris sphincter muscle, muscle of accommodation of ciliary body to cholinergic stimulation, resulting in dilation of pupil, paralysis of accommodation

Uses: Iritis, uveitis, cycloplegic refraction

Dosage and routes:

- *Adult:* Refraction (1%) instil 1 drop into each eye twice daily for 1 or 2 days before examination

Uveitis (1%) instil 1 or 2 drops into the eye(s) 4 times daily or as required

- *Children:* Refraction (1%) instil 1 drop twice daily for 1–3 days before examination and 1 hr before. Eye ointment 1% preferred for children under 5 yr—apply twice daily for 3 days before examination

Uveitis (1%) instil 1 drop into the eye(s) up to 3 times daily

Available forms include: Eye ointment 1%; eye drops 1% 5, 10 ml, Minim 1%

Side effects/adverse reactions:

SYST: Constipation, vomiting, giddiness, flushing, dry skin, dry mouth, abdominal discomfort (infants: abdominal distention), bradycardia followed by tachycardia, palpitations and arrhythmias, urinary urgency, difficulty and retention

EENT: Increased intraocular pressure, stinging, sensitivity to light. Prolonged use—irritation, hyperaemia, oedema, conjunctivitis

INTEG: Contact dermatitis, rash (in children)
Contraindications: Hypersensitivity, glaucoma or tendency to glaucoma, soft contact lenses (some preparations), pregnancy, lactation, children under 3 months
Precautions: Darkly pigmented iris more resistant to dilation
Pharmacokinetics:
Instil: Peak 30–40 min (mydriasis), 60–180 min (cycloplegia), duration 6–12 days
Interactions/incompatibilities:
Effects enhanced by other drugs with antimuscarinic properties
Treatment of overdose: Supportive treatment. Infants and small children—keep body surface moist. Accidental ingestion—induce emesis/gastric lavage

NURSING CONSIDERATIONS

Evaluate:
• Observe for resolution of inflammation, pupil dilation
• Withold dose if eye pain occurs and inform clinician

Teach patient/family:
• To report visual disturbances e.g. loss of sight, difficulty breathing, sweating, hot flushes
• That blurring is inevitable but will decrease with repeated use of drops and ointment
• How to administer eyedrops; protect eyes from bright illumination during dilation
• To avoid driving, operating machinery until able to see
• To wait 5 min before instilling other eyedrops
• Not to blink more than usual
• Not to get the preparation in a child's mouth and to wash their own hands and the child's hands following administration

auranofin

Ridaura
Func. class.: Antirheumatic
Chem. class.: Orally active gold complex
Legal class.: POM

Action: Anti-inflammatory action unknown, may decrease phagocytosis, lysosomal activity or decrease prostaglandin synthesis; decreases concentration of rheumatoid factor, immunoglobulins
Uses: Active progressive rheumatoid arthritis when NSAIDs ineffective alone
Dosage and routes: On expert advice
• *Adult:* By mouth 3 mg twice daily, single 6 mg dose if well tolerated, may increase to 9 mg/day in 3 divided doses after 6 months, discontinue if no effect after further 3 months
Available forms include: Tablets 3 mg
Side effects/adverse reactions:
HAEM: Thrombocytopenia agranulocytosis, aplastic anaemia, leucopenia, granulocytopenia
INTEG: Rash, pruritus, alopecia
GI: Diarrhoea, abdominal cramping, stomatitis, nausea, vomiting, other GI symptoms, metallic taste
GU: Proteinuria, haematuria
EENT: Conjunctivitis
RESP: Pulmonary fibrosis
Contraindications: Hypersensitivity to gold, necrotising enterocolitis, bone marrow aplasia, children, lactation, pregnancy, porphyria, pulmonary fibrosis, exfoliative dermatitis, systemic lupus erythematosus, blood dyscrasias, progressive renal disease, severe hepatic disease
Precautions: Elderly, allergic conditions, eczema, ulcerative colitis, renal impairment, rash, drugs

causing blood disorders, liver dysfunction, inflammatory bowel disease, history of bone marrow depression
Pharmacokinetics:
By mouth: Absorbed by GI tract, peak 2 hr, steady state 8–12 weeks, excreted in urine, faeces
Interactions/incompatibilities:
None known
Clinical assessment:
• Perform urine tests monthly. Proteinuria may necessitate withdrawal
• Annual chest X-ray—watch for breathlessness, dry cough
• Perform monthly full blood counts (including total and differential white cell and platelet counts) drug should be discontinued if platelets less than 100,000/mm^3. Monitor gold toxicity, e.g. decreased Hb, white blood count and platelets
• Perform liver function tests; renal function tests
• Monitor for GI bleeding, rash, pruritus, stomatitis, metallic taste
Treatment of overdose: Induce vomiting or gastric lavage. Supportive treatment; chelating agents may be indicated
NURSING CONSIDERATIONS
Assess:
• Fluid balance
Administer:
• With food
Evaluate:
• Therapeutic response to treatment; ability to move joints with less pain
• Urine for haematuria, proteinuria
• Stools for diarrhoea
• Respiratory status; inform clinician of dyspnoea, wheezing
• Allergic reaction, e.g. rash, dermatitis, pruritus. (Drug may be discontinued if side effects are pronounced.)
Teach patient/family:
• To use a mouthwash for mild stomatitis
• To avoid hot, spicy foods and those that are highly acidic
• A soft toothbrush should be used
• That drug must be taken exactly as prescribed to be effective
• That diarrhoea is common, but if blood appears in stools or urine, the clinician must be informed at once
• To report skin conditions, stomatitis, fatigue, jaundice; these may indicate blood dyscrasias
• That therapeutic effect may take 3–4 months
• To practice contraception and avoid becoming pregnant

azathioprine

Azamune, Berkaprine, Imuran, Immunoprin
Func. class.: Immunosuppressant
Chem. class.: Purine analogue
Legal class.: POM

Action: Produces immunosuppression by inhibiting purine synthesis in cells, interferes with nucleic acid synthesis
Uses: Organ transplants to prevent rejection, refractory rheumatoid arthritis and other refractory diseases, autoimmune conditions (when steroids inadequate), e.g. chronic active hepatitis, haemolytic anaemia, systemic lupus erythematosus
Dosage and routes:
Prevention of rejection
• *Adult and child:* By mouth or slow IV injection, loading dose of up to 5 mg/kg then maintenance 1.0–4.0 mg/kg daily; IV *only* if oral not practical
Other conditions
• *Adult and child:* Seek specialist

advice, starting dose seldom exceeds 3 mg/kg daily

Available forms include: Tablets 25, 50 mg; powder for injection IV 50 mg vial (as sodium salt)

Side effects/adverse reactions:

GI: Nausea, vomiting, stomatitis, anorexia, oesophagitis, pancreatitis, hepatotoxicity, jaundice

HAEM: Leucopenia, thrombocytopenia, anaemia, pancytopenia, increased mean corpuscular volume, red cell haemoglobin content, myelosuppression

INTEG: Rash

MS: Arthralgia, muscle wasting, muscle pain

CV: Cardiac dysrhythmia, hypotension

CNS: Malaise, dizziness, rigors

Transplant patients also receiving steroids: hair loss, increased susceptibility to infection

Contraindications: Hypersensitivity to azathioprine or 6-mercaptopurine, pregnancy (see literature)

Precautions: Renal disease, hepatic disease, elderly, recent/concommitant cytostatic agents

Pharmacokinetics: Metabolised in liver, excreted in urine (active metabolite)

Interactions/incompatibilities:

• Increased action of this drug: allopurinol, oxipurinol, thiopurinol

• Increased effect of: depolarising muscle relaxants

• Decreased effect of: non-depolarising muscle relaxants

Clinical assessment:

• Blood studies: complete blood counts (including platelets) at least weekly initially

• Watch for manifestations of bone marrow depression: infections, bruising, bleeding

• Examine skin for tumours regularly in transplant recipients

• Liver function studies

Treatment of overdose: (Chronic and acute) Symptomatic. Gastric lavage. Monitor blood picture and liver function

NURSING CONSIDERATIONS

Assess:

• Temperature, pulse baseline

Administer:

• Do not crush tablets

• Avoid inhaling or ingesting dust when breaking tablets

• Tablets should be taken with food if nausea occurs

• IV powder for injection should be reconstituted with 5–15 ml water for injection and further diluted with 20–200 ml sodium chloride 0.9% or dextrose–saline before IV infusion. If this is not practical, reconstituted injection may be administered by slow IV injection over at least 1 min followed immediately by not less than 50 ml sodium chloride 0.9% or dextrose–saline

• With prophylactic medication (e.g. oral nystatin for stomatitis) if required to protect against side effects

Evaluate:

• Temperature, pulse daily (for pyrexia)

• For signs of nausea, vomiting, damage to oral/oesophageal mucosae, rash, muscle-wasting pain arthralgia

• For signs of infection, bone marrow suppression

Teach patient/family:

• About all side effects and report immediately

• Increased potential risk of infection – avoid contact with people who have obviously infective illnesses

• Record daily temperature

• Inform prescribing clinician of any medication already taken, e.g. allopurinol

azelaic acid ▼

Skinoren
Func. class.: Anti-acne, topical
Chem. class.: Antibacterial, keratolytic
Legal class.: POM

Action: Inhibits growth of propionibacteria involved in acne and their production of acne-promoting fatty acids. Also reduces keratinocyte activity thereby reducing comedone formation
Uses: Topical treatment of acne vulgaris
Dosage and routes: Topically twice a day for up to 6 months. 4 cm (1 g) of cream will generally be sufficient for each application to the face; for larger areas a total daily application of 40 cm (10 g) should not normally be exceeded. Patients with sensitive skins should apply only in the evening for the first week
Available forms include: Cream (20%)
Side effects/adverse reactions:
INTEG: Skin irritation, erythema, scaling, photosensitivity
Contraindications: Hypersensitivity
Precautions: Pregnancy, breast-feeding
Treatment of overdose: Low toxicity; overdose not likely in normal use

Administer:
- After skin cleansing

Evaluate:
- Therapeutic effect, indicated by reduction in severity of acne

Teach patient/family:
- To avoid application to unaffected skin, nose, eyes, mucous membranes
- To discontinue if skin rash develops and to seek medical advice
- That cream may stain hair or clothing; to avoid contact with either if possible
- That patients with sensitive skin should apply cream only in the evening for the first week
- That dryness and peeling of skin are to be expected
- That treatment may last up to six months

azlocillin sodium

Securopen
Func. class.: Antipseudomonal antibiotic
Chem. class.: Ureidopenicillin
Legal class.: POM

Action: Interferes with cell wall replication of susceptible organisms; the cell wall, rendered osmotically unstable, swells, bursts from osmotic pressure
Uses: Infections due to *Pseudomonas aeruginosa* especially respiratory and urinary tract and septicaemia
Dosage and routes:
- *Adult:* IV injection 2 g every 8 hr, IV infusion 5 g 8 hrly
- *Premature infant:* IV injection 50 mg/kg 12 hrly
- *Neonate:* IV injection 100 mg/kg 12 hrly
- *Infant:* IV injection 7 days-1 yr 100 mg/kg 8 hrly
- *Child 1–14 yr:* IV injection 75 mg/kg 8 hrly
- Reduce dose in renal impairment

Available forms include: Powder for injection 500 mg, 1 g, 2 g. Powder for infusion 5 g. All as sodium salt
Side effects/adverse reactions:
HAEM: Increased bleeding time
INTEG: Local irritation, rashes, pruritus
GI: Nausea, vomiting, diarrhoea, pseudomembranous colitis
SYST: Anaphylaxis

Contraindications: Hypersensitivity to penicillins and cephalosporins
Precautions: Pregnancy, neonates, renal impairment
Pharmacokinetics: Half-life 55–70 min, metabolised in liver, (limited extent), excreted in urine, bile, breast milk (small amount)
Interactions/incompatibilities:
• Increased penicillin concentrations when used with: probenicid
• Prolonged neuromuscular blockade: vecuronium and other non-depolarising muscle relaxants
• Anti-coagulants: need more frequent monitoring
• Reduced contraceptive effect: oral contraceptives
• Incompatibility in solution: seek pharmacist's advice before mixing
Treatment of overdose: Standard monitoring and supportive measures. Reduce serum levels by dialysis
NURSING CONSIDERATIONS
Administer:
• Seek pharmacist's advice before mixing (incompatibility in solutions)
• For doses of 2 g or less administer as IV bolus injection. Larger doses infuse over 20–30 min
• Dilute injection in appropriate infusion solutions, e.g. glucose 5%, sodium chloride 0.9%
• IV as a 10% solution in water for injections; doses of 2 g or less are given by bolus injection, higher doses by infusion over 20–30 min. Adjust dose in renal impairment
Perform/provide:
• Check IV site for local irritation
• Observe for skin rashes and pruritus
Teach patient/family:
• To observe for bruising or bleeding if taking anti-coagulants

azithromycin ▼

Zithromax
Func. class.: Antibiotic
Chem. class.: Macrolide antibiotic
Legal class.: POM

Action: Interferes with bacterial protein synthesis
Uses: Infections caused by susceptible organisms including those of the upper and lower respiratory tract, skin and soft tissues; genital infections due to *Chlamydia trachomatis*
Dosage and routes:
Chlamydia trachomatis
• *Adult:* By mouth 1 g as a single dose
Other indications
• *Adult:* By mouth 500 mg daily for 3 days
• *Child (over 6 months):* By mouth 10 mg/kg once daily for 3 days; or body-weight 15–25 kg, 200 mg daily for 3 days; body weight 26–35 kg, 300 mg daily for 3 days; body weight 36–45 kg, 400 mg daily for 3 days
Available forms include: Capsules 250 mg (as dihydrate); oral liquid, powder for reconstitution, 200 mg/5 ml (as dihydrate)
Side effects/adverse reactions:
GI: Nausea, abdominal pain/cramps, vomiting, flatulence, diarrhoea, hepatotoxicity
HAEM: Transient reduction in neutrophil counts
Contraindications: Hypersensitivity, hepatic disease
Precautions: Severe renal impairment, pregnancy, breast-feeding
Interactions:
• Absorption reduced by antacids, give 1 hr before or 2 hr after
• Effects of the following drugs possibly enhanced: warfarin, digoxin, cyclosporin
• Ergotism possible with ergotamine

• Possible risk of cardiac arrhythmias with terfenadine

Treatment of overdose: Gastric lavage in the first few hours after ingestion, symptomatic and supportive treatment

NURSING CONSIDERATIONS

Assess:

• Vital signs (temperature pulse, respirations)
• Culture and sensitivity before treatment starts
• For known sensitivities and allergies
• Bowel pattern
• Fluid balance

Administer:

• An hour before food, on an empty stomach and with a full glass of water

Perform/provide:

• Adequate fluids increased if diarrhoea occurs

Evaluate:

• Therapeutic response; resolution of symptoms, fall in neutrophil count
• Nausea, abdominal pain and other side effects

Teach patient/family:

• Drug should be taken before food with a full glass of water
• To maintain an adequate fluid intake (2 l/day)
• To report any side effects, particularly diarrhoea
• To take the full course of treatment unless otherwise advised by nurse or clinician

aztreonam

Azactam

Func. class.: Antibiotic

Chem. class.: Monocyclic β-lactam (monolactam)

Legal class.: POM

Action: Bactericidal antibiotic which acts by inhibiting bacterial cell wall synthesis by binding to and inhibiting enzymes which catalyse the final steps in this synthesis

Uses: The treatment of serious infections caused by susceptible Gram-negative aerobes. It is often used for its antipseudomonal activity

Dosage and routes:

• *Adults:* By IM (doses up to 1 g only) or IV injection or infusion (0.5–2 g every 6–8 hr, maximum daily dose 8 g)
• *Children (over 1 week of age):* 30 mg/kg every 6–8 hr, increased to 50 mg/kg every 6–8 hr in severe infections in children over 2 yr of age, maximum daily dose 8 g

Renal impairment

• *Creatinine clearance 10–30 ml/min:* After the first dose, half the normal dose should be given
• *Creatinine clearance less than 10 ml/min:* After the first dose, one quarter of the normal dose should be given

Available forms include: Injection 500 mg, 1 g, 2 g; IV infusion bottle 2 g

Side effects/adverse reactions:

CNS: Confusion, dizziness, vertigo, malaise, headache

CV: Hypotension

EENT: Mouth ulcers, taste disturbances, halitosis, sneezing, nasal congestion

ELECT: Raised serum creatinine

GI: Diarrhoea, nausea, vomiting, abdominal cramps, jaundice, hepatitis, elevated liver enzymes

HAEM: Eosinophilia; increased prothrombin and partial thromboplastin time; thrombocytopenia; neutropenia; anaemia; bleeding

INTEG: Rash, pruritus, urticaria, erythema, petechiae, exfoliative dermatitis, sweating

MS: Muscle aches

SYST: Allergic reactions including anaphylaxis

MISC: Weakness, breast tenderness, fever
Contraindications: Hypersensitivity, pregnancy
Precautions: Hypersensitivity to other β-lactam antibiotics including penicillins and cephalosporins; hepatic impairment; severe renal impairment
Pharmacokinetics: Peak serum levels 1 hr after IM injection; mainly eliminated via the kidneys; elimination half-life 1.7 hr
Interactions:
• Oral anticoagulants: Prothrombin times should be monitored during concomitant therapy
Incompatibilities:
• Do not mix with metronidazole
Treatment of overdose: There have been no cases of overdose reported; symptomatic treatment would be appropriate
NURSING CONSIDERATIONS
Assess:
• Vital signs (temperature, pulse, respiration, BP); respiratory status, fluid balance, urine test (as appropriate)
• Known sensitivities
Administer:
• Only after culture and sensitivity tests
• IV: by infusion over 20–60 mins. Contents of each infusion bottle should be dissolved in 6–10 ml water for injection, before dilution with suitable volume (at least 50 ml per gram) of infusion fluid
• IV: by injection. The contents of each vial should be dissolved in at least 3 ml of water for injection
• IM: into large muscle mass; each gram of aztreonam should be dissolved in at least 3 ml of water for injection or 0.9% sodium chloride
Perform/provide:
• Adequate fluids
• Nursing techniques appropriate to underlying disease
Evaluate:
• Therapeutic effect; reduction in symptoms
• Vital signs 4-hourly or as appropriate
• For side effects
Teach patient/family:
• About side effects and to report these to nurse or clinician

---

bacampicillin HCl

Ambaxin
Func. class.: Broad spectrum antibiotic
Chem. class.: Aminopenicillin
Legal class.: POM

Action: Interferes with cell wall replication of susceptible organisms; the cell wall, rendered osmotically unstable, swells, bursts from osmotic pressure
Uses: Respiratory tract infections, skin, urinary tract infections; effective for Gram-positive cocci, Gram-negative cocci, Gram-negative bacilli
Dosage and routes:
• *Adult:* By mouth, 400 mg 2 or 3 times daily, doubled in severe infection
• *Child:* By mouth, over 5 yr 200 mg 3 times daily
Gonorrhoea
• *Adult:* By mouth, 1.6 g as a single dose with probenecid 1 g
Available forms include: Tablets, scored 400 mg
Side effects/adverse reactions:
Sensitivity reactions: (discontinue treatment) rashes, urticaria, fever, joint pain, angioedema, anaphylactic shock
HAEM: Anaemia, increased bleeding time, bone marrow depression, granulocytopenia
GI: Nausea, vomiting, diarrhoea, increased aspartate aminotrans-

ferase, rarely pseudomembranous colitis, increased alanine aminotransferase, abdominal pain, glossitis, colitis
GU: Oliguria, proteinuria, haematuria, vaginitis, moniliasis, glomerulonephritis
CNS: Lethargy, hallucinations, anxiety, depression, twitching, coma, convulsions
META: Hypokalaemia, alkalosis
Contraindications: Hypersensitivity to penicillins
Precautions: Pregnancy, renal impairment, history of allergy, lactation, risk of erythematous rashes particularly high in glandular fever, lymphatic leukaemia and HIV infection. Possibility of superinfection with mycotic organisms or bacterial pathogens. Renal, hepatic and haemopoietic function should be monitored during prolonged therapy
Pharmacokinetics:
Period of onset: 30–60 min, duration 5–6 hr, hydrolysed to ampicillin in gut wall and plasma, metabolised in liver, excreted in urine
Interactions/incompatibilities:
• Phenindione and warfarin: prothrombin time can be prolonged
• Small risk of reduced contraceptive effect with combined oral contraceptives
• Decreased antimicrobial effectiveness of this drug: tetracyclines, erythromycins
• Increased penicillin concentrations when used with: aspirin, probenicid
Lab. test interferences: Interferes with tests for amino acids, serum-albumin and glucose
Treatment of overdose: Problems of overdose unlikely to be encountered
NURSING CONSIDERATIONS
Assess:
• Bowel pattern
• Fluid balance
• Allergies before initiation of treatment; reaction of each medication; highlight allergies on chart
• Check for pregnancy, history of allergy, lactation, glandular fever, lymphatic leukaemia, HIV infection, other medication (see interactions)
• Any patient with compromised renal system, since drug is excreted slowly in poor renal system function; toxicity may occur rapidly
• Liver studies: aspartate aminotransferase, alanine aminotransferase
• Renal studies: urinalysis, protein, blood
• Culture, sensitivity before drug therapy; drug may be taken as soon as culture is taken
Administer:
• After culture and sensitivity completed
Perform/provide:
• Adrenaline, suction, tracheostomy set, endotracheal intubation equipment on unit
• Adequate intake of fluids (2 litres) during diarrhoea episodes
Evaluate:
• For therapeutic effectiveness:
• Bowel pattern before, during treatment
• Fluid balance; report haematuria, oliguria since penicillin in high doses is nephrotoxic
• Skin eruptions after administration of penicillin to 1 week after discontinuing drug
• Respiratory status: rate, character, wheezing, tightness in chest
Teach patient/family:
• Aspects of drug therapy: culture may be taken after completed course of medication
• To report sore throat, fever, fatigue (could indicate superimposed infection)

• To wear or carry a Medic Alert ID if allergic to penicillins
• To notify nurse of diarrhoea

---

baclofen

Lioresal

Func. class.: Skeletal muscle relaxant
Chem. class.: GABA chlorophenyl derivative
Legal class.: POM

Action: Antispastic agent acting at spinal level. GABA derivative. Depresses monosynaptic and polysynaptic reflex transmission probably by activating GABA neurotransmission. Neuromuscular transmission is unaffected. Reduces painful flexor spasms and spontaneous clonus. Antinociceptive effect

Uses: Spinal cord injury, spasticity in multiple sclerosis, motor neurone disease

Dosage and routes:

• *Adult:* By mouth, 5 mg 3 times daily, increased gradually to avoid sedation and hypotonia. Control usually achieved with 60 mg daily in divided doses but up to maximum of 100 mg daily may be required

• *Child:* By mouth, 0.75–2 mg/kg daily (over 10 yr maximum 2.5 mg/kg daily) or 2.5 mg 4 times daily increased gradually according to age to maintenance: 1–2 yr 10–20 mg daily, 2–6 yr 20–30 mg daily, 6–10 yr 30–60 mg daily

Available forms include: Tablets 10 mg; sugar-free liquid 5 mg/5 ml

Side effects/adverse reactions:

CNS: Dizziness, weakness, fatigue, drowsiness, headache, disorientation, insomnia, paraesthesiae, tremors, hallucinations, nightmares, convulsions, increased spasticity, muscular hypotonia, muscular pain, daytime sedation, mental confusion, euphoria, depressive states

MS: Myalgia, muscular weaknesses, ataxia

EENT: Nasal congestion, blurred vision, accommodation disorders

CV: Hypotension, chest pain, palpitations, cardiovascular depression

GI: Nausea, constipation, vomiting, increased aspartate aminotransferase, alkaline phosphatase, abdominal pain, dry mouth, anorexia, retching, diarrhoea, alteration in taste, deterioration in liver function tests

GU: Urinary frequency, dysuria, enuresis

INTEG: Rash, pruritus, hyperhidrosis

RESP: Respiratory depression

Contraindications: Hypersensitivity, peptic ulceration, porphyria

Precautions: Psychotic disorders, schizophrenia, confusional states, epilepsy, antihypertensive therapy, cerebrovascular accident, respiratory, hepatic or renal impairment, hypertonic bladder sphincter, diabetes mellitus, pregnancy, elderly, spastic states of cerebral origin. Treatment should be withdrawn gradually over 1–2 weeks

Pharmacokinetics:

Peak ½–1½ hr. Half life 3–4 hr Serum protein binding approximately 30%. Eliminated largely in unchanged form via kidneys

Interactions/incompatibilities:

Increased effect: tricyclic antidepressants. Increased sedation: alcohol, CNS depressants. Aggravation of hyperkinetic symptoms: lithium. Increased effect of: antihypotensives. Increased toxicity: ibuprofen, levodopa with carbidopa

Clinical assessment:

• Perform EEG for patients with history of epilepsy

Lab. test interferences:
Increase: Aspartate aminotransferase, alkaline phosphatase, blood glucose, SGOT
Treatment of overdose: No specific antidote. Induce vomiting, gastric lavage; comatose patients should be intubated prior to gastric lavage. Administration of activated charcoal. If necessary, saline aperient. In respiratory depression, administration of artificial respiration, also measures in support of cardiovascular functions. Generous quantities of fluid should be given, possibly with a diuretic. If convulsions occur, diazepam should be administered cautiously IV

NURSING CONSIDERATIONS

Administer:
- With food or milk to reduce gastric symptoms
- If muscle hypotonia is a problem it may often be relieved by reducing the daytime doses and increasing the night-time dose

Perform/provide:
- Mouthcare, mouthwashes for dry mouth
- Help during standing/walking if dizziness or drowsiness occurs

Evaluate:
- Effectiveness of drug indicated by decreased pain and spasticity
- Urinary output; watch for urinary retention, frequency, hesitancy
- Allergic reactions e.g. rash, fever, respiratory distress
- Weakness, numbness in extremities
- Psychological dependency e.g. increased need for medication, more frequent requests for medication, increased pain
- CNS depression; dizziness, drowsiness, psychiatric symptoms

Teach patient/family:
- Medication must not be discontinued suddenly; hallucinations, spasticity, tachycardia will occur. Drug must be discontinued slowly over 1–2 weeks
- Not to take with alcohol or other CNS depressants
- To avoid driving or operating machinery if dizzy or drowsy
- To avoid medicines that have not been prescribed, especially cough linctuses, antihistamines
- To take with food/milk
- Some benefits after 2–3 hr, but full benefits after several weeks
- To report any urinary problems
- Ask patient about fits/seizures if a known epileptic; this drug may induce seizures

---

bambuterol hydrochloride

Bambec ▼
Func. class.: Bronchodilator
Chem. class.: β_2-adrenergic agonist (terbutaline prodrug)
Legal class.: POM

Action: Converted *in vivo* to terbutaline which produces bronchodilatation by stimulating bronchial β-receptors
Uses: Management of obstructive airways disease including asthma
Dosage and routes:
- *Adult:* By mouth, 20 mg once daily, at bedtime; a starting dose of 10 mg can be used in patients receiving oral β_2-agonist therapy

Renal impairment
- Starting dose should be halved in patients with GFR less than 50 ml/min

Significant hepatic impairment
- Not recommended because of unpredictable conversion to terbutaline

Available forms include: Tablets 10, 20 mg
Side effects/adverse reactions:

CNS: Headache, anxiety
CV: Palpitations, arrhythmias
ELECT: Hypokalaemia, hyperglycaemia
MISC: Tremor
MS: Muscle cramps
Contraindications: Hypersensitivity
Precautions: Pregnancy; breast-feeding; cardiac disorders; thyrotoxicosis; diabetes mellitus; impaired hepatic function; patients with hypokalaemia or with conditions/receiving treatments predisposing them to hypokalaemia
Pharmacokinetics: Nearly 20% absorbed following oral administration; peak plasma concentrations 2–4 hr after dosing
Interactions:
• Prolonged action of: suxamethonium
• Antagonised by: β-blockers
• Increased risk of hypokalaemia with: diuretics, corticosteroids, aminophylline, theophylline
Treatment of overdose: Gastric lavage or the administration of activated charcoal if ingestion is recent; cardiovascular monitoring; supportive and symptomatic care; a cardioselective β-blocker may be helpful in arrhythmias, at the risk of inducing bronchospasm

NURSING CONSIDERATIONS

Assess:
• Vital signs (temperature, pulse, respiration, BP); ECG in those with underlying heart disease
• Degree of bronchospasm
Administer:
• Before bedtime for maximum effect
Perform/provide:
• Cardiac monitoring for patients with arrhythmias, angina, hypertension
Evaluate:
• Therapeutic effect; reduction in bronchospasm
• For side effects
Teach patient/family:
• Reason for taking drug before bedtime
• About side effects: headache, anxiety, muscle cramps, tremor and to report these to nurse or clinician
• Not to use OTC medicines

BCG (bacillus Calmette-Guérin vaccine)

Func. class.: Vaccine
Chem. class.: Live attenuated strain derived from bovine *Mycobacterium tuberculosis*
Legal class.: POM

Action: Stimulates the development of immunity to the bacillus *Mycobacterium tuberculosis*
Uses: Active immunisation against tuberculosis
Dosage and routes: Intradermal injection 0.1 ml (infants under 3 months, 0.05 ml) by operators skilled in the technique. Percutaneous vaccine *not* recommended
Available forms include:
• BCG vaccine
• BCG vaccine, Isoniazid-Resistant
• BCG vaccine, Percutaneous
Side effects/adverse reactions:
INTEG: Mild discomfort at injection site; prolonged ulceration or subcutaneous abscess formation due to faulty injection technique; rash, induration, pain
SYSTEM: Mild fever and malaise, lymphadenopathy. Anaphylactic reactions are rare
Contraindications: Tuberculoprotein hypersensitivity, HIV-positive and other immunocompromised patients, existing acute illness; pregnancy, systemic treatment with corticosteroids, immunosuppressive treatment, malignant disease, pyrexia, infected derma-

toses, eczema at injection site, radiotherapy and irradiation tumours of reticuloendothelial system, generalised septic skin conditions. For time lapse between stopping drug therapy and having BCG – refer to clinician

Precautions: Do not give within 3 weeks (or minimum 10 days) of other live vaccines; do not administer other vaccines in the same arm as BCG for at least 3 months

Pharmacokinetics: Seroconversion occurs within 8–14 weeks

Clinical assessment:

• Measles or rubella infection can cause tuberculin positive patients to revert temporarily and become tuberculin negative

• Perform skin test for sensitivity. Newborn infants require no skin test. When BCG is given to infants there is no need to delay primary immunisations including polio

NURSING CONSIDERATIONS

Administer:

• Nurses must be fully competent in the technique of intradermal injection

• After preparation according to manufacturer's instruction using sodium chloride or water for injection

• Do not shake. Allow to stand for 1 min. Draw up twice to ensure homogenous solution. Once prepared protect from light and use within 4 hr

• If the injection site is swabbed with alcohol, allow to dry before administration of vaccine to prevent contamination

• Use syringe fitted with a short bevel gauge 25 needle. The use of jet injectors is not recommended

• Give intradermally in the arm over the insertion of the deltoid muscle. The thigh can be used in females for cosmetic reasons but is not recommended in neonates

• Record date, name of vaccine, dose, route, site and batch number of vaccine and sodium chloride or water in patient's notes

Perform/provide:

• Incinerate excess vaccine or treat with disinfectant such as strong hypochlorite solution

Teach patient/family:

• To leave open to facilitate healing or, if discharging, cover with dry, non-occlusive dressing. Avoid abrasion, e.g. by tight clothing

• To expect some mild discomfort

• To expect small swelling after 1 week, ulcer at 3 weeks which heals after 6–12 weeks. Scar is initially red and later becomes white

• To see clinician in event of pain, swelling discharge or increasing fever

• High risk workers e.g. nurses, to contact clinician or occupational health department after 6 weeks for follow-up to confirm immunity, if indicated

---

beclomethasone dipropionate (inhaled)

Becotide 50, Becotide 100, Becotide 200, Becodisks, Becotide Rotacaps, Becloforte, AeroBec, AeraBec Fate Beclazone, Beclafone 250, Filair, Filair Forte

Func. class.: Synthetic corticosteroid

Chem. class.: Beclomethasone diester

Legal class.: POM

Action: Reduces inflammation by depression of migration of polymorphonuclear leucocytes, fibroblasts, reversal of increased capillary permeability and lysosomal stabilisation. At normal therapeutic doses the inhaled preparation lacks systemic side effects

Uses: Treatment and prophylaxis of asthma

Dosages and routes:

• *By inhalation of powder* Becodisks/Rotacaps: *Adult:* 200 mcg 3 to 4 times daily or 400 mcg twice daily. Maximum dose 1 mg daily

• *Child*: 100 mcg 2 to 4 times daily or 200 mcg twice daily

• *By aerosol inhalation: Adult:* 200 mcg twice daily or 100 mcg 3 to 4 times daily (in more severe cases, initially 600–800 mcg daily)

• *Child*: 50–100 mcg 2 to 4 times daily

• High dose aerosol inhaler (250 mcg/actuation): *Adult:* 500 mcg twice daily or 250 mcg 4 times daily. Maximum 500 mcg 3 to 4 times daily. Not indicated for children

• *By nebulisation: Child:* up to 1 year: 50 mcg 2 to 4 times daily; 1 to 12 years: 100 mcg 2 to 4 times daily, adjust according to response. Unsuitable for adults.

Available forms include:

Aerosol inhalation: 50 mcg, 100 mcg, 200 mcg, 250 mcg, per metered inhalation. Autohaler, 50 mcg, 200 mcg, 250 mcg per breath-activated metered inhalation

Rotacaps containing powder for inhalation: 100, 200, 400 mcg

Becodisks containing 8 powder blisters per disk: 100, 200, 400 mcg

Becloforte VM (2 Becloforte inhalers plus volumatic spacer)

Becotide for nebulisation, 50 mcg/ml

Side effects/adverse reactions:

EENT: Dry mouth, candidiasis of mouth and throat (treat with topical antifungal therapy whilst still continuing inhaler), hoarseness or throat irritation

RESP: Potential for paradoxical bronchospasm (discontinue treatment immediately and institute alternative therapy)

Contraindications: Hypersensitivity to beclomethasone, active or quiescent pulmonary tuberculosis, status asthmaticus (primary treatment), non-asthmatic bronchial disease

Precautions: Pregnancy, lactation, poor inhalation technique. After transfer from oral corticosteroid therapy may need to reinstate systemic therapy during periods of stress, infection or when airway obstruction or mucus prevent drug access to smaller airways. Use regularly. No adrenal suppression likely until doses of 1500 mcg per day. Reduced plasma cortisol levels reported at doses of 2000 mcg per day

Pharmacokinetics:

Inhalation: Onset 10 min, excreted in faeçes (metabolites), half-life 3–15 hr, metabolised in lungs, liver, GI system

Interactions: None significant

Incompatibilities: None significant

• Check inhalation technique, advise to use regularly

• Candidiasis is reduced with 'spacer' apparatus and also responds to antifungal lozenges without discontinuing treatment

• Assess adrenal function periodically

• Becloforte – advise carry steroid card. Do not stop abruptly

Treatment of overdose: Inhalation of large amounts of drug over a short time – no special emergency action needed. Continue treatment at recommended dose. Hypothalamic-pituitary-adrenal (HPA) function recovers in a day or two. Excessive use over a long time could lead to adrenal suppression, transfer to oral corticosteroid therapy and when condition is stabilised return to inhaled therapy at recommended dose. Then withdraw oral steroids gradually

NURSING CONSIDERATIONS

Administer:

• With correct technique and equipment, e.g. Spacer

• Use Rotacaps in Rotahaler device

• Dilute nebulisation solution up to 50% with sodium chloride 0.9%. Use with respirator or nebuliser

Perform/provide:

• Mouthcare, mouthwashes to counteract dryness and reduce risk of fungal colonisation

Evaluate:

• By recording peak flow pre- and post-administration. Assess for paradoxical bronchospasm

Teach patient/family:

• Correct technique of administration

• To wash inhaler with warm water after use and dry thoroughly

• If mouth and/or throat problems occur after use advise to rinse mouth thoroughly with water immediately after inhalation

• To carry identity as a steroid user

• To report if the drug no longer seems effective, as the dose may need readjusting

• All aspects of drug taking and side effects, including Cushingoid symptoms

• To recognise symptoms of adrenal insufficiency, e.g. nausea, anorexia, fatigue, dizziness, dyspnoea, weakness, joint pain, depression

• To seek advice if not well, particularly nausea, anorexia, joint pain

beclomethasone dipropionate (nasal)

Beconase

Func. class.: Synthetic corticosteroid

Chem. class.: Beclomethasone diester

Legal class.: POM

Action: Anti-inflammatory properties in nasal passages

Uses: Treatment and prophylaxis of seasonal or perennial rhinitis

Dosage and routes:

• *Adult and child over 6 yr:* Apply 100 mcg (2 puffs) into each nostril twice daily or 50 mcg (1 puff) 3 to 4 times daily. Maximum 8 puffs daily

Available forms include: Aerosol 50 mcg per inhalation, aqueous spray 50 mcg per spray

Side effects/adverse reactions:

EENT: Dryness, nasal irritation, burning, sneezing

Contraindications: Hypersensitivity to any components, children under 6 yr

Precautions: Pregnancy, lactation, infections of nasal passages and paranasal sinuses, systemic steroid therapy, prolonged use in children

Pharmacokinetics:

INSTIL: Readily absorbed; peak, concentration, other data have not been determined

Treatment of overdose: Inhalation of large amounts over a short time — no special emergency action needed. Continue treatment at the recommended dose. Hypothalamic-pituitary-adrenal (HPA) function recovers in a day or two

NURSING CONSIDERATIONS

Administer:

• After cleaning top of aerosol with warm water and drying thoroughly

• After cleaning/blowing nose

Perform/provide:
• Storage in a cool place, do not puncture or incinerate
Evaluate:
• Condition of nasal passages during long term treatment for changes in mucous membrane
Teach patient/family:
• To clear nasal passages before administration, use decongestant if needed, shake inhaler, invert, tilt head backwards, insert nozzle into nostril away from septum, hold other nostril closed, depress activator, inhale through nose and exhale through mouth
• When Beconase *Aerosol* administered as 2 puffs, the 1st puff should be directed at the upper and the 2nd puff at the lower part of the nasal cavity
• If sneezing occurs nasal passages should be cleared and dose repeated
• To continue treatment if mild nasal bleeding occurs; it is usually transient
• How to use and to read manufacturer's instructions

bendrofluazide

Aprinox, Berkozide Neo-NaClex, Centyl, combination product
Func. class.: Diuretic
Chem. class.: Thiazide
Legal class.: POM

Action: Acts on distal tubule by increasing excretion of water, sodium, chloride, potassium
Uses: Oedema, hypertension
Dosage and routes:
• *Adult:* By mouth: oedema, initially 5–10 mg in the morning, daily or on alternate days, maintenance 2.5–10 mg 1–3 times weekly; hypertension: 2.5 mg in the morning

Available forms include: Tablets 2.5, 5 mg
Side effects/adverse reactions:
GU: Polyuria, uraemia, glycosuria, impotence, thirst
CNS: Dizziness, weakness
GI: Nausea, vomiting, anorexia, hepatic encephalopathy, constipation, diarrhoea, cramps, pancreatitis, GI irritation
INTEG: Rash, purpura, photosensitivity
META: Hyperglycaemia, hyperuraemia, increased plasma cholesterol
HAEM: Neutropenia, thrombocytopenia
CV: Orthostatic hypotension
ELECT: Hypokalaemia, hypochloraemic alkalosis, hypercalcaemia, hyponatraemia, hypomagnesaemia, hyperuricaemia, gout
Contraindications: Hypersensitivity to thiazides or sulphonamides, anuria, lactation, lithium, pregnancy, hypercalcaemia, Addison's disease, porphyria, severe hepatic/renal failure, diabetic ketoacidosis
Precautions: Hypokalaemia, renal/hepatic impairment, elderly, gout, lupus erythematosus, diabetes mellitus, prostatic hypertrophy
Pharmacokinetics:
Period of onset: Onset 2 hr, peak 4 hr, duration 6–12 hr
Excreted some in urine 3–6 hr, excreted in breast milk
Interactions/incompatibilities:
• Increased effect/toxicity: lithium, non-depolarising skeletal muscle relaxants, NSAIDs, chlorpropamide
• Decreased effects of: antidiabetics
• Decreased absorption of thiazides: cholestyramine, colestipol (give at least 2 hr apart)
• Increased action of: halothane
• Enhanced hypotensive effects:

barbiturates, alcohol, MAOIs, narcotics, antihypertensives
• If hypokalaemia: Increased side effects/toxicity: amiodarone, disopyramide, flecainide, quinidine, pimozide, sotalol, cardiac glycosides, allopurinol. Decreased effect: lignocaine, mexiletine, tocainide
• Antagonise diuretic effect: NSAIDs, corticosteroids, oestrogens, combined oral contraceptives, carbenoxolone
• Increased risk of hypokalaemia: indapamide, corticosteroids, other diuretics, carbenoxolone ACTH, acetazolamide, NSAIDs
• Increased risk of postural hypotension: tricyclics
• Risk of hypercalcaemia: calcium salts

Clinical assessment:
• Electrolytes: potassium, sodium, calcium, magnesium, chloride; include blood urea nitrogen, blood sugar, serum creatinine, blood pH, and uric acid
• Potassium replacement if necessary
• Monitor renal function throughout therapy
• Monitor insulin requirement of diabetic patients
• Monitor blood lipids
• Test for glycosuria

Lab. test interferences:
• Estimation of serum protein-bound iodine
• Tests of parathyroid function

Treatment of overdose: Lavage if recently taken orally, activated charcoal. Monitor electrolyte and fluid balance, BP, renal function. Avoid cathartics. Symptomatic and supportive treatment. No specific antidote

NURSING CONSIDERATIONS

Assess:
• Baseline BP, weight, fluid balance

Administer:
• In the morning to avoid interference with sleep if using drug as a diuretic
• With food if nausea occurs; absorption may be decreased slightly

Evaluate:
• Weight, fluid balance daily to determine fluid loss; effect of drug may be decreased if used daily
• Rate depth, rhythm of respiration, effect of exertion
• BP lying, standing; postural hypotension may occur
• Glucose in urine if patient is diabetic
• Improvement in oedema of feet, legs, sacral area daily if medication is being used in congestive cardiac failure
• Improvement in CVP and BP recordings
• Signs of metabolic acidosis: drowsiness, restlessness
• Signs of hypokalaemia: postural hypotension, malaise, fatigue, tachycardia, leg cramps, weakness
• Rashes, pyrexia daily
• Confusion especially in elderly; observe carefully

Teach patient/family:
• To increase fluid intake to 2–3 litres daily unless contraindicated; to rise slowly from lying or sitting position
• To notify clinician of muscle weakness, cramps, nausea, dizziness, joint pain (gout)
• Drug may be taken with food or milk
• That blood sugar may be increased in diabetics
• To take early in day to avoid nocturia

benorylate

Benoral
Func. class.: Non-narcotic analgesic
Chem. class.: Aspirin and paracetamol ester
Legal class.: P

Action: Blocks pain impulses in CNS by inhibition of prostaglandin synthesis; antipyretic action results from inhibition of hypothalamic heat-regulating centre to produce vasodilation to allow heat dissipation
Uses: Mild to moderate pain and inflammation in rheumatic disease and other musculoskeletal disorders, including arthritis; fever
Dosage and routes:
Rheumatic diseases
• *Adult:* By mouth 4–8 g divided into 2–3 doses with food as needed
• ***Mild to moderate pain and pyrexia:*** 2 g twice daily with food
Available forms include: Tablets 750 mg, granules 2 g/sachet, suspension 2 g/5 ml. 2 g benorylate is equivalent to 1.15 g aspirin and 0.97 g paracetamol
Side effects/adverse reactions:
HAEM: Rare blood dyscrasias, increased prothrombin time
CNS: Stimulation, drowsiness, dizziness, confusion, convulsion, headache, flushing, hallucinations, coma (in large doses)
GI: Nausea, vomiting, GI bleeding, diarrhoea, heartburn, anorexia, hepatitis
INTEG: Rash, urticaria, bruising
EENT: Tinnitus, hearing loss
RESP: Wheezing
ENDO: Hypoglycaemia
Contraindications: Hypersensitivity to salicylates and paracetamol, GI ulceration, bleeding disorders, children under 12 yr (except for juvenile rheumatoid arthritis) association with Reye's syndrome, breast-feeding
Precautions: Anaemia, hepatic disease, renal disease, Hodgkin's disease, pregnancy, elderly, dehydration, peptic ulcer
Pharmacokinetics: Benorylate metabolised to salicylate and paracetamol by esterases after absorption. Metabolised by liver, excreted by kidneys, excreted in breast milk
Interactions/incompatibilities:
• Decreased effects of this drug: antacids, steroids, urinary alkalinisers
• Increased effects of salicylate: carbonic anhydrase inhibitors
• Increased blood loss: alcohol, heparin
• Increased effects of: anticoagulants, insulin, methotrexate
• Decreased effects of: probenecid, frusemide
• Decreased blood sugar levels: salicylates
Clinical assessment:
• Liver function tests: enzymes, aspartate aminotransferase, alanine aminotransferase, bilirubin, creatinine if problem anticipated
• Renal function studies: blood urea, urine creatinine if patient has renal impairment, problem anticipated
• Prior drug history; there are many drug interactions
Lab. test interferences:
Increase: Coagulation studies, liver function studies
Treatment of overdose: Measure serum levels of salicylate and paracetamol; lavage, activated charcoal, monitor electrolytes, vital signs, forced alkaline diuresis, correction of acid-base balance. May have to use IV acetylcysteine or oral methionine to correct paracetamol overdose if given within 10–12 hr of drug ingestion
NURSING CONSIDERATIONS

Assess:
• Fluid balance, weight
Administer:
• With food or milk to decrease gastric symptoms; give with or after meals
Perform/provide:
• Repositioning to decrease pain
• Cooling for fever
Evaluate:
• Fluid balance; decreasing output may indicate renal failure (long-term therapy)
• Hepatotoxicity: dark urine, clay-coloured stools, yellowing of skin, sclera, itching, abdominal pain, fever, diarrhoea if patient is on long-term therapy
• Oedema in feet, ankles, legs
Teach patient/family:
• To take with food or milk
• To report any symptoms of hepatotoxicity, renal toxicity, visual changes, ototoxicity, allergic reactions (long-term therapy)
• Not to exceed recommended dosage; acute poisoning may result
• To read label on other non-prescribed drugs; many contain aspirin or paracetamol
• That therapeutic response takes 2 weeks (arthritis)
• To avoid alcohol; GI bleeding may occur
• Report indigestion or black tarry stools

benzhexol

Artane, Broflex
Func. class.: Antimuscarinic
Chem. class.: Synthetic tertiary amine
Legal class.: POM

Action: Decreases cholinergic function in CNS, correcting the imbalance in cholinergic and dopaminergic function and reducing extrapyramidal effects
Uses: Parkinsonian symptoms, drug-induced extrapyramidal symptoms (except tardive dyskinesia)
Dosage and routes:
• *Adult:* By mouth 1 mg daily increased by 1–2 mg every 3–5 days until symptoms controlled, to a total of 5–15 mg daily in 3–4 divided doses
Available forms include: Tablets 2, 5 mg; elixir 5 mg/5 ml
Side effects/adverse reactions:
CNS: Confusion, anxiety, restlessness, irritability, delusions, hallucinations, dizziness
EENT: Blurred vision, photophobia, dilated pupils, difficulty swallowing
CV: Palpitations, tachycardia
GI: Dryness of mouth, constipation, nausea, vomiting, abdominal distress, paralytic ileus
GU: Urinary retention
Contraindications: Hypersensitivity, tardive dyskinesia, closed-angle glaucoma, prostatic hypertrophy, urinary retention (untreated), gastrointestinal obstruction
Precautions: Hypertension, cardiac disorders, liver or kidney disorders, elderly, arteriosclerosis, prostatic hypertrophy, narrow-angle glaucoma, myasthenia gravis, GI/GU obstruction, risk of abuse
Pharmacokinetics:
By mouth: Onset 1 hr, peak 2–3 hr, duration 6–12 hr, excreted in urine
Interactions/incompatibilities:
• Increased anticholinergic effects: antihistamines, tricyclic antidepressants, MAOIs, phenothiazines, amantadine, nefopam, disopyramide

NURSING CONSIDERATIONS
Assess:
• Fluid balance
• Bowel patterns

• Age of patient—over 65 yr slightly more sensitive and require smaller amounts of drugs

Administer:

• Orally following the dosage regimen for suitable gradual introduction

• At bedtime if a single daily dose is given

• After food to prevent nausea, or before food to reduce dry mouth

Perform/provide:

• Frequent drinks to prevent a dry mouth

Evaluate:

• Therapeutic response: decreased rigidity of muscle spasm, tremors slow movement, excessive salivation. Relieving depression and mental inertia

• Input and output of fluids, observe for retention

• Minor side effects—dryness of mouth, constipation, urinary retention, blurring of vision

• Optimal response with minimal side effects

Teach patient/family:

• Not to discontinue medication without medical advice. Dose changes by gradual increments and tapered off slowly

• Not to take any other drugs without medical advice

---

benzoyl peroxide

Acetoxyl, Acnecide, Acnegel, Benoxyl, Benzagel, Nericur, Panoxyl

Func. class.: Anti-acne agent

Legal class.: P

Action: Antibacterial activity especially against predominant bacteria causing acne. Also keratolytic and sebostatic

Uses: Acne vulgaris

Dosage and routes:

• *Adult:* Topical. Apply to affected area once or twice daily. Start with lower strengths

• *Child:* Under 12 yr, seek clinician's or pharmacist's advice

Available forms include: Topical cleansers, lotions, creams, gels 2.5%, 5%, 10%

Side effects/adverse reactions:

INTEG: Local skin irritation, reddening, scaling, increased peeling in first few weeks (discontinue temporarily)

Contraindications: Hypersensitivity to benzoic acid derivatives

Precautions: Avoid contact with eyes, mouth and mucous membranes; may bleach fabrics. Care on sensitive areas (e.g. neck)

Pharmacokinetics:

Topical: 50% absorbed through skin, metabolised to benzoic acid, excreted in urine

Interactions/incompatibilities: None known

NURSING CONSIDERATIONS

Administer:

• Use gloves to apply, then wash hands immediately to avoid irritation

• Avoid contact with eyes, mouth and mucous membranes

• May bleach fabrics

• With care to sensitive areas (e.g. neck)

Evaluate:

• Effectiveness, indicated by decreased acne

• Other factors which help or aggravate condition

• Allergic reaction e.g. rash, irritation, dermatitis; use should be discontinued

Teach patient/family:

• To avoid application to unaffected skin, nose, eyes, mucous membranes

• To discontinue if rash develops

• May cause transitory warmth or stinging over area treated

• May stain hair or clothing. Avoid contact

• Cosmetics may be used over treated area
• That some dryness and peeling is to be expected

benztropine

Cogentin
Func. class.: Antimuscarinic
Chem. class.: Tertiary amine
Legal class.: POM

Action: Antagonises central cholinergic activity, which decreases involuntary movements
Uses: Parkinsonism, drug-induced extrapyramidal symptoms (not tardive dyskinesia)
Dosage and routes:
Parkinsonism
• *Adult:* By mouth 0.5–1 mg daily usually at bedtime, gradually increased to maximum 6 mg daily as necessary. Usual maintenance dose 1–4 mg daily in single or divided doses
Extrapyramidal symptoms
• *Adult:* IM/IV injection 1–2 mg; repeated if symptoms reappear
Available forms include: Tablets 2 mg (scored); injection IM, IV 1 mg/ml (2 ml)
Side effects/adverse reactions:
CNS: Confusion, anxiety, numbness of fingers, disorientation memory impairment, listlessness, hallucinations, exacerbation of pre-existing psychotic symptoms, sedation, depression, dizziness
EENT: Blurred vision, dilated pupils
INTEG: Allergic rash, anhidrosis
CV: Tachycardia
GI: Dryness of mouth, constipation, nausea, vomiting
GU: Hesitancy, retention, dysuria
Contraindications: Hypersensitivity, closed-angle glaucoma, prostatic hypertrophy, urinary retention (untreated), gastro-intestinal obstruction
Precautions: Pregnancy, elderly, lactation, tachycardia, myasthenia gravis, abnormalities of sweating, children. May impair ability/alertness for driving etc. Cumulative action. Mental disorders, cardiovascular disease urinary retention, hepatic/renal impairment. Do not withdraw abruptly, liable to abuse
Pharmacokinetics:
IM/IV: Onset 15 min, duration 6–10 hr
Period of onset: Onset 1 hr, duration 6–10 hr
Interactions/incompatibilities:
• Antagonism of GI effect: cisapride, domperidone, metoclopramide
• Increased antimuscarinic side effects: other drugs with antimuscarinic effects, nefopam, disopyramide tricyclics, MAOIs, antihistamines, phenothiazines, amantadine
• Reduced absorption: ketoconazole
• Decreased plasma levels: phenothiazines
• Reduced effect: sublingual nitrates
Treatment of overdose: Induce emesis or gastric lavage if recent ingestion. Physostigmine salicylate to reverse anticholinergic symptoms. Symptomatic and supportive treatment. Possible use of short-acting barbiturate for CNS excitement (NB: subsequent depression, also avoid convulsant stimulants), artificial respiration, local miotic, ice bags, vasopressor, fluids, darkened room

NURSING CONSIDERATIONS

Administer:
• At bedtime to avoid drowsiness during day
• With or after meals to prevent gastric upset; may be given with fluids other than water

• Parenteral dose slowly. Patient should stay in bed for at least 1 hr afterwards

Perform/provide:

• Mouthcare and mouthwashes to relieve dry mouth

Evaluate:

• Response to drug; parkinsonism, extrapyramidal symptoms e.g. shuffling gait, muscle rigidity, involuntary movements should decrease

• Dose may need to be increased or changed in the event of tolerance or long term treatment

• Urinary output; retention may occur

• Fluid intake, fibre in diet and encourage exercise if constipation occurs

• GI problems—especially paralytic ileus

• Worsening of mental symptoms during early treatment, e.g. CNS depression, change in mood or affect

Teach patient/family:

• Drug must not be discontinued suddenly, but gradually over 1 week

• To avoid driving or operating machinery as drowsiness may occur

• To avoid medicines that have not been prescribed, especially those for coughs and colds and antihistamines

• Not to be taken with alcohol

---

benzylpenicillin (Penicillin G)

Crystapen, combination products

Func. class.: Antibiotic, broad-spectrum

Chem. class.: Penicillin

Legal class.: POM

Action: Interferes with cell wall replication of susceptible organisms; osmotically unstable cell wall swells, bursts from osmotic pressure

Uses: Bacterial infections due to susceptible organisms, including tonsillitis, otitis media, erysipelas, streptococcal endocarditis, meningococcal and pneumococcal meningitis, prophylaxis in limb amputation, diphtheria, gas gangrene, gonococcal infections, syphilis, tetanus

Dosage and routes:

Mild—moderate infections

• *Adult:* IM or slow IV injection 0.6–1.2 g daily in 2–4 divided doses, increased up to 2.4 g daily or more if necessary

• *Child:* 1 month–12 yr 10–20 mg/kg daily in 4 divided doses

• *Neonate:* 30 mg/kg daily in 2–4 divided doses

Bacterial endocarditis

• Slow IV injection or infusion up to 7.2 g daily in 4–6 divided doses

Meningitis

• *Child 1 month–12 yr:* Slow IV injection or infusion 180–300 mg/kg daily in 4–6 divided doses

• *Neonate:* Up to 7 days, 60–90 mg/kg daily in 2 divided doses; over 7 days old, 90–120 mg/kg daily in 3 divided doses

Available forms include: Injection IV/IM 600 mg

Side effects/adverse reactions:

HAEM: Haemolytic anaemia, increased bleeding time, granulocytopenia

GI: Nausea, diarrhoea, sore mouth, heartburn

INTEG: Rash, urticaria, angioedema (signs of hypersensitivity)

CNS: Convulsions, encephalopathy, and paralysis (high/intrathecal dosage)

META: Hypokalaemia, hypernatraemia

SYST: Anaphylaxis, joint pains, fever (hypersensitivity)

Contraindications: Hypersensitivity to penicillins

Precautions: History of allergy, renal impairment

Pharmacokinetics:

IM: Peak 12–24 hr, half-life 0.5 hr. Metabolised in liver, excreted in faeces, breast milk

Interactions/incompatibilities:

• Possibly decreased antimicrobial effectiveness of penicillin: tetracyclines, erythromycins, chloramphenicol
• Increased antimicrobial effectiveness of penicillin: aminoglycosides
• Increased penicillin concentrations when used with: aspirin, probenecid

Lab. test interferences:

False positive: Urine glucose, urine protein

Treatment of overdose: Supportive care; blood levels reduced by haemodialysis

NURSING CONSIDERATIONS

Assess:

• Bowel pattern
• Fluid balance

Administer:

• Drug after culture and sensitivity has been completed
• IM as a solution containing 600 mg dissolved in 1.6 to 2 ml water for injections; IV as a solution containing 600 mg in 4 to 10 ml water for injections or at least 10 ml of suitable infusion solution. IV doses should be given at a rate of no more than 300 mg/min

Perform/provide:

• Patch test to assess allergy, when penicillin is only drug of choice or history of allergy to penicillins
• Emergency resuscitation kit in case of anaphylaxis
• Adequate fluid intake (2 litres daily) during diarrhoea episodes
• Aseptic technique during IV/IM injection
• Observe IV injection site for inflammation

Evaluate:

• Therapeutic effectiveness: absence of fever, draining wounds
• Fluid balance, report haematuria, oliguria since penicillin in high doses is nephrotoxic
• Any patient with compromised renal system since drug is excreted slowly in poor renal system function; toxicity may occur rapidly
• Bowel pattern before and during treatment
• Skin eruptions after administration of penicillin to 1 week after discontinuing drug
• Respiratory status: rate, character, wheezing, tightness in chest
• Allergies before initiation of treatment, reaction of each medication; highlight allergies on nursing care plan

Teach patient/family:

• Aspects of drug therapy, including need to complete course of medication to ensure organism death; culture may be taken after completed course
• To report sore throat, fever, fatigue; could indicate superimposed infection
• To wear or carry Medic Alert ID if allergic to penicillins
• To notify nurse of diarrhoea
• To report any rash

---

betahistine hydrochloride

Serc

Func. class.: Vasodilator
Chem. class.: Histamine analogue
Legal class.: POM

Action: Reduces endolymphatic pressure

Uses: Vertigo, tinnitus, hearing loss associated with Meniere's disease

Dosage and routes:

• *Adult:* By mouth initially 16 mg 3 times daily, maintenance 24–48 mg daily in divided doses

Available forms include: Tablets, 8, 16 mg
Side effects/adverse reactions:
GI: Nausea
Contraindications: Phaeochromocytoma
Precautions: Asthma, pregnancy
Pharmacokinetics: Peak 3–5 hr. Excreted in urine (metabolites)
Interactions/incompatibilities: Antihistamines – antagonism (theoretical)
Treatment of overdose: Symptomatic management; gastric lavage may be indicated

NURSING CONSIDERATIONS

Administer:
- With or after food

Perform/provide:
- Storage in original package

Evaluate:
- Benefits of therapy
- Side effects

Teach patient/family:
- About side effects; headache, nausea and rash and need to inform clinician
- Not to remove from pack until just before taking dose (tablets are hygroscopic)

betamethasone dipropionate

Diprosone
Func. class.: Topical corticosteroid
Chem. class.: Synthetic fluorinated agent (potent)
Legal class.: POM

Action: Possesses antipruritic, anti-inflammatory actions
Uses: Psoriasis, eczema, severe dermatitis and inflammatory skin disorders
Dosage and routes:
- *Adult and child:* Apply thinly to affected area once or twice daily

Available forms include: Ointment 0.05%; cream 0.05%; lotion 0.05%
Side effects/adverse reactions:
INTEG: Acne, hypertrichosis, perioral dermatitis, hypopigmentation, atrophy, striae, secondary infection
Contraindications: Hypersensitivity, long-term therapy, rosacea, acne, perioral dermatitis, tuberculous and viral skin infection, untreated fungal or bacterial skin infection, peri-anal and genital pruritus, ulcerative conditions
Precautions: Pregnancy, large areas of broken skin, long-term use especially on face, psoriasis

NURSING CONSIDERATIONS

Administer:
- Only to affected areas; do not get in eyes
- Leave uncovered or use light dressing; do not cover with occlusive dressing
- Only to dermatoses; do not use on weeping, denuded, or infected area
- Apply thinly
- Apply thinly, wearing gloves, only to the affected areas. Do not cover with an occlusive dressing or apply to the skin of the face for more than 7 days unless specifically requested

Perform/provide:
- Cleansing before application of drug
- Treatment for a few days after area has cleared

Evaluate:
- Therapeutic response: absence of severe itching, patches on skin, flaking
- Temperature; if fever develops, drug should be discontinued

Teach patient/family:
- To avoid sunlight on affected area; burns may occur
- That ointment is not curative; rebound exacerbation may occur when discontinued

betamethasone valerate

Betnovate, Betnovate-RD
Func. class.: Topical corticosteroid
Chem. class.: Synthetic fluorinated agent (potent)
Legal class.: POM

Action: Possesses antipruritic, anti-inflammatory actions
Uses: Psoriasis, eczema, contact dermatitis, pruritus and other severe inflammatory skin disorders unresponsive to less potent corticosteroids
Dosage and routes:
• *Adult and child:* Apply thinly to affected area two or three times daily—for child see precautions
Available forms include: Ointment 0.025%, 0.1%; cream 0.025%, 0.1%; lotion 0.1%; scalp application 0.1%
Side effects/adverse reactions:
SYST: Prolonged use, large amounts, extensive area: hypercorticism, Hypothalamic-pituitary-adrenal (HPA) axis suppression
INTEG: Acne, hypertrichosis, perioral dermatitis, spread of untreated infection, thinning, dilatation of superficial blood vessels, striae, depigmentation, vellus hair
Contraindications: Dermatoses in children under 1 yr. Hypersensitivity to skin viral infections, rosacea, acne, perioral dermatitis, peri-anal and genital pruritus, ulcerative conditions, untreated fungal or bacterial skin infections
Precautions: Pregnancy, lactation, psoriasis, secondary infection, children, avoid long-term continuous therapy especially on face, large areas of broken skin
Interactions/incompatibilities:
None known

NURSING CONSIDERATIONS

Administer:
• To affected areas wearing gloves. Do not get in eyes
• Cover treated area with occlusive dressing (only if prescribed), change 12 hrly. Occlusive dressings will increase absorption and systemic side effects
• Apply only to affected area; avoid raw, weeping or infected areas
• Apply thinly, wearing gloves (if applying to patient), only to the affected areas. Do not cover with an occlusive dressing or apply to the skin of the face for more than 7 days unless specifically requested.
Perform/provide:
• Cleansing before application
• Continued treatment for a few days after inflammation has resolved
Evaluate:
• Temperature daily; if fever develops clinician should be informed and treatment should discontinue
• Monitor quantity of preparation used—more than 100 g per week of 0.1% likely to cause adrenal suppression
• In childhood or on face—limit use to 5 days, do not use occlusive dressings
• Monitor adrenal function if prolonged use
• Response to treatment; itching and flaking should subside
Teach patient/family:
• Must avoid exposing treated area to strong sunshine; sunburn may occur
• To use sparingly
• To avoid eyes
• That ointment is not curative; rebound exacerbation may occur when discontinued

betamethasone/ betamethasone sodium phosphate

Betnelan, Betnesol
Func. class.: Synthetic corticosteroid
Chem. class.: Glucocorticoid, long-acting
Legal class.: POM

Action: Decreases inflammation by suppression of migration of polymorphonuclear leucocytes, fibroblasts, reversal of increased capillary permeability and lysosomal stabilisation

Uses: Suppression of inflammatory, auto-immune, and allergic disease, adrenal hyperplasia, cerebral oedema, severe shock, immunosuppression

Dosage and routes:
- *Adult:* By mouth 0.5–5 mg/daily in divided doses; IM or IV infusion 4–20 mg (as sodium phosphate) up to 4 times in 24 hr
- *Child:* less than 1 yr: Slow IV injection 1 mg; 1–5 yr: 2 mg; 6–12 yr: 4 mg

Available forms include: Tablets 500 mcg (as base or sodium phosphate); Injection 4 mg/ml (as sodium phosphate)

Side effects/adverse reactions:
INTEG: Acne, poor wound healing, flushing, bruising, skin thinning
CNS: Depression, mental disturbances, headache, raised intracranial pressure, mood changes
CV: Thromboembolic disorders
MS: Fractures, osteoporosis, weakness, muscle wasting
GI: Gastrointestinal disturbances, peptic ulcer, increased appetite, pancreatitis
EENT: Oral fungal infections, increased intraocular pressure, cataract
ENDO: Hyperglycaemia, adrenal suppression, growth retardation (children)
MISC: Increased susceptibility to infection, moon face (Cushingoid symptoms)

Contraindications: Hypersensitivity (injection contains sodium metabisulphite), untreated systemic infection, live virus vaccine immunisation

Precautions: Psychosis, hypertension, congestive heart failure, surgery or intercurrent illness, elderly, peptic ulcer, pregnancy, diabetes mellitus, glaucoma, osteoporosis, seizure disorders, myasthenia gravis; withdrawal should be gradual

Pharmacokinetics:
Period of onset: Onset 1–2 hr, peak 1 hr, duration 3 days
IM/IV: Onset 10 min, peak 4–8 hr, duration 1–1½ days
Metabolised in liver, excreted in urine as steroids

Interactions/incompatibilities:
- Decreased action of betamethasone: cholestyramine, colestipol, barbiturates, rifampicin, ephedrine, phenytoin, theophylline
- Possibly decreased effects of: anticonvulsants, antidiabetics, antihypertensives, diuretics, non-steroidal anti-inflammatory agents
- Increased effects of anticoagulants

Clinical assessment:
- Assess blood potassium levels and blood sugar levels while on long term treatment
- Prescribe lowest effective dose
- Prescribe in a single dose to be given in the morning to prevent adrenal suppression

NURSING CONSIDERATIONS

Assess:
- Baseline BP, weight and fluid balance

Administer:

• Injections after shaking solution
• IM injections deeply into large muscle, rotate sites, use 19G needle
• Orally with food or milk to decrease GI symptoms

Evaluate:
• Weight daily. Inform clinician if weekly gain greater than 2 kg
• BP 4 hrly and pulse. Inform clinician of chest pain
• Fluid balance chart. Be alert for decreasing urinary output and oedema
• Response to treatment; decreased respiratory embarrassment, decreased inflammation
• Temperature; drug may mask signs of infection even after course has been completed
• Signs of potassium depletion, e.g. paraesthesiae, fatigue, nausea, vomiting, depression, polyuria, dysrhythmias, weakness
• Cardiac symptoms, e.g. oedema, hypotension
• Aggression, behavioural change, change in mood or affect

Teach patient/family:
• To carry identity as a steroid user
• Clinician must be informed if response to drug decreases; dose may need adjustment
• Drug must not be discontinued suddenly or adrenal crisis may result
• Medicines should be avoided unless prescribed, particularly aspirin, cough or cold mixtures containing alcohol
• All aspects of treatment and recognition of Cushingoid symptoms
• To recognise symptoms of adrenal insufficiency, e.g. nausea, anorexia, fatigue, dizziness, dyspnoea, weakness, joint pain

betaxolol (ophthalmic)

Betoptic
Func. class.: Antihypertensive, ocular; antiglaucoma agent
Chem. class.: Cardioselective β-blocker
Legal class.: POM

Action: Reduces intra-ocular pressure, probably by reducing the rate of production of aqueous humour
Uses: Chronic simple glaucoma, ocular hypertension
Dosage and routes:
• *Adult:* Instil one drop into affected eye(s) twice daily
Available forms include: Eyedrops 0.5% (as hydrochloride)
Side effects/adverse reactions:
EENT: Eye irritation, transitory dry eyes, tearing, allergic blepharo-conjunctivitis
Contraindications: Asthma, history of obstructive airways disease, bradycardia, heart block, heart failure
Precautions: Concurrent systemic beta-blocker or adrenergic psychotropic therapy, diabetes, thyrotoxicosis, general anaesthesia, soft contact lenses, pregnancy, lactation, asthma, history of obstructive air-ways disease, systemic absorption may occur
Pharmacokinetics: Systemic absorption may occur; extensively metabolised and excreted in urine; half-life 17 hr
Interactions/incompatibilities: If significant systemic absorption occurs:-
• Greatly enhances hypertensive effects of adrenaline, noradrenaline, amphetamines, phenylephrine, phenylpropanolamine and other sympathomimetic amines
• Increases toxicity of: calcium antagonists, anti-arrhythmic drugs,

rauwolfia alkaloids, mefloquine, cardiac glycosides, sotalol
• Increased risk of vasoconstriction with ergotamine
• Mydriasis when given with adrenaline
• Increased hypotensive effect: alcohol, anaesthetics, antihypertensives, anxiolytics, hypnotics, diuretics
• Increased effect of: antidiabetics
• Increased risk of withdrawal hypertension of clonidine
• Reduced effect of xamoterol and reduced β-blockade
Clinical assessment:
• Check history of cardiac conditions, asthma and chronic obstructive airways disease
Treatment of overdose: Flush from eye(s) with warm tap water
NURSING CONSIDERATIONS
Administer:
• Using correct technique to instil drops
Evaluate:
• Pulse 4 hrly, respirations
• Intra-ocular pressure every 4 weeks at different times of day
Perform/provide:
• Care for dryness of eyes
• Safe environment if visually handicapped
Evaluate:
• Side effects especially those affecting the eye
Teach patient/family:
• Correct method of instilling eye drops and care of equipment
• To report: eye irritation, visual changes, breathing problems, sweating, flushing, rashes
• Blurred vision will decrease with continued use. Withdraw slowly
• To discard after 4 weeks of opening eye-drops

betaxolol hydrochloride

Kerlone
Func. class.: Antihypertensive
Chem. class.: β-blocker
Legal class.: POM

Action: Preferentially blocks cardiac β-adrenergic receptors, reducing response to sympathetic stimulation
Uses: Hypertension
Dosage and routes:
• *Adult:* By mouth, 20 mg daily increased to 40 mg daily if required; elderly: initial dose 10 mg
Available forms include: Tablets, 20 mg
Side effects/adverse reactions:
RESP: Bronchospasm
CV: Bradycardia, heart failure, peripheral vasoconstriction, exacerbation of Raynaud's disease or intermittent claudication, paraesthesiae, hypotension, atrioventricular block, cardiac insufficiency
EENT: Dry eyes
GI: Disturbances
SYST: Fatigue
Contraindications: Uncontrolled heart failure, second or third degree heart block, cardiogenic shock, bradycardia (less than 50 beats/min); history of asthma or obstructive airways disease, metabolic acidosis
Precautions: Pregnancy, breast feeding; avoid abrupt withdrawal in angina; reduced dose in renal impairment; history of cardiovascular disease; diabetes mellitus; inform anaesthetist before general anaesthesia
Pharmacokinetics: Peak plasma concentration within 4–6 hr. Half-life 16–20 hr, excreted in urine as unchanged drug and metabolites
Interactions/incompatibilities:
Toxicity enhanced by myocardial

depressants or drugs which depress atrioventricular conduction such as verapamil and related calcium channel blockers

Treatment of overdose: Atropine for bradycardia; supportive care

NURSING CONSIDERATIONS

Assess:

- Baseline BP (lying and standing) and pulse, respirations
- For history of chronic obstructive airways disease/asthma

Administer:

- Orally with full glass of water

Perform/provide:

- BP (lying and standing), pulse for bradycardia

Evaluate:

- Therapeutic response: reduction in blood pressure to required level
- Side effects, e.g. headache, weight gain, bradycardia

Teach patient/family:

- Not to stop drug unless advised by clinician
- To change position slowly to avoid dizziness
- About possible sleep disturbances/nightmares, GI upsets and cold extremities

---

bezafibrate

Bezalip, Bezalip-Mono

Func. class.: Hypolipidaemic agent
Chem. class.: Clofibrate analogue
Legal class.: POM

Action: Decreases serum triglycerides, reduces LDL-cholesterol, raises HDL-cholesterol

Uses: Severe hyperlipidaemia or hypertriglyceridaemia resistant to modification of diet

Dosage and routes:

- By mouth, 200 mg 3 times daily; may be reduced to twice daily in hypertriglyceridaemia; modified-release tablets, 400 mg daily in evening

Available forms include: Tablets, 200 mg; modified-release tablets 400 mg

Side effects/adverse reactions:

GI: Nausea, abdominal discomfort
GU: Impotence (rare)
INTEG: Pruritus, urticaria
SYST: Hypersensitivity
MS: Myositis

Contraindications: Severe renal or hepatic impairment, primary biliary cirrhosis, hypoalbuminaemia, gallbladder disease, nephrotic syndrome, pregnancy, breast-feeding, hypersensitivity

Precautions: Anticoagulant therapy, moderate renal impairment

Pharmacokinetics: Peak plasma concentrations 2 hr, progressive hypolipidaemic response over several weeks. Half-life 2 hr, excreted in urine

Interactions/incompatibilities:

- May increase effects of: anticoagulant, antidiabetic agents

NURSING CONSIDERATIONS

Administer:

- In the evening with food, swallowed whole and not chewed if modified release

Perform/provide:

- Smaller meals if 'fullness' a problem

Evaluate:

- Side-effects including pruritus

Teach patient/family:

- To continue with other measures—maintain ideal weight, low fat diet, no smoking, stress management and reduce alcohol intake. Encourage compliance
- To avoid pregnancy

biphasic insulin

Rapitard MC
Func. class.: Antidiabetic
Chem. class.: Insulin (intermediate acting)
Legal class.: P

Action: Decreases blood sugar
Uses: Diabetes mellitus
Dosage and routes:
• *Adult and child:* Subcutaneous individualised dose; do not give IV
Available forms include: Subcutaneous injection 100 U/ml
Side effects/adverse reactions:
EENT: Blurred vision
INTEG: Erythema, induration, urticaria, rash, oedema and lipodystrophy at injection site
META: Hypoglycaemia
SYST: Anaphylaxis
Contraindications: Hypersensitivity, hypoglycaemia
Pharmacokinetics: Onset 30 min; peak 4–12 hr; duration up to 22 hr
Interactions:
• Increased hypoglycaemia: alcohol, β-blockers, oral hypoglycaemic MAOI's, octreotide
• Hyperglycaemia: thiazides, thyroid hormones, oral contraceptives, corticosteroids, lithium, diazoxide, loop diuretics, nifedipine
• Mask signs/symptoms of hypoglycaemia: β-blockers
Incompatibilities: Phosphate-containing insulins
Treatment of overdose: Glucose by mouth if conscious or glucose 50% IV if comatose; glucagon 1 mg IM, subcutaneous, IV if glucose not available
NURSING CONSIDERATIONS
Administer:
• By subcutaneous injection (avoiding vascular injection), not more than 30 min before meals
• Shake vial before withdrawing dose
Perform/provide:
• Storage: long term; refrigerated at 2–8°C, protected from light. Vials in use at constant temperature (room or refrigerator) for up to one month, protected from excessive heat
Evaluate:
• Therapeutic effect; satisfactory control of diabetes
• For side effects
Teach patient/family:
• How to give subcutaneous injection, including rotating injection sites
• Not to use discoloured suspensions
• To test urine regularly
• To store properly at constant temperature (refrigerator or room)
• To report any side effects promptly to nurse or clinician

bisacodyl

NHS Dulcolax
Func. class.: Laxative, stimulant
Chem. class.: Diphenylmethane
Legal class.: P

Action: Acts directly on intestine by increasing motor activity
Uses: Short-term treatment of constipation, bowel or rectal preparation for surgery, examination
Dosage and routes:
Constipation
• *Adult:* By mouth, 5–10 mg at night, increased if necessary to 15–20 mg; rectal 10 mg in the morning
• *Child:* By mouth, 5 mg at night; rectal 5 mg in the morning
Bowel preparation
• *Adult:* By mouth 10 mg at night for 2 days before procedure, plus 10 mg by rectum 1 hr before procedure if necessary
Available forms include: Enteric

coated tablets 5 mg; suppository 5 mg, 10 mg
Side effects/adverse reactions:
GI: Cramps, diarrhoea, rectal burning (suppositories)
META: Hypokalaemia, electrolyte and fluid imbalances (prolonged or excessive use)
Contraindications: Hypersensitivity; intestinal obstruction
Precautions: Children, inflammatory bowel disease, rectal fissures, ulcerated haemorrhoids
Pharmacokinetics:
Tablets taken after food act in 10–12 hr
Suppositories produce a motion within 20–60 min of insertion
Partially absorbed, metabolised by liver, excreted in urine, bile, faeces, breast milk

NURSING CONSIDERATIONS

Assess:
- Normal bowel function/pattern

Administer:
- Swallow whole, do not chew
- Alone to enhance absorption; should not be taken within an hour of other drugs, antacids, cimetidine or milk

Evaluate:
- Response; bowel action should result

Perform/provide:
- Inform clinician if cramping, rectal bleeding, nausea or vomiting occur; drug should be discontinued

Teach patient/family:
- Tablets should be swallowed whole; they should not be chewed
- Bowel movements do not always occur daily
- Laxatives should not be used long term; bowel tone will be lost
- Tablets should not be taken if there is abdominal pain, nausea, vomiting
- To tell clinician if constipation is not relieved or if symptoms of electrolyte imbalance occur: muscle cramps, pain, weakness, dizziness
- Of dietary changes to avoid constipation

---

bismuth chelate

De-Nol, De-Noltab
Func. class.: Anti-ulcer agent
Chem. class.: Metal chelate
Legal class.: P

Action: Has several relevant pharmacological actions including a direct toxic effect on gastric *Helicobacter (Campylobacter) pylori* and stimulation of gastric mucosal prostaglandin production and bicarbonate secretion
Uses: Treatment of benign gastric and duodenal ulcers
Dosage and routes:
- *Adult:* By mouth, 240 mg twice a day (30 min before breakfast and 30 min before the evening meal), or 120 mg four times a day (30 min before each main meal of the day and 2 hr after the evening meal)

Available forms include: Tablets, 120 mg (calculated as Bi_2O_3); oral solution; 120 mg (calculated as Bi_2O_3)/5 ml
Side effects/adverse reactions:
EENT: Darkening of the tongue
GI: Blackening of the stool; nausea; vomiting
Contraindications: Severe renal impairment; pregnancy
Precautions: Renal disease
Pharmacokinetics: Little systemic absorption
Interactions:
- Reduced absorption of: oral tetracyclines
- Reduced effect of bismuth chelate: taken within half an hour of antacids; large quantities of milk

Treatment of overdose: Little experience of overdose, contact manufacturer

NURSING CONSIDERATIONS

Assess:

• Pain from ulcer, particularly that related to food

Administer:

• Antacid 30 mins before or after bismuth chelate

• By mouth, on an empty stomach (30 min before or 2 hr after a meal); with a full glass of water

Evaluate:

• Therapeutic effect: reduction of gastric pain

• Side effects

Teach patient/family:

• About the drug; timing of dose relative to food and necessity for taking on an empty stomach

• That antacids and large quantities of milk should not be taken (reduces effectiveness)

• About the side effects, including blackening of stools and possible blackening of tongue (both to be considered normal whilst taking bismuth chelate)

---

bisoprolol fumarate

Emcor, Monocor

Func. class.: Antihypertensive, anti-anginal

Chem. class.: Cardioselective β-blocker

Legal class.: POM

Action: Preferentially blocks β-adrenoceptors in the heart, reducing response to sympathetic stimulation. Some action on peripheral vasculature

Uses: Hypertension, angina

Dosage and routes:

• *Adult:* By mouth, 10 mg daily (5 mg daily adequate in some patients); maximum 20 mg daily

Available forms include: Tablets, 5 mg, 10 mg

Side effects/adverse reactions:

RESP: Bronchospasm

CNS: Headache, dizziness, paraesthesia, sleep disturbances

CV: Bradycardia, exacerbation of Raynaud's disease or intermittent claudication, hypotension, atrioventricular block, cardiac insufficiency

EENT: Dry eyes

INTEG: Rashes, sweating

GI: Disturbances

SYST: Lassitude

Contraindications: Bronchospasm, asthma, history of obstructive airways disease, metabolic acidosis, sinus bradycardia, partial heart block, uncontrolled congestive heart failure

Precautions: Pregnancy, breast feeding, prolonged PR conduction interval, poor cardiac reserve, peripheral circulatory disease, diabetes mellitus, obstructive airways disease; avoid abrupt withdrawal in angina; reduce dose in renal or hepatic impairment; inform anaesthetist before general anaesthesia

Pharmacokinetics: Half-life 10–12 hr, metabolised in liver and excreted in urine as inactive metabolites and unchanged drug

Interactions/incompatibilities:

• Increased effects of bisoprolol: anaesthetics, other antihypertensives, diuretics, cimetidine

• Possibly increased toxicity: anti-arrhythmics, calcium channel blockers, cardiac glycosides, sympathomimetics (hypertension), ergotamine

• Increased effects of: antidiabetic agents

• Decreased effects of bisoprolol: NSAIDs, corticosteroids, oestrogens, oral contraceptives, rifampicin

Treatment of overdose: Supportive symptomatic care

NURSING CONSIDERATIONS

Assess:

• Baseline BP (lying and standing) and pulse

• Respirations

Administer:

• With a full glass of water
Perform/provide:
• BP (lying and standing), pulse (for bradycardia) 4-hrly
Evaluate:
• Weight gain, GI upsets and other side effects
• Therapeutic response: reduction in BP to required level
• Reduction in chest pain
Teach patient/family:
• Do not stop unless advised by clinician
• Sleep disturbances and nightmares may occur
• To report any side effects e.g. cold extremities

bleomycin sulphate

Func. class.: Antineoplastic
Chem. class.: Glycopeptide antibiotic
Legal class.: POM

Action: Inhibits synthesis of DNA, RNA, protein; replication is decreased by binding to DNA, which causes strand splitting; drug is phase specific in the G_2 and M phases
Uses: Squamous cell carcinoma, Hodgkin's disease and other lymphomas, malignant effusion of serous cavities, testicular teratoma, malignant melanoma
Dosage and routes: Doses are highly variable, and dependent on local treatment protocols, concomitant therapy and tumour type; the following dose schedules have been used:
• *Adult:* IM/IV 15–60 units weekly, total dose usually no greater than 500 units; IV infusion 15 units daily for 10 days or 30 units daily for 5 days; intracavity, for malignant effusions, 60 units/100 ml sodium chloride 0.9%
• *Elderly:* IM/IV 15–30 units weekly, total dose usually no greater than 100–300 units
Available forms include: Injection 15 units
Side effects/adverse reactions:
SYST: Anaphylaxis, fever
GI: Nausea, anorexia, stomatitis
INTEG: Rash, hyperkeratosis, nail changes, alopecia, hyperpigmentation
RESP: Fibrosis (potentially fatal), pneumonitis, wheezing
CV: Hypotension, thrombophlebitis
Contraindications: Hypersensitivity, pregnancy, breast-feeding, reduced lung function, pulmonary infection
Precautions: Renal impairment, respiratory disease, lymphoma (increased risk of anaphylaxis)
Pharmacokinetics: Half-life 2 hr when creatinine clearance is 35 ml/min; for lower clearance, half-life is increased. Metabolised in tissues (except lung, skin), 50% excreted in urine (unchanged)
Interactions/incompatibilities:
• Increased toxicity: other antineoplastics or radiation therapy
• Risk of respiratory failure if general anaesthetic given with high inspired oxygen concentrations; particularly if cummulative dose of bleomycin is more than 100 units
Clinical assessment:
• Obtain chest X-ray before treatment commences and weekly throughout treatment and for one month after

NURSING CONSIDERATIONS

Assess:
• Baseline temperature
Administer:
• HANDLING: take safety precautions appropriate to antineoplastic agents
• Following local antineoplastic (cytotoxic) policies
• After ensuring that clinician is aware of blood results

• IV, IM, intra-arterially, or intralesionally as prescribed
• By intracavity injection following drainage of effusion fluid
• Other medications, by mouth if possible. Avoid IV, IM, SC routes to prevent infection and bruising
• Anti-emetic 30–60 min before treatment
• All other medication as prescribed, including analgesics, antibiotics, anti-emetics, antispasmodics

Perform/provide:
• Encouragement for deep breathing exercises taught by physiotherapist
• Mouthwashes 3–4 times daily and gentle mouth care; a soft tooth brust and unwaxed dental floss should be used
• Support in bed to facilitate breathing

Evaluate:
• Dyspnoea, unproductive cough, chest pain, tachypnoea, fatigue, tachycardia, pallor, lethargy
• Food preferances
• Effects of alopecia on body image; discuss feelings about body changes
• Oral mucosa 8 hrly for dryness, sores, ulceration, white patches, bleeding, dysphagia
• Injection site for local irritation, pain, burning, discolouration
• Severe allergic reaction e.g. rash, pruritus, urticaria, purpuric skin lesions, itching, hot flushes can occur 3–5 hr post administration

Teach patient/family:
• Any side effects must be reported to clinician or nurse
• Any respiratory changes or coughing must be reported
• That hair may be lost during treatment but a wig or hair piece may be worn (available free on NHS). New hair may be different in colour or texture
• That mouth should be examined once a day; bleeding, white spots, ulcers should be reported
• That short-term pain can be experienced

botulism antitoxin

Func. class.: Trivalent antitoxin
Chem. class.: Antitoxin globulins
Legal class.: POM

Action: Neutralises toxins A, B and E produced by the bacterium *Clostridium botulinum* types A, B, and E

Uses: Post-exposure prophylaxis and treatment of botulism

Dosage and routes:
• *Prophylaxis:* IM injection 20 ml as soon as possible after exposure
• *Treatment:* Slow IV infusion, 20 ml diluted to 100 ml with 0.9% sodium chloride, then 10 ml 2–4 hr later if necessary; further doses at intervals of 12–24 hr

Available forms include: Available from designated holding centres

Side effects/adverse reactions:
SYST: Hypersensitivity

Precautions: Asthma, allergic rhinitis, other allergic conditions; ineffective in infantile botulism

Clinical assessment: Previous history of antitoxin administration or allergic conditions should be checked before administration; prior sensitivity test should be carried out (using diluted antitoxin if history of allergy)

NURSING CONSIDERATIONS

Administer:
• IM or slow IV infusion as directed by clinician

Teach patient/family:
• That there may be mild discomfort at the injection site

bretylium tosylate

Bretylate, Min-I-Jet Bretylium Tosylate
Func. class.: Anti-arrhythmic (class II/III)
Chem. class.: Quaternary ammonium compound
Legal class.: POM

Action: Inhibits release of noradrenaline in postganglionic nerve endings; prolongs duration of cardiac action potential
Uses: Ventricular arrhythmias resistant to other treatment
Dosage and routes:
• *Adult:* IM 5 mg/kg repeated after 6–8 hr if required then 5–10 mg/kg every 6–8 hr; slow IV injection 5–10 mg/kg over 8–10 min, repeated after 1–2 hr if required to maximum dose 30 mg/kg; maintenance 1–2 mg/min by IV infusion or IM dose as above
• *Adult:* Life-threatening situations in association with other resuscitation measures, rapid IV injection, initially 5 mg/kg; repeat or increase dose to 10 mg/kg after 5 min if no response; maximum 30 mg/kg
Available forms include: Injection 50 mg/ml
Side effects/adverse reactions:
GI: Nausea, vomiting
CV: Hypotension, transient hypertension, tachycardia, ectopic beats, bradycardia
MS: Tissue necrosis at injection site (restrict volume at any site to 5 ml)
Contraindications: Hypersensitivity, phaeochromocytoma
Precautions: Renal disease, pulmonary hypertension, severe aortic stenosis
Pharmacokinetics:
IV: Onset 5 min
IM: Onset ½–2 hr, peak 6–9 hr, duration 24 hr
Half-life 4–17 hr, excreted unchanged by kidneys (70%–80% in 24 hr), not metabolised
Interactions/incompatibilities:
• Increased effects of bretylium: other antiarrhythmics
• Increased effects of: sympathomimetics
• Toxicity: digitalis
Clinical assessment:
• Patient requires cardiac monitoring
Treatment of overdose: Supportive symptomatic care; extreme caution if catecholamines considered necessary for hypotension (effects may be enhanced, use only under expert supervision)

NURSING CONSIDERATIONS

Assess:
• Baseline vital signs and ECG
Administer:
• By slow injection 8–10 min or infusion as prescribed
• To patient on strict bed rest, under close supervision
Perform/provide:
• Resuscitation equipment in case of further cardiac arrhythmias
• In cardiac arrest, must continue resuscitation for further 20 min to ensure action
• Continuous ECG monitoring in high dependency area
Evaluate:
• For rebound hypertension after 1 hr
• Frequency of ventricular arrhythmia
• Response to treatment and continuation of arrhythmias
• BP and vital signs—correct hypovolaemia, hypotension or hypertension
• Electrolyte balance: as exacerbation of arrhythmias
• For side effects

bromocriptine mesylate

Parlodel

Func. class.: Dopamine agonist

Chem. class.: Ergot alkaloid derivative

Legal class.: POM

Action: Inhibits prolactin release by activating postsynaptic dopamine receptors; activation of dopamine receptors could be reason for improvement in Parkinson's disease

Uses: Female infertility, Parkinson's disease, suppression of post-partum lactation, galactorrhoea or hypogonadism caused by hyperprolactinaemia, cyclic mastalgia and menstrual disorders, acromegaly, prolactinoma

Dosage and routes:

Parkinson's disease

• By mouth: initially 1–1.25 mg at night for 1 week, then 2–2.5 mg at night for 1 week, increasing by 2.5 mg weekly increments as required to an optimum dosage range 10–40 mg daily in divided doses

Suppression of lactation

• By mouth: 2.5 mg daily for 2–3 days then 2.5 mg twice daily for 14 days

Galactorrhoea, infertility, hypogonadism

• By mouth: 1–1.25 mg at night increased by 1–2.5 mg at 2–3 day intervals to 7.5 mg daily in divided doses, maximum 30 mg daily

Cyclic benign breast disease, menstrual disorder

• By mouth: 1–1.25 mg at night, increased gradually to 2.5 mg twice daily

Acromegaly, prolactinoma

• By mouth: 1–1.25 mg at night increased by 2.5 mg daily at 2–3 day intervals up to maximum 30 mg daily

Available forms include: Capsules 5, 10 mg; tablets 1, 2.5 mg

Side effects/adverse reactions:

EENT: Blurred vision, diplopia, dry mouth, nasal congestion

CNS: Headache, dizziness, drowsiness, excitation, confusion, psychotic reactions, hallucinations, dyskinesias

GU: Incontinence

GI: Nausea, vomiting, constipation, dry mouth, GI haemorrhage, retroperitoneal fibrosis

RESP: Pleural effusions

CV: Orthostatic hypotension, cold-induced digital vasospasm, arrhythmias

Contraindications: Hypersensitivity to ergot, porphyria, toxaemia of pregnancy, post-partum hypertension

Precautions: Pregnancy, lactation, hepatic disease, cardiovascular disease, history of psychosis

Pharmacokinetics:

Period of onset: Peak 1–3 hr, duration 4–8 hr, 90%–96% protein bound, half-life 3–8 hr, metabolised by liver (inactive metabolites), excreted in urine, faeces

Interactions/incompatibilities:

• Decreased action of bromocriptine: phenothiazines, haloperidol, droperidol, domperidone, metoclopramide, oral contraceptives

• Possibly increased action of bromocriptine: erythromycin

• Increased toxicity: Alcohol

Clinical assessment:

• Monitor for pituitary enlargement, especially during pregnancy

• Gynaecological assessment including cervical/endometrial cytology every 6 months in post-menopausal and every 12 months in premenopausal women if on long-term therapy

• Assess acromegalic patients for peptic ulceration before therapy

• Observe patients on long-term high dose therapy for signs of retroperitoneal fibrosis or pleural effusion

NURSING CONSIDERATIONS

Assess:

- BP before, during and after treatment

Administer:

- Orally following the dosage regimen for suitable gradual introduction
- With food to prevent nausea and vomiting. Not suitable under 15 yr

Evaluate:

- Therapeutic responses:
  1) Parkinson's disease: decreased dyskinesia, slow movement, excessive salivation
  2) Female infertility: pregnancy
  3) Suppression of lactation
  4) Menstrual disorders
- Optimal response with minimum side effects

Teach patient/family:

- To stand-up slowly to prevent postural hypotension
- To use other forms of contraception if oral contraceptives have been used or if female of child-bearing age
- That gynaecological assessment is necessary including cervical and endometrial cytology; 6-monthly for post-menopausal, annually for regular menstruation
- That therapeutic response may not be immediate, up to 2 months galactorrhoea, amenorrhoea
- That alcohol should not be taken
- Not to driving or operate machinery if dizziness occurs

budesonide (inhaled)

Pulmicort, Pulmicort Respules
Func. class.: Synthetic Corticosteroid
Chem. class.: Non-halogenated synthetic corticosteroid
Legal class.: POM

Action: Reduces inflammation in bronchial mucosae, leading to reduction in oedema and mucus secretion. At normal therapeutic doses the inhaled preparation lacks systemic side effects

Uses: Chronic airways obstruction, especially in asthma not controlled by bronchodilators and/or anti-allergic agents

Dosage and routes:

Asthma

- *Adults:* Inhalation (metered dose) 200 mcg twice daily, increased if necessary to maximum 1600 mcg daily. Reduce for maintenance but should not go below 200 mcg daily
- By nebulisation inhalation 1–2 mg twice daily (maybe increased further in severe cases), reduced to 0.5–1 mg twice daily for maintenance
- *Children:* Inhalation (metered dose) 50–200 mcg twice daily, increased to 400 mcg twice daily if necessary; nebuliser inhalation 0.5–1 mg twice daily, reduced to 0.25–0.5 mg twice daily for maintenance

Available forms include: Aerosol inhaler 50 mcg, 200 mcg/inhalation with spacer; Turbohaler 100 mcg, 200 mcg, 400 mcg/inhalation Respules 250 mcg, 500 mcg/ml

Side effects/adverse reactions:

EENT: Candidiasis of mouth or throat, coughing, irritation, hoarseness, irritation of skin around mouth following nebulisation

META: Slight adrenal suppression (high dose)
Contraindications: Hypersensitivity
Precautions: Respiratory tract infection (especially tuberculosis), pregnancy, breast-feeding, steroid dependence
Pharmacokinetics: Therapeutic effect usually within 10 days

NURSING CONSIDERATIONS

Assess:
• Peak flow, respiration, wheezing before administration and 4 hrly after administration

Administer:
• Regularly
• With correct technique and equipment (space nebuliser, etc.)
• Shake gently before use
• When inhaled, bronchodilators are coprescribed; use these first
• Rinse mouth after use to minimise the risk of candidiasis
• Aerosol inhaler may be given via nebuhaler
• Wash face after use of nebuliser
• Respules solution can be diluted with sodium chloride 0.9%

Perform/provide:
• Mouth care, provide fluids and mouth washes for dry mouth
• Inspect mouth and throat for candidiasis, oedema, inflammation
• Use respules within 3 months once packaging opened and within 12 hr of opening respule
• Protect respule from light

Evaluate:
• Breathing: less wheezing and dyspnoea

Teach patient/family:
• Always to carry a steroid card for high dose.
• That improvement takes 3–7 days
• Not to stop unless advised by clinician and to maintain regular use
• To see clinician if condition worsens
• Proper administration techniques
• Care of equipment
• About side effects which include adrenal suppression
• That drug is not effective during an asthma attack
• Wash face after using nebuliser

---

budesonide (nasal)

Rhinocort, Rhinocort Aqua
Func. class.: Synthetic corticosteroid
Chem. class.: Non-halogenated synthetic corticosteroid
Legal class.: POM

Action: Reduces inflammation in bronchial or nasal mucosae, leading to reduction in oedema and mucus secretion. At normal therapeutic doses the inhaled preparation lacks systemic side effects
Uses: Seasonal and perennial allergic and vasomotor rhinitis
Dosage and routes:
Rhinitis
• *Adults and children over 12 yr:* (children over 6 yr for rhinocest 50 mcg). Nasal spray 100 mcg into each nostril twice daily or 200 mcg per nostril once daily, reduced to half these doses for maintenance
Available forms include: Nasal spray 50 mcg and 100 mcg/dose
Side effects/adverse reactions:
EENT: Irritation and dryness of nose and throat, sneezing and slight haemorrhage after intranasal administration
Contraindications: Hypersensitivity, children under 6 yr
Precautions: Respiratory tract infection (especially tuberculosis), nasal infection, pregnancy, breast-feeding, steroid dependence
Pharmacokinetics: Therapeutic effect usually within 10 days

NURSING CONSIDERATIONS

Assess:

• Inspect nasal mucosa for candidiasis, oedema, inflammation

Administer:

• Regularly
• Shake gently before use
• Start treatment before exposure to allergens if possible
• After cleaning/blowing nose
• With correct technique as directed

Perform/provide:

• Mouth care, provide fluids and mouth washes for dry mouth

Evaluate:

• Nasal symptoms

Teach patient/family:

• That improvement takes 3–7 days
• Not to stop unless advised by clinician and to maintain regular use
• To see clinician if condition worsens
• Proper administration techniques
• About side effects
• If sneezing occurs upon administration, to repeat dose

bumetanide

Burinex, combination products
Func. class.: Loop diuretic
Chem. class.: Sulphonamide derivative
Legal class.: POM

Action: Acts on ascending loop of Henle by increasing excretion of chloride, sodium

Uses: Oedema, oliguria such as that associated with renal failure

Dosage and routes:

• *Adult:* By mouth 1 mg in the morning repeated if required after 6–8 hr, refractory cases may need up to 5 mg or more daily; IV injection 1–2 mg repeated if necessary after 20 min; IV infusion 2–5 mg in 500 ml fluid over 30–60 min; IM 1 mg initially adjusted according to response
• *Elderly:* 0.5 mg daily may be sufficient

Available forms include: Tablets 1, 5 mg; injection 0.5 mg/ml; oral liquid 1 mg/5 ml

Side effects/adverse reactions:

GU: Gynaecomastia
META: Hypokalaemia, hypochloraemic alkalosis, hyponatraemia, hyperuricaemia, hypocalcaemia
CNS: Headache, fatigue, dizziness
GI: Nausea, diarrhoea, vomiting, cramps, upset stomach, abdominal pain, acute pancreatitis, altered liver enzyme values
EENT: Loss of hearing, tinnitus
INTEG: Rash, pruritus, Stevens-Johnson syndrome
MS: Cramps, arthralgia, myalgia
ENDO: Hyperglycaemia
HAEM: Thrombocytopaenia, granulocytopenia
CV: Hypotension, circulatory collapse

Contraindications: Hypersensitivity to sulphonamides, anuria or oliguria developing during treatment, hepatic coma

Precautions: Severe electrolyte depletion, severe renal disease, pregnancy, lactation, elderly, diabetes mellitus, gout, low-salt diets

Pharmacokinetics:

Period of onset: Onset ½–1 hr, duration 4 hr
IM: Onset 40 min, duration 4 hr
IV: Onset 5 min, duration 2–3 hr
Excreted by kidneys, liver

Interactions/incompatibilities:

• Increased toxicity: lithium, antiarrhythmics, aminoglycosides, carbenoxolone, cardiac glycosides, cephalosporins, corticosteroids, other diuretics, NSAIDs, tricyclic antidepressants, vancomycin

• Increased effects of: antihypertensives
• Decreased effects of: antidiabetics
• Decreased diuretic effect: corticosteroids, oestrogens, oral contraceptives, NSAIDs

Clinical assessment:
• Regular checks of serum electrolytes and electrolyte replacement where indicated

Treatment of overdose: Supportive symptomatic care

NURSING CONSIDERATIONS

Assess:
• Baseline BP, weight, fluid balance

Administer:
• In the morning to avoid nocturia
• With food if nausea occurs: absorption may decrease slightly

Evaluate:
• Response to drug; oedema in feet, legs, sacral area if drug is used for congestive cardiac failure
• Daily weight
• Fluid balance chart; effectiveness of drug may decrease if used every day
• Rate, depth, rhythm of respiration and effect of exertion
• BP lying and standing; postural hypotension may occur
• Urine for glucose if patient is diabetic
• Improvement in CVP and BP recordings
• For signs of myalgia, rashes, purpura, gynaecomastia joint pains (early gout)
• For signs of metabolic acidosis e.g. drowsiness, restlessness
• For signs of hypokalaemia e.g. postural hypotension, fatigue, tachycardia, leg cramps, weakness
• Elderly people are particularly likely to become confused: observe carefully

Teach patient/family:
• That fluid intake should be increased to 2–3 litres daily unless contraindicated.
• To rise slowly from sitting or lying position
• To inform prescribing clinician if taking any other medication
• Possible adverse reactions e.g. muscle cramps, weakness, nausea, dizziness
• That gastric symptoms may be counteracted by taking tablets with food or milk
• To take tablets early in day to prevent nocturia
• Blood sugar may rise in diabetes

---

bupivacaine HCl

Marcain
Func. class.: Local anaesthetic
Chem. class.: Amide
Legal class.: POM

Action: Competes with calcium for sites in nerve membrane that control sodium transport across cell membrane; decreases rise of depolarisation phase of action potential

Uses: Epidural anaesthesia, peripheral nerve block

Dosage and routes:
• As a 0.25–0.75% solution. Dose depends on route and nature of anaesthesia

Available forms include: Injection 0.25%, 0.5%, 0.75%; injection 0.25%, 0.5% with adrenaline 1 in 200,000; injection 5 mg/4 ml with glucose 80 mg/ml
• Test dose in epidural anaesthesia

Side effects/adverse reactions:
CNS: Lightheadedness, dizziness, convulsions, loss of consciousness, drowsiness
CV: Myocardial depression, cardiac arrest, arrhythmias, bradycardia, hypotension
GI: Nausea, vomiting

EENT: Numbness of tongue (warning sign of systemic toxicity)
INTEG: Rash, urticaria, allergic reactions
RESP: Respiratory arrest, anaphylaxis
Contraindications: Hypersensitivity, IV regional anaesthesia (Bier's block), hypovolaemia, complete heart block; porphyria; epidural use contraindicated in CNS disease, coagulation disorders, shock, pyogenic skin infection; solutions with adrenaline contraindicated for appendages and in thyrotoxicosis, severe heart disease, 0.75% solution for epidural use in obstetrics
Precautions: Elderly, debilitated, pregnancy, cardiovascular disease, epilepsy, respiratory impairment, hepatic disease
Pharmacokinetics:
Onset 4–17 min, duration 4–8 hr, excreted in urine (metabolites), metabolised by liver
Treatment of overdose: Supportive, symptomatic care; prolonged resuscitation may be needed in cardiac arrest

NURSING CONSIDERATIONS

Assess:
- If used as epidural infusion assess patient position; extent of anaesthesia and unilateral/bilateral effect depending on level of epidural cannula
- Baseline BP

Perform/provide:
- Nursing supervision to detect and provide assistance for daily living activities
- Hospital policy will indicate who may/may not refill epidurals/ epidural infusions
- Emergency equipment
- Discard any solution not used

Evaluate:
- BP, pulse, respiration throughout treatment, possibility of hypotension, tachycardia, respiratory depression and neurological disturbance
- Degree of anaesthesia throughout procedure
- For allergic reaction, e.g. rash, urticaria, itching

---

buprenorphine HCl

Temgesic
Func. class.: Opioid analgesic
Chem. class.: Thebaine derivative
Legal class.: POM (Sch 3) CD

Action: Inhibits ascending pain pathways in limbic system, thalamus, midbrain, hypothalamus
Uses: Moderate to severe pain
Dosage and routes:
- *Adult:* Sublingual 200–400 mcg every 6–8 hr as necessary; IM/ slow IV injection 300–600 mcg every 6–8 hr
- *Child:* Sublingual, 16–25 kg bodyweight: 100 mcg, 25–37.5 kg, 100–200 mcg, 37.5–50 kg, 200–300 mcg; IM/slow IV injection 3–6 mcg/kg every 6–8 hr, maximum 9 mcg/kg

Available forms include: Sublingual tablets 200, 400 mcg; injection 300 mcg/ml
Side effects/adverse reactions:
CNS: Drowsiness, dizziness, confusion, lightheadedness, headache, euphoria, depression, dependence, hallucinations
GI: Nausea, vomiting, cramps
RESP: Respiratory depression
INTEG: Sweating
Contraindications: Hypersensitivity, raised intracranial pressure, head injury
Precautions: History of drug abuse, opioid dependence (may provoke withdrawal due to partial antagonist action), respiratory depression, hepatic impairment, pregnancy, labour

Pharmacokinetics:
IM: Onset 10–30 min, peak ½ hr, duration 3–4 hr
IV: Onset 1 min, peak 5 min
Metabolised in liver, excreted in faeces, urine; half-life 2½–3½ hr
Interactions:
• Increased effect/toxicity: alcohol, other opioids, sedatives/hypnotics, antipsychotic agents, MAOIs, other CNS depressants
• Decreased effects of: cisapride, domperidone, metoclopramide
Treatment of overdose: Supportive symptomatic care; naloxone (other opioid antagonists) may not be completely effective in reversing symptoms
NURSING CONSIDERATIONS:
Assess:
• Respiratory function as potential respiratory depressant
• Pain control and appropriateness of analgesic
• Need for anti-emetic
Administer:
• Sublingually or by IM/IV route as prescribed
Perform/provide:
• Safe environment (potent analgesic). Patient to refrain from mobilising until drug has taken effect in case of dizziness
Evaluate:
• Effectiveness of pain control
• For CNS and respiratory depression: support and inform clinician
Teach patient/family:
• That tablets should not be swallowed or chewed
• Not to exceed recommended frequency of administration
• To report dizziness, drowsiness, etc., to medical staff

---

buserelin

Suprefact, Suprecur
Func. class.: Hormone antagonist
Chem. class.: Gonadotrophin-releasing hormone analogue
Legal class.: POM

Action: Causes initial stimulation of LH release by the pituitary gland followed by a decrease in LH secretion and reduced production of testosterone
Uses: Metastatic prostate cancer
Dosage and routes:
Prostate cancer
• *Adult:* SC 500 mcg 8-hrly for 7 days; then by nasal spray, 100 mcg into each nostril 6 times daily
Endometriosis
• *Adult:* Nasal spray 150 mcg into each nostril 3 times a day
Available forms include: Injection 1 mg/ml (as acetate); nasal spray 100 mcg, 150 mcg/metered spray (as acetate)
Side effects/adverse reactions:
CV: Hot flushes, thrombosis, pulmonary embolism
CNS: Headache, loss of libido, transient increase in pain, mental depression
EENT: Transient nasal irritation and nosebleed (nasal spray)
GU: Impotence, gynaecomastia
SYST: Disease flare, anaphylaxis
INTEG: Urticaria, erythema (hypersensitivity)
Contraindications:
General: Hypersensitivity
Males: Surgical removal of testes, tumours unresponsive to hormone manipulation
Precautions: Concomitant anti-androgen such as cyproterone acetate may be commenced 3 days before buserelin and continued for at least 3 weeks to prevent disease flare
Clinical assessment:

• Monitor testosterone levels for response to therapy
• Evaluate for possible spinal cord compression or ureteric obstruction if disease flare occurs

NURSING CONSIDERATIONS

Assess:
• Testerone level before and during initial treatment

Administer:
• Subcutaneously for 7 days. Then intranasal spray, one spray dose into each nostril before and after each meal (6 times a day) as maintenance therapy
• Prophylactic anti-androgen drugs if required to prevent disease flare

Perform/provide:
• Adequate pain relief

Evaluate:
• Therapeutic response: decreased pain often after an initial increase in pain which is transient
• If no improvement, but decreased testerone—shows tumours not sensitive to hormone therapy. Alternative therapy required
• Increased pain may include cord compression
• Side effects: hot flushes, nose bleeds, loss of potency, depressed libido growth of male breasts

Teach patient/family:
• How to spray into each nostril
• To discard container after 7 days use
• That regular administration is necessary for any benefits
• That body changes will occur, including enlarged breasts, loss of libido hot flushes
• That nose bleeds do not effect absorption and are usually transient
• To see clinician immediately if urinary difficulties or pain increases or altered sensations occurs; sign of cord compression

busulphan

Myleran
Func. class.: Antineoplastic alkylating agent
Chem. class.: Methane sulphonate derivative
Legal class.: POM

Action: Alkylates DNA, preventing cell replication; mode of action not completely established
Uses: Chronic myeloid leukaemia
Dosage and routes:
Doses are highly variable, and dependent on local treatment protocols, concomitant therapy and tumour type; the following dose schedules have been used:

Chronic myeloid leukaemia
• *Adult:* By mouth induction of remission: 60 mcg/kg daily to maximum 4 mg/day, discontinue when WBC 20,000–25,000/mm^3 or platelets less than 100,000/mm^3; maintenance 0.5–2 mg daily

Polycythaemia vera
• *Adult*: By mouth, 4–6 mg daily for 4–6 weeks

Myelofibrosis, essential
• *Adult:* By mouth, 2–4 mg daily

Available forms include: Tablets 500 mcg, 2 mg

Side effects/adverse reactions:
HAEM: Thrombocytopaenia, leucopenia, pancytopenia, haemorrhage, delayed or irreversible bone marrow depression
GI: Nausea, vomiting, diarrhoea, hepatotoxicity
GU: Sterility, amenorrhoea, gynaecomastia
INTEG: Hyperpigmentation, rash, erythema
RESP: Fibrosis, pneumonitis (may be progressive and fatal)
EENT: Cataracts
CNS: Convulsions (highdoses)
META: Pseudo-Addisonian syndrome

Contraindications: Pregnancy, breast-feeding

Precautions: Radiotherapy or concomitant chemotherapy, non-malignant disorders (probable carcinogen, mutagen), pregnancy (teratogen)

Pharmacokinetics: Well absorbed orally, excreted in urine, excreted in breast milk

Interactions/incompatibilities:

• Increased toxicity: other antineoplastics or radiation, oxygen (may exacerbate pulmonary effects)

Clinical assessment:

• Blood tests: total and differential blood count at least weekly

• Periodic monitoring of pulmonary function

Treatment of overdose: Supportive; monitor blood counts, give infusion products, filgrastim as appropriate

NURSING CONSIDERATIONS

Assess:

• Weight before treatment

• Fluid balance

• Full blood count before and weekly during treatment. Special attention to platelets and WBC

• Signs of infection, fever, cough, cold

Administer:

• HANDLING: take safety precautions appropriate to antineoplastic agents

• Following local antineoplastic (cytotoxic) policies

• After ensuring that clinician is aware of blood results

• By mouth, tailoring dosage and length of course to patient for induction and remission. Tablets should be swallowed whole, not crushed

• Other medications by mouth if possible. Avoid IV, IM, SC routes to prevent infection and bruising

• Anti-emetic 30–60 min before treatment and antacid immediately before busulphan

• All other medication as prescribed, including analgesics, antibiotics, anti-emetics, antispasmodics

Perform/provide:

• Protective isolation and medical asepsis if low WBC

• Dietary advice

Teach patient/family:

• Need for protective isolation

• To report any bleeding of skin, bowels and excessive bruising immediately

• That in females and gynaecomastia in males amenorrhoea may occur, but are reversible after treatment has been discontinued

• That regular blood tests are essential

• That changes in breathing, coughing must be reported

---

calcitriol (1,25-Dihydroxycholecalciferol)

Rocaltrol

Func. class.: Fat soluble vitamin

Legal class.: POM

Action: Increases intestinal absorption of calcium and phosphate, regulates bone mineralisation, increases renal tubular absorption of phosphate

Uses: Correction of calcium and phosphate abnormalities in renal osteodystrophy

Dosage and routes:

• *Adult:* initially 1–2 mcg/day increased by increments of 0.25–0.5 mcg to 2–3 mcg/day as required

Available forms include: Capsules 0.25, 0.5 mcg

Side effects/adverse reactions:

CVS: Cardiac arrhythmias

CNS: Headache, apathy, somnolence, overt psychosis (rarely)

HAEM: Hypercalcaemia

GI: Nausea, vomiting, anorexia, paralytic ileus, abdominal pain
GU: Polyuria, hypercalciuria, nocturia; dehydration; thirst
Contraindications: Hypercalcaemia, metastatic calcification
Precautions: Pregnancy (use not established, potential benefit versus possible hazard), lactation (not known if enters human milk)
Pharmacokinetics:
Period of onset: Peak 4 hr, duration 15–20 days, half-life 12–22 days
Interactions/incompatibilities:
• Phosphate binding agents; dosage may need to be modified
Clinical assessment:
• Blood urea nitrogen, urinary calcium, aspartate aminotransferase, alanine aminotransferase, cholesterol, creatinine, uric acid, chloride, magnesium, electrolytes, urine pH, phosphate. Serum calcium should be kept at 2.12–2.65 mmol/litre, vitamin D 3–30 ng/ml, phosphate 0.8–1.5 mmol/litre
• For increased blood level since toxic reactions may occur rapidly
Treatment of overdose: Gastric lavage up to 8 hr after ingestion; discontinue drug in hypercalcaemia; general supportive measures; rehydration and induced diuresis in severe hypercalcaemia
NURSING CONSIDERATIONS:
Assess:
• Fluid balance
• Calcium sufficiency
• Weight, rate and respirations
Administer:
• By mouth, may be adjusted pending on serum calcium level
Perform/provide:
• Restriction of sodium, potassium if required
• Restriction of fluids if required for chronic renal failure
Evaluate:
• For dry mouth, polyuria, bone pain, muscle weakness, headache, fatigue, tinnitus, change in loss of consciousness, irregular pulse, dysrhythmias, increased respirations, anorexia, nausea, vomiting, cramps, abdominal pain, constipation, tetany, fitting; may indicate hypercalcaemia
• Renal status: decreased urinary output (oliguria, anuria), oedema in extremities, weight gain, periorbital oedema, dyspnoea
• Changes in weight
• Nutritional status
Teach patient/family:
• The symptoms of hyper- and hypocalcaemia
• About foods rich in calcium
• To avoid products with sodium
• To avoid products with potassium in chronic renal failure
• To avoid non-prescribed medicines containing calcium, potassium, or sodium in chronic renal failure
• All aspects of drug: action, side effects, dose, when to notify clinician
• To avoid all preparations containing vitamin D
• To inform prescribing clinician of current medication
• To seek advice if pregnant

calcium chloride/calcium gluconate/calcium lactate

Cacit, Calcichew, Calcidrink, Calcium 500, Citrical, Sandocal, combination products, Min-I-Jet (injection)
Func. class.: Mineral supplement
Chem. class.: Calcium salt
Legal class.: Injection POM oral P/GSL

Action: Caution needed for maintenance of nervous, muscular and skeletal enzyme reactions, normal

cardiac contractility, coagulation of blood; affects secretory activity of endocrine, exocrine glands
Uses: Prevention and treatment of hypocalcaemia, hypermagnesaemia, hypoparathyroidism, neonatal tetany, cardiac toxicity caused by hyperkalaemia
Dosage and routes:
Osteoporosis
• 20 mmol calcium daily
Hypocalcaemic tetany
• IV initially 2.25 mmol then infusion IV 9 mmol daily
Cardiac arrest
• IV 10 ml 10% calcium chloride injection
Available forms include: Tablets (chewable/dispersible), granules, syrup, injection. Many strengths
Side effects/adverse reactions:
CVS: Bradycardia, arrhythmias
GI: Nausea, vomiting, anorexia, constipation
GU: Polyuria, thirst
CNS: Headache, coma, lethargy, muscle weakness
HAEM: Hypercalcaemia
MISC: Irritation after IV injection
Contraindications: Hypercalcaemia, digitalis toxicity, ventricular fibrillation, renal calculi
Precautions: Pregnancy, lactation, children, renal disease, respiratory disease, cor pulmonale, digitalised patient, respiratory failure
Interactions/incompatibilities:
• Large IV doses of calcium may precipitate arrhythmias; risk of hypercalcaemia with thiazides
• Antibacterials: reduced absorption of tetracyclines
• Biphosphonates; reduced absorption

NURSING CONSIDERATIONS
Assess:
• Continuous vital signs
Administer:
• Slowly through a large vein cannula. There is a risk of tissue necrosis if given via a peripheral vein.
• Calcium chloride should not be given through the same IV line as bicarbonate salts due to precipitation
• May be given IM in emergencies only when IV route unavailable
• Oral calcium to be given after meals or with milk
• Continuous ECG and blood pressure monitoring while administering
Perform/provide:
• Seizure precautions: padded side rails, decreased stimuli, (noise, light); place airway suction equipment, padded mouth gag if calcium levels are low
Evaluate:
• Cardiac status: rate, rhythm, CVP
• Therapeutic response: decreased twitching, paraesthesias, muscle spasms, absence of tremors, convulsions, dysrhythmias, dyspnoea, laryngospasm, negative Chvostek's sign, Trousseau's sign
• Baseline ECG for decreased QT and T wave inversion: hypercalcaemia, drug should be reduced or discontinued
• Total bound calcium levels during treatment (2.10–2.60 mmol/litre is normal level, providing albumin levels are normal)
Teach patient/family:
• To remain recumbent ½ hr after IV dose
• To add calcium-rich foods to diet: dairy products, shellfish, dark green leafy vegetables; and decrease oxalate-rich and zinc-rich foods: nuts, legumes, chocolate, spinach, soy, rhubarb

capreomycin

Capastat
Func. class.: Antitubercular
Chem. class.: Poly-peptide antibiotic
Legal class.: POM

Action: Inhibits RNA synthesis, decreases tubercle bacilli replication
Uses: Pulmonary tuberculosis resistant to first-line drugs, as adjunctive
Dosage and routes:
• *Adult:* IM 1 g daily (not more than 20 mg/kg) for 60–120 days then 1 g 2–3 times weekly
Available forms include: Powder for injection 1 g (1,000,000 units)
Side effects/adverse reactions:
INTEG: Pain, irritation, sterile abscess at injection site, rash, urticaria
CNS: Headache, vertigo, fever, neuromuscular blockade with large doses
EENT: Tinnitus, deafness, ototoxicity
GU: Proteinuria, decreased creatinine clearance, increased blood urea nitrogen, tubular necrosis, hypokalaemia, alkalosis, haematuria, albuminuria, nephrotoxicity
HAEM: Eosinophilia, leucocytosis, leucopaenia, thrombocytopenia (rarely)
Contraindications: Hypersensitivity, pregnancy
Precautions: Renal disease, hearing impairment, allergy history, hepatic disease, lactation
Pharmacokinetics:
IM: Peak 1–2 hr, half-life 4–6 hr; excreted in urine unchanged
Interactions/incompatibilities:
• Increased toxicity: aminoglycosides, polymyxin, colistin, vancomycin
• Cytotoxics: increased risk of nephrotoxicity and ototoxicity with cisplatin
Clinical assessment:
• Liver studies weekly: aspartate aminotransferase, alanine aminotransferase, bilirubin, potassium
• Renal status: before, therapy, weekly blood urea nitrogen, creatinine, output, urinalysis
• Blood levels of drug
• Audiometry and assessment of vestibular functions before and during treatment
Treatment of overdose: Symptomatic and supportive therapy is required. Activated charcoal rather than lavage or emesis. Rehydration and haemodialysis are effective

NURSING CONSIDERATIONS

Administer:
• Give IM in large muscle mass, rotating sites. Observe for pain or induration at injection site
• Reconstituted solutions may be stored for 14 days in a refrigerator or 48 hr at room temp
• With other antituberculars
• After sputum culture every month is completed (to detect resistance)
• Reduced dosage in renal impairment
• By deep IM injection over 2 to 3 min dissolved in 2 ml of 0.9% sodium chloride or water for injections. Reduce dose in renal impairment (consult data sheet)
Evaluate:
• Therapeutic response: decreased dyspnoea, fatigue
• Ototoxicity: tinnitus, vertigo, change in hearing; audiometric testing should be done before, during, after treatment
• Hepatic status: decreased appetite, jaundice, dark urine, fatigue
Teach patient/family:
• That compliance with dosage

schedule, length is necessary
• Side effects: hearing loss, change in urine or urinary habits

capsaicin

Axsain
Func. class.: Topical analgesic
Chem. class.: Alkaloid from chilli pepper
Legal class.: P

Action: Probably reduces transmission of pain impulses along nerves by depleting peripheral sensory nerves of the neurotransmitter substance P
Uses: Pain relief in post-herpetic neuralgia, after open skin lesions have healed
Dosage and routes: Topically, not more than 3–4 times daily
Available forms include: Cream (0.075%)
Side effects/adverse reactions:
INTEG: Transient burning at application site
Contraindications: Broken or irritated skin; tightly bandaged areas
Precautions: Lesions near the eyes
NURSING CONSIDERATIONS
Administer:
• Wearing protective gloves
• Only to areas where skin lesions have healed and not to those which are tightly bandaged
Perform/provide:
• Wash hands immediately after application
Evaluate:
• Therapeutic effect: reduction in pain
Teach patient/family:
• To apply by gentle massage, washing hands immediately after
• Not to apply to skin which is broken or inflamed, or to areas which are tightly bandaged
• To avoid eyes, mucous membranes
• That transient burning sensation may occur

captopril

Capoten, Acepril, combination product
Func. class.: Antihypertensive
Chem. class.: Angiotensin converting enzyme inhibitor
Legal class.: POM

Action: Selectively suppresses renin-angiotensin-aldosterone system; inhibits angiotensin converting enzyme, prevents conversion of angiotensin I to angiotensin II, reducing vasoconstriction
Uses: Mild to moderate hypertension, first-line treatment alone or with thiazide; severe resistant hypertension, where standard therapy is ineffective; adjunctive treatment of congestive heart failure with diuretics and digitalis where appropriate
Dosage and routes:
Diuretics should be stopped if possible for 2–3 days before starting treatment to minimise the risk of a rapid fall in blood pressure and hypotension
Hypertension
• *Adult:* Initial dose alone, 12.5 mg twice daily; with thiazide, in elderly or in renal impairment, initially 6.25 mg twice daily; maintenance 25–50 mg twice daily, maximum 50 mg twice daily (rarely 3 times daily in severe hypertension)
Congestive heart failure
• *Adult:* By mouth with thiazide, initially 6.25–12.5 mg under supervision in hospital, maintenance 25 mg 2–3 times daily (maximum 50 mg 3 times daily)

Available forms include: Tablets 12.5 mg, 25 mg, 50 mg

Side effects/adverse reactions:

CV: Tachycardia, hypotension

GU: Dysuria, nocturia, proteinuria, nephrotic syndrome, acute reversible renal failure, polyuria, oliguria, urinary frequency

HAEM: Neutropenia, anaemia, thrombocytopenia, hyperkalaemia

INTEG: Rash, pruritus, photosensitivity

RESP: Bronchospasm, cough

CNS: Paraesthesia of hands

MISC: Angioedema of face, lips mucous membranes, tongue and extremeties

Contraindications: Hypersensitivity, pregnancy, breast-feeding, aortic stenosis or outflow obstruction, renovascular disease, porphyria

Precautions: Dialysis patients, hypovolaemia, leukaemia, blood dyscrasias, congestive cardiac failure, renal disease, diuretics with first dose may cause hypotension, hypotension with low sodium diet, dialysis or dehydration

Pharmacokinetics:

Period of Onset: Peak 1 hr; duration 2–6 hr; half-life 6–7 hr, metabolised by liver, metabolites, excreted in urine; crosses placenta, excreted in breast milk

Interactions/incompatibilities:

• Increased hypotension: diuretics, other antihypertensives, ganglionic blockers, adrenergic blockers
• Increased toxicity: potassium-sparing diuretics, lithium, NSAIDs, cyclosporin
• Do not use with vasodilators, hydralazine, prazosin
• Allopurinol, procainamide: Stevens-Johnson syndrome reported
• Azathioprine, cyclophosphamide: blood dyscrasias in patients with renal failure
• Probenecid: reduced renal clearance

Clinical assessment:

• Blood studies: neutrophils, decreased platelets
• Renal studies: protein, blood urea nitrogen, creatinine, watch for increased levels that may indicate nephrotic syndrome
• Baselines in renal, liver function tests before therapy begins
• Potassium levels, although hyperkalaemia rarely occurs

Lab. test interferences

False positive: Urine acetone

Treatment of overdose: Monitor BP and if hypotensive give volume expansion. Removed by dialysis

NURSING CONSIDERATIONS

Assess:

• BP, apex/radial baselines

Administer:

• With patient in supine position if hypotensive
• IV infusion of sodium chloride 0.9% (as prescribed) to expand fluid volume if severe hypotension occurs

Perform/provide:

• Supine or Trendelenburg position for severe hypotension

Evaluate:

• BP ¼ hrly for 1½ hr, starting 1 hr after 1st dose. Continue if BP drops
• Apex/radial first dose. Report any significant change
• Daily urinalysis for protein (first morning specimen) 24 hr urine collection if positive.
• Assess ankle oedema daily
• Therapeutic response: decrease in BP in hypertensives, decreased signs of cardiac failure
• *Observe for:* Allergic reaction (rash, fever, pruritus, urticaria); drug should be stopped if antihistamines fail to help. Renal symptoms (polyuria, oliguria, frequency)

Teach patient/family:

• Not to discontinue drug abruptly
• Not to use non-prescribed (cough, cold, or allergy) products unless directed by clinician
• Prescribed doses should be continued even if the patient feels better. Rise to sitting/standing position slowly to reduce effect of postural hypotension
• Inform clinician if mouth ulcers, sore throat, fever, palpitations, chest pain, or ankle oedema occur
• May experience dizziness or fainting during first days of therapy

---

carbamazepine

Tegretol, Tegretol Chewtabs, Tegretol Liquid, Tegretol Retard
Func. class.: Anticonvulsant
Chem. class.: Iminostilbene derivative
Legal class.: POM

Action: Inhibits nerve impulses by limiting influx of sodium ions across cell membrane in motor cortex

Uses: Tonic-clonic, complex-partial, mixed seizures; trigeminal neuralgia; prophylaxis of manic depressive psychosis in patient unresponsive to lithium therapy

Dosage and routes:

Epilepsy
• *Adult:* By mouth, initially 100–200 mg 1–2 times daily; increase according to blood levels to 0.8–1.2 g daily in divided doses; maximum 1.6 g daily
• *Child:* By mouth, in divided doses, up to 1 yr, 100–200 mg daily; 1–5 yr, 200–400 mg daily; 5–10 yr, 400–600 mg daily; 10–15 yr, 0.6–1.0 g daily; over 15 yr, as for adults
• *Adult, child over 5 yr:* By mouth, modified-release, as above in 1–2 daily doses

Trigeminal neuralgia
• *Adult:* By mouth, initially 100 mg 1–2 times daily; increase according to response; usual effective dose 200 mg 3–4 times daily; maximum 1.6 g daily
• *Adult:* By mouth, modified-release, as above in 1–2 daily doses

Manic depression
• *Adult:* By mouth, initially 400 mg daily in divided doses; increase according to response; usual effective dose 400–600 mg daily; maximum 1.6 g daily

Available forms include: Tablets, 100 mg, 200 mg, 400 mg; tablets, chewtabs, 100 mg, 200 mg; tablets, modified-release, 200 mg, 400 mg; liquid, 100 mg/5 ml

Side effects/adverse reactions:
HAEM: Thrombocytopenia, agranulocytosis, leucocytosis, neutropenia, aplastic anaemia, eosinophilia, leucopenia, thromboembolism
CNS: Drowsiness, dizziness, confusion, fatigue, headache, somnolence, ataxia, states of confusion and agitation (in the elderly)
GI: Nausea, constipation, diarrhoea, anorexia, vomiting, increased liver enzymes, hepatitis
INTEG: Rash, Stevens-Johnson syndrome, urticaria
EENT: Tinnitus, dry mouth, blurred vision, diplopia, nystagmus, conjunctivitis
GU: Proteinuria, hyponatraemia
MISC: Lymph node enlargement, fever

Contraindications: Hypersensitivity, porphyria, atrio-ventricular conduction abnormality

Precautions: Hepatic disease, renal disease, cardiac disease, pregnancy, lactation, elderly, blood counts and liver function tests prior to initial therapy

Pharmacokinetics:
Period of onset: Onset slow, peak

4–8 hr, metabolised by liver, excreted in urine, faeces, excreted in breast milk, half-life 14–16 hr
Interactions/incompatibilities:
• Toxicity: erythromycin, cimetidine, isoniazid, dextropropoxyphene, lithium, verapamil
• Decreased effects of: oral anticoagulants, phenytoin, primidone, oral contraceptives, cyclosporin, theophylline
• Do not administer with or within 2 weeks of MAOI therapy
Clinical assessment:
• Renal studies: urinalysis, blood urea nitrogen, urine creatinine
• Blood studies: RBC, haematocrit, Hb, reticulocyte counts weekly for 4 weeks then monthly; if myelosuppression occurs, drug should be discontinued
• Hepatic studies: aspartate aminotransferase, alanine aminotransferase, bilirubin, creatinine
• Drug levels during initial treatment; should remain at 4–14 mg/litre (caution in the range of 8–14 mg/litre)
Lab. test interferences:
Decrease: Thyroid function tests
Treatment of overdose: Lavage, activated charcoal as appropriate
NURSING CONSIDERATIONS
Administer:
• Chewable tablets, sucked or chewed, after a meal
• Modified-release tablets whole, not chewed or crushed
Perform/provide:
• Hard sweets, frequent rinsing of mouth to relieve dryness of mouth
• Assistance with ambulation during early part of treatment if dizziness occurs
Evaluate:
• Therapeutic response: decreased seizure activity, record in care plan evaluation
• Side effects: usually disappear spontaneously 7–14 days after initiating therapy
• Mental status: mood, alertness, affect, behavioural changes; if mental status changes notify medical staff
• Eye problems: need for ophthalmic examinations before, during, after treatment (slit lamp, fundoscopy, tonometry)
• Allergic reaction: purpura, red raised rash, if these occur, medication should be discontinued
• Blood dyscrasias: fever, sore throat, bruising, rash, jaundice
• Toxicity: bone marrow depression, nausea, vomiting, ataxia, diplopia, cardiovascular collapse, Stevens-Johnson syndrome
Teach patient/family:
• To carry ID card or Medic-Alert bracelet
• To avoid driving, other activities that require alertness, early in treatment
• To avoid alcohol ingestion; convulsions may result
• Not to discontinue medication quickly after long-term use
• Urine may turn pink to brown depending on dose
• All aspects of drug: action, use, side effects, adverse reactions, when to notify clinician

---

carbaryl

Carylderm, Clinicide Derbac-C, Suleo-C
Func. class.: Parasiticide
Chem. class.: Carbamate
Legal class.: P

Action: Inhibits the enzyme cholinesterase in lice and mites resulting in a build up of the neurotransmitter acetylcholine which results in interference with neuromuscular transmission, paralysis and death
Uses: Eradication of head and pubic lice. Not for routine prophylactic use

Dosage and routes:
Treatment of head lice
• *Adult and child:* By single (most products) or multiple (Carylderm shampoo) topical application, following the manufacturer's instructions for individual products. Contact time required: 5 min (Carylderm shampoo); 2 hr (Carylderm lotion); 12 hr (Derbac-C and Suleo-C lotions)
Treatment of pubic lice
• *Adult:* By single topical application (Carylderm lotion; contact time 2 hr) or two 5 min applications separated by rinse (Carylderm shampoo)
Available forms include: Alcoholic lotion 0.5%; non-alcoholic lotion 1%; shampoo 1%
Side effects/adverse reactions:
INTEG: Skin irritation
MISC: May affect permed, coloured or bleached hair
RESP: Isopropyl alcohol in some products may cause wheezing in asthmatics
Contraindications: Hypersensitivity
Precautions: Children under 6 months of age should only be treated under medical supervision; pregnancy; breast-feeding
Pharmacokinetics: Little absorption when used correctly
Treatment of overdose: Gastric lavage; symptomatic and supportive treatment; atropine may be required to counteract cholinesterase inhibition. Some preparations are alcohol-based and will result in alcohol intoxication as well as malathion toxicity

NURSING CONSIDERATIONS

Assess:
• For signs of head and pubic lice
Administer:
• Staff should wear protective rubber or plastic gloves if using carbaryl regularly
• Keeping away from mouth and eyes
• Allow lotions to dry naturally—do not apply heat
• Leave on for recommended period of time; do not wash treated area before recommended contact time has elapsed
Perform/provide:
• Isolation until treatment completed
• Removal of lice by using a fine-toothed comb rinsed in vinegar after treatment
Evaluate:
• Eradication of head and/or pubic lice
Teach patient/family:
• To wash clothing of all residents. Preventative treatment may be required for all persons living in the same house
• Sexual contacts should be treated simultaneously
• Lotion/shampoo may affect permed, coloured or bleached hair
• May cause wheezing in asthmatics
• To seek medical advice if swallowed
• Alcohol-based lotion is flammable—do not use near sources of ignition
• Do not wash treated area before recommended contact time has elapsed

carbenicillin

Pyopen
Func. class.: Antibiotic, antipseudomonal
Chem. class.: Carboxypenicillin
Legal class.: POM

Action: Inhibits bacterial cell wall synthesis producing non-viable cell; bactericidal.
Uses: Infections due to *Pseudomonas aeruginosa* and *Proteus* spp

Dosage and routes:
• *Adult:* By slow IV injection or rapid IV infusion 5 g 4–6 hrly; by IM injection 1–2 g 6-hrly
• *Child:* By slow IV infusion or rapid IV infusion 250–400 mg/kg daily in divided doses; by IM injection 50–100 mg/kg daily in divided doses
• May be given by other routes in conjunction with systemic therapy
Available forms include: Vials 1 g, 5 g
Side effects/adverse reactions:
GI: Nausea, vomiting, diarrhoea
INTEG: Skin rashes, haemorrhage (rarely)
Contraindications: Penicillin hypersensitivity
Precautions: Pregnancy and lactation
Pharmacokinetics: Peak plasma concentration 15 min after IV injection; half-life 1–1.5 hr, excreted unchanged in the urine
Incompatibilities:
• Intravenous lipid emulsions
• Intravenous aminoglycosides
Clinical assessment:
• Dosage may need to be reduced when renal function impaired
• Monitor electrolytes; high sodium content in 5 g vial
Treatment of overdose: Removed by haemodialysis
NURSING CONSIDERATIONS:
Assess:
• Baseline observations
Administer:
• After samples have been sent for culture and sensitivity
• By IV infusion, slow or rapid depending on severity of condition
• Immediately after reconstitution NB. Must not be mixed with aminoglycosides
• For IV administration, dissolve 5 g in 20 ml water for injections and give by slow injection over 3 to 4 min, or add to 100–150 ml of infusion fluid and infuse over 30–40 min. For IM administration, dissolve 1 g in 2 ml water for injections or 0.5% lignocaine hydrochloride solution. Dosage may need to be adjusted in renal impairment
Evaluate:
• Therapeutic response
• For side effects
• Signs of anaphylaxis

carbenoxolone sodium

Bioral, Bioplex, Pyrogastrone
Func. class.: Anti-ulcer agent
Chem. class.: Synthetic liquorice derivative
Legal class.: POM/P (Preparations for the treatment of mouth ulcers in adults)

Action: Probably acts locally to exert its healing action by stimulating the synthesis of protective mucous and by prolonging the lifespan of mucosal epithelia
Uses: Treatment of oesophageal inflammation, erosions and ulcers due to hiatus hernia and other conditions causing gastro-oesophageal reflux; treatment of mouth ulcers, local application
Dosage and routes:
Gastric ulceration
• *Adult:* By mouth, 20 mg three times a day after meals and at bedtime
Mouth ulcers
• *Adult and child:* Apply 2% gel after meals and at bedtime, or rinse mouth with 20 mg three times a day and at bedtime
Available forms include: Oral gel (2%); mouthwash granules, 20 mg per 2 g sachet; chewable tablets, 20 mg (also contain aluminium hydroxide, magnesium trisilicate and alginic acid); oral liquid, powder for reconstitution 10 mg/

5 ml (also contains aluminium hydroxide, potassium bicarbonate and sodium alginate)

Side effects/adverse reactions:
CV: Hypertension secondary to sodium and fluid retention
ELECT: Sodium and water retention, hypokalaemia
GU: Renal damage secondary to hypokalaemia
MS: Muscle damage secondary to hypokalaemia
Note: These adverse effects would not be expected with preparations used to treat mouth ulcers when used at the recommended dosage and according to manufacturer's instructions, i.e. spitting out mouthwash after rinsing

Contraindications (to systemic treatment): Hypersensitivity; age over 75 yr; children; pregnancy; cardiac, renal or hepatic failure; hypokalaemia; patients being treated with cardiac glycosides unless it is possible to monitor serum electrolyte levels on a weekly basis and measures are taken to avoid hypokalaemia

Precautions (systemic treatment): Patients pre-disposed to sodium and water retention and those where this would present a particular risk, e.g. those with renal, hepatic or cardiac disease and the elderly

Pharmacokinetics: Absorbed from the stomach; plasma concentrations peak several hours after ingestion in non-fasted state; enterohepatically recycled and mainly excreted in the faeces via the bile; elimination half-life increases with age

Interactions:
• Increased toxicity of: digoxin, digitoxin, ouabain (by inducing hypokalaemia)
• Increased risk of hypokalaemia with: most diuretics, corticosteroids
• Reduced effect of carbenoxolone with: amiloride, spironolactone
• Reduced effect of: antihypertensives
Note: These interactions would not be expected to be significant when carbenoxolone is used for the treatment of mouth ulcers at the recommended dosage and according to manufacturer's instructions, i.e. spitting out mouthwash after rinsing

Treatment of overdose: Gastric lavage; monitor serum electrolytes and correct any hypokalaemia; administer diuretics if needed, for sodium and fluid retention

NURSING CONSIDERATIONS

Assess:
• BP, weight, fluid balance
• Age of patient (not suitable for children or people over 75 yr of age)
• Life-style (eating, drinking, smoking habits, stress)
• Possible problems with dentures in cases of mouth ulcers

Administer:
• By mouth; tablet to be chewed after meals, as prescribed
• Gel or granules (dissolved in warm water) as mouthwash for mouth ulcers

Perform/provide:
• Mouth care (for mouth ulcers), including dental assistance if indicated

Evaluate:
• Therapeutic effect: reduction in gastric pain, or in pain produced by mouth ulcers
• Side effects: fluid retention and overload of CV system

Teach patient/family:
• To chew the tablets, not swallow whole
• How to reconstitute granules for use as mouthwash and to rinse the mouth thoroughly
• About side effects, including fluid retention, ankle oedema,

shortness of breath; to report these to nurse or clinician
• About changes in diet, drinking or smoking to reduce incidence of GI ulceration
• About care of the mouth, teeth and dentures in patients with mouth ulcers. To visit dentist regularly

carbimazole

Neo-mercazole
Func. class.: Antithyroid agent
Chem. class.: Imidazoline
Legal class.: POM

Action: Inhibits production of thyroid hormones after metabolism to methimazole
Uses: Hyperthyroidism, preparation for thyroidectomy and radio-iodine treatment
Dosage and routes:
• *Adult:* By mouth initially 20–60 mg daily in 2–3 doses until euthyroid. Maintenance, 5–15 mg daily or, in combination with 50–150 mcg/day thyroxine, 20–60 mg daily. Maintenance therapy should be continued for up to 18 months
• *Child:* 15 mg daily according to response
Available forms include: Tablets, 5, 20 mg
Side effects/adverse reactions:
HAEM: Agranulocytosis, neutropenia
CNS: Headache
GI: Nausea, gastric distress
INTEG: Rashes, pruritus, alopecia
MS: Arthralgia
SYST: Jaundice
Contraindications: Hypersensitivity, breast-feeding
Precautions: Pregnancy
Pharmacokinetics: Converted to active metabolite, producing peak plasma concentration after 0.5–1 hr. Clinical improvement seen after 1–3 weeks. Half-life 3 hr, excreted in urine
Clinical assessment:
• Perform ECG
• Prescribe antihistamines for rashes
• Stop prior to thyroid surgery and prescribe iodine
• Evaluate level of thyroid function, be alert to hypothyroid states occurring
• Evaluate possibility of bone marrow suppression
• Full blood count and platelets (if sore throat reported)
• Measure thyroid function—T3, T4, TSH
Lab. test interferences:
Increase: aspartate aminotransferase, alanine aminotransferase

NURSING CONSIDERATIONS

Assess:
• Baseline ECG, pulse and BP
Administer:
• Once daily (same time) with food
• Discontinue prior to use of ^{131}I (3 or 4 weeks before) or thyroid surgery
Perform/provide:
• Measures to minimise pruritus e.g. cotton clothes
Evaluate:
• Pulse (sleeping), temperature 4 hrly, BP, daily weight, mouth and throat
• For hypothyroidism, oedema, weight gain in excess (weight daily for first week)
• Other side effects, e.g. sore throat, nausea, headaches, rashes, pruritus, arthralgia (rarely), alopecia, agranulocytosis, jaundice
Teach patient/family:
• Report sore throat, mouth lesions, fever, rashes
• That breast-feeding is contraindicated unless neonatal development is monitored closely
• To check pulse and increases in weight

carboplatin

Paraplatin
Func. class.: Antineoplastic agent
Chem. class.: Cisplatin analogue
Legal class.: POM

Action: Platinum forms cross-links between strands DNA. Not cell specific
Uses: Advanced ovarian carcinoma of epithelial origin, small cell carcinoma of lung, other sensitive tumours
Dosage and routes:
Doses are highly variable, and dependent on local treatment protocols, concomitant therapy and tumour type; the following dose schedules have been used:
• *Adult:* IV infusion 400 mg/m^2 as single dose every 4 weeks; reduce by 20–25% if risk factors (e.g. prior myelosuppression) present
Available forms include: Injection 50 mg, 150 mg, 450 mg
Side effects/adverse reactions:
EENT: High tone hearing loss, tinnitus
CNS: Peripheral neuropathy
META: Hypomagnesaemia, hypocalcaemia, hypokalaemia, abnormal liver function tests
GI: Nausea and vomiting, altered taste
GU: Nephrotoxity
HAEM: Thrombocytopenia, leucopenia, anaemia
SYSTEM: Fever, chills
Contraindications: Severe renal impairment (creatinine clearance less than 20 ml/min), severe myelosuppression, hypersensitivity to platinum compounds or mannitol, pregnancy, breast-feeding
Precautions: Reduce dose in renal impairment
Pharmacokinetics: Free platinum excreted in urine predominantly within 24 hr; half-life 24 hr nadir blood count 14–21 days post-treatment
Interactions/incompatabilities:
Toxicity enhanced by other nephrotoxic and myelosuppressive agents
Clinical assessment:
• Neurological assessment, hearing test. Check sensitivity to platinum and mannitol. Only used by experienced clinicians. Do not repeat under 4 weeks. Do not give if myellosuppression severe. Anti-emetics, anti-bacterial drugs, anti-uric acid drugs, Transfusion as required
• Evaluate blood results, tumour regression, extent of side effects
• *Renal function*: urea, creatinine clearance, uric acid. Full blood count at nadir and prior to treatment. Liver function tests: aspartate aminotransferase, alanine aminotransferase, bilirubin, alkaline phosphatase—monthly. Electrolytes—especially magnesium, calcium before each treatment
Treatment of overdose:
Monitor blood count, supportive therapy as required

NURSING CONSIDERATIONS

Assess:
• Temperature, pulse, respiration and BP, respiration and cough, fluid balance, test urine
• Weight
Administer:
• HANDLING: take safety precautions appropriate to antineoplastic agents
• Following local antineoplastic (cytotoxic) policies
• After ensuring that clinician is aware of blood results
• Other medications by mouth if possible. Avoid IV, IM, SC routes to prevent infection and bruising
• Anti-emetic 30–60 min before treatment
• All other medication as prescribed, including analgesics, anti-

biotics, anti-emetics, antispasmodics
• Reconstitute immediately before use with water for injection, sodium chloride 0.9% or dextrose 5%
• By IV infusion over 15–60 min

Perform/provide:
• Reconstituted drug stable for 8 hr at room temperature, 24 hr refrigerated
• Avoid subcutaneous and IM injections where possible
• Other drugs as prescribed, e.g. anti-emetics, pre-medication, antimicrobials
• Nausea: severe with initial therapy
• Anti-emetics before and during treatment
• Protection from infection: asepsis/isolation as required
• Fluids (2–3 l), toast, dry biscuits as vomiting subsides. Ascertain food preferences and provide diet low in purines
• Mouth care: fizzy mouth washes, teeth cleaning and oral toilet
• Help with mobilisation if neurological side effects exist

Evaluate:
• For infection (temperature, pulse, respiration)
• Mouth 8 hrly (infection)
• Other signs of infection/inflammation
• Bruising or bleeding
• Tetany: corpopedal spasm
• Report urine output less than 30–60 ml hrly
• Extent of side effects and effectiveness of measures to minimise them

Teach patient/family:
• Reasons for protective isolation and high standard of hygiene
• Importance of reporting side effects
• Mouth examination for infection, ulcers, etc.
• Signs of cytopenia

carmustine (BCNU)

BiCNU
Func. class.: Antineoplastic alkylating agent
Chem. class.: Nitrosourea
Legal class.: POM

Action: Alkylates DNA, RNA; is able to inhibit enzymes that allow synthesis of amino acids in proteins
Uses: Brain tumours such as glioblastoma, brainstem glioma, medulloblastoma, astrocytoma, ependymoma and metastatic brain tumours, multiple myeloma, Hodgkin's disease, other lymphomas
Dosage and routes:
Doses are highly variable, and dependent on local treatment protocols, concomitant therapy and tumour type; the following dose schedules have been used:
• *Adult:* IV 200 mg/m^2 every 6 weeks, adjusted according to WBC, other drugs
Available forms include: Injection 100 mg
Side effects/adverse reactions:
HAEM: Delayed myelosuppression, thrombocytopenia, leucopenia, anaemia
GI: Nausea, vomiting, hepatic toxicity
GU: Decrease in kidney size, azotaemia, renal failure
RESP: Pulmonary infiltrate, fibrosis
INTEG: Burning, intense flushing, suffusion of the conjunctiva
Contraindications: Hypersensitivity, leucopenia, thrombocytopenia, pregnancy, breast-feeding
Pharmacokinetics: Degraded within 15 min, crosses blood-brain barrier, 70% excreted in urine as metabolites within 96 hr, 10% excreted as CO_2, fate of 20% is unknown
Interactions/incompatibilities:

• Increased toxicity: other antineoplastics, or radiation

Clinical assessment:

• Pulmonary function tests, chest X-ray films before, during therapy; chest film should be obtained regularly during treatment

• Renal function studies: blood urea nitrogen, serum uric acid, urine creatinine clearance before, during therapy

Treatment of overdose:

Monitor blood count, supportive therapy as required—transfusion products, filgrastim

NURSING CONSIDERATIONS

Assess:

• Full blood count, differential, platelet count weekly; withhold drug if WBC is less than 4000 or platelet count is less than 75,000; notify clinician of results

Administer:

• HANDLING: take safety precautions appropriate to antineoplastic agents

• Following local antineoplastic (cytotoxic) policies

• After ensuring that clinician is aware of blood results

• By IV infusion over 1–2 hours, immediately after reconstitution

• Other medications by mouth if possible. Avoid IV, IM, SC routes to prevent infection and bruising

• Anti-emetic 30–60 min before treatment

• All other medication as prescribed, including analgesics, antibiotics, anti-emetics, antispasmodics

Perform/provide:

• Storage in refrigerator

• Avoid contact with skin. Wash off thoroughly if contact occurs

• Strict medical asepsis, protective isolation if WBC levels are low

• Administer as an infusion. Painful as a bolus injection

• Increase fluid intake to 2–3 litres daily to prevent urate deposits, calculi formation

• Rinsing of mouth 3 or 4 times daily with water, prescribed mouthwashes; brushing of teeth 2 or 3 times daily with soft brush or cotton tipped applicators for stomatitis; use unwaxed dental floss

• Warm compresses at injection site for inflammation if indicated

Evaluate:

• Monitor temperature 4 hrly (in neutrophic patients only, may indicate beginning infection)

• Bleeding: haematuria due to thrombocytopenia, bruising or petechiae, mucosa or orifices 8 hrly

• Dyspnoea, rales, unproductive cough, chest pain, tachypnoea

• Food preferences; list likes, dislikes

• Inflammation of mucosa, breaks in skin

• Severity of nausea/vomiting (often severe)

Teach patient/family:

• Of protective isolation precautions if indicated due to neutropenia

• To report any complaints or side effects to nurse or clinician

• To report any changes in breathing or coughing

• Good mouth care and to report any bleeding, white spots, or ulceration in mouth to clinician; tell patient to examine mouth daily

---

carteolol hydrochloride (opthalmic)

Teoptic

Func. class.: Anti-hypertensive, ocular; antiglaucoma agent

Chem. class.: Non-selective β-blocker

Legal class.: POM

Action: Non-selective β-adrenergic blocking agent

Uses: Ocular hypertension, chronic

open-angle glaucoma, some secondary glaucomas
Dosage and routes:
• *Adult:* One drop of the 1% solution instilled into the affected eye(s) twice daily; if inadequate use 2% solution
Available forms include: Eye-drops 1%, 2%
Side effects/adverse reactions:
SYST: May cause systemic effects if absorbed
EENT: Ocular irritation, burning, pain, dryness, blurred vision, hyperaemia, diffuse superficial keratitis
Contraindications: Asthma, history of obstructive airways disease, bradycardia, heart block, heart failure
Precautions: Sinus bradycardia, 2nd or 3rd degree atrioventricular block, cardiogenic shock, right ventricular insufficiency due to pulmonary hypertension or congestive heart failure, diabetes mellitus

NURSING CONSIDERATIONS

Assess:
• Ability of patient to instil drops
Administer:
• Into lacrimal sac
Perform/provide:
• Storage in refrigerator
Evaluate:
• Therapeutic response
• For allergic reactions-occular-irritation, pain, burning
Teach patient/family:
• Instillation method
• That drop must not be used by anyone else
• To discard drops after 28 days
• To store in refrigerator

cefotaxime sodium

Claforan
Func. class.: Antibiotic, broad-spectrum
Chem. class.: Cephalosporin (3rd generation)
Legal class.: POM

Action: Inhibits bacterial cell wall synthesis, rendering cell wall osmotically unstable
Uses: Septicaemia, infections of respiratory tract, urinary tract, soft tissue, bone and joint, gonococcal infections, meningitis, surgical prophylaxis, obstetric and gynaecological infections
Dosage and routes:
• *Adult:* IM/IV 1 g 8–12 hrly, life-threatening infection 2 g 8 hrly or more, maximum 12 g daily
• *Neonate:* 50 mg/kg daily in 2–4 doses, severe infections 150–200 mg/kg daily
• *Child:* 100–150 mg/kg daily in 2–4 doses, severe infections up to 200 mg/kg daily
Gonorrhoea
• *Adult:* IV/IM 1 g as a single dose
Available forms include: Powder for injection IM/IV, 500 mg, 1 g, 2 g
Side effects/adverse reactions:
CNS: Fever
GI: Diarrhoea, rises in liver transaminase and alkaline phosphatase
GU: Candidiasis
HAEM: Eosinophilia, leucopenia, neutropenia, haemolytic anaemia, granulocytopenia, agranulocytosis
INTEG: Rash, injection site pain, phlebitis
Contraindications: Hypersensitivity to cephalosporins
Precautions: Hypersensitivity to penicillins, severe renal dysfunction, pregnancy, lactation
Pharmacokinetics:
IV: Onset 5 min
IM: Onset 30 min

Half-life 1 hr, 35%–65% is bound to plasma proteins, 40%–65% is eliminated unchanged in urine in 24 hr, 25% eliminated as metabolites excreted in breast milk (small amounts)

Interactions/incompatibilities:

• Increased toxicity: aminoglycosides, frusemide, probenecid, vancomycin

Clinical assessment:

• Nephrotoxicity: increased blood urea nitrogen, creatinine

• Blood studies: aspartate aminotransferase, alanine aminotransferase, full blood count, haematocrit, bilirubin, lactic dehydrogenase, alkaline phosphatase, Coombs' test monthly if patient is on long-term therapy

• Electrolytes: potassium, sodium, chloride monthly if the patient is on long-term therapy

Lab. test interferences: False positive to glucose with reducing methods

Treatment of overdose: Serum levels decreased by peritoneal dialysis or haemodialysis

NURSING CONSIDERATIONS

Assess:

• Fluid balance

• Bowel pattern

Administer:

• For IM/IV injection, dissolve 1 g in 4 ml water for injections or 2 g in 10 ml; for IV infusion, dissolve 1–2 g in 40–100 ml of suitable diluent and infuse over 20–60 min.

• After culture and sensitivity completed

Evaluate:

• Therapeutic response

• Bowel pattern daily; if severe diarrhoea occurs, drug should be discontinued; may indicate pseudomembranous colitis

• IV site for extravasation or phlebitis, change site 72 hrly

• Urine output; if decreasing, notify clinician; may indicate nephrotoxicity

• Allergic reactions: rash, urticaria, pruritus, chills, fever, joint pain, angioneurotic oedema; may occur few days after therapy begins

• Bleeding: ecchymosis, bleeding gums, haematuria, blood in faeces daily

• Overgrowth of infection: perineal itching, fever, malaise, redness, pain, swelling, drainage, rash, diarrhoea, change in cough, sputum

Teach patient/family:

• To use live yogurt to maintain intestinal flora, decrease diarrhoea

• To report sore throat, bruising, bleeding, joint pain; may indicate blood dyscrasias (rare)

• To be aware of side effects

• Diabetics may get false values when testing urine

---

cefoxitin

Mefoxin

Func. class.: Antibiotic, broad spectrum

Chem. class.: Cephamycin

Legal class.: POM

Action: Inhibits bacterial cell wall synthesis rendering cell wall osmotically unstable

Uses: Susceptible bacterial infections causing: peritonitis, intra-abdominal and intrapelvic infections, gonorrhoea and septicaemia; infections of: female genital tract, urinary tract, respiratory tract, bones, joints, skin and soft tissues. Gram-negative and Gram-positive susceptible pathogens both aerobic and anaerobic

Dosage and routes:

• IM, slow IV, or IV infusion, 1–2 g every 6–8 hr, maximum 12 g daily

• *Child:* Up to 1 week, 20–40 mg/kg every 12 hr; 1–4 weeks, 20–40 mg/kg every 8 hr; over 1 month, 20–40 mg/kg every 6–8 hr

Urinary tract infections

• *Adult:* IM 1 g every 12 hr

Gonorrhoea

• *Adult:* IM 2 g as a single dose plus probenecid 1 g by mouth

Prophylaxis

• *Adult:* IM/IV 2 g before surgery then every 6 hr if necessary

• *Child:* IM/IV 30–40 mg/kg before surgery and every 6 hr if necessary

Available forms include: Powder for injections; 1, 2 g vial

Side effects/adverse reactions:

CNS: Fever

GI: Nausea and vomiting, pseudomembranous colitis, transient increased aspartate aminotransferase, alanine aminotransferase, alkaline phosphatase and jaundice

GU: Increased creatinine and blood urea, acute renal failure

HAEM: Eosinophilia, leucopenia, granulocytopenia; neutropenia, thrombocytopenia, and bone marrow depression

CV: Hypotension

INTEG: Thrombophlebitis, pain, induration, tenderness, rash, exfoliative dermatitis, urticaria, pruritus, anaphylaxis

Contraindications: Hypersensitivity to cephalosporins, porphyria

Precautions: Hypersensitivity to penicillins, pregnancy, lactation, renal disease (dosage reduction necessary) GI disease

Pharmacokinetics:

IV: Peak 3 min

IM: Peak 15–60 min

Half-life 1–2 hr, 33%–55% bound by plasma proteins, 90%–100% eliminated unchanged in urine; crosses blood-brain barrier, eliminated in milk, not metabolised

Interactions:

Probenecid: reduced excretion of cefoxitin

Lab. test interferences:

• False positive reaction to glucose in the urine

• False high creatinine with Jaffe technique

• False high corticosteroid level with Porter Silber method

• Positive Coombs' test

Treatment of overdose: Not absorbed from GI tract so reaction on accidental ingestion is unlikely. After injection no known antidote is available, give supportive treatment

NURSING CONSIDERATIONS

Assess:

• Bowel pattern

• Fluid balance

Administer:

• After samples taken for culture and sensitivity

• Via IV route by slow bolus injection

• For IM use reconstitute 1 g with 2 ml water for injection or lignocaine 0.5–1.0% and give by deep injection into a large muscle mass; for IV injection reconstitute 1 or 2 g in 10 ml water for injections and give over 3–5 min, or add to solution for IV infusion

Evaluate:

• Fluid balance daily

• Bowel pattern daily; if severe diarrhoea occurs, drug may be discontinued, (risk of pseudomembranous colitis)

• IV site for extravasation or phlebitis; change site every 72 hr

• Urine output; if decreasing, notify clinician as may indicate nephrotoxicity

• For allergic reactions; rash, urticaria, pruritus, chills, fever, joint pain, angioneurotic oedema; may occur a few days after therapy begins

• For bleeding; ecchymosis, bleed-

ing gums, haematuria, stool Hb daily
• False positive Coombs' test (diabetics)
• For overgrowth of infection; perineal itching, fever, malaise, pain redness, swelling, drainage, rash, diarrhoea, change in cough, sputum
• Therapeutic response:
Teach patient/family:
• To report sore throat, bruising, bleeding, joint pain; may indicate blood dyscrasias (rare)

cefpodoxine

Orelox
Func. class.: Antibiotic, broad-spectrum
Chem. class.: Cephalosporin (3rd generation)
Legal class.: POM

Action: Bactericidal through inhibition of bacterial cell wall synthesis. Resistant to majority of beta-lactamases
Uses: Infections caused by susceptible organisms including bronchitis, bacterial pneumonia, sinusitis. Should only be used in tonsillitis and laryngitis when infection is chronic, recurrent or caused by organisms resistant to commonly used antibiotics
Dosage and routes:
Sinusitis
• *Adult:* By mouth 200 mg twice daily
Upper respiratory tract infections (other than sinusitis)
• *Adult:* By mouth 100 mg twice daily
Lower respiratory tract infections
• *Adult:* By mouth 100–200 mg twice daily
Renal impairment: If creatinine clearance is less than 40 ml/min reduce dose by half, and administer as a single daily dose
Available forms include: Tablets 100 mg (as cefpodoxine proxetil)
Side effects/adverse reactions:
CNS: Headache
GI: Diarrhoea, nausea, vomiting, abdominal pain, colitis, raised liver enzymes
GU: Raised serum creatinine and urea
INTEG: Rash pruritis
HAEM: Thrombocytosis, thrombocytopenia, leucopenia, eosinophilia, neutropenia, agranulocytosis
MISC: Superinfection with fungi or resistant bacteria
Contraindications: Hypersensitivity to cephalosporins
Precautions: Penicillin hypersensitivity, severe renal impairment, pregnancy, breast feeding
Interactions: Reduced absorbtion given with: antacids, omeprazole, ranitidine, cimetidine, other H_2 antagonists
Lab. test interferences: False positive reaction for glucose with Fehling's or Benedict's solutions or copper sulphate test tablets but not with glucose oxidase test strips. False positive Coomb's test leading to interference with blood cross-matching
Treatment of overdose: Symptomatic and supportive treatment

NURSING CONSIDERATIONS

Assess:
• Vital signs (temperature pulse, respirations)
• Culture and sensitivity before treatment starts
• For known sensitivities and allergies
• Bowel pattern
• Fluid balance
Administer:
• During meals for optimum absorption

Perform/provide:
• Adequate fluids increased if diarrhoea occurs
Evaluate:
• Therapeutic response; resolution of symptoms, fall in neutrophil count
• Nausea, abdominal pain and other side effects
Teach patient/family:
• Drug should be taken with food and a full glass of water
• To maintain an adequate fluid intake (2 l/day)
• To report any side effects, particularly diarrhoea, sore throat, bruising, unexpected bleeding, joint pain
• Not to take alcohol or medications with alcohol whilst taking Cefpodoxine
• To take the full course of treatment unless otherwise advised by nurse or clinician

---

ceftazidime

Fortum
Func. class.: Antibiotic, broad-spectrum
Chem. class.: Cephalosporin (3rd generation)
Legal class.: POM

Action: Bactericidal through inhibition of bacterial cell wall synthesis. Resistant to majority of beta-lactamases
Uses: Active against a wide range of organisms including:
Gram-negative: *Haemophilus influenzae, Escherichia coli, Proteus mirabilis, Proteus vulgaris, Proteus rettgeri, Klebsiella pneumoniae, Klebsiella* spp, *Citrobacter* spp, *Enterobacter* spp, *Salmonella* spp, *Shigella* spp, *Actinobacter* spp, *Neisseria gonorrhoeae, Neisseria meningitidis, Serratia* spp, *Pseudomonas aeruginosa, Pseudomonas* spp (other), *Morganella morganii, Providencia* spp, *Yersinia enterocolitica, Pasteurella multocida*
Gram positive: *Streptococcus pneumoniae, Streptococcus pyogenes, Streptococcus* spp, *Staphylococcus aureus, Staphylococcus epidermitis, Micrococcus* spp
Anaerobic strains: *Streptococcus* spp, *Peptostreptococcus* spp, *Propionibacterium* spp, *Fusobacterium* spp, *Bacteroides* spp, *Clostridium perfringens*
Upper, lower, serious respiratory tract, urinary tract, skin, gonococcal, intra-abdominal infections, septicemia, meningitis
Dosage and routes:
• *Adult:* IM, IV or infusion 1 g 8 hrly or 2 g every 12 hr, severe infections 2 g every 8–12 hr, less severe infections e.g. urinary tract infections 500 mg–1 g 12 hrly. Elderly usual maximum 3 g daily
• *Child:* up to 2 months, IV 25–60 mg/kg daily in 2 divided doses; over 2 months, 30–100 mg/kg daily in 2–3 divided doses. Meningitis, immunocompromised or fibrocystic children up to 150 mg/kg daily in 3 divided doses
Cystic fibrosis: Pseudomonal lung infection
• *Adult:* IM/IV 100–150 mg/kg daily in 3 divided doses
• *Child:* IV Up to 150 mg/kg daily in 3 divided doses
Available forms include: Injection vials of 250 mg, 500 mg, 1 g and 2 g
Side effects/adverse reactions:
CNS: Headache, dizziness, weakness, paraesthesia, hyperactivity, confusion
GI: Nausea, vomiting, diarrhoea, pain, bad taste, colitis (possibly pseudomembranous colitis) transient hepatitis and cholestatic jaundice
GU: Vaginitis, candidiasis, reversible interstitial nephritis

HAEM: Leucopenia, thrombocytopenia, neutropenia, lymphocytosis, agranulocytosis, eosinophilia, transient elevation of blood urea, blood urea nitrogen and/or serum creatinine
INTEG: Maculopapular or urticarial rash
MISC: Allergic reactions: fever, pruritus, etc., rarely angioedema, anaphylaxis
Contraindications: Hypersensitivity to cephalosporins, porphyria
Precautions: Penicillin allergy, renal impairment (reduce dosage—see data sheet), pregnancy, breast-feeding, concurrent treatment with nephrotoxic drugs, overgrowth of non-susceptible organisms, possible antagonism with concurrent treatment with chloramphenicol
Pharmacokinetics:
IV/IM: Peak 1 hr, half-life ½–1 hr, 90% bound by plasma proteins, 80% eliminated unchanged in urine, excreted in breast milk
Interactions/incompatibilities:
• Possible increased toxicity with aminoglycosides
• Do not mix with vancomycin, aminoglycosides in same giving set
Lab. test interferences:
• *False positive:* Coombs' test (about 5% patients) leading to interference with blood cross matching
• *Slight interference:* with Benedict's, Fehling's and Clinitest
Treatment of overdose: Supportive measures. Dialysis reduces serum levels

NURSING CONSIDERATIONS

Assess:
• Fluid balance
• Bowel pattern
Administer:
• IM as a solution containing 210–260 mg/ml by deep IM injection into a large muscle mass; IV as a solution containing about 90 to 170 mg/ml, or by infusion of a solution containing 2 g in 50 ml of diluent over up to 30 min.
• After specimens have been obtained for bacteriological culture and sensitivity
Evaluate:
• Response to treatment indicated by apyrexia and resolution of all signs and symptoms of infection
• Bowel pattern daily. If severe diarrhoea occurs the drug must be discontinued as this may be indicative of pseudomembranous colitis
• Intravenous site for extravasation, infection and phlebitis
• Urinary output. Inform clinician of oliguria as this may indicate nephrotoxicity
• Allergic reactions: rash, urticaria, pruritus, chills and fever which may develop within a few days of commencement of treatment
• Bleeding: ecchymosis, bleeding gums, haematuria, melaena
• Secondary infection indicated by perineal irritation, pyrexia, malaise, inflammation, discharge, rash, diarrhoea, productive cough
Teach patient/family:
• To inform clinician/nurse of sore throat, bruising, bleeding and joint pain which may indicate blood dyscrasias

---

ceftriaxone ▼

Rocephin
Func. class.: Antibiotic, broad spectrum
Chem. class.: Cephalosporin (3rd generation)
Legal class.: POM

Action: Bactericidal through inhibition of bacterial cell wall synthesis. Resistant to majority of beta-lactamases

Uses: Treatment of infections caused by susceptible organisms, including those occurring in neutropenic patients; peri-operative prophylaxis of infection

Dosage and routes:

• *Adult and child over 12 yr:* By IV/deep IM injection or IV infusion 1 g once daily, increased to 2–4 g once daily in severe infections

• *Child under 12 yr:* By IV/deep IM injection or IV infusion 20–50 mg/kg once daily

Acute, uncomplicated gonorrhoea

• *Adult:* By deep IM injection 250 mg as a single dose

Peri-operative prophylaxis

• *Adult:* By IV/deep IM injection 1 g as a single dose, increased to 2 g and combined with a suitable agent against anaerobic organisms in colorectal surgery

Pre-terminal renal failure: Limit daily dosage to 2 g if creatinine clearance is less than 10 ml/min

Available forms include:

Injection 250 mg, 1, 2 g (as hydrated disodium ceftriaxone) vials

Side effects/adverse reactions:

CNS: Headache, dizziness

EENT: Stomatitis, glossitis

ENDO: Glycosuria

GI: Diarrhoea, nausea, vomiting, raised liver enzymes, pseudomembranous colitis

GU: Oliguria, haematuria, precipitation of drug in urine

HAEM: Anaemia, leucopenia, neutropenia, thrombocytopenia, eosinophilia, agranulocytosis, prolonged prothrombin time

INTEG: Rash, pruritis, oedema

CV: Phlebitis following IV injection

MISC: Deposits of precipitated drug in gallbladder visible on sonograms. Superinfection with fungi or resistant bacteria

MS: Pain at injection site after IM injection

RESP: Bronchospasm

SYST: Fever, anaphylaxis

Contraindications: Hypersensitivity to cephalosporins; premature infants and full-term infants during the first 6 weeks of life

Precautions: Pregnancy; hypersensitivity to penicillins; severe renal impairment combined with hepatic impairment; pre-terminal renal failure; patients undergoing haemodialysis

Incompatibilities: Calcium-containing solutions including Hartmann's and Ringer's

Lab. test interferences:

False positive: Coomb's test leading to interference with blood cross-matching

Treatment of overdose: Symptomatic and supportive

NURSING CONSIDERATIONS

Assess:

• Vital signs (temperature pulse, respirations)

• Culture and sensitivity before treatment starts

• For known sensitivities and allergies (sensitivity to penicillins)

• Bowel pattern

• Fluid balance

Administer:

• IV infusion: 2 g should be dissolved in 40 ml of dextrose 5%, sodium chloride 0.9% or sodium chloride and dextrose and infused over at least 30 min

• IV injection: 250 mg should be dissolved in 5 ml of water or 1 g in 10 ml of water; to be given slowly over 2–4 min

• IM: 250 mg to be dissolved in 2 ml of 1% lignocaine hydrochloride or 1 g in 3.5 ml of 1% lignocaine hydrochloride. Doses of more than 1 g should be divided and injected deeply at more than one site

Perform/provide:

• Adequate fluids increased if diarrhoea occurs

• Storage: reconstituted solutions are stable at room temperature for 5 hr and for 24 hr if refrigerated

Evaluate:

• Therapeutic response; resolution of symptoms, fall in neutrophil count

• Urinary output; if less than 30–50 ml/hr inform clinician (may indicate nephrotoxicity)

• Nausea, abdominal pain and other side-effects

• Pain and phlebitis at injection site

Teach patient/family:

• About the drug and possible side-effects

• To maintain an adequate fluid intake (2 litres/day)

• To report any side effects, particularly diarrhoea, sore throat, bruising or unexpected bleeding

• Not to take alcohol or medications with alcohol

• That the full course of treatment must be given unless otherwise advised by nurse or clinician

• That diabetics may get false readings for blood sugar results (unless clinistix is used)

cefuroxime sodium/ cefuroxime axetil

Zinacef, Zinnat

Func. class.: Antibiotic, broad-spectrum

Chem. class.: Cephalosporin (2nd generation)

Legal class.: POM

Action: Bactericidal through inhibition of bacterial cell wall synthesis, resistant to majority of beta-lactamases

Uses: Active against a wide range of organisms including:

Gram negative: *Haemophilus influenzae, Escherichia coli, Neisseria* spp, *Proteus mirabilis, Klebsiella* spp, *Proteus rettgeri, Enterobacter* spp, *Salmonella typhi, Salmonella typhimurium, Salmonella* spp, *Shigella* spp, *Bordetella pertussis*

Gram positive: *Staphylococcus aureus, Staphylococcus epidermitis, Streptococcus pyogenes, Streptococcus mitis, Clostridium* spp

Respiratory tract, urinary tract, skin, bone, joint, soft tissue, gynaecological and obstetric, ear, nose and throat, gonococcal infections, septicaemia, meningitis, surgical prophylaxis

Dosage and routes:

• *Adult:* By mouth, with or after food, 250 mg twice daily doubled in more severe infections, e.g. pneumonia; IM, IV 750 mg every 6–8 hr, increased in severe infections 1.5 g IV every 6–8 hr

• *Child:* By mouth 125 mg twice daily increased in children over 2 yrs of age with otitis media to 250 mg twice daily. IM, IV 30–100 mg/kg daily in 3–4 divided doses (2–3 divided doses in neonates)

Gonorrhoea:

• Uncomplicated, by mouth 1 g as a single dose; IM 1.5 g as a single dose (divided between 2 sites)

Meningitis

• *Adult:* 3 g IV every 8 hr

• *Child:* IV 200–240 mg/kg daily in 3–4 divided doses reduced to 100 mg/kg daily after 3 days or on clinical improvement

• *Neonate:* 100 mg/kg daily reduced to 50 mg/kg daily

Surgical prophylaxis

• 1.5 g IV at induction, then supplemented depending on surgery—see BNF

Available forms include:

Injection: IM, IV 250, 750 mg, 1.5 g cefuroxime as cefuroxime sodium
Tablets: 125, 250 mg cefuroxime as cefuroxime axetil

Side effects/adverse reactions:
CNS: Headache, dizziness, confusion, agitation
GI: Nausea, vomiting, diarrhoea, pseudomembranous colitis, transient hepatitis, cholestatic jaundice
GU: Candidiasis, reversible interstitial nephritis
HAEM: Eosinophilia, leucopenia, neutropenia, thrombocytopenia
INTEG: Maculopapular and urticarial rash
MISC: Allergic reactions, fever, anaphylaxis, pruritus, erythema multiforme, toxic epidermal necrolysis

Contraindications: Hypersensitivity to cephalosporins, porphyria

Precautions: Penicillin sensitivity, renal impairment (reduce dosage), pregnancy, breast-feeding, concurrent treatment with potent diuretics, aminoglycosides and other nephrotoxic drugs, overgrowth of non-susceptible organisms

Pharmacokinetics:
IV: Peak 3 min
IM: Peak 30–45 min
Half-life 1–2 hr, 33%–50% bound to plasma proteins, 90%–100% eliminated unchanged in urine, crosses blood-brain barrier, excreted in breast milk, not metabolised

Interactions/incompatibilities:
- Possible increased toxicity with aminoglycosides
- Do not mix with aminoglycosides in same giving set

Lab. test interferences:
- *False positive:* Coombs' test leading to interference with blood cross matching
- *Slight interference:* with Benedict's, Fehling's, and Clinitest

Treatment of overdose: Supportive measures. Dialysis reduces serum levels

NURSING CONSIDERATIONS

Assess:
- Bowel pattern
- Fluid balance

Administer:
- For IM administration add 1 ml water for injections per 250 mg; for IV injection add at least 2 ml per 250 mg. For IV infusion 1.5 g may be dissolved in 50 ml water for injections and infused over up to 30 min. Oral doses should be given with or after food
- With food
- After specimens have been obtained for culture and sensitivity

Evaluate:
- Therapeutic response
- Bowel pattern daily; if severe diarrhoea occurs, drug should be discontinued; may indicate pseudomembranous colitis
- IV site for extravasation, phlebitis; change site 72 hrly
- Urine output: if decreasing, notify clinician may indicate nephrotoxicity
- Allergic reactions: rash, urticaria, pruritus, chills, fever, joint pain, angioneurotic oedema; may occur few days after therapy begins
- Bleeding: ecchymosis, haematuria, stools daily
- Overgrowth of infection: perineal itching, fever, malaise, redness, pain, swelling, drainage, rash, diarrhoea, change in cough, sputum

Teach patient/family:
- Be aware of side effects
- To use yoghurt to maintain intestinal flora, decrease diarrhoea
- To take all medication prescribed for length of time ordered
- To report sore throat, bruising, bleeding, joint pain; may indicate blood dyscrasias (rare)

celiprolol ▼

Celectol
Func. class.: Antihypertensive
Chem. class.: Cardioselective β-blocker
Legal class.: POM

Action: Preferentially blocks β-adrenoceptors in the heart, reducing response to sympathetic stimulation. Also has partial β_2-agonist action which probably accounts for its mild vasodilating action

Uses: Mild to moderate hypertension

Dosage and routes:

- *Adult:* By mouth, 200–400 mg once daily, on rising

Available forms include: Tablets, 200 mg

Side effects/adverse reactions:

CNS: Headache, dizziness, fatigue, somnolence

CV: Bradycardia

GI: Nausea

Contraindications: Hypersensitivity; second or third degree heart block; severe bradycardia; overt heart failure; cardiogenic shock; severe renal impairment with creatinine clearance less than 15 ml per min; reversible obstructive airways disease; breast feeding

Precautions: Pregnancy; mild to moderate renal impairment; hepatic impairment; well controlled congestive cardiac failure. Avoid abrupt withdrawal in patients with ischaemic heart disease

Interactions:

- Increased effects of celiprolol: alcohol; anaesthetics; other antihypertensives; anxiolytics; hypnotics; diuretics
- Reduced effects of celiprolol: NSAIDs, corticosteroids, sex hormones, xamoterol
- Severe hypertension with: adrenaline, noradrenaline, other sympathomimetics including possibly those in cough and cold remedies
- Risk of myocardial depression, bradycardia, arrhythmias with: antiarrhythmics, verapamil
- Risk of bradycardia, heart block with: diltiazem, cardiac glycosides
- Reduced effect of: xamoterol, theophylline
- Increased effects of: antidiabetic agents
- Increased peripheral vasoconstriction: ergotamine

Treatment of overdose: Gastric lavage; atropine 1–2 mg IV to counter bradycardia; glucagon 10 mg IV as cardiac stimulant, repeated if needed; β-agonist by slow infusion if glucagon fails

NURSING CONSIDERATIONS

Assess:

- Vital signs (pulse, respirations, BP); ECG, peak flow, fluid balance
- Existing chest conditions, especially asthma

Administer:

- By mouth, 30 min before food in the morning with a full glass of water

Evaluate:

- Vital signs (blood pressure and pulse)
- For side effects, particularly if patient complains of feeling faint or unwell, or is wheezy or breathless (inform medical staff of hypotension, bradycardia, wheeziness or difficulty in breathing)

Teach patient/family:

- About the drug and side effects
- To inform nurse or clinician about dizziness, faintness or headaches (side effects)
- To avoid hazardous activities, including driving, until stabilised on medication
- Not to discontinue taking celiprolol without medical advice

cephalexin monohydrate

Ceporex, Keflex
Func. class.: Antibiotic, broad-spectrum
Chem. class.: Cephalosporin (1st generation)
Legal class.: POM

Action: Inhibits bacterial cell wall synthesis, rendering cell wall osmotically unstable
Uses: Active against a wide range of organisms including:
Gram negative: *Haemophilus influenzae, Escherichia coli, Proteus mirabilis, Klebsiella* spp, *Moraxella catarrhalis*
Gram positive: *Streptococcus pneumoniae, Streptococcus* spp, *Staphylococcus* spp
Respiratory tract, urinary tract, skin, bone, joint, soft tissue, gynaecological and obstetric, dental, ear, nose and throat and gonococcal infections
Dosage and routes:
• *Adult:* By mouth 250 mg 6 hrly or 500 mg every 8–12 hr increasing to 1–1.5 g every 6–8 hr for severe infections
• *Child:* By mouth under 1 yr 125 mg every 12 hr, 1–5 yr 125 mg every 8 hr, 6–12 yr 250 mg every 8 hr, or 25 mg/kg daily in divided doses, doubled for severe infections
Available forms include: Capsules 250, 500 mg, tablets 250, 500 mg, 1 g, syrup 125, 250, 500 mg/5 ml, suspension 125, 500 mg/5 ml, drops 125 mg/1.25 ml
Side effects/adverse reactions:
CNS: Headache, dizziness, agitation, confusion, hallucinations
GI: Nausea, vomiting, diarrhoea, pain, dyspepsia, pseudomembranous colitis, transient hepatitis and cholestatic jaundice
GU: Vaginitis, candidiasis, reversible interstitial nephritis
HAEM: Thrombocytopenia, eosinophilia, neutropenia
INTEG: Maculopapular or urticarial rash
MISC: Allergic reactions: fever, pruritus, angioedema, anaphylaxis, erythema multiforme, toxic epidermal necrolysis
Contraindications: Hypersensitivity to cephalosporins, porphyria
Precautions: Penicillin sensitivity, renal impairment (reduce dosage), overgrowth of non-susceptible organisms, pregnancy, breast-feeding, concurrent treatment with nephrotoxic drugs
Pharmacokinetic:
Period of onset: Peak 1 hr, duration 6–8 hr, half-life 30–72 min, 5%–15% bound to plasma proteins, 90%–100% eliminated unchanged in urine, excreted in breast milk
Interactions/incompatibilities:
• Possible increased toxicity with aminoglycosides, probenecid
Lab. test interferences:
False positive: Coombs' test leading to interference with blood cross matching, Benedict's test, Fehling's test and Clinitest
Treatment of overdose: Supportive measures, dialysis reduces serum levels

NURSING CONSIDERATIONS

Assess:
• Bowel pattern
• Fluid balance
Administer:
• With food if needed, for GI symptoms
• After specimens have been obtained culture and sensitivity
• Adjust dose in renal impairment
Evaluate:
• Therapeutic response
• Bowel pattern daily, if severe diarrhoea occurs, drug should be discontinued; may indicate pseudomembranous colitis
• IV site for extravasation, phlebitis; change site 72 hrly

• Urine output: if decreasing, notify clinician; may indicate nephrotoxicity
• Allergic reactions: rash, urticaria, pruritus, chills, fever, joint pain, angioneurotic oedema, may occur few days after therapy begins
• Bleeding: ecchymosis, bleeding gums, haematuria, melaena
• Overgrowth of infection: perineal itching, fever, malaise, redness, pain, swelling, drainage, rash, diarrhoea, change in cough, sputum

Teach patient/family:
• To use yoghurt or buttermilk to maintain intestinal flora, decrease diarrhoea
• To take all medication prescribed for length of time ordered
• To report sore throat, bruising, bleeding, joint pain; may indicate blood dyscrasias (rare)
• To be aware of side effects
• Diabetics may get false values when testing urine

---

cephazolin sodium

Kefzol
Func. class.: Antibiotic, broad-spectrum
Chem. class.: Cephalosporin (1st generation)
Legal class.: POM

Action: Inhibits bacterial cell wall synthesis rendering cell wall osmotically unstable

Uses: Active against a wide range of organisms including:
Gram negative: *Escherichia coli, Klebsiella* spp, *Proteus mirabilis, Haemophilus influenzae, Enterobacter aerogenes*
Gram positive: *Streptococcus pneumoniae, Staphylococcus aureus, Staphylococcus epidermidis*
Upper, lower respiratory tract, genito-urinary tract, skin and soft tissue, bone and joint, biliary tract infections, septicaemia, endocarditis and surgical prophylaxis

Dosage and routes:
• *Adult:* IM, IV 0.5–1 g every 6–12 hr
• *Child:* 25–50 mg/kg daily in divided doses, increasing to 100 mg/kg daily in severe infections

Available forms include: Injection IM, IV 500 mg, 1 g cephazolin as sodium salt

Side effects/adverse reactions:
CNS: Headache, dizziness, paraesthesia
GI: Nausea, vomiting, diarrhoea, anorexia, oral candidiasis, symptoms of pseudomembranous colitis, transient hepatitis, cholestatic jaundice
GU: Candidiasis, vaginitis, pruritus
HAEM: Leucopenia, thrombocytopenia, neutropenia, eosinophilia
INTEG: Rash
MISC: Allergic reactions, fever, anaphylaxis

Contraindications: Hypersensitivity to cephalosporins, porphyria

Precautions: Penicillin allergy, renal impairment (reduce dosage), pregnancy, breast feeding, concurrent treatment with potent diuretics, aminoglycosides and other nephrotoxic drugs, overgrowth of non-susceptible organisms, safety in prematures and infants under 1 month not established

Pharmacokinetics:
IM: Peak ½–2 hr, half-life 1–2 hr
IV: Peak 10 min, half-life 30 min, eliminated unchanged in urine

Interactions/incompatibilities:
• Possible increased toxicity with aminoglycosides, probenecid, potent diuretics
• Do not mix with other antibiotics, including aminoglycosides in same giving set

Lab. test interferences:
False positive: Coombs' test (leading to interference with blood cross matching), Benedict's, Fehling's and Clinitest
Treatment of overdose: Supportive measures. Dialysis reduces serum levels

NURSING CONSIDERATIONS

Assess:
• Bowel pattern
• Fluid balance

Administer:
• IM diluted in 2–4 ml of diluent; IV diluted in at least 10 ml water for injections and injected over 3–5 min, or diluted in 50–100 ml of fluid and given by infusion. Adjust dose in renal impairment.
• After culture and sensitivity completed

Evaluate:
• Therapeutic response: decreased fever, malaise, chills
• Bowel pattern daily; if severe diarrhoea occurs drug should be discontinued; may indicate pseudomembranous colitis
• IV site for extravasation or phlebitis, change site 72 hrly
• Urine output: if decreasing, notify clinician (may indicate nephrotoxicity)
• Allergic reactions: rash, urticaria, pruritus, chills, fever, joint pain, angioedema; may occur few days after therapy begins
• Bleeding: ecchymosis, bleeding gums, haematuria, melaena
• Overgrowth of infection: perineal itching, fever, malaise, redness, pain, swelling, drainage, rash, diarrhoea, change in cough, sputum

Teach patient/family:
• To use yoghurt or buttermilk to maintain intestinal flora, decrease diarrhoea
• To report sore throat, bruising, bleeding, joint pain; may indicate blood dyscrasias (rare)
• To be aware of other side effects
• Diabetics may get false values when testing urine

---

cephradine

Velosef
Func. class.: Antibiotic, broad-spectrum
Chem. class.: Cephalosporin (1st generation)
Legal class.: POM

Action: Inhibits bacterial cell wall synthesis, rendering cell wall osmotically unstable
Uses: Active against a wide range of organisms including:
Gram negative: *Haemophilus influenzae, Escherichia coli, Proteus mirabilis, Klebsiella* spp, *Shigella* spp, *Salmonella* spp, *Neisseria* spp
Gram positive: *Staphylococcus aureus, Streptococcus pneumoniae, Streptococcus pyogenes, Streptococcus faecalis*
Respiratory tract, urinary tract, skin and soft tissue, gastrointestinal tract infections, surgical prophylaxis, septicaemia, endocarditis, bone and joint infections
Dosage and routes:
• *Adult:* By mouth 250–500 mg every 6 hr or 0.5–1 g every 12 hr
• *Child:* By mouth 25–50 mg/kg daily in divided doses
• *Adult:* IM, IV or by IV infusion 0.5–1 g every 6 hr, severe infections increase to 8 g daily
• *Child:* IM IV or by IV infusion 50–100 mg/kg daily in 4 divided doses
Available forms include: Injection 500 mg, 1 g; capsules 250, 500 mg; syrup 250 mg/5 ml
Side effects/adverse reactions:
CNS: Headache, dizziness, confusion, nervousness
GI: Nausea, vomiting, diarrhoea,

dyspepsia, pseudomembranous colitis, abdominal pain, transient hepatitis, cholestatic jaundice
GU: Vaginitis, candidiasis, reversible interstitial nephritis
HAEM: Leucopenia, eosinophilia, thrombocytopenia
INTEG: Skin rashes
MISC: Allergic reactions: fever, pruritus, anaphylaxis, erythema multiform, toxic epidermal necrolysis
Contraindications: Hypersensitivity to cephalosporins, porphyria
Precautions: Penicillin sensitivity, renal impairment (reduce dosage) overgrowth of non-susceptible organisms, pregnancy, breast-feeding, concurrent treatment with nephrotoxic drugs
Pharmacokinetics:
Period of asset: By mouth: Peak 1 hr
IV: Peak 5 min
IM: Peak 1 hr
Half-life 36–54 min, 20% bound to plasma proteins, 60%–90% eliminated unchanged in urine, excreted in breast milk
Interactions/incompatibilities:
• Possible increased toxicity with aminoglycosides, probenecid
Lab. test interferences:
False positive: Coomb's test leading to interferance with blood cross matching, Benedict's test, Fehling's test and Clinitest
Treatment of overdose: Supportive measures. Dialysis reduces serum levels

NURSING CONSIDERATIONS

Assess:
• Bowel patterns
• Fluid balance
Administer:
• For IM administration, dissolve in 2 ml water for injections or 0.9% sodium chloride per 500 mg and give by deep IM injection; for IV solutions add 5 ml water for injections per 500 mg and inject over 3–5 min, or add to IV infusion fluid. Adjust dose in renal impairment.
• With food if needed, for GI symptoms
• After specimens have been obtained for culture and sensitivity
Evaluate:
• Therapeutic response
• Bowel pattern daily; if severe diarrhoea occurs, drug should be discontinued; may indicate pseudomembranous colitis
• IV site for extravasation, phlebitis; change site 72 hrly
• Urine output: if decreasing, notify clinician; may indicate nephrotoxicity
• Allergic reactions: rash, urticaria, pruritus, chills, fever, joint pain, angioneurotic oedema; may occur few days after therapy begins
• Bleeding: ecchymosis, bleeding gums, haematuria, stool haem daily
• Overgrowth of infection: perineal itching, fever, malaise, redness, pain, swelling, drainage, rash, diarrhoea, change in cough, sputum
Teach patient/family:
• Management of diet
• Not to discontinue medication except on medical instruction
• To report sore throat, bruising, bleeding, joint pain; may indicate blood dyscrasias (rare)
• To be aware of other side effects
• Diabetics may get false values when testing urine

cetirizine

Zirtek
Func. class.: Antihistamine
Chem. class.: Active metabolite of hydroxyzine
Legal class.: POM

Action: Potent antihistamine; a selective H_1-antagonist for symptomatic relief of allergy
Uses: Allergic rhinitis, urticaria
Dosage and routes:
• *Adult:* By mouth 10 mg daily or 5 mg twice daily
Available forms include: Tablets, 10 mg
Side effects/adverse reactions:
EENT: Dry mouth
CNS: Drowsiness, headache, dizziness, agitation
GI: Discomfort
Contraindications: Not recommended in children under 12; breast-feeding; pregnancy; history of hypersensitivity; porphyria
Precautions: Do not exceed the recommended dose if driving or operating machinery, halve dose in renal impairment
Pharmacokinetics: Peak plasma concentration at 0.5–1 hr; half-life 9 hr
Interactions/incompatabilities:
• Drowsiness potentiated by alcohol
Treatment of overdose: Gastric lavage with the usual supportive measures

NURSING CONSIDERATIONS
Evaluate:
• Nasal secretions/rash, level of side effects
Perform/provide:
• Fluids, boiled sweets, fruit for dry mouth
• Safe environment if drowsiness occurs
Teach patient/family:
• May cause drowsiness, if this occurs not to drive or operate machinery
• To avoid alcohol.

chenodeoxycholic acid

Chendol, Chenofalk, combination products
Func. class.: Dissolution of gallstones
Chem. class.: Natural human bile acid
Legal class.: POM

Action: Reduces biliary cholesterol secretion and saturation of cholesterol in bile allowing solubilisation of gallstones
Uses: Dissolution of radiolucent gallstones
Dosage and routes:
• By mouth 10–15 mg/kg daily in divided doses or single dose at bedtime. Treatment is from 3 months to 2 yr depending on gallstone size and continued for 3 months after dissolution
Available forms include: Tablets 250 mg; capsules 125 mg, 250 mg
Side effects/adverse reactions:
GI: Diarrhoea, transient rises in liver transaminases
INTEG: Pruritus
Contraindications: Radio-opaque gallstones; non-functioning gall bladder; chronic liver disease, inflammatory bowel disease; biliary colic, biliary obstruction; gastric or duodenal ulcer; liver cirrhosis; pregnancy; children; breast-feeding
Precautions: Consider other methods of contraception by women than oral contraceptives as they may increase the lithogenicity of bile
Pharmacokinetics: Metabolised by liver, excreted in faeces (metabolite/unchanged drug)

Interactions/incompatibilities:
• Concurrent administration of cholestyramine, colestipol, aluminium antacids, charcoal may bind chenodeoxycholic acid and interfere with absorption

NURSING CONSIDERATIONS

Assess:
• Baseline vital signs and fluid balance

Administer:
• With meals for better absorption
• Antidiarrhoeals if necessary

Perform/provide:
• Increased fluids, fibre, encouragement to exercise, to decrease constipation

Evaluate:
• Therapeutic response; absence of epigastric pain, gallstones on diagnostic testing
• Assess cardiac status; check for dysrhythmias, increased rate, palpitations
• Fluid balance; check for urinary retention or hesitancy
• For GI complaints; nausea, vomiting, anorexia, diarrhoea; (if diarrhoea is severe, drug may need to be decreased)

Teach patient/family:
• That stone dissolution may take 3 months–2 yr; therapy is discontinued after 18 months if gallstones still intact
• To notify clinician if pregnancy is likely

---

chloral betaine

Welldorm (tablets)
Func. class.: Hypnotic
Chem. class.: Chloral hydrate derivative
Legal class.: POM

Action: CNS depressant
Uses: Short-term treatment of insomnia
Dosage and routes: By mouth
• *Adult:* By mouth, 1–2 tablets (equivalent to 414–828 mg of chloral hydrate) at night; maximum 5 tablets (3.5 g, equivalent to 2 g chloral hydrate) daily
Available forms include: Tablets 707 mg (equivalent to chloral hydrate 414 mg)
Side effects/adverse reactions:
CNS: Drowsiness the following day; headache, excitement, delirium, dependence
GI: Gastric irritation, flatulence
GU: Renal damage on prolonged use, ketonuria
INTEG: Rashes
Contraindications: Gastritis, severe cardiac disease, marked hepatic or renal impairment
Precautions: History of drug abuse or personality disorder; respiratory disease; pregnancy, lactation; reduce dose in elderly or debilitated patients; avoid prolonged use and abrupt withdrawal
Pharmacokinetics: Converted to chloral hydrate and ultimately to trichlorethanol (half-life 7–11 hr). Onset of action within 30 minutes
Interactions/incompatibilities:
• Effects enhanced by: other CNS depressants, including alcohol
• May increase the effects of: coumarin anticoagulants
Treatment of overdose: Gastric lavage, haemoperfusion; supportive treatment

NURSING CONSIDERATIONS

Administer:
• With water or milk 20 min prior to bedtime
• Avoid contact with skin/mucous membranes

Perform/provide:
• Safe environment: cot sides, help with mobilisation

Evaluate:
• Rashes
• Observe for any abnormal bleeding

• Signs of dependence
• Sleep pattern improvement

Teach patient/family:
• They may be drowsy next day; if affected not to drive or operate machinery
• Report side effects—rash, headache
• That nightmares may occur
• To take with full glass of water
• That tolerance may occur
• About encouraging normal sleep patterns: exercise in day, milk drink, warm bath, relaxation techniques, books/TV etc.
• Not to discontinue medication abruptly

---

chloral hydrate

Noctec, Welldorm (elixir)
Func. class.: Hypnotic
Chem. class.: Chloral derivative
Legal class.: POM

Action: Metabolite trichlorethanol believed to have central depressant effect which induces sleep

Uses: Short-term treatment of insomnia

Dosage and routes:
• *Adult:* 0.5–1 g, 15–30 min before bedtime with plenty of water. Maximum 2 g
• *Child:* 30–50 mg/kg, maximum 1 g per day

Available forms include: Capsules 500 mg; elixir 143 mg/5 ml

Side effects/adverse reactions:
HAEM: Eosinophilia, leucopenia
CNS: Excitement, headache, delirium, lightheadedness, ataxia, paranoia
INTEG: Allergic skin reactions
CV: Hypotension, dysrhythmias
RESP: Depression (in children)
GI: Gastric irritation, abdominal distension, flatulence

Contraindications: Marked hepatic or renal impairment, severe cardiac disease, gastritis, hypersensitivity to chloral hydrate

Precautions: Causes drowsiness, possibility of habituation

Pharmacokinetics:
Period of onset: Onset 30 min–1 hr, duration 4–8 hr. Metabolised by liver, excreted by kidneys (inactive metabolite) and faeces, excreted in breast milk; half-life 8–11 hr; metabolite is highly protein bound

Interactions/incompatibilities:
• Increased action of anticoagulants, increased action of both drugs with alcohol, benzodiazepines, other hypnotics and anxiolytics
• When chloral hydrate is followed by IV frusemide variable blood pressure including hypertension, sweating, hot flushes may result

Clinical assessment:
• Monitor prothrombin time if patients on anticoagulants. Watch for habituation if on long-term treatment and delirium on sudden withdrawal

Lab. test interferences: Possible false positive results in some tests for glucose, measurement of urinary 17-hydroxycorticosteroids, possible raised results in blood urea determinations

Treatment of overdose: Gastric lavage or induction of vomiting to empty the stomach. Supportive measures must be used; in severe poisoning haemoperfusion or dialysis may be beneficial

NURSING CONSIDERATIONS

Administer:
• After trying conservative measures for insomnia
• ½–1 hr before bedtime for insomnia
• With milk or plenty of water

Perform/provide:
• Checking to see oral medication swallowed

• Assistance with ambulation after receiving dose
• Safety measure: siderails, nightlight, callbell within easy reach

Evaluate:
• Therapeutic response: ability to sleep at night, decreased amount of early morning awakening if taking drug for insomnia
• Mental status: mood, alertness, affect, memory (long, short)
• Physical dependency: more frequent requests for medication, shakes, anxiety
• Respiratory dysfunction: respiratory depression, character, rate, rhythm; hold drug if respirations are less than 12/min or if pupils are dilated (rare)
• Blood dyscrasias: fever, sore throat, bruising, rash, jaundice, epistaxis (rare)
• Previous history of substance abuse, cardiac disease, or gastritis

Teach patient/family:
• To avoid driving or other activities requiring alertness
• To avoid alcohol ingestion or CNS depressants; serious CNS depression may result
• Not to discontinue medication quickly after long-term use; drug should be tapered over 1–2 weeks
• That effects may take 2 nights for benefits to be noticed
• Alternate measures to improve sleep (reading, exercise several hours before bedtime, warm bath, warm milk, TV, self-hypnosis, deep breathing)

chlorambucil

Leukeran
Func. class.: Antineoplastic alkylating agent
Chem. class.: Nitrogen mustard
Legal class.: POM

Action: Interferes with cell replication by alkylating DNA, RNA; inhibits enzymes that allow synthesis of proteins

Uses: Chronic lymphocytic leukaemia, Hodgkin's disease, certain forms of non-Hodgkin's lymphoma, Waldenstrom's macroglobulinaemia, advanced ovarian adenocarcinoma, breast cancer

Dosage and routes:
Doses are highly variable, and dependent on local treatment protocols, concomitant therapy and tumour type; the following dose schedules have been used:
• *Adult and child:* By mouth, usually 100–200 mcg/kg daily for 4–8 weeks as a single agent

Available forms include: Tablets 2.5 mg

Side effects/adverse reactions:
CNS: Seizures, peripheral neuropathy
HAEM: Bone marrow suppression, jaundice
GI: Nausea, vomiting, diarrhoea, oral ulceration
MISC: Hypersensitivity
RESP: Fibrosis, pneumonia
GU: Sterile cystitis

Contraindications: Teratogenic, avoid in first trimester if possible, use balanced against benefit; avoid breast-feeding; patients given other cytotoxic agents or recent radiotherapy

Precautions: Used only by experienced physicians, monitor blood counts, impaired renal function

Pharmacokinetics: Well absorbed orally, metabolised in liver, excreted in urine; half-life 2 hr

Interactions/incompatibilities:
• Increased toxicity: other antineoplastics or radiation
• Reduce dosage if patients receiving phenylbutazone

Clinical assessment:
• Ensure full blood count, differential, platelet count weekly; notify clinician of results

• Pulmonary functions test, chest X-ray films before, during therapy; chest film should be obtained at intervals during treatment
• Renal function studies: blood urea nitrogen, serum uric acid, urine creatinine clearance before, during therapy
• Liver function tests before, during therapy (bilirubin, aspartate aminotransferase, alanine aminotransferase, lactic dehydrogenase) as needed or monthly

Treatment of overdose: Monitor blood picture, institute general supportive measures; blood transfusion, filgrastim if necessary

NURSING CONSIDERATIONS

Administer:
• HANDLING: take safety precautions appropriate to antineoplastic agents
• Following local antineoplastic (cytotoxic) policies
• After ensuring that clinician is aware of blood results
• By mouth, with or after food
• Other medications by mouth if possible. Avoid IV, IM, SC routes to prevent infection and bruising
• Anti-emetic 30–60 min before treatment and antacid immediately before chlorambucil
• All other medication as prescribed, including allopurinal, analgesics, antibiotics, anti-emetics, antispasmodics

Perform/provide:
• Strict medical asepsis, protective isolation if WBC levels are low
• Special skin care
• Increase fluid intake to 2–3 litres daily to prevent urate deposits, calculi formation
• Diet low in purines: offal (kidney, liver), dried beans, peas, to maintain alkaline urine

Evaluate:
• Fluid balance; report fall in urine output of 30 ml/hr
• Monitor temperature and BP 4 hrly in bone marrow depression
• Unexpected bleeding: e.g. haematuria, bruising or petechiae
• Yellowing of skin, sclera, dark urine, clay-coloured stools, itchy skin, abdominal pain, fever, diarrhoea
• Signs and symptoms of infection, particularly in the chest
• Effects of alopecia on body image; discuss feelings about body changes (rare)

Teach patient/family:
• Protective isolation precautions
• To report any complaints or side effects to nurse or clinician
• To report any changes in breathing or coughing
• That hair may be lost during treatment; a wig or hairpiece may make patient feel better (obtainable free on NHS); new hair may be different in colour, texture (rare)
• That impotence or amenorrhoea can occur but is generally reversible after discontinuing treatment

---

chloramphenicol (ear drops)

Func. class.: Broad-spectrum antibiotic
Chem. class.: Dichloroacetic acid derivative
Legal class.: POM

Action: Interferes with protein synthesis in intact bacterial cells

Uses: Bacterial infection in external ear (otitis externa)

Dosage and routes:
• *Adult and child:* Instil into ear 2–3 drops 2–3 times daily

Available forms include: Ear drops 5%, 10% in propylene glycol

Side effects/adverse reactions:
EENT: Itching, irritation in ear
INTEG: Rash, urticaria, contact dermatitis, burning

Contraindications: Hypersensitivity, perforated eardrum
Precautions: Avoid prolonged use, high incidence of sensitivity reactions to vehicle

NURSING CONSIDERATIONS

Administer:

- After removing impacted cerumen by irrigation with 0.5% bicarbonate of soda or 0.9% sodium chloride
- After cleaning stopper with alcohol
- After warming solution to body temperature
- Avoid use for longer than about a week

Evaluate:

- Therapeutic response: decreased ear pain
- For redness, swelling, pain in ear, which indicates superimposed infection

Teach patient/family:

- Method of instillation, using aseptic technique, including not touching dropper to ear
- That dizziness may occur after instillation
- To avoid prolonged use
- About side effects

chloramphenicol (ophthalmic)

Chloromycetin, Snophenicol, Minims chloramphenicol
Func. class.: Broad spectrum antibiotic
Legal class.: POM

Action: Bacteriostatic action by interference with protein synthesis in intact bacterial cells. Antibacterial action effective against virtually all bacterial pathogens causing eye disease
Uses: Infection of eye
Dosage and routes:

- *Adult and child:* Instil 2 drops every 2 hr then reduce frequency as infection controlled; continue for 48 hr after healing. Apply ointment at night if drops are being used or 3–4 times daily if ointment used alone

Available forms include: Eye drops 0.5%, eye ointment 1%
Side effects/adverse reactions:
EENT: Transient stinging, burning sensations, overgrowth of non-susceptible organisms
HAEM: Aplastic anaemia (rare)
Contraindications and precautions: Hypersensitivity

NURSING CONSIDERATIONS

Administer:

- After washing hands, cleanse crusts or discharge from eye before application
- Apply pressure to lacrimal sac for 1 min to prevent systemic absorption
- Apply ointment topically inside lower eye lid (to conjunctival sac)

Perform/provide:

- Storage at room temperature, protect from light

Evaluate:

- Therapeutic response: absence of redness, inflammation, tearing
- Allergy: itching, lacrimation, redness, swelling

Teach patient/family:

- To use drug exactly as prescribed
- That drug container tip should not be touched to eye
- To use separate applicator for each eye
- Wash hands between applications to reduce risk of cross-infection
- Not to use eye makeup, towels, washcloths, eye medication of others; reinfection may occur
- That drug may cause blurred vision when ointment is applied
- To report itching, increased redness, burning, stinging, swelling; drug should be discontinued

chloramphenicol/ chloramphenicol palmitate/ chloramphenicol sodium succinate

Chloromycetin, Kemicetine
Func. class.: Broad spectrum antibiotic
Chem. class.: Dichloroacetic acid derivative
Legal class.: POM

Action: Interferes protein synthesis in intact bacterial cells to exert a mainly bacteriostatic effect

Uses: Active against a wide range of organisms including:
Gram-negative, particularly *Salmonella typhi, Haemophilus influenzae, Neisseria meningitidis*
Gram-positive, *Streptococcus pneumoniae, Rickettsia* spp, *Mycoplasma* spp, *Vibro* spp., *Chlamydia* spp of the Psittacosis–Lymphogranuloma group

Dosage and routes:
- *Adults and children over 2 weeks:* By mouth, IV 50 mg/kg daily in 4 divided doses
- For severe infections—septicaemia, meningitis—may be doubled. Reduce high doses as soon as clinically indicated
- *Infants under 2 weeks:* 25 mg/kg daily in 4 divided doses

Available forms include: Injection IV 300 mg, 1.0, 1.2 g; capsules 250 mg; oral suspension 125 mg/5 ml

Side effects/adverse reactions:
HAEM: Aplastic anaemia, bone marrow depression, hypoplastic anaemia, thrombocytopenia, agranulocytosis, leucopenia
EENT: Optic neuritis, blindness
GI: Nausea, vomiting, diarrhoea, dry mouth, glossitis, stomatitis, enterocolitis, pruritus ani
INTEG: Erythema multiforme
CU: Haemoglobinuria (nocturnal)
MISC: Grey's syndrome in newborn: abdominal distension with or without vomiting, pallid cyanosis, vasomotor collapse, irregular respiration

Contraindications: Hypersensitivity, previous toxic reaction to drug, pregnancy, breast-feeding, porphyria, trivial infections, administration IV during labour

Precautions: Reduce dose in impaired hepatic or renal function, overgrowth of non-susceptible organisms, carry out blood studies

Pharmacokinetics:
Period of onset: IV: Peak 1–2 hr, duration 8 hr, half-life 1½–4 hr, conjugated in liver, excreted in urine (up to 15% as free drug), breast milk, faeces

Interactions/incompatibilities:
- Enhanced effects of: coumarin anticoagulants (nicoumalone, warfarin), some hypoglycaemic agents (e.g. tobutamide), phenytoin
- Reduced action of chloramphenicol: rifampicin, phenobarbitone
- Half-life prolonged by: paracetamol
- Avoid myelossuppressive drugs, increased risks of blood disorders

Treatment of overdose: Empty stomach if oral dosage (excess of 12 capsules or 120 ml suspension), then supportive measures as necessary. After IV dosage, supportive measures as necessary

NURSING CONSIDERATIONS

Assess:
- Allergies before treatment, reaction of each medication; note allergies on chart, in bright red letters; alert all people giving medication
- Bowel patterns
- Fluid balance

Administer:

• If IV, as a solution containing 25 or 100 mg/ml, by injection over at least 1 min, or by infusion after further dilution in a suitable quantity of fluid. Adjust dose in renal or hepatic impairment. Plasma concentrations should be monitored in neonates and ideally under 4 yrs of age: peak concentration 1 hr after administration should be about 15–25 mg/l, pre-dose concentrations should be less than 15 mg/l
• After specimens have been obtained for culture and sensitivity
• IV slowly over at least 1 min
• Reconstituted solution should be used once only
• Oral form on empty stomach with full glass of water

Perform/provide:
• Storage: reconstituted solution at room temperature for up to 30 days
• Ensure emergency equipment available should anaphylaxis occur
• Adequate intake of fluids (2 litres daily) during diarrhoea episodes
• Record/be aware of fluid balance in view of possible renal impairment
• Care of IV site: look for phlebitis extravasation, etc

Evaluate:
• Therapeutic response: decreased temperature, negative culture and sensitivity
• Bowel pattern before, during treatment
• Skin eruptions, itching
• Respiratory status: rate, character, wheezing, tightness in chest
• Signs of bone marrow suppression. Ensure blood studies reviewed at regular intervals
• Neonates for beginning of Grey's syndrome: cyanosis, abdominal distention, irregular respiration, failure to feed; drug should be discontinued immediately

Teach patient/family:
• Aspects of drug therapy: need to complete entire course of medication to ensure organism death; culture may be taken after complete course of medication
• To report sore throat, fever, fatigue, unusual bleeding, bruising; could indicate bone marrow depression (may occur weeks or months after termination of drug)
• That drug must be taken in equal intervals around clock to maintain blood levels
• To wear or carry identification if allergic to this drug
• To notify nurse of diarrhoea
• To be aware of all side effects

---

chlordiazepoxide

NHS Librium, Tropium
Func. class.: Anxiolytic
Chem. class.: Benzodiazepine
Legal class.: CD (Sch 4) POM

Action: Action via GABA receptors depressing subcortical levels of CNS, including limbic system, reticular formation

Uses: Short term management of anxiety, adjunct in acute alcohol withdrawal

Dosage and routes:

Anxiety
• *Adult:* By mouth, 10 mg 3 times daily; up to 60–100 mg daily in divided doses if necessary; elderly, debilitated, half adult dose

Muscle spasm
• *Adult:* By mouth, 10–30 mg daily in divided doses; elderly, debilitated, half adult dose

Alcohol withdrawal
• *Adult:* By mouth, 25–100 mg, repeated 2–4 hrly if required; elderly, debilitated, half adult dose

Available forms include: Capsules

(hydrochloride), 5 mg, 10 mg; tablets (base), 5 mg, 10 mg, 25 mg

Side effects/adverse reactions:

CNS: Drowsiness, sedation, unsteadiness, ataxia, confusion, headache, vertigo

GI: Upsets—diarrhoea, constipation, salivation changes

INTEG: Rashes

EENT: Visual disturbances

HAEM: Blood disorders and jaundice reported

GU: Urinary retention

MISC: Changes in libido

Contraindications: CNS depression, coma, respiratory depression, sleep apnoea

Precautions: Chronic pulmonary insufficiency, psychosis, marked personality disorder, muscle weakness, drug abuse, pregnancy, lactation. Reduce dose in elderly, debilitated, hepatic and renal impairment. Avoid prolonged use and sudden withdrawal. Alteration of performance at skilled tasks e.g. driving

Pharmacokinetics:

Period of onset: Onset 30 min, peak ½ hr, duration 4–6 hr, metabolised by liver, excreted by kidneys, in breast milk, half-life 5–30 hr

Interactions/incompatibilities:

• Increased effects of this drug: CNS acting drugs: neuroleptics, tranquillisers, antidepressants, hypnotics, analgesics, anaesthetics, alcohol, disulfiram, ulcer healing drugs e.g. cimetidine

Treatment of overdose: Gastric lavage if soon after ingestion. In hospital IV flumazenil as antidote in emergency situations. Take supportive measures. Do not use barbiturates if excitation occurs

NURSING CONSIDERATIONS

Assess:

• Baseline BP and fluid balance

Administer:

• Crush tablets if patient is unable to swallow medication whole

• Boiled sweets, frequent sips of water for dry mouth

Perform/provide:

• Check to see oral medication has been swallowed

• Assistance with ambulation during initial therapy, since drowsiness/dizziness occurs

• Safety measure, including siderails

Evaluate:

• Therapeutic response: decreased anxiety, restlessness, sleeplessness

• BP (lying, standing), pulse; if systolic BP drops 20 mmHg, withhold drug, notify clinician

• Fluid balance, may indicate renal dysfunction

• Mental status: mood, alertness, affect, sleeping pattern, drowsiness, dizziness

• Physical dependency, withdrawal symptoms: headache, nausea, vomiting, muscle pain, weakness after long-term use

• Suicidal tendencies

Teach patient/family:

• That drug may be taken with food

• Not to be used for everyday stress or used longer than 4 months, unless directed by clinician

• Avoid non-prescribed preparations unless approved by clinician

• To avoid driving, activities that require alertness; drowsiness may occur

• To avoid alcohol ingestion or other psychotropic medications, unless prescribed by clinician

• Not to discontinue medication abruptly after long-term use

• To rise slowly or fainting may occur

• That drowsiness might worsen at beginning of treatment

chlorhexidine gluconate chlorhexidine acetate

Bacticlens, Chlorasept, CX Antiseptic Dusting Powder, Hibitane Obstetric, Hibidil, Hibiscrub, Hibisol, Hibitane 5% concentrate, Hibitane gluconate 20% Phiso-med, Rotersept, Sterexidine, Steripod, Unisept

Func. class.: Antiseptic and disinfectant

Chem. class.: Polychlorinated phenol derivative

Legal class: GSL, P

Action: Antimicrobial agent effective against a wide range of vegetative Gram-positive and Gram-negative bacteria

Uses: Surgical scrub, skin cleanser, bladder irrigation, wound cleanser, disinfection of surfaces, instruments, obstetrics

Dosage and route:

• *Adult and child:* Use as product directions indicate

Available forms include: Soap, solution, spray, cream, bladder irrigation, powder

Side effects/adverse reactions:

INTEG: Irritation, sensitivity, dryness, dermatitis

MISC: Rare generalised allergic reactions

Contraindications: Hypersensitivity to chlorhexidine; use on brain, meninges, middle ear, eye, body cavities or other sensitive tissues

Precautions: Bladder irrigations of concentrated solutions may cause haematuria

Interactions/incompatibilities: Soaps and other anionic materials

Treatment of overdose: Ingestion: gastric lavage using milk, gelatin or mild soap. Supportive measures as necessary

NURSING CONSIDERATIONS

Administer:

(Refer to information provided by pharmacist)

• Topically to body areas only. Avoid contact with face, lips, eyes and mouth and all mucous membranes

• Surgical scrub-rinse and dry hands thoroughly after treatment to prevent irritation

• Bladder irrigation—administer under aseptic conditions

• Only to adults; repeated use may lead to systemic absorption

Evaluate:

• Area of body involved; irritation, rash, breaks, redness, dryness, itching

Teach patient/family:

• To report itching, irritation, dizziness, headache, confusion; discontinue use immediately

chlorinated solutions

Chlorasol, Chloros, Milton

Non-proprietary names: Chlorinated lime and boric acid solution (Eusol), surgical chlorinated soda solution (Dakin's solution), sodium hypochlorite solution

Func. class.: Disinfectant and antiseptic

Chem. class.: Inorganic chlorine compounds

Legal class.: GSC

Action: Act as a source of chlorine which is a powerful oxidising agent with bactericidal, fungicidal and viracidal properties

Uses: Chlorinated solutions are widely used as disinfectants for cleaning hospital and food equipment where they have the advantage of low residual toxicity. They were once extensively used in wound care but are no longer routinely used for this purpose because they are rapidly inactivated in the wound and interfere with the healing process, they are still occasionally used for debriding necrotic wounds

Dosage and routes:

As a cleansing agent for necrotic wounds

• *Adult and child:* Topically by direct application of a lotion or a saturated gauze dressing. Eusol (2500 ppm available chlorine) and Dakin's solution (5000–5500 ppm available chlorine) are the most common chlorine sources for this application. Chlorinated solutions are not suitable for routine wound care

As a disinfectant

• As with all disinfectants chlorinated solutions should only be used in accordance with any local disinfectants policy. Typically solutions containing 200–250 ppm available chlorine are used for the disinfection of relatively clean, impervious surfaces such as babies' bottles, baths, trolleys; solutions containing 250–300 ppm available chlorine are used for food equipment where organic contamination is likely and solutions containing 10,000 ppm available chlorine are used for disinfecting equipment and surfaces contaminated by blood

Available forms include:

As wound cleansing agents

Chlorinated lime and boric acid solution (Eusol; 2500 ppm available chlorine); surgical chlorinated soda solution (Dakin's solution; 5000–5500 ppm available chlorine)

As general disinfectants

Sodium hypochlorite solutions of various strengths, some stabilised by the addition of other agents

Side effects/adverse reactions:

Used as wound cleansing agents:

INTEG: Irritation of wound and surrounding healthy skin; delayed wound healing; irritation of mucous membranes

Precautions: Renal impairment (eusol)

Interactions: N/A

Incompatibilities:

• Readily inactivated by: organic material

• Dangerous liberation of chlorine gas when mixed with some other cleaning agents

• Concentrated solutions capable of bleaching dyed materials

Treatment of overdose: Seek specialist advice if ingested; contact Poisons Centre

NURSING CONSIDERATIONS

Assess:

As a cleansing agent for necrotic wounds

• Woundsite for necrotic tissue

As a disinfectant

• Area/equipment to be disinfected

Administer:

As wound cleansing agent

• To necrotic tissue only; keep away from healthy skin

• In dilution recommended (irritant)

• Protect wound margins with soft paraffin

As a disinfectant

• Remove all organic material from site to be disinfected before using solution

• Use correct strength according to manufacturer's guidelines and local policy

Perform/provide:

As wound cleansing agent

• Plastic or rubber gloves

As a disinfectant

• Staff should wear protective rubber or plastic gloves

• Disinfect in accordance with local policy

Evaluate:

As wound cleansing agent

• For signs of wound healing

• Discontinue use as soon as wound is debrided
• For side effects; reddening, irritation of skin (discontinue use)

Teach patient/family

As wound cleansing agent

• Reason for using solution
• Not to use for routine wound care
• Not to use undiluted, as this is now considered too irritant
• Discontinue use if irritation occurs

As a disinfectant

• Not to use with other cleaning agents
• Solutions may bleach dyed materials
• Keep substance away from skin, eyes, mucous membranes
• Use strong solutions only in well-ventilated areas
• Wear protective gloves

chlormethiazole

Heminevrin
Func. class.: Hypnotic
Chem. class.: Non-benzodiazepine
Legal class.: POM

Action: Hypnotic, sedative and anticonvulsant properties via effects on catecholaminergic and GABAergic systems

Uses: Alcohol withdrawal, severe insomnia, restlessness and agitation in the elderly

IV Infusions: Pre-eclamptic toxaemia, eclampsia, status epilepticus, acute alcohol withdrawal, sedation during regional anaesthesia

Dosage and routes:

Severe insomnia

• By mouth, 1–2 capsules at bedtime, 5–10 ml syrup

Restlessness/agitation in elderly

• By mouth, 1 capsule or 5 ml syrup 3 times a day

Alcohol withdrawal

• *Adult:* By mouth, initially 2–4 capsules, repeated if necessary in several hours; day 1, 9–12 capsules in 3 or 4 divided doses; day 2, 6–8 capsules in 3 or 4 divided doses; day 3, 4–6 capsules in 3 or 4 divided doses; then gradually reduced. Total treatment not to exceed 9 days. 5 ml of syrup can be substituted for each capsule. IV infusion, dose controlled by patient's response. See data sheet for recommendations. Not recommended for use in children

Available forms include: Capsules, 192 mg base; syrup (as edisylate), 250 mg/5 ml, (therapeutically equivalent to 1 capsule); intravenous infusion 8 mg/ml as edisylate

Side effects/adverse reactions:

RESP: Respiratory depression
HAEM: Thrombophlebitis
EENT: Sneezing, conjunctival irritation
CNS: Headache, confusion, paradoxical excitement, dependence
GI: Gastrointestinal disturbances
CV: Cardiovascular depression
SYSTEM: Hypersensitivity

Contraindications: Sensitivity to chlormethiazole, acute pulmonary insufficiency, alcoholics who continue to drink

Precautions: Cardiac or respiratory disease, chronic respiratory insufficiency, reduce dose in elderly, debilitated and in patients with hepatic or renal impairment, history of drug abuse, personality disorder, avoid prolonged use or abrupt withdrawal. Causes drowsiness; patients so affected should not drive or operate machinery

Pharmacokinetics: Peak plasma concentration within 15–45 min; extensively metabolised in liver

Interactions/Incompatibilities:

• Increased effects: CNS depressants e.g. tranquillisers, alcohol, anaesthetics, etc
• Increase in blood/plasma levels given with: cimetidine
• Sinus bradycardia: propranolol
• Adverse neonatal reactions: maternal administration of chlormethiazole and diazoxide

Clinical assessment:
• Monitor constantly when continuously infused. Danger in high doses as patient may pass into deep unconsciousness with risk of mechanical airway obstruction

Treatment of overdose: Symptomatic basis, similar principles as barbiturate overdosage. Secure airway, give oxygen, take supportive measures

NURSING CONSIDERATIONS

Assess:
• Establish baseline of BP, pulse and respiration rates

Administer:
• Orally—ensuring patient's compliance with treatment
• Use glass equipment for small children, in adults use Teflon IV cannula and change giving set every 24 hr

Perform/provide:
• Safe environment: cot sides, help with mobilisation
• Facilities for intubation and resuscitation
• Eye care; if irritation occurs check that no alcohol is consumed
• Constant monitoring of vital signs when given IV

Evaluate:
• Therapeutic effect
• Vital signs and conscious level (check by reducing IV rate during prolonged treatment) and continuous heart monitoring
• For acute confusion states resulting from hypoxia
• Side effects
• Thrombophlebitis at administration site

Teach patient/family:
• Not to take any alcohol
• That drug may cause drowsiness which persists into the next day. If this occurs not to drive or operate machinery
• That side effects include GI upsets, sneezing, headache
• About encouraging normal sleep patterns: exercise in day, milk drink, warm bath, relaxation techniques, TV/books
• Ensure patient is aware of importance of regime

---

chloroquine phosphate, chloroquine sulphate

Avloclor, Nivaquine

Func. class.: Antimalarial

Chem. class.: Synthetic 4-aminoquinoline derivative

Legal class.: POM but if for the prophylaxis of malaria P

Action: Inhibits parasite replications. Mechanism is unclear but there is interference with parasitic synthesis of nucleoproteins and influence on haemoglobin digestion

Uses: Treatment, prophylaxis and suppression of malaria caused by *Plasmodium vivax*, *Plasmodium ovale* and *Plasmodium falciparum* (some strains), rheumatoid arthritis, discoid and systemic lupus erythematosus, light sensitive skin eruptions, amoebic hepatitis and abscess

Dosage and routes:

Malaria prophylaxis
• *Adult:* By mouth 300 mg (base) weekly on same day; begin 2 weeks before journey and continue for 4 weeks after return
• *Child less than 5 weeks:* 12.5% adult dose; 6 weeks–11 months, 25% adult dose; 1–5 yr, 50% adult

dose; 6–12 yr, 75% adult dose

Malaria (benign) treatment

- *Adult:* By mouth 600 mg (base) then 300 mg after 6–8 hr, and 300 mg on subsequent 2 days
- *Child:* By mouth 10 mg/kg then 5 mg/kg after 6–8 hr, and 5 mg/kg on subsequent 2 days
- *Adult and child:* Slow IV infusion in sodium chloride 0.9% injection 10 mg/kg base over 8 hr followed by three 8-hr infusions of 5 mg/kg base; consult data sheet and BNF for further information

Amoebic hepatitis

- *Adult:* By mouth 600 mg (base) daily for 2 days then 150 mg twice daily for 2–3 weeks

Rheumatoid arthritis

- *Adult:* By mouth 150 mg (base) daily at bedtime
- *Child:* 3 mg/kg (base) per day

Systemic lupus erythematosus

- *Adult:* By mouth 150 mg (base) daily until maximum improvement then smaller maintenance dosage
- *Child:* 3 mg/kg (base) per day

Light sensitive skin eruptions

- *Adult:* By mouth 150–300 mg (base) daily
- *Child:* By mouth 3 mg/kg (base) daily

Available forms include: Tablets (phosphate) 250 mg; tablets (sulphate) 200 mg; both approximately equivalent to chloroquine base 150 mg. Syrup (sulphate) 68 mg/5 ml; equivalent to base 50 mg/5 ml. Injection (sulphate) 54.5 mg/1 ml; equivalent to base 40 mg/1 ml

Side effects/adverse reactions:

CV: ECG changes, hypotension, cardiac arrhythmias

INTEG: Pruritus, depigmentation, skin eruptions, alopecia, bleaching of hair pigment

CNS: Headache, psychosis, anxiety, personality changes

EENT: Blurred vision, irreversible retinal damage, difficulty in accommodation, corneal opacities, retinal degeneration

GI: Disturbances including nausea, vomiting, diarrhoea

HAEM: Thrombocytopenia, agranulocytosis, aplastic anaemia, neutropenia

Contraindications: No absolute contraindications

Precautions: Porphyria, hepatic and renal impairment, alcoholism, pregnancy (when malaria treatment outweighs the risks), irreversible retinal damage, psoriasis, neurological disorders especially epilepsy, G6PD deficiency, children, hypersensitivity, avoid concurrent therapy with hepatoxic drugs

Pharmacokinetics:

Period of onset: Peak 1–2 hr, half-life 3–5 days, metabolised in the liver, excreted in urine, faeces, breast milk

Interactions/incompatibilities:

- Reduced absorption: antacids
- Increased plasma concentration: cimetidine
- Chloroquine possibly increases plasma concentration of digoxin
- Antagonism of effects of: neostigmine and pyridostigmine

Clinical assessment:

- Ensure blood counts taken and examination for ocular disturbances if patient on extended treatment

Treatment of overdose: Induce vomiting, gastric lavage urgently. Institute resuscitation measures: protect airway and if necessary provide artificial ventilation. Reduce absorption of remaining chloroquine using activated charcoal. Consult data sheet for further information

NURSING CONSIDERATIONS

Administer:

- IV by slow infusion over 8 hours
- Before or after meals at same time each day to maintain drug level

Perform/provide:
• Storage in tight, light-resistant containers at room temperature; injection should be kept in cool environment
Evaluate:
• Allergic reactions: pruritus, rash, urticaria
• Blood dyscrasias: malaise, fever, bruising, bleeding (rare)
• For ototoxicity (tinnitus, vertigo, change in hearing)
• For toxicity: blurring vision, difficulty focusing, headache, dizziness, knee, ankle reflexes; drug should be discontinued immediately
Teach patient/family:
• To use sunglasses in bright sunlight to decrease photophobia
• To report hearing, visual problems, fever, fatigue, bruising, bleeding, which may indicate blood dyscrasias
• Warn against driving or operating machinery on first taking drug as visual disturbances can occur
• About side-effects that should be reported immediately
• The importance of continuing drug therapy for 4 weeks, after return, for malaria prophylaxis
• To seek immediate replacement if medication is misplaced
• To be aware of malarial risk in area of travel (also quinine resistance)

chlorothiazide

Saluric
Func. class.: Diuretic
Chem. class.: Thiazide; sulphonamide derivative
Legal class.: POM

Action: Increases excretion of water by inhibiting sodium reabsorption at beginning of distal tubule
Uses: Oedema, hypertension
Dosage and routes:
Oedema
• *Adult:* By mouth initially 250 mg–1 g once or twice a day (max. 2 g daily), maintenance 0.5–1 g daily or on alternate days, or less frequently
Oedema of premenstrual tension
• *Adult:* By mouth, 250–500 mg once or twice a day, from the first morning of symptoms to the onset of menses
Hypertension
• *Adult*: By mouth, 250–500 mg daily in single or divided doses (max 1 g daily)
Available forms include: Tablets 500 mg
Side effects/adverse reactions:
GU: Impotence, glycosuria
CNS: Paraesthesia, headache, dizziness, vertigo, weakness
GI: Nausea, vomiting, anorexia, constipation, diarrhoea, cramps, pancreatitis, gastric irritation, jaundice, salivary gland inflammation
EENT: Yellow vision, blurred vision
INTEG: Rash, urticaria, purpura, photosensitivity
HAEM: Aplastic anaemia, haemolytic anaemia, leucopenia, agranulocytosis, thrombocytopenia
CV: Hypotension, orthostatic hypotension
MISC: Hypokalaemia, hypochloraemia, hyponatraemia, hyperglycaemia, hyperuricaemia, renal dysfunction, interstitial nephritis, renal failure, muscle spasm, anaphylactic reactions
RESP: Respiratory distress: pneumonitis, pulmonary oedema
Contraindications: Hypersensitivity to thiazides or sulphonamides, anuria, severe renal or hepatic impairment, Addison's

disease, hypercalcaemia, breast feeding, porphyria

Precautions: Fluid and electrolyte imbalance, hypokalaemia, diabetes, gout, pregnancy, renal and hepatic impairment, lupus erythematosus, allergy, bronchial asthma

Pharmacokinetics:

Period of onset: Onset 2 hr, peak 4 hr, duration 6–12 hr; excreted in breast milk

Interactions/Incompatibilities:

- Increased toxicity: lithium, non-depolarising skeletal muscle relaxants, digitalis, NSAIDs, amiodarone, disopyramide, flecainide, quinidine, corticosteroids, corticotrophin
- Decreased effects of: antidiabetics
- Decreased absorption of chlorothiazide: cholestyramine, colestipol
- Decreased hypotensive response: indomethacin
- Enhanced hypotensive response: angiotensin-converting enzyme inhibitors
- Hypercalcaemia: calcium salts
- Potentiate orthostatic hypotension: alcohol, barbiturates, narcotics
- Additive effect: other hypertensives
- Decreased arterial responsiveness to pressor amines, e.g. adrenaline

Clinical assessment:

- Monitor for signs of electrolyte depletion: hypokalaemia, hypochloraemia, hyponatraemia, dehydration

Lab. test interferences: Parathyroid function tests: possibility of interference as thiazides may affect calcium metabolism

Treatment of overdose: Symptomatic and supportive therapy. Recent ingestion: emesis or gastric lavage. Treat dehydration, electrolyte imbalance, hepatic coma and hypotension. Oxygen or artificial respiration if impaired respiration

NURSING CONSIDERATIONS

Assess:

- Baseline BP, weight, fluid balance

Administer:

- In morning to avoid interference with sleep if using drug as a diuretic
- Potassium replacement as prescribed if potassium is less than 3.0
- With food if nausea occurs; absorption may be decreased slightly

Evaluate:

- Weight, fluid balance daily to determine fluid loss; effect of drug may be decreased if used daily
- BP lying, standing; postural hypotension may occur
- Glucose in urine if patient is diabetic
- Improvement in oedema of feet, legs, sacral area daily if medication is being used in congestive cardiac failure
- Improvement in CVP 8 hrly
- Signs of metabolic acidosis: drowsiness, restlessness
- Signs of hypokalaemia: irregular pulse, postural hypotension, malaise, fatigue, tachycardia, leg cramps, weakness
- Rashes, raised temperature
- Confusion, especially in elderly; take safety precautions if needed

Teach patient/family:

- To increase fluid intake 2–3 litres daily unless contraindicated
- To rise slowly from lying or sitting position
- To report muscle weakness, cramps, nausea, dizziness
- Drug may be taken with food or milk
- That blood sugar may be increased in diabetics
- To take early in day to avoid nocturia

chlorpheniramine maleate

Piriton
Func. class.: Antihistamine
Chem. class.: Alkylamine derivative
Legal class.: P (oral); POM (injection)

Action: Acts on blood vessels, GI system, respiratory system, by competing with histamine for H_1-receptor site; decreases allergic response by blocking histamine

Uses: By oral route for symptomatic relief from allergic conditions responsive to antihistamines such as hay fever, rhinitis, urticaria. By injection for emergency treatment of anaphylactic reactions

Dosage and routes:

• *Adult:* By mouth, 4 mg four to six hrly (maximum daily: 24 mg), SC/IM 10–20 mg, maximum 40 mg/24 hr; IV 10–20 mg diluted in syringe with 5–10 ml blood over 1 min

• *Children by mouth 6–12 yr:* 2 mg four to six hrly (maximum daily 12 mg), 2–5 yr: 1 mg four to six hrly (maximum daily 6 mg), 1–2 yr: 1 mg twice daily

Available forms include: Tablets 4 mg; syr 2 mg/5 ml; injection IM, SC, IV 10 mg/ml

Side effects/adverse reactions:

CNS: Various degrees of sedation; dizziness, poor coordination, inability to concentrate, excitation, headaches

CV: Hypotension, palpitations, tachycardia, arrhythmias

RESP: Increased thick secretions, chest tightness

HAEM: Haemolytic and other blood dyscrasias

INTEG: Urticaria, photosensitivity, exfoliative dermatitis

GI: Dry mouth, nausea, vomiting, diarrhoea, anorexia, constipation

EENT: Blurred vision

GU: Urinary retention

Contraindications: Hypersensitivity to H_1-receptor antagonists; patients treated with monoamine oxidase inhibitors within 14 days; premature infants; neonates

Precautions: Pregnancy, breast feeding, narrow angle glaucoma, urinary retention, prostatic hypertrophy, hepatic or cardiovascular disorders

Pharmacokinetics:

Period of onset: Onset 20–60 min, duration 8–12 hr; detoxified in liver, excreted by kidneys, (metabolites/free drug), half-life 20–24 hr

Interactions/incompatibilities:

• Increased CNS depression: alcohol, tricyclic antidepressants, anxiolytics, hypnotics

• Antagonism: betahistine—theoretical

• Enhancement of antimuscarinic effects: MAOIs. Avoid within 2 weeks of MAOI treatment.

• Additive antimuscarinic action: atropine, tricyclic antidepressants

• Causes drowsiness; patients so affected should not drive or operate machinery

Clinical assessment:

• Monitor response and watch for side effects

Lab. test interferences: May suppress positive skin test results and hence stopped several days before the test

Treatment of overdose: Administer ipecacuanha syrup or perform gastric lavage, then activated charcoal or cathartics to minimise absorption, take supportive measures

NURSING CONSIDERATIONS

Administer:

• IV; slowly over 1 min after diluting in syringe with 5–10 ml blood

• With meals if GI symptoms

occur; absorption may slightly decrease

Perform/provide:

• Frequent sips of water, rinsing of mouth for dryness

Evaluate:

• Therapeutic response: absence of running or congested nose or rashes

• Fluid balance; be alert for urinary retention, frequency, dysuria; drug should be discontinued if these occur

• Blood dyscrasias: thrombocytopenia, agranulocytosis (rare)

• Respiratory status: rate, rhythm, increase in bronchial secretions, wheezing, chest tightness

• Cardiac status: palpitations, increased pulse, hypotension, CNS stimulation

Teach patient/family:

• All aspects of drug use; to notify clinician if confusion, sedation, hypotension occurs

• To avoid driving or other hazardous activity if drowsiness occurs

• To avoid concurrent use of alcohol or other CNS depressants

chlorpromazine hydrochloride

Largactil

Func. class.: Neuroleptic

Chem. class.: Phenothiazine/antipsychotic; anti-emetic

Legal class.: POM

Action: Depresses cerebral cortex, hypothalamus, limbic system, which control activity aggression; blocks neurotransmission produced by dopamine at synapse; exhibits antagonism of α-adrenergic, cholinergic effects

Uses: Schizophrenia and other psychoses, mania and hypomania, short term adjunctive management of violent or dangerously impulsive behaviour, severe anxiety, psychomotor agitation, excitement, intractable hiccup, nausea and vomiting, induction of hypothermia

Dosage and routes:

Psychoses

• *Adult:* By mouth initially 25 mg 3 times daily or 75 mg at night increasing as required to 75–300 mg daily, maximum 1 g daily; deep IM 25–50 mg 6–8 hrly; rectal 100 mg 6–8 hrly

• *Child:* IM, by mouth 1–5 yr, 500 mcg/kg 4–6 hrly, maximum 40 mcg daily; 6–12 yr, 33%–50% adult dose, maximum 75 mg daily

Nausea and vomiting of terminal illness

• *Adult:* By mouth 10–25 mg 4–6 hrly; deep IM 25 mg initially then 25–50 mg 3–4 hrly; rectal 100 mg every 6–8 hr as needed

• *Child:* By mouth 1–5 yr, 0.5 mg/kg 4–6 hrly, maximum 40 mg daily, IM 0.5 mg/kg 6–8 hrly; 6–12 yr by mouth 0.5 mg/kg 4–6 hrly, maximum 75 mg daily, IM 0.5 mg/kg 6–8 hrly

Intractable hiccups

• *Adult:* By mouth 25–50 mg 3 or 4 times a day; IM 25–50 mg (used only if oral dose does not work); and if this fails IV infusion 25–50 mg in 500–1000 ml sodium chloride injection infused slowly

Induction of hypothermia

• *Adult:* Deep IM 25–50 mg every 6–8 hr

• *Child:* 1–12 yr, deep IM initially 0.5–1 mg/kg; maintenance 500 mcg/kg every 4–6 hr

Available forms include: Tablets 10, 25, 50, 100 mg; syrup 25 mg/5 ml, 100 mg/5 ml; suppositories 100 mg (special order); injection IM, IV 25 mg/ml

Side effects/adverse reactions:

RESP: Nasal stuffiness, respiratory depression

CNS: Extrapyramidal symptoms: pseudoparkinsonism, acute dystonias or dyskinesias, akathisia, tardive dyskinasia, agitation, drowsiness, apathy
HAEM: Leucopenia, agranulocytosis, anaemia
INTEG: Contact skin sensitisation, rash, photosensitivity
CV: Arrhythmias, ECG changes, tachycardia
GI: Dry mouth, constipation
ENDO: Galactorrhoea, gynaecomastia, amenorrhoea, impotence, weight gain
EENT: Blurred vision
MISC: Impaired liver function, hypothermia

Contraindications: Pregnancy unless clinician considers essential, bone-marrow depression, coma caused by CNS depressants

Precautions: Pregnancy, breast feeding, cardiovascular and cerebrovascular disease, elderly, respiratory disease, hepatic or renal dysfunction, epilepsy, Parkinson's disease, hypothyroidism, phaeochromocytoma, myasthenia gravis, prostate hypertrophy, leucopenia, acute infections, history of jaundice. Monitor for eye defects and abnormal skin pigmentation on prolonged use. Avoid abrupt withdrawal. May cause drowsiness, do not drive or operate machinery

Pharmacokinetics:
Period of onset: By mouth: onset erratic, peak 2–4 hr. Duration: may be detected for up to 6 months after last dose
IM: Onset 15–30 min, peak 15–20 min. Duration: may be detected for up to 6 months after last dose
IV: Onset 5 min, peak 10 min. Duration: may be detected for up to 6 months after last dose
REC: Onset erratic, peak 3 hr
Metabolised by liver, excreted in urine (metabolites), enters breast milk; 95% bound to plasma proteins; elimination half-life 10–20 hr

Interactions/incompatibilities:
- Oversedation: other CNS depressants, alcohol, barbiturates, other sedatives
- Enhanced hypotensive effect: antihypertensive drugs, anaesthetics
- Decreased absorption with: antacids
- Increased anticholinergic effects: other anticholinergics
- Decreased effects of: levadopa, amphetamine, clonidine, guanethidine, adrenaline, antiparkinsonian agents
- Reduced antipsychotic effect: anticholinergics
- Reduced response to hypoglycaemic agents
- Possible transient metabolic encephalopathy with simultaneous administration of desferrioxamine
- Increased toxicity with lithium

Lab. test interferences:
False positive: Pregnancy tests, thyroid function tests, Coombs' test
Interferes with: Adrenal medullary tests
Interferes with estimation for: 5-hydroxyindole-acetic acid, blood urea, urinary ketones and steroids, porphobilinogen and vitamin B_{12}

Treatment of overdose: Gastric lavage up to 6 hr after ingestion. Induction of vomiting unlikely to be any use. Give activated charcoal and supportive measures. Seek specialist advice

NURSING CONSIDERATIONS

Assess:
- Baseline BP (lying and standing)
- For hoarding or giving of medication to other patients

Administer:
- Being aware that drug can cause

contact sensitisation
- Drug in liquid form if hoarding is suspected (ensure drug is swallowed)

Perform/provide:
- Decreased noise input by dimming lights, avoiding loud noises
- Supervised ambulation until stabilised on medication; do not involve in strenuous exercise because fainting is possible; patient should not stand still for long periods of time
- Increased fluids to prevent constipation
- Sips of water, frequent rinsing for dry mouth

Evaluate:
- Therapeutic response: decrease in emotional excitement, hallucinations, delusions, paranoia, reorganisation of patterns of thought, speech
- Effect, orientation, loss of consciousness, reflexes, gait, coordination, sleep pattern disturbances
- BP standing and lying; report drops of 30 mmHg; pulse and respirations 4 hrly during initial treatment
- Dizziness, faintness, palpitations, tachycardia on rising
- Extrapyramidal symptoms including akathisia (inability to sit still, no pattern to movements), tardive dyskinesia (bizarre movements of the jaw, mouth, tongue, extremities), pseudoparkinsonism (rigidity, tremors, pill rolling, shuffling gait)
- Skin turgor daily
- Constipation, urinary retention daily; if these occur, increase bulk, water in diet

Teach patient/family:
- That orthostatic hypotension occurs often, and to rise from sitting or lying position gradually
- To remain lying down after IM injection for at least 30 min
- To avoid saunas, hot showers, or hot baths since hypotension may occur
- To avoid abrupt withdrawal of this drug
- To avoid non-prescribed preparations (cough, hayfever, cold) unless approved by clinician since serious drug interactions may occur; avoid use with alcohol or CNS depressants; increased drowsiness may occur
- To use a sunscreen during sun exposure to prevent photosensitivity
- Regarding compliance with drug regimen
- About necessity for meticulous oral hygiene since oral candidiasis may occur
- To report sore throat, malaise, fever, bleeding, mouth sores

---

chlorpropamide

Diabinese, Glymese
Func. class.: Oral hypoglycaemic
Chem. class.: Sulphonylurea
Legal class.: POM

Action: Causes functioning β-cells in pancreas to synthesise and release insulin, leading to drop in blood glucose levels; not effective if patient lacks functioning β-cells; effects outside the pancreas may also play a role in action

Uses: Stable, mild to moderately severe maturity onset diabetes (diabetes mellitus, type II diabetes), diabetes insipidus

Dosage and routes:

Diabetes mellitus
- *Adult:* By mouth 250 mg daily initially, with breakfast, adjusted according to response. Recommended maximum daily dose is 500 mg
- *Elderly:* By mouth 100–125 mg

daily initially but alternative drug used if possible

Diabetes insipidus

- *Adult:* up to 350 mg daily
- *Child:* up to 200 mg daily

Available forms include: Tablets 100, 250 mg

Side effects/adverse reactions:

CNS: Headache, weakness, dizziness

GI: Cholestatic jaundice, nausea, vomiting, diarrhoea

HAEM: Leucopenia, thrombocytopenia, agranulocytosis, aplastic anaemia, pancytopenia, haemolytic anaemia

INTEG: Sensitivity reactions leading to transient rashes, dermatitis, photosensitivity

ENDO: Hypoglycaemia

Contraindications: Hypersensitivity to sulphonylureas, breast feeding, insulin dependent (juvenile) diabetes mellitus, diabetic ketoacidosis, pregnancy, surgery, severe infection or trauma, serious impairment of hepatic, renal or thyroid function; porphyria

Precautions: Severe hypoglycaemic reactions, lactation

Pharmacokinetics:

Period of onset: Completely absorbed by GI route, onset 1 hr, peak 3–6 hr, duration 24 hr, half-life 36 hr, metabolised in liver, excreted in urine (metabolites and unchanged drug), breast milk, 90%–95% is plasma protein bound

Interactions/incompatibilities:

- Increased effects of chlorpropamide by drugs that are highly protein bound: NSAIDs, salicylates, sulphonamides, chloramphenicol, probenecid, coumarins, also MAOIs, β-blockers
- Alcohol intolerance with chlorpropamide may produce a disulfiram–alcohol interaction
- Decreased effectiveness and hyperglycaemia may be caused by calcium channel blockers, corticosteroids, oral contraceptives, thiazide and other diuretics, isoniazid, oestrogens, thyroid preparations, phenytoin, nicotinic acid and symphathomimetics
- Cyclophosphamide may alter diabetic control in some patients

Treatment of overdose: Acute poisoning, empty the stomach by aspiration and lavage; no loss of consciousness treat with oral glucose; severe reaction with coma use 50% glucose intravenously followed by 10% glucose as a continuous infusion; blood glucose level to be maintained above 5.6 mmol/l. In case hypoglycaemia recurs monitor patient over several days

NURSING CONSIDERATIONS

Assess:

- Blood glucose prior to administration

Administer:

- Drug 30 min before breakfast and ensure dietary allowance is consumed to prevent hypoglycaemia

Evaluate:

- Therapeutic response: decrease in polyuria, polydipsia, polyphagia, clear alertness, absence of dizziness, stable gait
- Hypoglycaemic/hyperglycaemic reaction that can occur soon after meals

Teach patient/family:

- That all food included in diet plan must be eaten in order to prevent hypoglycaemia
- To take drug in morning to prevent hypoglycaemic reactions at night
- That this drug must be continued on daily basis; explain consequence of discontinuing drug abruptly
- Symptoms of hypo- and hyperglycaemia, what to do about each
- To test urine glucose levels with

reagent strip approximately 2 hr after each meal as appropriate
• To use capillary blood glucose test while on this drug as appropriate
• To check for symptoms of cholestatic jaundice: dark urine, pruritus, yellow sclera; if these occur, clinician should be notified
• That diabetes is life-long illness, drug will not cure disease
• To carry Medic-Alert ID and/or Diabetic card for emergency purposes
• To seek clinician's advice about taking other medicines

chlortetracycline HCl

Aureomycin
Func. class.: Broad spectrum antibiotic
Chem. class.: Tetracycline
Legal class.: POM

Action: Interferes with bacterial cell synthesis
Uses: Respiratory tract infection; sexually-transmitted disease, acne; infection due to *Chlamydia*, *Brucella*, *Mycoplasma*, *Rickettsia* spp
Dosage and routes:
• *Adult:* By mouth 250–500 mg 6 hrly; topical apply 3 times a day; eye apply 2-hrly
Available forms include: Capsules 250 mg; eye ointment 1%; ointment, cream 3%
Side effects/adverse reactions:
Side effects following topical application are mild and transient.
• *GU:* Nephrotoxicity
• *CNS:* Headache, benign intracranial hypotension
• *GI:* Nausea, vomiting, diarrhoea, anorexia, hepatotoxicity, enterocolitis
• *HAEM:* Eosinophilia, neutropenia, thrombocytopenia, haemolytic anaemia
INTEG: Rash, urticaria, photosensitivity; stinging, burning at site of topical application
Contraindications: Hypersensitivity to tetracyclines, children under 12 yr, severe renal insufficiency, pregnancy, lactation, systemic lupus erythematosus
Precautions: Over growth of resistant organisms may occur with long-term use
Interactions/incompatibilities:
• Decreased absorption of tetracycline: antacids, dairy products, iron, quinalpril, calcium salts, sucralfate, bismuth, zinc
• Increased effect of: oral anticoagulants
• Decreased effect: penicillins
• Nephrotoxicity enhanced by: methoxyflurane
• Reduced effect of: oral contraceptives
Treatment of overdose:
After oral ingestion: Gastric lavage, administer milk or antacid, supportive treatment

NURSING CONSIDERATIONS

Administer:
• Enough medication to completely cover lesions (topical)
• After cleansing with soap and water and drying well before each topical application
• Orally 1 hr before or 2 hr after ferrous or milk products; 3 hr after antacid
• By mouth an hour before food or on an empty stomach; not to be taken with milk, iron preparations or antacids
Evaluate:
• Allergic reaction: burning, stinging, swelling, redness (topical)
• Therapeutic response: decrease in size, number of lesions (topical)
• Negative blood cultures following oral therapy
Teach patient/family:

For topical application:
• To use gloves when applying a cream ointment
• To avoid use of non-prescribed creams, ointments, lotions unless directed by clinician
• To wash hands before, after each application
• To avoid touching or squeezing lesions to prevent spread of infection
For oral medication:
• To avoid milk products administered at same time as tetracycline
• Avoid sun exposure since burns may occur; sunscreen does not decrease photosensitivity
• That all prescribed medication must be taken to prevent superimposed infection

chlorthalidone

Hygroton
Func. class.: Diuretic
Chem. class.: Thiazide-related; sulphonamide derivative
Legal class.: POM

Action: Acts on distal tubule by increasing excretion of water, sodium, chloride, potassium
Uses: Oedema, hypertension, diabetes insipidus
Dosage and routes:
Oedema
• By mouth: Initially 50 mg daily or 100–200 mg alternate days, reduced for maintenance
Hypertension
• By mouth: 25–50 mg daily
Diabetes insipidus
• By mouth: Initially 100 mg twice a day reduced to 50 mg daily for maintenance, where possible
Available forms include: Tablets 50 mg
Side effects/adverse reactions:
GU: Uraemia, glycosuria
CNS: Drowsiness, paraesthesia, dizziness
GI: Nausea, vomiting, anorexia, constipation, diarrhoea, cramps, pancreatitis, hepatitis
EENT: Blurred vision
INTEG: Rash, urticaria
META: Hyperglycaemia, hyperuraemia, increased creatinine
HAEM: Aplastic anaemia, haemolytic anaemia, leucopenia, agranulocytosis, thrombocytopenia
CV: Irregular pulse, orthostatic hypotension
ELECT: Hypokalaemia, hypercalcaemia, hyponatraemia, hypochloraemia, hypomagnesaemia
Contraindications: Hypersensitivity to thiazides or sulphonamides, severe renal or hepatic disease, hypercalcaemia, Addison's disease, symptomatic hyperuricaemia
Precautions: Hypokalaemia, renal disease, pregnancy, hepatic disease, gout, lupus erythematosus, diabetes mellitus, coronary or cerebral arteriosclerosis, lactation, hyperlipidaemia
Pharmacokinetics:
Period of onset: Onset 2 hr, peak 6 hr, duration 24–72 hr; excreted unchanged by kidneys, enters breast milk, half-life 35–55 hr
Interactions/incompatibilities:
• Increased toxicity: lithium, digitalis, carbenoxolone, corticosteroids, corticotrophin, NSAIDs
• Increased effects of: antihypertensive drugs (e.g. guanethidine, methyldopa, β-blockers, vasodilators, calcium antagonists and angiotensin-converting enzyme inhibitors), non-depolarizing skeletal muscle relaxants
• Decreased effects of: antidiabetics, disopyramide
• Decreased absorption of thiazides: cholestyramine, colestipol

• Decreased hypotensive response: NSAIDs

Clinical assessment:

• Electrolytes: potassium, sodium, chloride; include blood urea nitrogen, blood sugar, full blood count, serum creatinine, blood lipids (in hyperlipidaemic patients)

Treatment of overdose: Lavage, emesis or activated charcoal, monitor electrolytes and blood pressure, and give supportive treatment

NURSING CONSIDERATIONS

Assess:

• Baseline BP standing, lying; respirations, weight, fluid balance

Administer:

• Orally. In morning to avoid interference with sleep if using as a diuretic

• Potassium replacement may be required in severe cases of oedema, hepatic cirrhosis and in long-term therapy

• With food if nausea occurs; absorption may be decreased slightly

Evaluate:

• Weight during initial treatment: fluid balance to determine fluid loss.

• Initial effect of drug, increase or decreasing—then reduce where possible to a maintenance dose

• Rate, depth, rhythm of respiration, effect of exertion

• Effect of any other drugs taken e.g. digoxin may need to be reduced in congestive cardiac failure

• BP lying, standing; postural hypotension may occur

• Regular urinalysis

• Improvement in oedema of feet, legs, sacral area daily if medication is being used in congestive heart failure

• Improvement in CVP 8 hrly

• Signs of metabolic acidosis: infrequent and mild; usually resolve spontaneously or following temporary reduction of dosage

• Signs of hypokalaemia: postural hypotension, malaise, fatigue, tachycardia, leg cramps, weakness

• Rashes

• Confusion, especially in elderly; electrolyte balance (precarious)

Teach patient/family:

• To increase fluid intake to 2–3 litres daily unless contraindicated. To rise slowly from lying or sitting position

• To notify clinician of muscle weakness, cramps, nausea, dizziness, gout, increase in oedema

• Drug may be taken with food or milk if nausea occurs

• To take in morning for oedema

• To test urine

---

cholera vaccine

Func. class.: Vaccine
Chem. class.: Killed suspension of *Vibrio cholerae*
Legal class.: POM

Action: Stimulates antibodies to causative organism of cholera

Uses: Provides some protection against the bacterium *Vibrio cholerae*

Dosage and routes:

• Two doses, minimum 1 week, preferably 4 weeks apart; deep subcutaneous or IM injection

• *Adult:* First dose, 0.5 ml; 2nd dose, 1.0 ml

• *Child 1–5 yr:* First dose, 0.1 ml; 2nd dose, 0.3 ml

• *Child 5–10 yr:* First dose, 0.3 ml; 2nd dose, 0.5 ml

Available forms include: Multidose injection 10 ml, single dose 1.5 ml

Side effects/adverse reactions:

CNS: Headache

INTEG: Mild discomfort at injection site

NERV: Neuritis, polyneuritis

SYST: Mild fever and malaise
Contraindications: Existing acute illness hypersensitivity, infants less than 1 yr
Precautions: Pregnancy
Pharmacokinetics: Immunity persists for 6 months
Clinical assessment:
- Immune status

NURSING CONSIDERATIONS
Assess:
- Active or suspected infection
- History of allergies or known hypersensitivity to any component

Administer:
- Deep subcutaneous or IM route. To reduce reactions use the intradermal route after repeated doses
- At least 1 week between doses and preferably 4 weeks
- Shake well prior to use
- Discard unused vaccine at the end of session

Perform/provide:
- Store at 2–8°C, protect from light. Record details (lot numbers) of vaccine and patient
- Ensure correct documentation completed
- Facilities for dealing with anaphylaxis

Evaluate:
- Reaction to vaccination
- Level of patient understanding for further precautions against cholera

Teach patient/family:
- That general food/water hygiene is still required
- That full immunity is not immediate, unless it is a booster dose
- Remind that documents needed in some countries
- Recommend further dose in 6 months if living in endemic area
- Warn about general malaise, raised temperature and mild discomfort at site

cholestyramine

Questran, Questran A
Func. class.: Hypolipidaemic
Chem. class.: Bile acid sequestrant
Legal class.: POM

Action: Adsorbs, combines with bile acids to form insoluble complex that is excreted through faeces; loss of bile acids lowers cholesterol levels
Uses: Primary hyperlipidemia; pruritus associated with biliary obstruction; diarrhoea caused by ileal resection, radiation, vagotomy, Crohn's disease, vagal neuropathy
Dosage and routes:
- *Adult:* By mouth. Hyperlipidaemia, diarrhoea 12–24 g daily, maximum 36 g daily. Pruritus 4–8 g daily
- *Child 6–12 yrs:* Initial dose based on following calculation (child's weight in kg × adult dose) ÷ 70. Subsequent dosage adjustment may be necessary where clinically indicated

Available forms include: Powder 4 g
Side effects/adverse reactions:
GI: Constipation, abdominal pain, nausea, faecal impaction, aggravation of haemorrhoids, flatulence, vomiting, diarrhoea
INTEG: Rash, irritation of perianal area
HAEM: Decreased vitamin A, D, K leading to increased bleeding tendency, hyperchloremic acidosis
Contraindications: Hypersensitivity, complete biliary obstruction
Precautions: Pregnancy, lactation, children under 6 yr
Pharmacokinetics:
Period of onset: Maximum effect in 2 weeks; excreted in faeces
Interactions/incompatibilities:
- Decrease absorption of phenyl-

butazone, warfarin, thiazides, digitalis, penicillins, tetracyclines, phenobarbitone, folic acid, corticosteroids, iron, thyroxine, clindamycin, trimethoprim, chenodeoxycholic acid, anticoagulants, paracetamol, vitamins A, D, K
• Decreased activity of oral vancomycin

Clinical assessment:
• Cardiac glycoside level, if both drugs are being administered
• Clotting time if anticoagulants are being co-administered
• Serum cholesterol, triglyceride levels, electrolytes if on extended therapy

NURSING CONSIDERATIONS

Assess:
• For signs of vitamin A, D, K deficiency

Administer:
• Drug before meals, at bedtime; give all other medications 1 hr before cholestyramine or 4–6 hr after cholestyramine to avoid poor absorption
• Drug sprinkled on foodor stirred into beverage; let stand for 2 min
• May result in excess foaming if mixed with carbonated drinks (use large glass)

Evaluate:
• Bowel pattern daily; increase bulk, water in diet if constipation develops
• Therapeutic response: decreased triglyceride, cholesterol level (hyperlipidaemia); diarrhoea, pruritus (excess bile)

Teach patient/family:
• Symptoms of hypothrombinaemia: bleeding mucous membranes, dark tarry stools, petechiae; report immediately
• Stress patient compliance since toxicity may result if doses are missed
• That risk factors should be decreased: high fat diet, smoking, alcohol consumption, absence of exercise
• That non-prescribed preparations should be avoided unless directed by clinician

---

choline magnesium trisalicylate

Trilisate

Func. class.: Anti-inflammatory analgesic
Chem. class.: Salicylate
Legal class.: P

Action: Prevents inflammation and pain impulse production by peripheral and CNS inhibition of prostaglandin synthesis; antipyretic action results from inhibition of hypothalamic heat-regulating centre

Uses: Rheumatoid arthritis, osteoarthritis

Dosage and routes:
• *Adult:* By mouth 0.5–1.5 g twice a day

Available forms include: Tablets 500 mg

Side effects/adverse reactions:
HAEM: Thrombocytopenia, agranulocytosis, leucopenia, neutropenia, haemolytic anaemia, increased bleeding time
CNS: Stimulation, drowsiness, dizziness, confusion, convulsions, headache, flushing, hallucinations, coma
GI: Nausea, vomiting, GI bleeding, diarrhoea, heartburn, anorexia, hepatitis
INTEG: Rash, urticaria, bruising
EENT: Tinnitus, hearing loss
CV: Rapid pulse, pulmonary oedema
RESP: Wheezing, hyperpnoea
ENDO: Hypoglycaemia, hyponatraemia, hypokalaemia

Contraindications: Hypersensitivity

to salicylates, GI bleeding, haemophilia, active peptic ulcer, children less than 12 yr
Precautions: Anaemia, hepatic disease, renal disease, Hodgkin's disease, pregnancy, lactation, gastritis
Pharmacokinetics:
Period of onset: Onset 15–30 min, peak 1–2 hr, duration 4–6 hr, metabolised by liver, excreted by kidneys, excreted in breast milk, half-life 1–3½ hr
Interactions/incompatibilities:
• Decreased effects of this drug: antacids, steroids, urinary alkalinisers
• Increased effects of this drug: metoclopramide
• Increased blood loss: alcohol, heparin
• Increased effects of: anticoagulants, insulin, methotrexate, phenytoin, sulphonylurea hypoglycaemics
• Decreased effects of: probenecid, spironolactone, sulfinpyrazone
• Toxic effects: Digoxin, acetazolamide
Clinical assessment:
• Liver function studies: aspartate aminotransferase, alanine aminotransferase, bilirubin, if patient is on long-term therapy
• Renal function studies: blood urea nitrogen, serum creatinine if patient is on long-term therapy
• Blood studies: Full blood count, Hb, prothrombin-time if patient is on long-term therapy
Lab. test interferences:
Increase: Coagulation studies, liver function studies, serum uric acid, amylase, CO_2, urinary protein
Decrease: Serum potassium, protein bound iodine, cholesterol
Treatment of overdose: Lavage with sodium bicarbonate solution 5%, monitor electrolytes and vital signs

NURSING CONSIDERATIONS
Assess:
• Baseline weight and fluid balance
Administer:
• Crushed or whole; chewable tablets may be chewed
• 30 min before or 2 hr after meals
Perform/provide:
• Repositioning to decrease pain
• Cool cloth for fever
Evaluate:
• Fluid balance; decreasing output may indicate renal failure (long-term therapy)
• Hepatotoxicity: dark urine, clay-coloured stools, yellowing of skin, sclera, itching, abdominal pain, fever, diarrhoea if patient is on long-term therapy
• Allergic reactions: rash, urticaria; if these occur, drug may need to be discontinued
• Renal dysfunction: decreased urine output
• Ototoxicity: tinnitus, ringing, roaring in ears
• Visual changes: blurring, halos, corneal, retinal damage
• Oedema in feet, ankles, legs
• Prior drug history; there are many drug interactions
• Weight changes
Teach patient/family:
• To report any symptoms of hepatotoxicity, renal toxicity, visual changes, ototoxicity, allergic reactions (long-term therapy)
• Not to exceed recommended dosage; acute poisoning may result
• To read label on other non-prescription drugs; many contain aspirin and should not be taken
• That therapeutic response takes 2 weeks (arthritis)
• To avoid alcohol ingestion; GI bleeding may occur
• To record weight daily

choline theophyllinate

Choledyl, Sabidal SR
Func. class.: Bronchodilator
Chem. class.: Choline salt of theophylline
Legal class.: P

Action: Relaxes smooth muscle of respiratory system by blocking phosphodiesterase, which increases cyclic-AMP; 64% theophylline
Uses: Relief and prevention of bronchospasm in asthma, chronic bronchitis and emphysema
Dosage and routes:
• *Adult and child over 12 yr:* By mouth 100–400 mg 4 times a day; modified-release tablets 424 mg, one twice daily increasing after 3 days to one morning and two evening
• *Child 3–6 yr:* By mouth 62.5–125 mg 8 hrly
• *6–12 yr:* 300–400 mg daily in divided doses. Adjust doses to desired response, and therapeutic level
Narrow margin between therapeutic and dose, plasma levels must be monitored: optimum theophylline level 10–20 mg/l
Available forms include: Elixir 62.5 mg/5 ml; tablets 100 mg, 200 mg, modified-release tablets 424 mg
Side effects/adverse reactions:
CNS: Anxiety, restlessness, insomnia, dizziness, convulsions, headache, lightheadedness
CV: Palpitations, sinus tachycardia, hypotension
GI: Nausea, vomiting, anorexia, diarrhoea, bitter taste, dyspepsia
RESP: Increased rate
INTEG: Flushing, urticaria
Contraindications: Hypersensitivity to xanthines, tachydysrhythmias; porphyria; concurrent use of other xanthines; concurrent use of ephedrine in children
Precautions: Elderly, congestive cardiac failure, cor pulmonale, hepatic disease, active peptic ulcer disease, hyperthyroidism, hypertension, children, cardiac disease
Pharmacokinetics:
Rapid absorbtion, metabolised in liver, excreted in urine, breast milk
Interactions/incompatibilities:
• Decreased action of this drug: phenytoin, rifampicin, aminoglutethimide, carbamazepine smoking, alcohol
• Increased action of this drug: cimetidine, erythromycin, allopurinol, propranolol, oral contraceptives, influenza vaccine, β-adrenergic agonists
• Cardiotoxicity: ephedrine and other sympathomimetics
Clinical assessment:
• Assess therapeutic blood levels; toxicity may occur with small increase above therapeutic level peak serum levels not greater than 20 mcg/ml, optimum is 10–20 mcg/ml
Treatment of overdose: Induced emesis or gastric lavage, activated charcoal, saline laxative and in severe cases (usually serum theophylline of 40 mg/litre or more) charcoal haemoperfusion. For fall in blood pressure nurse in head down position. Monitor and correct electrolyte imbalances

NURSING CONSIDERATIONS

Administer:
• After meals to decrease GI symptoms; swallow monitored release tablets whole with water
Evaluate:
• Therapeutic response: absence of dyspnoea, wheezing
• Fluid balance: if diuresis occurs, dehydration may result in elderly or children
• Respiratory rate, rhythm, depth; notify clinician of abnormalities

• Allergic reactions: rash, urticaria; if these occur, inform clinician and withhold further doses

Teach patient/family:

• To check non-prescribed medications, current prescription medications for ephedrine, which will increase stimulation

• To avoid hazardous activities; dizziness may occur

• On all aspects of drug therapy: dosage, routes, side effects, when to notify the clinician

• If GI upset occurs, to take drug with 200 ml water; avoid food; absorption may be decreased

chorionic gonadotrophin, human

Gonadotrophon LH, Profasi, Pregnyl

Func. class.: Human chorionic gonadotrophin

Chem. class.: Polypeptide hormone

Legal class.: POM

Action: Stimulates production of gonadal steroids, stimulates ovulation from developed follicles

Uses: Infertility, anovulation, hypogonadism, non-obstructive cryptorchidism

Dosage and routes:

Infertility/anovulation

• *Adult:* IM 10,000 U 1 day after last dose of menotrophin

Hypogonadism

• *Adult:* IM 500–2000 U 2 or 3 times a week for minimum 4 months, when menotrophin may be added if required

Cryptorchidism

• *Child (boy 4–9 yr):* IM 500–1000 U alternate days for several weeks

Available forms include: Powder for injection 500, 1000, 2000, 5000 U

Side effects/adverse reactions:

CNS: Headache, depression, fatigue, anxiety, irritability

GU: Gynaecomastia, early puberty, oedema, ectopic pregnancy, multiple pregnancy

INTEG: Pain at injection site

Contraindications: Hypersensitivity, pituitary hypertrophy/tumour, early puberty, prostatic cancer

Precautions: Where fluid retention may be dangerous: asthma, migraine, convulsive disorders, cardiac disease, renal disease

Pharmacokinetics:

IM: Peak 6 hr, half-life 11–24 hr, excreted by kidneys

Interactions/incompatibilities:

None known

Treatment of overdose: Conservative support required for ovarian hyperstimulation

NURSING CONSIDERATIONS

Assess:

• Baseline BP, weight, fluid balance

Administer:

• Only after clomiphene citrate has been tried on anovulatory client

• After reconstitution with solvent enclosed in package

Evaluate:

• Weight weekly; notify clinician if weekly weight gain is more than 2 kg

• BP

• Be alert for decreasing urinary output, increasing oedema

• Oedema, hypertension

Teach patient/family:

• All aspects of drug usage

• That some lower abdominal pain may occur 36 hr after administration

• Advise best time to have intercourse – about 36 hr after injection

• To report persistent or severe abdominal pain, abdominal distension or breathlessness immediately

• To report symptoms of ectopic pregnancy: dizziness, pain on one side or shoulder, pallor, weak thready pulse, haemorrhage (shock may proceed rapidly)
• To report facial, axillary, pubic hair, change in voice, penile enlargement, acne in male, abdominal pain, distention, vaginal bleeding in women. (Changes only for long-term use)

cilazapril ▼

Vascace
Func. class.: Antihypertensive
Chem. class.: Angiotensin converting enzyme (ACE); inhibitor
Legal class.: POM

Action: Selectively suppresses renin-angiotensin-aldosterone system; inhibits angiotensin converting enzyme (ACE); prevents conversion of angiotensin I to angiotensin II, reducing vasoconstriction
Uses: All grades of essential hypertension and renovascular hypertension where standard therapy is ineffective or inappropriate because of adverse effects
Dosage and routes:
• *Adult:* By mouth, initially 1 mg (500 mcg in patients with congestive heart failure) once daily; usual range 2.5–5 mg once daily
• *Elderly:* Initiate therapy with 500 mcg once daily and adjust according to response
Available forms include: Tablets 0.25, 0.5, 1, 2–5 mg
Side effects/adverse reactions:
CNS: Headache, dizziness, fatigue
CV: Hypotension
GI: Dyspepsia, nausea
GU: Raised serum creatinine/urea
HAEM: Decreased haemoglobin, haematocrit and/or white cell count
INTEG: Rash
RESP: Cough
SYST: Allergic reactions including angioneurotic oedema
Contraindications: Hypersensitivity; ascites; pregnancy; breast-feeding
Precautions: Cardiac failure; renal impairment; liver cirrhosis; dehydration; low-sodium diet
Interactions:
• Exaggerated hypotensive response: other antihypertensives, diuretics, general anaesthetics
• Hyperkalaemia: Potassium sparing diuretics; potassium supplements; cyclosporin
• Reduced antihypertensive effect: NSAIDs. Raised blood levels of lithium: give concomitantly
Treatment of overdose: Symptomatic and supportive treatment. Hypotension should be treated by volume expansion. Can be removed from the body by haemodialysis if indicated

NURSING CONSIDERATIONS

Assess:
• Vital signs (temperature, pulse, respiration, BP), ECG, renal function, fluid balance, weight
Administer:
• By mouth
• With patient under supervision, preferably in bed (profound hypotension often occurs in early stages of medication)
Perform/provide:
• Monitoring of BP, pulse
• Reduced potassium supplements to prevent hyperkalaemia
Evaluate:
• Therapeutic effect over several months (dependent on reason for medication)
• Side effects
• Fluid balance
Teach patient/family:
• About the drug

• About side effects, particularly hypotension. Dry cough may occur (clinician prescribing another ACE inhibitor may deal with this)
• To report any side effects to nurse or clinician
• Not to discontinue taking tablets without medical advice
• To rise slowly to standing to reduce postural hypotension
• If dizziness occurs, to avoid hazardous activities, including driving, until stabilised on medication

cimetidine

Tagamet, Dyspamet, Peptimax, Phimetin, Galenamet, combination product
Func. class.: H_2 receptor antagonist
Chem. class.: Imidazole derivative
Legal class.: POM

Action: Antagonises histamine at H_2 receptor site in parietal cells, which inhibits gastric acid secretion
Uses: Treatment and prophylaxis of benign gastric and duodenal ulcer; Zollinger-Ellison syndrome; reflux oesophagitis, prophylaxis for stress ulcer, Mendelson's syndrome
Dosage and routes:
Gastric/duodenal ulcer
• *Adult:* By mouth, 400 mg twice a day or 800 mg at night for 4–6 weeks (8 weeks in NSAID associated ulceration), maximum 2.4 g daily in divided doses
• *Child:* By mouth or injection, 20–30 mg/kg daily in divided doses
Prophylaxis
• *Adult:* By mouth, 400 mg at night or twice a day
Reflux oesophagitis
• *Adult:* By mouth, 400 mg 4 times a day for 4–8 weeks
Zollinger-Ellison syndrome
• *Adult:* By mouth, 400 mg 4 times a day increased as required, normal maximum 2.4 g daily in divided doses
Acid aspiration syndrome:
• *Adult:* Tablet 400 mg at start of labour or 90–120 min before induction of anaesthesia
Before pancreatic enzyme supplements:
• *Adult:* By mouth, 800–1600 mg daily or divided doses an hour before meals
Prophylaxis of stress ulceration:
• *Adult:* By mouth IV/IM 200–400 mg 4–6 hourly (maximum direct IV dose 200 mg)
Injection:
• *Adult: IM 200 mg 4–6 hourly*
• *IV infusion 400 mg in 100 ml 4–6 hourly*
• *IV injection: if unavoidable consult data sheet*
Available forms include: Tablets 200 mg, 400 mg, 800 mg; liquid/suspension 200 mg/5 ml; injection 200 mg; infusion 400 mg in 100 ml 0.9% sodium chloride; chewable tablets 200 mg; soluble tablets 400 mg
Side effects/adverse reactions:
CNS: Headache, depression, dizziness, anxiety, weakness, psychosis, tremors, convulsions, confusion
GI: Diarrhoea, abdominal cramps, paralytic ileus, jaundice, altered bowel habit
GU: Gynaecomastia, galactorrhoea, impotence, interstitial nephritis
CV: Bradycardia, tachycardia
HAEM: Agranulocytosis, thrombocytopenia, neutropenia, aplastic anaemia, increase in bleeding time
INTEG: Urticaria, rash, alopecia, sweating, flushing, exfoliative dermatitis
Contraindications: Hypersensitivity to cimetidine
Precautions: Pregnancy, lactation,

hepatic disease, renal disease
Pharmacokinetics:
Period of onset: Peak 1–1½ hr after oral administration, half-life 1½ hr; metabolised by liver, excreted in urine (unchanged), enters breast milk
Interactions/incompatibilities:
• Increased toxicity: fluorouracil, flecainide, disopyramide, pethidine, metronidazole, quinine, metformin, metoprolol, propranolol, phenytoin, quinidine, theophylline, tricyclic antidepressants, lignocaine, anticoagulants, carbamazepine
• Decreased action of this drug: rifampicin
Clinical assessment:
• Blood urea nitrogen, creatinine; plasma phenytoin levels in patients on both drugs
Treatment of overdose: Gastric lavage or forced emesis
NURSING CONSIDERATIONS
Assess:
• Fluid balance ratio
• Temperature, pulse, respiration and BP
Administer:
• With meals for prolonged drug effect
• Only the direct IV injection if unavoidable IV slowly (maximum 200 mg over at least 2 mins); arhrythmias may occur infusion is preferable
• Give infusion over 30 min–1 hr)
Teach patient/family:
• About side effects
• That gynaecomastia, impotence may occur, but is reversible after treatment is ended
• Avoid driving or other hazardous activities until patient is stabilised on this medication
• Give dietary advice
• To avoid non-prescribed preparations: aspirin, cough, cold preparations
• Inform clinician if pregnancy is suspected

---

ciprofibrate ▼

Modalim
Func. class.: Hypolipidaemic agent
Chem. class.: Isobutyric acid derivative
Legal class.: POM

Action: Decreases serum triglycerides, LDL and VLDL cholesterol and raises HDL cholesterol levels
Uses: Hyperlipidaemias of Frederickson types IIa, IIb, III and IV in patients who have not responded adequately to diet
Dosage and routes:
• *Adult:* By mouth; initially 100 mg once daily adjusted according to therapeutic response, maximum 200 mg once daily
Available forms include: Tablets, 100 mg
Side effects/adverse reactions:
CNS: Headache, vertigo
GI: Diarrhoea, dyspepsia
GU: Impotence
INTEG: Hair loss
MS: Myalgia
Contraindications: Hypersensitivity, severe hepatic impairment, severe renal impairment, pregnancy, breast-feeding
Precautions: Impaired renal or hepatic function
Interactions:
• Enhanced effect of: oral anticoagulants, antidiabetic agents
Treatment of overdose: Symptomatic and supportive treatment, gastric lavage if recently ingested
NURSING CONSIDERATIONS
Assess:
• Vital signs (temperature, pulse, respiration, BP); ECG, weight, diabetic status

• Life-style: eating, drinking, smoking, work habits

Administer:

• By mouth after food; dose adjusted according to therapeutic response. Nocturnal administration may help to reduce GU symptoms

Perform/provide:

• Recording of weight regularly
• Appropriate diet
• Counselling/advice about side effects such as hair loss and impotence

Evaluate:

• Therapeutic response
• Wide range of side effects

Teach patient/family:

• About the drug
• About side effects and to report any of these to nurse or clinician
• About other methods of reducing heart disease factors: diet, smoking, exercise, stress
• Importance of adhering to low-fat diet
• To monitor diabetic and/or anticoagulant control regularly (may be desirable to visit clinic more often)

---

ciprofloxacin

Ciproxin
Func. class.: Broad spectrum antibiotic
Chem. class.: 4-quinolone
Legal class.: POM

Action: Inhibits the enzyme DNA gyrase, preventing bacterial synthesis of functional DNA

Uses: Infection due to Gram-negative or Gram-positive bacteria, including those resistant to other antibiotics. Anaerobic bacteria, *Ureaplasma* and some *Mycobacteria* are normally less susceptible

Dosage and routes:

Uncomplicated urinary tract infections

• *Adult:* By mouth 250 mg 12 hrly; IV 100 mg 12 hrly

Complicated/severe urinary tract infections

• *Adult:* By mouth 500 mg 12 hrly; IV 200 mg 12 hrly

Respiratory, bone, skin, joint infections

• *Adult:* By mouth 250–750 mg 12 hrly; IV 200 mg 12 hrly

Gonorrhoea

• *Adult:* By mouth 250 mg as a single dose; IV, 100 mg as a single dose

Available forms include: Tablets 250, 500 mg (as hydrochloride); injection 100, 200 mg (as lactate)

Side effects/adverse reactions:

CNS: Headache, dizziness, fatigue, insomnia, depression, restlessness, confusion, convulsions

GI: Nausea, abdominal pain, flatulence, heartburn, vomiting, diarrhoea, oral candidiasis, dysphagia, increased alanine aminotransferase, aspartate aminotransferase

INTEG: Rash, pruritus, urticaria, photosensitivity, flushing, fever, chills

MS: Blurred vision, tinnitus

Contraindications: Hypersensitivity to quinolones, children, adolescents

Precautions: Pregnancy, lactation, children, severe renal disease, history of convulsive disorder

Pharmacokinetics:

Period of onset: Peak 1 hr, half-life 3–4 hr; excreted in urine as active drug, metabolites

Interactions/incompatibilities:

• Decreased absorption: magnesium antacids, aluminium hydroxide, iron salts
• Increased serum levels of ciprofloxacin: probenecid
• Increased theophylline levels when used with ciprofloxacin

• Prolonged bleeding time when administered with anticoagulants
Clinical assessment:
• Serum theophylline levels in patients receiving both drugs
Treatment of overdose: Gastric lavage

NURSING CONSIDERATIONS

Assess:
• Fluid balance and urinary pH. pH of less than 5.5 is ideal

Administer:
• IV, by direct infusion over 30–60 min. Adjust dose in severe renal impairment.
• After a clean midstream specimen of urine has been obtained for bacterial culture and sensitivity tests
• Advise patient to limit intake of highly alkaline foods, drugs, and dairy products, peanuts, vegetables, antacids and sodium bicarbonate

Evaluate:
• Response to treatment indicated by decreased dysuria, frequency, urgency and negative bacteriological test results, which suggest that infection has resolved
• Allergic reactions: fever, rash, urticaria, pruritus
• CNS symptoms: headache, dizziness, fatigue, insomnia, depression

Teach patient/family:
• Avoid antacids containing magnesium or aluminium until at least 4 hr after taking the drug
• To avoid sunlight or use suncare preparations as photosensitivity occurs
• Fluid intake must be increased to 3 litres daily to avoid crystallisation and renal calculi
• If dizziness occurs ambulant patients require careful supervision
• The full course of treatment must be completed
• The clinician must be informed if adverse reactions occur
• Medication must be taken with food or milk to reduce gastric irritation
• Effects of alcohol can be enhanced

cisapride

Prepulsid, Alimix
Func. class.: Gastrointestinal prokinetic agent
Chem. class.: Methoxybenzamide
Legal class.: POM

Action: Cisapride probably acts by enhancing the release of acetylcholine at the level of the myenteric plexus in the gut wall
Uses: Treatment of symptoms (e.g. heartburn, regurgitation) and mucosal lesions associated with gastro-oesophageal reflux. Relief of symptoms (e.g. nausea, early satiety, anorexia, bloating, epigastric pain) of impaired gastric motility secondary to disturbed and delayed gastric emptying associated with diabetes, systemic sclerosis and autonomic neuropathy
Dosage and routes:
Gastro-oesophageal reflux
• *Adult:* By mouth 10 mg 3 or 4 times a day for 12 weeks, maintainance usually 20 mg at bedtime or 10 mg twice a day
Impaired gastric motility
• *Adult:* By mouth 10 mg 3 or 4 times a day for at least 6 weeks
Non-ulcer dyspepsia
• *Adult:* By mouth 10 mg 3 times a day for usually 4 weeks
• *Children (below 12 yr):* Not recommended
Available forms include: Tablets 10 mg, suspension 5 mg/5ml

Side effects/adverse reactions:
CNS: Headache, lightheadedness, convulsions
GI: Abdominal cramps, borborygmi, diarrhoea
Contraindications: Pregnancy; gastrointestinal haemorrhage; mechanical obstruction; perforation.
Precautions: Elderly, renal or hepatic impairment, lactation. Accelerates gastric emptying so gastric absorption of concomitant drugs can be diminished, while intestinal absorption is increased. Plasma levels of drugs needing careful titration, e.g. anticonvulsants
Pharmacokinetics: Rapidly absorbed, peak 1–2 hr, elimination half-life 10 hr, metabolised by liver, excreted in urine, faeces. Cisapride is extensively bound to plasma proteins
Treatment of overdose: Gastric lavage, close observation and general supportive measures

NURSING CONSIDERATIONS

Assess:
- Bowel pattern before treatment

Administer:
- 15 to 30 min before a meal. When an additional dose is required to control night-time symptoms, the tablet should be taken at bedtime

Evaluate:
- Reduction of symptoms.
- Bowel pattern during treatment

Teach patient/family:
- Not to take non-prescribed medicines
- To inform clinician if pregnancy occurs

cisplatin

Func. class.: Antineoplastic alkylating agent
Chem. class.: Platinum complex
Legal class.: POM

Action: Alkylates DNA, RNA; inhibits enzymes that allow synthesis of proteins
Uses: Advanced bladder cancer, lung cancer, stomach cancer, adjunctive in metastatic testicular cancer, adjunctive in metastatic ovarian cancer
Dosage and routes:
Doses are highly variable, and dependent on local treatment protocols, concomitant therapy and tumour type; the following dose schedules have been used:
- *Adult:* IV infusion 50–120 mg/m^2 every 3–4 weeks as a single agent, or 15–20 mg/m^2 daily for 5 days every 3–4 weeks as a single agent

Available forms include: Injection 1.0 mg/ml; powder for preparing IV solution, 50 mg
Side effects/adverse reactions:
EENT: Tinnitus, hearing loss, vestibular toxicity
HAEM: Thrombocytopenia, leucopenia, pancytopenia
CV: Cardiac abnormalities
GI: Nausea, vomiting, diarrhoea, weight loss
GU: Renal tubular damage, renal insufficiency, impotence, sterility, amenorrhoea, gynaecomastia, hyperuraemia
INTEG: Alopecia, dermatitis, peripheral neuropathy
CNS: Convulsions
RESP: Fibrosis
META: Hypomagnesaemia, hypocalcaemia, hypokalaemia, hypophosphataemia
Contraindications: Hypersensi-

tivity, dehydration, renal impairment, hearing disorders, depressed bone marrow function, pregnancy, breast-feeding

Precautions: Live vaccines, radiation therapy within 1 month, chemotherapy within 1 month, thrombocytopenia

Pharmacokinetics: Mainly excreted in urine; half-life of unbound, active drug 1 hr

Interactions/incompatibilities:

• Increased toxicity: aminoglycosides

Clinical assessment:

• Full blood count, differential, platelet count weekly; withhold drug if WBC is less than 2000, or platelet count is less than 75,000; notify clinician of results

• Renal function studies: blood urea nitrogen, serum uric acid, urine creatinine clearance before, during therapy

Treatment of overdose:

Monitor blood count, renal function, electrolytes. Correct electrolyte imbalances; transfusion products, filgrastim as needed

NURSING CONSIDERATIONS

Assess:

• Baseline vital signs

Administer:

• HANDLING: take safety precautions appropriate to antineoplastic agents

• Following local antineoplastic (cytotoxic) policies

• After ensuring that clinician is aware of blood results

• IV: by slow IV infusion over 2–8 hours following 1–2 hours prehydration and preceding 8–12 hours post-hydration

• Avoid use of aluminium equipment as cisplatin is degraded on contact

• Other medications by mouth if possible. Avoid IV, IM, SC routes to prevent infection and bruising

• Anti-emetic 30–60 min before treatment

• Sedation during treatment (usually haloperidol and lorazepam)

• All other medication as prescribed including analgesics, antibiotics, anti-emetics, antispasmodics

Perform/provide:

• Strict medical asepsis, protective isolation if WBC levels are low

• Strict fluid balance with forced diuresis for patients on high doses

• Anti-emetics before and during treatment

• Sedation during treatment (usually haloperidol and lorazepam)

• Storage protected from light, at room temperature, for 20 hr once reconstituted

• Special skin care

• Increase fluid intake to 2–3 litre/daily to prevent urate deposits, calculi formation

• Diet low in purines: offal (kidney, liver), dried beans, peas to maintain alkaline urine

Evaluate:

• Weight

• Temperature and blood pressure 4 hrly when neutropenic. Changes may indicate start of infection

• Fluid balance; report fall in urine output of 30 ml/hr

• Bruising, bleeding due to thrombocytopenia, cytopenia

• Nausea and vomiting

• Diarrhoea

• Fluid overload

• Signs of infection

• Dyspnoea, râles, unproductive cough, chest pain, tachypnoea

• Urinalysis changes indicate nephrotoxicity

• Effects of alopecia on body image, discuss feelings about body changes

• Yellowing of skin, sclera, dark

urine, clay-coloured stools, itchy skin, abdominal pain, fever, diarrhoea
- Joint or stomach pain, oedema in feet and legs, shaking
- Inflammation of mucosa, breaks in skin

Teach patient/family:
- Protective isolation precautions
- To report any complaints or side effects to clinician
- That impotence or amenorrhoea can occur, reversible after discontinuing treatment
- To report any changes in breathing or coughing
- That hair may be lost during treatment; a wig or hairpiece may make patient feel better (available free on NHS); new hair may be different in colour, texture
- The possibility of tinnitus and peripheral neuropathy
- Good mouth care
- Bland diet due to metallic taste
- That a bland diet may reduce the metallic taste

---

clarithromycin ▼

Klaricid
Func. class.: Antibiotic
Chem. class.: Macrolide antibiotic
Legal class.: POM

Action: Interacts with phospholipids in the cell wall of a broad spectrum of gram-positive and gram-negative bacteria to produce bacteriostatic action

Uses: Respiratory tract infections and mild to moderate skin and soft tissue infections caused by susceptible organisms

Dosage and routes:
- *Adult and child over 12 yr:* By mouth 250–500 mg twice daily
- *Child 1–12 yr:* By mouth 75 mg/kg twice daily

Available forms include: Tablets 250 mg; oral liquid, powder for reconstitution, 125 mg/5 ml

Side effects/adverse reactions:
CNS: Headache
GI: Nausea, vomiting, diarrhoea, abdominal pain
INTEG: Rash

Contraindications: Hypersensitivity to macrolide antibiotics

Precautions: Impaired hepatic or renal function

Interactions:
- Increased action of: oral anticoagulants, digoxin, theophylline, carbamazepine

Treatment of overdose: Symptomatic and supportive treatment, gastric lavage if recently ingested

NURSING CONSIDERATIONS

Assess:
- Vital signs (temperature, pulse, respiration)
- Culture and sensitivity before treatment starts
- For known sensitivities and allergies (sensitivity to penicillins)
- Bowel pattern
- Fluid balance

Administer:
- By mouth with a full glass of water or with food if GI symptoms occur

Perform/provide:
- Increase adequate fluids if diarrhoea occurs

Evaluate:
- Therapeutic response; resolution of symptoms; fall in neutrophil count
- Nausea, abdominal pain and other side effects

Teach patient/family:
- Drug should be taken with food and a full glass of water or with food if GI symptoms occur
- To maintain an adequate fluid intake (2 l/day)

• To report any side effects, particularly diarrhoea
• To take the full course of treatment unless otherwise advised by nurse or clinician

---

clemastine fumarate

Tavegil
Func. class.: Antihistamine H_1-receptor antagonist
Chem. class.: Ethanolamine derivative
Legal class.: P

Action: Acts on blood vessels, GI tract, respiratory system by competing with histamine for H_1-receptor site; decreases allergic response by blocking histamine
Uses: Allergy symptoms, rhinitis, angioneurotic oedema, urticaria
Dosage and routes:
• *Adult and child over 12 yr:* By mouth 1 mg twice a day
• *Child 1 to 3 yr:* By mouth 250–500 mcg twice a day; 3 to 6 yr 500 mcg twice a day; 6 to 12 yr: 500–1000 mcg twice a day
Available forms include: Tablets 1 mg; elixir 500 mcg/5 ml
Side effects/adverse reactions:
CNS: Dizziness, drowsiness, poor coordination, fatigue, anxiety, euphoria, confusion, paraesthesia, neuritis
CV: Hypotension, palpitations, tachycardia
RESP: Increased thick secretions, wheezing, chest tightness
GI: Dry mouth, nausea, vomiting, anorexia, constipation, diarrhoea
INTEG: Rash, urticaria, photosensitivity
GU: Retention
EENT: Blurred vision, dilated pupils, tinnitus, nasal stuffiness, dry nose, throat, mouth
Contraindications: Hypersensitivity to H_1-receptor antagonists; pregnancy; breast-feeding; hepatic disease; children below 1 year of age; porphyria
Precautions: Increased intraocular pressure, renal disease, bronchial asthma, stenosed peptic ulcers, prostatic hypertrophy, bladder neck obstruction, acute asthma attack, lower respiratory tract disease
Pharmacokinetics:
Period of onset: Peak 5–7 hr, duration 10–12 hr or more; metabolised in liver, excreted by kidneys
Interactions/incompatibilities:
• Increased CNS depression: barbiturates, narcotics, hypnotics, tricyclic antidepressants, alcohol, betahistine, anticholinergics, antiparkinsonian drugs, e.g. benzhexol
• Increased effect of this drug: MAOIs
Treatment of overdose: Administer ipecacuanha syrup or lavage, diazepam for convulsions, vasopressors

NURSING CONSIDERATIONS

Administer:
• With meals if GI symptoms occur; absorption may slightly decrease
• Elixir may be diluted with syrup BP or Sorbitol syrup (10%)
• One diluted use within 14 days
Perform/provide:
• Boiled sweets, gum, frequent rinsing of mouth for dryness
Evaluate:
• Therapeutic response: absence of running or congested nose or rashes
• Fluid balance; be alert for urinary retention, frequency, dysuria; drug should be discontinued if these occur
• Blood dyscrasias: thrombocytopaenia, agranulocytosis (rare)
• Respiratory status: rate, rhythm, increase in bronchial secretions,

wheezing, chest tightness

• Cardiac status: palpitations, increased pulse, hypotension

Teach patient/family:

• All aspects of drug use; to notify clinician if confusion, sedation, hypotension occur

• To avoid driving or other hazardous activity if drowsiness occurs

• To avoid concurrent use of alcohol or other CNS depressants

• To change position slowly, as drug may cause dizziness, hypotension (elderly)

---

clindamycin HCl/ clindamycin palmitate HCl/clindamycin phosphate

Dalacin C, Dalacin T

Func. class.: Antibiotic

Chem. class.: Lincosamide derivative

Legal class.: POM

Action: Binds to 50S subunit of bacterial ribosomes, suppresses protein synthesis

Uses: Infections caused by staphylococci, streptococci, pneumococci, *Rickettsia* spp, *Fusobacterium* spp, *Actinomyces*, spp, *Peptostreptococcus*, spp, *Bacteroides* spp, topically in acne vulgaris

Dosage and routes:

• *Adults:* By mouth 150–450 mg 6-hrly; IM IV 0.6–4.8 g daily in 2–4 doses

• *Child:* By mouth 3–6 mg/kg, 6 hrly, IM/IV 15–40 mg/kg daily (minimum 300 mg daily) in 3–4 doses

Acne

• Topical, apply a thin film twice daily

Available forms include: Injection 150 mg/ml; capsules 75, 150 mg; oral suspension 75 mg/5ml; topical lotion and solution 0.1%

Side effects/adverse reactions:

HAEM: Leucopenia, eosinophilia, agranulocytosis, thrombocytopenia

GI: Nausea, vomiting, abdominal pain, diarrhoea, pseudomembranous colitis. Increased aspartate aminotransferase, alanine aminotransferase, bilirubin, alkaline phosphatase, jaundice

GU: Vaginitis

INTEG: Rash, urticaria, pruritus, erythema, pain, abscess at injection site, skin irritation, contact dermatitis, Gram-negative folliculitis and stinging of the eyes after topical administration

Contraindications: Hypersensitivity to this drug or lincomycin, diarrhoeal states, neonates under 1 month of age

Precautions: Renal disease, liver disease, GI disease, pregnancy, lactation

Pharmacokinetics:

Period of onset: Oral: peak 45 min

IM: Peak 3 hr. Half-life 2½ hr, metabolised in liver, excreted in urine, bile, faeces as active/ inactive metabolites, crosses placenta, excreted in breast milk

Interactions/incompatibilities:

• Increased neuromuscular blockade: non-depolarising muscle relaxants

• Decreased action of: pyridostigmine, neostigmine

Clinical assessment:

• Any patient with compromised renal system; drug is excreted slowly in poor renal system function; toxicity may occur rapidly

• Liver studies: aspartate aminotransferase, alanine aminotransferase. Drug excreted more slowly in hepatic impairment and may be hepatotoxic

• Blood studies: During long-term

therapy WBC, RBC, platelets; drug should be discontinued if bone marrow depression occurs
Treatment of overdose: No specific treatment. Not removable from circulation by dialysis

NURSING CONSIDERATIONS

Assess:
• Bowel patterns
• Fluid balance
• Allergies before treatment, reaction of each medication; note allergies on chart in bright red letters; notify all people giving drugs
• Culture and sensitivity before drug therapy; drug may be used as soon as culture is taken
• BP, pulse in patient receiving drug parenterally

Administer:
• IV by infusion only; do not administer bolus dose
• IM deep injection; rotate sites
• Orally with at least 250 ml water
• By mouth, to be taken with plenty of water. IM, as a solution containing 150 mg/ml, by deep IM injection in single doses up to 600 mg – higher doses should be given IV. If IV it should be diluted to a solution of not more than 12 mg/ml and infused at not more than 30 mg/min in single doses up to 1.2 g

Perform/provide:
• Storage at room temperature (capsules) and up to 2 weeks (reconstituted solution)
• Adrenaline, suction, endotracheal intubation, equipment on unit/ward
• Adequate intake of fluids (2 litres) during diarrhoea episodes

Evaluate:
• Therapeutic response: decreased temperature, negative culture and sensitivity
• Bowel pattern during treatment
• Skin eruptions, itching, dermatitis after administration
• Respiratory status: rate, character, wheezing, tightness in chest

Teach patient/family:
• To take oral drug with full glass of water; may be taken with food if GI symptoms occur
• Aspects of drug therapy: need to complete entire course of medication to ensure organism death
• To report sore throat, fever, fatigue; could indicate superimposed infection
• That drug must be taken in equal intervals around clock to maintain blood levels
• To wear or carry ID if allergic to this drug
• To notify nurse of diarrhoea

---

clobetasol propionate

Dermovate
Func. class.: Topical corticosteroid
Chem. class.: Synthetic fluorinated agent, group I potency (very potent)
Legal class.: POM

Action: Antipruritic and anti-inflammatory properties
Uses: Psoriasis, eczema, contact dermatitis, lichen planus, discoid lupus erythematosus; usually reserved for short-term treatment of severe dermatoses that have not responded to less potent formulation
Dosage and routes:
• *Adult and child:* Apply sparingly to affected area twice daily for up to 4 weeks, reducing frequency according to response
Available forms include: Ointment 0.05%; cream 0.05%; scalp application 0.05%
Side effects/adverse reactions:
INTEG: Burning, irritation, acne, folliculitis, hypertrichosis, perioral dermatitis, hypopigmentation,

atrophy, striae, miliaria, allergic contact dermatitis, secondary infection
METAB: Adrenocortical suppression
Contraindications: Hypersensitivity, skin infection, rosacea, acne, perioral dermatitis
Precautions: Pregnancy, lactation, viral infections, bacterial infections
NURSING CONSIDERATIONS
Administer:
- Only to affected areas; do not get in eyes
- Leaving uncovered or lightly covered; occlusive dressing is not recommended
- Only to dermatoses; do not use on weeping, denuded, or infected area

Perform/provide:
- Cleansing to remove bacteria and cream before application of drug
- Treatment for a few days after area has cleared

Evaluate:
- Therapeutic response: absence of severe itching, patches on skin flaking
- Temperature, if fever develops, drug should be discontinued

Teach patient/family:
- To avoid sunlight on affected area; photosensitivity may occur
- To limit treatment to 14 days using less than 50 g a week
- To report any side effects

---

clofibrate

Atromid-S
Func. class.: Hypolipidaemic
Chem. class.: Aryloxyisobutyric acid derivative
Legal class.: POM

Action: Reduces blood levels of very low density lipoproteins, low density lipoproteins and triglycerides by reducing synthesis or increasing clearance. Increases high density lipoprotein-cholesterol
Uses: Type III hyperlipidaemia, severe hypertriglyceridaemia in types IIb, IV and V
Dosage and routes:
- *Adult:* By mouth over 65 kg, 2 g daily in divided doses (50–65 kg, 1–5 g daily)

Available forms include: Capsules 500 mg
Side effects/adverse reactions:
GI: Nausea, vomiting, dyspepsia, increased liver enzymes, flatulence, hepatomegaly, gastritis, increased cholelithiasis
INTEG: Rash, urticaria, pruritus, dry hair and skin, alopecia
HAEM: Leucopenia, anaemia, eosinophilia
CNS: Fatigue, weakness, headache
GU: Decreased libido, impotence, dysuria, proteinuria, oliguria
MS: Myalgias, arthralgias, myositis
CV: Angina, dysrhythmias, thrombophlebitis, pulmonary emboli
Contraindications: Severe hepatic disease, severe renal disease, primary biliary cirrhosis, pregnancy, breast-feeding, gall bladder disease, gall stones
Precautions: Peptic ulcer, nephrotic syndrome
Pharmacokinetics:
Period of onset: Peak 2–6 hr, plasma protein binding greater than 90%; half-life 6–25 hr, excreted in urine, metabolised in liver
Interactions/incompatibilities:
- Increased effects of: sulphonylureas, anticoagulants, phenytoin

Clinical assessment:
- Renal and hepatic function in patients on long-term therapy

Lab. test interferences:

Increase: Serum protein-bound iodine
Decrease: Urinary VMA
Treatment of overdose:
Symptomatic
NURSING CONSIDERATIONS
Evaluate:
• A wide range of adverse reactions; including nausea, vomiting, rashes, fatigue, weakness, angina, headaches
Teach patient/family:
• To take tablets regularly, toxicity may occur from missed doses
• To report bleeding mucous membranes or dark tarry stools immediately (signs of hypothrombinaemia)
• To report GU symptoms i.e. decreased libido, impotence, dysuria, proteinuria, oliguria
• That birth control should be practiced whilst taking the drug
• To reduce other risk factors i.e. high fat diet, smoking, lack of exercise

---

clomiphene citrate

Clomid, Serophene
Func. class.: Ovulation stimulant
Chem. class.: Non-steroidal triethylamine derivative
Legal class.: POM

Action: Increases LH, FSH, which increase maturation of ovarian follicle, ovulation, development of corpus luteum
Uses: Anovulatory infertility
Dosage and routes:
• *Adult:* By mouth 50 mg daily for 5 days from 5th day of cycle; if no ovulation occurs double dose for next cycle; 3 cycles should constitute an adequate therapeutic trial
Available forms include: Tablets 50 mg

Side effects/adverse reactions:
EENT: Blurred vision, diplopia, photophobia, scotomata
HAEM: Haemolytic anaemia
CNS: Headache, depression, restlessness, anxiety, nervousness, fatigue, insomnia
GI: Nausea, vomiting, constipation, increased appetite, abdominal pain
INTEG: Rash, dermatitis, urticaria, alopecia, hot flushes
GU: Polyuria, frequency, birth defects, spontaneous abortions, multiple ovulation, breast pain, oliguria, ovarian hyperstimulation
Contraindications: Hypersensitivity, pregnancy, hepatic disease, undiagnosed vaginal bleeding, endometrial cancer, ovarian cyst
Precautions: Depression
Pharmacokinetics: Readily absorbed; metabolised in liver, excreted in faeces, stored in fat, half-life 5–7 days
Interactions/incompatibilities:
None known
NURSING CONSIDERATIONS
Administer:
• At same time each day to maintain drug level
Teach patient/family:
• That multiple births are slightly more common after drug is taken
• To notify clinician if low abdominal pain occurs, may indicate ovarian cyst, cyst rupture (miscarriage rate is slightly higher)
• Visual symptoms (blurring, spots) may occur rarely and should be reported to clinician; drug will be stopped
• Mucus awareness (temperature taking is rarely accurate)
• Suggest intercourse alternate days when mucus appears ovulatory
• If pregnancy is suspected, clinician must be notified immediately

clomipramine hydrochloride

Anafranil, Anafranil SR
Func. class.: Antidepressant
Chem. class.: Tricyclic antidepressant
Legal class.: POM

Action: Inhibits neuronal reuptake of neurotransmitters noradrenaline and serotonin within CNS; precise mechanism of antidepressive action uncertain
Uses: Depressive illness, adjunctive treatment of obsessional/phobic states, cataplexy associated with narcolepsy
Dosage and routes:
• By mouth, initially 10 mg daily, increased gradually as necessary to 30–150 mg in divided doses or as single dose at bedtime, higher doses may be required; elderly patients 10 mg daily, up to 30–75 mg maximum
• IM injection: initially 25–50 mg, increased by 25 mg daily; maximum 150 mg daily
• IV infusion: initially 25–50 mg to test tolerance, then approximately 100 mg daily for 7–10 days
Available forms include: Capsules, 10, 25 mg; syrup, 25 mg/5 ml; injection, 25 mg/2 ml; tablets modified-release 75 mg
Side effects/adverse reactions:
HAEM: Agranulocytosis, leucopenia, eosinophilia, purpura, thrombocytopenia, jaundice
CNS: Sedation, blurred vision, tremor, confusion, hypomania, behavioural disturbances, convulsions
META: Blood sugar level changes in diabetics or weight changes
GI: Nausea, dry mouth, black tongue, paralytic ileus
GU: Difficulty with micturition, changes in sexual function
INTEG: Sweating, rashes
CV: Arrhythmias, postural hypotension, tachycardia, syncope
Contraindications: Recent myocardial infarction, heart block, cardiac failure, any cardiac arrhythmia, severe liver impairment, concurrent use of MAOIs, narrow angle glaucoma, urinary retention, mania, porphyria
Precautions: Diabetes, cardiac disease, epilepsy, pregnancy, hepatic impairment, thyroid disease, psychoses; avoid abrupt cessation of therapy; caution in anaesthesia, elderly, bladder neck obstruction, lactation
Pharmacokinetics: Onset of effect over 2–4 weeks. Half-life 17–28 hr. Converted in liver to active metabolite; excreted in urine
Interactions/incompatibilities:
Increased toxicity: MAOIs within 3 weeks of stopping therapy, anaesthetic agents
• Decreased effects of guanethidine, bethanidine, debrisoquine, clonidine, methyldopa
• Potentiation of adrenaline, ephedrine, isoprenaline, noradrenaline, phenylephrine, phenylpropanolamine
• Sedation potentiated by alcohol, other CNS depressants
• Plasma levels decreased by barbiturates, and increased by methylphenidate, neuroleptics
• Effects enhanced by thyroid hormones
Clinical assessment:
• Check that MAOIs have not been taken in last 3 weeks
• Caution prescribing with anaesthesia
• Full blood count, white cell differential montly for first 4 months, thereafter if problems suspected
Treatment of overdose: Gastric lavage, activated charcoal; nurse in intensive therapy unit monitor-

ing ECG. Supportive treatment

NURSING CONSIDERATIONS

Assess:

• Baseline BP; all vital signs in patient with cardiovascular disease
• Weight

Administer:

• IV infusion in 0.9% sodium chloride or 5% dextrose and mix well
• Orally at bedtime if drowsiness occurs, check dose taken. Divide dose in the elderly. Not with alcohol

Perform/provide:

• Counselling for sexual problems
• Fluids and fibre for constipation
• Mouth care as required for dryness
• Measures to minimise effects of sweating e.g. change linen
• Checks that retention has not occurred
• Safe environment; get patient up slowly; help with mobilisation

Evaluate:

• BP (lying and standing) 4 hrly plus other vital signs in cardiovascular disease
• Weight weekly (may lose/gain)
• Other side effects
• Mood, sleeping pattern
• Suicidal tendencies

Teach patient/family:

• To swallow whole, not to be chewed
• Patient must not drive or operate machinery if drug causes drowsiness
• To avoid alcohol
• That medication takes 2–3 weeks to work; not to stop taking drug suddenly
• The importance at reporting side effects such as sore throat, mouth lesions and fever
• About problems with sexual functions

clonazepam

Rivotril

Func. class.: Anticonvulsant
Chem. class.: Benzodiazapine
Legal class.: CD Benz POM

Action: Prevents generalisation of convulsive activity and raises seizure threshold

Uses: All clinical forms of epilepsy including; absence, atypical absence, akinetic, myoclonic seizures, status epilepticus

Dosage and routes:

Epilepsy, myoclonus

• *Adult:* By mouth, initially, 1 mg at night; increase according to response over 2–4 weeks to 4–8 mg daily in divided doses
• *Elderly:* By mouth, initially, 0.5 mg at night; increase according to response over 2–4 weeks to 4–8 mg daily in divided doses
• *Child:* By mouth, daily in divided doses, up to 1 yr, initially 250 mcg increased to 0.5–1.0 mg; 1–5 yr, initially 250 mcg increased to 1–3 mg; 5–12 yr, initially 0.5 mg increased to 3–6 mg

Status epilepticus

• *Adult:* Slow IV injection or IV infusion, 1 mg
• *Child:* Slow IV injection or IV infusion, 500 mcg

Available forms include: Tablets 0.5 mg, 2 mg; injection 1 mg/ml

Side effects/adverse reactions:

HAEM: Thrombocytopenia, leucocytosis, eosinophilia
CNS: Drowsiness, dizziness, confusion, behavioural changes, tremors, insomnia, headache, suicidal tendencies
GI: Nausea, constipation, polyphagia, anorexia, abnormal liver function tests, diarrhoea
INTEG: Rash, alopecia, hirsutism
EENT: Increased salivation, nystagmus, diplopia, abnormal

eye movements, sore gums
RESP: Respiratory depression, dyspnoea, congestion
CV: Palpitations, bradycardia
Contraindications: CNS depression, coma, respiratory depression, sleep apnoea
Precautions: Open-angle glaucoma, chronic respiratory disease, lactation, pregnancy, porphyria
Pharmacokinetics:
Period of onset: Peak 1–2 hr, metabolised by liver, excreted in urine, half-life 18–50 hr
Interactions/incompatibilities:
• Increased CNS depression: alcohol, barbiturates, narcotics, antidepressants, other anticonvulsants
• Decreased effect of this drug: carbamazepine phenytoin, phenobarbitone
Clinical assessment
Assess:
• Renal studies: blood urea nitrogen, urine creatinine
• Blood studies: RBC, haematocrit, Hb, WBC, platelet
• Hepatic studies: alanine aminotransferase, aspartate aminotransferase, bilirubin
Treatment of overdose: Lavage. Supportive treatment. Antagonism with flumazenil in non-epileptic patients
NURSING CONSIDERATIONS
Administer:
• IV injection slowly over 30 seconds after diluting in water for injection
• IV infusion in glucose 5%, 10%, or sodium chloride 0.9%, suggested volume 250 ml
Perform/provide:
• Assistance with ambulation during early part of treatment; dizziness occurs
Evaluate:
• Therapeutic response: decreased seizure activity, document on patient's chart
• Mental status: mood, alertness, affect, behavioural changes; if mental status changes, notify clinician
• Allergic reaction: red raised rash; if this occurs, drug should be discontinued
• Blood dyscrasias: may cause fever, sore throat, bruising, rash, jaundice
• Toxicity: bone marrow depression, nausea, vomiting, ataxia, diplopia, cardiovascular collapse
Teach patient/family:
• To avoid driving, other activities that require alertness
• To avoid alcohol ingestion or CNS depressants, increased sedation may occur
• Not to discontinue medication quickly after long-term use; taper off over several weeks
• All aspects of the drug: action, use, side effects, adverse reactions, when to notify clinician

---

clonidine hydrochloride

Catapres, Dixarit, Catapres Perlongets
Func. class.: Antihypertensive antimigraine agent
Chem. class.: Central α-adrenergic agonist
Legal class.: POM

Action: Inhibits sympathetic vasomotor centre in CNS, which reduces impulses in sympathetic nervous system; blood pressure decreases, pulse rate, cardiac output decreases
Uses: Hypertension, migraine prophylaxis, menopausal flushing
Dosage and routes:
Hypertension
• *Adult:* By mouth 50–100 mcg 3 times a day increased every 2–3 days, usual maximum 1.2 mg daily;

modified-release capsules, 250 mcg daily increased if necessary to 500–750 mcg daily; slow IV injection 150–300 mcg, maximum 750 mcg in 24 hr for hypertensive crisis
Migraine prophylaxis, menopausal flushing
• *Adult:* 50 mcg twice daily increased after 2 weeks to 75 mcg twice a day if required
Available forms include: Tablets 25 mcg, 100 mcg, 300 mcg; capsules, modified-release tablets 250 mcg; injection 150 mcg/ml
Side effects/adverse reactions:
CV: Hypotension, orthostatic palpitations, rebound hypertension after sudden withdrawal
CNS: Drowsiness, sedation, headache, fatigue, nightmares, insomnia, mental changes, anxiety, depression, hallucinations, delirium
GI: Nausea, vomiting, malaise, constipation, dry mouth
INTEG: Rash, alopecia, facial pallor, pruritus, oedema, chilblains
EENT: Taste change, parotid pain
ENDO: Hyperglycaemia
MS: Muscle/joint pain, leg cramps
GU: Impotence, dysuria, nocturia, gynaecomastia
Contraindications: Hypersensitivity, porphyria
Precautions: Myocardial infarction (recent), chronic renal failure, Raynaud's disease, thyroid disease, depression, pregnancy, lactation
Pharmacokinetics:
Period of onset: Peak 3–5 hr; half-life 6–20 hr, metabolised by liver, 70% excreted in urine (50% unchanged, 20% inactive metabolites), crosses blood-brain barrier, excreted in breast milk
Interactions/incompatibilities:
• Increased CNS depression: narcotics, sedatives, alcohol, anaesthetics
• Decreased hypotensive effects: tricyclic antidepressants, MAOIs, α-adrenergic blockers
• Increased hypotensive effects: diuretics
• Increased bradycardia: β-blockers, cardiac glycosides
Clinical assessment:
• Increased risk of withdrawal hypertension: β-blockers, tricyclic antidepressants
• Baselines in renal, liver function tests before therapy begins
Treatment of overdose: Gastric lavage, supportive treatment, administer an α-adrenergic blocking drug e.g. phentolamine for severe overdose

NURSING CONSIDERATIONS

Administer:
• 1 hr before meals
• IV infusion of 0.9% sodium chloride (as prescribed) to expand fluid volume if severe hypotension occurs. (For nurses practicing extended role)
Evaluate:
• Therapeutic response: decrease in BP
• Signs of chronic cardiac failure
• Renal symptoms: polyuria, oliguria, frequency
Teach patient/family:
• To take dose 1 hr before meals
• Not to discontinue drug abruptly; rebound rise in BP may follow causing raised BP, anxiety, headache, insomnia, tachycardia, tremors, nausea, sweating
• That drug may cause dizziness, fainting, lightheadedness during first few days of therapy
• Stress patient compliance with dosage schedule even if feeling better
• Not to use non-prescription (cough, cold, or allergy) products unless directed by clinician
• Not to stop drug unless directed by clinician
• Patient to avoid sunlight or wear

sunscreen if in sunlight, photosensitivity may occur
• Notify clinician of: mouth sores, sore throat, fever, swelling of hands or feet, irregular heartbeat, chest pain, signs of angioneurotic oedema
• Excessive perspiration, dehydration, vomiting; diarrhoea may lead to fall in BP—consult clinician if these occur
• May cause skin rash or impaired perspiration

clotrimazole (topical)

Canesten
Func. class.: Antifungal
Chem. class.: Imidazole derivative
Legal class.: P

Action: Interferes with fungal DNA replication; binds sterols in fungal cell membrane, which increases permeability, leaking of cell nutrients
Uses: Tinea pedis, tinea cruris, tinea corporis, tinea versicolor, *Candida albicans* infection of the vagina, vulva. Dermatophyte infections of the skin
Dosage and routes:
• *Adult and child:* Topical: apply to affected area twice a day for at least 2 weeks for candidal infections and 1 month for dermatophyte infections; Intravaginal: 1 tablet at night for 1 (500 mg), 3 (200 mg) or 6 (100 mg) nights, or 1 application of cream (10%) at night for 1 night or application of cream (2%) twice daily for 3 days or 1 application of cream (2%) for 6 nights
Available forms include: Cream, powder, solution, spray 1%; vaginal tablets 100, 200, 500 mg, vaginal cream 2%, 10%
Side effects/adverse reactions:
INTEG: Rash, urticaria, stinging, burning
Contraindications: Hypersensitivity
Precautions: Pregnancy, lactation
NURSING CONSIDERATIONS
Administer:
• After cleansing with soap, water before each application, dry well
• Enough medication to cover lesions completely
• 1 filled applicator or 1 tablet deep-intravaginally each night; 500 mg as a single dose
Evaluate:
• Allergic reaction: burning, stinging, swelling, redness
• Therapeutic response: decrease in size, number of lesions, in itching or white patches around vulva
Teach patient/family:
• To wash hands before, after each application
• To apply with glove to prevent further infection
• To avoid use of non-prescription creams, ointments, lotions unless directed by clinician
• Cream should be applied daily to the partner's penis to prevent re-infection in vaginal, vulval infections

clozapine

Clozaril
Func. class.: Antipsychotic neuroleptic
Chem. class.: Dibenzodiazepine
Legal class.: POM

Action: Rapid acting sedative antipsychotic. Weak dopamine antagonist properties, potent α-adrenergic blocker, anticholinergic, antihistaminic
Uses: In patients who are non-responsive to, or intolerant of, conventional neuroleptics; hos-

pital use only, registration with manufacturer required

Dosage and routes:

• *Adult:* The dose must be adjusted individually. By mouth 25–50 mg on the first day. The dose may then be increased in daily increments of 25–50 mg to a maximum of 300 mg daily. Judicious increments (not exceeding 100 mg) are permissible up to 900 mg daily. In most patients, efficacy can be expected with 200–450 mg daily in divided doses. After achieving maximum therapeutic benefit many patients can be maintained on a lower dose. Careful downward titration to 150–300 mg daily in divided doses is recommended. Up to 200 mg can be given as a single evening dose

• *Elderly:* By mouth initial dose 25 mg, increasing in increments of 25 mg daily

Available forms include: Tablets 25, 100 mg

Side effects/adverse reactions:

INTEG: Skin reactions

GI: Hypersalivation, gastrointestinal disturbances, dry mouth, cholestasis, increases in hepatic enzymes

CV: Tachycardia, ECG changes, arrhythmias, postural hypotension

CNS: Drowsiness, fatigue, transient autonomic reactions, EEG changes and lowering of the seizure threshold, rarely delirium, extrapyramidal symptoms, neuroleptic malignant syndrome, disturbances in temperature regulation

HAEM: Neutropenia, unexplained leucocytosis

Contraindications: History of drug-induced neutropenia/agranulocytosis; myeloproliferative disorders; alcoholic and toxic psychoses; drug intoxication; comatose conditions and other forms of severe CNS depression; severe hepatic or renal disease; pregnancy; breast-feeding; children; coadministration drugs causing agranulocytosis

Precautions: Prostatic enlargement, narrow-angle glaucoma, paralytic ileus, renal disease

Pharmacokinetics: 90–95% absorption of oral doses 50–60% first pass metabolism. Peak plasma levels 2.1 hr post-dose. Hepatic metabolism. Half life 6–26 hr

Interactions/incompatibilities:

• Enhanced toxicity to blood: co-trimoxazole, chloramphenicol, sulphonamides, pyrazolone analgesics, phenylbutazone, penicillamine, carbamazepine, cytotoxic agents

• Enhanced risk of neuroleptic malignant syndrome: lithium

• Enhanced toxicity of: warfarin

• Enhanced CNS effects of: narcotics, benzodiazepines, alcohol, antihistamines MAOIs

• Enhanced activity of: anticholinergic, hypotensive drugs

Clinical assessment:

• If the white blood cell count falls below 3000/mm^3 and/or the absolute neutrophil count drops below 1500/mm^3 the drug must be withdrawn and the patient closely monitored

• In the event of an infection, or routine WBC count between 3000 and 3500/mm^3 and/or a neutrophil count between 1500 and 2000/mm^3 the patient should be re-evaluated immediately

• Should either count decline further, clozapine must be withdrawn at once. Otherwise, treatment may continue provided that leucocytes and granulocytes are checked at least twice weekly until it is certain that they are stable

• If the WBC count falls below 1000/mm^3 after drug withdrawal and/or neutrophils decrease below

500/mm^3 the patient should be referred immediately for specialised care

• In patients with a history of seizures, or with cardiovascular, renal or liver disease, the initial dose should be low and any increase should be slow

• Regular monitoring of liver function tests in patients with liver disease

• Warfarin levels in patients receiving both drugs

Treatment of overdose: Gastric lavage, activated charcoal, supportive measures. Close medical supervision for at least 4 days; possible delayed reactions

NURSING CONSIDERATIONS

Assess:

• Patients must be registered with the Clorazil Patient Monitoring Service

• Initiation of treatment must be in hospital inpatients, who must have a normal white blood cell and differential blood count

• Only patients with normal findings may receive the drug

Perform/provide:

• Blood count should be repeated every week for the first 18 weeks, and then at 2 weeks intervals for the duration of the therapy

Teach patient/family:

• If treatment is to be stopped, a gradual dose reduction over 1 to 2 weeks is recommended. Abrupt discontinuation carries the risk of rebound psychosis

• That they must ensure regular blood test undertaken whilst on this medication this may restrict holidays

• To contact the clinician immediately if any kind of infection begins to develop

co-beneldopa (benserazide levodopa)

Madopar, Madopar CR

Func. class.: Antiparkinson agent

Chem. class.: Combination of dopamine precursor (levodopa) with an inhibitor of the enzyme dopadecarboxylase (benserazide)

Legal class.: POM

Action: Levodopa is decarboxylated in the brain to dopamine, reducing dopamine deficit. Benserazide prevents peripheral breakdown of levodopa

Uses: Parkinsonism

Dosage and routes:

• *Adult:* By mouth, initially 50–100 mg twice daily, adjusted according to response; usual maintenance dose 400–800 mg daily in divided doses

When transferring patients from levodopa, 3 capsules of co-beneldopa 25/100 (Madopar 125) should be substituted for 2 g levodopa

Note: Dosage requirements are very variable

Available forms include: Capsules (mg benserazide/mg levodopa) 12.5/50, 25/100, 50/200; tablets, dispersible 12.5/50, 25/100; capsules, modified release 25/100

Side effects/adverse reactions:

CV: Arrhythmias, postural hypotension, gastrointestinal bleeding, flushing, elevated liver enzymes

CNS: Elation, anxiety, agitation, insomnia, depression, aggression, delusions, hallucinations, unmasking of psychoses, involuntary movements, fluctuation in therapeutic response after prolonged use, drowsiness

ELECT: Raised serum uric acid and urea

GI: Nausea, vomiting, anorexia

GU: Red urine
HAEM: Haemolytic anaemia, mild transient leucopenia
INTEG: Sweating
Contraindications: Narrow angle glaucoma; uncontrolled wide angle glaucoma; severe psychoneuroses or psychoses; severe endocrine, renal, hepatic or cardiac disorders; patients under 25; active melanoma or history of melanoma; pregnancy; breast feeding
Precautions: Treatment with co-beneldopa should not be discontinued abruptly
Interactions:
• Hypertensive crisis with: MAOIs (except selegiline) or within 21 days of stopping
• Cardiac arrhythmias with: cyclopropane, halogenated hydrocarbon anaesthetics
• Increased effect of: guanethidine, methyldopa, other antihypertensives
• Decreased effect of: antipsychotics
• Effects of co-beneldopa reduced by: benzodiazepines, antipsychotics, iron
• Increased blood levels of levodopa with: domperidone, metoclopramide
Lab. test interferences:
False positive: Urine ketones (dipstick)
False negative: Urine glucose (glucose oxidase method)
Treatment of overdose: Gastric lavage, ECG monitoring, supportive treatment
NURSING CONSIDERATIONS
Assess:
• Baseline vital signs, particularly BP
• Age of patient (smaller doses are needed by elderly)
Administer:
• With or immediately after food, particularly if gastrointestinal effects are severe
• Precise timing of doses may be important in optimising therapeutic response
Perform/provide:
• Storage protection from moisture
Evaluate
• Therapeutic improvement within 1–3 weeks. Dosage requirements are very variable
• For side effects, particularly hypotension and gastrointestinal effects (less than with levodopa)
• Colour of urine. Darkening or a reddish tinge is an expected side effect and does not imply renal disease
Teach patient/family:
• To take medication with or after food to avoid nausea and vomiting
• About side effects. Nausea, vomiting, anorexia, weakness and postural hypotension will occur at the start of treatment and at some time during treatment with this drug for most patients (often dose-related and very commonly in the elderly)
• That urine will change colour, becoming dark with a reddish tinge. This is to be expected
• Not to discontinue the drug abruptly or without consultation

co-careldopa (levodopa/carbidopa)

Sinemet, Sinemet LS, Sinemet-Plus, Sinemet CR
Func. class.: Antiparkinsonian agent
Legal class.: POM

Action: Decarboxylation of levodopa to dopamine, which increases dopamine levels in brain. Carbidopa prevents peripheral breakdown of levodopa
Uses: Parkinsonism

Dosage and routes:

• *Adult:* By mouth initially, 100–125 mg (expressed as levodopa) 3–4 times daily adjusted according to response; usual maintenance 0.75–1.5 g daily in divided doses after food

Sinemet-Plus: By mouth initially 1 tablet 3 times daily, adjusted according to response up to 8 daily; larger doses by gradual substitution of Sinemet for Sinemet-Plus

Available forms include: Tablets (mg carbidopa/mg levodopa) 10/100, 12.5/50, 25/100; modified-release 50/200

Side effects/adverse reactions:

HAEM: Haemolytic anaemia, transient leucopenia/thrombocytopenia

CNS: Choreiform involuntary movements, fatigue, headache, anxiety, twitching, numbness, weakness, confusion, agitation, insomnia, nightmares, psychosis, hallucinations, hypomania, depression, dizziness, peripheral neuropathy

GI: Nausea, vomiting, anorexia, abdominal distress, bitter taste, transient rises in liver enzymes, GI bleeding

INTEG: Sweating, alopecia, flushing

CV: Orthostatic hypotension, tachycardia, hypertension, palpitation, arrythmias

MISC: Reddish colouration of urine and other body fluids

Contraindications: Concurrent use of MAOIs (except selegiline), hypersensitivity, narrow-angle glaucoma, previous history of or active malignant melanoma, drug-induced parkinsonism

Precautions: Renal disease, cardiovascular disease, hepatic disease, peptic ulcer, diabetes, pregnancy, psychosis

Pharmacokinetics (of levodopa component):

By mouth: Peak 1–3 hr, metabolised in gut, liver, kidney, excreted in urine (metabolites), plasma half-life 45–65 min. Dose required 20–40% of that given without carbidopa

Interactions/incompatibilities:

• Hypertensive crisis: MAOIs (except selegiline) or within 21 days of stopping

• Dysrhythmias: cyclopropane, halogenated hydrocarbon anaesthetics

• Increased effects of: guanethidine, methyldopa, other antihypertensives

• Decreased effect of: antipsychotics

• Effects of co-careldopa reduced by: benzodiazepines, metoclopramide, domperidone, iron

Clinical assessment:

• Adjust dosage depending on patient response

• Hepatic, haematological, renal, cardiovascular, psychiatric surveillance during prolonged therapy

• Domperidone for nausea

Lab. test interferences:

False positive: Urine ketones (dipstick)

False negative: Urine glucose (glucose oxidase method)

Treatment of overdose: Gastric lavage, ECG monitoring, supportive treatment

NURSING CONSIDERATIONS

Administer:

• Drug to be given until patient is starved (before surgery)

• Follow exact prescribing times to ensure maximum therapeutic effect

• With meals; limit protein taken with drug

• If transferring to modified release preparation from levodopa, stop levodopa 8 hr beforehand (12 hours for modified release levodopa)

Perform/provide:

• Assistance with ambulation during beginning therapy
• Testing for diabetes mellitus, acromegaly if on long-term therapy

Evaluate:
• Mental status: affect, mood, behavioural changes, depression, assess suicidal tendencies
• Therapeutic response: decrease in involuntary movements; diminution of early morning stiffness

Teach patient/family:
• To change positions slowly to prevent orthostatic hypotension
• To report side effects: twitching, eye spasms; indicate overdose
• To use drug exactly as prescribed; if drug is discontinued abruptly, parkinsonian crisis may occur
• That urine, sweat may darken

co-danthramer

Codalax (Co-danthramer suspension)
Codalax Forte (strong co-danthramer suspension)
Func. class.: Laxative
Chem. class.: Combination of an anthraquinone compound (danthron) and synthetic surface active agent (poloxamer 188)
Legal class.: POM

Action: Facilitates bowel movement by stimulating muscle activity in the large intestine, increasing the water content of the stool and softening it and lubricating the contents of the distal colon

Uses: Relief of constipation in geriatric patients, patients suffering from terminal illness, and patients with cardiac failure or coronary thrombosis in whom straining to defaecate would be hazardous

Dosage and routes:
• *Adult:* By mouth; starting doses, 5–10 ml of co-danthramer suspension or 2.5–10 ml strong co-danthramer suspension at bedtime. This dose may be increased until the desired effect is achieved
• *Child:* By mouth, starting dose, 2.5–5 ml of co-danthramer suspension at bedtime

Available forms include: Oral suspension (poloxamer 188, 200 mg; and danthron, 25 mg/5 ml); oral suspension, strong (poloxamer 188, 1000 mg; danthron, 75 mg/5 ml)

Side effects/adverse reactions:
GI: Nausea, griping, staining and sloughing of the buttocks in incontinent and/or bedridden patients
GU: Pinkish colouration of urine

Contraindications: Intestinal obstruction. *Note* Based on animal studies there is a small, theoretical risk that co-danthramer may be carcinogenic. Therefore its use should be confined to those groups of patients listed under 'indications'

Precautions: Incontinent patients and babies in nappies (increased risk of staining and damage to peri-anal skin); pregnancy

Pharmacokinetics: Danthron is absorbed from the small intestine to some extent. It is excreted in the faeces and urine

Treatment of overdose: Patients should be given plenty of fluids; anticholinergic agents may help reduce excessive intestinal motility

NURSING CONSIDERATIONS

Assess:
• Bowel habit (frequency, type of stool, straining)
• Fluid intake
• Life-style including amount of exercise, diet

Administer:
• At bedtime (takes 6–12 hr to work)
• Graduated dosage until 'normal'

stool is achieved

Perform/provide:
- Plenty of fluids
- Appropriate diet
- Storage away from strong light
- Support and counselling for underlying disease (in patients with carcinoma, etc.)

Evaluate:
- Therapeutic response
- For side effects
- Fluid balance
- Staining of perianal skin in incontinent patients

Teach patient/family:
- About side effects, including pink colouration of urine and discolouration of perianal skin
- That 6–12 hr elapse before medication takes effect
- About other methods for reducing constipation (diet, fluids, exercise)

co-phenotrope, diphenoxylate HCl with atropine sulphate (diphenoxylate HCl 2.5 mg with atropine sulphate 25 mcg)

Lomotil, Diarphen

Func. class.: Antidiarrhoeal
Chem. class.: Diphenoxylate—phenylpipeoridine derivative, opiate agonist. Atropine—antimuscarinic alkaloid
Legal class.: POM

Action: Inhibits gastric motility by acting on mucosal receptors responsible for peristalsis

Uses: Adjunct to rehydration in acute diarrhoea; control of stool formation after colostomy/ileostomy; relief of symptoms in chronic mild ulcerative colitis

Dosage and routes: By mouth
- *Adult:* 4 tablets or 20 ml followed by 2 tablets or 10 ml every 6 hr
- *Children under 4:* not recommended
- *4–8 yr:* 1 tablet or 5 ml 3 times a day
- *9–12 yr:* 1 tablet or 5 ml 4 times a day
- *13–16 yr:* 2 tablets or 10 ml 3 times a day

Available forms include: Tablets 2.5/0.025 mg; liquid 2.5/0.025 mg in 5 ml

Side effects/adverse reactions:
CNS: Malaise, lethargy, sedation, somnolence, confusion, dizziness, depression, restlessness, euphoria, hallucinations, headache, flushing, hyperthermia
ALLERGIC: Anaphylaxis, angioedema, urticaria, pruritus
GI: Paralytic ileus, toxic megacolon, nausea, vomiting, anorexia, abdominal discomfort
EENT: Blurred vision, dry mouth
INTEG: Dry skin and mucous membranes
CVS: Tachycardia
GU: Urinary retention

Contraindications: Hypersensitivity; severe liver disease; pseudomembranous enterocolitis; acute ulcerative colitis; diverticular disease; intestinal obstruction; glaucoma; children less than 4 yr; electrolyte imbalances; severe dehydration

Precautions: Ulcerative colitis, lactation, Down's syndrome, renal disease

Pharmacokinetics dynamics:
Period of onset: Onset 45–60 min, peak 2 hr, duration 3–4 hr, half-life 2½ hr; metabolised in liver to active, inactive metabolites; excreted in urine, faeces, breast milk

Interactions/incompatibilities:
- Do not use with or within 14 days of MAOIs; hypertensive crisis may occur
- Increased action of: alcohol,

narcotics, barbiturates, other CNS depressants
Clinical assessment:
• Electrolyte balance (potassium, sodium, chloride and appropriate fluid intake)
Treatment of overdose: Danger of narcosis (respiratory depression) or atropine poisoning (i.e. hyperthermia, tachycardia, lethargy, coma). Treat respiratory depression with naloxone and consider gastric lavage and activated charcoal. Observe for at least 48 hr
NURSING CONSIDERATIONS
Assess:
• Bowel pattern
• Fluid balance
Administer:
• For 48 hr only
Evaluate:
• Therapeutic response: return to normal bowel habit
• Bowel pattern before; for rebound constipation after termination of medication
• Response after 48 hr; if no response, drug should be discontinued
• Hydration status—if unable to produce adequate urinary output, IV fluids may be necessary
• Dehydration in children
• Abdominal distention, toxic megacolon, which may occur in ulcerative colitis
Teach patient/family:
• Avoid non-prescribed products unless directed by clinician; may contain alcohol
• Inform of side effects and advise to contact clinician if any occur
• Not to exceed recommended dose

co-trimoxazole (sulphamethoxazole and trimethoprim)

Bactrim, Septrin, Comixco, Fectrim, Laratrim, Comox
Func. class.: Antibiotic
Chem. class.: Combined sulphonamide and synthetic pyrimidine derivative
Legal class.: POM

Action: Sulphamethoxazole interferes with bacterial biosynthesis of proteins by competitive antagonism of PABA when adequate levels are maintained; trimethoprim blocks synthesis of tetrahydrofolic acid; this combination blocks 2 consecutive steps in bacterial synthesis of essential nucleic acids, protein
Uses: Urinary tract infections, otitis media, chronic prostatitis, shigellosis, *Pneumocystis carinii* pneumonitis, chronic bronchitis
Dosage and routes:
• *Adult:* By mouth 960 mg 12-hrly, maximum 1.44 g 12-hrly, 480 mg 12 hrly if treated for more than 14 days; IM, IV infusion 960 mg twice a day, maximum 1.44 g 12 hrly, 960 mg 8 hrly
• *Child:* By mouth 6 weeks–6 months, 120 mg twice a day, 6 months–6 yr, 240 mg twice a day, 6–12 yr, 480 mg twice a day; IV infusion 36 mg/kg daily in 2 divided doses, maximum 54 mg/kg daily
Pneumocystis carinii pneumonitis
• *Adult and child:* 120 mg/kg daily in divided doses
Available forms include: Tablets 20 mg trimethoprim 100 mg sulphamethoxazole (120 mg); 80 mg trimethoprim/400 mg sulphamethoxazole (480 mg), 160 mg trimethoprim/800 mg sulphamethoxazole (960 mg); suspension

240 mg/5 ml, 480 mg/5 ml; IV injection 96 mg/ml, IM 320 mg/ml

Side effects/adverse reactions:

SYST: Anaphylaxis

GI: Nausea, vomiting, abdominal pain, stomatitis, hepatitis, glossitis, pancreatitis, diarrhoea, enterocolitis

CNS: Headache, confusion, insomnia, hallucinations, depression, vertigo, fatigue, anxiety, convulsions, drug fever, chills

HAEM: Leucopenia, neutropenia, thrombocytopenia, agranulocytosis, haemolytic anaemia, megaloblastic anaemia (due to trimethoprim)

INTEG: Rash, dermatitis, urticaria, Stevens-Johnson syndrome, erythema multiforme, photosensitivity, pain, inflammation at injection site

GU: Renal failure, toxic nephrosis, increased blood urea nitrogen, creatinine, crystalluria

CV: Allergic myocarditis

Contraindications: Hypersensitivity to trimethoprim or sulphonamides, pregnancy megaloblastic anaemia, liver damage, blood disorders, severe renal insufficiency, infants up to 6 weeks, premature infants

Precautions: Pregnancy, lactation, renal disease, elderly, G-6-PD deficiency, impaired hepatic function, possible folate deficiency, severe allergy, bronchial asthma

Pharmacokinetics:

Period of onset: Rapidly absorbed, peak 1–4 hr; half-life 8–13 hr, excreted in urine (metabolites and unchanged), breast milk, highly bound to plasma proteins

Interactions/incompatibilities:

- Increased effect of: sulphonylurea hypoglycaemic agents, phenytoin, methotrexate, thiopentone
- Increased anticoagulant effects: oral anticoagulants
- Decreased renal excretion of: methotrexate
- Decreased hepatic clearance of: phenytoin
- Increased nephrotoxic effect: cyclosporin
- Increased anti-folate effect: pyrimethamine

Clinical assessment:

- Kidney function studies: blood urea nitrogen, creatinine, urinalysis if on long-term or high dose therapy

Treatment of overdose:

- Gastric lavage within 1 hr. Calcium folinate, general supportive measures

NURSING CONSIDERATIONS

Assess:

- Fluid balance

Administer:

- By mouth, with fluid, preferably after meals. IM by deep injection alternately into each buttock. IV, by dilution of one 5-ml ampoule to 125 ml infusion solution (2 ampoules to 250 ml or 3 to 500 ml) directly before use, and infusion usually over about 1.5 hours. Adjust dose in renal impairment
- After specimens taken for culture and sensitivity
- With resuscitative equipment available; severe allergic reactions may occur
- With full glass of water to maintain adequate hydration; increase fluids to 2 litres daily to decrease crystallisation in kidneys
- Medication after culture and sensitivity; repeat culture and sensitivity after full course of medication completed (allow 5 days after end of course before re-culture)

Evaluate:

- Therapeutic response: absence of pain, fever, culture and sensitivity negative
- Blood dyscrasias: skin rash, fever, sore throat, bruising,

bleeding, fatigue, joint pain
• Allergic reaction: rash, dermatitis, exfoliation, urticaria, pruritus, dyspnoea
• Note colour, character, pH of urine if drug administered for urinary tract infections; if urine is highly acidic, alkalinisation may be needed

Teach patient/family:
• To take each oral dose with full glass of water to prevent crystalluria
• To complete full course of treatment to prevent superimposed infection
• To avoid non-prescription medications (aspirin, vitamin C) unless directed by clinician
• To notify clinician if skin rash, sore throat, fever, mouth sores, unusual bruising, bleeding occur
• To seek advice if there is any possibility of pregnancy

cocaine HCl (opthalmic)

Cocaine Eye-drops, Combination product
Func. class.: Local anaesthetic
Chem. class.: Ester
Legal class.: CD POM

Action: Prevents generation and transmission of pain impulses along neurones; produces local vasoconstriction
Uses: Local anaesthetic
Dosage and routes: Topical solutions of 1–4% (greater than 4% not recommended due to systemic effects)
Available forms include: Eye-drops, 4%
Side effects/adverse reactions:
SYSTEM: Absorption after topical application, hypersensitivity
CNS: Dependence, stimulation, excitement, tremor, convulsions
CV: Bradycardia, tachycardia, hypotension, hypertension, ventricular fibrillation
EENT: Blurred vision, corneal damage, ulceration
Contraindications: Hypersensitivity to ester local anaesthetics
Precautions: Cardiovascular disease, thyrotoxicosis, hypertension, porphyria
Pharmacokinetics: Rapid onset of anaesthesia, duration at least 30 min
Interactions/incompatibilities:
• Toxicity increased by: sympathomimetics (adrenaline), MAOIs
Clinical assessment:
• Evaluate effects on eye such as keratitis

NURSING CONSIDERATIONS
Perform/provide:
• Proper storage and administration according to CD regulations (abuse/misuse)
• Storage in a cool place
Evaluate:
• Therapeutic effect
• Side effects
Teach patient/family:
• Effects of drug
• Not to attempt to drive until effects of drug have worn off

codeine phosphate

Func. class.: Narcotic analgesic
Chem. class.: Opioid, phenanthrene derivative
Legal class.: P or POM (tablets, syrup), CD POM (injection)

Action: Inhibits ascending pain pathways in CNS, increases pain threshold, alters pain perception
Uses: Moderate to severe pain, non-productive cough, diarrhoea
Dosage and routes:
Pain

• *Adult:* By mouth 30–60 mg 4-hrly, maximum 240 mg daily; IM 30–60 mg every 4 hr when necessary
• *Child (1–12 yr):* By mouth 3 mg/kg daily in divided doses 4-hrly

Cough
• *Adult:* By mouth 15–30 mg 3 or 4 times a day
• *Child (1–5 yr):* By mouth 3 mg 3 or 4 times a day

Available forms include: Injection IM, 60 mg/ml; tablets 15, 30, 60 mg, linctus 15 mg/5 ml, 3 mg/5 ml, syrup 25 mg/5 ml

Side effects/adverse reactions:
CNS: Drowsiness, sedation, dizziness, agitation, dependency, lethargy, restlessness
GI: Nausea, vomiting, anorexia, constipation
RESP: Respiratory depression, respiratory paralysis
CV: Bradycardia, palpitations, orthostatic hypotension, tachycardia
GU: Urinary retention
INTEG: Flushing, rash, urticaria

Contraindications: Hypersensitivity to opioids, respiratory depression, increased intracranial pressure, head injury, severe respiratory disorders

Precautions: Elderly, cardiac dysrhythmias

Pharmacokinetics: Onset 15–30 min, peak 1–2 hr, duration 4–6 hr; metabolised by liver, excreted by kidneys, excreted in breast milk, half-life 2½–4 hr

Interactions/incompatibilities:
• CNS depression may be increased with other CNS depressants: alcohol, narcotics, sedative/hypnotics, antipsychotics, skeletal muscle relaxants

NURSING CONSIDERATIONS

Administer:
• With antiemetic if nausea, vomiting occur
• With milk or food for less severe GI symptoms

Perform/provide:
• Assistance with walking
• Safety measures: call bell, cot sides

Evaluate:
• Level of pain
• Need for analgesia
• Cough: type, duration, ability to expectorate
• CNS changes, dizziness, drowsiness, hallucinations, restlessness, agitation, mood changes, level of consciousness
• Fluid balance; check for decreasing output; may indicate urinary retention
• Skin rashes, itching, facial flushing
• Respiratory changes: respiratory depression, check rate and depth
• Physical dependence

Teach patient/family:
• To report any symptoms of CNS changes
• To observe for itching, rashes, facial flushing
• That physical dependency may result when used for extended periods of time
• To change position slowly as hypotension may occur
• To avoid hazardous activities such as driving or operating machinery if drowsiness or dizziness occurs
• To avoid alcohol unless directed by clinician
• To take a high fibre diet as constipation may occur

colchicine

Func. class.: Antigout agent
Chem. class.: Colchicum autumnale alkaloid
Legal class.: POM

Action: Inhibits microtubule formation in leucocytes, which decreases phagocytosis in joints
Uses: Acute gout, short-term prophylaxis of gout when commencing allopurinol therapy
Dosage and routes:
Prophylaxis
• *Adult:* By mouth 500 mcg twice or three times a day
Treatment
• *Adult:* By mouth, initially 1 mg, then 500 mcg every 2–3 hr until pain relief, max total dose 10 mg; do not repeat within 3 days
Available forms include: Tablets 500 mcg
Side effects/adverse reactions:
HAEM: Agranulocytosis, thrombocytopenia, aplastic anaemia, pancytopaenia
CNS: Headache, drowsiness, neuritis, dizziness
GI: Nausea, vomiting, anorexia, malaise, metallic taste, cramps, peptic ulcer, diarrhoea, abdominal pain
GU: Renal damage
EENT: Retinopathy, cataracts
INTEG: Stomatitis, fever, chills, dermatitis, pruritus, purpura, erythema, alopecia
Contraindications: Hypersensitivity
Precautions: Severe cardiac, GI or renal disease, blood dyscrasias, pregnancy, lactation
Pharmacokinetics:
Period of onset: Peak ½–2 hr, half-life 20 min, deacetylated in liver, excreted in faeces (metabolites/active drug)
Clinical assessment:
• Full blood count, platelets, reticulocytes before, 3 monthly during therapy
NURSING CONSIDERATIONS
Administer:
• With a full glass of water
Evaluate:
• Therapeutic response: decreased stone formation on x-ray, decreased pain in kidney region, absence of haematuria; decreased pain in joints
• Fluid balance; observe for decrease in urinary output
Teach patient/family:
• To avoid alcohol, non-prescription preparations that contain alcohol; skin rashes may occur
• To report any pain, redness, or hard area often in lower limb joints; any signs of toxicity
• Stress patient compliance with medical regimen; bone marrow depression may occur

colistin sulphate

Colomycin
Func. class.: Antibiotic
Chem. class.: Polymyxin
Legal class.: POM

Action: Interacts with phospholipids, penetrates cell wall; changes occur immediately in bacterial cytoplasmic membrane causing leakage of essential intracellular metabolites
Uses: Infections caused by *Pseudomonas* spp, *Enterobacter* spp, *E. coli*, *Klebsiella* spp, *Shigella* spp, *Haemophilus* spp, *Salmonella* spp, *Serratia* spp, *Bordetella* spp, *Vibrio cholerae*, bowel sterilisation in neutropenic patients
Dosage and routes:
• *Adult:* IM/IV nebulised 2 million units 8-hrly. By mouth (for bowel sterilisation) 1.5–3 million units

every 8 hr. Topically as 1% powder, solution, or ointment.

• *Child:* By mouth 15–30 kg, 0.75–1.5 million units 8-hrly; under 15 kg body-weight, 0.25–0.5 million units 8-hrly

Available forms include: Tablets 1.5 million units; oral powder for suspension 250,000 units/5 ml; powder for IM, IV injection 500,000 units/vial, 1 million units/vial; powder for topical administration 1 g

Side effects/adverse reactions:

INTEG: Pruritus, urticaria, rash, pain at injection site

RESP: Arrest, dyspnoea

GU: Nephrotoxicity

CNS: Paresthaesia, dizziness, ataxia, slurred speech, psychosis, coma, drug fever, confusion

EENT: Blurred vision

Contraindications: Hypersensitivity, myasthenia gravis, porphyria

Precautions: Elderly pregnancy, renal failure

Pharmacokinetics:

Poorly absorbed by mouth

IM: Peak 2 hr, duration less than 12 hr

IV: Peak 2 hr, duration less than 12 hr Half-life 1½–8 hr IM, IV; excreted in urine (active drug, metabolites)

Interactions/incompatibilities:

• Increased neurotoxicity, nephrotoxicity: cephalothin, aminoglycosides, amphotericin B, polymixin, vancomycin

• Increased neuromuscular blockade: tubocurarine, decamethonium, suxamethonium, gallamine

Clinical assessment:

• Liver studies: aspartate aminotransferase, alanine aminotransferase

• Renal studies: urinalysis, protein, blood, blood urea nitrogen, creatinine

• Drug level in impaired hepatic, renal systems (10–15 mcg/ml)

Treatment of overdose: Renal insufficiency, muscle weakness and apnoea may result. Supportive treatment. Increase drug elimination by mannitol diuresis, prolonged haemodialysis or peritoneal dialysis

NURSING CONSIDERATIONS

Assess:

• Fluid balance

• Bowel pattern

• Allergies before treatment, reaction of each medication; note allergies on chart, in bright red letters; advise all people giving medication

• Any patient with compromised renal system; drug is excreted slowly in poor renal system function; toxicity may occur rapidly

• Culture and sensitivity before drug therapy; drug may be used as soon as culture is taken

Administer:

• IV by slow injection or by infusion over up to 6 hr; topically diluted to 1% with lactose, Biosorb, a suitable ointment basis or as 1% solution in saline or water

• IV by infusion only; do not administer bolus dose

• IM deep injection; rotate sites

• Orally with at least 200 ml water

• Nebuliser: 2 million units 8 hrly nebulised for 10–20 min. Mix with 2–4 ml sterile water or sodium chloride 0.9% (nebulise with compressor to generate a flow of at least 8 litres/min)

• If nebulised: isolate patient and use an aerosol concentration device (e.g. Mizer System 22) to prevent general contamination of ward environment and protect other patients/staff from exposure

Perform/provide:

• Colistin oral solution; can be stored in refrigerator for up to 2 weeks, protect from light

• Ensure that emergency equip-

ment is available on unit; respiratory arrest has occurred following IM dose
• Adequate intake of fluids (2 litres) during diarrhoea episodes
Evaluate:
• Therapeutic response: decreased temperature, negative culture and sensitivity
• BP, pulse in patient receiving drug parenterally
• Bowel pattern during treatment
• Skin eruptions, itching, dermatitis
• Respiratory status: rate, character, wheezing, tightness in chest
Teach patient/family:
• To take oral drug with full glass of water, may be taken with food if GI symptoms occur
• Aspects of drug therapy: need to complete entire course of medication to ensure organism death; culture may be taken after completed course of medication
• To report sore throat, fever, fatigue; could indicate superimposed infection
• That drug must be taken in equal intervals around clock to maintain blood levels
• To notify nurse of diarrhoea

---

cortisone acetate

Cortistab, Cortisyl
Func. class.: Corticosteroid, synthetic
Chem. class.: Glucocorticoid, short-acting
Legal class.: POM

Action: Decreases inflammation by suppression of migration of polymorphonuclear leucocytes, fibroblasts, reversal of increased capillary permeability and lysosomal stabilisation
Uses: Adrenal insufficiency
Dosage and routes:
• *Adult:* 12.5–50 mg daily in divided doses
• *Child:* 5–25 mg daily in divided doses
Available forms include: Tablets 5, 25 mg
Side effects/adverse reactions:
INTEG: Acne, poor wound healing, ecchymosis, bruising, petechiae
CNS: Depression, flushing, sweating, headache, mood changes, euphoria, insomnia
CV: Thrombophlebitis, embolism, tachycardia, congestive cardiac failure, hypertension
HAEM: Thrombocytopenia
MS: Fractures, osteoporosis, weakness, proximal myopathy, growth retardation in children
GI: Diarrhoea, nausea, abdominal distention, GI haemorrhage, increased appetite, pancreatitis
EENT: Fungal infections, increased intraocular pressure, blurred vision
METAB: Hyperglycaemia, hypokalaemia
Contraindications: Systemic fungal infection, hypersensitivity
Precautions: Psychosis, idiopathic thrombocytopenia, pregnancy, diabetes mellitus, glaucoma, osteoporosis, epilepsy, peptic ulceration, congestive cardiac failure, myasthenia gravis, hypertension
Pharmacokinetics:
Period of onset: Peak 2 hr, duration 1½ days
Interactions/incompatibilities:
• Decreased action of this drug: cholestyramine, barbiturates, rifampicin, phenytoin
• Decreased effects of: anticoagulants, anticonvulsants, anti diabetics, toxoids, vaccines
• Increased side effects: alcohol, salicylates, indomethacin, amphotericin B

Clinical assessment:
• Plasma cortisol levels during long-term therapy
• Potassium, blood glucose; hypokalaemia and hyperglycaemia

NURSING CONSIDERATIONS

Assess:
• BP, pulse, fluid balance, weight

Administer:
• Titrated dose, use lowest effective dose
• In one dose in morning to prevent adrenal suppression
• With food or milk to decrease GI symptoms

Perform/provide:
• Assistance with ambulation in patient with bone tissue disease to prevent fractures

Evaluate:
• Therapeutic response: ease of respirations, decreased inflammation
• Glycosuria while on long-term therapy
• Weight daily, notify clinician of weekly gain greater than 2 kg
• BP 4 hrly, pulse, notify clinician if chest pain occurs
• Fluid balances; be alert for decreasing urinary output and increasing oedema
• Infection: increased temperature; drug masks symptoms of infection
• Potassium depletion: paraesthesias, fatigue, nausea, vomiting, depression, polyuria, dysrhythmias, weakness
• Oedema, hypotension, cardiac symptoms
• Mental status: affect, mood, behavioural changes, aggression

Teach patient/family:
• That a steroid medication card should be carried at all times
• To notify clinician if therapeutic response decreases; dosage adjustment may be needed
• Not to discontinue this medication abruptly or adrenal crisis can result
• To avoid non-prescription products: salicylates, alcohol in cough products, cold preparations unless directed by clinician
• Teach patient all aspects of drug usage, including Cushingoid symptoms
• Symptoms of adrenal insufficiency: nausea, anorexia, fatigue, dizziness, dyspnoea, weakness, joint pain

---

crisantaspase

Erwinase

Func. class.: Antineoplastic
Chem. class.: Asparaginase enzyme
Legal class.: POM

Action: Indirectly inhibits protein synthesis in tumour cells; breaks down L-asparagine which tumour cells are unable to synthesise

Uses: Acute lymphoblastic leukaemia in combination with other antineoplastics

Dosage and routes:
Doses are highly variable, and dependent on local treatment protocols, concomitant therapy, and tumour type; the following dose schedules have been used
• *Adult:* IM, subcutaneous, IV 200 IU/kg (5000–6000 IU/m^2 body surface area)

Available forms include: Injection 10,000 IU

Side effects/adverse reactions:
HAEM: Thrombocytopenia, leucopenia, anaemia
GI: Nausea, vomiting, anorexia, cramps, stomatitis, hepatotoxicity, pancreatitis
GU: Urinary retention, renal failure, glycosuria, polyuria, azotaemia
INTEG: Rash, urticaria, chills, fever

ENDO: Hyperglycaemia
RESP: Anaphylaxis
CNS: Neuritis, dizziness, headache, coma, depression, fatigue, confusion, hallucinations
Contraindications: Hypersensitivity, pregnancy, pancreatitis
Precautions: Renal disease, hepatic disease, lactation
Pharmacokinetics: Half-life 4–9 hr, terminal 1.4–1.8 hr
Clinical assessment:
• Perform full blood count and platelet count weekly
• Perform tests for blood urea, uric acid, electrolytes and creatinine clearance before and during treatment
• Perform liver function tests before and during treatment
• Obtain blood for Hb and haematocrit as these may be reduced
• Prescribe anti-emetics
• Prescribe allopurinol to maintain uric acid levels
• Prescribe antibiotics as prophylaxis against infection

NURSING CONSIDERATIONS

Assess:
• Baseline observations including BP and weight
• Urinalysis for hyperglycaemia if pancreatitis suspected
Administer:
• HANDLING: take safety precautions appropriate to antineoplastic agents
• Following local antineoplastic (cytotoxic) policies
• After ensuring that clinician is aware of blood results
• IV:IM; after 50 IU intradermal test dose for hypersensitivity
• Other medications by mouth if possible. Avoid IV, IM, SC routes to prevent infection and bruising
• Anti-emetic 30–60 min before treatment
• All other medication as prescribed including analgesics, antibiotics, anti-emetics, antispasmodics
Perform/provide:
• Strict hygienic precautions; protective isolation may be necessary if white blood cell count becomes low
• Encouragement for deep breathing exercises as taught by physiotherapist
• Increased fluid intake to 2–3 litres daily to prevent formation of renal calculi (urate deposits)
• Diet low in purines, e.g. offal, pulses to maintain alkaline urine
• Nutritious diet with iron and vitamin supplements. Advice of dietician may be sought
• Mouthcare. Encourage frequent mouthwashes and the use of a soft toothbrush to avoid stomatitis. Unwaxed dental floss should be used
• Care of skin
• Support in bed to facilitate breathing
Evaluate:
• Fluid balance; report decrease in urinary output to 30 ml/min to clinician
• Temperature and BP 4 hrly if neutropenic
• 8 hrly for signs of bleeding e.g. haematuria, occult blood in stools, melaena, bruising, petechiae, perianal lesions
• Signs of chest infection e.g. dyspnoea, increased respiratory rate, fatigue, lethargy
• Food preferences
• Joint and abdominal pain, shaking, oedema in feet and legs
• Jaundice e.g. skin discolouration, yellow sclera, dark urine, clay-coloured stools, itchy skin, fever, diarrhoea
• Oral mucosa 8 hrly for dryness, sores or ulceration, infection, pain, bleeding, dysphagia
• Inflammation at injection site
• Symptoms of severe allergic

reaction e.g. rash, pruritus, urticaria, purpuric skin lesions, itching, hot flushes
• Diarrhoea, signs of acidosis and dehydration
• General malaise
• Observe for anaphylaxis

Teach patient/family:
• Need for protective isolation
• To report side effects to nurse or clinician
• To report any changes in respiration, breathing
• To avoid foods containing citric acid, and those that are very spicy
• Good mouthcare
• Possibility of side effects

---

cyclizine HCl, cyclizine lactate

Valoid
Func. class.: Anti-emetic
Chem. class.: Antihistamine
Legal class.: Tablets P; Injection POM

Action: Acts centrally by blocking chemoreceptor trigger zone, which is turn acts on vomiting centre
Uses: Nausea, vomiting, including drug-induced, radiation-induced, post-operative; vertigo, motion sickness, labyrinthine disorders
Dosage and routes:
• *Adult:* By mouth IM/IV 50 mg 3 times a day
• *Child 6–12 yr:* By mouth 25 mg 3 times a day
Available forms include: Tablets 50 mg as hydrochloride: injection 50 mg/ml as lactate
Side effects/adverse reactions:
CNS: Drowsiness, dizziness, restlessness, insomnia
EENT: Dry mouth, blurred vision
MISC: tachycardia, urinary retention, constipation
Contraindications: Hypersensitivity to cyclizine
Precautions: Children, narrow-angle glaucoma, urinary retention, lactation, prostatic hypertrophy, elderly, pregnancy, shock
Pharmacokinetics:
Duration 4–6 hr, other pharmacokinetics not known
Interactions/incompatibilities:
• May increase effect of: alcohol, tranquilisers, narcotics, anticholinergic agents
• Decreased effects of: betahistine
Treatment of overdose: Gastric lavage and general supportive measures

NURSING CONSIDERATIONS

Assess:
• Temperature, pulse, respiration, BP; check patients with cardiac disease regularly

Administer:
• Intramuscularly, intravenously, orally; subcutaneously in infusion pumps especially in terminal symptom control (not a licensed indication)

Perform/provide:
• If in subcutaneous pump observe at least 4 hrly for skin irritation

Evaluate:
• Signs of toxicity of other drugs or masking of symptoms of disease: brain tumour, intestinal obstruction
• Observe for drowsiness, dizziness
• May be irritant to skin especially if used as subcutaneous route

Teach patient/family:
• To avoid hazardous activities or activities requiring alertness including driving as drug can cause drowsiness; dizziness may occur; that assistance with ambulation may be needed
• That a false negative result may occur with skin testing; skin testing procedures should not be scheduled for 4 days after discontinuing use

• Avoid alcohol, other CNS depressants

---

cyclopenthiazide

Navidrex, combination products
Func. class.: Diuretic
Chem. class.: Thiazide
Legal class.: POM

Action: Inhibits reabsorption of sodium chloride and water at the distal tubule; reduces peripheral vascular resistance
Uses: Oedema, hypertension, congestive heart failure
Dosage and routes:
Oedema, congestive heart failure
• *By mouth* initially 0.5–1 mg in morning, maintenance 500 mcg on alternate days
Oedema of pre-menstrual tension:
• *Adult:* By mouth, 250–500 mcg daily from onset of symptoms to menstruation
Hypertension
• 250–500 mcg in morning. Maximum dose, 1.5 mg daily
Available forms include: Tablets, 500 mcg
Side effects/adverse reactions:
HAEM: Thrombocytopenia, hypokalaemia
EENT: Photosensitivity
META: Hyperuricaemia, hyperglycaemia
GU: Impotence, glycosuria
INTEG: Rashes
Contraindications: Hypercalcaemia, renal failure, Addison's disease, porphyria, concurrent lithium therapy
Precautions: Pregnancy, diabetes, gout, renal or hepatic impairment, hyperlipidaemia
Pharmacokinetics: Diuresis induced within 1–2 hr, duration 12 hr
Interactions/incompatibilities:
• Increased cardiac glycoside toxicity due to hypokalaemia
• Antagonism of insulin and oral antidiabetic agents
• Antagonism of effects by NSAIDs
• Increased hypokalaemia with ACTH, corticosteroids
Clinical assessment:
• Frequent checks on potassium levels
• Review of hypoglycaemic requirement in known diabetics
Treatment of overdose: Induction of vomiting and gastric lavage, check BP and electrolytes, IV fluids and electrolyte replacement

NURSING CONSIDERATIONS

Administer:
• In the morning with food
Perform/provide:
• Potassium rich diet, high fibre to avoid constipation
• Help with getting up, patient should rise slowly
• Monitor diabetics carefully
• Counselling for sexual problems
Evaluate:
• Fluid balance, pulse 4 hrly; risk of potassium depletion
• Weight daily, BP (lying/standing) daily; possibility of postural hypotension
• Test urine for glucose
• Irregular heart rate
• Muscle fatigue/spasm
• Oedema/dry skin
• Bruising
• Rashes
• Effects on urinary output/oedema
• Insulin requirements in known diabetics
Teach patient/family:
• About possibility of impotence (reversible)
• To use a sunscreen
• To rise slowly
• To report side effects including painful joints

• Dietary advice on potassium, salt, fibre intake
• To seek advice about drug interactions

cyclopentolate HCl (opthalmic)

Mydrilate, Minims
Func. class.: Mydriatic, cycloplegic, anticholinergic
Legal class.: POM

Action: Dilates the pupil and paralyses the ciliary muscle
Uses: Diagnostic purposes for fundoscopy and cycloplegic refraction, dilating the pupil in inflammatory conditions of the iris and uveal tract
Dosage and routes:
Refraction
• *Adults:* Instil one drop of a 0.5% solution and repeat after 15 min if necessary
• *Child: 6–16 yr* Instil one drop of a 1% solution 40 min before examining the eye; under 6 yr, instil one or two drops as above
Uveitis
• *Adult:* Instil one or two drops of a 0.5% solution up to 4 times a day
• *Child:* At the discretion of the prescriber
Deeply pigmented eyes may require a 1% solution
Available forms include: 0.5%, 1% solution in multi-use bottles; 0.5%, 1% Minims
Side effects/adverse reactions:
CV: Tachycardia, flushing (infants: abdominal distention, irregular pulse, respiratory depression)
EENT: Blurred vision, temporary burning sensation on instillation, eye dryness, photophobia, conjunctivitis, increased intraocular pressure
CNS: (In children), psychotic reaction, behavior disturbances, ataxia, restlessness, hallucinations, somnolence, disorientation, grand mal seizures; confusion, fever
GI: Abdominal distention, vomiting, dry mouth
Contraindications: Hypersensitivity, infants less than 3 months, local or systemic glaucoma, conjunctivitis, paralytic ileus, soft contact lenses (Minims may be used)
Precautions: Prostatic enlargement, coronary insufficiency, cardiac failure
Pharmacokinetics:
INSTIL: Peak 30–60 min (mydriasis), 25–74 min (cyclopegia), duration ¼–1 day
Interactions/incompatibilities:
• Enhanced effects with: other anti-muscarinic agents
Treatment of overdose: Supportive measures, induce vomiting and gastric lavage if accidentally ingested

NURSING CONSIDERATIONS

Evaluate:
• Therapeutic response
• Side effects particularly in very young and elderly
Perform/provide:
• Storage in a cool place
• Clear explanation of effect of drug
Teach patient/family:
• To report change in vision, blurring, or loss of sight, trouble breathing, sweating, flushing
• Method of instillation: pressure on lacrimal sac for 1 min, do not touch dropper to eye
• That blurred vision will decrease with repeated use of drug
• That drug may sting when instilled
• Wear dark sunglasses for photophobia
• Not to do hazardous tasks until able to see clearly (up to 4 hr)

cyclophosphamide

Endoxana

Func. class.: Cytotoxic alkylating agent

Chem. class.: Nitrogen mustard

Legal class.: POM

Action: Alkylates DNA, RNA; inhibits enzymes that allow synthesis of proteins; is also responsible for cross linking DNA strands

Uses: Leukaemias, lymphomas and a wide range of solid tumours. May be used alone or in combination with other cytotoxic agents

Dosage and routes:

Doses are highly variable, and dependent on local treatment protocols, concomitant therapy and tumour type; the following dose schedules have been used

• *Adult:* Variable, depending on patient's condition, regimen and tumour

Available forms include: Injection 100 mg, 200 mg, 500 mg, 1 g; tablets 50 mg

Side effects/adverse reactions:

CV: Cardiotoxicity (high doses)

HAEM: Thrombocytopenia, leucopenia, pancytopenia

GI: Nausea, vomiting, diarrhoea, weight loss, colitis, hepatotoxicity

GU: Haemorrhagic cystitis, haematuria, neoplasms, amenorrhoea, azoospermia, impotence, sterility, ovarian fibrosis

INTEG: Alopecia, dermatitis

RESP: Fibrosis, pneumonitis

CNS: Headache, dizziness

Contraindications: Hypersensitivity, haemorrhagic cystisis, porphyria, acute infections, bone marrow aplasia

Precautions: Radiation therapy, pregnancy, bone marrow depression, renal failure, liver failure

Pharmacokinetics: Metabolised by liver to active compound, excreted in urine; half-life 4–6½ hr; 50% bound to plasma proteins

Interactions/incompatibilities:

• Increased hypoglycaemic effects of sulphonylurea compounds

• Potentiation of suxamethonium effects

• Increased bone marrow depression: allopurinol

Clinical assessment:

• Full blood count, differential, platelet count weekly

• Pulmonary function tests, chest X-ray films before, during therapy

• Renal function studies: blood urea nitrogen, serum uric acid, urine creatinine clearance before, during therapy

• Liver function test before during therapy

• Prescribe mesna (with high dose therapy), anti-emetics

Treatment of overdose: Early gastric lavage if drug in tablet form. Supportive measures, e.g. broad-spectrum antibiotics, blood transfusions, IV mesna (if recognised early), maintenance of fluid balance

NURSING CONSIDERATIONS

Assess:

• Urinalysis for blood

• Weight, fluid balance

Administer:

• HANDLING: take safety precautions appropriate to antineoplastic agents

• Following local antineoplastic (cytotoxic) policies

• After ensuring that clinician is aware of blood results

• IV: By slow IV injection over 2–3 min or by IV infusion

• By mouth: with plenty of water and with food if GI disturbance is severe

• Antacid before oral administration and prescribed mesna with high dose therapy

• Other medications by mouth if possible. Avoid IV, IM, SC routes

to prevent infection and bruising
- Anti-emetic 30–60 min before treatment
- All other medication as prescribed including analgesics, antibiotics, anti-emetics, antispasmodics

Perform/provide:
- Protective isolation if/when neutropenic
- Deep breathing exercises with patient 3 or 4 times a day
- Increase fluid intake to 3 litres daily to prevent urate deposits, calculi formation
- Mouth care; brushing of teeth with soft brush or cotton-tipped applicators for stomatitis; use unwaxed dental floss
- Warm compresses at injection site for inflammation
- Urinalysis for blood

Evaluate:
- Fluid balance (report fall in urine output of 30 ml/hr)
- Monitor temperature and BP 4 hrly when neutropenic; hourly if temperature is above 38°C
- Bleeding in any site or tissue
- Signs and symptoms of cytopenia and haemorrhagic cystitis
- Dyspnoea, rales, unproductive cough, chest pain, tachypnoea
- Food preferences; list likes, dislikes
- Effects of alopecia on body image, discuss feelings about body changes
- Yellowing of skin, sclera, dark urine, clay-coloured stools, itchy skin, abdominal pain, fever, diarrhoea
- Oedema in feet, joint pain, stomach pain, shaking
- Inflammation of mucosa, breaks in skin
- Buccal cavity 8 hrly for dryness, sores or ulceration, white patches, oral pain, bleeding, dysphagia
- Symptoms indicating severe allergic reaction: rash, pruritus, urticaria, purpuric skin lesions, itching, flushing
- Tachypnoea, ECG changes, dyspnoea, oedema, fatigue

Teach patient/family:
- Protective isolation precautions
- To report any complaints or side effects to nurse or clinician
- That impotence or amenorrhoea can occur, but is reversible after discontinuing treatment
- To report any changes in breathing or coughing
- That hair may be lost during treatment; a wig or hairpiece may make patient feel better (available free on NHS); new hair may be different in colour, texture
- Dietary advice
- To report any bleeding, white spots or ulcerations in mouth to clinician; tell patient to examine mouth 6 hrly

---

cycloserine

Func. class.: Antibiotic, antitubercular
Chem. class.: D-alanine analogue
Legal class.: POM

Action: Inhibits cell wall synthesis, decreases tubercle bacilli replication

Uses: In combination with other drugs, tuberculosis resistant to first-line drugs

Dosage and routes:
- *Adult:* By mouth 250 mg 12-hrly, maximum 1 g daily
- *Children:* Start at 10 mg/kg daily and adjust according to blood levels and clinical response

Available forms include: Capsules 250 mg

Side effects/adverse reactions:
INTEG: Dermatitis, photosensitivity

CV: Congestive cardiac failure, dysrhythmias
CNS: Headache, anxiety, drowsiness, tremors, convulsions, lethargy, depression, confusion, psychosis, aggression
METAB: Changes in liver function tests
HAEM: Megaloblastic anaemia
Contraindications: Hypersensitivity, severe renal disease, alcoholism (chronic), depression, severe anxiety or neurosis, epilepsy, porphyria
Precautions: Pregnancy, children
Pharmacokinetics:
Period of onset: Peak 3–4 hr; excreted unchanged in urine, excreted in breast milk
Interactions/incompatibilities:
• May increase toxicity: ethionamide, isoniazid, alcohol
• Increased plasma level of: phenytoin
Clinical assessment:
• Liver studies every week: aspartate aminotransferase, alanine aminotransferase, bilirubin
• Renal status: before therapy and every month: blood urea nitrogen, creatinine, output, specific gravity, urinalysis
• Blood levels of drug; keep below 30 mcg/ml or toxicity may occur
Lab. test interferences:
Increase: Aspartate aminotransferase, alanine aminotransferase
Treatment of overdose: Administer vitamin B_6, anticonvulsants, O_2, assisted respiration, activated charcoal to reduce absorption, haemodialysis in life-threatening acute toxicity
NURSING CONSIDERATIONS
Administer:
• Reduce dosage in renal impairment; maintain blood levels below 30 mcg/ml
• After culture and sensitivity is completed every month to detect resistance
Evaluate:
• Mental status often: affect, mood, behavioural changes, psychosis may occur
• Hepatic status: decreased appetite, jaundice, dark urine, fatigue
Teach patient/family:
• Avoid alcohol while taking drug
• That compliance with dosage schedule, length is necessary
• To report neurotoxicity: confusion, headache, drowsiness, tremors, paraesthesia, mental changes
• To avoid hazardous activities if drowsiness or dizziness occurs

---

cyclosporin

Sandimmun
Func. class.: Immunosuppressant
Chem. class.: Fungus-derived peptide
Legal class.: POM

Action: Produces immunosuppression by blocking resting lymphocytes and inhibiting lymphokine production and release
Uses: Organ transplants (including allogeneic bone marrow transplants) to prevent rejection, prophylaxis and treatment of graft-versus-host disease
Dosage and routes:
Organ transplants
• *Adult and child:* By mouth 10–15 mg/kg several hours before surgery then daily for 1–2 weeks, reduce daily dosage to 2–6 mg/kg a day; dose can be adjusted according to blood levels and renal function; maintenance doses are lower and reached sooner with concomitant immunosuppressant therapy (e.g. corticosteroids)
Bone marrow transplant, graft-versus-host disease

• IV initially 3–5 mg/kg on the day before transplantation and continuing until oral therapy starts within 2 weeks; by mouth 12.5 mg/kg daily for 3–6 months then gradually decrease to zero

Psoriasis

• *Adult and child:* By mouth, initially 2.5 mg/kg daily in 2 divided doses, increased gradually to a maximum of 5 mg/kg if no improvement within 1 month

Available forms include: Oral solution 100 mg/ml; injection (concentrate for IV infusion) 50 mg/ml (1 ml, 5 ml ampoules); capsules 25, 50, 100 mg

Side effects/adverse reactions:

GI: Nausea, vomiting, diarrhoea, anorexia, oral candidiasis, gum hyperplasia, hepatotoxicity

INTEG: Rash, acne, hirsutism

ELEC: Hyperkalaemia

CNS: Tremors, headache

GU: Albuminuria, haematuria, proteinuria, renal impairment

Contraindications: Hypersensitivity, breast-feeding. For treating psoriasis: abnormal renal function, uncontrolled hypertension, uncontrolled infection

Precautions: Severe renal disease, severe hepatic disease

Pharmacokinetics: Peak 4 hr, highly protein bound, half-life (biphasic) 1.2 hr, 25 hr; metabolised in liver, excreted in faeces, excreted in breast milk

Interactions/incompatibilities:

• Increased action of this drug: diltiazem, erythromycin, nicardipine, progestogens, verapamil, ketoconazole, itraconazole, danazol

• Decreased action of this drug: phenytoin, rifampicin, phenobarbitone, carbamazepine, primidone, octreotide

• Increased nephrotoxicity: amphotericin B, aminoglycosides

• Increased hyperkalaemia: enalapril, captopril, potassium supplements, potassium-sparing diuretics

• Increased myopathy: simvastatin, pravastatin

Clinical assessment:

• Renal function, urea and electrolytes, creatinine at least monthly during treatment, 3 months after treatment

• Liver function studies: alkaline phosphatase, aspartate aminotransferase, alanine aminotransferase, bilirubin

• Drug blood levels during treatment

NURSING CONSIDERATIONS

Administer:

• As part of immunosuppressive regime

• Oral solution should be diluted with cold milk, cold chocolate drink or fruit juice in a glass (not plastic) immediately before taking

• Injection should be diluted 1:20 to 1:100 with sodium chloride 0.9% of dextrose 5%, and given by slow IV infusion over 2–6 hr

• At prescribed time for accurate monitoring of serum levels and taking account of these values

• With oral nystatin for potential *Candida* infections (at least 6 weeks of therapy)

Perform/provide:

• Store and administer liquid preparation in glass containers

Evaluate:

• Toxicity: reduced urinary output and/or dark urine, jaundice, pruritus, pale stools

• Hypersensitivity; severe tremor of hands, nausea, vomiting, diarrhoea

Teach patient/family:

• To report any signs of infection immediately (fever, sore throat general malaise)

• Importance of minimising exposure to infection

• Importance of continuity and

accurate administration of medication
• Not to breast feed
• To use contraceptive measures during treatment, and for 12 weeks after ending therapy
• To avoid direct sunlight; use sunscreen and protective measures

---

cyproheptadine HCl

Periactin
Func. class.: Antihistamine
Chem. class.: H_1-receptor antagonist, piperidine derivative
Legal class.: P

Action: Acts on blood vessels, GI, respiratory system by competing with histamine for H_1-receptor site; decreases allergic response by blocking histamine
Uses: Allergy symptoms, rhinitis, pruritus, stimulation of appetite, migraine
Dosage and routes:
Allergy and pruritus
• *Adult:* By mouth 4 mg, 3 or 4 times a day, maximum 32 mg daily
• *Child 7–14 yr:* By mouth 4 mg 2 or 3 times a day, not to exceed 16 mg daily
• *Child 2–6 yr:* By mouth 2 mg 2 or 3 times a day, not to exceed 12 mg daily
Appetite stimulation
• *Adult:* By mouth 4 mg 3 times a day or 12 mg in the evening
• *Child 7–14 yr:* Not more than 12 mg daily
• *Child 2–6 yr:* Not more than 8 mg daily
Migraine
• *Adult:* By mouth, 4 mg repeated after 30 min if required; maintenance 4 mg every 4–6 hr
Available forms include: Tablets 4 mg; syrup 2 mg/5 ml
Side effects/adverse reactions:
CNS: Dizziness, drowsiness, poor coordination, fatigue, anxiety, euphoria, confusion, paraesthesia, neuritis, increased appetite
CV: Hypotension, palpitations, tachycardia
RESP: Increased thick secretions, wheezing, chest tightness
GI: Dry mouth, nausea, vomiting, anorexia, constipation, diarrhoea
INTEG: Rash, urticaria, photosensitivity
GU: Retention, dysuria, frequency
EENT: Blurred vision, dilated pupils, tinnitus, nasal stuffiness, dry nose, throat, mouth
Contraindications: Hypersensitivity to H_1-receptor antagonists; acute asthma attack; lower respiratory tract disease; stenosing peptic ulcer; glaucoma; neonate; premature infant; children under 2 yr of age; breast-feeding; symptomatic prostatic hypertrophy; bladder neck obstruction; GI obstruction; elderly or debilitated patients; urinary retention; MAOIs; porphyria
Precautions: Increased intraocular pressure, renal disease, cardiac disease, hypertension, bronchial asthma, seizure disorder, hyperthyroidism, pregnancy
Pharmacokinetics:
By mouth: duration 4–6 hr, metabolised in liver, excreted by kidneys, excreted in breast milk
Interactions/incompatibilities:
• Increased CNS depression: barbiturates, narcotics, hypnotics, tricyclic antidepressants, alcohol
• Increased effect of this drug: MAOIs
Clinical assessment:
• Full blood count during long term therapy
Lab. test interferences: Reduces hypoglycaemia-induced growth hormone secretion
Treatment of overdose: Induce

emesis or gastric lavage, plus supportive therapy

NURSING CONSIDERATIONS

Administer:

• With meals if GI symptoms occur; absorption may slightly decrease
• Syrup may be diluted with syrup BP and used within 14 days; do not freeze

Perform/provide:

• Frequent drinks and mouth washes for dryness

Evaluate:

• Therapeutic response: absence of running or congested nose or rashes
• Fluid balance: observe for urinary retention, frequency, dysuria; drug should be discontinued if these occur
• Respiratory status: rate, rhythm, increase in bronchial secretions, wheezing, chest tightness
• Cardiac status: palpitations, increased pulse, hypotension

Teach patient/family:

• All aspects of drug use; notify the clinician if confusion, sedation, hypotension occurs
• Driving or operation of machinery may be impaired
• To avoid concurrent use of alcohol or other CNS depressants

---

cyproterone acetate

Androcur, Cyprostat

Func. class.: Anti-androgen with progestogenic activity
Chem. class.: Steroid
Legal class.: POM

Action: Antagonises the effects of androgens by blocking androgen receptors; reduces gonadotrophin secretion by negative feedback

Uses: Control of severe hypersexuality or sexual deviation in men; palliative treatment of prostatic carcinoma

Dosage and routes:

• *Hypersexuality:* 50 mg twice daily, prostatic carcinoma: 200–300 mg daily in 2–3 doses

Prostatic carcinoma

By mouth, 300 mg daily in 2–3 divided doses. Reduce dose if side effects occur, but should aim for 200–300 mg daily

Available forms include: Tablets, 50 mg

Side effects/adverse reactions:

META: Weight gain, changes in hair pattern, gynaecomastia, galactorrhoea, benign breast nodules
GU: Inhibition of spermatogenesis, abnormal sperm, reduced menstrual flow, intermenstrual bleeding
GI: Liver abnormalities, hepatic tumours, nausea, vomiting
MS: Osteoporosis, may arrest bone maturation in young men
SYST: Severe fatigue, lassitude
CNS: Headache, changed libido, depression
INTEG: Chloasma, patchy body hair growth, lightening of hair colour

Contraindications: Patients under 18 yr; liver disease, malignant or wasting disease (excluding prostatic cancer), severe depression, history of thromboembolic disorders (ineffective in chronic alcoholism), pregnancy, lactation, sickle cell anaemia, abnormal vaginal bleeding of unknown cause.

Precautions: Diabetes mellitus, adrenocortical insufficiency, hypertension, abnormal liver function

Pharmacokinetics: Peak plasma concentration within 3–10 hr, excreted as metabolites in faeces and urine

Interactions/incompatibilities:

• Effects diminished by: alcoholism
• Risk of chloasma increased by: UV light and strong sunlight

Clinical assessment:
• Full blood count, Hb (hypochronic anaemia)
• Liver function tests, adrenal function, blood glucose (especially diabetics)
• Check history of alcohol abuse, hepatic tumours and thromboembolic conditions
• Obtain fully informed consent

Treatment of overdose: Gastric lavage, symptomatic treatment

NURSING CONSIDERATIONS

Assess:
• Baseline weight

Administer:
• With or after food

Evaluate:
• Weight—weekly; fluctuations may occur

Teach patient/family:
• That reversible male infertility may occur
• To avoid alcohol
• That ability to drive or operate machinery may be impaired; causes drowsiness at first
• That hair pattern may change, skin becomes dry and gynaecomastia may occur.
• Tiredness may be a problem

cytarabine (ARA-C, cytosine arabinoside)

Alexan, Cytosar

Func. class.: Antineoplastic agent, antimetabolite
Chem. class.: Pyrimidine nucleoside
Legal class.: POM

Action: Competes with physiological substrate, inhibits DNA synthesis; interferes with cell replication at S phase, directly before mitosis

Uses: Acute myeloid leukaemia, acute lymphoblastic leukaemia, chronic myeloid leukaemia, and in combination for non-Hodgkin's lymphomas

Dosage and routes:
Doses are highly variable, and dependent on local treatment protocols, concomitant therapy and tumour type

Available forms include: Injection 20 mg/ml, 100 mg/ml; powder for IV solution 100 mg, 500 mg

Side effects/adverse reactions:
HAEM: Thrombophlebitis, bleeding, thrombocytopenia, leucopenia, myelosuppression, anaemia
GI: Nausea, vomiting, anorexia, diarrhoea, stomatitis, hepatotoxicity, abdominal pain, haematemesis, GI haemorrhage
EENT: Sore throat, conjunctivitis
GU: Urinary retention, renal failure, hyperuricaemia
INTEG: Rash, fever, freckling, cellulitis
RESP: Pneumonia, dyspnoea
CV: Chest pain
CNS: Neuritis, dizziness, headache, personality changes, coma
CYTARABINE SYNDROME: Fever, myalgia, bone pain, chest pain, rash, conjunctivitis, malaise (6–12 hr after administration)

Contraindications: Hypersensitivity, pregnancy, breast-feeding

Precautions: Renal disease, hepatic disease, bone marrow depression

Pharmacokinetics:
IV: Distribution half-life 10 min, elimination half-life 1–3 hr

Interactions/incompatibilities:
• Increased toxicity: radiation or other antineoplastics
• Decreased effects of: oral digoxin
• Increased risk of cardiomyo-

pathy with cyclophosphamide

Clinical assessment:

- Full blood count (RBC, PCV, Hb), differential, platelet count weekly
- Renal function studies: blood urea nitrogen, serum uric acid, urine creatinine clearance, electrolytes before and during therapy
- Liver function tests before and during therapy: bilirubin, alanine aminotransferase, aspartate aminotransferase, alkaline phosphatase, as needed or monthly
- Blood uric acid levels during therapy

NURSING CONSIDERATIONS

Administer:

- HANDLING: take safety precautions appropriate to antineoplastic agents
- Following local antineoplastic (cytotoxic) policies
- After ensuring that clinician is aware of blood results
- IV; continuous IV infusion over 5–10 days
- Intrathecally: solutions for this must be isotonic, unpreserved
- Subcutaneously: change sites for each injection
- Other medications by mouth if possible. Avoid IV, IM, SC routes to prevent infection and bruising
- Anti-emetic 30–60 min before treatment and as prescribed throughout the course of treatment
- All other medication as prescribed, including analgesics, antibiotics, anti-emetics, antispasmodics

Perform/provide:

- Good aseptic technique when administering and/or connecting to IV line
- Subcutaneous injection: charge site for each injection
- Increase fluid intake to 2–3 litres a day to prevent urate deposits and calculi formation, unless contraindicated
- Mouthcare, brushing of teeth with soft brush or cotton-tipped applicators for stomatitis; use unwaxed dental floss
- Observe subcutaneous injection sites for skin irritation
- Warm compresses at injection site for inflammation, pain

Evaluate:

- Fluid balance; report fall in urine output to below 30–50 ml/hr
- Temperature, pulse, respiration and BP if neutropenic 4 hrly; fever may indicate infection
- Fever, flu-like symptoms, myalgia, bone pain, chest pain, rash, conjunctivitis, malaise
- Bleeding in any site or tissue
- Dyspnoea, unproductive cough, chest pain, tachypnoea, fatigue, increased pulse, pallor, lethargy, personality changes, with high doses
- Oedema in feet, joint pain, abdominal pain, shaking
- Inflammation of mucosa, breaks in skin
- Yellowing of skin, sclera, dark urine, clay-coloured stools, itchy skin, abdominal pain, diarrhoea
- Signs of stomatitis
- GI symptoms: frequency of stools, cramping
- Acidosis, signs of dehydration: rapid respirations, poor skin turgor, decreased urine output, dry skin, restlessness, weakness

Teach patient/family:

- Protective isolation precautions
- To report signs of stomatitis, bleeding from any source, or feelings of malaise
- Dietary advice
- Major side effects of drug

dacarbazine

DTIC-Dome
Func. class.: Antineoplastic, alkylating agent
Chem. class.: Cytotoxic triazine
Legal class.: POM

Action: Alkylates DNA, RNA; inhibits enzymes that allow synthesis of proteins; also responsible for cross-linking DNA strands

Uses: Hodgkin's disease, sarcomas, neuroblastoma, malignant melanoma. Also used in combination with other cytotoxic agents; carcinoma—colon, ovary, breast, lung, testicular teratoma, solid tumours in children

Dosage and routes:
Doses are highly variable, and dependent on local treatment protocols, concomitant therapy and tumour type; the following dose schedules have been used
• *Adult:* IV 2–4.5 mg/kg daily for 10 days repeated after 4 weeks, or 250 mg/m^2 for 5 days repeated after 3 weeks, or total dose on first day. Other schedules are used

Available forms include: Injection 100 mg, 200 mg

Side effects/adverse reactions:
HAEM: Thrombocytopenia, leucopenia, anaemia
GI: Nausea, anorexia, vomiting, diarrhoea, hepatotoxicity
CNS: Facial paraesthesia, flushing, fever, malaise, anaphylaxis
INTEG: Alopecia, dermatitis, pain at injection site, photosensitivity reactions

Contraindications: Breast-feeding, hypersensitivity, pregnancy

Precautions: Radiation therapy

Pharmacokinetics: Metabolised by liver, excreted in urine; half-life 35 min, terminal 5 hr, 5% protein bound

Clinical assessment:
• Full blood count, differential, platelet count weekly; withhold drug if WBC is less than 4.0 × 10^9/litre or platelet count is less than 75 × 10^9/litre
• Liver function tests before, during therapy (bilirubin, aspartate aminotransferase, alanine aminotransferase, lactic dehydrogenase) as needed or monthly

NURSING CONSIDERATIONS

Assess:
• Temperature, pulse, respiration

Administer:
• HANDLING: take safety precautions appropriate to antineoplastic agents
• Following local antineoplastic (cytotoxic) policies
• After ensuring that clinician is aware of blood results
• IV: by infusion over 15–20 min
• Other medications by mouth if possible. Avoid IV, IM, SC routes to prevent infection and bruising but only if thrombocytopenic. IV route used if central line *in situ*
• Anti-emetic 30–60 min before treatment
• All other medication as prescribed including analgesics, antibiotics, anti-emetics, antispasmodics

Perform/provide:
• Strict medical asepsis, protective isolation if WBC levels are low
• Special skin care
• Increase fluid intake to 2–3 litres daily to prevent urate deposits, calculi formation
• Warm compresses at injection site for inflammation

Evaluate:
• Bleeding: haematuria, bruising or petechiae, mucosa or orifices 8 hrly
• Food preferences; list likes, dislikes
• Effects of alopecia on body image, discuss feelings about changes in body image

• Yellowing of skin, sclera, dark urine, clay-coloured stools, itchy skin, abdominal pain, fever, diarrhoea
• Inflammation of mucosa, breaks in skin

Teach patient/family:
• Of protective isolation precautions
• To report any complaints or side effects to nurse or clinician

dactinomycin (actinomycin D)

Cosmegen Lyovac
Func. class.: Antineoplastic
Chem. class.: Cytotoxic antibiotic
Legal class.: POM

Action: Inhibits DNA, RNA, protein synthesis; derived from *Streptomyces parrullus*; replication is decreased by binding to DNA, which causes strand splitting; cell cycle nonspecific

Uses: Sarcomas, melanomas, trophoblastic tumours in women, testicular cancer, Wilms' tumour, rhabdomyosarcoma, experimental indication include Ewing's sarcoma, oestrogenic sarcoma

Dosage and routes: (Other schedules may be used)
Doses are highly variable, and dependent on local treatment protocols, concomitant therapy, and tumour type; the following dose schedules have been used
• *Adult:* IV 500 mcg daily for 5 days, repeat after 3 weeks if required
• *Child:* IV 15 mcg/kg daily for 5 days, or a total dose of 2500 mcg/m^2 given IV over 1 week
• Dose for adults and children not to exceed 15 mcg/kg or 400–600 mcg/m^2 daily for 5 days; stop drug until bone marrow recovery, then repeat cycle (not within 3 weeks)
• Isolated limb perfusion: 35 mcg/kg (upper extremity), 50 mcg/kg (lower extremity or pelvis). Seek specialist advice

Available forms include: Injection 500 mcg

Side effects/adverse reactions:
HAEM: Thrombocytopenia, leucopenia, myelosuppression, aplastic anaemia
GI: Nausea, vomiting, anorexia, stomatitis, hepatotoxicity, abdominal pain, diarrhoea, gastrointestinal ulceration
INTEG: Rash, alopecia, pain at injection site, folliculitis, acne
EENT: Cheilitis, ulcerative stomatitis, dysphagia, oesophagitis
CNS: Malaise, fatigue, lethargy, fever
MS: Myalgia
META: Hypocalcaemia

Contraindications: Hypersensitivity, chickenpox, herpes zoster infections, children under 12 months

Precautions: Renal disease, hepatic disease, pregnancy, lactation, bone marrow depression

Pharmacokinetics: Half-life 36 hr
IV: onset 2–5 min, concentrates in kidneys, liver, spleen; does not cross blood-brain barrier, excreted in bile and urine

Interactions/incompatibilities:
• Increased toxicity: other antineoplastics or radiation

Clinical assessment:
• Full blood count, differential, platelet count weekly; withhold drug if WBC is less than 4.0×10^9/litre or platelet count is 75×10^9/litre; notify clinician of these results
• Renal function studies: urea, serum uric acid, creatinine clearance, electrolytes before, during therapy
• Liver function tests before,

during therapy: bilirubin, aspartate aminotransferase, alanine aminotransferase, alkaline phosphatase, as needed or monthly

NURSING CONSIDERATIONS

Assess:

• Baseline vital signs and fluid balance

Administer:

• HANDLING: take safety precautions appropriate to antineoplastic agents

• Following local antineoplastic (cytotoxic) policies

• After ensuring that clinician is aware of blood results

• IV: by IV injection, preferably into tubing of fast-running IV infusion, taking care to avoid extravasation

• Other medications by mouth if possible. Avoid IV, IM, SC routes to prevent infection and bruising

• Anti-emetic 30–60 min before treatment

• All other medication as prescribed including analgesics, antibiotics, anti-emetics, antispasmodics

Perform/provide:

• Strict medical asepsis, protective isolation if WBC levels are low

• Nutritious diet (as tolerated by the patient)

• Scrupulous care of the mouth

• Warm compresses at injection site for inflammation; check for extravasation

Evaluate:

• Fluid balance; report fall in urine output to less than 30–50 ml/hr

• Temperature, pulse, respiration 4 hrly; fever may indicate infection

• Bleeding: haematuria, bruising, petechiae, mucosa or orifices 8-hrly

• Food preferences; nutritional status

• Effects of alopecia on body image; discuss feelings about in body image changes

• Oedema in feet; joint, abdominal pain; shaking

• Inflammation of mucosa, breaks in skin

• Yellowing of skin, sclera, dark urine, clay-coloured stools, itchy skin, abdominal pain, fever, diarrhoea

• Buccal cavity for dryness, sores, ulceration, white patches, oral pain, bleeding, dysphagia; 8-hrly

• Local irritation, pain, burning at injection site

• Symptoms indicating severe allergic reaction: rash, pruritus, urticaria, purpuric skin lesions, itching, flushing

• GI symptoms: frequency of stools, cramping

• Acidosis, signs of dehydration: rapid respirations, poor skin turgor, decreased urine output, dry skin, restlessness, weakness

Teach patient/family:

• Why protective isolation precautions are necessary

• To report any complaints, side effects to nurse or clinician

• That hair may be lost during treatment and wig or hairpiece may make patient feel better (available free on NHS); tell patient that new hair may be different in colour, texture

• To avoid foods which irritate mucosa

• To report any bleeding, white spots, ulcerations in mouth to clinician; tell patient to examine mouth daily

---

dalteparin

Fragmin

Func. class.: Anticoagulant

Chem. class.: Low molecular weight heparin

Legal class.: POM

Action: Prevents conversion of

fibrinogen to fibrin, with a longer duration of action than normal heparin

Uses: Prevention of deep vein thrombosis in patients undergoing surgery, and prevention of clotting in extracorporeal circulation of patients undergoing haemodialysis or haemofiltration

Dosage and routes:

Prophylaxis of peri-operative deep vein thrombosis

Moderate thromboembolic risk

• *Adult:* By SC injection 2500 IU 1–2 hr prior to surgery, then 2500 IU daily for 5 days or until the patient is fully ambulant

High thromboembolic risk

• *Adult:* By SC injection 2500 IU 1–2 hr prior to surgery repeated 12 hr later, then 5000 IU daily for 5 days or until the patient is fully ambulant

Prophylaxis during extracorporeal circulation during haemodialysis/haemofiltration:

Haemodialysis/haemofiltration lasting longer than 4 hr

• *Adult:* By IV injection 35 IU/kg body weight, followed by 13 IU/kg body weight/hr by IV infusion

Haemodialysis/haemofiltration lasting less than 4 hr

• *Adult:* By IV injection 5000 IU, *or* use infusion schedule above

Acute renal failure, or chronic renal failure in patients at high risk of bleeding

• *Adult:* By IV injection 8 IU/kg body weight, followed by 5 IU/kg body weight/hr by IV infusion

Available forms include: Prefilled syringes for SC injection 2500, 5000 IU; ampoules for IV injection 10,000 IU in 1 ml, 10,000 IU in 4 ml

Side effects/adverse reactions:

GI: Raised liver enzymes

Haem: Thrombocytopenia, haemorrhage

Contraindications: Hypersensitivity

Precautions: Patients at high risk of haemorrhage, e.g. following trauma, haemorrhagic stroke, severe liver or renal impairment, thrombocytopenia; defective platelet function; subacute endocarditis; uncontrolled hypertension; diabetic retinopathy; pregnancy, breast-feeding

Pharmacokinetics: Around 87% absorbed after SC administration; elimination half life 3½–4 hr and 2 hr after SC and IV administration respectively; metabolised in liver, excreted in urine

Interactions:

• Increased risk of bleeding: aspirin, dipyridamole, NSAIDs, oral anticoagulants, dextran

Treatment of overdose: Withdraw dalteparin therapy; in an emergency give protamine to neutralise dalteparin (1 mg of protamine per 100 IU dalteparin)

NURSING CONSIDERATIONS

Assess:

• Previous history of haemorrhage

• Baseline vital signs particularly BP

• Full blood count

Administer:

• IV infusion diluted only with 0.9% sodium chloride or 5% dextrose solutions and used within 24 hr of dilution

• SC injections into the abdominal wall with the patient lying supine. The entire length of the needle should be introduced vertically into a skinfold held between the forefinger and thumb throughout the injection

Perform/provide:

• Regular monitoring for signs of bleeding anywhere

• Measures to counteract risk of deep vein thrombosis

Evaluate:

• Therapeutic effect

Teach patient/family:

• Reasons for giving drug and about side effects
• Other action to take to avoid the risk of deep vein thrombosis and unwanted clotting (movement, deep breathing)

danaparoid ▼

Orgaran
Func. class.: Antithrombotic
Chem. class.: Heparinoid, low-molecular weight
Legal class.: POM

Action: Inhibits thrombus formation mainly by inhibiting coagulation factor Xa, but has little anticoagulant effect as a result of relatively weak inhibition of factor IIa (thrombin), hence its use is associated with a low risk of bleeding
Uses: Prevention of deep vein thrombosis in patients undergoing surgery. It can safely be used in most patients with heparin-induced thrombocytopenia
Dosage and routes:
• *Adult:* By SC injection 750 anti-factor Xa units twice daily for 7–10 days. The last pre-operative dose should be given not later than one hour before surgery
Available forms include: Injection, 750 anti-factor Xa units
Side effects/adverse reactions:
GI: Elevated liver enzymes
HAEM: Enhanced bleeding or haematoma at operation site, thrombocytopenia
INTEG: Pain and/or bruising at injection site, rash
MISC: Hypersensitivity reactions
Contraindications: Hypersensitivity, including sulphite hypersensitivity; severe haemorrhagic diathesis, e.g. haemophilia and idiopathic thrombocytopenic purpura; haemorrhagic stroke in the acute phase; uncontrollable active bleeding; severe renal or hepatic impairment; severe hypertension; active gastroduodenal ulcer, unless it is the reason for surgery; diabetic retinopathy; acute bacterial endocarditis; pregnancy; breast-feeding; positive *in vitro* aggregation test in the presence of danaparoid in patients with a history of thrombocytopenia induced by heparin-like anticoagulants
Precautions: Moderate renal or hepatic impairment with impaired haemostasis; GI ulceration; diseases which lead to increased risk of haemorrhage; patients with a thrombocytopenic response to heparin
Pharmacokinetics: Completely bioavailable after SC injection; peak plasma levels 4–5 hr after administration; largely eliminated by renal excretion; elimination half-lives of anti-factor Xa and thrombin generation inhibiting components 25 hr and 7 hr respectively
Interactions: Increased risk of GI bleed: Aspirin, corticosteroids, NSAIDs
Lab. test interferences: Monitoring of the anticoagulant activity of oral anticoagulants by prothrombin time and thrombotest is unreliable in the 5 hr after danaparoid administration
Treatment of overdose: Withdraw treatment, administer blood products if necessary

NURSING CONSIDERATIONS

Assess:
• Clotting time, other blood patterns
Administer:
• SC injection only
• Not less than one hour pre-operatively or post-surgery
Perform/provide:
• Storage: protected from light

Evaluate:
- Therapeutic effect
- For side effects
- For bleeding, bruising at operation or injection sites

Teach patient/family:
- To report any signs of bleeding, bruising or rash
- Not to take aspirin or other nonprescribed medicines without seeking medical advice

---

danazol

Danol

Func. class.: Androgen
Chem. class.: α-Ethinyl testosterone derivative
Legal class.: POM

Action: Decreases FSH, LH, which are controlled by pituitary; this leads to amenorrhoea/anovulation, atrophy of endometrial tissue. Inhibition of enzymes of steroidgenesis

Uses: Endometriosis, benign breast disorders, menorrhagia, gynaecomastia, mastalgia

Dosage and routes:

Endometriosis
- *Adult:* By mouth initial dose 400 mg in 2–4 doses, adjusted as required, for 6 months. Up to 9 months therapy may be necessary

Benign breast disorders
- *Adult:* By mouth initially 300 mg daily, adjusted according to response, for 3–6 months

Gynaecomastia
- *Adolescents:* 200 mg daily for 6 months, increased to 400 mg if no response after 2 months
- *Adults:* 400 mg, daily in divided doses for 6 months

Mastalgia
- 200–300 mg daily according to symptoms for 3–6 months

Menorrhagia
- 200 mg daily for 3 months

Available forms include: Capsules 100, 200 mg

Sides effects/adverse reactions:
HAEM: Erythrocytosis, polycythaemia, eosinophillia, leucopenia
INTEG: Rash, acneiform lesions, oily hair, skin, flushing, sweating, acne vulgaris, alopecia, hirsutism
CNS: Dizziness, headache, fatigue, tremors, paraesthesias, flushing, sweating, anxiety, lability, insomnia
MS: Cramps, spasms
CV: Increased BP, tachycardia, hypertension
GU: Haematuria, amenorrhoea, vaginitis, decreased libido, decreased breast size, clitoral hypertrophy, testicular atrophy
GI: Nausea, vomiting, constipation, weight gain, cholestatic jaundice
EENT: Carpal tunnel syndrome, conjunctival oedema, nasal congestion, voice changes, visual disturbances
ENDO: Abnormal glucose tolerance test

Contraindications: Hypersensitivity, pregnancy—ensure patients with amenorrhoea are not pregnant, breast-feeding, genital bleeding (abnormal), porphyria, androgen dependant tumour, thromboembolic disease

Precautions: Migraine headaches, seizure disorders, diabetes mellitus, renal disease, cardiac disease, hepatic disease

Pharmacokinetics: Half life 4.5 hr, metabolised in liver, metabolites excreted in urine

Interactions/incompatibilities:
- Increased effects of: oral antidiabetics, cyclosporin, alphacalcidol, carbamazepine
- Increased prothrombin time: anticoagulants potentiated
- Reduced effect of: anti-

hypotensives due to promotion of fluid retention
• Decreased effects of: insulin
Clinical assessment:
• Potassium, blood sugar, urine glucose while on long-term therapy
• Haematological monitoring
• Liver function studies: aspartate aminotransferase, alanine aminotransferase, alkaline phosphatase
Lab. test interferences:
Increase: LDL-cholesterol; uptake of tri-iodothyronine
Decrease: HDL-cholesterol, thyroid binding globulin
NURSING CONSIDERATIONS
Assess:
• Baseline weight and fluid balance
Administer:
• With food or milk to decrease GI symptoms
Perform/provide:
• Physiotherapy exercise for patients who are immobile
Evaluate:
• Therapeutic response: decreased pain in endometriosis, decreased size, pain in benign breast disorders
• Weight daily; notify clinician if weekly weight gain more than 2.5 kg
• Fluid balance; observe for urine retention, increasing oedema
• Oedema, hypertension, cardiac symptoms, jaundice
• Mental status: affect, mood, behavioural changes, aggression, sleep disorders, depression
• Signs of virilisation: deepening of voice, decreased libido, facial hair (may not be reversible)
Teach patient/family:
• Notify clinician if therapeutic response decreases
• Not to discontinue medication abruptly but to taper over several weeks
• All aspects of drug usage
• Women to report menstrual irregularities, that amenorrhoea usually occurs but menstruation resumes 2–3 months after termination of therapy
• Routine breast self-examination, report any increase in nodule size
• Drug should induce anovulation; reversible within 60–90 days after drug is discontinued

---

dantrolene sodium

Dantrium, Dantrium Intravenous
Func. class.: Skeletal muscle relaxant
Legal class.: POM

Action: Interferes with the release of calcium in muscle therefore preventing contraction
Uses: Spasticity in multiple sclerosis, stroke, spinal cord injury, cerebral palsy. Intravenously for malignant hyperthermia
Dosage and routes:
Spasticity
• *Adult:* By mouth initially 25 mg daily increasing weekly over 7 weeks, to maximum of 100 mg 4 times a day; use lowest dose compatible with response. Discontinue after 45 days if no response
• *Child:* Not recommended
Malignant hyperthermia
• *Adult and child:* IV 1 mg/kg, may repeat to total dose of 10 mg/kg; if relapse occurs, repeat administration at last effective dose. Average total dose commonly required is 2.5 mg/kg
Available forms include: Capsules 25, 100 mg; powder for injection IV 20 mg/vial
Side effects/adverse reactions:
CNS: Dizziness, fatigue, drowsiness, malaise, headache, seizures, insomnia
EENT: Visual disturbance

MS: Muscle weakness
GI: Nausea, constipation, vomiting, transient diarrhoea, increased aspartate aminotransferase, alkaline phosphatase, hepatotoxicity, hepatitis
GU: Urinary frequency, incontinence, urinary retention, haematuria, crystalluria
INTEG: Acneiform rash
Contraindications: Hepatic dysfunction, hypersensitivity, children, where spasticity is useful, acute skeletal muscle spasm
Precautions: Impaired cardiac, renal disease, hepatic disease, obstructive lung disease, pregnancy
Pharmacokinetics:
Period of onset: Peak 5 hr, highly protein bound, half-life 8 hr, metabolised in liver, excreted in urine (metabolites)
Interactions/incompatibilities:
• Increased CNS depression: alcohol, tricyclic antidepressants, narcotics, barbiturates, sedatives, hypnotics
• Increased risk of liver damage: oestrogens
• Hyperkalaemia: verapamil with IV dantrolene
Clinical assessment:
• EEG in epileptic patients; poor seizure control has occurred in patients taking this drug
• Hepatic function by frequent determination of aspartate aminotransferase, alanine aminotransferase, bilirubin, alkaline phosphate
Treatment of overdose: Induce emesis in conscious patient, gastric lavage, dialysis

NURSING CONSIDERATIONS

Assess:
• Fluid balance
• Liver function before, after 6 weeks and periodically
• Attainable therapeutic goals
Administer:
• Intravenously (usually in hospital) for malignant hyperthermia; inject directly into vein rapidly take care to prevent extravasation as high pH
• Orally with meals. To increase dosages at recommended rate until optimum response with minimum side effects
Perform/provide:
• Help with mobility
Evaluate:
• Therapeutic response: attained physical goal, decreased pain, spasticity
• Fluid balance, retention, frequency, hesitancy
• For increased epileptic seizure activity
• Any adverse effects: drowsiness, dizziness, malaise, headache, nausea, diarrhoea usually transient
• Incontinence more common in elderly
• Signs of jaundice, report immediately
• Psychological dependency: increased need for medication, frequent requests for medication, increased pain
Teach patient/family:
• Not to discontinue medication without medical advice. Drug should be tapered off slowly
• To take other medication only if directed by clinician
• That alcohol should not be taken
• To avoid driving or use of machinery until therapy is established
• To notify clinician if there is any yellowing in skin, clay coloured stools, dark urine

dapsone

Func. class.: Antibiotic, leprostatic
Chem. class.: Sulphone
Legal class.: POM

Action: Competitive inhibition of bacterial replication of folic acid from PABA

Uses: Leprosy, dermatitis herpetiformis

Dosage and routes:

Leprosy

• *Adult:* By mouth 1–2 mg/kg daily with rifampicin and/or clofazimine for at least 2 yr (multibacillary) or 6 months (paucibacillary)

Dermatitis herpetiformis

• 50 mg daily increased to 300 mg or more if necessary

Available forms include: Tablets 50, 100 mg; combination product with pyrimethamine, *Maloprim*, for malaria prophylaxis

Side effects/adverse reactions:

INTEG: Allergic dermatitis, Stevens-Johnson syndrome, exfoliative dermatitis

CV: Tachycardia

CNS: Headache, anxiety, insomnia, tremors, lethargy, depression, confusion, psychosis, aggression

EENT: Blurred vision, optic neuritis, photophobia

HAEM: Haemolytic anaemia, agranulocytosis, methaemoglobinaemia

GI: Anoxeria, nausea, vomiting, hepatitis

Contraindications: Hypersensitivity to sulphones, severe anaemia, porphyria

Precautions: Cardiac or pulmonary disease, hepatic disease, glucose-6-phosphate dehydrogenase deficiency, pregnancy, breast-feeding

Pharmacokinetics: Complete absorption, half-life 20–30 hr; metabolite highly protein bound

Interactions/incompatibilities:

• Increased action of dapsone: probenecid, folic acid antagonists

• Decreased action of dapsone: rifampicin

Clinical assessment:

• Liver function weekly; aspartate aminotransferase, alanine aminotransferase, bilirubin

• Renal function, urea, creatinine

• Blood levels of drug

• Full blood count

Treatment of overdose: Gastric lavage, aspiration. Administration of activated charcoal. Treat methaemoglobinaemia with methylene blue 1–2 mg/kg IV

NURSING CONSIDERATIONS

Assess:

• Baseline temperature

• Fluid balance, specific gravity, urinalysis

Administer:

• With meals to decrease GI symptoms

• Anti-emetic if vomiting occurs

• After culture and sensitivity is completed; repeat monthly to detect resistance

Perform/provide:

• Infants to be kept with mothers infected with leprosy, breast-feeding during drug therapy is encouraged. NB: Small risk of haemolytic anaemia in infants

Evaluate:

• Temperature, if less than 38°C, drug should be reduced

• Mental status often: affect, mood, behavioural changes; psychosis may occur

• Hepatic status: decreased appetite, jaundice, dark urine, fatigue

• Urinalysis, specific gravity monthly

Teach patient/family:

• That therapeutic effects may occur after 3–6 months of drug therapy

• That compliance with dosage schedule, length is necessary

• That scheduled appointments must be kept or relapse may occur

dehydrocholic acid

Func. class.: Biliary stimulant
Chem. class.: Unconjugated oxidised acid
Legal class: P

Action: Facilitates drainage from gallbladder by increasing volume, water content, flow of low-viscosity diluted bile
Uses: Post biliary tract surgery, to flush common duct and drainage tube and wash away small calculi obstructing bile flow
Dosage and routes:
• *Adult:* By mouth 250–750 mg 3 times a day
Cholecystography
• 500–750 mg 4 hrly for 12 hr before and after procedure
Available forms include: Tablets 250 mg
Contraindications: Complete biliary obstruction, chronic liver disease, occlusive hepatitis
Precautions: Asthma, prostatic hypertrophy, hepatitis, child under 12 years, elderly, pregnancy
Pharmacokinetics:
Period of onset: Concentrated in liver, excreted in bile
NURSING CONSIDERATIONS
Administer:
• With fluids
Teach patient/family:
• About effect of drug and use before and after cholecystography

demeclocycline HCl

Ledermycin, combination products
Func. class.: Antibiotic, broad-spectrum
Chem. class.: Tetracycline
Legal class.: POM

Action: Inhibits protein synthesis, phosphorylation in microorganisms by binding to 30S ribosomal subunits, reversibly binding to 50S ribosomal subunits
Uses: Gram-positive/Gram-negative bacteria, protozoa, rickettsia, mycoplasma, infections; inappropriate ADH syndrome, acne
Dosage and routes:
• *Adult:* By mouth 150 mg 6 hrly or 300 mg 12 hrly, atypical pneumonia 900 mg daily in 3 divided doses, 6 days total
Inappropriate ADH syndrome
• *Adult:* 900–1200 mg daily in divided doses then 600–900 mg daily as maintenance
Available forms include: Tablets 300 mg; capsules 150 mg
Side effects/adverse reactions:
HAEM: Eosinophilia, neutropenia, thrombocytopenia, leucocytosis, haemolytic anaemia
EENT: Dysphagia, glossitis, decreased calcification of deciduous teeth, abdominal pain, oral candidiasis
GI: Nausea, vomiting, diarrhoea, anorexia, enterocolitis, hepatotoxicity, flatulence, abdominal cramps, epigastric burning, stomatitis, pseudomembranous colitis
CV: Pericarditis
GU: Increased blood urea nitrogen, polyuria, polydipsia, renal failure, nephrotoxicity
INTEG: Rash, urticaria, photosensitivity, increased pigmentation, exfoliative dermatitis, pruritus, angioedema, exacer-

bation of systemic lupus erythematosus

Contraindications: Hypersensitivity to tetracyclines, children under 12 yr, pregnancy, severe renal insufficiency, lactation, systemic lupus erythematosus

Precautions: Renal disease, hepatic disease, lactation

Pharmacokinetics:

Period of onset: Peak 3–6 hr, half-life 10–17 hr, excreted in urine and faeces, excreted in breast milk, 36%–91% bound to serum protein

Interactions/incompatibilities:

• Decreased effect of this drug: antacids, sodium bicarbonate, dairy products, oral iron, calcium, zinc, magnesium, aluminium

• Increased effect: anticoagulants

• Decreased effect: penicillins, oral contraceptives

Clinical assessment:

• Blood studies, full blood count, urea, creatinine, prothrombin time, aspartate aminotransferase, alanine aminotransferase

Treatment of overdose: No antidote. Gastric lavage, administration of milk, antacids

NURSING CONSIDERATIONS

Assess:

• Fluid balance

Administer:

• By mouth, an hour before food or on an empty stomach; not to be taken with milk, iron preparations, or antacids. Doses may need to be adjusted in renal impairment

• On empty stomach 1 hr before, or 2 hr after meals with a glass of water

• After culture and sensitivity obtained

• 2 hr before or after laxative or iron (ferrous) products; 3 hr after antacid

Evaluate:

• Therapeutic response: decreased temperature, absence of lesions, negative culture and sensitivity

• Allergic reactions: rash, itching, pruritus, angioedema

• Nausea, vomiting, diarrhoea; administer anti-emetic, antacids as ordered

(NB: antacids reduce absorption of tetracyclines)

• Overgrowth of infection: increased temperature, malaise, redness, pain, swelling, drainage, perineal itching, diarrhoea, changes in cough, sputum

Teach patient/family:

• To avoid sun exposure since burns may occur; sunscreen does not seem to decrease photosensitivity

• That diabetics should avoid use of Clinistix Diastix for urine glucose testing

• All prescribed medication must be taken to prevent superimposed infection

• To avoid milk products

desferrioxamine mesylate

Desferal

Func. class.: Chelating agent
Chem. class.: Siderochrome
Legal class.: POM

Action: Binds iron ions (ferric ions), and aluminium ions to form water-soluble complex that is removed by kidneys

Uses: Acute iron intoxication, chronic iron overload, aluminium overload, corneal rust stains and occular siderosis

Dosage and routes:

Acute

• *Adult and child:* By mouth 50–100 ml 10% solution after lavage, then IM 1–2 g every 3–12 hrly, to maximum 6 g in 24 hr, or IV 15 mg/kg/hr to maximum 80 mg/kg in 24 hr

Chronic

• *Adult and child:* IM 500 mg—1 g daily initially, usual daily dose 20–40 mg/kg. Subcutaneous infusion 20–40 mg/kg over 8–24 hr 3–7 times a week. All dosage regimens and routes dependent on individual needs

Aluminium overload

• Individual doses determined by patient's needs

Haemodialysis/haemofiltration

• IV 1 g over 1 hr during last hr of third dialysis

CAPD

• IV, subcutaneous, IM, intraperitoneal, 1 g once or twice a week

Corneal rust stains and occular siderosis

• 10% eye drop prepared from injection, applied 4–6 times daily

Available forms include: Powder for injection IV, IM, subcutaneous 500 mg/vial

Side effects/adverse reactions:
INTEG: Urticaria, erythema, pruritus, pain at injection site, fever
CNS: Dizziness, convulsions
MS: Leg cramps
HAEM: Thrombocytopenia
CV: Hypotension, tachycardia
GI: Diarrhoea, abdominal cramps
EENT: Blurred vision, night or colour blindness, visual field defects, hearing disturbance
GU: Dysuria, pyelonephritis
SYST: Anaphylaxis, infection

Contraindications: Hypersensitivity, renal impairment (dialysis may be necessary)

Precautions: Pregnancy, lactation

Pharmacokinetics: Excreted by kidneys as complex, unchanged drug

Interactions/incompatibilities:

• Prolonged unconsciousness with prochlorperazine
• Vitamin C: enhanced excretion of iron

Clinical assessment:

• Renal function tests: urea, creatinine, creatinine clearance
• Monitor serum iron levels

Treatment of overdose:
Supportive measures, reduce dose, remove excess by dialysis

NURSING CONSIDERATIONS

Assess:

• Vital signs. Observe for hypotension
• Fluid balance
• Weight
• Monitor disturbance in vision, hearing

Administer:

• Injection diluted according to each route of administration. Follow dosage regimen appropriate to each patient; duration depends on condition
• When adrenaline and resuscitation equipment available for acute therapy in case of anaphylaxis

Perform/provide:

• Drugs and equipment for resuscitation

Evaluate:

• Allergic reactions: rash, urticaria; if these occur, drug should be discontinued
• Side effects
• For hypotension

Teach patient/family:

• That blood tests and treatment may continue for several months with chronic iron overload
• How to manage subcutaneous infusion for long-term therapy

---

desipramine HCl

Pertofran

Func. class.: Antidepressant, tricyclic

Chem. class.: Dibenzazepine, secondary amine

Legal class.: POM

Action: Blocks reuptake of noradrenaline, serotonin into nerve endings, increasing action of noradrenaline, serotonin in nerve cells

Uses: Depression

Dosage and routes:

• *Adult:* By mouth initially 75 mg daily, increasing to 150–200 mg daily if required in divided doses or single dose at night

• *Elderly:* By mouth initial dose 25 mg daily

Available forms include: Tablets 25 mg

Side effects/adverse reactions:

HAEM: Agranulocytosis, thrombocytopenia, eosinophilia, leucopenia

CNS: Dizziness, drowsiness, confusion, headache, anxiety, tremors, agitation, weakness, insomnia, nightmares, increased psychiatric symptoms

GI: Constipation, dry mouth, nausea, vomiting, increased appetite, cramps, epigastric distress, jaundice, hepatitis, stomatitis

GU: Retention, disturbance in sexual function

INTEG: Rash, urticaria, sweating, pruritus, photosensitivity

CV: Orthostatic hypotension, ECG changes, tachycardia, hypertension, palpitations

EENT: Blurred vision, tinnitus, mydriasis, ophthalmoplegia

Contraindications: Recovery phase of myocardial infarction, heart block or other cardiac arrhythmias, narrow-angle glaucoma, severe liver disease, porphyria, mania, child less than 12 yr, urinary retention

Precautions: Suicidal patients, severe depression, convulsive disorders, prostatic hypertrophy, elderly, pregnancy, lactation, avoid abrupt cessation of therapy

Pharmacokinetics:

Period of onset: Steady state 2–11 days; metabolised by liver, excreted by kidneys, half-life 7–62 hr

Interactions/incompatibilities:

• Increased effect of this drug: neuroleptics, methylphenidate

• Decreased effects of this drug: barbiturates

• Decreased effects of: guanethidine, clonidine, indirect acting sympathomimetics (ephedrine)

• Increased effects of: direct acting sympathomimetics (adrenaline), alcohol, benzodiazepines, CNS depressants

• Hyperpyretic crisis, convulsions, hypertensive episode: MAOIs

• Anaesthetics: increased effects of arrhythmia and hypotension

Clinical assessment:

• Blood studies; full blood count WBC and differential cardiac enzymes (if receiving long term therapy)

• Hepatic studies; aspartate aminotransferase, alanine aminotransferase, bilirubin, creatinine

• ECG for flattening of T-wave, bundle branch block, atrioventricular block, dysrhythmias in cardiac patients

Treatment of overdose: ECG monitoring, induce emesis, lavage, activated charcoal, administer IV diazepam for convulsions

NURSING CONSIDERATIONS

Assess:

• Baseline pulse, weight

Administer:

• Increased fluids, fibre in diet if constipation, urinary retention occur

• With food or milk for GI symptoms

• Dosage at bedtime if oversedation occurs during day; may take entire dose at bedtime; elderly may not tolerate once daily dosing

• Frequent sips of water for dry mouth

Perform/provide:

• Assistance with ambulation during beginning therapy since drowsiness/dizziness may occur

Evaluate:

• BP (lying, standing), pulse; take vital signs 4 hrly in patients with cardiovascular disease
• Weight weekly, appetite may increase with drug
• Blurred vision
• Mental status: mood, alertness, affect, suicidal tendencies, an increase in psychiatric symptoms: depression, panic
• Urinary retention, constipation
• Withdrawal symptoms: headache, nausea, vomiting, muscle pain, weakness; do not usually occur unless drug was discontinued abruptly
• Alcohol consumption; increases sedative effect

Teach patient/family:
• That therapeutic effects may take 2–3 weeks
• Use caution in driving or other activities requiring alertness because of drowsiness, dizziness, blurred vision
• To avoid alcohol ingestion, other CNS depressants
• Do not discontinue medication quickly after long-term use, may cause nausea, headache, malaise
• Wear sunscreen or large hat since photosensitivity occurs

---

desmopressin acetate

DDAVP, Desmospray
Func. class.: Pituitary hormone
Chem. class.: Synthetic antidiuretic hormone analogue peptide
Legal class.: POM

Action: Promotes reabsorption of water by action on renal tubular epithelium, contracts smooth muscles, causing vasoconstriction with a pressor

Uses: Haemophilia, von Willebrand's disease prior to surgery, pituitary diabetes insipidus, nocturnal enuresis

Dosage and routes:

Diabetes insipidus
• *Diagnosis: Adult and Child:* Intranasally 20 mcg, IM, subcutaneous 2 mcg

Treatment:
• *Adult:* Intranasally 10–40 mcg daily as a single dose or in divided doses; IM/IV subcutaneous 1–4 mcg daily
• *Child:* Intranasally 5–30 mcg daily; IM/IV subcutaneous 0.4 mcg daily

Haemophilia/von Willebrand's disease
• 0.3–0.4 mcg/kg IV infusion ½–1½ hr before surgery

Primary nocturnal enuresis
• *Adult and child over 7 yr:* Intranasally 20–40 mcg at bedtime; withdraw for a least one week for reassessment after 3 months

Renal function testing
• *Adult:* Intranasally 40 mcg
• *Child:* (1–15 years) 20 mcg, (under 1 year), 10 mcg

Available forms include: Intranasal spray 10 mcg/metered dose and drops 100 mcg/ml; injection IV, IM 4 mcg/ml

Side effects/adverse reactions:
EENT: Nasal irritation, congestion, rhinitis (all after intranasal use)
GI: Nausea, cramps
CV: Increased BP
SYST: Water retention, hyponatraemia, hypersensitivity reactions
INTEG: Pallor

Contraindications: Hypersensitivity, nephrogenic diabetes insipidus

Precautions: Pregnancy, asthma, hypertension, renal impairment, cystic fibrosis, cardiovascular disease

Pharmacokinetics:
NASAL: Onset 1 hr, peak 1–5 hr, duration 8–20 hr, half-life

0.4–4 hr, excreted in breast milk

Interactions/incompatibilities:

• Decreased response to desmopressin: alcohol

• Increased response to desmopressin: carbamazepine, chlorpropamide, fludrocortisone

Clinical assessment:

• Withdraw for at least 1 week for reassessment after 3 months' treatment of enuresis

• Monitor fluid balance when starting therapy; body weight, serum electrolytes at regular intervals during treatment

NURSING CONSIDERATIONS

Assess:

• Baseline BP and pulse when to be given IV

Evaluate:

• Therapeutic response: absence of severe thirst, decreased urine output, osmolality

• Pulse, BP when giving drug IV

• Weight daily, check for oedema in extremities

• Intranasal use: nausea, congestion, cramps, headache, usually decreased with decreased dose

Teach patient/family:

• Technique for nasal instillation: to insert tube into nasal cavity to instil drug

• Avoid non-prescribed products: response; do not use with alcohol

• All aspects of drug: action, side effects, dose, when to notify clinician

---

dexamethasone (opthalmic)

Maxidex, combination products

Func. class.: Anti-inflammatory, ophthalmic

Legal class.: POM

Action: Anti-inflammatory, resulting in decreased pain, photophobia

Uses: Inflammation of eye, lids, conjunctiva, cornea, uveitis, iridocyclitis, allergic conditions, burns, foreign bodies. May be combined with antibiotics

Dosage and routes:

• *Adult and child:* Instil 1–2 drops into conjunctival sac ½–4 hrly depending on condition

Available forms include: Ophthalmic suspension 0.1%, several combination products

Side effects/adverse reactions:

EENT: Increased intraocular pressure, poor corneal wound healing, increased possibility of corneal infection, decreased acuity, visual field defects, cataracts

MISC: Systemic glucocorticoid action may be seen with intensive use

Contraindications: Hypersensitivity, acute superficial herpes simplex, fungal/viral diseases of the eye or conjunctiva, ocular tuberculosis, infections of the eye, undiagnosed red eye

Precautions: Corneal abrasions, glaucoma

Clinical assessment:

• Check intraocular pressure and lens clarity regularly during long-term therapy

NURSING CONSIDERATIONS

Administer:

• Only to dermatoses; do not use on weeping, denuded or infected areas

• Only to affected areas

• After thoroughly cleansing area to be treated

• Apply wearing gloves; wash hands well before and after application

Perform/provide:

• Treatment for a few days after area has cleared

Evaluate:

• Therapeutic response: improved vision, decrease inflammation

• Temperature; if pyrexia de-

velops, treatment should be discontinued
• Allergic reactions: redness, itching, swelling, lacrimation
• Therapeutic response: absence of swelling, redness, exudate
• Development of side effects such as increased intraocular pressure

Teach patient/family:
• Not to use other non-prescribed products unless approved by clinician
• Instillation method: pressure on lacrimal sac for 1 min
• Not to share eye medications with others
• Discard eyedrops 28 days after opening

---

dexamethasone/ dexamethasone phosphate/ dexamethasone sodium phosphate

Decadron, Decadron Shock-Pak
Func. class.: Corticosteroid
Chem. class.: Glucocorticoid, long-acting
Legal class.: POM

Action: Decreases inflammation by suppression of migration of polymorphonuclear leucocytes, fibroblasts, reversal of increase capillary permeability and lysosomal stabilisation; anti-emetic

Uses: Inflammation, allergies, neoplasms, cerebral oedema, shock, arthritis, chemotherapy-induced nausea and vomiting

Dosage and routes:

Inflammation
• *Adult:* By mouth 0.5–9 mg daily preferably as a single morning dose; IM or IV 0.5–20 mg
• *Child:* IM or IV 200–500 mcg/kg daily

Shock
• *Adult:* IV 2–6 mg/kg repeated after 2–6 hr if required

Cerebral oedema
• *Adult:* IV 10 mg initially, then IM 4 mg 6 hrly for 2–10 days, reduce dose gradually
Acute life-threatening cerebral oedema, use high dose IV schedule. (See data sheet)

Intra-articular/intrabursally/into tendon sheaths
• *Adult:* 0.4–4 mg every 3 days–3 weeks depending on response and condition being treated

Anti-emesis with chemotherapy
• *Adult:* IV 5–20 mg 30 min prior to chemotherapy then 2–4 mg 2 or 3 times a day by mouth as required
Note: Many other treatment schedules in use
Therapy longer than 5 days should be reduced slowly, not stopped abruptly

Available forms include: Tablets 0.5 mg, 2 mg; injection IV (as sodium phosphate) 5 mg/ml, (as phosphate) 4 mg/ml, (as dexamethasone) 20 mg/ml

Side effects/adverse reactions:
INTEG: Acne, poor wound healing, ecchymosis, petechiae, striae, skin atrophy, hirsutism, increased sweating, allergic skin reactions, tingling in perineum after rapid IV injection
CNS: Depression, flushing, headache, mood changes, convulsions, vertigo, psychosis
CV: Hypertension, circulatory collapse, thrombophlebitis, embolism
MS: Fractures, osteoporosis, weakness, growth retardation (children), myopathy
GI: Nausea, abdominal distention, GI haemorrhage, increased appetite, pancreatitis,

gastric/duodenal ulcer, dyspepsia
EENT: Increased intraocular pressure, blurred vision, cataracts
ENDO: Cushingoid state, adrenocortical suppression, decreased glucose tolerance
GU: Menstrual irregularities, fluid retention, sodium retention, hypokalaemia
Contraindications: Hypersensitivity
Precautions; Psychosis, amoebiasis, fungal and certain viral infections, live viral vaccines, gastro-intestinal ulceration, pregnancy, diabetes mellitus, glaucoma, osteoporosis, seizure disorders, ulcerative colitis, chronic cardiac failure, myasthenia gravis, Cushing's syndrome, renal impairment, hypertension, migraine, latent tuberculosis, incomplete growth, lactation, cerebral malaria
Pharmacokinetics: Well absorbed by mouth, metabolised in liver and kidneys, excreted in urine, plasma half-life 190 min
Dexamethasone 4 mg/ml = dexamethasone phosphate 4.8 mg/ml = dexamethasone sodium phosphate 5 mg/ml
Interactions/incompatibilities:
• Decreased action of dexamethasone: barbiturates, rifampicin, ephedrine, phenytoin, aminoglutethimide
• Decreased effects of: antidiabetics, antihypertensives, isoniazid, vaccines
• Increased side effects of: salicylates, indomethacin, amphotericin B, digitalis preparations, diuretics, live viral vaccines
• Increased action of dexamethasone: oestrogens
Clinical assessment:
• Electrolytes especially potassium in patients on potassium-lowering drugs or cardiac glycosides
• Review requirements for hypoglycaemic agents/oral anti-coagulants in co-treated patients
Treatment of overdose: Symptomatic treatment
NURSING CONSIDERATIONS
Assess:
• Baseline vital signs
Administer:
• Titrated dose, use lowest effective dose
• IM injection deeply in large mass
• Rotate sites, avoid deltoid, use 19G needle
• By mouth as one morning dose to prevent adrenal suppression
• Avoid subcutaneous administration, damage may be done to tissue
• If treatment lasts more than 5 days reduce dose slowly when stopping
Perform/provide:
• Assistance with ambulation in patient with bone tissue disease to prevent fractures
Evaluate:
• Weight daily, notify clinician of weekly gain more than 2 kg
• BP and pulse, 4 hrly
• Fluid balance; be alert for decreasing urinary output and increasing oedema
• Therapeutic response: ease of respirations, decreased inflammation
• Infection: increased temperature, WBC even after withdrawal of medication; drug masks symptoms of infection
• Potassium depletion: parasthesia, fatigue, nausea, vomiting, depression, polyuria, dysrhythmias, weakness
• Oedema hypotension, cardiac symptoms
• Blood/urine glucose especially in diabetic patients
• Mental status: affect, mood behavioural changes, aggression
Teach patient/family:

• That steroid user card must be carried
• Notify clinician if therapeutic response decreases; dosage adjustment may be needed
• Not to discontinue this medication abruptly or adrenal crisis can result
• Avoid non-prescribed products: salicylates, alcohol in cough products, cold preparations unless directed by clinician
• All aspects of drug usage, including Cushingoid symptoms
• Symptoms of adrenal insufficiency: nausea, anorexia, fatigue, dizziness, dyspnoea, weakness, joint pain
• To report any chest pain
• Inform any clinician, dentist or therapist of drug regimen

---

dexamphetamine sulphate

Dexedrine
Func. class.: Cerebral stimulant
Chem. class.: Amphetamine
Legal class.: CD (Sch 2) POM

Action: Increases release of noradrenaline, dopamine from neurones
Uses: Narcolepsy; attention deficit disorder with hyperactivity in children under the supervision of a clinician specialising in child psychiatry
Dosage and routes:
Narcolepsy
• *Adult:* By mouth 10 mg daily in divided doses; increase by 10 mg daily at 1-week intervals according to response; maximum 60 mg daily
• *Elderly:* By mouth 5 mg daily in divided doses; increase by 5 mg daily at 1-week intervals according to response; maximum 60 mg daily
Hyperactivity
• *Child over 6 yr:* 5–10 mg each morning; increase by 5 mg at 1-week intervals; usual maximum 20 mg daily
Available forms include: Tablets 5 mg
Side effects/adverse reactions:
CNS: Hyperactivity, insomnia, restlessness, talkativeness, dizziness, headache, chills, stimulation, dysphoria, irritability, aggresiveness, dependence, psychosis, tremor
GI: Nausea, vomiting, anorexia, dry mouth, diarrhoea, constipation, weight loss, cramps
GU: Impotence, change in libido
CV: Palpitations, tachycardia, hypertension, cardiomyopathy
INTEG: Urticaria, sweating
ENDO: Growth retardation in children
Contraindications: Hypersensitivity to sympathomimetic amines, hyperthyroidism, moderate to severe hypertension, glaucoma, parkinsonism, drug abuse, cardiovascular disease, anxiety, porphyria, pregnancy, breast-feeding
Precautions: Gilles de la Tourette's disorder, anorexia, unstable personality, mild hypertension
Pharmacokinetics:
Period of onset: Onset 30 min, peak 1–3 hr, duration 4–20 hr, metabolised by liver, excreted by kidneys, breast milk, elimination half-life 12–13 h
Interactions/incompatibilities:
• Hypertensive crisis: MAOIs or within 14 days of MAOIs inhibitors
• Increased effect of dexamphetamine: acetazolamide, antacids, sodium bicarbonate
• Decreased effects of dexamphetamine: ascorbic acid, ammonium chloride
• Decreased effects of: guanethidine, other antihypertensives
Treatment of overdose: Gastric

lavage, no specific antidote, supportive treatment including diazepam for convulsions. Elimination increased by forced acid diuresis

NURSING CONSIDERATIONS

Assess:

• Weight and height in children and monitor growth rates
• Diet, check for food allergies especially 'E' numbers in children
• Pulse, blood pressure and respiration, before treatment

Administer:

• Orally following the dosage regimen for suitable gradual introduction
• Optimum response at smallest dose
• Do not give late in the day to avoid interference with sleep

Perform/provide:

• Frequent drinks to prevent a dry mouth

Evaluate:

• Therapeutic response: increased mental attention, decreased drowsiness
• Over stimulation; hyperactivity insomnia, restlessness, talkativeness, palpitation, tachycardia
• Drug dependency may occur as tolerance develops. Larger dose for some effect. Treatment should be stopped gradually
• Growth rate, height in children (maybe decreased)

Teach patient/family:

• To follow suitable diet, avoiding foods that may increase irritability, combined with rest and exercise
• That alcohol should be avoided
• Not to discontinue medication without medical advise. Drug should be tapered off slowly
• To take other medication only if directed by clinician. The effect of dexamphetamine is increased and decreased by several drugs
• To avoid driving or use of machinery until therapy established

dextran

Gentran, Rheomacrodex, Macrodex
Func. class.: Plasma volume expander
Chem. class.: Low molecular weight polysaccharide
Legal class.: POM

Action: Similar to human albumin, expands plasma volume

Uses: Expand plasma volume, prophylaxis of embolism, thrombosis, emergency blood substitute in haemorrhage

Dosage and routes:

• *Adult:* IV infusion initially 500–1000 ml, up to 2500–3000 ml over several days according to patient's needs. Consult specialist literature for treatment regimens

Available forms include: 10% dextran 40 in 0.9% sodium chloride or 5% dextrose; 6% dextran 70 in 0.9% sodium chloride or 5% dextrose; 6% dextran 110 in 0.9% sodium chloride or 5% dextrose

Side effects/adverse reactions:

HAEM: Decreased haematocrit, increased bleeding/coagulation times
INTEG: Rash, urticaria, pruritus, angioneurotic oedema
RESP: Wheezing, dyspnoea, bronchospasm, pulmonary oedema
GU: Renal failure
GI: Nausea, vomiting
SYST: Anaphylaxis, other allergic reactions

Contraindications: Hypersensitivity, renal failure, severe congestive cardiac failure, extreme dehydration, bleeding disorders such as thrombocytopenia, hypofibrinogenaemia

Precautions: Bleeding disorders, pregnancy

Pharmacokinetics:

IV: Expands blood volume 1–2 times the amount infused, excreted in urine and faeces, low molecular weight dextrans largely excreted unchanged. Dextran 110 metabolised in tissues, half-life depends on product

Interactions/incompatibilities:

• May precipitate weak acid drugs, avoid adding drugs to dextrans if possible

Clinical assessment:

• Blood grouping and crossmatching, biochemical tests prior to administration of dextran to avoid interference

Lab. test interferences:

False increase: Blood glucose (using acid reagents), urinary protein

Interferes: Blood typing/crossmatching, some bilirubin assays, total protein using Biuret reagent

Treatment of overdose: Stop or slow infusion, supportive treatment

NURSING CONSIDERATIONS

Assess:

• Baseline vital signs including ECG and CVP (if possible)

• Fluid balance

Administer:

• After crossmatching, if blood is to be given also

• Do not administer through same set as blood unless finished first with saline

Perform/provide:

• Discard part-used units

Evaluate:

• Vital signs every 5 min for 30 min

• CVP during infusion

• Urine output hrly; watch for increase in urinary output which is common; if output does not increase, infusion should be decreased or discontinued

• Allergy: rash, urticaria, pruritus, wheezing, dyspnoea, bronchospasm, drug should be discontinued immediately

• Circulatory overload: increased pulse, respiration, dyspnoea, wheezing, chest tightness, chest pain

• Dehydration after infusion: decreased output, increased temperature, poor skin turgor, increased specific gravity, dry skin

---

dextromoramide

Palfium

Func. class.: Narcotic analgesic

Chem. class.: Pyrrolidine derivative

Legal class.: CD (Sch 2) POM

Action: Potent narcotic analgesic acting at CNS opiate receptors

Uses: Severe acute pain, short duration of action makes it unsuitable for chronic pain control

Dosage and routes:

• By mouth, 5 mg increasing to 20 mg when required

• Rectal suppositories, 10 mg, when required

Available forms include: Tablets, 5, 10 mg (as tartrate); suppositories, 10 mg (as tartrate)

Side effects/adverse reactions:

RESP: Respiratory depression, cough suppression

CNS: Drowsiness, alteration of pupillary responses, hallucinations, vertigo, mood changes

GI: Nausea, reduced motility, constipation

GU: Urinary retention

INTEG: Pain and tissue damage at injection site, sweating, rashes

SYST: Tolerance, dependence

CV: Hypotension, palpitation

Contraindications: Childbirth, respiratory depression, within 21 days of taking MAOIs, head injury, raised intracranial pressure

Precautions: History of drug abuse, dosage may need to be reduced for elderly or debilitated patients, hypothyroidism, pregnancy, lactation, hypotension, decreased respiratory reserve, asthma, renal impairment, liver damage

Pharmacokinetics: Onset of analgesia within 20–30 min, duration 2–3 hr

Interactions/incompatibilities:

• Risk of hypertensive crisis with: MAOIs or within 21 days of stopping them

• Increased effect of: hypnotics, other CNS depressants

Clinical assessment:

• Co-prescribe laxatives, antiemetic if needed

• Switch to longer acting agent if prolonged analgesia needed

Treatment of overdose: Gastric lavage if recently ingested; specific antagonist: naloxone; supportive treatment

NURSING CONSIDERATIONS

Assess:

• Baseline vital signs

• Pain levels

• Respirations, BP, pulse, pupils and conscious level 4 hrly

Administer:

• With an antiemetic if needed

Perform/provide:

• Proper storage and administration of drug according to CD regulations (abuse/misuse)

• Physiotherapy as required

• Fluids and fibre for constipation

• Safe environment: assist with mobilisation, cot sides

• Local treatment to site of injection

Evaluate:

• Side effects

• Response (short duration only, 2–3 hr)

Teach patient/family:

• Not to use machinery or mobilise without assistance

• To take no alcohol.

• Warn about dependence.

• May cause dizzy turns and sweating if ambulant. To rest supine after first few doses

• To store securely

---

dextrose (D-glucose)

Func. class.: Caloric
Chem. class.: Monosaccharide
Legal class.: POM (injection) GSL (powder)

Action: Essential component of carbohydrate metabolism

Uses: Increases intake of calories, maintains fluid balance in patients unable to maintain adequate intake orally

Dosage and routes:

• *Adult and child:* By mouth, IV depends on individual requirements

Available forms include: Injection 5%, 10%, 20%, 25%, 50% IV; powder

Side effects/adverse reactions:

NB: Seen mainly in diabetic patients or with hypertonic (greater than 5%) solutions; 5% dextrose infusion/oral dextrose are without adverse effects

CNS: Confusion, loss of consciousness, dizziness

CV: Hypertension, congestive cardiac failure, pulmonary oedema

GU: Glycosuria, osmotic diuresis with hypertonic solutions

META: Hyperglycaemia, rebound hypoglycaemia, hyperosmolar syndrome, hyperosmolar hyperglycaemic nonketotic syndrome, electrolyte disturbances

INTEG: Chills, flushing, warm feeling, extravasation necrosis with hypertonic solutions

Contraindications: Hyperglycaemia. Hypertonic solutions: delirum tremens with dehydration, haemorrhage (cranial/spinal), anuria

Clinical assessment:

• Electrolytes (potassium, sodium, calcium, chloride, magnesium), blood glucose, ammonia, phosphate for acute therapy

NURSING CONSIDERATIONS

Assess:

• Respiratory function 4-hrly

• Temperature 4 hrly for increased fever, indicating infection; if infection suspected, infusion is discontinued, tubing, infusion bag/container cultured

• Urine glucose 6 hrly using Clinistix, Keto-Diastix, which are not affected by infusion substances

• Nutritional status: consult dietician

Administer:

• Solutions stronger than 5% by central venous line; use peripheral route for stronger solutions only under direction of clinician

Perform/provide:

• Care of central line using aseptic technique

• Infusion of these solutions should not be rapid or very prolonged

Evaluate:

• Injection site for extravasation: redness along vein, oedema at site, necrosis, pain, hard tender, area; site should be changed immediately

• Therapeutic response: increased weight

Teach patient/family:

• Reason for dextrose infusion

---

diamorphine hydrochloride

Diaphine

Func. class.: Narcotic analgesic

Chem. class.: Diacetyl derivative of morphine

Legal class.: CD (Sch 2) POM

Action: Potent narcotic analgesic acting at CNS opiate receptors. Inhibits ascending pain pathways in CNS, increases pain threshold, alter pain perception

Uses: Severe pain, particularly in terminal illness; acute pulmonary oedema; myocardial infarction

Dosage and routes:

Acute pain

• *Adult:* Subcutaneous/IM injection, 5 mg (maximum 10 mg for large patients) repeated 4 hrly if necessary; by slow IV injection quarter to half of corresponding IM dose

Chronic pain

• *Adult:* By mouth, subcutaneous, IM; 5–10 mg 4 hrly, may be increased according to need; IM dose should be approximately half oral dose for treating same level of pain

Pulmonary oedema

• *Adult:* Slow IV injection (1 mg/min) 2.5–5 mg

Myocardial infarction:

• *Adult:* Slow IV injection (1 mg/min), 5 mg followed by 2.5–5 mg if necessary; reduce dose by half in elderly or frail patients

Available forms include: Tablets, 10 mg; injection, powder for reconstitution, 5, 10, 30, 100, 500 mg ampoules; extemporaneously prepared oral liquids

Side effects/adverse reactions:

RESP: Respiratory depression, cough suppression

EENT: Miosis

META: Hypothermia

CNS: Drowsiness, alteration of pupillary responses, hallucinations, vertigo, mood changes

GI: Nausea, reduced motility, constipation, vomiting, anorexia, cramps, dry mouth

GU: Urinary retention

INTEG: Pain and tissue at injection site, sweating, urticaria, pruritis, flushing

SYST: Tolerance, dependence

CV: Hypotension, palpitations, bradycardia

Contraindications: Respiratory depression, within 21 days of taking MAOIs, head injury, raised intracranial pressure, paralytic ileus, hypersensitivity
Precautions: History of drug abuse, pregnancy, childbirth, lactation, hypotension, hypothyroidism, decreased respiratory reserve, asthma, renal impairment, liver damage; dosage may need to be reduced for elderly or debilitated patients
Pharmacokinetics: Ultimately converted by hepatic metabolism to morphine, excreted in urine, duration of action about 4 hr
Interactions/incompatibilities:
• Risk of hypotensive crisis given within 21 days of: monoamine-oxidase inhibitors
• Potentiation of: Hypnotics, other CNS depressants, alcohol
• Absorption of mexiletine may be delayed by opiates and cisapride action antagonised
Clinical assessment:
• Must be given 4 hrly in chronic pain
• IV route no more than 1 mg/min
• Prescribe anti-emetic as required
• Prescribe prophylactic laxative
Treatment of overdose: Gastric lavage; specific antagonist: naloxone 0.4–2 mg IV at 2 to 3 min intervals up to 10 mg, supportive treatment

NURSING CONSIDERATIONS

Assess:
• Baseline pulse, respirations, BP
• Fluid balance
• When pain is beginning to return; determine dosage interval by patient response
Administer:
• With an anti-emetic if nausea and vomiting
Perform/provide:
• Safe environment: help with mobilisation
• Fluids and fibre (constipation)
Evaluate:
• Side effects
• Changes in BP and respiratory rate
• Need for additional analgesia, physical dependence
• Therapeutic response: decrease in pain
Teach patient/family:
• Effects of drug
• No alcohol
• May cause dizziness
• That dependency may result if dose taken is more than that required to relieve pain
• Withdrawal symptoms may occur if high dosage reduced too quickly: nausea, vomiting, cramps, fever, faintness, anorexia
• Need for secure storage
• Not to mobilise without assistance

---

diazepam

Tensium, Rimapam, Atensine, Diazemuls, Stesolid, Valium
Func. class.: Anxiolytic, hypnotic, anticonvulsant, muscle relaxant
Chem. class.: Benzodiazepine
Legal class.: CD (Sch 4) POM (oral preparations only prescribable generically on NHS

Action: Depresses subcortical levels of CNS, including limbic system, reticular formation
Uses: Anxiety, insomnia, acute alcohol withdrawal, adjunct in seizure disorders, induction and IV sedation, muscle spasm
Dosage and routes:
Anxiety
• *Adult:* 2 mg 3 times daily; increase according to response to 15–30 mg daily in divided doses if required
• *Adult:* IM or slow IV injection, severe anxiety, panic attacks,

10 mg; repeat after 4 hr if required
• *Adult, child over 3 yr:* By rectal route (solution) 10 mg; child 1–3 yr 5 mg; repeat after 5 min if required
• *Child:* By mouth, night terrors, somnambulism, 1–5 mg at bedtime
• *Elderly:* half adult dose

Insomnia
• *Adult:* 5–15 mg at bedtime

Status epilepticus
• *Adult:* IV injection 10–20 mg at a rate of 5 mg/min; repeat after 30–60 min if required or use IV infusion maximum 3 mg/kg in 24 hr
• *Adult:* By rectum (solution) 10 mg; elderly, 5 mg; repeat after 5 min if required
• *Child:* IV injection 200–300 mcg/kg
• *Child:* By rectum (solution) 1–3 yr 5 mg; over 3 yr 10 mg; repeat after 5 min if required

Muscle spasm
• *Adult:* By mouth 2–15 mg daily in divided doses; increase according to response to 60 mg daily
• *Adult:* IM or slow IV injection 10 mg; repeat after 4 hr if required

Cerebral spasticity
• *Child:* 2–40 mg daily in divided doses

Tetanus
• *Adult, child:* IV injection 100–300 mcg/kg; repeat every 1–4 hr if required
• *Adult, child:* IV infusion or by nasoduodenal tube, 3–10 mg/kg in 24 hr adjusted to response

Sedation and premedication
• *Adult:* By mouth 5 mg at bedtime, on waking and 2 hr before procedure
• *Adult:* Slow IV injection, sedation, 10–20 mg over 2–4 min; premedication, 100–200 mcg/kg
• *Adult:* By rectum (solution) 10 mg; elderly 5 mg
• *Child:* By rectum (solution) 1–3 yr, 5 mg; over 3 yr, 10 mg

Febrile convulsions
• *Child:* Slow IV 250 mcg/kg; by rectum (solution) 500 mcg/kg (preferred)

Acute alcohol withdrawal
• *Adult:* IM or slow IV injection, 10 mg; repeat after 4 hr if required

Available forms include: Tablets 2 mg, 5 mg, 10 mg; injection (solution) 5 mg/ml; injection (emulsion) 5 mg/ml; suppositories 10 mg; oral solution 2 mg/5 ml, 5 mg/5 ml; rectal solution 5 mg, 10 mg

Side effects/adverse reactions:
CNS: Dizziness, drowsiness, confusion, headache, anxiety, tremors, stimulation, fatigue, depression, insomnia, hallucinations, ataxia, dependence, amnesia, vertigo, changed libido
GI: Constipation, dry mouth, nausea, anorexia, diarrhoea
INTEG: Rash, dermatitis, itching, pain and thrombophlebitis after injection
CV: Orthostatic hypotension, hypotension
EENT: Blurred vision
RESP: Respiratory depression, apnoea
HAEM: Blood dyscrasias

Contraindications: CNS depression, coma, respiratory depression, sleep apnoea, phobias, obsessions, chronic psychosis

Precautions: Elderly, debilitated, hepatic disease, renal disease, respiratory disease, muscle weakness, history of drug abuse, pregnancy, lactation

Pharmacokinetics:
By mouth: Onset 30 min, peak 1–2 hr
IM: Onset 15–30 min, absorption erratic
IV: Onset 1–5 min
Metabolised by liver, excreted by kidneys, breast milk, half-life 20–50 hr, active metabolite, half-life 30–200 hr

Interactions/incompatibilities:
- Increased effects of diazepam with: CNS depressants, alcohol, cimetidine, disulfiram
- Incompatible with all drugs in solution or syringe

Clinical assessment:
- Dependence potential, use for shortest possible period

Treatment of overdose: Gastric lavage, specific antidote: flumazenil, supportive care, vital signs

NURSING CONSIDERATIONS

Assess:
- Baseline vital signs
- BP, pulse, respiration if IV administration

Administer:
- IM only when oral or IV route not available
- IV into large vein at a maximum of 5 mg/min
- IV emulsion preparation to reduce risk of thrombophlebitis
- IV infusion (solution) in glucose 5% or sodium chloride 0.9% to maximum 40 mg/500 ml
- IV infusion (emulsion) in glucose 5% or 10% to maximum 200 mg/500 ml
- IV (emulsion) via drip tubing into an infusion of glucose 5%, 10% or sodium chloride 0.9%
- Small IV doses or use rectal solution instead in status epilepticus if resuscitation facilities are not available.
- Rectally if unable to take oral medication

Perform/provide:
- Frequent sips of water for dry mouth
- Help with walking during beginning therapy, since drowsiness/dizziness occurs
- Safety measures, including cot sides
- Check to see oral medication has been swallowed

Evaluate:
- Therapeutic response: decreased anxiety, restlessness, insomnia, muscular spasm, spasticity
- Mental status: mood, sensorium, affect, sleeping pattern, drowsiness, dizziness
- Physical dependency, withdrawal symptoms: headache, nausea, vomiting, muscle pain, weakness after long-term use
- Suicidal tendencies in depressed patients

Teach patient/family:
- Not to be used for everyday stress or used longer than 4 months, unless directed by clinician
- Avoid non-prescribed preparations unless approved by clinician
- Avoid driving, activities that require alertness; drowsiness may occur
- Avoid alcohol ingestion or other psychotropic medications, unless prescribed by clinician
- Do not discontinue medication abruptly after long-term use
- Rise slowly or fainting may occur
- Drowsiness might worsen at beginning of treatment
- To seek psychiatric help if depressed

---

diazoxide

Eudemine

Func. class.: Antihypertensive
Chem. class.: Benzothiadiazine
Legal class.: POM

Action: Vasodilation of arteriolar smooth muscle by direct relaxation producing a reduction in blood pressure with concomitant increases in heart rate, cardiac output

Uses: Hypertensive crisis when urgent decrease of diastolic pressure required

Dosage and routes:
• *Adult:* Rapid IV injection 1–3 mg/kg, maximum 150 mg as a single dose; may be repeated after 5–15 min
Available forms include: Injection 15 mg/ml
Side effects/adverse reactions:
CV: Hypotension, T wave changes, angina pectoris, palpitations, supraventricular tachycardia, oedema, rebound hypertension, bradycardia
CNS: Extrapyramidal symptoms, cerebral infarction
GI: Nausea, vomiting, dry mouth
INTEG: Rash, burning at injection site
HAEM: Thrombocytopenia, leucopenia, haemolytic anaemia
ENDO: Hyperglycaemia, ketoacidotic coma
META: Sodium, water retention
Contraindications: Hypersensitivity
Precautions: Pregnancy, labour, aortic coarctation or arteriovenous shunt, dissecting aortic aneurysm, lactation, impaired cerebral or cardiac circulation, children, impaired renal function, low plasma proteins
Pharmacokinetics:
IV: Onset 1–2 min, peak 5 min, duration 3–12 hr
Half-life 20–36 hr, metabolised in liver excreted slowly in urine, crosses blood-brain barrier, placenta
Interactions/incompatibilities:
• Do not mix with any drug in syringe or solution
• Increased effects of: warfarin, other coumarins, antihypertensives, diuretics
• Increased hyperglycaemia/hyperuricaemia when given with: thiazides, diuretics
• Decreased pharmacological effects of: hypoglycaemic agents
Clinical assessment:
• Electrolytes (potassium, sodium, chloride), glucose, carbon dioxide, full blood count
• Treat hypoglycaemia with tolbutamide, exceptionally insulin
• Control sodium, water retention with diuretic
Treatment of overdose: Supportive treatment including insulin for hypoglycaemia, IV fluids for hypotension

NURSING CONSIDERATIONS

Assess:
• Baseline BP and weight
Administer:
• IV injection must be administered rapidly and not exceed 30 seconds
• Patient in recumbent position, keep in that position for 1 hr after administration
Evaluate:
• Therapeutic response: decreased BP, primarily diastolic pressure
• BP every 5 min for 2 hr, then hrly for 2 hr, then 4 hrly
• Pulse, jugular venous distention 4 hrly
• Fluid balance
• Oedema in feet, legs daily
• Skin turgor, dryness of mucous membranes for hydration status
• Rales, dyspnoea, orthopnoea
• IV site for extravasation
• Signs of congestive cardiac failure, dyspnoea, oedema wet rales
• Postural hypotension, take BP sitting, standing 4 hrly

diclofenac sodium

Voltarol, Rhumalgan, Valenac, Volraman, Diclozip
Func. class.: Non-steroidal anti-inflammatory drug
Chem. class.: Phenylacetic acid derivative
Legal class.: POM

Action: Inhibits prostaglandin

synthesis; possesses analgesic, anti-inflammatory, antipyretic properties

Uses: Acute, chronic rheumatoid arthritis, renal colic, osteoarthrosis, ankylosing spondylitis, gout, acute musculoskeletal disorders; post-operative pain, juvenile chronic arthritis

Dosage and routes:

• *Adult:* By mouth 25–50 mg 8–12 hrly; modified-release, 100 mg daily or 75 mg once or twice daily; rectal, 100 mg daily, usually at night; IM 75 mg once or twice a day for 2 days maximum. Total daily dose should not exceed 150 mg

• *Child over 1 yr:* 1–3 mg/kg daily in divided doses

Available forms include: Tablets enteric coated 25 mg, 50 mg; modified-release, 75 mg, 100 mg; dispersible 50 mg (as base); suppositories 12.5 mg, 100 mg; injection IM 75 mg/3 ml

Side effects/adverse reactions:

GI: Nausea, anorexia, vomiting, diarrhoea, jaundice, hepatitis, constipation, flatulence, cramps, dry mouth, peptic ulcer, GI bleeding, dyspepsia, colitis, pancreatitis, stomatitis

CNS: Dizziness, drowsiness, fatigue, tremors, confusion, insomnia, anxiety, depression, paraesthesia, muscle weakness, headache, psychosis

CV: Peripheral oedema, palpitations, hypertension, fluid retention, chest pain

INTEG: Purpura, rash, pruritus, sweating, erythema, petechiae, photosensitivity, alopecia; suppositories only: ano-rectal irritation. Pain at injection site

GU: Nephrotoxicity: haematuria, oliguria, azotaemia, nephrotic syndrome, papillary necrosis

HAEM: Blood dyscrasias, epistaxis, bruising

EENT: Tinnitus, hearing loss, blurred vision, taste disturbances

RESP: Dyspnoea, haemoptysis, pharyngitis, bronchospasm, laryngeal oedema, rhinitis

Contraindications: Hypersensitivity to aspirin or other NSAIDs; active or suspected peptic ulcer or gastrointestinal bleeding; asthma; porphyria, 3rd trimester of pregnancy. Do not use suppositories in inflammatory conditions of anus, rectum, sigmoid colon.

Precautions: Pregnancy, bleeding disorders, history of GI disorders, cardiac, hepatic or renal disorders, recovery from major surgery, elderly

Pharmacokinetics:

By mouth: Peak 1–4 hr, elimination half-life 1–2 hr, 90% bound to plasma proteins, metabolised in liver excreted in urine

Interactions/incompatibilities:

• Increased anticoagulant effect: oral anticoagulants (low risk)

• Increased toxicity of: cyclosporin

• Increased plasma levels of diclofenac: probenecid

• Increased plasma levels of: methotrexate, lithium, cardiac glycosides

• Reduced effects of: antihypertensives

• Altered requirements for: oral antidiabetics

Clinical assessment:

• Renal, hepatic function at intervals during long-term therapy

• Changes in clotting parameters if diclofenac started/stopped during treatment with oral anticoagulants

Treatment of overdose: Gastric lavage, activated charcoal, symptomatic and supportive treatment

NURSING CONSIDERATIONS

Administer

• With food and/or milk

• Swallow whole except dispersible tablets which should be dissolved

in a glass of water and stirred
- Do not take indigestion mixtures at the same time as the enteric coated tablets

Evaluate:
- Effectiveness of drug regarding movement of joints and stiffness
- Bruising, fatigue, bleeding and impaired healing, indigestion or black tarry stool (indicates possible blood dyscrasia)

Teach patient/family:
- To be effective drug must be taken until the course is complete
- To inform clinician/nurse of bleeding bruising, fatigue and malaise—blood dyscrasias could occur
- To avoid aspirin and alcohol
- To take with food, milk or antacids to avoid gastric irritation
- To be careful/avoid driving as drowsiness and dizziness may occur
- To report any unresolved indigestion
- How to administer suppositories

diclofenac (topical)

Voltarol Emulgel
Func. class.: Non-steroidal anti-inflammatory agent, topical
Legal class.: POM

Action: Inhibits prostaglandin synthesis; possesses analgesic and anti-inflammatory properties
Uses: Local symptomatic relief of pain and inflammation in trauma of tendons, ligaments, muscles and joints; localised forms of soft tissue rheumatism
Dosage and routes:
- 2–4 g (circular mass of 2.0–2.5 cm diameter) rubbed gently into the skin 3–4 times a day
- Review after 14 days

Available forms include: Gel containing equivalent to 1% diclofenac sodium
Side effects/adverse reactions:
INTEG: Local irritation, erythema, pruritis, dermatitis, photosensitivity, bullous or vesicular eruptions, urticaria.
Systemic side effects are unlikely
Contraindications: Hypersensitivity or asthma induced by diclofenac, aspirin or other NSAIDs; hypersensitivity to propylene glycol or isopropanol; children
Precautions: Do not apply to damaged or broken skin; do not use an occlusive dressing; keep away from eyes, lips and mucous membranes; pregnancy; lactation
Pharmacokinetics: 6% of the dose applied topically is absorbed through the skin
Interactions: None known with topical use
Treatment of overdose: Overdose unlikely. If ingested in large quantities treatment consists of supportive and symptomatic measures

NURSING CONSIDERATIONS

Assess:
- Hypersensitivity or asthma

Perform/provide:
- Gloves for professional applicant

Administer:
- By rubbing gently into skin

Evaluate:
- Therapeutic response
- For side effects

Teach patient/family:
- Correct method of application
- Not to apply to broken skin, mucous membranes, lips, near eyes
- To wash hands after application (unless hands are being treated)
- To discontinue if local reaction occurs or pregnancy is likely
- To store in a cool place

dienoestrol

Ortho Dienoestrol
Func. class.: Oestrogen
Chem. class.: Non-steroidal synthetic oestrogen
Legal class.: POM

Action: Applied topically, reverses post-menopausal and other atrophic changes to vagina and vulva

Uses: Atrophic vaginitis, kraurosis vulvae; pruritus vulvae and dysparenia when associated with atropic vaginal epithelium

Dosage and routes:

• *Adult:* Vaginal cream 0.01% 1–2 applicatorfuls daily for 1–2 weeks, then gradually reduce to half dose for 1–2 weeks then to 1 application 1–3 times weekly

Available forms include: Vaginal cream 0.01%

Side effects/adverse reactions:

CNS: Dizziness, headache, migraines, depression

CV: Hypertension, thrombophlebitis, oedema, thromboembolism, stroke, pulmonary embolism, myocardial infarction. Risks of CV effects small in post-menopausal women

GI: Nausea, vomiting, diarrhoea, pancreatitis, cramps, increased appetite, cholestatic jaundice

EENT: Contact lens intolerance, increased myopia, astigmatism

GU: Amenorrhoea, cervical erosion, breakthrough bleeding, dysmenorrhoea, vaginal candidiasis, endometrial hypertrophy/carcinoma, irritation at administration site, change in cervical secretions, increase in size of fibromyomata

INTEG: Rash, urticaria, acne, oily skin, seborrhoea, purpura, melasma

META: Folic acid deficiency, weight gain, hypercalcaemia, hyperglycaemia

ENDO: Breast tenderness, enlargement, secretion

Contraindications: Breast cancer, thromboembolic disorders, oestrogen-dependent cancer, genital bleeding (abnormal, undiagnosed), pregnancy, severe liver disease, porphyria, uterine fibromyomata, endometrosis, history of pemphigoid gestation

Precautions: Hypertension, asthma, gall-bladder disease, congestive cardiac failure, diabetes mellitus, bone disease predisposing to hypercalcaemia, depression, migraine headache, convulsive disorders, hepatic disease, family history of cancer of the breast or reproductive tract, contact lenses

Pharmacokinetics:

Topical: Significant absorption, degraded in liver, excreted in urine, excreted in breast milk

Interactions/incompatibilities:

• Decreased action of: oral anticoagulants, oral hypoglycaemics, antihypertensives

• Increased toxicity of: tricyclic antidepressants, cyclosporin, (raised blood levels)

• Increased action of: corticosteroids

Clinical assessment:

• Liver function studies

• Regular measurement of blood pressure

NURSING CONSIDERATIONS

Assess:

• Baseline weight and fluid balance

Administer:

• At bedtime for better absorption

• Titrated dose, use lowest effective dose, to prevent adverse reactions

• Dosage reduction should continue at 3–6 month intervals

Evaluate:

• Weight daily; notify clinician of weekly weight gain more than 2 kg
• BP 4 hrly
• Fluid balance, be alert for decreasing urinary output and increasing oedema
• Oedema, hypertension, cardiac symptoms, jaundice
• Mental status; affect, mood, behavioural changes, aggression
• Hypercalcaemia

Teach patient/family:

• How to fill applicator and insert cream
• Report breast lumps, vaginal bleeding, oedema, jaundice, dark urine, clay coloured stools, dyspnoea, headache, blurred vision, abdominal pain, numbness or stiffness in legs, chest pain

---

diflunisal

Dolobid

Func. class.: Non-steroid anti-inflammatory drug
Chem. class.: Salicylate
Legal class.: POM

Action: Inhibits prostaglandin synthesis; possesses analgesic, anti-inflammatory, antipyretic actions

Uses: Mild to moderate pain including osteoarthritis and rheumatoid arthritis

Dosage and routes:

Pain/fever

• *Adult:* By mouth 500–1500 mg daily in 2–3 divided doses
• Osteoarthritis, rheumatoid arthritis
• *Adult:* By mouth 500 mg–1 g daily as a single dose or in 2 divided doses

Available forms include: Tablets 250 mg, 500 mg

Side effects/adverse reactions:

HAEM: Thrombocytopenia, granulocytosis, haemolytic anaemia, increased prothrombin time
GU: Renal impairment, dysuria
CNS: Stimulation, drowsiness, dizziness, confusion, convulsions, headache, flushing, hallucinations, coma, insomnia, anxiety, paraesthesia
GI: Nausea, vomiting, GI bleeding, diarrhoea, heartburn, anorexia, hepatitis, ulceration, liver damage, stomatitis
INTEG: Rash, urticaria, exfoliative dermatitis
EENT: Tinnitus, hearing loss, blurred vision
CV: Rapid pulse, oedema
RESP: Wheezing, bronchospasm

Contraindications: Hypersensitivity; hypersensitivity to salicylates or NSAIDs; active or suspected peptic ulcer or G.I. bleeding; children; pregnancy; asthma; breast-feeding

Precautions: Bleeding disorders, hepatic disease, renal disease, Hodgkin's disease, history of GI ulceration

Pharmacokinetics:

Period of onset: Onset 30–60 min, peak 2–3 hr, metabolised by liver, excreted by kidneys, 99% protein bound, excreted in breast milk, plasma half-life 7–11 hr (dose dependent)

Interactions/incompatibilities:

• Decreased effects of diflunisal: aluminium antacids
• Increased effects of: anticoagulants
• Decreased effects of: antihypertensives, diuretics
• Increased toxicity of: methotrexate, cyclosporin, lithium, indomethacin

Clinical assessment:

• Liver function studies if toxicity suspected

• Renal function studies: blood urea creatinine if impairment suspected
• Changes in clotting parameters in patients already receiving oral anticoagulants, or if diflunisal withdrawn from such patients

Treatment of overdose: Gastric lavage, activated charcoal, monitor electrolytes, vital signs, supportive treatment

NURSING CONSIDERATIONS:

Assess:
• Baseline fluid balance
• Prior drug history; there are many drug interactions

Administer:
• Swallow whole: not to be crushed or chewed
• With food or milk
• Not with aluminium containing antacids

Perform/provide:
• Repositioning to decrease pain
• Cool cloth for fever

Evaluate:
• Fluid balance; decreasing output may indicate renal failure (long-term therapy)
• Hepatotoxicity: dark urine, clay-coloured stools, yellowing of skin, sclera, itching, abdominal pain, fever, diarrhoea if patient is on long-term therapy
• Allergic reactions: rash, urticaria; if these occur, drug may need to be discontinued
• Ototoxicity: tinnitus, ringing, roaring in ears; audiometric testing is needed before, after long-term therapy
• Visual changes: blurring, halos, corneal, retinal damage
• Oedema in feet, ankles, legs

Teach patient/family:
• To report any symptoms of hepatotoxicity, renal toxicity, visual changes ototoxicity, allergic reactions (long-term therapy)
• Not to exceed recommended dosage; acute poisoning may result
• To read label on other non-prescribed drugs; many contain aspirin
• That therapeutic response takes 2 weeks (arthritis)
• To avoid alcohol ingestion; GI bleeding may occur

digitoxin

Func. class.: Cardiac inotropic agent
Chem. class.: Cardiac glycoside
Legal class.: POM

Action: Acts by influx of calcium ions from extracellular to intracellular cytoplasm, increasing force of contraction and cardiac output

Uses: Congestive heart failure, atrial fibrillation, atrial flutter, atrial tachycardia

Dosage and routes:
• *Adult:* By mouth, maintenance 50–200 mcg daily
• *Adult:* Digitalisation, by mouth, 600 mcg, then 400 mcg after 4–6 hr, then 200 mcg every 6 hr, up to maximum 1.6 mg
• *Adult:* Slower digitalisation, by mouth, 200 mcg twice daily for 4 days
• *Adult:* Maintenance, by mouth, 50–200 mcg daily
• *Child:* Seek specialist advice

Available forms include: Tablets 100 mcg

Side effects/adverse reactions:
CNS: Headache, drowsiness, apathy, confusion, disorientation, fatigue, depression, hallucinations
CV: Dysrhythmias, bradycardia, atrioventricular block
GI: Nausea, vomiting, anorexia,

abdominal pain, diarrhoea, intestinal ischaemia/necrosis
EENT: Blurred vision, yellow-green halos, photophobia, diplopia
MS: Muscular weakness
ENDO: Gynaecomastia
INTEG: Skin rashes
Contraindications: Hypersensitivity to digitalis, supraventricular arrhythmias caused by Wolff-Parkinson-White syndrome
Precautions: Renal disease, hepatic disease, acute myocardial infarction, atrioventricular block, severe respiratory disease, hypothyroidism, elderly (reduce dose), electrolyte disturbances (especially hypokalaemia), cardioversion
Pharmacokinetics:
By mouth: Onset about 120 min, peak effect about 12 hr, duration variable, half-life 5–7 days, metabolised in liver, excreted in urine
Interactions/incompatibilities:
• Drugs increasing hypokalaemia and risk of digitoxin toxicity: diuretics, amphotericin B, corticosteroids, lithium, carbenoxolone
• Blood levels of digitoxin increased: spironolactone, verapamil, diltiazem, possibly other calcium antagonists
• Decreased blood levels of digitoxin: aminoglutethimide, barbiturates, anti-epileptics, rifampicin, cholestyramine, colestipol
• Increased risk of cardiac toxicity: β-blockers, suxamethonium, verapamil
• *Caution advised for those drugs interacting with digoxin*
Clinical assessment:
• Electrolytes (prior to treatment; if toxicity suspected; if patient at risk of renal/electrolyte abnormalities): potassium, sodium, chloride, calcium; renal function studies: urea, creatinine
• Monitor drug levels (therapeutic level 10–30 mcg/litre) once treatment stabilised; if toxicity suspected
Treatment of overdose: Gastric lavage if ingestion recent, activated charcoal, correct any hypokalaemia, treat arrhythmias with non-cardiac glycoside drugs, consider administration of specific antibody fragments, monitor ECG continuously

NURSING CONSIDERATIONS:
Assess
• BP, respiration, pulse
• Pulse is taken prior to each dose of digitoxin. If radial or apex pulse is less than 60 withhold drug and retake pulse after 1 hr; if pulse less than 60 notify clinician
• Weigh before and regularly during treatment
• Fluid balance; check for oedema and retention
Administer:
• Orally using the lowest effective dose
• Potassium supplements if prescribed for potassium levels less than 3.0 mmol/litre
Evaluate:
• Cardiac status: apical pulse, character, rate, rhythm
• Therapeutic response: decreased weight, oedema, pulse, respiration and increased urine output
Teach patient/family:
• Visual changes, headache
• To report symptoms of toxicity, oedema
• To only take other medication on clinicians advice
• To take own pulse and contact clinician if it falls below 60
• Not to take antacid at the same time
• Not to stop drug abruptly; teach all aspects of drug

digoxin

Lanoxin, Lanoxin-PG
Func. class.: Cardiac inotropic agent
Chem. class.: Cardiac glycoside
Legal class.: POM

Action: Acts by influx of calcium ions from extracellular to intracellular cytoplasm; increases cardiac contractility and cardiac output
Uses: Congestive heart failure, atrial fibrillation, atrial flutter, atrial tachycardia
Dosage and routes:
• *Adult:* Rapid digitalisation, by mouth, 750–1000 mcg, then 250 mcg every 6 hr until desired effect; usual total dose 1.5 mg in 24 hr
• *Adult:* Slower digitalisation, by mouth, 250 mcg once or twice daily until steady state levels, usually about 7 days
• *Adult:* Maintenance, by mouth, 62.5–500 mcg daily, usually 125–250 mcg daily
• *Adult:* Urgent treatment, IV infusion, 0.5–1.0 mg over more than 2 hr, followed by maintenance by mouth as above
• *Elderly:* Initiate gradually and with smaller doses
• *Child:* Doses based on body weight, response, and developmental age; seek specialist advise
Available forms include: Elixir 50 mcg/ml; tablets 62.5 mcg, 125 mcg, 250 mcg; injection 100 mcg/ml (hospital only), 250 mcg/ml
Side effects/adverse reactions:
CNS: Headache, drowsiness, apathy, confusion, disorientation, fatigue, depression, hallucinations
CV: Dysrhythmias, bradycardia, atrioventricular block
GI: Nausea, vomiting, anorexia, abdominal pain, diarrhoea, intestinal ischaemia/necrosis
EENT: Blurred vision, yellow-green halos, photophobia, diplopia
MS: Muscular weakness
ENDO: Gynaecomastia
INTEG: Skin rashes
Contraindications: Hypersensitivity to digitalis, supraventricular arrhythmias caused by Wolff-Parkinson-White syndrome
Precautions: Renal disease, acute myocardial infarction, atrioventricular block, hypothyroidism, elderly (reduce dose), electrolyte disturbances (especially hypokalaemia), cardioversion
Pharmacokinetics:
IV: Onset 5–30 min, peak 1–5 hr, duration variable, half-life 1.5 days excreted in urine, therapeutic range in plasma 1.5–3 mcg/litre
Interactions/incompatibilities:
• Drugs increasing risk of hypokalaemia and digoxin toxicity: diuretics, amphotericin B, corticosteroids, lithium, carbenoxolone
• Increased blood levels of digoxin: spironolactone, quinidine, verapamil, nifedipine, diltiazem, amiodarone, quinine, prazosin, erythromycin, tetracyclines, quinine, nicardipine
• Decreased blood levels of digoxin: anticholinergics, neomycin, sulphasalazine, certain cytotoxics, cholestyramine, colestipol
• Increased risk of cardiotoxicity: β-blockers, verapamil, suxamethonium, IV calcium
Clinical assessment:
• Electrolytes (prior to treatment; if toxicity suspected; if patient at risk of renal/electrolyte abnormality): potassium, sodium, chloride, calcium; renal function studies, urea, creatinine
• Drug levels (therapeutic levels 1.5–3.0 mcg/litre) once therapy stabilised; if toxicity suspected
Treatment of overdose: Gastric

lavage if ingestion recent, correct any hypokalaemia, treat arrhythmias with non-cardiac glycoside drugs, consider administration of digoxin-specific antibody fragments, monitor ECG continuously

NURSING CONSIDERATIONS

Assess:

- BP, respiration, pulse
- Apex and radical pulse for 1 min before each dose: if below than 60, take again in 1 hr; if greater than 60, call clinician and withhold drug
- Fluid balance, weight; check for oedema and retention

Administer:

- Orally using the lowest effective dose
- Potassium supplements if prescribed for potassium levels less than 3.0 mmol/litre

Evaluate:

- Cardiac status: pulse, character, rate, rhythm at least once a day
- Therapeutic response: decreased weight, oedema, pulse, respiration and increased urine output
- For weight gain
- Apex beat and pulse: inform clinician of discrepancy

Teach patient/family:

- Not to stop drug abruptly; teach all aspects of drug
- Visual changes, headache
- To report symptoms of toxicity, oedema
- To only take other medication on clinician's advice
- To take own pulse and contact clinician if it falls below 60
- Not to take antacid at the same time

digoxin-specific antibody fragments (Fab)

Digibind

Func. class.: Antidote

Chem. class.: Fragments of sheep antibody to digoxin

Legal class.: POM

Action: Fragments bind to free digoxin; reverses digoxin toxicity by enhancing excretion and removal from site of action

Uses: Life-threatening digoxin or digitoxin toxicity, overdose with other digitalis derivatives

Dosage and routes:

- *Adult:* IV dosage used to counteract digoxin or digitoxin overdose is calculated depending on the time lapsed following ingestion and the total body load of digoxin (one vial of Digibind will neutralise 0.6 m digoxin). For an unknown overdose, 10 vials of Digibind may be administered initially and then patient's response observed before further doses given

Available forms include: Injection 40 mg/vial

Side effects/adverse reactions:

CV: Return of symptoms controlled by cardiac glycoside

INTEG: Hypersensitivity, allergic reactions

SYST: Anaphylactic or other allergic reactions possible

Contraindications: None known

Precautions: Renal disease, pregnancy, allergy to sheep products; concurrent digoxin or digitoxin therapy

Pharmacokinetics:

IV: Peaks after completion of infusion, onset 30 min (variable); half-life biphasic 14–20 hr; prolonged in renal disease; excreted by kidneys

Lab. test interferences:

Interfere: Digoxin immunoassay

NURSING CONSIDERATIONS

Administer:

• By a bolus injection if cardiac arrest is imminent, otherwise by slow intravenous injection over 30 min using a 0.22 micron millipore filter

Perform/provide:

• Nursing in ICU preferable

• Continuous monitoring of cardiac status

• Reconstituted solution should not be stored for more than 24 hr, even in refrigerator

Evaluate:

• Response to treatment: correction of digoxin toxicity. Digoxin levels must be checked

• Watch for unmasking of symptoms controlled by cardiac glycosides

dihydrocodeine tartrate

DHC Continus, combination products.

Func. class.: Narcotic analgesic
Chem. class.: Opioid
Legal class.: POM, CD (oral formulation Sch 5; Injection Sch 2.)

Action: Narcotic analgesic acting at opiate receptors in the CNS. Inhibits ascending pain pathways in CNS, increases pain threshold, alter pain perception

Uses: Moderate to severe pain

Dosage and routes:

• *Modified-release:* 120–240 mg daily in 2 divided doses

• *Deep subcutaneous/IM injection*: up to 50 mg every 4–6 hr

• *Adult:* By mouth, 30 mg every 4–6 hr required

• *Child over 4 yr:* By mouth 0.5–1 mg/kg every 4–6 hr

Available forms include: Tablets, 30 mg; modified-release tablets, 60, 90, 120 mg; elixir, 10 mg/5 ml; injection 50 mg/ml

Side effects/adverse reactions:

RESP: Respiratory depression, cough suppression, exacerbation/precipitation of asthma

CNS: Drowsiness, alteration of pupillary responses, hallucinations, mood changes

GI: Nausea, reduced motility, constipation, gastric irritation, vomiting, anorexia, cramps, dry mouth

EENT: Miosis

CV: Hypotension, palpatations, bradycardia

META: Hypothermia

GU: Urinary retention

INTEG: Pain at injection site, rashes

SYST: Tolerance, dependence

Contraindications: Respiratory depression, head injury, raised intracranial pressure

Precautions: History of drug abuse, asthma, pregnancy, childbirth, lactation, hypotension, hypothyroidism, renal impairment, liver damage; dosage may need to be reduced for elderly or debilitated patients

Pharmacokinetics: Well absorbed orally, metabolised in liver, excreted in urine. Elimination half-life 3.4–5.5 hr. Excreted in breast milk

Interactions/incompatibilities:

• Risk of hypertensive crisis with: MAOIs or within 21 days of stopping them

• Increased effects of: hypnotics, other CNS depressants, alcohol

Clinical assessment:

• Co-prescribe laxatives, antiemetic if needed

• Evaluate degree of pain control

Treatment of overdose: Gastric lavage; specific antagonist: naloxone 0.4–2 mg IV at 2 to 3 min intervals up to 10 mg; supportive treatment

NURSING CONSIDERATIONS

Assess:

• Pain; to determine dosage interval appropriate for patient

• BP, pulse, respirations, pupils and conscious level

• Fluid balance

Administer:

• With an anti-emetic if nausea, vomiting

• With or after food (oral)

Perform/provide:

• Storage and administration, according to CD regulations; diluted elixir should be protected from light; has a 14 day "life"

• Fibre/fluids (constipation)

• Safe environment: cot sides, help with mobilisation

• Local treatment for injection site

• Assistance with ambulation

Evaluate:

• Need for additional analgesia, physical dependence

• Side effects

• Therapeutic response: decrease in pain

Teach patient/family:

• That dizziness/drowsiness may occur, if affected on't drive or operate machinery

• To take with food and not to have alcohol.

• About side effects, tolerance and dependence

---

diltiazem hydrochloride

Tildiem, Britiazem, Adizem, Tildiem Retard, Adizen-SR, Angiozem, Adizem-XL, Tildiem LA

Func. class.: Antihypertensive, anti-langinal

Chem. class.: Benzothiazepine, calcium-channel blocker

Legal class.: POM

Action: Inhibits calcium ion influx across cell membrane during cardiac depolarisation; produces relaxation of coronary vascular smooth muscle, dilates coronary arteries

Uses: Prophylaxis and treatment of angina, hypotension

Dosage and routes:

Diltiazem preparations are modified-release. In addition, some are formulated to further increase duration of action (longer-acting preparations). Care should be taken not to confuse preparations

Hypertension

• *Adult:* By mouth, longer-acting preparations, 90–120 mg twice daily; increase to 360 mg daily if required

Angina

• *Adult:* By mouth, standard modified-release preparations, 60 mg 3 times daily; increase gradually to 360 mg daily if required; maximum 480 mg daily in divided doses; elderly: initial dose 60 mg twice daily

• *Adult:* By mouth, longer-acting preparations, use once or twice daily, usually after initial dose titration; consult manufacturer datasheet

Available forms include: Tablets, modified-release, 60 mg; tablets, longer acting 90 mg, 120 mg, capsules, longer acting, 90 mg, 120 mg, 180 mg, 300 mg

Side effects/adverse reactions:

CV: Bradycardia, hypotension, heart block

GI: Nausea, vomiting, gastric upset, deranged liver function studies

INTEG: Rash, pruritus, flushing, photosensitivity

CNS: Headache, fatigue, drowsiness, dizziness, anxiety, depression

Contraindications: Sick sinus syndrome, 2nd or 3rd degree heart block, severe hypotension, severe

bradycardia, pregnancy, porphyria
Precautions: Congestive cardiac failure, mild hypotension, hepatic impairment, lactation, renal disease, mild bradycardia
Pharmacokinetics:
By mouth: Rapidly and completely absorbed, approximately 50% first-pass metabolism, half-life 3½–9 hr; metabolised by liver, excreted in urine (96% as metabolites)
Interactions/incompatibilities:
• Increased blood levels of: β-blockers, digitalis glycosides, cyclosporin, carbamazepine
• Increased cardiac toxicity given with: amiodarone, β-blockers
• Increased effects of: theophylline, antihypertensives
Treatment of overdose: Gastric lavage, observation in coronary care unit, supportive treatment
NURSING CONSIDERATIONS
Assess:
• Baseline vital signs, ECG
Administer:
• Before meals, bed time
Evaluate:
• Therapeutic response: decreased anginal pain, reduction in BP to required level
• Cardiac status: BP, pulse, respiration, ECG
Teach patient/family:
• How to take pulse before taking drug; record or graph should be kept
• To avoid hazardous activities until stabilised on drug and dizziness is no longer a problem
• To limit caffeine consumption
• To avoid non-prescribed drugs unless directed by a clinician
• Importance of compliance to all areas of medical regimen: diet, exercise, stress reduction, drug therapy

dimercaprol (BAL)

Func. class.: Chelating agent
Chem. class.: Dithiol compound
Legal class.: POM

Action: Binds ions from arsenic, gold, mercury, lead, copper to form water-soluble complex removed by kidneys
Uses: Heavy metal poisoning
Dosage and routes:
• *Adult:* IM 2.5–3 mg/kg 4-hrly, for 2 days, 2–4 times on the 3rd day then once or twice a day for 10 days or until recovery
Available forms include: Injection 50 mg/ml
Side effects/adverse reactions:
CNS: Headache, paraesthesia, convulsions, coma
INTEG: Urticaria, erythema, pruritus, pain at injection site, sweating, fever (especially in children), burning sensation of lips, mouth, throat, eyes
EENT: Lachrymation, conjunctivitis, rhinorrhoea
MS: Myalgia, muscle spasm
CV: Hypertension, tachycardia
GI: Nausea, vomiting, salivation, abdominal pain
Contraindications: Hypersensitivity, hepatic insufficiency, poisoning by iron or cadmium, severe renal disease, hepatic impairment due to arsenic
Precautions: Hypertension, pregnancy, lactation
Pharmacokinetics: Metabolised by plasma enzymes, excreted by kidneys and bile as complex of heavy metal and unchanged drug. Peak plasma levels 1 hr after IM injection
Interactions/incompatibilities:
• Increased toxicity: iron, selenium, uranium, cadmium
• Urinary alkalinisers may reduce nephrotoxicity by stabilising dimercaprol-metal complexes

Clinical assessment:
• Kidney function studies: blood urea nitrogen, creatinine, creatinine clearance
• Urine: pH albumin, casts and blood
• Metal levels daily

NURSING CONSIDERATIONS

Assess:
• Baseline BP, fluid balance

Administer:
• IM in deep muscle mass; rotate injection sites
• Only when adrenaline 1:1000 is on unit for anaphylaxis
• In conjunction with the general treatment for each particular metal poison

Perform/Provide:
• If ampoule appears cloudy in cold weather, warm slightly before use
• Drugs and equipment for resuscitation
• Acetazolamide or sodium citrate to decrease pH of urine, which decreases renal damage

Evaluate:
• BP, increasing BP or tachycardia
• Monitor fluid balance, report decreases in output, weight changes
• Urine: pH, albumin, blood
• Therapeutic effect: decreased levels of metal in blood
• Increased renal impairment; renal failure will reduce effectiveness of drug
• Side effects; usually reversible, rarely necessary to stop treatment
• Severity of poisoning; determines duration of therapy

Teach patient/family:
• That breath may smell

dimethicone

Infacol, Windcheaters, many combination products
Func. class.: Antiflatulent
Legal class.: GSL/P (depending on product)

Action: Disperses, prevents gas pockets in GI system
Uses: Flatulence, gripes, colic or wind pains
Dosage and routes:
• *Adult and child over 12 yr:* Up to 2 g daily in divided doses after meals and at bedtime
• *Infants:* 20–40 mg before feeds
Available forms include: Capsules 100 mg; liquid 40 mg/ml
Side effects/adverse reactions:
GI: Belching, rectal flatus
Contraindications: Hypersensitivity
Pharmacokinetics: By mouth, not absorbed

NURSING CONSIDERATIONS:

Administer:
• Before each feed for infants

Evaluate:
• Therapeutic response: absence of flatulence, colic

dinoprost trometamol

Prostin F_2 alpha
Func. class.: Oxytocic
Chem. class.: Prostaglandin F_2 alpha
Legal class.: POM (hospital only)

Action: Stimulates uterine contractions causing abortion
Uses: Abortion during 2nd trimester
Dosage and routes:
Therapeutic abortion
• Intra-amniotic injection 40 mg, slowly

Available forms include: Intra-amniotic injection 5 mg/ml
Side effects/adverse reactions:
CNS: Headache, dizziness, fainting, convulsions, EEG changes
CV: Hypotension, cardiovascular collapse
GI: Nausea, vomiting, diarrhoea, cramps, epigastric pain
INTEG: Flushing, hot flushes, shivering, irritation at injection site
GU: Uterine rupture
RESP: Wheezing, bronchospasm
Contraindications: Hypersensitivity, uterine fibrosis, cervical stenosis, pelvic surgery, pelvic inflammatory disease (PID), hypotonic arterie inertia, placenta praevia, severe toxaemia, history of Caesarean section, fetal malpresentation, history of difficult delivery, major cephalopelvic mismatch
Precautions: Hepatic disease, renal disease, cardiac disease, asthma, anaemia, convulsive disorders, hypotension, glaucoma, multiple pregnancy, multiparity
Treatment of overdose: Symptomatic, supportive
NURSING CONSIDERATIONS
Assess:
• Baseline vital signs
Administer:
• With emergency resuscitation equipment available on unit
Evaluate:
• BP, pulse; watch for change that may indicate haemorrhage
• For length, duration of contraction; notify clinician of contractions lasting over 1 min or absence of contractions, blood loss and products passed per vaginum
Teach patient/family:
• To report increased blood loss, abdominal cramps, increased temperature, foul-smelling lochia or any side effects

dinoprostone

Prepidil, Prostin E_2
Func. class.: Oxytocic
Chem. class.: Prostaglandin E_2
*Legal class.:*POM

Action: Stimulates uterine contractions and causes vasodilation
Uses: Induction of labour, fetal death *in utero*, termination of pregnancy, missed abortion and hydatidiform mole
Dosage and routes:
Cervical softening and dilation
• *Cervical gel:* 500 mcg as a single dose
Induction of labour
• *Tablets:* by mouth 500 mcg followed by 0.5–1 mg (maximum 1.5 mg) at hrly intervals
• *IV infusion:* 1 mg/1 ml, dilute and infuse at 0.25 mcg/minute for 30 min and then maintain or increase
• *Vaginal gel:* 1 or 2 mg followed after 6 hr by 1–2 mg if required. Maximum 3 or 4 mg depending on induction features
• *Vaginal tablets:* posterior fornix 3 mg followed after 6–8 hr by 3 mg if labour not established, maximum 6 mg
Termination of pregnancy, missed abortion, hydatidiform mole
• By IV infusion 10 mg/1 ml–dilute and infuse at 2.5 mcg/min for 30 min and then maintain or increase to 5 mcg/min. Maintain rate for at least 4 hr before increasing further
Termination of pregnancy
• *Extra-amniotic:* 10 mg/1 ml. Dilute to produce 100 mcg/ml and instil 1 ml then depending on response instil 1 or 2 ml at 2-hrly intervals
Note: Vaginal tablets and gel are not bioequivalent
Available forms include: Cervical

gel 200 mcg/1 ml; tablets 500 mcg; intravenous solution 1 mg/ml, 10 mg/ml; extra-amniotic solution 10 mg/ml; vaginal gel 400 mcg/1 ml; vaginal tablets 3 mg

Side effects/adverse reactions:
CNS: Headache, dizziness, flushing
GI: Nausea, vomiting, diarrhoea
GU: Vaginitis, vaginal pain, vulvitis, vaginismus, shivering, uterine hypertonus
MS: Leg cramps, joint swelling, weakness, severe uterus contractions
HAEM: Raised blood cell
All dose related and more common after intravenous therapy; local tissue reaction and erythema after intravenous administration

Contraindications: No absolute contraindications, but not recommended where oxytoxic drugs generally contraindication, ruptured membranes, hypersensitivity to prostaglandins, unexplained vaginal bleeding, non-vertex presentations, pelvic infection/vaginal infections/PID

Precautions: Glaucoma, asthma, hypotonus, fetal distress

Pharmacokinetics:
Metabolised in spleen, kidney, lungs, excreted in urine

Treatment of overdose:
Supportive measures, appropriate obstetric measures as indicated

NURSING CONSIDERATIONS

Assess:
- Cervical ripening (i.e. Bishop's score)
- Fetal well-being (CTG tracing)
- Presentation
- Gestation

Administer:
- With bladder empty
- Do not give if BP high (risk of cord prolapse)
- Tablets are inserted high into posterior fornix of vagina
- Useful to dip pessary in water before inserting (starts dissolving process)
- Do not use chlorhexidine obstetric cream

Perform/provide:
- Call bell (patient to remain supine for 30 min)
- CTG tracing 20 min after insertion
- Refrigerated storage for gel

Evaluate:
- Cervical assessment according to treatment regimen as necessary (e.g. 4–8 hr)
- CTG (fetal well-being)

Teach patient/family:
- Stay supine for ½ hr
- Report spontaneous rupture of membranes or rapid fetal movements
- Painful contractions, backache may ensue

diphtheria vaccines

Diptheria, adsorbed
Diptheria vaccine for adults, adsorbed
Component of:-
Trivax-AD (Adsorbed Diptheria, Tetanus and Pertusis Vaccine)
Adsorbed Diptheria and Tetanus Vaccine
Trivax (Diptheria, Tetanus and Pertussis Vaccine)
Diptheria and Tetanus Vaccine

Func. class.: Vaccine (bacterial toxoid)
Chem. class.: Denatured bacterial toxin
Legal class.: POM

Action: Stimulates production of specific antibodies against the toxin produced by *Corynebacterium diptheriae*

Uses: Prevention of diptheria

Dosage and routes:
Routine childhood vaccination

• *Child:* By IM or deep SC injection 0.5 ml of Adsorbed Diptheria, Tetanus and Pertussis vaccine at 2 months of age followed by 2 further doses at intervals of 4 weeks. A further reinforcing dose of Adsorbed Diptheria and Tetanus Vaccine should be given at school entry. In children where immunisation against whooping cough is contraindicated, Adsorbed Diptheria and Tetanus Vaccine can be substituted using the same schedule

Protection of child contacts of diptheria case or carrier

• *Child under 10 yr previously immunised:* By IM or deep SC injection, single 0.5 ml dose of Diptheria Vaccine Adsorbed

• *Child under 10 yr not previously immunised:* By IM or deep SC injection, 0.5 ml Diptheria Vaccine Adsorbed, repeated twice at 4-week intervals

Primary vaccination of adults and children over 10 yr

• *Adult and child over 10 yr:* By IM or deep SC injection, 0.5 ml Diptheria Vaccine for Adults, Adsorbed, repeated twice at 4-week intervals

Reinforcement of immunity in previously vaccinated adults and children over 10 yr at special risk (e.g. case contacts or microbiology laboratory workers)

• *Adult and child over 10 yr:* By IM or deep SC injection, a single 0.5 ml dose of Diptheria Vaccine for Adults, Adsorbed

Note: Non-adsorbed formulations of Diptheria, Tetanus and Pertussis Vaccine and Diptheria and Tetanus Vaccines are available, but the Adsorbed formulations are preferred

Available forms include: Adsorbed Diptheria, Tetanus and Pertussis Vaccine: Injection 0.5 ml ampoule, 5 ml vial
Diptheria, Tetanus and Pertussis Vaccine: Injection 0.5 ml ampoule, 5 ml vial
Adsorbed Diptheria and Tetanus Vaccine: Injection 0.5 ml ampoule, 0.5 ml prefilled syringe
Diptheria and Tetanus Vaccine: Injection 5 ml vial
Diptheria Vaccine, Adsorbed: Injection 0.5 ml ampoule
Diptheria Vaccine for Adults, Adsorbed: Injection 0.5 ml ampoule

Side effects/adverse reactions:
CNS: Malaise, headache, polyradicular neuritis, peripheral neuropathy
INTEG: Swelling, redness and tenderness at injection site, urticaria
SYST: Transient fever, anaphylaxis and other allergic reactions

Contraindications: Hypersensitivity; acute infection; adults and children over 10 yr unless first shown to lack immunity using the Schick test; pertussis-containing vaccines should be avoided in children with a personal or family history of epilepsy or other familial or hereditary diseases of the CNS

Precautions: Pregnancy, breast-feeding

Interactions:

• Reduced effect with: immunosuppressive agents including high-dose corticosteroids, cytotoxic chemotherapy, azathioprine

Incompatibilities:

• Do not mix with any other vaccine or drug

NURSING CONSIDERATIONS

Assess:

• Previous history of diphtheria vaccination; a Schick test may be indicated

• For history of hypersensitivity, especially to previous vaccines containing diphtheria

• For acute illness, infection, pregnancy or breast-feeding

• For personal or family history of epilepsy or CNS disease if the vaccine containing pertussis is to be used

Administer:
- After checking expiry date
- After shaking vial
- 0.5 ml dose by IM or deep SC injection
- Diphtheria vaccine for adults (low dose) adsorbed, for adults and children over 10 yr old
- Do not mix with other drugs or vaccines
- With adrenaline 1:1000 to hand in case of anaphylactic reaction

Perform/provide:
- Record name, date, dose, route, site used, batch number of vaccine in patient's notes
- Store in refrigerator (2°–8°C) protected from light
- Discard part-used vials at end of clinic
- Patient with written record of name and date of vaccination

Evaluate:
- For anaphylactic reaction
- For local/systemic reactions

Teach patient/family:
- About possible side-effects
- Of the need to complete course of vaccine. Children may need booster dose at time of school entry; advice should be sought at the appropriate time
- That a Schick test may be indicated 3 months after vaccination for those exposed to diphtheria

---

dipipanone hydrochloride

Diconal

Func. class.: Narcotic analgesic (with anti-emetic)

Chem. class.: Opioid

Legal class.: CD (Sch 2) POM

Action: Narcotic analgesic acting at opiate receptors in CNS. Inhibits ascending pain pathways in CNS, increases pain threshold, alter pain perception

Uses: Moderate to severe pain in patients not responding to pethidine or morphine

Dosage and routes:
- *Adults:* By mouth 1 tablet 6-hrly, gradually increased to 3 tablets 6-hrly if required

Available forms include: Tablets, dipipanone hydrochloride 10 mg, cyclizine hydrochloride 30 mg

Side effects/adverse reactions:

RESP: Respiratory depression, cough suppression

CV: Hypotension, bradycardia, palpatations

CNS: Drowsiness, alteration of pupillary responses, blurred vision, hallucinations, vertigo

GI: Nausea, reduced motility, constipation, dry mouth, vomiting, cramps, dry mouth

GU: Difficulty in micturition

SYST: Tolerance, dependence

Contraindications: Respiratory depression, obstructive airways disease, concurrent use of MAOIs, head injury, raised intracranial pressure

Precautions: Severe liver or kidney disease. Possibility of addiction, impaired respiration. Use of other CNS depressants, pregnancy, lactation

Pharmacokinetics: Onset of effect within 1 hr, duration 6 hr

Interactions/incompatibilities:
- Risk of hypotensive crisis given within 21 days of: Monoamine-oxidase inhibitors

Clinical assessment
- Prescribe anti-emetic as required (preparation contains cyclizine)
- Prescribe prophylactic laxative if constipated

Treatment of overdose: Respiratory depression—use naloxone 0.4–2 mg IV at 2 to 3 min intervals up to 10 mg, gastric lavage, oxygen and respiratory support if necessary

NURSING CONSIDERATIONS

Assess:

• Base line vital signs: blood pressure, pulse, respiration, pupils, consciousness level

• Fluid balance

• When pain is beginning to return; determine dosage interval by patient response

Perform/provide:

• Fluids/fibre (constipation)

• Assistance with ambulation

Evaluate:

• For changes in vital signs

• Pain, side effects (blurred vision, drowsiness)

• Therapeutic response: decrease in pain

Teach patient/family:

• That it may cause drowsiness, if affected not to drive/operate machinery. Take no alcohol

• About side effects, tolerance and dependence

• To report side effects

• Withdrawal symptoms may occur if high, long term dosage reduced too quickly: nausea, vomiting, cramps, fever, faintness, anorexia

dipivefrin hydrochloride/ (opthalmic)

Propine

Func. class.: Antihypertensive, ocular; antiglaucoma agent

Chem. class.: Diesterified adrenaline

Legal class.: POM

Action: Converted to adrenaline which decreases aqueous humour production and increases outflow

Uses: Chronic open angle glaucoma or occular hypertensive patient with anterior chamber open angle

Dosage and routes:

• *Adult:* Instil 1 drop into affected eye(s) 12 hrly

Available forms include: Eye drops 0.1%

Side effects/adverse reactions:

CV: Hypertension, tachycardia, arrhythmias

EENT: Burning, stinging, mydriasis, photophobia, corneal deposits, conjunctivitis

Contraindications: Closed angle glaucoma, soft contact lenses

Precautions: Aphakia, narrow angles

Pharmacokinetics:

Instil: Onset 30 min, duration 1 hr

NURSING CONSIDERATIONS

Perform/provide:

• Storage of drug at room temperature

Teach patient/family:

• To report stinging, burning, itching, lacrimation, puffiness

• Method of instillation, including pressure on lacrimal sac for 1 min and not to touch dropper to eye

• To discard 28 days after opening

• Not to wear soft (hydrophilic) contact lenses

dipyridamole

Persantin

Func. class.: Coronary vasodilator, antiplatelet agent

Chem. class.: Pyrimidine derivative

Legal class.: POM

Action: Decreases platelet aggregation, adhesion and survival when given orally. Intravenous use causes coronary vasodilatation

Uses: Prophylaxis of thrombo-

embolism associated with prosthetic heart valves (tablets)
Injection – myocardial imaging

Dosage and routes:
• *Adult:* By mouth 300–600 mg daily in 3 or 4 divided doses
• *Adult:* IV injection 0.56 mg/kg over 4 min

Available forms include: Tablets 25 mg, 100 mg; injection 10 mg/2 ml

Side effects/adverse reactions:
CV: Postural hypotension, increased anginal attacks, myocardial ischaemia
CNS: Headache, dizziness, weakness, fainting, syncope
GI: Nausea, vomiting, anorexia, diarrhoea, dyspepsia
INTEG: Rash, flushing

Contraindications: Hypersensitivity; injection: aortic stenosis, hypotension in recent myocardial infarction, significant valvular disease, uncompensated heart failure, cardiac conduction defects, dysrhythmias

Precautions: Pregnancy, unstable angina, aortic coagulation disorders, stenosis

Pharmacokinetics:
Period of onset: Onset 30 sec, peak 2–2½ min. Therapeutic response may take several months, metabolised in liver, excreted in bile, undergoes enterohepatic recirculation

Interactions/incompatibilities:
• Enhance effects of: anticoagulants
• Decreased effects: antacids

Treatment of overdose: Administer aminophylline for coronary vasolidatation

NURSING CONSIDERATIONS

Assess:
• Baseline vital signs, ECG

Administer:
• On an empty stomach: 1 hr before meals or 2 hr after

Evaluate:
• BP, pulse during treatment until stable; take BP lying, standing; ECG monitor may be necessary; orthostatic hypotension is common
• Therapeutic response: decreased chest pain (angina)
• Cardiac status: chest pain, what aggravates or ameliorates condition

Teach patient/family:
• That medication is not cure, may need to be taken continuously; therapeutic response may not be evident for 2–3 months
• That it is necessary to stop smoking to prevent excessive vasoconstriction
• To avoid hazardous activities until stabilised on medication; dizziness may occur

Clinical assessment:
• Blood urea nitrogen, creatinine, phosphate, urine hydroxyproline uric acid, chloride, electrolytes, pH, urine calcium, magnesium, alkaline phosphatase, urinalysis, calcium, vitamin D
• Muscle spasm, laryngospasm, paraesthesia, facial twitching, nutritional status with regard calcium and phosphate, colic; may indicate hypocalcaemia

Treatment of overdose: Symptoms of hypocalcaemia; withdraw drug and correct hypocalcaemia with IV calcium gluconate

disopyramide

Dirythmin, SA, Rythmodan, Rythmodan Retard
Func. class.: Anti-arrhythmic (Class Ia)
Chem. class.: Synthetic butyramide
Legal class.: POM

Action: Decreases myocardial contractility. Shortens sinus node recovery time, increases atrial/ventricular refractory time, suppresses ectopic focal activity, reduces duration of action potential between normal, infracted myocardium

Uses: Atrial or ventricular ectopic beats. Paroxysmal atrial or ventricular tachycardia. Arrhythmias post—myocardial infarction. Wolf-Parkinson-White syndrome. Maintains sinus rhythm after electro-cardioversion. Control of glycoside induced arrhythmias

Dosage and routes:

• *Adult:* By mouth 300–800 mg daily in divided doses; modified-release tablets 250–375 mg daily maximum oral dose 800 mg daily

• *Adult:* Slow IV injection, 2 mg/kg; maximum 150 mg; patients should respond within 10–15 min; then by mouth 200 mg every 8 hr for 24 hr *or* IV infusion 0.4 mg/kg/hr, maximum 300 mg in first hour, total daily maximum 800 mg

Available forms include: Capsules 100 mg, 150 mg; modified-release tablets 150 mg, 250 mg (as phosphate); injection 10 mg/ml (as phosphate)

Side effects/adverse reactions:

GU: Retention, hesitancy
CNS: Headache, dizziness, psychosis
GI: Dry mouth, constipation, nausea, flatulence, cholestatic jaundice
CV: Hypotension, bradycardia, angina, premature ventricular contraction, tachycardia, increases QRS, QT segments, cardiac arrest, oedema, weight gain, atrioventricular block
META: Hypoglycaemia
MS: Weakness, pain in extremities
EENT: Blurred vision, dry nose, throat, eyes, narrow-angle glaucoma
HAEM: Thrombocytopenia, agranulocytosis, anaemia (rare)

Contraindications: Hypersensitivity, 2nd/3rd degree atrioventricular block, cardiogenic shock, congestive cardiac failure (uncompensated), series node disease without pacemaker

Precautions: Widening of QRS or prolonging of QT internal. Atrial flutter/tachycardia with block, significant heart failure, hypocalcaemia will reduce patient response. Digitalis intoxication, bundle branch block. Hypoglycaemia

Pharmacokinetics:

IV: Onset 30 min-3½ hr, peak 1–2 hr, duration 1½–8½ hr
IM: Onset 30 min, peak 60–90 min, duration 6–8 hr
Half-life 4–10 hr, metabolised in liver, excreted in faeces, urine, breast milk

Interactions/incompatibilities:

• Amiodarone—increased risk of ventricular arrhythmias

• Anti-arrhythmics – myocardial depression
• Disopyramide – plasma level increased by erythromycin, plasma level decreased by rifampicin, phenobarbitone, phenytoin
• Antimuscarinics – increased antimuscarinics side effects
• Diuretics – hypokalaemia will increase disopyramide toxicity

Clinical assessment:
• Blood levels during treatment
• Electrolytes (sodium, chloride potassium)
• Liver, kidney function studies: aspartate amino transferase alonine aminotransferase bilirubin, urea, creatinine during treatment
• ECG, check for increased QT, widening QRS; drug should be discontinued

Treatment of overdose: O_2, artificial ventilation, ECG, administer dopamine or isoprenaline for circulatory depression; administer diazepam or thiopentone for convulsions. Possibility of haemodialysis or haemoperfusion in poor renal function

NURSING CONSIDERATIONS

Assess:
• Baseline weight, pulse rate
• Consider fluid balance in heart failure
• Diabetics for signs of hypoglycaemia – regular BM stix

Administer:
• Frequent sips of water for dry mouth
• Reduced dosage slowly with ECG monitoring

Evaluate:
• BP regularly for hypotension, hypertension
• Increase in QRS, QT; report to clinician
• For rebound hypertension after 1–2 hr
• For constipation; consider increasing fibre content of diet; possible need of laxatives
• Heart rate; respiration; rate, rhythm, character
• Assess for urinary hesitancy, frequency or retension daily
• Check for oedema daily; daily weight

Teach patient/family:
• Take drug exactly as prescribed
• Avoid alcohol or severe hypotension may occur; to avoid non-prescribed drugs or serious drug interactions may occur
• Change position slowly during early therapy to prevent fainting
• Avoid hazardous activities if dizziness or blurred vision occurs
• Stress patient compliance with drug regimen; explain to patient that this drug does not cure condition

---

distigmine bromide

Ubretid

Func. class.: Anticholinesterase, cholinergic

Chem. class.: Quaternary ammonium compound

Legal class.: POM

Action: Long-acting inhibition of the enzymic degradation of the neurotransmitter acetylcholine and enhances neuromuscular transmission in voluntary and involuntary transmission

Uses: Post-operative urinary retention. Post-operative ileus and intestinal atony. Emptying of neurogenic bladder. Myasthenia gravis

Dosage and routes:

Myasthenia gravis
• *Adult:* By mouth initially 5 mg daily 30 min before breakfast, increase at intervals of 3–4 days as necessary to maximum 20 mg daily
• *Child:* Maximum 10 mg by mouth daily, according to age

Urinary retention, ileus or intestinal atony post surgery

• *Adult:* By mouth, 5 mg 30 min before breakfast, daily; IM injection, 500 mcg 12 hr after surgery, repeat every 24 hr if necessary

Neurogenic bladder

• *Adult:* By mouth, 5 mg daily or on alternate days 30 min before breakfast. IM: injection may be given in place of tablets for the first few days

Available forms include: Tablets 5 mg; IM injection 500 mcg/ml

Side effects/adverse reactions:

GI: Nausea, increased salivation, vomiting, diarrhoea, abdominal cramps, intestinal colic

CNS: Blurred vision

INTEG: Sweating

CV: Bradycardia

SYST: Cholinergic crisis caused by accumulation of acetylcholine

Contraindications: Intestinal or urinary obstruction; recent anastomosis; severe post-operative shock; spastic or mechanical ileus; severe circulatory insufficiency; pregnancy

Precautions: Elderly patients, epilepsy, parkinsonism, asthma, cardiovascular disease, peptic ulcer, vagotonia, lactation

Pharmacokinetics: Cholinesterase maximally inhibited 9 hr after single IM dose, duration 24 hr; normal function within 48 hr

Interactions/incompatibilities:

• Absorption impaired by food

• Adverse effects enhanced by other anticholinergic agents

Clinical assessment:

• Check recent history of cardiac disease (myocardial infarction), check mechanical obstruction not cause of retention, check ileus not due to mechanical obstruction. Recent bowel anastomosis

Treatment of overdose: Atropine for 24 hr, up to 2 mg IM, symptomatic treatment

NURSING CONSIDERATIONS

Assess:

• BP, pulse, respiration

• Fluid balance

• Extent of underlying pathology to enable accurate evaluation

Administer:

• 30 min before breakfast; absorption impaired by food

• Diluent for ampoules: water for injection

Perform/provide:

• Close supervision in early stages if used for myasthenia gravis ('crisis')

• Toilet facilities in case of disturbance in bowel habit

• Wash/change linen for sweating

• Atropine always available

• Safe environment: Cot side, Help with mobilisation directed by individual patient assessment

Evaluate:

• Side effects, e.g. BP or slowed pulse, colic, problems passing urine, abdominal distention; salivation

• Improvement in urinary function, bowel movement, micturition, etc.

• Bowel sounds

• Therapeutic effect as elicited by formal assessment

Teach patient/family:

• About blurred vision. That effects last for up to 24 hr, returning to normal within 48 hr

• To take as prescribed

• Change position slowly. To report increased salivation

• About sweating, breathing (potential) problems. To wear medialer and bracelet if they have myasthenia gravis

• To seek medical advice if adverse reactions occur

disulfiram

Antabuse 200
Func. class.: Alcohol deterrent
Chem. class.: Aldehyde dehydrogenase inhibitor
Legal class.: POM

Action: Blocks oxidation of alcohol at acetaldehyde stage
Uses: Chronic alcoholism with appropriate supportive treatment
Dosage and routes:
• *Adult:* By mouth after a 24 hr alcohol-free period:
Day 1: no more than 4 tablets as one dose
Day 2: 3 tablets
Day 3: 2 tablets
Day 4 and 5: 1 tablet
Subsequent dose as 1 or ½ tablet daily
Available forms include: Tablets 200 mg
Side effects/adverse reactions:
CNS: Headache, drowsiness, restlessness, dizziness, fatigue, tremors, psychosis, libido reduction
GI: Nausea, vomiting, anorexia, hepatotoxicity, halitosis
INTEG: Rash, dermatitis, urticaria, peripheral neuritis
GU: Severe thirst
Contraindications: Hypersensitivity, alcohol intoxication, psychoses, hypertension, cardiac failure, coronary artery disease, history of CVA
Precautions: Hypothyroidism, hepatic disease, diabetes mellitus, seizure disorders, respiratory disease, diabetes mellitus, renal failure
Pharmacokinetics:
By mouth: Onset 12 hr, oxidized by liver, excreted unchanged in faeces
Interactions/incompatibilities:
• Increased effects of: tricyclic antidepressants, theophylline, oral anticoagulants, phenytoin, diazepam, chlordiazepoxide, narcotics, amphetamines
• Disulfiram reaction: alcohol, chlorpromazine, amitriptyline—both may increase intensity of alcohol reactions
• Psychosis: metronidazole, paraldehyde, isoniazid
Clinical assessment:
• Liver function studies every 2 weeks during therapy: aspartate aminotransferase, alanine aminotransferase
• Full blood count sequential multiple analysis every 3–6 months to detect any abnormality including increased cholesterol
Treatment of overdose: Low toxicity—symptomatic with gastric lavage or observation

NURSING CONSIDERATIONS

Administer:
• Once per day in the morning or bedtime if drowsiness occurs
• Only after patient has not had alcohol for more than 12 hr
• Only after a 24 hr alcohol-free period
Evaluate:
• Mental status: affect, mood, drug history, ability to follow treatment, abstain from alcohol
Teach patient/family:
• Effect of this drug if alcohol is taken—check patient understanding and record in nursing documentation
• That shaving lotions, creams, cough preparations, skin products must be checked for alcohol content; even in small amount, alcohol can produce a reaction
• That tolerance will not develop if treatment is prolonged
• That reaction may occur for 2 weeks after last dose
• Carry medication record card listing disulfiram therapy

• Avoid driving or hazardous tasks if drowsiness occurs
• That disulfiram reaction occurs 10 min after drinking alcohol; characterised by by violent flushing, dyspnoea, headache, palpitations, tachycardia, nausea and vomiting

dithranol/dithranol triacetate

Alphodith, Anthranol, Dithocream, Psoradra, Exolam, combination products

Func. class.: Antipsoriatic agent
Legal class.: POM/P depending on strength

Action: Inhibits epidermal cell replication by decreasing mitosis by halting nucleic protein synthesis
Uses: Subacute and chronic psoriasis
Dosage and routes:
• *Adult and child:* Topical, apply to affected area for 30–60 min. Start with low concentrations and build up
Available forms include: Cream 0.1%, 0.2%, 0.25%, 0.4%, 0.5%, 1%, 2%; ointment 0.1%, 0.25%, 0.4%, 1%, 2%, 3%
Side effects/adverse reactions:
INTEG: Rash on normal skin, discolouration of nails, hair, skin, clothing, burning sensation and irritation
Contraindications: Hypersensitivity, acute and pustular psoriasis
Precautions: Excessive soreness—reduce frequency. Avoid eyes and mucous membranes
Pharmacokinetics:
Topical: Absorption poor, absorbed amount excreted in urine
Interactions/incompatibilities: None known
NURSING CONSIDERATIONS
Assess:
• Urinalysis weekly for albumin and casts
Administer:
• Apply sparingly, avoid hair, area near eyes, eyes, mucous membranes
• Avoid contamination of healthy surrounding skin by protection with barrier cream, e.g. zinc oxide, vaseline (petroleum jelly)
• Cover with dressing to avoid staining of clothes
• Apply to the scalp after the application of olive oil or liquid paraffin. Remove scales with comb
• Apply at bedtime to ensure contact time of 10–12 hr if required
• Continue treatment for 2–4 weeks, as required
Evaluate:
• Therapeutic response: decreased itching, redness, dryness and scaling
• Observe the skin involved carefully, noting any agents that appear to aggravate the condition
Teach patient/family:
• To avoid application to surrounding healthy skin, mucous membranes and eyes
• Skin, nails and hair may assume a brown-yellow tinge if cream is applied to them
• To discontinue use if rash, urticaria or folliculitis develop

dobutamine HCl

Dobutrex

Func. class.: Adrenergic direct-acting β-agonist
Chem. class.: Sympathomimetic amine
Legal class.: POM

Action: Causes increased contractility and heart rate by acting on β-1 receptors in heart

Uses: Low output cardiac failure due to myocardial infarction, open heart surgery, sepsis, shock, possible alternative to exercise in stress testing

Dosage and routes:

• *Adult:* IV infusion 2.5–10 mcg/kg/min, may increase to 40 mcg/kg/min if needed. Should be given diluted and adjust according to patient response

Available forms include: Injection IV solution 12.5 mg (as hydrochloride)/ml

Side effects/adverse reactions:

CV: Palpitations, tachycardia, hypertension, angina

GI: Nausea, vomiting

Contraindications: Hypersensitivity

Precautions: Pregnancy, lactation, ventricular filling or outflow obstruction. Hypotension due to cardiogenic shock

Pharmacokinetics:

IV: Onset 1–5 min, peak 10 min, half-life 2 min, metabolised in liver (inactive metabolites), excreted in urine

Interactions/incompatibilities:

• Incompatible with alkaline solutions: sodium, bicarbonate

Treatment of overdose: Withdraw dobutamine until condition stabilises

NURSING CONSIDERATIONS

Assess:

• Heart rate, rhythm, BP, ECG, cardiac output

• Fluid balance

• Hrly urine measurement—patient may need urinary catheter. Inform clinician if output less than 30 ml/hr

• Continuous cardiac monitoring during administration

• BP and pulse after parenteral route half hrly initially. Assess dependency on stability of patient's condition and therapeutic response

Administer:

• Patients usually managed on a cardiac or intensive care unit

• May be given peripherally but ideally through a central line with pressure monitoring (or such a central line or Swan Ganz catheter) in situ

• Must be diluted as prescribed and given via intravenous pump (usually to 50 mls and given via a syringe pump)

Perform/provide:

• Storage of reconstituted solution, if refrigerated, for no longer than 48 hr

Evaluate:

• Therapeutic response: increased BP with stabilisation, increase in urinary output and effect on heart rate—or inform medical staff of lack of response

Teach patient/family:

• Reason for drug administration

• Explanation of equipment and monitors to allay fear

---

docusate sodium

Dioctyl, Norgalax Micro-enema, Fletchers' Enemette, combination products

Func. class.: Laxative

Chem. class.: Anionic surfactant

Legal class.: P

Action: Increases water penetration to soften stools for easier passage

Uses: Prevent and treat chronic constipation

Dosage and routes:

• *Adult:* By mouth up to 500 mg a day in divided doses; initial doses should be larger and gradually reduced; enema 5 ml as needed; with barium meal 400 mg

• *Child over 3 yr:* Fletcher's Enemette enema as adult (Norgalax in children over 12 yr only)

• *Child 2–12 yr:* By mouth 12.5–25 mg 3 times a day

• *Infant over 6 months:* By mouth 12.5 mg 3 times a day

Available forms include: Tablets 100 mg; oral solution 50 mg/5 ml, paediatric solution 12.5 mg/5 ml; enema 90 mg/5 ml, 120 mg/10 g

Side effects/adverse reactions:

GI: Nausea, anorexia, cramps atonic colon, hypocalcaemia

Contraindications: Intestinal obstruction; abdominal pain; nausea/vomiting; infants under 6 months; rectal preparations: haemorrhoids; anal fissures; recto colitis bleeding: inflammatory bowel disease

Precautions: Breast-feeding

Pharmacokinetics: By mouth onset 1–2 days; enema onset 5–20 minutes

Interactions/incompatibilities:

• Mineral oil; Anthraquinones, increased absorption

Clinical assessment:

• Urine/blood electrolytes

Treatment of overdose: Fluids to replace excessive loss

NURSING CONSIDERATIONS

Assess:

• Cause of constipation; identify whether fluids, fibre or exercise is missing from lifestyle

• Fluid balance to identify fluid loss

Administer:

• Alone for better absorption; do not take within 1 hr of other drugs or within 1 hr of antacids, milk, or cimetidine

• Take tables and solution with a full glass of water

• Swallow tablets whole

• Do not use undue force when giving enema

• Use paediatric solution for children

Evaluate:

• Therapeutic response: decrease in constipation – if diarrhoea, discontinue and seek advice

• Cramping, rectal bleeding, nausea, vomiting; if these symptoms occur, drug should be discontinued

Teach patient/family:

• Health education: to other possible means of avoiding constipation

• Swallow tablets whole; do not chew

• That normal bowel movements do not always occur daily

• Do not use in presence of abdominal pain, nausea, vomiting

• Notify clinician if constipation unrelieved or if symptoms of electrolyte imbalance occur: muscle cramps, pain, weakness, dizziness

domperidone

Motilium

Func. class.: Antiemetic

Chem. class.: Substituted imidazoline

Legal class.: POM

Action: Dopamine antagonist which blocks chemoreceptor trigger zone and acts upon upper GI tract

Uses: Acute treatment of nausea and vomiting of any aetiology in adults; nausea and vomiting associated with L-dopa and bromocriptine. *Children:* Only for nausea and vomiting due to cancer chemotherapy or radiation

Dosage and routes:

• *Adults:* By mouth 10–20 mg, by rectum 30–60 mg every 4–8 hr

• *Children:* 0.2–0.4 mg/kg 4–8 hrly orally, by rectum 2–12 yr, 30–120 mg a day depending on weight

Available forms include: Tablets, 10 mg; sugar-free suspension, 5 mg/5 ml; suppositories, 30 mg

Side effects/adverse reactions:

META: Raised prolactin levels, possible galactorrhoea, gynaecomastia

Precautions: Pregnancy/lactation

Pharmacokinetics: Excreted in faeces and urine as metabolites
Interactions/incompatibilities: Effects reduced by anticholinergic agents, opioid analgesics
• Antagonises hyperprolactinaemic action of bromocriptine
• Possible enhanced GI absorption of concurrent oral drugs
Lab. test interferences: *Increase:* prolactin

NURSING CONSIDERATIONS

Assess:
• Fluid balance (renal disease)
• Degree of nausea and vomiting
• Weight of children

Administer:
• Limit to short-term treatment only
• Orally as tablets or suspension but as suppository if frequent vomiting
• Underlying medical cause of nausea/vomiting

Perform/provide:
• Cool storage for suppositories
• Mouth washes as required
• Adequate fluids by mouth or IV

Evaluate:
• Side effects related to concurrent drug therapy
• Therapeutic response: decrease in nausea/vomiting

Teach patient/family:
• About side effects of increased prolactin, e.g. galactorrhoea
• That therapy is for short term use only. Maximum usually 12 weeks

---

dopamine hydrochloride

Intropin
Func. class.: Dopaminergic
Chem. class.: Sympathomimetic amine
Legal class.: POM

Action: At low doses causes renal and mesenteric vascular dilatation, improving renal blood flow, glomerular filtration rate and urine output. At higher doses, exerts positive inotropic effect and increases blood pressure and urine output. At very high doses, increases blood pressure by peripheral vasoconstriction
Uses: Correction of poor perfusion, low cardiac output, renal failure and shock due to myocardial infarction, trauma, endotoxin septicaemia, open heart surgery, heart failure
Dosage and routes:
• *Adult:* IV infusion 2–5 mcg/kg/min titrated upwards in increments of 5–10 mcg/kg/min up to 20–50 mcg/kg/min if required
Side effects/adverse reactions:
CNS: Headache
CV: Palpitations, tachycardia, hypertension, hypotension, ectopic beats, angina, dyspnoea resp
GI: Nausea, vomiting
Contraindications: Hypovolaemia, ventricular fibrillation, tachydysrhythmias, phaeochromocytoma, hyperthyroidism
Precautions: Hypersensitivity to sulphites, extravasation-use large vein, occlusive vascular disease
Pharmacokinetics:
IV: Onset 5 min, duration up to 10 min, metabolised in liver, excreted in urine (metabolites)
Interactions/incompatibilities:
• Do not use within 2 wks of monoamine oxidase inhibitors, or hypertensive crisis may result; starting dose 1/10 of normal dose
• Dysrhythmias: general anaesthetics
• Incompatible with alkaline solutions: sodium bicarbonate
Clinical assessment:
• Therapeutic level, cardiovascular and renal parameters
• ECG during administration continuously

• CVP during infusion if possible to measure cardiac output

Treatment of overdose:
Dose reduction or discontinue; if fails consider phentolamine mesylate

NURSING CONSIDERATIONS

Assess:
• To exclude hypovolaemia: administer prescribed plasma expanded
• BP, pulse and respiration prior to administration: CVP is also valuable
• Baseline electrolytes, renal function and fluid balance

Administer:
• By infusion pump having calculated prescribed dose in mcg/kg/min
• Via central line access or large peripheral versus access as last resort
• No other medications through same line to avoid bolus doses

Perform/provide:
• Continuous cardiac monitoring: report elevations in heart rate and blood pressure, dose may require adjustment tiltrated against effect
• Hrly vital sign recording and fluid balance
• Resuscitation equipment available

Evaluate:
• Therapeutic response: increased urine output for example
• IV site: observe for extravasation at least hrly
• Peripheral circulation as may cause vasoconstriction

dothiepin hydrochloride

Prothiaden, Dothapax, Prepadine
Func. class.: Antidepressant
Chem. class.: Tricyclic antidepressant
Legal class.: POM

Action: Blocks reuptake of noradrenaline and serotonin into nerve endings, increasing action of noradrenalin, serotonin in nerve cells

Uses: Depressive illness, particularly where sedation and an anxiolytic action is required

Dosage and routes:
• *Adult:* By mouth, initially 75 mg daily in divided doses or as single dose at bedtime, increased as necessary to maximum 225 mg; elderly patients 75 mg maximum

Available forms include: Capsules 25 mg; Tablets 75 mg

Side effects/adverse reactions:
HAEM: Agranulocytosis, depression of bone marrow, jaundice
CNS: Sedation, blurred vision, tremor, confusion, hypomania, behavioural disturbances, convulsions
GI: Nausea, dry mouth, paralytic ileus
GU: Difficulty with micturition, changes in sexual function
INTEG: Sweating, rashes
CV: Arrhythmias, postural hypotension, tachycardia

Contraindications: Recent myocardial infarction, heart block; mania; liver disease, porphyria

Precautions: Diabetes, cardiac disease, epilepsy, pregnancy, hepatic impairment, psychoses, urinary retention, elderly, narrow angle glaucoma, prostatic hypertrophy; avoid abrupt cessation of therapy; caution in anaesthesia

Pharmacokinetics:
Converted in liver to active metab-

olite; half-life 19–33 hr, excreted in urine. Onset of antidepressant effect 2–4 weeks, anxiolytic effect apparent within several days

Interactions/incompatibilities:
- Increased effect: alcohol, antihistamines, anxiolytics, disulfiram
- Risk of hypertension: anaesthetics, anti-hypotensives, sympathomimetics, diuretics
- Reduced effect: antiepileptics
- Risk of hypertension: MAOIs, other antidepressants

Clinical assessment:
- ECG and cardiac status
- Check no urinary retention or glaucoma
- Full blood count, WBC and differential every 4 weeks. Blood glucose

Treatment of overdose: Gastric lavage, activated charcoal, ECG, intubate, treatment for convulsions or arrhythmias

NURSING CONSIDERATIONS

Assess:
- Blood pressure (lying/standing), pulse, temperature
- Weight, fluid balance

Administer:
- At bedtime with food or as a divided dose. Ensure dose taken
- Not with alcohol
- Withdraw therapy gradually

Perform/provide:
- Fluids/fibre for constipation
- Fluids, sips of water for dry mouth
- Safe environment: Cot sides
- Help with mobilisation

Evaluate:
- Sleeping patterns
- Retention of urine
- Mood, level of confusion, mental state

Teach patient/family:
- That drug may cause drowsiness, if affected don't drive or operate machinery
- No alcohol. Warn that response may take 2–4 weeks, encourage them to persist and not stop abruptly
- About side effects: dry mouth, sore throat, weight gain, blurred vision, retention, sweating, rapid pulse, sexual problems; these should be reported
- That they must report these to doctor
- To get up slowly to avoid fainting

---

doxapram HCl

Dopram

Func. class.: Respiratory stimulant
Chem. class.: Analeptic agent
Legal class.: POM

Action: Respiratory stimulation through action on peripheral chemoreceptors

Uses: Acute respiratory failure, postanaesthesia respiratory stimulation

Dosage and routes:

Acute respiratory failure
- *Adult:* IV infusion 1.5 mg/min to 4.0 mg/min
- Rapid production of steady state blood levels has been achieved by: 4 mg/min for 15 mins, then 3 mg/min for 15 mins, then 2 mg/min for 30 mins, then 1.5 mg/min thereafter but should be tailored to patient response and minimum effective dose used

Following anaesthesia
- *Adult:* IV injection, 1.0–1.5 mg/kg over 30 secs or more, repeated at 1 hrly intervals if necessary; IV infusion, 2–3 mg/min according to response

Available forms include: Injection IV 20 mg/ml 5 ml ampoule; infusion 2 mg/ml, 500 ml infusion in 5% glucose

Side effects/adverse reactions:

CNS: Headache, restlessness, dizziness, confusion, paraesthesia,

flushing, sweating, rigidity (clonus/generalised), depression
GI: Nausea, vomiting, anorexia, diarrhoea, hiccups
GU: Retention, incontinence
CV: Chest pain, hypotension, change in heart rate, lowered T waves, tachycardia
INTEG: Pruritus, irritation at injection site
EENT: Pupil dilation, sneezing
RESP: Laryngospasm, bronchospasm, rebound hypoventilation, dyspnoea
Contraindications: Hypersensitivity; epilepsy, severe hypertension, severe bronchial asthma; severe dyspnoea; coronary artery disease physical, obstruction of respiratory tract; pneumothorax; pulmonary embolism; severe respiratory disease; thyrotoxicosis; children
Precautions: Bronchial asthma, hyperthyroidism, phaeochromocytoma, severe tachycardia, dysrhythmias, cerebral oedema, increased cerebrospinal fluid
Pharmacokinetics:
IV: Onset 20–40 sec, peak 1–2 hr, duration 5–10 hr; metabolised by liver, excreted by kidneys (metabolites)
Interactions/incompatibilities:
- Synergistic pressor effect: monoamine oxidase inhibitors, sympathomimetics
- Cardiac dysrhythmias: halothane, cyclopropane, enflurane
- Do not mix in alkaline solution including aminophylline, frusemide
- Increased skeletal muscle activity and agitation with aminophylline

Clinical assessment:
- Heart rate, blood gases before administration, every 30 mins
- Arterial oxygen tension, arterial carbon dioxide tension, oxygen saturation during treatment

Treatment of overdose:
Lavage, activated charcoal, monitor electrolytes, vital signs

NURSING CONSIDERATIONS

Assess:
- B/P, pulse and other vital signs

Administer:
- IV use only
- IV at prescribed infusion rate, adjust for desired respiratory response
- Using infusion pump IV
- IV injection slowly over 30 seconds or more
- Only after adequate airway is established
- With oxygen, resuscitation equipment available
- In patients with bronchoconstriction, use in conjunction with a β-adrenoreceptor bronchodilator

Perform/provide:
- Discontinue infusion if side effects occur
- Frequent arterial blood gas studies and pH measurements

Evaluate:
- Therapeutic effect
- For hypertension, dysrhythmias, tachycardia, dyspnoea, skeletal muscle hyperactivity; may indicate overdosage; discontinue if these occur
- For signs of respiratory stimulation: increased respiratory rate
- Extravasation, change IV site 48 hrly
- If unsuccessful further respiratory support should be considered, i.e. ventilation

---

doxazosin

Cardura
Func. class.: Antihypertensive
Chem. class.: α-blocker
Legal class.: POM

Action: Selective competitive antagonist at post-synaptic alpha$_1$-

receptor, causing vasodilatation
Uses: Hypertension, if necessary in conjunction with thiazide or beta-blocker
Dosage and routes:
• *Adult:* By mouth, 1 mg daily, if necessary increased after 1–2 weeks to 2 mg daily and thereafter to 4 mg daily; maximum dose 16 mg daily
Available forms include: Tablets, 1 mg, 2 mg, 4 mg (as mesylate)
Side effects/adverse reactions:
CNS: Dizziness, vertigo, headache, fatigue, asthenia
CV: Postural hypotension, oedema
Contraindications: Hypersensitivity, breast-feeding
Precautions: Pregnancy
Pharmacokinetics:
Peak plasma concentration within 2 hr; metabolised in liver and excreted in faeces as metabolites; half-life 22 hr. Maximum hypotensive effect 2–6 hr after administration. Highly protein bound
Clinical assessment:
• Introduce slowly
• Thiazides and β-blockers may be required as additional treatment
Treatment of overdose: Supine position, IV-volume expanders, vasopressors with care. Not removed by dialysis

NURSING CONSIDERATIONS

Assess:
• Baseline blood pressure (lying/standing), pulse, fluid balance, weight
Administer:
• First dose at bedtime
Perform/provide:
• Safe environment: get up slowly, help with mobilisation
Evaluate:
• Side effects: postural hypotension particularly at start of therapy
• Therapeutic response: reduction in BP to required level
Teach patient/family:
• Take first dose in bed
• Get up slowly to avoid postural hypotension
• Not to drive or operate machinery after first dose

doxepin HCl

Sinequan
Func. class.: Antidepressant, tricyclic
Chem. class.: Dibenzoxepin, tertiary amine
Legal class.: POM

Action: Blocks reuptake of noradrenaline, serotonin into nerve endings, increasing action of noradrenaline serotonin in nerve cells
Uses: Endogenous depression, especially where sedation is required
Dosage and routes:
• *Adult:* By mouth, initially 75 mg (elderly 10–50 mg) daily in 3 divided doses, increased gradually to maximum 300 mg daily in divided doses; up to 100 mg may be given as a single dose at bedtime
Available forms include: Capsules 10, 25, 50, 75 mg
Side effects/adverse reactions:
HAEM: Agranulocytosis, thrombocytopenia, eosinophilia, leucopenia
CNS: Dizziness, drowsiness, confusion, headache, anxiety, tremors, agitation, weakness, insomnia, nightmares, increased psychiatric symptoms
GI: Diarrhoea, dry mouth, nausea, vomiting, paralytic ileus, increased appetite, cramps, epigastric distress, jaundice, hepatitis, stomatitis
GU: Retention, acute renal failure
INTEG: Rash, urticaria, sweating, pruritus, photosensitivity
CV: Orthostatic hypotension,

ECG changes, tachycardia, hypertension, palpitations
EENT: Blurred vision, tinnitus, mydriasis, ophthalmoplegia, glossitis
Contraindications: Hypersensitivity to tricyclic antidepressants, porphyria, urinary retention, narrow-angle glaucoma, prostatic hypertrophy, recent myocardial infarction, severe hepatic disease, mania
Precautions: Suicidal patients, elderly, recent myocardial infarction, epilepsy, pregnancy, lactation
Pharmacokinetics:
Period of onset: Steady state 2–8 days; metabolised by liver, excreted by kidneys, excreted in breast milk, half-life 8–24 hr
Interactions/incompatibilities:
• Decreased effects of: guanethidine, debrisoquine, clonidine, indirect acting sympathomimetics (ephedrine)
• Increased effects of: direct acting sympathomimetics (adrenaline), alcohol, barbiturates, benzodiazepines, CNS depressants, thyroxine
• Hyperpyretic crisis, convulsions, hypertensive episode: monoamine oxidase inhibitors
Clinical assessment:
• Blood studies: full blood count, WBCs and differential, cardiac enzymes if patient is receiving long-term treatment
• ECG for flattening of T wave, bundle branch block, AV block, dysrhythmias in cardiac patients
Treatment of overdose
ECG monitoring, induce emesis, gastric lavage, activated charcoal, administer anticonvulsant

NURSING CONSIDERATIONS

Assess:
• Pulse and B/P, check for postural hypotension
• Weight wkly, appetite may increase with drug

Administer:
• Orally, increase dose slowly according to clinical response; dose reduction may be possible for maintenance
• With food or milk for GI symptoms
• Dosage at bedtime if oversedation occurs during day; may take entire dose at bedtime elderly may not tolerate once/day dosing
• Frequent sips of water for dry mouth

Perform/provide:
• Assistance with walking during beginning therapy since drowsiness/dizziness occurs
• Safety measures, including cot sides, primarily in elderly
• Checking to see oral medication swallowed

Evaluate:
• Therapeutic response: improved mental state
• Side effects such as dizziness, drowsiness, dry mouth, blurred vision, skin rashes
• For extrapyramidal symptoms primarily in elderly: rigidity, dystonia, akathisia
• Mental status: mood, alertness, affect; for suicidal tendencies, an increase in psychiatric symptoms: depression, panic
• Alcohol consumption; if alcohol is consumed, withhold dose until morning

Teach patient/family:
• That therapeutic effects may take 2–3 wks
• To only take other medication if directed by clinician
• To use caution in driving or other activities requiring alertness because of drowsiness, dizziness, blurred vision
• To avoid alcohol and other CNS depressants
• Not to discontinue medication without medical supervision; gradual dosage reduction necessary

• To wear sunscreen or large hat in sunshine since photosensitivity can occur

doxorubicin HCl

Doxorubicin Rapid Dissolution, Doxorubicin Solution for Injection
Func. class.: Antineoplastic
Chem. class.: Antibiotic, cytotoxic
Legal class.: POM

Action: Inhibits DNA synthesis, primarily; derived from *Streptomyces peucetius;* replication is decreased by binding to DNA, which causes strand splitting; active throughout entire cell cycle

Uses: Antimitotic and cytotoxic. Produces regression in acute leukaemia, lymphomas, soft-tissue and oestrogenic sarcomas, paediatric malignancies and adult solid tumours, in particular breast and lung carcinomas. Frequently used in combination therapy

Dosage and routes: Doses are highly variable, and dependent on local treatment protocols, concomitant therapy and tumour type; the following dose schedules have been used

• *Adult:* IV injection 60–75 mg/m^2 every 3 weeks as a single dose when used alone. Reduce to 30–40 mg/m^2 every 3 weeks if used in combination therapy. Calculated on basis of body weight: 1.2–2.4 mg/kg as a single dose every 3 weeks. Weekly administration 20 mg/m^2 leads to reduced cardiotoxicity. Reduce dose in elderly and impaired hepatic function

• Intra-arterial or intravesical administration is used for certain disorders. Seek specialist advice

Available forms include: Injection 10, 50 mg; powder for preparing IV solution 10, 50 mg

Side effects/adverse reactions:

HAEM: Thrombocytopenia, leucopenia, myelosuppression, anemia
GI: Nausea, vomiting, anorexia, mucositis, hepatotoxicity
GU: Impotence, sterility, amenorrhoea, gynaecomastia, hyperuricaemia
INTEG: Rash, necrosis at injection site, dermatitis, reversible alopecia, cellulitis, thrombophlebitis at injection site
CV: Cardiomyopathy, CCF
CNS: Fever, chills

Contraindications: Hypersensitivity, pregnancy, breast-feeding, systemic infections sensitivity to hydroxybenzoates

Precautions: Renal, hepatic, cardiac disease, gout, bone marrow depression (severe). Accumulative dose of 450–500 mg/m^2 should only be exceeded with extreme caution due to cardiac toxicity

Pharmacokinetics: Triphasic pattern of elimination; half-life 12 min, 3⅓ hr, 29⅔ hr, metabolised by liver, appears in breast milk, excreted in urine, bile

Interactions/incompatibilities:

• Increased toxicity: other antineoplastics or radiation
• Do not mix with other drugs in solution or syringe

Clinical assessment:

• Full blood count, differential, platelet count weekly
• Blood, urine uric acid levels
• Renal function studies: blood urea nitrogen serum uric acid, urine creatinine clearance electrolytes before, during therapy
• Liver function tests before, during therapy: bilirubin, aspartate aminotransferase, alanine aminotransferase, alkaline phosphatase as needed or monthly
• ECG; for ST-T wave changes, low QRS and T, possible dysrhythmias (sinus tachycardia, heart block)

Treatment of overdose: Supportive

measures, blood transfusions, barrier nursing. Look for signs of cardiac failure

NURSING CONSIDERATIONS

Assess:

• Baseline signs, weight, fluid balance

Administer:

• HANDLING: take safety precautions appropriate to antineoplastic agents
• Following local antineoplastic (cytotoxic) policy
• After ensuring that clinician is aware of blood results
• Other medication by mouth if possible, avoiding IV, IM or SC routes to prevent infection and bruising
• Anti-emetic 30–60 min before treatment
• By slow IV injection, preferably into tubing of a fast-running IV infusion, taking cae to avoid extravasation
• Allopurinol or sodium bicarbonate to maintain uric acid levels, alkalinisation of urine
• All other medication as prescribed including antibiotics, antiemetics, antispasmodics and analgesics

Perform/provide:

• Strict medical asepsis and protective isolation if WBC levels are low
• Diet as tolerated
• Increased fluid intake to 2–3 L/day to prevent urate, calculi formation
• Diet low in purines: omit offal (kidney, liver), dried beans, peas to maintain alkaline urine
• Mouth care
• Warm compresses at injection site for inflammation; check for extravasation

Perform/provide:

• Storage at room temperature for 24 hr after reconstituting infusion or 48 hr refrigerated

Evaluate:

• Bleeding: haematuria, bruising or petechiae, mucosa or orifices 8 hrly
• Food preferences; list likes, dislikes
• Effects of alopecia on body image; discuss feelings about body changes
• Oedema in feet, joint, abdominal pain, shaking
• Inflammation of mucosa, breaks in skin
• Yellowing of skin, sclera, dark urine, clay-coloured stools, itchy skin, abdominal pain, fever, diarrhoea
• Buccal cavity 8 hrly for dryness, sores, ulceration, white patches, oral pain, bleeding, dysphagia
• Local irritation, pain, burning at injection site
• GI symptoms: frequency of stools, cramping
• Acidosis, signs of dehydration: rapid respirations, poor skin turgor, decreased urine output, dry skin, restlessness, weakness
• Cardiac status: B/P, pulse, character, rhythm, rate

Teach patient/family:

• Why protective isolation precautions are necessary
• To report any complaints, side effects to nurse or clinician
• That hair may be lost during treatment and wig or hairpiece may make the patient feel better (available free on NHS); tell patient that new hair may be different in colour, texture
• To avoid foods with citric acid, hot or rough texture
• To report any bleeding, white spots, ulcerations in mouth to physician; tell patient to examine mouth daily
• That urine may be red-orange for 48 hr

doxycycline hydrochloride

Vibramycin, Nordox, Vibramycin-D
Func. class.: Antibiotic broad spectrum
Chem. class.: Tetracycline
Legal class.: POM

Action: Inhibits protein synthesis, prosphorylation in microorganisms by binding to 30S ribosomal subunits, reversibly binding to 50S ribosomal subunits

Uses: Effective against a wide range of Gram-positive and Gram-negative bacteria. Chlamydia trachomatis, gonorrhoea, lymphogranuloma venereum, mycoplasma, brucellosis (with rifampicin), exacerbations of chronic bronchitis, severe acne vulgaris, prostatitis and sinusitis, traveller's diarrhoea, leptospirosis

Dosage and routes:
- *Adult:* By mouth 200 mg on first day, then 100 mg daily; severe infections 200 mg daily

Acne
- 50 mg daily for 6–12 weeks

STD
- 100 mg twice daily for 7 days

Acute epididymoorchitis
- 100 mg twice daily for 10 days

Primary/secondary syphilis
- 300 mg daily in divided doses for at least 10 days

Available forms include: Tablets dispersible 100 mg; capsules 50, 100 mg

Side effects/adverse reactions:
CNS: Fever, headache, paraesthesia
HAEM: Eosinophilia, neutropenia, thrombocytopenia, leucocytosis, haemolytic anaemia
EENT: Dysphagia, glossitis, decreased calcification of deciduous teeth, abdominal pain, oral candidiasis
GI: Nausea, vomiting, diarrhoea, anorexia, enterocolitis, hepatotoxicity, flatulence, abdominal cramps, gastric burning, stomatitis, pseudomembranous colitis
CV: Pericarditis
GU: Increased blood urea nitrogen, polyuria, polydipsia, renal failure, nephrotoxicity
INTEG: Rash, urticaria, photosensitivity, increased pigmentation, exfoliative dermatitis, pruritus, angioedema

Contraindications: Hypersensitivity to tetracyclines, children less than 12 yr, pregnancy, lactation, porphyria

Precautions: Hepatic disease, lactation

Pharmacokinetics:
Period of onset: Peak 1½–4 hr, half-life 15–22 hr; excreted in bile, 25%–93% protein bound

Interactions/incompatibilities:
- Decreased effects of this drug: antacids, sodium bicarbonate, dairy products, alkali products
- Increased effect: anticoagulants (chronic treatment)
- Decreased effects: penicillins
- Nephrotoxicity: methoxyflurane

Clinical assessment:
- Blood studies: full blood count, Pathrombin time, blood urea nitrogen, aspartate aminotransferase, alanine aminotransferase, creatinine

Treatment of overdose: Supportive measure, gastric lavage

NURSING CONSIDERATIONS

Assess:
- Baseline fluid balance

Administer:
- By mouth to be taken with food and washed down with plenty of water; should be taken while sitting or standing (i.e. not recumbent), and well before retiring for the night; not to be taken with iron preparations or antacids.
- With food and plenty of fluids

• After culture and sensitivity obtained
• Not at the same time as antacids, calcium, iron; all decrease absorption

Perform/provide:
• Storage in tight, light-resistant container at room temperature

Evaluate:
• Therapeutic response: decreased temperature, absence of lesions, negative culture and sensitivity
• Allergic reactions: rash, itching, pruritus, angioneurotic oedema
• Nausea, vomiting, diarrhoea; administer antiemetic, antacids as ordered
• Overgrowth of infection: increased temperature, malaise, redness, pain, swelling, drainage, perineal itching, diarrhoea, changes in cough or sputum

Teach patient/family:
• Avoid sun exposure since burns may occur; sunscreen does not seem to decrease photosensitivity
• Of diabetic to avoid use of Clinistix, Diastix, for urine glucose testing
• That all prescribed medication must be taken to prevent superimposed infection
• When to take milk products in relation to dose

droperidol

Droleptan

Func. class.: Antipsychotic neuroleptic; anti-emetic
Chem. class.: Butyrophenone derivative
Legal class.: POM

Action: Acts on CNS at subcortical levels, produces tranquilisation, sleep

Uses: Premedication for surgery, neuroleptanalgesia, anti-emetic, emergency sedation or rapid calming the manic, agitated patient

Dosage and routes:
Neuroleptanalgesia
• *Adult:* IV 5–15 mg with narcotic analgesic at induction
• *Child:* IV 0.2–0.3 mg/kg

Premedication in anaesthesia
• *Adult:* IM up to 10 mg 60 min before procedure
• *Child:* IM 0.2–0.5 mg/kg

Anti-emetic
• *Adult:* IV, IM 5 mg post-operative
• *Child:* IV, IM 0.02–0.075 mg/kg post-operative

In cancer chemotherapy for anti-emesis
• *Adults:* IM/IV 1–10 mg loading dose 30 min before therapy then IV infusion 1–3 mg/hr or IV/IM 1–5 mg every 1–6 hr as required
• *Child:* IV/IM 20–75 mcg/kg according to requirements

Emergency sedation
• *Adult:* By mouth 5–20 mg every 4–8 hr; IV 5–15 mg every 4–6 hr; IM up to 10 mg every 4–6 hr
• *Child:* By mouth, IM 0.5–1 mg daily adjusted according to response

Available forms include: Injection IM, IV 5 mg/ml, 2 ml ampoules; Tablets 10 mg, Oral liquid 1 mg/ml

Side effects/adverse reactions:
RESP: Laryngospasm, bronchospasm
CNS: Dystonia, akathisia, flexion of arms, fine tremors, dizziness, anxiety, drowsiness, restlessness, hallucination, depression
GI: Nausea, loss of appetite, dyspepsia
ENDO: Galactorrhoea, gynaecomastia, and oligo-or amenorrhoea
CV: Tachycardia, hypotension
EENT: Upward rotation of eyes, oculogyric crisis
SYST: Chills, facial sweating, shivering

Contraindications: Hypersensitivity, pregnancy, coma caused by CNS depressants, bone-marrow depression, basal ganglia disease
Precautions: Elderly, cardiovascular disease (hypotension, bradydysrhythmias), epilepsy, renal disease, liver disease, Parkinson's disease, lactation
Pharmacokinetics:
IM/IV: Onset 3–10 min, peak ½ hr, duration 3–6 hr; metabolised in liver, excreted in urine as metabolites
Interactions/incompatibilities:
• Increased CNS depression: alcohol, narcotics, barbiturates, anti-psychotics, methyldopa or other CNS depressants
• Decreased effects of: amphetamines, anticonvulsants, anticoagulants, levadopa, when given with this drug
• Increased intraocular pressure: anticholinergics, antiparkinson drugs
• Increased side effects of: lithium
Clinical Assessment:
• Fluid balance and blood pressure when used in anaesthesia
• Liver and renal function
Treatment of overdose: Supportive measures combined with sedative or anti-Parkinsonian drugs, as required
NURSING CONSIDERATIONS
Assess:
• Baseline vital signs including temperature
Administer:
• Only with resuscitation equipment nearby
• IV slowly only
Perform/provide:
• Slow movement of patient to avoid orthostatic hypotension
Evaluate:
• Changes in vital signs every 10 min during IV administration, every 30 min after IM dose
• Therapeutic response: decreased anxiety, absence of vomiting during surgery
• Extrapyramidal reactions: tremor dystonia, akathisia
• For increasing heart rate or decreasing B/P, notify clinician at once; do not place patient in Trendelenburg position or sympathetic blockade may occur causing respiratory arrest
Teach patient/family:
• Drug must not be discontinued suddenly (may cause acute withdrawal syndrome or rapid relapse)

dydrogesterone

Duphaston
Func. class.: Progestogen, orally active
Chem. class.: Progesterone analogue
Legal class.: POM

Action: Produces secretory endometrium in oestrogen-primed uterus but lacks androgenic or oestrogenic activity and does not inhibit ovulation
Uses: All cases of endogenous progesterone deficiency: Endometriosis, infertility, irregular menstruation, amenorrhoea, dysmenorrhoea, premenstrual syndrome, dysfunctional uterine bleeding, habitual abortion, HRT, threatened abortion
Dosage and routes:
Endometriosis
• *Adult:* By mouth 10 mg 2–3 times daily from 5th–25th day of cycle or continuously
Infertility, irregular cycles
• 10 mg twice daily from days 11–25 of cycle until conception, for at least 6 cycles
Amenorrhoea
• 10 mg twice daily from days 11–25 of cycle, with oestrogen therapy from days 1–25 of cycle

Dysmenorrhoea
• 10 mg twice daily from days 5–25 of cycle
Premenstrual syndrome
• 10 mg twice daily from days 12–26 of cycle, increased if necessary
Dysfunctional uterine bleeding
• 10 mg twice daily (with an oestrogen) for 5–7 days to arrest bleeding; 10 mg twice daily from days 11–25 of cycle (together with an oestrogen) to prevent bleeding
Habitual abortion
• 10 mg twice daily from days 11–25 of cycle until conception, then continuously until 20th week of pregnancy and then gradually reduced
Hormone replacement therapy
• With continuous oestrogen therapy, 10 mg twice daily for first 12–14 days of each calendar month; with cyclical oestrogen therapy, 10 mg twice daily for last 12–14 days of each treatment cycle
Threatened abortion
• 40 mg at once then 10 mg 8-hrly until symptoms remit; increase dose by 10 mg every 8 hr if symptoms return. Continue for 1 week after remission and gradually withdraw
Primary dysmenorrhoea
• *Child:* By mouth 10 mg twice daily at discretion of the physician
Available forms include: Tablets 10 mg
Side effects/adverse reactions:
META: Oedema, weight gain, changes in libido, breast discomfort; in treatment of habitual abortion
GU: Breakthrough bleeding may occur (increase dose)
GI: Disturbances, jaundice
Contraindications: Undiagnosed vaginal bleeding, severe congestive heart disease, porphyria
Precautions: Diabetes, liver, cardiac or renal disease, hypertension, history of thrombo-embolism, mammary carcinoma
Pharmacokinetics: 50% of dose excreted in urine within 24 hr
Clinical assessment:
• Liver function tests, aspartate aminotransferase, alanine aminotransferase, bilirubin during long term treatment
• Renal function—urea, creatinine
Lab. test interferences: No false positive in any diagnostic urine tests
Treatment of overdose: Gastric lavage, symptomatic treatment

NURSING CONSIDERATIONS

Assess:
• Blood pressure (at start of treatment), weight, fluid balance
• History of thrombo-embolic disorders
Administer:
• With food
Perform/provide:
• Counselling for sexual problems
• Breast examination
Evaluate:
• Oedema, weight gain
• Bleeding per vagina
• Rise in BP
• Side effects
Teach patient/family:
• Explain drug regimen in full and warn about side effects such as 'breakthrough' bleeding
• Report any of the following: weight gain, breast discomfort, pain in legs or chest sexual problems
• About breast examination
• Diabetics should monitor glucose more often
• Need for regular follow-up and examination

econazole nitrate

Ecostatin, Gyno-Pevaryl, Pevaryl, combination product
Func. class.: Antifungal
Chem. class.: Imidazole derivative
Legal class.: P or POM (vaginal route)

Action: Interferences with fungal DNA replication; binds sterols in fungal cell membrane, which increases permeability, leaking of cell nutrients
Uses: *Tinea pedis*, *tinea cruris*, *tinea corporis*, *tinea versicolor*, candida infection
Dosage and routes:
• *Adult and child:* Topical, apply to affected area 2 or 3 times a day depending on condition; intravaginal, 150 mg as a single dose or nightly for 3 nights
Available forms include: Cream, 1%; pessaries 150 mg; lotion, powder, spray 1%
Side effects/adverse reactions:
INTEG: Rash, urticaria, stinging, burning, pruritus
Contraindications: Hypersensitivity

NURSING CONSIDERATIONS

Administer:
• After cleansing with soap, water before each application, dry well
• Enough medication to cover lesions completely
Perform/provide:
• Storage at room temperature in dry place
Evaluate:
• Allergic reaction: burning, stinging, swelling, redness
• Therapeutic response: decrease in size, number of lesions
Teach patient/family:
• Use medical asepsis (hand washing) before, after each application
• Avoid use of non-prescribed creams, ointments, lotions unless directed by clinician

edrophonium chloride

Tensilon
Func. class.: Anticholinesterase, cholinergic
Chem. class.: Quaternary ammonium compound
Legal class.: POM

Action: Inhibits destruction of acetylcholine, which increases concentration at sites where acetylcholine is released; this facilitates transmission of impulses across myoneural junction
Uses: To diagnose myasthenia gravis, antagonist of non-depolarising muscle relaxants such as tubocurarine, differentiation of myasthenic crisis from cholinergic crisis
Dosage and routes:
Tensilon test
• *Adult:* IV 1–2 mg, then after 30 seconds a further 8 mg if no response; IM 10 mg
• *Child:* 20 mcg/kg then after 30 seconds a further 80 mcg/kg if no response
Reversal of neuromuscular blockade
• *Adult and child:* IV 0.5–0.7 mg/kg
• After or with atropine 0.6 mg over several minutes
Diagnosis of dual block
• *Adult:* IV 10 mg with atropine
Differentiation of myasthenic crisis from cholinergic crisis
• *Adult:* IV 2 mg 1 hr after last dose of anticholinergic agent
Available forms include: Injection IV 10 mg/ml
Side effects/adverse reactions:
INTEG: Rash, urticaria
CNS: Dizziness, headache, sweating, confusion, weakness, convulsions, incoordination, paralysis
GI: Nausea, diarrhoea, vomiting, cramps
CV: Tachycardia
GU: Frequency, incontinence

RESP: Respiratory depression, bronchospasm, constriction
EENT: Miosis, blurred vision, lacrimation
Contraindications: Hypersensitivity; hypotension; obstruction of intestine; renal system
Precautions: Bradycardia, seizure disorders, bronchial asthma, coronary occlusion, hyperthyroidism, dysrhythmias, peptic ulcer, megacolon, poor GI motility, Parkinsonism
Pharmacokinetics:
IV: Onset 30–60 sec, duration 6–24 min
IM: Onset 2–10 min, duration 12–45 min
Interactions/incompatibilities:
• Decreased action of this drug: procainamide, quinidine
• Bradycardia: digoxin

NURSING CONSIDERATIONS

Assess:
• Baseline vital signs, respiration
Administer:
• Only with atropine sulphate available for cholinergic crisis
• Only after all other cholinergics have been discontinued
NB: only in the presence of a person skilled in intubation
Perform/provide:
• Storage at room temperature
• Resuscitation equipment available on unit
Evaluate:
• Vital signs and respiratory rate
• Therapeutic response: increased muscle strength, hand grasp, improved gait, absence of laboured breathing (if severe)
Teach patient/family:
• Wear Medicare ID specifying myasthenia gravis, and prescribed therapy

enalapril maleate

Innovace, combination product
Func. class.: Antihypertensive
Chem. class.: Angiotensin converting enzyme inhibitor
Legal class.: POM

Action: Selectively suppresses renin-angiotensin-aldosterone system; inhibits angiotensin-converting enzyme, prevents conversion of angiotensin I to angiotensin II
Uses: Hypertension not responsive to other hypertensive medications; adjunct to diuretics/digoxin for congestive heart failure
Dosage and routes:
Diuretics should be stopped if possible for 2–3 days before starting treatment to minimise the risk of a rapid fall in blood pressure and hypotension
Hypertension
• *Adult:* By mouth, initial dose 5 mg daily; with diuretics, in elderly, renal impairment, initial dose 2.5 mg daily; maintenance 10–20 mg daily, maximum dose 40 mg daily
Congestive heart failure
• *Adult:* By mouth, initial dose 2.5 mg under hospital supervision; maintenance 10–20 mg daily
Available forms include: Tablets 2.5 mg, 5 mg, 10 mg, 20 mg
Side effects/adverse reactions:
CV: Hypotension, chest pain, tachycardia, dysrhythmias
CNS: Insomnia, dizziness, paraesthesia, headache, fatigue, anxiety
GI: Nausea, vomiting, colitis, cramps, diarrhoea, constipation flatulence, dry mouth
INTEG: Rash, purpura, alopecia
HAEM: Agranulocytosis
EENT: Tinnitus, visual changes, sore throat, double vision, dry burning eyes, angioneurotic oedema

GU: Proteinuria, renal failure, increased frequency of polyuria or oliguria
RESP: Dyspnoea, cough, rales
Contraindications: Hypersensitivity, pregnancy, breast-feeding, aortic stenosis or outflow obstruction, renovascular disease, porphyria
Precautions: Renal disease, hyperkalaemia, lactation
Pharmacokinetics:
Period of onset: Peak 4–6 hr; half-life 1½ hr; metabolised by liver to active metabolite, excreted in urine
Interactions/incompatibilities:
• Severe hypotension: diuretics, other antihypertensives
• Decreased effects when used with: aspirin
• Increased potassium levels: salt substitutes, potassium-sparing diuretics, potassium supplements
• May increase effects of: ergot derivatives, neuromuscular blocking agents, antihypertensives, hypoglycaemics, barbiturates, lithium, reserpine, levodopa
• Effects may be increased by: phenothiazines, diuretics, phenytoin, quinidine
Clinical assessment:
• Electrolytes: potassium, sodium chloride
• Baselines in renal liver function tests, before therapy begins
Lab. test interferences:
Interferences: Glucose/insulin tolerance tests
Treatment of overdose: Gastric lavage, IV atropine for bradycardia, IV theophylline for bronchospasm, digoxin, O_2, diuretic for cardiac failure, haemodialysis
NURSING CONSIDERATIONS
Assess:
• Baseline BP, apical/radial pulse
Administer:
• With patient in supine position if hypotension
• First dose under supervision, monitor BP for hypotension
Evaluate:
• BP, pulse 4 hrly, note rate, rhythm, quality
• Apical/radial pulse before administration; notify clinician of any significant changes
• Oedema in feet, legs daily
• Skin turgor, dryness of mucous membranes for hydration status
• Symptoms of congestive cardiac failure: oedema, dyspnoea
Teach patient/family:
• Not to discontinue drug abruptly
• Rise slowly to sitting or standing position to minimise postural hypotension
• Benefits of therapy in heart failure (such as reduction in fatigue) are often long-term rather than immediate

---

enflurane

Func. class.: Inhalation anaesthetic
Chem. class.: Halogenated ether
Legal class.: P

Action: Produces central nervous system depression and loss of consciousness
Uses: Induction and maintenance of general anaesthesia. Rapid onset of, and recovery from, anaesthesia make it suitable for dental and outpatient use
Dosage and routes:
Induction
• *Adult and child:* By inhalation from specially calibrated vaporiser 0.4 to maximum of 4.8% in air, oxygen or nitrous oxide–oxygen, according to response. Minimum anaesthetic concentration decreases with advancing age
Maintenance
• *Adult and child:* By inhalation from specially calibrated vaporiser 0.5–3% in nitrous oxide–oxygen.

Minimum anaesthetic concentration decreases with advancing age
Available forms include: Bottles, 250 ml
Side effects/adverse reactions:
CNS: Seizures
CV: Hypotension, cardiac arrhythmias
ELECT: Elevated serum fluoride
ENDO: Elevated blood glucose
GI: Nausea and vomiting during recovery, hepatotoxicity
HAEM: Elevated white blood cell count
MISC: Hiccups and shivering during recovery
MS: Muscle twitching and jerking
RESP: Hyperventilation, respiratory depression
Contraindications: Sensitivity to enflurane; known or suspected genetic susceptibility to malignant hyperthermia; porphyria
Precautions: Patients susceptible to cerebral stimulation by virtue of their medical or drug history; renal impairment; pregnancy; obstetric anaesthesia
Pharmacokinetics: Readily absorbed on inhalation; mostly excreted unchanged through the lungs; small amounts are excreted in the urine as inorganic fluoride
Interactions:
• Potentiation of: non-depolarising muscle relaxants
• Risk of cardiac arrhythmias with: adrenaline (including, possibly, topical preparations), isoprenaline, levodopa, tricyclic antidepressants, verapamil
• Enhanced hypotensive effect with: antihypertensives, antipsychotics, β-blockers, verapamil

NURSING CONSIDERATIONS
Assess:
• Baseline vital signs
Administer:
• With adequate concentrations of oxygen to avoid hypoxia
• With all other supporting equipment appropriate for general anaesthesia
Perform/provide:
• Regular monitoring and recording of vital signs
• Storage: with bottles tightly closed, protected from light and stored below 25°C
Evaluate:
• Effect of drug and any side effects, including those occurring during recovery
Teach patient/family:
• About the drug and the side effects, particularly those occurring during recovery

---

enoxaparin

Clexane
Func. class.: Anticoagulant
Chem. class.: Low molecular weight heparin
Legal class.: POM

Action: Prevents conversion of fibrinogen to fibrin, with a longer duration of action than normal heparin
Uses: Prevention of deep vein thrombosis, and prevention of clotting in extracorporeal circulation
Dosage and routes:
Prophylaxis of deep-vein thrombosis
Low-moderate thromboembolic risk
• *Adult:* By deep SC injection 20 mg (2000 IU) once daily. First dose should be given 2 hr preoperatively in patients undergoing surgery
High thromboembolic risk
• *Adult:* By deep SC injection 40 mg (4000 IU) once daily. First dose should be given 12 hr preoperatively in patients undergoing surgery
Prophylaxis during extracorporeal circulation during haemodialysis

• *Adult:* By injection into the arterial line of the dialysis circuit 1 mg/kg (100 IU/kg) at the beginning of dialysis; a further 500 to 1000 mcg/kg (50 to 100 IU/kg) may be given if fibrin rings are found. In patients at high risk of haemorrhage, the dose should be reduced to 500 mcg/kg for double vascular access or 750 mcg/kg for single vascular access

Available forms include: Prefilled syringes 20 mg (2000 IU), 40 mg (4000 IU)

Side effects/adverse reactions:
GI: Raised liver enzymes
HAEM: Thrombocytopenia, haemorrhage

Contraindications: Acute bacterial endocarditis; major bleeding disorders; thrombocytopenia in patients with a positive *in vitro* aggregation test in the presence of enoxaparin; active peptic ulcer; stroke (except if due to systemic emboli); increased risk of haemorrhage; hypersensitivity

Precautions: Hepatic impairment; uncontrolled arterial hypertension; history of gastrointestinal ulceration; pregnancy; breast-feeding

Pharmacokinetics: Completely absorbed after SC injection, peak plasma activity 1–4 hr after injection, elimination half-life 4–5 hr; metabolised in liver, excreted in urine

Interactions:
• Increased risk of bleeding: aspirin, dipyridamole, NSAIDs, oral anticoagulants, dextran

Incompatibilities: Enoxaparin should not be mixed with other drugs or infusion solutions

Treatment of overdose: Withdraw enoxaparin therapy; in an emergency give protamine to neutralise enoxaparin (1 anti-heparin unit of protamine per unit of enoxaparin given)

NURSING CONSIDERATIONS

Assess:
• Previous history of haemorrhage
• Baseline vital signs, particularly BP
• Full blood count

Administer:
• Must NOT be given IM
• Into the arterial line of the dialysis circuit at the start of dialysis
• SC injections into the left and right anterolateral and left and right posteriolateral abdominal wall. The entire length of the needle should be introduced vertically into a skinfold held between the forefinger and thumb throughout the injection. Syringes should not be purged of air

Perform/provide:
• Regular monitoring for signs of bleeding anywhere
• Other measures to counteract risk of deep vein thrombosis

Evaluate:
• Therapeutic effect

Teach patient/family:
• Reasons for giving drug and about side effects
• Other action to take to avoid the risk of deep vein thrombosis and unwanted clotting (movement, deep breathing)

---

enoximone

Perfan
Func. class.: Cardiac inotropic agent
Chem. class: Phosphodiesterase inhibitor
Legal class.: POM

Action: Phosphodiesterase inhibitor

Uses: Congestive heart failure where cardiac output reduced and filling pressure increased

Dosage and routes:
• *Adult:* Slow IV injection, initially 0.5–1 mg/kg, then 500 mcg/kg every 30 min until satisfactory response or total of 3 mg/kg given; maintenance, initial dose of up to 3 mg/kg may be repeated every 3–6 hr as required
• *Adult:* IV infusion: initially 90 mcg/kg/min over 10–30 min, followed by continuous or intermittent infusion of 5–20 mcg/kg/min; total dose over 24 hr should not normally exceed 24 mg/kg
Available forms include: Injection 5 mg/ml
Side effects/adverse reactions:
CV: Ectopic beats, less frequently ventricular tachycardia or supraventricular arrhythmias (more likely in patients with pre-existing arrhythmias), hypotension, chills, fever
CNS: Headache, insomnia, upper and lower limb pain
GU: Oliguria, urinary retention
GI: Nausea, vomiting, diarrhoea
Precautions: Heart failure associated with hypertrophic cardiomyopathy, stenotic or obstructive valvular disease or other outlet obstruction, renal impairment
NURSING CONSIDERATIONS
Assess:
• Baseline vital signs, ECG, CPV
Administer:
• Dilute before use with water for injection or sodium chloride 0.9%.
• Use immediately post dilution
• Do not use if diluted solution is not a clear yellow colour
• Avoid extravasation
• Plastic containers and syringes should be used as crystal formation occurs when glass is used
Evaluate:
• For side effects
• BP, heart rate, ECG, central venous pressure, fluid and electrolyte status, platelet count, hepatic enzymes
Perform/provide:
• Continuous monitoring (preferably in coronary care unit or intensive care unit

ephedrine hydrochloride

Func. class.: Adrenergic, indirect and direct acting
Chem. class.: Sympathomimetic amine
Legal class.: P

Action: Direct bronchodilatation, relaxes bladder detrusor muscle and increases bladder sphincter tone
Uses: Nocturnal enuresis, bronchodilation
Dosage and routes:
Nocturnal enuresis
• *Child 7–8 yr:* By mouth 30 mg at night
• *9–12 yr:* 45 mg at night
• *13–15 yr:* 60 mg at night
Bronchodilator
• *Adult:* By mouth 15–60 mg 3 times a day
• *Child up to 1 yr*: By mouth 7.5 mg 3 times a day
• *1–5 yr:* 5 mg 3 times a day
• *6–12 yr:* 30 mg 3 times a day
Available forms include: Tablets 15, 30, 60 mg; syrup 4 mg/5 ml, 15 mg/5 ml
Side effects/adverse reactions:
CNS: Tremors, anxiety, insomnia, headache, dizziness, confusion, hallucinations, convulsions, CNS depression
EENT: Dry nose, irritation of nose and throat
CV: Palpitations, tachycardia, hypertension, chest pain, dysrhythmias
GI: Anorexia, nausea, vomiting
RESP: Depression
Contraindications: Hypersensitivity to sympathomimetics,

narrow-angle glaucoma, elderly
Precautions: Pregnancy, cardiac disorders, hyperthyroidism, diabetes mellitus, prostatic hypertrophy
Pharmacokinetics:
By mouth: Onset 15–60 min, duration 2–4 hr
Metabolised in liver, excreted in urine (unchanged), excreted in breast milk
Interactions/incompatibilities:
• Hypertensive crisis: MAOIs or tricyclic anti-depressants
• Decreased effect of this drug: methyldopa, urinary acidifiers, rauwolfia alkaloids
• Increased effect of this drug: urinary alkalinisers
Treatment of overdose: Administer an α-blocker, then noradrenaline for severe hypotension

NURSING CONSIDERATIONS

Assess:
• Fluid balance
• Frequency of nocturnal enuresis
Perform/provide:
• Do not use discoloured solutions
Evaluate:
• For paraesthesias and coldness of extremities, peripheral blood flow may decrease
• Therapeutic response: increased BP with stabilisation
• For hypovolaemia; plasma expanders may be ordered
Teach patient/family:
• Reason for drug administration
• Avoid drinks at bedtime if nocturnal enuresis

ephedrine hydrochloride (nasal)

Func. class.: Nasal decongestant
Chem. class.: Sympathomimetic amine
Legal class.: P

Action: Vasoconstriction of mucosal blood vessels reduces thickness of nasal mucosa
Uses: Nasal congestion associated with colds, hayfever, sinusitis, other allergic conditions, adjunct in middle ear infections
Dosage and routes:
• *Adult and child:* Instil 1–2 drops when required
Available forms include: Solution 0.5%, 1%
Side effects/adverse reactions:
EENT: Irritation, burning, sneezing, stinging, dryness, rebound congestion
INTEG: Contact dermatitis
CNS: Anxiety, restlessness, tremors, weakness, insomnia, dizziness, fever, headache
Contraindications: Hypersensitivity to sympathomimetic amines
Precautions: Child under 3 months, cardiovascular disease
Interactions/incompatibilities:
Minimal systemic absorption, interactions rare
• Hypertension: MAOIs, β-adrenergic blockers
• Hypotension: methyldopa, reserpine

NURSING CONSIDERATIONS

Administer:
• No more than 4 hrly and 4 consecutive days maximum
Perform/provide:
• Environmental humidification to decrease nasal congestion, dryness
Evaluate:
• Redness, swelling, pain in nasal passages
Teach patient/family:
• Stinging may occur for a few applications; drying of mucosa may be decreased by environmental humidification
• Notify clinician if irregular pulse, insomnia, dizziness, or tremors occur
• Proper administration to avoid systemic absorption

ergometrine maleate

Syntometrine (combination product)
Func. class.: Oxytocic
Chem. class.: Ergot alkaloid
Legal class.: POM

Action: Stimulates uterine contractions, decreases bleeding
Uses: Treatment of haemorrhage associated with postpartum or postabortion
Dosage and routes:
• *Adult:* IM 200–500 mcg; IV 100–500 mcg; by mouth 500 mcg–1 mg
Available forms include: Injection 500 mcg/ml; tablets 250 mcg, 500 mcg
Side effects/adverse reactions:
CNS: Headache, dizziness, fainting
CV: Hypertension, chest pain, vasoconstriction
GI: Nausea, vomiting
INTEG: Sweating
RESP: Dyspnoea
EENT: Tinnitus
GU: Cramping
Contraindications: Hypersensitivity to ergot derivatives, 1st and 2nd stages of labour, before delivery of placenta, spontaneous abortion (threatened), pelvic inflammatory disease (PID), renal, hepatic impairment
Precautions: Cardiac disease, asthma, anaemia, convulsive disorders, hypertension, glaucoma, toxaemia
Pharmacokinetics:
Metabolised in liver, excreted in urine
NURSING CONSIDERATIONS
Assess:
• Baseline BP and pulse
Administer:
• IM in deep muscle mass; rotate injection sites if additional doses are given
Evaluate:
• For side effects
• BP and pulse
• For length, duration of contraction
• Amount of blood loss per vaginum
Teach patient/family:
• To report increased blood loss, abdominal cramps, increased temperature or foul-smelling lochia when used at home

ergotamine tartrate

Lingraine, Medihaler-Ergotamine, combination products
Func. class.: Antimigraine agent
Chem. class.: Ergot alkaloid
Legal class.: POM

Action: Constricts smooth muscle in periphery, cranial blood vessels
Uses: Vascular headache attack, migraine
Dosage and routes:
• *Adult:* Sublingual 2 mg at onset of headache; repeat after 30 min if required; maximum 6 mg in 24 hr or 12 mg weekly
• *Adult:* Inhalation 1 puff (360 mcg) at onset of headache; repeat after 5 min if required; maximum 6 puffs in 24 hr or 15 puffs weekly
Available forms include: Tablets, sublingual, 2 mg; aerosol 360 mcg/inhalation
Side effects/adverse reactions:
CNS: Numbness in fingers, toes, headache
CV: Transient tachycardia, chest pain, bradycardia
GI: Increase or decrease in BP, nausea, vomiting
MS: Muscle pain
Contraindications: Hypersensitivity to ergot preparations, peripheral vascular disease, coronary

artery disease, pregnancy, breast-feeding, septic conditions, hypertension, renal, hepatic, cardiovascular disease, prophylatic treatment

Pharmacokinetics:

Period of onset: Peak 30 min–3 hr; metabolised in liver, excreted as metabolites in faeces, crosses blood-brain barrier, excreted in breast milk

Interactions/incompatibilities:

- Effects of ergotamine may be potentiated by: erythromycin
- Increase vasoconstriction may occur with: concurrent use of β-blockers

NURSING CONSIDERATIONS

Assess:

- Baseline weight
- Cardiac rate and rhythm

Administer:

- At beginning of headache, dose must be titrated to patient response
- Sublingual tablets under the tongue
- Aerosol inhalation using correct method
- At the recommended dose; maximum dose must not be exceeded
- Only to women who are not pregnant; harm to foetus may occur

Perform/provide:

- Quiet, calm environment with decreased stimulation for noise, or bright light or excessive talking

Evaluate:

- Weight daily
- Peripheral oedema in feet, legs
- Therapeutic response: decrease in frequency, severity of headache
- For stress level, activity, recreation, coping mechanisms of patient
- Neurological status: level of consciousness blurring vision, nausea, vomiting, tingling in extremities that can precede the headache
- Ingestion of tyramine foods (pickled products, beer, wine, some cheese), food additives, preservatives, colourings, artificial sweeteners, chocolate, caffeine, which may precipitate these types of headaches

Teach patient/family:

- Not to use non-prescribed medications, serious drug interactions may occur
- Maintain dose at approved level, not to increase even if drug does not relieve headache
- Report side effects including increased vasoconstriction starting with cold extremities, then paraesthesia, weakness
- That an increase in headaches may occur when this drug is discontinued after long-term use

---

erythromycin (topical)

Stiemycin, Zineryt (combination product)

Func. class.: Antibacterial

Chem. class.: Macrolide antibiotic

Legal class.: POM

Action: Interferes with bacterial DNA replication to disrupt bacterial cell wall formation bacteriostatic

Uses: Acne vulgaris

Dosage and routes:

- *Adult and child:* Topical, apply to affected area twice daily

Available forms include: Topical solution 2%

Side effects/adverse reactions:

INTEG: Rash, urticaria, stinging, burning, pruritus, dry or oily skin

Contraindications: Hypersensitivity

Precautions: Pregnancy, lactation

NURSING CONSIDERATIONS

Administer:

- Apply after washing

• Enough medication to cover lesions completely
• After cleansing with soap, water before each application, dry well

Evaluate:
• Allergic reaction: burning, stinging, swelling, redness
• Therapeutic response: decrease in size, number of lesions

Teach patient/family:
• To apply wearing gloves to prevent further infection
• Avoid use of non-prescribed creams, ointments, lotions unless directed by clinician
• To wash hands before and after each application

---

erythromycin base, erythromycin ethylsuccinate, erythromycin lactobionate, erythromycin stearate, erythromycin estolate

Erythrocin, Erythroped, Erymax, Ilosone

Func. class.: Antibiotic
Chem. class.: Macrolide
Legal class.: POM

Action: Broad spectrum bacteriostatic; interacts with phospholipids, penetrates cell wall; changes occur immediately in membrane

Uses: Wide range of infections due to Gram-positive and Gram-negative organisms in penicillin-sensitive patients or when due to *M. pneumoniae*, *B. pertussis*, *L. monocytogenes*, syphilis, Legionnaire's disease, *C. trachomatis Branhamella catarrhalis*

Dosage and routes:
• *Adult and child over 8 yr:* By mouth 250–500 mg 6 hrly, up to 4 g daily in severe infection; IV 25 mg/kg daily in 4 divided doses. Increase to 50 mg/kg daily in severe infection.
• *Child 2–8 yr:* By mouth 250 mg 6 hrly
• *Up to 2 yr:* 125 mg 6 hrly

Available forms include: Base: tablets enteric-coated 250, 500 mg; tablets film-coated 250, 500 mg; capsules enteric-coated 250 mg; estolate: tablets 500 mg, capsules 250 mg; suspension 125, 250 mg/5 ml; stearate: tablets, film-coated 250, 500 mg; ethylsuccinate: tablets, film-coated, 500 mg suspension 125, 250, 500 mg/5 ml, sachets 125, 250, 500 mg
Lactobionate: injection 1 g

Side effects/adverse reactions:
INTEG: Rash, urticaria, pruritus
GI: Nausea, vomiting, diarrhoea, hepatotoxicity, abdominal pain, stomatitis, heartburn, anorexia, pruritus ani
GU: Vaginitis, moniliasis
EENT: Hearing loss, tinnitus

Contraindications: Hypersensitivity, porphyria, estolate contraindicated in hepatic disease

Precautions: Pregnancy, hepatic disease

Pharmacokinetics: Peak 4 hr, duration 6 hr, half-life 1–3 hr, metabolised in liver, excreted in bile, faeces

Interactions/incompatibilities:
• Increased action of: oral anticoagulants, digoxin, theophylline, carbamazepine methylprednisolone, cyclosporin
• Decreased action of: clindamycin, penicillins

Clinical assessment:
• Liver studies: aspartate aminotransferase, alanine aminotransferase

Treatment of overdose: Withdraw drug, general supportive measures

NURSING CONSIDERATIONS

Assess:

- Bowel pattern
- Fluid balance
- Allergies before treatment; record allergies on drug chart, nursing documentation; notify all people giving drugs
- Culture and sensitivity before drug therapy is commenced; both may be repeated after treatment

Administer:

- Enteric-coated tablets may be given with food
- If IV, preferably by continuous infusion as a solution containing 1 mg/ml; alternatively as a solution containing up to 5 mg/ml by infusion over 20–60 min. Solution is reconstituted to 50 mg/ml with water for injections and then further diluted before administration.

Perform/provide:

- Adequate intake of fluids (2 litres) during diarrhoea episodes

Evaluate:

- Fluid balance report haematuria, oliguria in renal disease
- Urinalysis, protein, blood
- Bowel pattern, during treatment
- Skin eruptions, itching
- Respiratory status: rate, character, wheezing, tightness in chest; discontinue drug if these occur

Teach patient/family:

- Take oral drug with full glass of water; with food if GI symptoms occur
- Do not take with fruit juice
- Report sore throat, fever, fatigue; could indicate superimposed infection
- Notify nurse of diarrhoea
- Take at evenly spaced intervals; complete dosage regimen

erythropoietin

eprex (epoietin-α)
recormon (epoietin-β)
Func. class.: Hormone
Chem. class.: Human recombinant erythropoietin-glycoprotein
Legal class.: POM

Action: Stimulation of erythropoiesis by imitating the actions of endogenous erythropoietin on the mesenchymal stem cells in the bone marrow

Uses: Treatment of anaemia associated with chronic renal failure of dialysis and also for the treatment of severe anaemia of renal origin accompanied by clinical symptoms in patients with renal insufficiency not yet undergoing dialysis

Dosage and routes:

- Initially 20–50 U/kg by subcutaneous injection three times a week for four weeks
- IV injection 40 U/kg for four weeks. The dose of epoietin should be increased if necessary by 25 U/kg every four weeks when administered subcutaneously to achieve a Hb rise at a rate not greater than 2 g/dl per month
- Maintenance—reduce dose by half and adjust to once weekly therapy and adjusting subsequent doses according to response and the desired Hb concentration
- *Child over 2 yr of age:* Administer according to adult regimen
- *Newborn:* Doses of 20–50 U/kg subcutaneously 3 times weekly for anaemia of end-stage renal disease

Available forms include: Epoietin alfa solution in vials 1000 iu/0.5 ml, 2000 iu/ml, 4000 iu/ml, 10,000 iu/ml
Epoietin beta lyophilisate + water for injection for reconstituting freeze-dried erythropoietin,

1000 iu ampoules, 2000 iu ampoules, 5000 iu vial

Side effects/adverse reactions:

CV: Dose-dependent increase in blood pressure or aggravation of existing hypertension

CNS: Hypertensive crises with encephalopathy-like symptoms, e.g. headaches, confused state and generalised tonic clonic seizures. Sudden, stabbing, migraine-like headaches

SYST: 'Flu-like' symptoms such as headaches, joint pains and feelings of weakness, dizziness and tiredness may occur, usually at the start of treatment

ELEC: Serum potassium levels should be monitored in pre-dialysis patients. If a rising potassium is noted and causality is not established, consideration of cessation of epoietin therapy should be considered until the hyperkalaemia has been corrected

HAEM: Moderate dose dependent rise in the platelet count (regresses during the course of continued therapy)

Contraindications: Uncontrolled hypertension

Precautions: Sickle-cell anaemia, myelodysplastic syndromes or hypercoagulable states. Untreated, inadequately treated or uncontrolled hypertension in patients with ischaemic vascular disease, presence of malignancy, epilepsy, thrombocytosis, chronic hepatic failure; pregnancy; breast-feeding. Clotting in arteriovenous fistulae particularly in hypotensive patients or patients in whom packed cell volume rises too rapidly

Pharmacokinetics: In response to 3 times weekly administration, reticulocyte count increases within 10 days, followed by increases in red blood cell count, packed cell volume and Hb within two to six weeks

Volume of distribution is 0.033–0.055 l/kg. Clearance is about 0.00282 l/h/kg in adults. Half-life (initial dosing) 9.3 ± 3.3 h, multiple dosing 6.2 ± 1.8 hr

Interactions:

• No evidence currently exists indicating that treatment with epoietin alters the pharmacokinetics of other drugs. However, since cyclosporin is bound extensively in erythrocytes, cyclosporin levels should be monitored closely in patients receiving concomitant therapy with epoietin and cyclosporin

Incompatibilities:

• Do not administer as intravenous infusion or in conjunction with other drug solutions

NURSING CONSIDERATIONS

Assess:

• Baseline vital signs (temperature, pulse, respiration, BP)

• Complete blood pattern, including iron status

• Urine tests

• Condition of fistula (in dialysed patients)

Administer:

• SC injection

• IV bolus injection, not as infusion

• Alone, not in conjunction with other drug solutions

• Iron supplements

Perform/provide:

• Storage: refrigerated at 2–8°C

Evaluate:

• Blood patterns

• Therapeutic effect; rise in haemoglobin (10 days to 6 weeks)

• BP regularly, particularly at start of therapy

• Side effects, including hypotension, headaches, confusion, migraine-like pains, seizures

• Condition of arteriovenous fistulae for clotting

Teach patient/family:

• About the drug and reasons for administration

• Side effects; particularly those affecting CV and CNS systems

• To report any side effects promptly to nurse or clinician

• That iron supplement must also be taken as prescribed

---

esmolol ▼

Brevibloc

Func. class.: Anti-arrhythmic (Class II), antihypertensive

Chem. class.: Short-acting, cardio-selective β-blocker

Legal class.: POM

Action: Preferentially blocks β-adrenoceptors in the heart, reducing response to sympathetic stimulation, restores normal cardiac rhythm

Uses: Treatment of supraventricular tachyarrhythmias including atrial fibrillation, atrial flutter and sinus tachycardia; control of peri-operative tachycardia and hypertension

Dosage and routes:

• *Adult:* By IV infusion usually within the range 50–200 mcg/kg/min (consult manufacturer's data sheet for details of dose titration)

Available forms include: Injection 10, 250 mg/ml

Side effects/adverse reactions:

CNS: Confusion, somnolence, dizziness, fatigue, agitation, headache, anxiety, anorexia, speech disorder

CV: Hypotension, peripheral ischaemia, thrombophlebitis, bradycardia

EENT: Abnormal vision

GI: Nausea, constipation

GU: Urinary retention

INTEG: Inflammation, induration, burning, skin discoloration at infusion site, local skin necrosis following extravasation

RESP: Bronchospasm, wheezing, dyspnoea

SYST: Sweating, rigor, fever

Contraindications: Sinus bradycardia; heart block greater than first degree; cardiogenic shock; overt heart failure; pregnancy; breast feeding

Precautions: Reversible obstructive airways disease; renal impairment; infusion of longer than 24 hr duration; diabetes mellitus; low systolic blood pressure

Pharmacokinetics: Steady state blood-levels reached within 30 min at infusion rate of 50–300 mcg/kg body weight/min; elimination half-life 9 min, metabolised by esterases in red blood cells; de-esterified metabolite excreted in the urine

Interactions:

• Increased hypotension with: inhalational anaesthetics, other antihypertensives, diuretics

• Reduced hypotensive effect with: Corticosteroids

• Bradycardia and AV block with: amiodarone, diltiazem, cardiac glycosides

• Hypotension and heart failure with: nifedipine, verapamil

• Severe hypertension with: adrenaline, noradrenaline, other sympathomimetics

• Enhanced effects of: digoxin, oral hypoglycaemics, morphine, succinyl choline

• Antagonism of: Xamoterol

Incompatibilities: Sodium bicarbonate iv solution

NURSING CONSIDERATIONS

Assess:

• Baseline vital signs and fluid balance

• Patient's normal baseline cardiac pattern

Administer:

• IV 250 mg/ml solution must be diluted to 10 mg/ml before infusion. 10 mg/ml solution may be administered undiluted

Perform/provide:

• Cardiac monitoring during and after administration

• Local treatment to infusion site if extravasation occurs

Evaluate:

• Therapeutic effect of drug (reversion to cardiac pattern normal for the patient)

• Side effects

Teach patient/family:

• Reasons for giving the drug

• About side effects

---

estramustine phosphate

Estracyt

Func. class.: Antineoplastic

Chem. class.: Alkylating agent, oestrogen

Legal class.: POM

Action: Complex delivers mustine (alkylating agent) to oestrogen receptors

Uses: Prostate cancer

Dosage and routes:

Doses are highly variable, and dependent on local treatment protocols, concomitant therapy, and tumour type; the following dose schedules have been used

• *Adult:* By mouth 0.14–1.4 g daily

Available forms include: Capsules 140 mg (as disodium salt)

Side effects/adverse reactions:

HAEM: Thrombocytopenia, leucopenia

GI: Nausea, vomiting, diarrhoea, hepatotoxicity

GU: Impotence, gynaecomastia, fluid retention

INTEG: Rash

CV: Myocardial infarction, hypertension, angina

Contraindications: Peptic ulcer, severe hepatic or cardiac disease

Precautions: Oedema, thromboembolic disorders, cardiac disorders, epilepsy, hypertension, diabetes mellitus

Pharmacokinetics:

Period of onset: Peak 1–2 hr, metabolised in liver, excreted in bile, half-life 20 hr (terminal)

Interactions/incompatibilities:

Should not be taken with milk, dairy products

Clinical assessment:

• Periodic blood count

• Liver function tests

• ECG before, during treatment

Treatment of overdose:

Blood products if necessary indicated by low blood count

NURSING CONSIDERATIONS

Assess:

• Fluid balance

• Weight before initial treatment then at regular intervals

• ECG and blood count

Administer:

• HANDLING: take safety precautions appropriate to antineoplastic agents

• Following local antineoplastic (cytotoxic) policies

• After ensuring that clinician is aware of blood results

• By mouth with food, but excluding milk and dairy products

• Anti-emetic 30–60 mins before treatment

• All other medication as prescribed including analgesics, antiemetics, antibiotics and diuretics

Perform/provide:

• Diet suitable to enhance each patient's good health

Evaluate:

• Therapeutic response; destruction of malignant cells, decreased malignant grown

• Input and output of fluids check for retention
• Side effects: nausea, vomiting, diarrhoea, impotence, slight enlargement of breasts, fluid retention, rash, angina, myocardial infarction

Teach patient/family:
• That additional analgesia is available when required
• To report any chest pains or retention of urine immediately
• Not to take the drugs with milk or dairy products
• That nausea is often transient
• That body changes occur; impotence and sometimes breast enlargement in men

ethacrynic acid

Edecrin
Func. class.: Loop diuretic
Chem. class.: Ketone derivative
Legal class.: POM

Action: Acts on loop of Henle by increasing excretion of chloride, sodium
Uses: Pulmonary oedema, oedema in congestive cardiac failure, liver disease, renal disease
Dosage and routes:
• *Adult:* By mouth 50–150 mg daily may give up to 400 mg daily; given as 2 equally divided doses
• *Child over 2 yr:* By mouth 25 mg, increased by 25 mg a day until desired effect occurs

Pulmonary oedema
• *Adult:* IV 50–100 mg given over several min or 0.5–1 mg/kg as a single dose

Available forms include: Tablets 50 mg; powder for injection 50 mg
Side effects/adverse reactions:
GU: Polyuria, gynaecomastia, ejaculatory problems, renal failure, glycosuria
ELECT: Hypokalaemia, hypochloraemic alkalosis, hypomagnesaemia, hyperuricaemia, hypocalcaemia, hyponatraemia
CNS: Headache, fatigue, weakness, vertigo
GI: Nausea, diarrhoea, dry mouth, vomiting, anorexia, cramps, upset stomach, abdominal pain, acute pancreatitis, jaundice, GI bleeding
EENT: Loss of hearing, ear pain, tinnitus, blurred vision
INTEG: Rash, pruritus, purpura, Stevens-Johnson syndrome, sweating
MS: Cramps, arthritis, stiffness
ENDO: Hyperglycaemia
HAEM: Thrombocytopenia, agranulocytosis, leucopenia, neutropenia
CV: Chest pain, hypotension, circulatory collapse, ECG changes
Contraindications: Hypersensitivity to sulphonamides, anuria, hypovolaemia, children less than 2 yr, lactation, electrolyte depletion
Precautions: Dehydration, ascites, severe renal disease, pregnancy
Pharmacokinetics:
Period of onset: Onset ½ hr, peak 2 hr, duration 6–8 hr
IV: Onset 5 min, peak 15–30 min, duration 2 hr
Excreted by kidneys, half-life 30–70 min
Interactions/incompatibilities:
• Increased toxicity: lithium, nondepolarising skeletal muscle relaxants, digitalis, aminoglycosides, corticosteroids
• Increased anticoagulant activity

Clinical assessment:
• Electrolytes: potassium, sodium, chloride urea, blood sugar, serum creatinine, full blood count, pH and blood gases

Treatment of overdose: Gastric lavage if taken orally, monitor electrolytes, administer dextrose in saline

NURSING CONSIDERATIONS

Assess:

• Baseline vital signs, weight, fluid balance

Administer:

• Usually one dose of injection required, but if second dose required use new injection site to avoid thrombophlebitis

• In morning to avoid interference with sleep if using drug as a diuretic

• Potassium replacement if potassium is less than 3.0 mmol/litre

• With food, if nausea occurs, absorption may be decreased slightly

Evaluate:

• Weight, fluid balance daily to determine fluid loss; effect of drug may be decreased if used daily

• Rate, depth, rhythm of respiration, effect of exertion

• BP lying, standing; postural hypotension may occur

• Glucose in urine if patient is diabetic

• Improvement in oedema of feet, legs, sacral area daily if medication is being used in congestive cardiac failure

• Improvement in CVP 8 hrly

• Signs of metabolic acidosis: drowsiness, restlessness

• Signs of hypokalaemia: postural hypotension, malaise, fatigue, tachycardia, leg cramps, weakness

• Rashes, temperature elevation daily

• Confusion, especially in elderly, take safety precautions if needed

Teach patient/family:

• Increase fluid intake 2–3 litres daily unless contraindicated: to rise slowly from lying or sitting position

• Adverse reactions: muscle cramps, weakness, nausea, dizziness

• Take with food or milk for GI symptoms

• Take early in day to prevent nocturia

ethambutol hydrochloride

Myambutol, combination products

Func. class.: Antitubercular

Chem. class.: Di-isopropylethylene diamide derivative

Legal class.: POM

Action: Inhibits RNA synthesis, decreases tubercle bacilli replication

Uses: Pulmonary tuberculosis as an adjunctive. Should only be used in conjunction with other antitubercular drugs

Dosage and routes:

• *Adult:* By mouth 15 mg/kg daily as a single dose

• *Child over 6 yr:* Initially 25 mg/kg daily for 60 days then 15 mg/kg daily

• In impaired renal function the dose may need to be reduced according to blood levels (2–5 mcg/1 ml)

Retreatment

• *Adult and child:* By mouth 25 mg/kg daily as single dose for 60 days then decrease to 15 mg/kg daily as single dose

Available forms include: Tablets 100, 400 mg; in combination with isoniazid, tablets 200, 250, 300, 365 mg

Side effects/adverse reactions:

INTEG: Dermatitis, photosensitivity

CV: Congestive cardiac failure, dysrhythmias

CNS: Headache, anxiety, drowsiness, tremors, convulsions, lethargy, depression, confusion, psychosis, aggression, numbness, paraesthesia

EENT: Blurred vision, optic neuritis, photophobia, colour blindness

HAEM: Megaloblastic anaemia, vitamin B_{12}, folic acid deficiency

Contraindications: Hypersensitivity, optic neuritis, child less than 6 yr
Precautions: Pregnancy, renal disease, diabetic, retinopathy, cataracts, ocular defects
Pharmacokinetics:
Period of onset: Peak 2–4 hr, half-life 3 hr; metabolised in liver, excreted in urine (unchanged drug/inactive metabolites, faeces)
Interactions/incompatibilities:
• Increased toxicity: aminoglycosides, cisplatin, aluminium salts
Clinical assessment:
• Liver studies every week
• Renal status before therapy and every month: urea, creatinine
• Full ophthalmic examination including ophthalmoscopy, colour vision, periphery and visual acuity before and during treatment
NURSING CONSIDERATIONS
Assess:
• Urinalysis: output, specific gravity
Administer:
• As a single daily dose
• After samples sent for culture and sensitivity every month to detect resistance
• With meals to decrease GI symptoms
• Anti-emetic if vomiting occurs
Perform/provide:
• Storage of drug at controlled room temperature (15–30°C); prevent access of moisture
Evaluate:
• Ocular toxicity: blurred vision, colour blindness
• Mental status often: affect, mood, behavioural changes; psychosis may occur
• Hepatic status: decreased appetite, jaundice, dark urine, fatigue
Teach patient/family:
• That compliance with dosage schedule, length is necessary
• That scheduled appointments must be kept or relapse may occur
• Report any visual changes at once

ethinyloestradiol ▼

Func. class.: Oestrogen
Chem. class.: Synthetic oestrogen
Legal class.: POM

Action: Oestrogens are needed for adequate functioning of female reproductive system; affects release of pituitary gonadotrophins, inhibits ovulation, promotes adequate calcium use in bone structures
Uses: Menopause, primary amenorrhoea, hereditary haemorrhagic telangiectasia
Dosage and routes:
Menopause
• *Adult:* By mouth 10–20 mcg daily 3 weeks on, 1 week off, with progestogen from day 17 to day 26 of cycle if uterus intact
Primary amenorrhoea
• *Adult:* By mouth 10 mcg on alternate days to maximum 50 mcg daily, with progestrogen for last days of the month
Haemorrhagic telangiectasia
• *Adult:* By mouth 0.5–1 mg daily
Available forms include: Tablets 10 mcg, 20 mcg, 50 mcg, 1 mg
Side effects/adverse reactions:
CNS: Dizziness, headache, migraine, depression
CV: Hypertension, thrombophlebitis, oedema, thromboembolism, stroke, pulmonary embolism, myocardial infarction
GI: Nausea, vomiting, diarrhoea, anorexia, pancreatitis, cramps, constipation, increased appetite, increased weight, cholestatic jaundice
EENT: Contact lens intolerance, increased myopia, astigmatism
GU: Amenorrhoea, cervical

erosion, breakthrough bleeding, dysmenorrhoea, vaginal candidiasis, breast changes, gynaecomastia, testicular atrophy, impotence
INTEG: Rash, urticaria, acne, hirsutism, alopecia, oily skin, seborrhoea, purpura, chloasma
META: Folic acid deficiency, hypercalcaemia, hyperglycaemia
Contraindications: Breast cancer, thromboembolic disorders, oestrogen-dependent neoplasm, genital bleeding (abnormal, undiagnosed), pregnancy
Precautions: Hypertension, asthma, blood dyscrasias, gallbladder disease, congestive cardiac failure, diabetes mellitus, bone disease, depression, migraine headache, convulsive disorders, hepatic disease, renal disease, family history of cancer of breast or reproductive tract lactation
Pharmacokinetics: Metabolised in the liver, excreted in urine, excreted in breast milk
Interactions/incompatibilities:
• Decreased action of: anticoagulants, oral hypoglycaemics
• Toxicity: tricyclic antidepressants
• Decreased action of this drug: anticonvulsants, barbiturates, phenylbutazone, rifampicin
• Increased action of: corticosteroids

NURSING CONSIDERATIONS

Assess:
• Baseline BP, weight, urinalysis (in diabetics)
Administer:
• Titrated dose, use lowest effective dose
• With food or milk to decrease GI symptoms
Evaluate:
• BP 4 hrly, watch for increase caused by water and sodium retention
• Fluid balance, be alert for decreasing urinary output and increasing oedema
• Therapeutic response: absence of breast engorgement, reversal of menopause, or decrease in tumour size in prostatic cancer
• Oedema, hypertension, cardiac symptoms, jaundice, hypercalcaemia
• Mental status: affect, mood, behavioural changes, aggression
Teach patient/family:
• To weigh weekly, report gain more than 2.5 kg

---

ethosuximide

Zarontin, Emeside
Func. class.: Anticonvulsant
Chem. class.: Succinimide
Legal class.: POM

Action: Inhibits spike wave formation in absence seizures (petit mal), decreases amplitude, frequency, duration, spread of discharge in minor motor seizures
Uses: Absence seizures, myoclonic seizures, atypical seizures
Dosage and routes:
• *Adult:* By mouth, initially 500 mg daily; increase according to response by 250 mg every 4–7 days; usual range 1–1.5 g daily, up to 2 g may be needed
• *Child:* By mouth, under 6 yr, initially 250 mg daily, over 6 yr, initially 500 mg daily; increase gradually according to response to a maximum of 1 g daily
Available forms include: Capsules 250 mg; syrup 250 mg/5 ml
Side effects/adverse reactions:
HAEM: Agranulocytosis, aplastic anaemia, thrombocytopenia, leucocytosis, eosinophilia, pancytopenia
CNS: Drowsiness, dizziness, fatigue, euphoria, lethargy, anxiety,

aggressiveness, irritability, depression, insomnia
GI: Nausea, vomiting, heartburn, anorexia, diarrhoea, abdominal pain, cramps, constipation
GU: Vaginal bleeding, haematuria, renal damage
INTEG: Urticaria, pruritic erythema, hirsutism, Stevens-Johnson syndrome, systemic lupus erythematosus
EENT: Myopia, gum hypertrophy, tongue swelling, blurred vision
Contraindications: Hypersensitivity to succinimide derivatives, porphyrias
Precautions: Lactation, pregnancy, hepatic disease, renal disease
Pharmacokinetics:
Period of onset: Peak 1–7 hr, steady state 4–7 days, metabolised by liver, excreted in urine, bile, faeces, half-life 24–60 hr
Interactions/incompatibilities:
- Antagonist effect: tricyclic antidepressants (imipramine, doxepin)
- Decreased effects of: oestrogens, oral contraceptives

Clinical assessment:
- Renal studies: urinalysis, blood urea nitrogen, urine creatinine
- Blood studies: full blood count, haematocrit, Hb, reticulocyte counts every week for 4 weeks, then every month
- Hepatic studies: aspartate aminotransferase, alanine aminotransferase, bilirubin, creatinine
- Drug levels during initial treatment, therapeutic range (40–80 mcg/ml)

Lab. test interferences:
Increase: Coombs' test
Treatment of overdose: Lavage, activated charcoal, monitor electrolytes, vital signs

NURSING CONSIDERATIONS

Assess:
- Eye problems: need for ophthalmic examinations before, during, after treatment (slit lamp, ophthalmoscopy, tonometry)

Perform/provide:
- Frequent sips of water, mouthwashes to relieve dry mouth
- Assistance with ambulation during early part of treatment; dizziness occurs

Evaluate:
- Allergic reaction: red raised rash, exfoliative dermatitis; if these occur, drug should be discontinued
- Blood dyscrasias: fever, sore throat, bruising, rash, jaundice
- Toxicity: bone marrow depression, nausea, vomiting, ataxia, diplopia, cardiovascular collapse, Stevens-Johnson syndrome
- Therapeutic response: decreased seizure activity, document on patient's care plan
- Mental status: mood, alertness, affect, behavioural changes; if mental status changes notify clinician

Teach patient/family:
- To carry ID card or Medic-Alert bracelet stating drugs taken, condition, GP's name, phone number
- To avoid driving, other activities that require alertness
- To avoid alcohol ingestion, CNS depressants; increased sedation may occur
- Not to discontinue medication quickly after long-term use
- All aspects of drug: action, use, side effects, adverse reactions, when to notify clinician

---

etidronate disodium

Didronel
Func. class.: Parathyroid agent (calcium regulator)
Chem. class.: Diphosphonate
Legal class.: POM

Action: Reduces bone resorption of calcium

Uses: Paget's disease, hypercalcaemia of malignancy

Dosage and routes:

Paget's disease

• *Adult:* By mouth 5 mg/kg as single daily dose for up to 6 months. Doses above 10 mg/kg daily for up to 3 months. Doses above 20 mg/kg daily are not recommended

Hypercalcaemica of malignancy

• *IV infusion:* 7.5 mg/kg daily for 3 days, repeat course once if necessary after at least 7 days

• *By mouth:* On day after last IV dose 20 mg/kg as single daily dose for 30 days, maximum treatment period is 90 days

Available forms include: Tablets 200 mg; injection 50 mg/ml, 6 ml ampoule

Side effects/adverse reactions:

GI: Nausea, diarrhoea

MS: Bone pain, hypocalcaemia, decreased mineralisation of non-affected bones

INTEG: Angioneurotic oedema/urticaria, pruritus rush

Contraindications: Moderate/severe renal impairment, pregnancy, breast-feeding, oral administration in acute GI inflammatory disorders

Precautions: Pregnancy, lactation, enterocolitis, children, fractures, restricted vitamin D/calcium

Pharmacokinetics: Not metabolised, excreted in urine/faeces, therapeutic response: 1–3 months

Interactions/incompatibilities:

• Antacids reduced absorption

• Aminoglycoside: severe hypocalcaemia

Clinical assessment:

• Blood urea nitrogen, creatinine, phosphate, urine hydroxyproline uric acid, chloride, electrolytes, pH, urine calcium, magnesium, alkaline phosphatase, urinalysis, calcium, vitamin D

• Muscle spasm, laryngospasm, paraesthesia, facial twitching, nutritional status with regard calcium and phosphate, colic; may indicate hypocalcaemia

Treatment of overdose: Symptoms of hypocalcaemia; withdraw drug and correct hypocalcaemia with IV calcium gluconate

NURSING CONSIDERATIONS

Administer:

• On empty stomach with water

• Keep patient well hydrated when giving IV infusion

• IV infusion diluted to at least 250 ml in sodium chloride 0.9% and given over not less than 2 hours

• Avoid food for at least 2 hr before and after oral treatment—particularly calcium-containing products

Evaluate:

• Fluid balance check for decreased output in renal patients

• Nutritional status, diet for sources of vitamin D (milk, some seafood), calcium (dairy products, dark green vegetables), phosphate—adequate intake is necessary

• Persistent nausea or diarrhoea

Teach patient/family:

• Avoid non-prescribed products

• All aspects of drug: action, side effects, dose, when to notify clinician

• Therapeutic response may take 1–3 months, effects persist for months after drug is discontinued

• Adequate intake of calcium, vitamin D is necessary

• Teach patient about dietary requirements

etodolac

Lodine
Func. class.: Non-steroidal anti-inflammatory drug
Chem. class.: Indoleacetic acid derivative
Legal class.: POM

Action: Inhibits prostaglandin synthesis by decreasing enzyme needed for biosynthesis; possesses analgesic and anti-inflammatory, antipyretic actions

Uses: Acute or long-term treatment of rheumatoid arthritis

Dosage and routes:
- By mouth 200 mg twice daily or 400 mg once daily; maximum dose 600 mg daily

Available forms include: Tablets 200 mg; capsules 200 mg, 300 mg

Side effects/adverse reactions:
GI: Discomfort, bleeding, nausea, diarrhoea
CV: Angioneurotic oedema; congestive cardiac failure in elderly
CNS: Headache, dizziness, vertigo
RESP: Asthma
INTEG: Rashes
EENT: Hearing disturbances, tinnitus
META: Fluid retention
RENAL: Acute renal failure; papillary necrosis or interstitial fibrosis leading to chronic renal failure

Contraindications: Hypersensitivity; hypersensitivity to aspirin or other NSAIDS; active or suspected peptic ulcer or G.I. bleed; pregnancy; breast-feeding

Precautions: Elderly patients, asthma, renal or hepatic impairment, pregnancy

Interactions/incompatibilities:
Increased effect of: salicylates, anticoagulants, antihypertensives, cardiac glycocides, diuretics, captopril, enalpril, methotrexate

Clinical assessment:
- Hearing tests
- Check history of asthma, peptic ulcer, allergies
- H_2 receptor blockers if essential for patient with peptic ulcer
- Evaluate response and level of side effects
- Liver function tests, aspartate aminotransferase, alanine aminotransferase
- Renal function—urea, creatinine, Hb

Lab. test interference:
False positive: Bilirubin in urine

Treatment of overdose: No data available. Gastric lavage, activated charcoal and supportive treatment

NURSING CONSIDERATIONS

Administer:
- With or after food
- Lowest effective dose

Perform/provide:
- Help with mobility
- Safe environment (dizzy/vertigo)

Evaluate:
- Side effects such as tinnitus, bleeding
- Toxicity
- Swelling, mobility, stiffness and pain

Teach patient/family:
- To take with or after food
- Not to take other drugs unless specifically prescribed, especially aspirin or other NSAID
- No alcohol to be taken
- Report ringing in the ears, reduced urine output, abdominal pain, joint pain increase
- Report unresolved indigestion or black tar-like stools

etomidate

Hypnomidate
Func. class.: Anaesthetic, general
Chem. class.: Nonbarbiturate hypnotic
Legal class.: POM

Action: Acts at level of reticular-activating system to produce anaesthesiä
Uses: Induction of general anaesthesia
Dosage and routes:
• *Adult and child:* Slow IV 300 mcg/kg; high-risk patients 100 mcg/kg/min until anaesthetised
Available forms include: Injection IV 2, 125 mg/ml
Side effects/adverse reactions:
GI: Nausea, vomiting (postoperatively)
CNS: Tonic movements, myoclonic movements, averting movements, pain on injection
CV: Tachycardia, hypotension, hypertension, bradycardia
ENDO: Decreases steroid production
RESP: Laryngospasm
Contraindications: Hypersensitivity, labour/delivery, reduced adrenocortical function
Precautions: Pregnancy, lactation
Pharmacokinetics:
IV: Onset 20 sec, peak 1 min, duration 3–5 min; half-life 75 min, metabolised in liver, excreted in urine
Clinical assessment:
• Plasma cortisol levels if administered over several hours (5–20 mcg/100 ml normal level of cortisol)
• Corticosteroids for severe hypotension
• Etomidate should not be used for maintenance anaesthesia
Treatment of overdose: General supportive measures

NURSING CONSIDERATIONS
Assess:
• Starvation status
• Degree of pain during administration
• Do not mix with any other drug
Administer:
• IV slowly under anaesthetic supervision
• Dilute injection before use, about NaCl 0.9% infusion or dextrose solutions
• Only with emergency trolley/resuscitation equipment at hand
Evaluate:
• Vital signs every 10 min during IV administration
• Degree of extraneous muscle movement following injection
• Level of anaesthesia after 3–5 mins
• Cardiac and respiratory status
• Observe ECG for dysrhythmias
• IV slowly only, muscular twitching is reduced with fentanyl before anaesthesia induction
• Increasing or decreasing heart rate or dysrhythmias shown on ECG
Teach/patient:
• Effect of drug; drowsiness followed by sleep

etoposide

Vepesid
Func. class.: Antineoplastic
Chem. class.: Semisynthetic podophyllotoxin
Legal class.: POM

Action: Inhibits mitotic activity through metaphase to mitosis; also inhibits cells from entering mitosis, depresses DNA, RNA synthesis
Uses: Leukaemias, lung, testicular cancer, lymphomas, neuroblastoma
Dosage and routes:
Doses are highly variable, and

dependent on local treatment protocols, concomitant therapy and tumour type; the following dose schedules have been used

• *Adult:* IV 60–120 mg/m^2 daily for 5 days. Do not repeat within 3 weeks. Dilute injection to 0.25 mg/ml with sodium chloride 0.9% and give over 30 min

• *Adult:* By mouth 120–240 mg/m^2 daily for 5 days. Do not repeat within 3 weeks

Available forms include: Injection 20 mg/ml; capsules 50 mg, 100 mg

Side effects/adverse reactions:

HAEM: Thrombocytopenia, leucopenia, myelosuppression, anaemia

GI: Nausea, vomiting, anorexia, hepatotoxicity

INTEG: Rash, alopecia, phlebitis

RESP: Bronchospasm

CV: Hypotension

CNS: Headache, fever

Contraindications: Hypersensitivity, myelosuppression, severe hepatic disease, severe renal disease, bacterial infection

Precautions: Renal disease, hepatic disease, lactation, pregnancy, children, gout

Pharmacokinetics: Half-life 3 hr, terminal 15 hr, metabolised in liver, excreted in urine

Interactions/incompatibilities:

• Do not use with radiation

• Do not dilute injection with dextrose solution

Clinical assessment:

• Full blood count, differential, platelet count weekly; withhold drug if WBC is less than 4000 or platelet count is less than 100,000; notify clinician of results

• Pulmonary function tests, chest X-ray studies before, during therapy; chest X-ray film should be obtained every 2 weeks during treatment

• Renal function studies: blood urea nitrogen, serum uric acid, urine creatinine clearance, electrolytes before, during therapy

• Antibiotics, antispasmodics, analgesics as appropriate

• Liver function tests before, during therapy (bilirubin, aspartate aminotransferase, alanine aminotransferase, lactic dehydrogenase) as needed or monthly

• Transfusion for anaemia

NURSING CONSIDERATIONS

Administer:

• HANDLING: take safety precautions appropriate to antineoplastic agents

• Following local antineoplastic (cytotoxic) policies

• After ensuring that clinician is aware of blood results

• IV: as an IV infusion in sodium chloride 0.9% over not less than 30 min and a concentration not greater than 0.25 mg/ml

• All other medications by mouth if possible. Avoid IV, IM, SC routes to prevent infection and bruising

• Anti-emetic 30–60 min before treatment

• All other medication as prescribed including analgesics, antibiotics, anti-emetics, antispasmodics

Perform/provide:

• Strict asepsis for all procedures; protective isolation if WBC levels are low

• Special care of skin

• Increase fluid intake to 2–3 litres daily to prevent urate deposits, calculi formation

• Warm compresses at injection site for inflammation, avoid extravasation

• Pain relief as required

Evaluate:

• Nausea and vomiting (worse with oral medication)

• Fluid balance, report fall in urine output of 30 ml/hr

• Bleeding: haematuria, bruising

or petechiae, mucosa or orifices 8 hrly
• Dyspnoea, rales, unproductive cough, chest pain, tachypnoea, fatigue, increased pulse, pallor, lethargy
• Food preferences; list likes, dislikes
• Effects of alopecia on body image; discuss feelings about body changes
• Oedema in feet, joint pain, stomach pain, shaking
• Inflammation of mucosa, breaks in skin
• Yellowing of skin and sclera, dark urine, clay-coloured stools, itchy skin, abdominal pain, fever, diarrhoea
• Buccal cavity 8 hrly for dryness, sores or ulceration, white patches, oral pain, bleeding, dysphagia
• Local irritation, pain, burning, discolouration at injection site
• Symptoms indicating severe allergic reaction: rash, pruritus, urticaria, purpuric skin lesions, itching, flushing

Teach patient/family:
• About protective isolation precautions and rationale
• To report any complaints or side effects to nurse or clinician
• To report any changes in breathing or coughing
• That hair may be lost during treatment; a wig or hairpiece may be available on NHS; tell patient that new hair may be different in colour, texture

---

etretinate

Tigason
Func. class.: Antipsoriatic, systemic
Chem. class.: Retinoid
Legal class.: POM

Action: Reverses hyperkeratotic skin changes

Uses: Severe, extensive resistant psoriasis; palmo-plantar pustular psoriasis; severe congenital ichthyosis; keratosis follicularis

Dosage and routes:
• *Adult:* By mouth, starting dose 0.75 mg/kg daily in divided doses for 2–4 weeks, increased up to 1 mg/kg daily if needed. Total daily dose not to exceed 75 mg; maintenance dose 0.25–0.5 mg/kg daily

Available forms include: Capsules 10, 25 mg

Side effects/adverse reactions:
INTEG: Alopecia; peeling of palms, soles, fingertips; itching; rash; dryness; red scaling face; bruising; sunburn; pyogenic granuloma; paronychia; onycholysis; perspiration change
CNS: Fatigue, headache, dizziness, fever, pain, anxiety, amnesia, depression
EENT: Eye irritation, pain, double vision, change in lacrimation, earache, otitis externa
GI: Anorexia, abdominal pain, nausea, hepatitis, constipation, diarrhoea, flatulence
CV: Oedema, CV obstruction, atrial fibrillation, chest pain, coagulation disorders
RESP: Dyspnoea, cough
GU: WBC in urine, proteinuria, glycosuria, increased blood urea nitrogen, creatinine, haematuria, casts, ketonuria, haemoglobinuria
ELECT: Increase or decrease potassium, calcium, phosphate, sodium, chloride
MS: Hyperostosis, bone pain, cramps, myalgia, gout, hypertonia

Contraindications: Pregnancy, breast-feeding, hepatic or renal impairment

Precautions: Women of childbearing age; exclude possibility of pregnancy in subsequent 2 yr, children

Pharmacokinetics: 99% plasma

protein binding; excreted in bile, urine; terminal half-life 120 days; accumulates in fatty tissue

Interactions/incompatibilities:

• Increased absorption of etretinate: milk or high lipid diet

Clinical assessment:

• Liver function and blood lipids (fasting value) measured at start of therapy, after first month of administration and at 3 monthly intervals thereafter

• Blood sugar levels should be checked frequently at beginning of treatment period

• Investigate any atypical musculo-skeletal symptoms; possible etretinate-induced bone changes

NURSING CONSIDERATIONS

Administer:

• With or after food

Evaluate:

• Neurological status: headache, nausea, vomiting, visual disturbance, papilloedema

• Visual disturbance: blurring, poor nocturnal vision, decreased visual acuity. If these symptoms develop the drug must be discontinued and ophthalmic opinion sought

• Response to treatment indicated by decrease in scaling, itching and resolution of psoriasis

Teach patient/family:

• To take with food

• Not to take if pregnancy is suspected. A reliable form of contraception must be used for 2 yr after treatment is complete for women of child bearing age

• Not to take vitamin A supplements

• Wearing contact lens may be difficult/uncomfortable

• Not to donate blood either during or for at least 2 yr following discontinuation of therapy

famotidine

Pepcid PM

Func. class.: H_2-receptor antagonist

Chem. class.: Substituted thiazole

Legal class.: POM

Action: Competitively inhibits histamine at histamine H_2 receptor site, decreasing gastric secretion while pepsin remains at stable level

Uses: Short-term treatment of active duodenal and benign gastric ulcer, maintenance therapy for duodenal ulcer, Zollinger-Ellison syndrome, multiple endocrine adenomas

Dosage and routes:

Duodenal and gastric ulcer

• *Adult:* By mouth 40 mg at night for 4–8 weeks

Prophylaxis of duodenal ulcer relapse

• *Adult:* By mouth 20 mg at night

Reflux oesophagitis

• *Adult:* By mouth 20–40 mg twice a day for 6–12 weeks

Zollinger-Ellison syndrome

• *Adult:* By mouth 20 mg 4 times a day increasing to maximum 800 mg daily as necessary

Available forms include: Tablets 20 mg 40 mg

Side effects/adverse reactions:

HAEM: Thrombocytopenia

CNS: Headache, dizziness, paraesthesia, seizure, depression, anxiety, somnolence, insomnia, fever

GI: Constipation, nausea, vomiting, anorexia, cramps, abnormal liver enzymes

RESP: Bronchospasm

EENT: Taste change, tinnitus, orbital oedema

INTEG: Rash

MS: Myalgia, arthralgia

GU: Decreased libido

Contraindications: Hypersensitivity

Precautions: Pregnancy, breast-feeding, children, severe renal disease (reduce dose), severe hepatic function, can mask symptoms of gastric cancer
Pharmacokinetics:
Period of onset: Peak 1–3 hr, plasma protein-binding 15%–20%; metabolised in liver (active metabolites), excreted by kidneys, half-life 2.5–3.5 hr
Clinical assessment:
• Blood counts during therapy, watch for decreasing platelets, if low, therapy may need to be discontinued and restarted after haematologic recovery

NURSING CONSIDERATIONS

Assess:
• Baseline pulse
• Fluid balance
Evaluate:
• Blood dyscrasias (thrombocytopenia): bruising, fatigue, bleeding, poor healing
Perform/provide:
• Monitor pulse frequently during administration
Teach patient/family:
• That drug must be continued for prescribed time to be effective
• To report bleeding, bruising, fatigue, malaise since blood dyscrasias do occur
• Discuss possibility of decreased libido, reversible after discontinuing therapy
• Appropriate dietary advice

fat emulsions

Intralipid, Lipofundin MCT/LCT, Lipofundin S, Soyacal
Func. class.: Nutrition, caloric
Chem. class.: Fatty acid, long chain
Legal class.: POM

Action: Required for energy, heat production; consist of neutral triglycerides, primarily unsaturated fatty acids plus variable amounts of vitamin E
Uses: Increase calorie intake as part of balanced feeding regimen
Dosage and routes:
Adjunct to total parenteral nutrition
• *Adult:* IV infusion 500–1000 ml/24 hr 10%–20% maximum rate, 500 ml/5 hr 20%, 500 ml/3 hr 10%. Maximum 3 g fat/kg/24 hr
• *Infant:* 0.02–0.17 g fat/kg/hr; small for age/low birthweight, initially 0.5 g fat/kg/24 hr, maximum 2 g fat/kg/24 hr. Administer over 20 hr; measure blood electrolytes 4 hr later
Available forms include: Injection IV 10%, 20%
Side effects/adverse reactions:
CNS: Dizziness, headache, drowsiness, focal seizures, pyrexia
CV: Shock
GI: Nausea, vomiting, hepatomegaly, abnormal liver function tests
RESP: Dyspnoea, fat in lung tissue
HAEM: Hyperlipidaemia, hypercoagulation, thrombocytopenia, leucopenia, leucocytosis
Contraindications: Hypersensitivity, hyperlipidaemia, lipid necrosis, acute pancreatitis accompanied by hyperlipidaemia
Precautions: Severe liver disease, diabetes mellitus, thrombocytopenia, gastric ulcers, premature, term newborns
Interactions/incompatibilities:
• Do not mix with any drug, electrolytes, solutions, vitamin unless prepared by pharmacy e.g. TPN solutions
Clinical assessment:
• Triglycerides, free fatty acid levels, platelet counts daily to prevent fat overload, thrombocytopaenia
• Liver function studies: aspartate aminotransferase, alanine aminotransferase

NURSING CONSIDERATIONS

Administer:

• Alone; do not mix with any drug, solution vitamin or electrolyte

• Carefully due to tendency of solution to coagulate and clog IV line

• Use infusion pump: do not use in-line filter; clogging will occur

Perform/provide:

• Change IV tubing at each infusion: infection may occur with old tubing

Evaluate:

• Therapeutic response: increased weight

• Nutritional status: calorie count by dietician

Teach patient/family:

• Reason for use of lipids

• How to care for parenteral feeding and IV line if on long-term therapy, e.g. TPN

felbinac (topical)

Traxam

Func. class.: Topical non-steroidal anti-inflammatory agents

Chem. class.: Propionic acid derivatives

Legal class.: POM

Action: Active metabolite of ferlufer; inhibits prostaglandin synthesis, possesses analgesic and anti-inflammatory properties

Uses: Soft-tissue injuries such as sprains, strains and contusions

Dosage and routes:

• *Adult:* Topical foam, gently rub one golf-ball size (4 cm diameter or about 1 gram) into the affected area 2–4 times a day. Do not exceed 25 g/day

• *Adult:* Topical gel, gently rub into affected area 2–4 times a day. Do not exceed 25 g/day. Review after 14 days if symptoms not resolved

Available forms include: Foam 3.17%; Gel 3%

Side effects/adverse reactions:

Mild local erythema, dermatitis or pruritus. Systemic side effects are unlikely after topical use, but the following have been reported when ferlufer is taken by mouth and are theoretically possible:

CNS: Headache, dizziness, vertigo, fatigue, parasthesia, depression, malaise

CV: Fluid retention, angioneurotic oedema, cardiac failure in elderly

EENT: Tinnitus, hearing disturbances

GI: GI haemorrhage, peptic ulcer, gastritis, nausea, diarrhoea, dyspepsia, stomatitis, altered liver function, jaundice, hepatitis

GU: Acute renal failure, interstitial nephritis, nephrotic syndrome

HAEM: Blood dyscrasias

INTEG: Rash, urticaria, angioedema, purpura, photosensitive

RESP: Bronchospasm, asthma, allergic interstitial lung disorders

SYS: Hypersensitivity, anaphylaxis

Contraindications: Hypersensitivity ingredients; hypersensitivity or asthma precipitated by aspirine or other NSAIDs; children

Precautions: For tropical use only, use on intact skin, do not use on mucus membranes, lips or near eyes, do not use occlusive dressings; pregnancy, lactation, asthma

Pharmacokinetics: Serum levels are very low after topical administration

Interactions/incompatibilities:

• Clinically significant drug interactions are unlikely

Treatment of overdose: Unlikely to cause adverse systemic effects even if accidentally ingested. If a large quantity is ingested give symptomatic and supportive treatment

Pharmaceutical precautions:

Foam: Pressurized container, keep out of sunlight and temperatures above 50°C, do not refrigerate, do not use near naked flame or fire, do not smoke while using

Gel: Replace cap after use, dilution not recommended

NURSING CONSIDERATIONS:

Assess:

• Check for history of hypersensitivity

Administer:

Foam: Shake well before use, dispense onto hand and rub in gently; a clear liquid is formed in contact with the skin. Wash hands after use

Gel: Rub gently into affected area, wash hands after use

Evaluate

• Clinical response
• Side effects

Teach patient/family:

• Wash hands after use unless hands are being treated
• How to apply
• Not to apply to broken skin, mucous membrane, lips or near eyes
• Stop using if skin reaction occurs
• Do not use foam near naked flame
• Do not smoke while using
• Do not refrigerate
• Replace cap after use

---

felodipine ▼

Plendil

Func. class.: Antihypertensive
Chem. class.: Calcium channel blocker, dihydropyridine derivative
Legal class.: POM

Action: Inhibits calcium ion flux across cell membranes relaxing arterial smooth muscle, resulting in arterial vasodilation and reduction in blood pressure

Uses: Management of all grades of hypertension

Dosage and routes:

• *Adult:* By mouth, initially 5 mg in the morning; usual maintenance 5–10 mg once daily; doses above 20 mg daily rarely needed

Available forms include: Tablets, modified-release 5 mg, 10 mg

Side effects/adverse reactions:

CNS: Headache, dizziness, fatigue
CV: Flushing, palpitations, ankle swelling
EENT: Gingival hyperplasia
INTEG: Rash, pruritus

Contraindications: Hypersensitivity; women of child-bearing potential; children

Precautions: Hepatic impairment; lactation

Interactions:

• Effect of felodipine reduced by: carbamazepine, phenobarbitone, phenytoin, primidone
• Effect of felodipine enhanced by: cimetidine, other antihypertensives

Lab. test interferences: None known

Treatment of overdose: Treat hypotension by placing patient supine with legs elevated. Bradycardia, if present, should be treated with atropine 0.5–1 mg IV. If this is insufficient plasma volume should be increased by infusion of glucose, saline or dextran. Sympathomimetics acting predominantly on the alpha-1 adrenoceptor may be given, e.g. metaraminol, phenylephrine

NURSING CONSIDERATIONS

Assess:

• Vital signs (temperature, pulse, respiration, BP); ECG, weight

Administer:

• By mouth; tablets to be swallowed whole, not crushed

Evaluate:
• Therapeutic effect
• BP, pulse regularly, frequency depending on pre-therapy BP and response to medication
• Weight daily (risk of heart failure)
• Other side effects

Teach patient/family:
• That tablets are to be swallowed whole, not crushed or chewed
• Avoid hazardous activities, including driving, until stabilised on medication
• About side effects and to inform nurse or clinician if these occur
• Not to discontinue tablets without medical advice

fenbufen

Lederfen, Lederfen F
Func. class.: Non-steroidal anti-inflammatory drug
Chem. class.: Propionic acid derivative
Legal class.: POM

Action: Has both analgesic and anti-inflammatory effects
Uses: Pain and inflammation in rheumatic disease and other acute musculoskeletal disorders
Dosage and routes:
Adult: By mouth 300 mg in morning and 600 mg at night or 450 mg twice daily
Available forms include: Tablets 300 mg, 450 mg; effervescent tablets 450 mg; capsules 300 mg
Side effects/adverse reactions:
GI: Discomfort, bleeding, nausea, diarrhoea
CV: Angioneurotic oedema, congestive cardiac failure in elderly
CNS: Headache, dizziness, vertigo
RESP: Asthma
INTEG: Rashes
EENT: Hearing disturbances, tinnitus
META: Fluid retention
RENAL: Acute renal failure; papillary necrosis or interstitial fibrosis leading to chronic renal failure
Contraindications: Hypersensitivity; hypersensitivity to aspirin or other NSAIDS; active or suspected peptic ulcer or G.I. haemorrage; 3rd trimester of pregnancy
Precautions: Elderly patients, history of peptic ulceration, allergic disorders, asthma, renal or hepatic impairment, pregnancy
Pharmacokinetics: Converted to active metabolites with half-lives of approximately 10 hr; these undergo hepatic metabolism before excretion in the urine
Interactions/incompatibilities:
• Increased risk of side effects: salicylates, anticoagulants, antihypertensives, cardiac glycosides, diuretics, captopril, enalapril, methotrexate

Clinical assessment:
• Hearing tests in impaired patients
• Check history of peptic ulcer, asthma and any allergies
• Renal function: urea, creatinine before, during treatment if problem anticipated
• Liver function tests: aspartate aminotransferase, alanine, bilirubin, alkaline phosphatase before, during treatment if problem anticipated

Treatment of overdose: Gastric lavage, symptomatic treatment

NURSING CONSIDERATIONS

Assess:
• Fluid balance (renal failure/ oedema)
• Hepatic and renal studies, including fluid balance and oedema
• Respiration (asthma)
• Audio and visual ability, before and during treatment

Administer:
• With food or milk. Effervescent tablets in half a glass of water
Perform/provide:
• Help with mobility
Evaluate:
• Therapeutic response: decreased pain, stiffness, swelling in joints; increased mobility
• Signs of toxicity
• Rashes, erythema multiforme, tinnitus
Teach patient/family:
• That therapeutic response may not be immediate (2–4 weeks)
• To take other medication only if directed by clinician especially aspirin and other NSAIDs
• To report any rashes, ringing in ears, blood in stools or vomiting
• To report changes in urinary patterns

fenfluramine hydrochloride

Ponderax, Pacaps
Func. class.: Appetite suppressant
Chem. class.: Sympathomimetic
Legal class.: POM

Action: Increases release of noradrenaline, dopamine in cerebral cortex to reticular activating system
Uses: Treatment of severe obesity, including severe obesity associated with maturity-onset diabetes
Dosage and routes:
• *Adult:* By mouth 60 mg capsule daily, ½ hr before a meal
Available forms include: Capsules 60 mg
Side effects/adverse reactions:
CNS: Insomnia, talkativeness, dizziness, drowsiness, headache, irritability
GI: Nausea, vomiting, anorexia, dry mouth, diarrhoea, constipation, abdominal pain
GU: Impotence, change in libido, dysuria, urinary frequency
CV: Palpitations, tachycardia, hypertension, hypotension
INTEG: Urticaria, rash, burning, sweating, chills, fever
Contraindications: Hypersensitivity to sympathomimetic amines, glaucoma, drug abuse, cardiovascular disease, alcoholism, epilepsy, depression, pregnancy, breast-feeding, personality disorders, children
Precautions: Diabetes mellitus, hypertension, pregnancy, lactation, elderly
Pharmacokinetics:
Period of onset: Onset 1–2 min, duration 4–6 hr, metabolised by liver, excreted by kidneys
Interactions/incompatibilities:
• Hypertensive crisis: MAOIs or within 21 days of MAOIs
• Increased effect of this drug: acetazolamide, antacids, sodium bicarbonate, ascorbic acid, ammonium chloride, phenothiazines, haloperidol, antidepressants
• Decreased effects of this drug: barbiturates
• Decrease effects of: guanethidine, other antihypertensives
Clinical assessment:
• Full blood count; urinalysis; in diabetes, blood sugar, urine sugar, insulin changes may need to be made since eating will increase
• Height, growth rate in children (may be decreased)
Treatment of overdose: Administer fluids, haemodialysis or peritoneal dialysis; antihypertensive for increased BP; ammonium chloride for increased excretion

NURSING CONSIDERATIONS

Assess:
• Pulse, blood pressure and respirations before treatment
• Weight before, during and after treatment

• Diet
• Effect due to other drugs taken; antihypertensives check these patients more often

Administer:

• For obesity only if patient is on weight reduction programme, including dietary changes, exercise; patient will develop tolerance and weight loss won't occur without additional methods
• Orally ½ hour before a meal
• Do not give late in the day to avoid interference with sleep

Perform/provide:

• Frequent drinks to prevent a dry mouth
• Close support and supervision, especially with diet regime. (Weight reducing programme)

Evaluate:

• Therapeutic response: effective weight loss
• Side effects: insomnia, talkativeness dry mouth, diarrhoea palpitation, tachycardia
• If no weight loss occurs discontinue drug slowly
• Mental status: mood, alertness, affect, stimulation, insomnia, aggressiveness may occur
• Physical dependency: should not be used for extended time; dose should be discontinued gradually
• Withdrawal symptoms: headache, nausea, vomiting, muscle pain, weakness
• Drug tolerance will develop after long-term use
• Dosage should not be increased if tolerance develops
• Any other medication, the effect of fenfluamine may be increased or decrease or it may decrease to effects of other drug—antihypertensives

Teach patient/family:

• To follow suitable diet and seek support if necessary
• Avoid foods that may increase irritability, e.g. coffee, chocolate
• To combine diet with exercise and rest
• That alcohol should be avoided
• To avoid driving or use of machinery until therapy established
• To take other medication only if directed by clinician
• To discontinue treatment *after* six months. Drug should be tapered off slowly over several weeks

---

fenofibrate

Lipantil
Func. class.: Hypolipidaemic agent
Chem. class.: Isobutyric acid derivative
Legal class.: POM

Action: Precise mechanism of action is unclear. Lowers LDL- and VLDL-cholesterol and triglycerides. Increases HDL-cholesterol

Uses: Treatment of patients with severe hyperlipidaemia (Types IIa, IIb, III, IV, V) unresponsive to diet

Dosage and routes:

• *Adult:* By mouth initially 300 mg daily in divided doses with food. Maintenance dose usually in the range 200–400 mg daily
• *Children:* 5 mg/kg body-weight daily

Available forms include: Capsules 100 mg

Side effects/adverse reactions:

GI: Gastro-intestinal disturbances, elevated liver enzymes
INTEG: Skin reactions
CNS: Headache, fatigue, vertigo
MS: Muscle cramps
GU: Sexual asthenia

Contraindications: Severe liver dysfunction, existing gall bladder disease, severe renal disorders, pregnancy, breast-feeding, hypersensitivity

Precautions: Renal impairment. Discontinue if an adequate response is not achieved in 3 months
Pharmacokinetics: Rapidly and well absorbed; rapidly metabolised in liver to active metabolites, chiefly fenofibric acid. Drug and metabolites extensively protein bound. Plasma half-life 27 hr. Excreted in urine
Interactions/incompatibilities:
• Increased effect of oral anticoagulants and, possibly, other protein-bound drugs
Clinical assessment:
• Lipid profile
Treatment of overdose: Gastric lavage and supportive care

NURSING CONSIDERATIONS

Assess:
• Serum lipids
Administer:
• With food
Evaluate:
• For nausea and abdominal discomfort
Teach patient/family:
• That other risk factors should be decreased: high-fat diet, smoking, lack of exercise

fenoprofen calcium

Progesic, Fenopron
Func. class.: Non-steroidal anti-inflammatory drug
Chem. class.: Propionic acid derivative
Legal class.: POM

Action: Inhibits prostaglandin synthesis by inhibiting enzyme needed for biosynthesis; possesses analgesic, anti-inflammatory, antipyretic properties
Uses: Mild to moderate pain, osteoarthritis, rheumatoid arthritis, ankylosing spondylitis, pyrexia
Dosage and routes:
• *Adult:* By mouth 200–600 mg 3 or 4 times a day, maximum 3 g daily
Available forms include: Tablets 200 mg, 300 mg, 600 mg
Side effects/adverse reactions:
GI: Nausea, anorexia, vomiting, diarrhoea, jaundice, constipation, flatulence, cramps, dry mouth, peptic ulcer, bleeding, dyspepsia, jaundice, hepatitis, oral ulceration, pancreatitis, metallic taste
CNS: Dizziness, drowsiness, fatigue, tremors, confusion, insomnia, anxiety, depression
CV: Tachycardia, peripheral oedema, palpitations, dysrhythmias
INTEG: Purpura, rash, pruritus, sweating, exfoliative dermatitis, alopecia
GU: Nephrotoxicity: dysuria, haematuria, oliguria, azotaemia, cystitis, nephrotic syndrome
HAEM: Blood dyscrasias
EENT: Tinnitus, hearing loss, blurred vision
RESP: Bronchospasm in patients with history of asthma/allergy
Contraindications: Hypersensitivity; hypersensitivity to aspirin or other NSAIDs; active or suspected peptic ulcer or G.I. haemorrhage; 3rd trimester of pregnancy; breast-feeding; severe renal disease
Precautions: Pregnancy, lactation, asthma, anaemia, bleeding disorders, cardiac disorders, hypersensitivity to other NSAIDs, history of peptic ulcer, gastrointestinal haemorrhage, ulcerative colitis
Pharmacokinetics:
Period of onset: Peak 2 hr, half-life 3–3½ hr, metabolised in liver, excreted in urine (metabolites), 90% protein bound, enters breast milk
Interactions/incompatibilities:
• May increase the action of: oral anticoagulants, sulphonylurea hypoglycaemics, phenytoin

• Decreased effect of: diuretics
• Enhanced toxicity of: methotrexate, lithium, cyclosporin

Clinical assessment:
• Patient at high risk of peptic ulceration or GI bleeding
• Renal and hepatic function if impairment anticipated
• Eye examinations if visual disturbances occur
• Regular hearing tests in impaired patients

Treatment of overdose: Gastric lavage, supportive treatment, correct serum electrolytes

NURSING CONSIDERATIONS

Administer:
• With or after food

Evaluate:
• Decreased pain and stiffness in joints. Ability to move more easily
• For tinnitus, hearing loss, blurred vision, indigestion and black tarry stools

Teach patient/family:
• Report indigestion and black tarry stools
• Take with food or milk
• Report changes in vision or hearing

fenoterol (inhaled)

Berotec

Func. class.: β_2-adrenergic stimulant
Chem. class.: Isoprenaline analogue
Legal class.: POM

Action: Causes bronchodilatation by acting on β-receptors in bronchus and lung; has relatively little effect on cardiac receptors

Uses: Relief of bronchospasm associated with reversible obstructive airways disease

Dosage and routes:
• *Adult:* By metered-dose inhalation, 100–200 mcg up to 4 times a day. By nebulisation or via an intermittent positive pressure ventilator 0.5–1.25 mg (exceptionally, and under close medical supervision up to 5 mg) up to 4 times a day
• *Child (6–12 yr):* By metered-dose inhalation, 100 mcg (exceptionally 200 mcg) up to 4 times a day. By nebulisation or via an intermittent positive pressure ventilator up to 1.0 mg 3 times a day

Available forms include: Metered-dose inhaler 100, 200 mcg/inhalation; nebuliser solution 5 mg/ml

Side effects/adverse reactions:
CNS: Headache, anxiety
CV: Palpitations, tachycardia
ELECT: Hypokalaemia, cardiac arrhythmias secondary to hypokalaemia
MISC: Tremor

Contraindications: Hypersensitivity

Precautions: Thyrotoxicosis; myocardial insufficiency; angina; history of cardiac arrhythmias; hypertension; hypokalaemia and patients whose treatment or condition predispose then to hypokalaemia; pregnancy

Pharmacokinetics: Poorly absorbed after inhalation, extensively metabolised in the liver, excreted in urine and faeces; elimination half-life 6–7 hr

Interactions:
• Increased effect/toxicity of both drugs: other sympathomimetics
• Reduced action of both agents: β-blockers
• Increased risk of hypokalaemia: aminophylline, corticosteroids, diuretics, theophylline

Treatment of overdose: Supportive and symptomatic treatment with biochemical and ECG monitoring. The administration of cardioselective β-blockers to antagonise cardiac effects should only be done with extreme caution because of the risk of inducing bronchoconstriction

NURSING CONSIDERATIONS

Assess:

• Vital signs (temperature, pulse, respirations, BP); ECG, respiratory function, peak flow

Administer:

• By metered dose (inhalation) using nebuliser or via intermittent positive pressure ventilator, to be diluted with 0.9% sodium chloride solution

Perform/provide:

• Storage: inhalers and nebuliser solution protected from heat; nebuliser solution also from light

Evaluate:

• Therapeutic effect; relief of bronchospasm

• Tachycardia, palpitations and other side effects

Teach patient/family:

• Proper use and storage of inhaler and nebuliser solution

• About side effects and to report any of these to nurse or clinician

fentanyl citrate/ droperidol combination

Thalamonol

Func. class.: General anaesthetic/ opioid analgesic

Chem. class.: Phenylpiperone derivative

Legal class.: CD(Sch 2), POM

Action: Action at subcortical levels to reduce motor activity, produces neuroleptanalgesia

Uses: Premedication, adjunct to general and regional anaesthesia, maintenance of anaesthesia. Also for rapid relief of symptoms in intractable labyrinthine vertigo.

Dosage and routes:

Induction

• *Adult:* IV 6–8 ml followed by assisted ventilation

• *Child:* IM 0.4–1.5 ml

Premedication

• *Adult:* IM 1–2 ml 5–15 min before surgery or procedure

• *Child:* IM 0.03–0.045 ml/kg 5–15 min before surgery or procedure

Available forms include: Injection IM, IV 50 mcg fentanyl, 2.5 mg droperidol/ml

Side effects/adverse reactions:

RESP: Laryngospasm, bronchospasm, respiratory arrest

CNS: Dystonia, akathisia, flexion of arms, fine tremors, dizziness, anxiety, drowsiness, restlessness, hallucination, depression

CV: Tachycardia, hypotension, circulatory depression

EENT: Upward rotation of eyes, oculogyric crisis, blurred vision

INTEG: Chills, facial sweating, shivering, diaphoresis

GI: Nausea, vomiting

Contraindications: Hypersensitivity, severe depression, obstructive airways disease, treatment with MAOIs within 14 days, respiratory depression

Precautions: Elderly, increased intracranial pressure, cardiovascular disease (bradydysrhythmias), renal disease, liver disease, hypothyroidism Parkinson's disease, chronic obstructive airways disease

Pharmacokinetics:

IV: Onset 20 sec, peak 2–5 min, duration ½–2 hr

IM: Onset 7 min, duration 1–2 hr, metabolised in liver, excreted in urine metabolites (90%)

Interactions/incompatibilities:

• Increased CNS depression: alcohol, narcotics, barbiturates, antipsychotics or other CNS depressants

• Decreased effects of: amphetamines; anticonvulsants, anticoagulants

• Increased intraocular pressure: anticholinergics, antiparkinsonism drugs
• Increased side effects of: lithium
Treatment of overdose:
Administer naloxone 0.1–0.2 mg IV/IM as required to reverse effects. Respiratory support

NURSING CONSIDERATIONS

Assess:
• Baseline vital signs
Administer:
• Do not mix with barbiturates in solution
• Anticholinergics for extrapyramidal reaction
• Adult: IV followed by assisted ventilation or IM 5–15 minutes before surgery
• Child: IM route preferred
Perform/provide:
• Storage as Controlled Drug regulations and local procedures
Evaluate:
• Vital signs every 10 min during IV administration, every 30 min after IM dose
• Respiratory rate and function
• Observe for bradycardia, nausea, vomiting
• Therapeutic response: decreased anxiety, absence of vomiting, maintenance of anaesthesia
• Rigidity of skeletal muscles
• Extrapyramidal reactions: dystonia, akathisia
Teach patient/family:
• About effects of drug; drowsiness, lightheadedness
• To use deep breathing, coughing after surgery to prevent increased secretions in lungs

ferrous fumarate

Fersaday, Fersamal, many combination products
Func. class.: Haematinic
Chem. class.: Iron compound
Legal class.: P

Action: Replaces iron stores needed for red blood cell development, energy and O_2 transport, utilisation; drug contains 33% iron
Uses: Iron deficiency anaemia
Dosage and routes:
• *Adult:* By mouth 300–600 mg of ferrous fumarate (100–200 mg of elemental iron) daily
• *Full-term infant and child:* By mouth 2.5–5 ml of Fersamal syrup (22.5–45 mg of elemental iron) twice daily
• *Premature infant:* 0.6 ml/kg daily of Fersamal syrup (5.4 mg/kg of elemental iron). Increase to 2.4 ml/kg daily (21.6 mg/kg of elemental iron)
Available forms include: Tablets 200 mg (65 mg iron), 304 mg (100 mg iron); capsules 290 mg (100 mg iron); modified-release capsules 330 mg (110 mg iron); syrup 140 mg (45 mg iron) in 5 ml
Side effects/adverse reactions:
GI: Nausea, constipation, epigastric pain, black and red tarry stools, vomiting, diarrhoea
Contraindications: Hypersensitivity, ulcerative colitis/regional enteritis, haemosiderosis/haemochromatosis, active peptic ulcer disease, haemolytic anaemia, anaemia (long-term)
Precautions: Treated or controlled peptic ulcer
Pharmacokinetics:
By mouth: Excreted in faeces, urine, skin, breast milk
Interactions/incompatibilities:
• Decreased absorption of tetra-

cycline, ciprofloxacin, quinolones, penicillamine
• Decreased absorption of iron preparations: chloramphenicol, antacids
• Increased absorption of iron preparation: ascorbic acid

Clinical assessment:
• Blood studies: haematocrit, Hb reticulocytes, bilirubin before treatment, at least monthly
• Cause of iron loss or anaemia, including salicylates, sulphonamides, antimalarials, quinidine

Lab. test interferences:
False-positive: Occult blood

Treatment of overdose: Induce vomiting; give eggs, milk until lavage can be done. Administer desferroxamime IM and orally to remove iron. Fluid replacement essential

NURSING CONSIDERATIONS

Assess:
• Nutritional status, amount of iron in diet

Administer:
• Between meals for best absorption, may give with juice; do not give with antacids or milk, delay at least 1 hr; if GI symptoms occur, give with food, absorption may be decreased
• Syrup through plastic straw to avoid discolouration of tooth enamel; dilute thoroughly
• At least 1 hr before bedtime to avoid GI pain

Evaluate:
• Therapeutic response: improvement in haematocrit, Hb, reticulocytes, decreased fatigue, weakness
• Toxicity: nausea, vomiting, diarrhoea (green then tarry stools), haematemesis, pallor, cyanosis, shock, coma
• Elimination; if constipation occurs, increase fluid intake, bulk, activity

Teach patient/family:
• That iron will change colour of stools to black or dark green
• That iron poisoning may occur if increased beyond recommended level
• Not to crush; swallow tablet whole to prevent staining of teeth
• Keep out of reach of children
• Do not substitute one iron salt for another; elemental iron content differs (e.g. 300 mg ferrous fumarate contains about 100 mg elemental iron whereas 300 mg ferrous gluconate contains only about 30 mg elemental iron)
• Avoid reclining position for 15–30 min after taking drug to avoid oesophageal corrosion
• That medication may be needed for 6 months or more
• To increase amount of iron in diet (meat, dark green leafy vegetables, dried beans, dried fruits, eggs)

ferrous gluconate

Fergon
Func. class.: Haematinic
Chem. class.: Iron compound
Legal class.: P

Action: Replaces iron stores needed for red blood cell development; drug contains 11.6% iron

Uses: Iron deficiency anaemia

Dosage and routes:

Therapeutic
• *Adult:* By mouth 300–600 mg 3 times a day
• *Child 6–12 yr:* By mouth 300–900 mg daily

Prophylactic
• *Adult:* By mouth 600 mg daily
• *Child 6–12 yr:* By mouth 300–400 mg daily

Available forms include: Tablets 300 mg

Side effects/adverse reactions:
GI: Nausea, constipation, epigastric pain, black and red tarry stools, vomiting, diarrhoea
INTEG: Temporarily discoloured tooth enamel, eyes
Precautions: Hypersensitivity, ulcerative colitis/regional enteritis, haemosiderosis/haemochromatosis, peptic ulcer disease, haemolytic anaemia, cirrhosis, anaemia (long-term)
Pharmacokinetics:
Period of onset: Excreted in faeces, urine, through skin, breast milk
Interactions/incompatibilities:
- Decreased absorption of both drugs: tetracycline, zinc salts
- Decreased absorption of iron preparations: chloramphenicol, antacids
- Decreased absorption of: penicillamine, quinolone antibiotics
- Increased absorption of iron preparation: ascorbic acid

Clinical assessment:
- Blood studies: haematocrit, Hb, reticulocytes, bilirubin before treatment, at least monthly
- Only with vitamin E supplements to infants or haemolytic anaemia may occur
- Cause of iron loss or anaemia including salicylates, sulphonamides, antimalarials, quinidine
- Therapeutic response: improvement in haematocrit, Hb, reticulocytes, decreased fatigue, weakness

Lab. test interferences:
False positive: occult blood
Treatment of overdose: Induce vomiting; give eggs, milk until lavage can be done

NURSING CONSIDERATIONS

Assess:
- Cause of iron loss or deficiency
- Blood tests for haematocrit, Hb, reticulocytes, bilirubin before and monthly during treatment
- Prophylactic or therapeutic treatment

Administer:
- Orally about 1 hr before meals with water or juice; do not give with antacids or milk. Decreased absorption if stomach not empty
- After food if gastrointestinal symptoms occur
- At least 1 hr before bed time to diminish GI irritation

Perform/Provide:
- Store in childproof, light resistant container
- Mouth care, regular brushing teeth/dentures

Evaluate:
- Therapeutic response: improvement of haematocrit, Hb, reticulocytes, decreased fatigue, weakness
- Signs of toxicity: nausea, vomiting, diarrhoea (dark green tarry stools), haematemesis, pallor, cyaniosis, shock, coma
- Elimination—for constipation, increase fluids, fibre and bulk in diet, physical activity
- Diet: increase amount of iron rich foods

Teach patient/family:
- That iron will change stools to dark green or black and often cause constipation
- That iron poisoning is dangerous, never increase recommended doses
- Keep safe from children
- To swallow whole as iron stains teeth/dentures
- Not to replace their iron tablets for others as iron contents differ
- To avoid lying down for 15–30 min after taking drug as oesophageal corrosion can occur
- To eat an iron-rich diet

ferrous sulphate

Feospan, Ferrograd, Slow-Fe
Func. class.: Haematinic
Chem. class.: Iron compound
Legal class.: P

Action: Replaces iron stores needed for red blood cell development. Drug contains 20% iron
Uses: Iron deficiency anaemia, prophylaxis for iron deficiency in pregnancy
Dosage and routes:
Therapeutic
• *Adult:* By mouth 200–600 mg daily in divided doses
• *Child 6–12 yr:* By mouth 400 mg in divided doses
• *1–5 yr:* By mouth 240 mg in divided doses
• *Less than 1 year:* By mouth 120 mg in divided doses
Prophylactic
• *Adult:* By mouth 200 mg daily
Available forms include: Tablets 200 mg; modified-release tablets 160, 325 mg; modified-release capsules 150 mg; Paediatric Ferrous Sulphate Mixture 1.2%
Side effects/adverse reactions:
GI: Nausea, constipation, epigastric pain, black and red tarry stools, vomiting, diarrhoea
INTEG: Temporarily discoloured tooth enamel, eyes
Precautions: Hypersensitivity, ulcerative colitis/regional enteritis, haemosiderosis/haemochromatosis, peptic ulcer disease, haemolytic anaemia, cirrhosis, anaemia (long-term)
Pharmacokinetics:
By mouth: Excreted in faeces, urine, through skin, breast milk
Interactions/incompatibilities:
• Decreased absorption of both drugs: tetracycline, zinc salts
• Decreased absorption of iron preparations: chloramphenicol, antacids
• Decreased absorption of: penicillamine
• Increased absorption of iron preparation: ascorbic acid
Clinical assessment:
• Blood studies: haematocrit, Hb, reticulocytes, bilirubin before treatment, at least monthly
• Only with vitamin E supplements to infants or haemolytic anaemia may occur
• Only after determining cause of anaemia
Lab. test interferences:
False-positive: Occult blood
Treatment of overdose: Induce vomiting, give eggs, milk until lavage can be done

NURSING CONSIDERATIONS

Assess:
• Cause of iron loss or deficiency
• Blood tests for Hb, reticulocytes, haematocrit, bilirubin before and monthly during treatment
• Prophylactic or therapeutic treatment
Administer:
• Orally about 1 hr before meals with water or juice; do not give with antacids or milk. Decreased absorption if stomach is not empty
• At least 1 hr before bed time to diminish GI irritation
• After food if gastrointestinal symptoms occur
• Mixture to be taken well diluted with water
Perform/provide:
• Store in childproof, light-resistant container
• Mouth care, regular brushing of teeth/dentures
Evaluate:
• Therapeutic response: improvement of Hb, reticulocytes, haematocrit, decreased fatigue, weakness
• Signs of toxicity: nausea, vomiting, diarrhoea (dark green tarry

stools) cynanosis, pallor, haematemesis, shock, coma
• Elimination: for constipation increase fluids, fibre and bulk in diet, physical activity
• Diet: increase amount of iron rich foods

Teach patient/family:
• That iron will change stools to dark green or black and often causes constipation
• That iron poisoning is dangerous, never increase recommended doses
• Keep safe from children
• To swallow whole as iron stains teeth
• Not to replace their iron tablets for others as the iron contents differ
• To avoid lying down for 15–30 min after taking drug as oesophageal corrosion can occur
• To eat an iron-rich diet

filgrastim (granulocyte-colony stimulating factor; G-CSF) ▼

Neupogen
Func. class.: Haematopoietic growth factor
Chem. class.: Peptide
Legal class.: POM

Action: Stimulates the production and release of functioning neutrophils from the bone marrow
Uses: Reducing the duration and severity of neutropenia associated with cytotoxic chemotherapy of non-myeloid malignancies; reducing the duration of neutropenia in myeloablative therapy followed by bone-marrow transplantation
Dosage and routes:
Cytotoxic-induced neutropenia
• *Adult:* By subcutaneous injection or IV infusion 500,000 units (5 mcg)/kg daily started not less than 24 hr after cytotoxic chemotherapy, continued until neutrophil count in normal range
Myeloablative therapy followed by bone marrow transplantation
• *Adult:* By IV infusion over 30 min or 24 hr or by SC infusion over 24 hr 1 million units (10 mcg)/kg daily, started not less than 24 hr following cytotoxic chemotherapy after bone marrow infusion, and continued until sustained neutrophil recovery is seen
Available forms include: Injection, 30 million units (300 mcg)/ml; 1, 1.6 ml vials
Side effects/adverse reactions:
CV: Transient hypotension
ELECT: Raised serum uric acid levels
GI: Transient elevation of liver enzymes
GU: Dysuria
MS: Musculoskeletal pain
Contraindications: Hypersensitivity
Precautions: Pregnancy; breastfeeding; myelodysplasia; myeloid leukaemias
Interactions:
• Possibly enhanced myelosuppression if given within 24 hr of cytotoxic chemotherapy
Incompatibilities: Sodium chloride 0.9% iv solutions
Treatment of overdose: Supportive and symptomatic treatment. Discontinuation of treatment usually results in a 50% decrease in circulating neutrophils within 1–2 days, with a return to normal levels in 1–7 days

NURSING CONSIDERATIONS

Assess:
• Vital signs (temperature, pulse, respiration, BP), fluid balance

• Full blood count including platelets

Administer:

• IV infusion (started not less than 24 hr after antineoplastic chemotherapy)

• By subcutaneous injection

• If dilution is required 5% Dextrose should be used. If diluted to a final concentration of less than 200,000 U (2 mcg), 1 ml human serum albumin should first be added to a final concentration of 2 mg/ml to prevent drug absorption to infusion apparatus

Perform/provide:

• Platelet count twice weekly

• Storage: in a refrigerator or at room temperature for a single period of up to 7 days

• All supportive measures for primary disease

Evaluate:

• Therapeutic effect, reduction/absence of infection

• Side effects including enhanced myelosuppression, musculoskeletal pain, tumour growth

• Urinary output (dysuria occurs occasionally)

Teach patient/family:

• About the drug and its side effects

• To report any side effects promptly to nurse or clinician

• Technique for administration (if being carried out by patient or family member)

• To store the drug in a refrigerator

---

finasteride

Proscar

Func. class.: Anti-androgen
Chem. class.: Enzyme inhibitor
Legal class.: POM

Action: Inhibits the action of the enzyme 5-alpha reductase, preventing the conversion of testosterone to the more potent androgen, dihydrotestosterone

Uses: Treatment and control of benign prostatic hyperplasia

Dosage and routes:

• By mouth 5 mg once daily

Available forms include: Tablets, 5 mg

Side effects/adverse reactions:

GU: Impotence, decreased libido, decreased ejaculatory volume

Contraindications: Hypersensitivity

Precautions: Some signs of prostate cancer may be masked by finasteride; disease should be screened for before commencing therapy; large residual urinary volume/severely diminished urine flow (risk of obstructive uropathy until benefit of therapy seen); men with sexual partners who are pregnant or capable of becoming so should avoid exposing partner to semen (e.g. by use of a condom)

Interactions: N/A

Incompatibilities: N/A

Lab. test interferences: Reduces levels of serum markers of prostatic cancer such as prostate specific antigen

Treatment of overdose: Supportive and symptomatic treatment, single doses of up to 400 mg have been well tolerated

NURSING CONSIDERATIONS

Assess:

• Known sensitivities

• Levels of sexual activity

• Fluid balance, urinary flow

Perform/provide:

• Storage in a lightproof container

Evaluate:

• Therapeutic effect, improved urinary flow, reduction in size of prostatic tissue

• Side effects

Teach patient/family:

• About the drug and side effects

• That women who are pregnant or might become pregnant should

not crush or break tablets
- That impotence, decreased libido and decreased ejaculatory volume will occur but improve after treatment finishes
- That despite the GU side effects a condom should be worn if the woman is pregnant or likely to become pregnant (drug is excreted in semen)

flavoxate hydrochloride

Urispas
Func. class.: Antimuscarinic; smooth muscle relaxant
Chem. class.: Flavone derivative
Legal class.: POM

Action: Relaxes smooth muscles in urinary tract
Uses: Relief of nocturia, incontinence, suprapubic pain, dysuria, frequency associated with urologic conditions (symptomatic only)
Dosage and routes:
- *Adult:* By mouth 200 mg 3 times a day

Available forms include: Tablets 100 mg, 200 mg
Side effects/adverse reactions:
HAEM: Leucopenia, eosinophilia
CNS: Anxiety, restlessness, dizziness, convulsions, headache, drowsiness, confusion
CV: Palpitations, sinus tachycardia, hypotension
GI: Nausea, vomiting, anorexia, abdominal pain, constipation
GU: Dysuria
INTEG: Urticaria, dermatitis
EENT: Blurred vision, increased intraocular tension, dry mouth, throat
Contraindications: Hypersensitivity, intestinal obstruction or atony, severe ulcerative colitis, toxic megacolon, bladder outflow obstruction, glaucoma
Precautions: Pregnancy, lactation, suspected glaucoma, children under 12 yr
Pharmacokinetics: Excreted in urine

NURSING CONSIDERATIONS

Evaluate:
- Urinary status: dysuria, frequency, nocturia, incontinence
- Allergic reactions: rash, urticaria; if these occur, drug should be discontinued

Teach patient/family:
- To avoid hazardous activities; dizziness may occur
- On all aspects of drug therapy: dosage, routes, side effects, when to notify clinician

flecainide acetate

Tambocor
Func. class.: Anti-arrhythmic (Class Ic)
Chem. class.: Lignocaine analogue

Action: Increases electrical stimulation threshold of ventrical HIS-Purkinje system, which stabilises cardiac membrane
Uses: Ventricular tachyarrhythmias unresponsive to other therapy
Dosage and routes:
- *Adult:* Ventricular arrhythmias, by mouth 100 mg twice daily, maximum 400 mg daily, reduce after 5 days
- *Adult:* Supraventricular arrhythmias, 50 mg twice daily, maximum 300 mg daily
- *Adult:* Slow IV injection 2 mg/kg, maximum 150 mg; then IV infusion 15 mg/kg/hr for up to 24 hr; maximum total daily dose 600 mg; oral maintenance may be used instead of IV infusion

Available forms include: Tablets 50 mg, 100 mg; injection 10 mg/ml
Side effects/adverse reactions:

CNS: Headache, dizziness, involuntary movement, confusion, psychosis, restlessness, irritability, paraesthesia
EENT: Tinnitus, blurred vision, hearing loss
GI: Nausea, vomiting, anorexia
CV: Hypotension, bradycardia, angina, premature ventricular contraction, heart block, cardiovascular collapse, arrest, dysrhythmias
RESP: Dyspnoea, respiratory depression
INTEG: Rash, urticaria, oedema, swelling

Contraindications: Hypersensitivity, heart failure, asymptomatic ventricular ectopics, asymptomatic arrhythmias with history of myocardial infarction, long-standing atrial fibrillation where no attempt has been made to convert to sinus rhythm, significant valvular heart disease, sinus node dysfunction, 2nd/3rd degree atrioventricular block, bundle branch block, distal block unless pacing and resuscitation available

Precautions: Pregnancy, lactation, children elderly (reduce dose) renal disease, liver disease, congestive cardiac failure, respiratory depression, myasthenia gravis, cardiac pacemaker

Pharmacokinetics:
Period of onset: Peak 1 hr; half-life 7–20 hr; metabolised by liver, excreted unchanged by kidneys (10%), excreted in breast milk

Interactions/incompatibilities:
- May increase effects when used with: aminodarone cimetidine, propranolol, quinidine
- May decrease effects when used with: phenytoin

Lab. test interferences:
Increase: Creatinine phosphokinase

Treatment of overdose: O_2, artificial ventilation, ECG, administer dopamine for circulatory depression, administer diazepam or thiopentone for convulsions

NURSING CONSIDERATIONS

Assess:
- Baseline vital signs including temperature
- ECG before commencing drug

Administer:
- IV infusion diluted with 5% dextrose solution
- Cardiac monitoring in a specialist unit or ITU for IV administration
- Close observation for potential convulsions
- 4–6 hrly BP, TPR for oral use

Perform/provide:
- ECG continuously to determine increased PR or QRS segments; if these develop, discontinue

Evaluate:
- Blood levels of drug
- Malignant hyperthermia: tachypnoea, tachycardia
- Cardiac rate, respiration: rate, rhythm, character, continuously
- Respiratory status: rate, rhythm, lung fields for rales
- CNS effects: dizziness, confusion, psychosis, paraesthesia, convulsions; drug should be discontinued
- Lung fields, bilateral rales may occur in congestive cardiac failure patient
- Increased respiration, increased pulse; drug should be discontinued
- BP continuously for fluctuations
- Temperature and pulse rate. Report changes to clinician

Teach patient/family:
- To report any nausea, shortness of breath, dizziness, palpitations, rash or hearing loss to clinician
- To avoid hazardous activities if dizziness occurs

flucIorolone acetonide

Topilar

Func. class.: Corticosteroid, topical

Chem. class.: Fluorinated corticosteroid (potent)

Legal class.: POM

Action: Reduces inflammation

Uses: Severe inflammatory skin disorders, e.g. eczema in patients unresponsive to less potent corticosteroids

Dosage and routes:

- Apply sparingly twice daily; reduce strength and frequency as condition responds
- Undiluted: potent; Diluted: moderately potent

Available forms include: Cream, ointment 0.025%

Side effects/adverse reactions:

INTEG: Spread and worsening of untreated infection; thinning of the skin; irreversible striae atrophicae; perioral dermatitis; acne at site of application; mild depigmentation and vellus hair; increased hair growth

Contraindications:

- Untreated bacterial, fungal or viral skin infections
- Avoid if possible in infants

Clinical assessment:

- Reduce dose slowly

NURSING CONSIDERATIONS

Assess:

- Possibility of pregnancy
- Temperature

Administer:

- With appropriate anti-infective therapy for bacterial/fungal skin infections
- As a thin smear twice daily
- Use occlusion dressings if prescribed
- Avoid the eyes

Perform/provide:

- Store in cool place

Evaluate:

- Temperature 4-hrly
- Response to treatment
- Side effects
- Infection, worsening of condition

Teach patient/family:

- To apply sparingly. That nappies/plastic pants may increase absorption
- To report infection or worsening at once
- Avoid the eyes
- Not to use any other preparations
- Warn about skin changes, increased hair growth, etc.

flucloxacillin

Floxapen, Ladropen, Stafoxil, Staphlipen

Func. class.: Antibiotic antistaphylococcal

Chem. class.: Penicillinase-resistant penicillin

Legal class.: POM

Action: Bactericidal, interferes with bacterial cell wall synthesis. Resistant to degradation by bacterial penicillinases

Uses: Treatment of infections due to Gram-positive organisms, especially β-lactamase-producing staphylococci, including skin, soft tissue and respiratory tract infections, osteomyelitis, endocarditis, meningitis and septicaemia caused by sensitive organisms

Dosage and routes:

- *Adult:* By mouth 250 mg 6 hrly, at least 30 min before food; IM, 250 mg every 6 hr; IV, 0.25–1 g every 6 hr. Doses may be doubled in severe infection
- Osteomyelitis, endocarditis: up to 8 g daily in 3 or 4 divided doses
- Surgical prophylaxis: 1–2 g IV

at induction of anaesthesia followed by 500 mg by mouth, IV, IM 6-hrly for up to 72 hr
• In conjunction with systemic therapy: by nebuliser 125–250 mg 4 times a day; intrapleural 250 mg once daily; intra-articular 250–500 mg once daily
• *Child:* Under 2 yr, quarter adult dose; 2–10 yr, half adult dose
Available forms include: Capsules 250, 500 mg; oral mixture 125 mg/5 ml, 250 mg/5 ml; powder vials for preparing IV, IM, intra-articular, intrapleural injections, nebulisation solutions 250, 500 mg, 1 g
Side effects/adverse reactions:
GI: Nausea, diarrhoea, hepatitis, cholestatic jaundice, pseudomembranous colitis
INTEG: Skin rashes
CNS: Encephalopathy (in renal impairment, excessive doses)
Contraindications: Hypersensitivity to penicillins, ocular administration, porphyria
Precautions: Pregnancy, lactation
Pharmacokinetics: Peak plasma concentration about 1 hr after oral administration, after IM injection within 30 min. Half-life 1 hr, prolonged in neonates, 50–90% excreted in urine with 6 hr
Interactions/incompatibilities:
• Do not mix with aminoglycoside antibiotics in syringe, infusion bag or giving set, or with blood products, proteinaceous solutions, lipid emulsions for IV use
Clinical assessment:
• Sensitivity of bacterial cultures
Treatment of overdose: Symptomatic

NURSING CONSIDERATIONS
Assess:
• Site of infection: take specimens for culture and sensitivity before administration
• Check previous allergic response to penicillins; identify in red on patient's notes if any known allergies
• Temperature and other vital signs
• Bowel pattern
• Fluid balance
Administer:
• By mouth, to be taken at least 30 min before food. IV doses should be dissolved in 5 ml water for injections for each 250 mg, and injected over 3 to 4 min or added to IV infusion
• By mouth: 30 min before food with full glass of water
• IV: diluted with water for injection
Perform/provide:
• Monitor for allergic response: rashes, pyrexia, airway obstruction
Evaluate:
• Therapeutic response
• Reduction of temperature
• Effectiveness of treatment
• IV site for extravasation, phlebitis
Teach patient/family:
• To take before food
• To take all medication prescribed for length of time ordered

---

fluconazole

Diflucan
Func. class.: Antifungal
Chem. class.: Triazole
Legal class.: POM

Action: Inhibits fungal enzymes necessary for the synthesis of ergosterol
Uses: Acute or recurrent vaginal candidiasis, oropharyngeal candidiasis (including in immunocompromised patients), atrophic oral candidiasis associated with dentures, systemic candidiasis, mucosal candidiasis and cryptococciosis (including cryptococcal

meningitis). Prevention of relapse of cryptococcal disease in AIDS patients

Dosage and routes:

Vaginal candidiasis

• Doses for all indications can be given IV/by mouth without adjustment depending on condition of patient

• *Child over 1 yr with normal renal function:* superficial candidial infection, 1–2 mg/kg daily; systemic candidial/cryptococcal infection, 3–6 mg/kg or more daily, maximum 400 mg daily

• *Adult:* By mouth or IV 150 mg as single dose

Mucosal candidiasis

• Oropharyngeal candidiasis 50 mg daily for 7–14 days; other mucosal candidal infections, 50 mg daily for 14–30 days, maximum 100 mg daily.

Systemic candidiasis

• By mouth or IV 400 mg on day one then 200–400 mg daily according to response

Cryptococcosis

• Cryptococcal meningitis and other cryptococcal infections: 400 mg on day one then 200–400 mg daily; duration in meningitis usually 6–8 weeks

• Prevention of relapse of cryptococcal meningitis in patients with AIDS: at least 100 mg daily

Available forms include: Capsules 50, 150, 200 mg; powder for oral suspension, 50 or 200 mg/5 ml; injection 2 mg/ml, 25 ml, 100 ml vials

Side effects/adverse reactions:

GI: Nausea, abdominal discomfort, diarrhoea, flatulence, abnormalities of liver function

INTEG: Rash

Contraindications: Hypersensitivity to triazoles, lactation, pregnancy

Precautions: Renal impairment, toxicity, children

Pharmacokinetics: Rapidly and completely absorbed orally, 80% excreted unchanged in urine. Plasma half-life 30 hr

Interactions/incompatibilities:

• Potentiates effects of anticoagulants

• Increases blood levels of sulphonylurea oral hypoglycaemics and phenytoin

• Effectiveness reduced by rifampicin

Clinical assessment:

• Culture and sensitivity

• Anti-emetics for nausea

• Consider stopping if liver function tests abnormal, rash develops

Treatment of overdose: Gastric lavage and supportive treatment. Removable by haemodialysis if considered necessary

NURSING CONSIDERATIONS

Assess:

• Fluid balance (renal impairment), temperature

Administer:

• Increase dosage interval or reduce dosage in patients with impaired renal function receiving multiple dose therapy

• With food, avoid alkalis within 2 hr

Perform/provide:

• Adequate oral hygiene if used for oral conditions

Evaluate:

• Side effects, e.g. rashes, signs of liver toxicity (jaundice, pale stools)

• Therapeutic response, improvement

Teach patient/family:

• To take at regular intervals and always finish course unless told otherwise

• That long-term treatment is sometimes required

• To avoid other medicines

• Inform about side effects especially jaundice, pale stools etc. See clinician if side effects occur.

Warn not to take at same time as indigestion medicines

flucytosine

Alcobon

Func. class.: Antifungal

Chem. class.: Pyrimidine (fluorinated)

Legal class.: POM

Action: Converted to fluorouracil within fungal cell and interferes with protein synthesis

Uses: Infections with *Candida* spp (septicaemia, endocarditis, pulmonary, urinary tract infections), *Cryptococcus* spp (meningitis, pulmonary, urinary tract infections), *Torulopsis glabrata*, *Hansenula* spp

Dosage and routes:

• *Adult and child:* By mouth or IV 200 mg/kg daily in 4 doses

Available forms include: Tablets 500 mg; IV infusion 10 mg/ml, 250 ml bottle

Side effects/adverse reactions:

INTEG: Rash

CNS: Headache, confusion, dizziness, sedation, hallucinations

GI: Nausea, vomiting, anorexia, diarrhoea, cramps, enterocolitis, altered liver function tests, hepatitis, bowel perforation (rare)

HAEM: Thrombocytopenia, agranulocytosis, anaemia, leucopenia, pancytopenia

GU: Increased blood urea nitrogen, creatinine

Contraindications: Hypersensitivity, pregnancy

Precautions: Renal, hepatic disease, bone marrow depression, blood dyscrasias, radiation/ chemotherapy

Pharmacokinetics:

Period of onset: Peak 2½–6 hr, half-life 3–6 hr, excreted in urine (unchanged), well-distributed to CSF, aqueous humour, joints

Interactions/incompatibilities:

• Synergism: Amphotericin B

Clinical assessment:

• Blood studies: full blood count, including platelets at regular intervals

• Drug level during treatment in renal impairment; therapeutic level 25–50 mcg/ml, maximum 80 mcg/ml

• Prescribe drug only after culture and sensitivity confirms organism, drug needed to treat condition

• Few tablets at a time to decrease nausea, vomiting over 15 min

• Therapeutic response: decreased fever, malaise, rash, negative culture for infecting organism

• For renal toxicity: increasing blood urea nitrogen, serum creatinine; if serum creatinine greater than 1.7 mg/100 ml, dosage may be reduced

• For hepatotoxicity: check regularly for increasing aspartate aminotransferase, alanine aminotransferase, alkaline phosphatase

• For blood dyscrasias, fatigue, bruising, malaise, dark urine

NURSING CONSIDERATIONS

Assess:

• Baseline vital signs

• After samples taken for culture and sensitivity tests

Administer:

• Infuse via a giving set incorporating a 15 micron filter, over 20 to 40 min; may be given directly into a vein, through a central venous catheter, or by intraperitoneal infusion

Perform/provide:

• Symptomatic treatment as ordered for adverse reactions: aspirin, antihistamines, antiemetics, antispasmodics

Evaluate:

• Vital signs every 15–30 min during first infusion, note changes in

pulse and BP
- Therapeutic response
- For side effects

Teach patient/family:
- That long-term therapy may be needed to clear infection (1–2 months depending on type of infection)
- To report symptoms of blood dyscrasias; fatigue, bruising, malaise, dark urine

fludrocortisone acetate

Florinef

Func. class.: Corticosteroid
Chem. class.: Mineralocorticoid
Legal class.: POM

Action: Mimics endogenous adrenal hormones, promotes increased reabsorption of sodium and loss of potassium from the renal tubules

Uses: Adrenal insufficiency, salt-losing adrenogenital syndrome

Dosage and routes:
- *Adult:* By mouth 50–300 mcg daily
- *Child:* By mouth 5 mcg/kg daily

Available forms include: Tablets 100 mcg

Side effects/adverse reactions:

INTEG: Acne, poor wound healing, ecchymosis, petechiae, hirsutism, skin thinning, increased sweating, flushing

CNS: Depression, headache, mood changes, vertigo, convulsions, raised intracranial pressure, paraesthesia

CV: Hypertension, circulatory collapse, thrombophlebitis, embolism, tachycardia

HAEM: Thrombocytopenia

MS: Fractures, osteoporosis, weakness, proximal myopathy

GI: Diarrhoea, nausea, abdominal distention, GI haemorrhage, increased appetite, pancreatitis, ulcerative oesophagitis, peptic ulcer

EENT: Fungal infections, increased intraocular pressure, blurred vision, cataracts

ELECT: Sodium and fluid retention, hypokalaemia, hypokalaemic alkalosis

ENDO: Cushingoid states, menstrual irregularities, precipitation of diabetes mellitus, reduced adrenocortical stress response

METAB: Hyperglycaemia

SYST: Weight gain

Contraindications: Diseases causing sodium retention

Precautions: Psychosis, hypersensitivity, idiopathic thrombocytopenia, acute glomerulonephritis, amoebiasis, myasthenia gravis, exathematous disease, recent intestinal anastomoses, chronic nephritis, diuretic colitis, viral or fungal infection, peptic ulcer, metastatic cancer, osteoporosis, diverticulitis, hypertension, previous steroid myopathy, pregnancy, diabetes mellitus, glaucoma, seizure disorders, ulcerative colitis hypothyroidism, cirrhosis, congestive cardiac failure

Pharmacokinetics:
Rapid and complete absorption, plasma peak 1–2 hr, half-life 30 min, metabolised by liver, excreted in urine

Interactions/incompatibilities:
- Decreased action of this drug: cholestyramine, colestipol, barbiturates, rifampicin, phenytoin, carbamazepine
- Decreased effects of: anticonvulsants, antidiabetics, toxoids, vaccines, antihypertensives, diuretics
- Increased side effects: salicylates, indomethacin, amphotericin B, digitalis preparations, diuretics, carbenoxolone

Clinical assessment:
- Potassium, blood sugar, urine

glucose while on long-term therapy; hypokalaemia and hyperglycaemia

Lab. test interferences:

False negative: Skin allergy tests

Treatment of overdose: Plenty of water by mouth. Monitor serum electrolytes; restrict and supplement intake accordingly

NURSING CONSIDERATIONS

Assess:

• Baseline weight

Administer:

• With food or milk to decrease GI symptoms

Perform/provide:

• Assistance with ambulation in patient with bone tissue disease to prevent fractures

• Assistance with other activities of living as required

Evaluate:

• Weight daily, notify clinician of weekly gain greater than 2 kg

• Temperature

• BP pulse 4 hrly, notify clinician if chest pain occurs

• Fluid balance, be alert for decreasing urinary output and increasing oedema

• Infection: increased temperature, WBC, even after withdrawal of medication; drug masks symptoms of infection

• Potassium depletion: paraesthesia, fatigue, nausea, vomiting, depression, polyuria, dysrhythmias, weakness

• Oedema, hypotension, cardiac symptoms

• Mental status: affect, mood, behavioural changes, aggression

Teach patient/family:

• That identity card as steroid user should be carried

• To notify clinician if therapeutic response decreases; dosage adjustment may be necessary

• That medication must not be stopped abruptly or adrenal crisis can result

• To avoid non-prescribed drugs: salicylates, alcohol in cough products, cold preparations unless directed by clinician

• All aspects of drug use, including Cushingoid symptoms

• Symptoms of adrenal insufficiency: nausea, anorexia, fatigue, dizziness, dyspnoea, weakness, joint pain

---

flumazenil

Anexate

Func. class.: Specific benzodiazepine antagonist

Chem. class.: Benzodiazepine analogue

Legal class.: POM

Action: Competes with benzodiazepines for receptors and reverses their anxiolytic and sedative effects

Uses: Reversal of benzodiazepine sedation in intensive care, after anaesthesia and short diagnostic procedures

Dosage and routes:

• *Adults:* Slow IV injection 200 mcg over 15 seconds, then 100 mcg at 1 min intervals if required (usual range 300–600 mcg; maximum total dose 1 mg or, in intensive care, 2 mg)

• IV infusion if drowsiness recurs after injection, 100–400 mcg/hr according to level of arousal

Available forms include: Injection, 100 mcg/ml 5 ml ampoule

Side effects/adverse reactions:

CNS: Over-rapid wakening leading to anxiety, fear, agitation; convulsions, symptoms of benzodiazepine withdrawal (anxiety attacks, tachycardia, sweating, dizziness) in long-term benzodiazepine users

GI: Nausea, vomiting

INTEG: Flushing

CV: Transient increase in heart

rate, BP, in intensive care patients

Contraindications: Epileptics who have received prolonged benzodiazepine therapy, hypersensitivity to benzodiazepines

Precautions: Benzodiazepine dependence, anxiety, after major surgery ensure neuromuscular blockade is cleared before giving drug, avoid rapid administration; hepatic impairment, pregnancy, lactation

Pharmacokinetics: Metabolised in liver, half-life 50 min, excreted in urine as inactive metabolites

Interactions/incompatibilities:

- Decreased effects of: benzodiazepines, zopiclone
- May unmask toxic effects of drugs taken in overdose (e.g. tricyclic antidepressants)

NURSING CONSIDERATIONS

Assess:

- Ensure patient is not receiving Benzodiazepine therapy
- Baseline vital signs

Administer:

- Repeat doses may be necessary as drug is short acting
- IV very slowly or by continuous infusion
- Can be diluted in saline or dextrose
- Infusion solution must be discarded after 24 hr

Perform/provide:

- Continuous monitoring for 6 hr after a dose
- Respiratory rate and level of awareness; these may vary during treatment

Evaluate:

- Pulse, BP—tachycardia and hypertension may occur intensive care
- Avoid rapid administration
- For therapeutic action—reversal of sedative effects of benzodiazepines
- Need for repeat dose if drug effect is wearing off

Teach patient/family:

- Essential to avoid operating machinery or driving a vehicle for 24 hr

flunitrazepam

Rohypnol ~~NHS~~

Func. class.: Hypnotic

Chem. class.: Benzodiazepine

Legal class.: CD Benz POM

Action: Depresses CNS with sedative effect

Uses: Short-term treatment of insomnia

Dosage and routes:

- By mouth, 0.5–1 mg half an hour before bedtime; may be increased to 2 mg in severe insomnia; reduce starting dose to 0.5 mg and maximum to 1 mg in elderly patients

Available forms include: Tablets, 1 mg

Side effects/adverse reactions:

GI: GI upsets, jaundice

CVS: Hypotension, thromboembolic effects

HAEM: Blood dyscrasias (rare)

INTEG: Skin rashes

GU: Urinary retention

CNS: Drowsiness and lightheadedness the following day; ataxia, confusion, especially in elderly; headaches, vertigo, dependence, paradoxical aggression, excitement, unmasking of depression, changes in libido, visual disturbances

Contraindications: Acute pulmonary insufficiency, respiratory depression, porphyria, phobic or obsessional states, psychoses, hypersensitivity to benzodiazepines

Precautions: History of drug abuse or personality disorder; renal or hepatic impairment; pregnancy,

lactation; reduce dose in elderly or debilitated patients; avoid prolonged use and abrupt withdrawal; where morning alertness important
Pharmacokinetics: Extensively metabolised in the liver; half-life 22 hr, excreted as metabolites in urine, 80% protein bound
Interactions/incompatibilities:
• Increased action of both drugs: alcohol, CNS depressants
• Increased toxicity of: antiepileptics
Treatment of overdose: Gastric lavage if performed promptly, supportive treatment, flumazenil may be used to antagonise
NURSING CONSIDERATIONS
Assess:
• Pulse and blood pressure
• All drugs patient is on for compatibility. (Elderly often hoard drugs)
Administer:
• Drug to be taken before retiring
• Use lowest dose possible to relieve symptoms
• Avoid long-term use
Perform/provide:
• Assist with mobility (mainly elderly)
Evaluate:
• Therapeutic response; decreased insomnia
• For suicidal tendencies which may be released in depressed patients
• Side effects, drowsiness, ataxia, headaches, changes in libido and urinary retention
• Drug dependency if used long term
Teach patient/family:
• To use the lowest dose
• Not to discontinue medication without medical advice. Drug should be tapered off slowly
• Not to sleep during the day
• That suitable physical activity may aid sleep
• To avoid driving or hazardous activity if drowsiness occurs
• Not to drink coffee, take or do anything at night to interfere with sleep

---

fluocinolone acetonide

Synalar, Synalar 1 in 4 dilution, Synalar 1 in 10 dilution, Synalar C, Synalar N combination products
Func. class.: Corticosteroid, topical
Chem. class.: Fluorinated corticosteroid, potent
Legal class.: POM

Action: Reduces inflammation
Uses: Inflammatory skin disorders, e.g. eczema, seborrhoeic dermatitis, psoriasis
Dosage and routes: Apply topical preparations sparingly, 2–3 times daily; reduce strength and frequency as condition responds
Available forms include: Cream, 0.025%, 0.00625%, 0.0025%, 0.025% with clioquinol 3%, 0.025% with neomycin sulphate 0.5%, all in water-miscible base; gel, 0.025% in water miscible base; ointment, 0.025%, 0.00625%
Side effects/adverse reactions:
INTEG: Spread and worsening of untreated infection, thinning of the skin, irreversible striae atrophicae, perioral dermatitis, acne at site of application, mild depigmentation, increased hair growth
ENDO: Suppression of hypothalamic-pituitary-adrenal axis producing growth retardation and suppressed plasma cortisol, Cushing's syndrome, reduced glucose tolerance
Contraindications: Untreated bacterial (except Synalar C/N), fungal (except Synalar C) or viral skin infections, napkin eruptions, perioral dermatitis

Precautions: Pregnancy, lactation, occlusive dressings

Clinical assessment:

• Prescribe for not more than 5 days for treatment of face or children

• Use for shortest possible time on smallest possible area

NURSING CONSIDERATIONS

Administer:

• Cleanse area thoroughly before application especially if occlusive dressing required

• Apply sparingly

• Use occlusive dressings with care (increase side effects, whilst increasing effect)

Observe:

• For local atrophic skin changes in long-term therapy: striae, thinning skin

• For systemic signs of adrenal suppression

Evaluate:

• Unfavourable reactions: cease treatment at once if these occur

• Therapeutic response: less inflammation, itching, etc.

Teach patient/family:

• To avoid drug contact with eyes

• To avoid sunlight on treated areas as burns may occur

• About proper use of cream

• About side effects

• That cream is not a cure but alleviates symptoms

fluorescein sodium

Fluorets, Minims Fluorescein Sodium

Func. class.: Diagnostic agent, opthalmic

Chem. class.: Fluorescent dye

Legal class.: POM

Action: Allows breaks in the corneal tissue to absorb dye and show up as bright green under cobalt blue light

Uses: Diagnostic aid in identifying foreign bodies, fitting hard contact lenses, fundus photography, tonometry, identifying corneal abrasions, retinal angiography

Dosage and routes:

• *Adult:* Instil 1 drop of eye drops, or enough to stain damaged area, or wet strip with sterile water and touch conjunctiva or fornix, flush eye with irrigating solution

Available forms include: Eye drops 1%, 2%; impregnated paper strips 1 mg

Side effects/adverse reactions:

EENT: Stinging, burning, conjunctival redness

Contraindications: Hypersensitivity, Soft contact lenses

Interactions/incompatibilities: None known

NURSING CONSIDERATIONS

Administer:

• Solution, encourage patient to close eyelids for 1 min if possible

Evaluate:

• Eye colour after application: defects are green under normal light or bright yellow under cobalt blue light

Teach patient/family:

• Solution may sting or burn

fluorometholone (ophthalmic)

FML

Func. class.: Anti-inflammatory, ophthalmic

Chem. class.: Corticosteroid

Legal class.: POM

Action: Decreases inflammation, resulting in decreased pain, photophobia, hyperaemia, cellular infiltration

Uses: Steroid-responsive inflammation of conjunctiva, cornea and anterior globe

Dosage and routes:

• *Adult and child:* Instil 1–2 drops into conjunctival sac hrly for 2 days then reduce frequency to 2 to 4 times a day

Available forms include: Ophthalmic suspension 0.1%

Side effects/adverse reactions:

EENT: Increased intraocular pressure, poor corneal wound healing, increased possibility of corneal infections, glaucoma, cataract, optic nerve damage, decreased acuity, visual field defects, thinning of facial skin, striae, telangiectasia around eye

Contraindications: Hypersensitivity, acute superficial herpes simplex, fungal/viral diseases of the eye or conjunctiva, active diabetes mellitus, ocular tuberculosis, infections of the eye, soft contact lenses

Precautions: Corneal abrasions, glaucoma, thinning of the cornea/sclera, pregnancy

Interactions/incompatibilities:
Soft contact lenses

Clinical assessment:

• Intraocular pressure and signs of fungal infection should be checked during prolonged therapy

NURSING CONSIDERATIONS

Administer:

• After shaking

Evaluate:

• Allergic reactions: redness, itching, swelling, lacrimation

• Therapeutic response: absence of swelling, redness, exudate

Teach patient/family:

• Instillation method: pressure on lacrimal sac for 1 min

• Not to share eye medications with others

• If both eyes being treated do not interchange right eye/left eye drops

• That soft contact lenses may not be used

fluorouracil (systemic)

Fluoro-uracil
Func. class.: Antineoplastic, antimetabolite
Chem. class.: Pyrimidine analogue
Legal class.: POM

Action: Inhibits DNA synthesis; interferes with cell replication by competitively inhibiting thymidylate synthesis

Uses: Cancer of breast, colon, rectum, stomach, pancreas

Dosage and routes:
Doses are highly variable, and dependent on local treatment protocols, concomitant therapy and tumour type; the following dose schedules have been used

• *Adult:* By mouth 15 mg/kg daily for 6 days, then 15 mg/kg once weekly

• *Adult:* IV/intra-arterial toxicity highly schedule-dependent; doses very variable, seek specialist advice

Available forms include: Capsules 250 mg; IV/intra-arterial injection 25 mg/ml

Side effects/adverse reactions:

HAEM: Thrombocytopenia, leucopenia, myelosuppression, anaemia

GI: Anorexia, stomatitis, diarrhoea, nausea, vomiting, haemorrhage

CVS: Angina, ECG changes, myocardial infarction, spasm of vein used for infusion

EENT: Epistaxis, lacrimation, photophobia

INTEG: Rash, alopecia, fever

CNS: Lethargy, malaise, weakness confusion, headache, acute cerebellar syndrome, nystagmus

Contraindications: Hypersensitivity, myelosuppression, pregnancy, serious infections, lactation

Precautions: Renal disease, hepatic disease, bone marrow depression, cardiovascular disease, radiation, chemotherapy, probable carcinogen

Pharmacokinetics: Half-life 10–20 min, 20 hr terminal, metabolised in the liver, excreted in the urine, crosses blood-brain barrier, oral absorption erratic

Interactions/incompatibilities:

- Increased toxicity/therapeutic potency: radiation, other antineoplastics, calcium folinate, α-interferon
- Decreased effect: allopurinol

Clinical assessment:

- Full blood count, differential white cell count, platelet count weekly; withhold drug if WBC is less than 3500/mm^3 or platelet count is less than 100,000/mm^3. Cancer treatment centres may have different guidelines

Lab. test interferences:

Increase: Thyroxine and liothyronine

Treatment of overdose: Supportive

NURSING CONSIDERATIONS

Assess:

- Baseline temperature, pulse, respirations, BP

Administer:

- HANDLING: take safety precautions appropriate to antineoplastic agents
- Following local antineoplastic (cytotoxic) policies
- After ensuring that clinician is aware of blood results
- IV infusion
- By mouth with or after food (capsules)
- Other medication by mouth if possible. Avoid IV, IM, SC routes to prevent infection and bruising
- Anti-emetics 30–60 min before treatment
- All other medications as prescribed including analgesics, antibiotics, anti-emetics, antispasmodics
- Injection solution may be given by mouth and added to fruit juice to mask taste if a liquid formulation is required

Perform/provide:

- Strict asepsis, protective isolation if WBC levels are low
- Strict fluid balance—or daily weight to indicate fluid overload
- Rinsing of mouth 3 or 4 times a day with water, or prescribed mouth washes, brushing of teeth 2 or 3 times a day with soft brush or cotton-tipped applicators for stomatitis; use unwaxed dental floss
- Nutritious diet with iron, vitamin supplements as ordered
- Consider patient's likes/dislikes and preferences
- Offer smaller meals more often if desirable

Evaluate:

- Bleeding due to thrombocytopenia: haematuria, bruising or petechiae, mucosa or orifices 8 hrly
- Food preferences; list likes, dislikes
- Inflammation of mucosa, breaks in skin
- Buccal cavity 8 hrly for dryness due to stomatitis, sores or ulceration, white patches, oral pain, bleeding, dysphagia
- Symptoms indicating severe allergic reaction: rash, urticaria, itching, flushing
- GI symptoms: frequency of stools, cramping
- Acidosis, signs of dehydration: rapid respirations, poor skin turgour, decreased urine output, dry skin, restlessness, weakness

Teach patient/family:

- Why protective isolation precautions are necessary, only if indicated
- To report any complaints, side effects to the nurse or clinician
- To avoid foods with citric acid, hot or rough texture if stomatitis is present

• Avoid highly spiced or salty foods
• Good mouth care and to report stomatitis

fluorouracil (topical)

Efudix
Func. class.: Antineoplastic, antimetabolite
Chem. class.: Pyrimidine analogue
Legal class.: POM

Action: Inhibits synthesis of DNA, RNA in susceptible cells
Uses: Topical for malignant skin conditions including keratoses, superficial basal cell carcinoma, Bowen's disease
Dosage and routes:
• *Adult:* Topical, apply to affected area once or twice a day, under occlusive dressing if lesion malignant
Available forms include: Cream 5%
Side effects/adverse reactions:
INTEG: Erythema and irritation of healthy skin around lesions
Contraindications: Hypersensitivity, pregnancy, breast-feeding
Pharmacokinetics: Systemic absorption normally negligible
NURSING CONSIDERATIONS
Administer:
• Gloves or applicator must be used; avoid spillage
• To affected area only
Evaluate:
• Therapeutic response: decreased size of lesion
• Area of body involved for redness, swelling
• Check oral cavity daily for stomatitis; if present discontinue drug, indicates systemic absorption
Perform/provide:
• An occlusive dressing if required
• Thorough washing of hands after application
Teach patient/family:
• To apply with care; care with washing of skin
• To avoid application on normal skin or getting cream in eyes
• To wash hands after application
• To discontinue use if rash or irritation occurs
• Not to change application; use exactly as prescribed
• To avoid sunlight or use sunscreen, photosensitivity may occur
• Lesion will disappear in 1–2 months

fluoxetine hydrochloride

Prozac
Func. class.: Antidepressant, serotonin reuptake inhibitor
Chem. class.: Phenylpropylamine derivative
Legal class.: POM

Action: Inhibits CNS neurone uptake of serotonin, but not of noradrenaline
Uses: Depression, bulimia nervosa
Dosage and routes:
• *Adult:* By mouth, depression 20 mg daily; bulimia 60 mg daily
Available forms include: Capsules 20 mg; liquid 20 mg/5 ml
Side effects/adverse reactions:
CNS: Headache, nervousness, insomnia, drowsiness, anxiety, tremor, dizziness, fatigue, sedation, poor concentration, abnormal dreams, agitation, convulsions, apathy, euphoria, hallucinations, delusions, psychosis, dyskinesia
GI: Nausea, diarrhoea, dry mouth, anorexia, dyspepsia, constipation, cramps, vomiting, taste changes, pancreatitis
INTEG: Sweating, rash, pruritus, urticaria
RESP: Infection, pharyngitis,

sinusitus, cough, dyspnoea, bronchitis, pulmonary inflammation/ fibrosis
CV: Vasculitis, cerebral vascular accident
MS: Pain, arthritis, twitching
GU: Dysmenorrhoea, decreased libido, urinary frequency, urinary tract infection, amenorrhoea, cystitis, impotence
SYST: Asthenia, fever
ENDO: Hyperprolactinaemia
HAEM: Thrombocytopenia
ELECT: Hyponatraemia
Contraindications: Hypersensitivity, severe renal failure, breast-feeding, unstable epilepsy, MAOIs within last 14 days
Precautions: Pregnancy, children, elderly, epilepsy, renal or hepatic impairment
Pharmacokinetics:
Period of onset: Peak 6–8 hr; metabolised in liver, excreted in urine; half-life 2–7 days, protein bound
Interactions/incompatibilities:
• Do not use MAOIs until at least 5 weeks after discontinuing fluoxetine, do not use fluoxeline for 14 days after discontinuing MAOIs
• Increased agitation: L-tryptophan
• Increased side effects: highly protein bound drugs (e.g. anticoagulants, hypoglycaemics), cyclic antidepressants, diazepam
• Changes in lithium levels
Clinical assessment:
• Perform ECG: flattening of the T wave, bundle branch block, atrioventricular block and dysrhythmias may occur in cardiac patients
Treatment of overdose: Gastric lavage, activated charcoal, then supportive measures

NURSING CONSIDERATIONS

Assess:
• Baseline observations including neutral status
Administer:
• Increase fluid intake and dietary fibre if constipation or urinary retention occur
• Give with food or milk to avoid gastric irritation
• Give at bedtime if sedation occurs during the day: the entire dose may be taken before retiring, although this regime may not be tolerated well by the elderly
• Provide frequent mouth care
• Store at room temperature: avoid freezing
• Supervise ambulant patients carefully once the drug has been administered, as drowsiness and dizziness occur
• Check to ensure that all capsules have been swallowed
Evaluate:
• Mental status: mood, affect, suicidal tendencies, increase in psychiatric symptomatology, depression, panic attacks
• Blood pressure lying and standing and pulse 4 hrly. If systolic blood pressure falls by 20 mmHg drug should be withheld and clinician informed. For patients with cardiovascular disease vital signs must be reported 4 hrly
• Weigh 4 times a week, as appetite may decrease
• Extrapyramidal symptoms in the elderly, indicated by rigidity, dystonia and akathisia
• Urinary retention, constipation
• Withdrawal symptoms: headache, nausea, vomiting, muscular pain and weakness; usually if drug is discontinued suddenly
• If alcohol is taken the drug must be withheld until the following morning
Teach patient/family:
• The drug may not be effective for 2–3 weeks
• Caution must be taken when driving or performing other activities requiring mental alertness as

drowsiness, dizziness and blurred vision may develop
• The drug must not be discontinued suddenly after long-term treatment as this may result in nausea, headache and malaise
• Alcohol and other CNS depressants must be avoided
• The clinician must be informed if patient/client becomes pregnant or if pregnancy and breast-feeding are planned

flupenthixol

Depixol, Depixol-Conc, Fluanxol
Func. class.: Antipsychotic/neuroleptic; antidepressant
Chem. class.: Thioxanthene
Legal class.: POM

Action: Dopamine antagonist
Uses: Schizophrenia and related disorders (but not mania or psychomotor hyperactivity), depressive illness, short-term adjunctive treatment of severe anxiety
Dosage and routes:
Schizophrenia and related disorders
• *Adult:* By mouth, 3–9 mg daily adjusted according to response; maximum 18 mg daily
• Depot injection, deep IM, 20–40 mg repeated at intervals of 2–4 weeks, adjusted according to response; maximum 400 mg weekly
Depression
• *Adult:* By mouth, initially 1 mg in morning, increased after 1 week to 2 mg if necessary; maximum dose, 3 mg; elderly patients, half standard dose, maximum dose, 2 mg; daily doses above 2 mg (1 mg in elderly) to be divided and second portion to be given before 4 pm
Available forms include: Tablets, 0.5, 1, 3 mg (as dihydrochloride) Injection (oily), 20 mg/ml, 100 mg/ml (both as decanoate)
Side effects/adverse reactions:
CNS: Reversible extrapyramidal symptoms, tardive dyskinesia, drowsiness, apathy, insomnia, nightmares, depression, agitation, aggression, restlessness, dizziness, headache, mental dulling, convulsions
HAEM: Agranulocytosis, leucopenia, leucocytosis, haemolytic anaemia
EENT: Dry mouth, nasal congestion, corneal and lens opacities, purple pigmentation of cornea, conjunctiva and retina, blurred vision
META: Menstrual disturbances, galactorrhoea, gynaecomastia, weight gain, hyperprolactinaemia, impaired thermoregulation
GI: Constipation, nausea, changes in liver function tests
GU: Difficulty with micturition, impotence, impaired ejaculation, urinary incontinence and frequency, changes in libido
INTEG: Rashes, purple pigmentation of skin, pain, nodule formation at injection site, photosensitisation
CV: Hypotension, tachycardia, arrhythmias, oedema, ECG changes
SYSTEM: Lupus erythematosus-like syndrome, jaundice, hypersensitivity, neuroleptic malignant syndrome
Contraindications: Porphyria, bone marrow depression, coma caused by CNS depressants, hypersensitivity, excitation, agitation, mania, severe depression requiring hospitalisation or electroconvulsive therapy, pregnancy, breast-feeding, hypersensitivity
Precautions: Cardiovascular or severe respiratory disease, renal or hepatic impairment, epilepsy, parkinsonism, phaeochromocy-

toma, hypothyroidism, myasthenia gravis, prostatic hypertrophy, history of jaundice or leucopenia; prescribe with caution in elderly particularly in very hot or cold weather, avoid abrupt withdrawal, senile state, alcohol withdrawal, brain damage

Pharmacokinetics: After depot injection, plasma concentrations maximal after 4–7 days; after oral administration, peak concentration within 3–8 hours. Metabolised in liver

Interactions/incompatibilities:

• Reduced effects of: antiepileptics, dopamine agonists (e.g. bromocriptine, levodopa, lysuride), adrenaline and other sympathomimetics, guanethidine, clonidine

• Increased anticholinergic effects: tricyclic antidepressants, anticholinergics

• Effects of the following possibly increased: digoxin, quinidine, diazoxide, neuromuscular blockers

Clinical assessment:

• Try test dose of injection before treatment as undesirable side effects are prolonged

• Titrate dose and dose interval according to individual response

• Perform blood counts if prolonged, unexpected fever

• Prescribe anticholinergic drugs if extrapyramidal symptoms are a problem

• Avoid abrupt withdrawal

• Short course/lowest dose possible

• Close supervision

• Monitor symptoms of tardive dyskinesia, diabetic control, concurrent anticoagulant treatment

Treatment of overdose:

• Gastric lavage following tablet ingestion

• Symptomatic and supportive therapy, treat extrapyramidal symptoms with anticholinergics

NURSING CONSIDERATIONS

Assess:

• Baseline pulse and BP

Administer:

After test dose is given

• With care as contact sensitisation may occur

• Ensure by aspiration before injecting, that drug not given intravascularly

• Not more than 2–3 ml oily injection at any one site

• Do not withdraw drug abruptly

Perform/provide:

• For extrapyramidal symptoms, give anticholinergic drugs as prescribed

• Boiled sweets, sips of water for dry mouth

Evaluate:

• Check to ensure patient swallowed tablets

• Patient may need help with walking and other tasks if blurred vision occurs

• Therapeutic response: improvement in schizophrenic state, depressed state, etc.

• For side effects

• BP – hypotension may occur

• Pulse – tachycardia and arrhythmias may occur

NB: Stop drug and inform clinician at once if signs of neuroleptic malignant syndrome occur (hyperthermia, fluctuating loss of consciousness, muscular rigidity, pallor, tachycardia, labile BP, sweating, urinary incontinence)

Teach patient/family:

• To rise slowly as fainting may occur

• To avoid alcohol

• To avoid driving and other activities requiring alertness until certain that drowsiness does not occur

• Check with clinician before taking non-prescribed preparations

• Side effects may include menstrual disturbances or impotence

• Not to discontinue the medi-

cation abruptly
• Report any side effects to clinician

fluphenazine

Modecate, Modeten
Func. class.: Antipsychotic/ neuroleptic
Chem. class.: Phenothiazine
Legal class.: POM

Action: Dopamine antagonist with α-adrenergic and cholinergic blocking action
Uses: Psychotic disorders, schizophrenia, short-term adjunct in severe anxiety
Dosage and routes:
Decanoate
• *Adult:* IM schizophrenia, other psychosis initially 12.5 mg test dose (6.25 mg in elderly) then 12.5–100 mg after 4–7 days; repeat after 14–35 days, adjusted to response
HCl
• *Adult:* By mouth, severe anxiety 1–2 mg twice daily, increasing to 2 mg twice daily if required; psychoses 2.5–10 mg daily in 2–3 doses; maximum 20 mg daily (10 mg in elderly)
Available forms include: Hydrochloride tablets 1, 2.5, 5 mg; injection IM, decanoate 25, 100 mg/ml
Side effects/adverse reactions:
RESP: Laryngospasm, dyspnoea, respiratory depression
CNS: Extrapyramidal symptoms: pseudoparkinsonism, akathisia, dystonia, tardive dyskinesia, drowsiness, headache, seizures
HAEM: Anaemia, leucopenia, leukocytosis, agranulocytosis
INTEG: Rash, dermatitis
EENT: Blurred vision, glaucoma, lens opacities
GI: Dry mouth, nausea, vomiting, anorexia, constipation, diarrhoea, jaundice, weight gain, changes in liver function tests
GU: Urinary retention, urinary frequency, enuresis, impotence, amenorrhoea, gynaecomastia
CV: Orthostatic hypotension, hypertension, cardiac arrest, ECG changes, tachycardia, oedema
SYST: Hyperthermia, hypothermia, neuroleptic malignant syndrome
Contraindications: Hypersensitivity, circulatory collapse, cerebral arteriosclerosis, coma, cardiac insufficiency, bone marrow depression, renal failure, severe depression, phaeochromocytoma, liver failure
Precautions: Pregnancy, lactation, seizure disorders, hypertension/ hypotension, hepatic disease, thyrotoxicosis, Parkinson's disease, narrow angle glaucoma, hypothyroidism, prostatic hypertrophy, myasthenia gravis, brain damage, alcohol withdrawal, severe respiratory disease, diabetes, epilepsy, very hot weather
Pharmacokinetics:
By mouth (HCl): Onset 1 hr, peak 2–4 hr, duration 6–8 hr
IM (Decanoate): Onset 1–3 days, peak 1–2 days, duration over 4 weeks, half-life 2.5–16 weeks. Metabolised by liver, excreted in urine (metabolites), enters breast milk
Interactions/incompatibilities:
• Enhanced CNS depression with: alcohol, hypnotics, strong analgesics, other CNS depressants
• Reduced effects of: antiepileptics, dopamine agonists (e.g. bromocriptine, levodopa, pergolide, lysuride), adrenaline and other sympathomimetics, guanethidine, clonidine
• Increased anticholinergic effects: anticholinergics, tricyclic antidepressants

• Increased toxicity of: quinidine, digoxin, neuromuscular blocking agents, lithium, anticoagulants
• Decreased absorbtion (HCl): antacids

Clinical assessment:
• Prescribe drugs for extra-pyramidal symptoms
• Blood counts if prolonged, unexplained fever
• Control of diabetes, symptoms of tardive dyskinesia, concurrent anticoagulant treatment
• Inspect for lens/corneal opacities during prolonged use

Treatment of overdose: Lavage, if orally ingested. Symptomatic treatment, treat extrapyramidal symptoms with antimuscarinics

NURSING CONSIDERATIONS

Administer:
• Withdraw treatment gradually
• Short course/lowest dose possible
• Under close supervision
• Not more than 2–3 ml injection at any one site

Perform/provide:
• Decreased noise input by dimming lights, avoiding loud noises
• Supervised ambulation until stabilised on medication; do not involve in strenuous exercise programme because fainting is possible; patient should not stand still for long periods of time
• Increased fluids to prevent constipation
• Frequent sips of water for dry mouth to encourage salivation

Evaluate:
• Swallowing of oral medication; check for hoarding or giving of medication to other patients
• Skin turgor daily
• Constipation, urinary retention daily; if these occur, increase fibre, fluids in diet
• All side effects

Teach patient/family:
• That orthostatic hypotension occurs often, to rise from sitting or lying position gradually
• To avoid hot baths, hot showers, since hypotension may occur
• To avoid abrupt withdrawal of this drug or extrapyramidal symptoms may result; drug should be withdrawn slowly on graduated doses
• To avoid non-prescribed preparations (cough, hayfever, cold) unless approved by clinician since serious drug interactions may occur; avoid use with alcohol or CNS depressants; increased drowsiness may occur
• To use a sunscreen during sun exposure to prevent burns
• Regarding compliance with drug regimen
• About extrapyramidal symptoms and necessity for meticulous oral hygiene since oral candidiasis may occur
• To report sore throat, malaise, fever, bleeding, mouth sores; if these occur, full blood count should be performed and drug discontinued

---

flurandrenolone

Haelan, Haelan-C
Func. class.: Corticosteroid, topical
Chem. class.: Fluorinated corticosteroid, moderately potent
Legal class.: POM

Action: Reduces inflammation

Uses: 0.05% preparations, severe inflammatory skin disorders, e.g. eczema unresponsive to less potent corticosteroids; 0.0125% preparations, milder inflammatory skin disorders

Dosage and routes: Apply topical preparations, except tape, sparingly, 2–3 times daily; reduce strength and frequency as condition responds

Available forms include: Cream, 0.0125%, in water-miscible basis; 0.0125% with clioquinol 3%. Ointment, 0.0125%, in anhydrous greasy basis; 0.0125% with clioquinol 3%.

Side effects/adverse reactions:
INTEG: Spread and worsening of untreated infection; thinning of the skin; irreversible striae atrophicae; perioral dermatitis; acne at site of application; depigmentation; increased hair growth, telangiectasia
ENDO: Suppression of hypothalamic-pituitary-adrenal axis producing growth retardation and suppressed plasma cortisol, Cushing's syndrome, reduced glucose tolerance
CNS: Cranial hypertension in children

Contraindications: Untreated bacterial, fungal or viral skin infections, hypersensitivity to clioquinol (Haelan-C)

Precautions: Pregnancy, lactation, use with great care under occlusive dressings including nappies

Pharmacokinetics: Significant absorption can occur, especially under occlusive dressings

NURSING CONSIDERATIONS

Administer:
• Cleanse before applying drug
• Only to affected areas, avoid contact with eyes
• Apply cream to weeping lesions, ointment to scaly lesions
• Only to dermatoses, not to surrounding or infected areas
• Apply sparingly

Evaluate:
• Temperature if fever develops, discontinue drug
• Therapeutic response: absence of severe itching, patches on skin, flaking
• Systemic absorption: fever, infection, irritation

Teach patient/family:
• Apply sparingly to affected area only
• Avoid contact with eyes
• Avoid sunlight on skin, burns may occur

flurazepam

~~NHS~~ Dalmane
Func. class.: Hypnotic
Chem. class.: Benzodiazepine
Legal class.: CD (Sch. 4) POM

Action: Produces CNS depression at the limbic, thalamic, hypothalamic levels of CNS; may be mediated by neurotransmitter gamma aminobutyric (GABA); results are sedation, hypnosis, skeletal muscle relaxation anxiolytic action

Uses: Insomnia, short-term treatment

Dosage and routes:
• *Adult:* By mouth 15–30 mg at night
• *Geriatric:* By mouth 15 mg at night

Available forms include: Capsules 15, 30 mg

Side effects/adverse reactions:
HAEM: Leucopenia, granulocytopenia (rare)
CNS: Lethargy, drowsiness, daytime sedation, dizziness, confusion, lightheadedness, headache, anxiety, irritability, dependence potential, changes in libido, paradoxical aggression, excitement, unmasking of depression
GI: Nausea, vomiting, diarrhoea, heartburn, abdominal pain, constipation, bitter taste
CV: Chest pain, pulse changes
GU: Urinary retention

Contraindications: Hypersensitivity to benzodiazepines, acute pulmonary insufficiency, respiratory depression, phobic or obsessional states, chronic psychosis, porphyria

Precautions: Anaemia, hepatic

disease, renal disease, suicidal individuals, drug abuse, elderly, psychosis, child, lactation, pregnancy, where morning alertness important

Pharmacokinetics:
Period of onset: Onset 15–45 min, duration 7–8 hr; metabolised by liver, excreted by kidneys (inactive/active metabolites), excreted in breast milk; half-life 47–100 hr, additional 100 hr for active metabolites

Interactions/incompatibilities:
• Increased effects of this drug: cimetidine
• Increased action of both drugs: alcohol, CNS depressants

Clinical assessment:
• Continued requirement for treatment

Lab. test interferences:
False increase: Urinary 17-hydroxycorticosteroids

Treatment of overdose: Lavage, activated charcoal, monitor electrolytes, vital signs, flumazenil may be used to antagonise

NURSING CONSIDERATIONS

Administer:
• After trying conservative measures for insomnia
• ½–1 hr before bedtime for sleeplessness

Perform/provide:
• Assistance with mobilisation after receiving dose
• Safety measure: cot sides, call-bell within easy reach
• Checking to see oral medication has been swallowed

Evaluate:
• Therapeutic response: ability to sleep at night, decreased amount of early morning awakening if taking drug for insomnia
• Mental status: mood, alertness, affect, memory (long, short)
• Type of sleep problem: falling asleep, staying asleep
• Effectiveness of treatment by sleep patterns

Teach patient/family:
• To avoid driving or other activities requiring alertness until drug is stabilised
• To avoid alcohol ingestion or CNS depressants; serious CNS depression may result
• Alternative measures to improve sleep: reading, exercise several hours before bedtime, warm bath, warm milk, TV, self-hypnosis, deep breathing
• That hangover is common in elderly

flurbiprofen

Froben
Func. class.: Non-steroidal anti-inflammatory drug
Chem. class.: Propionic acid derivative
Legal class.: POM

Action: Inhibits prostaglandin synthesis; possesses analgesic, anti-inflammatory, antipyretic properties

Uses: Rheumatoid arthritis, osteoarthritis, ankylosing spondylitis

Dosage and routes:
• *Adult:* By mouth if by rectum 150–200 mg daily in divided doses, increased in acute conditions to 300 mg daily in divided doses; modified-release, 200 mg daily

Available forms include: Tablets 50 mg, 100 mg; modified-release capsules 200 mg; suppositories 100 mg

Side effects/adverse reactions:
GI: Nausea, anorexia, vomiting, diarrhoea, cholestatic jaundice, peptic ulcer, dyspepsia, indigestion, glossitis, gastrointestinal bleeding, local irritation after rectal administration
CNS: Dizziness, drowsiness, myalgia, headache
CV: Peripheral oedema

INTEG: Rash, urticaria, angio-oedema, exfoliative dermatitis (rare), alopecia
GU: Nephrotoxicity: dysuria, haematuria, oliguria, azotaemia, cystitis, nocturia, renal insufficiency
HAEM: blood dyscrasias, bone marrow depression
EENT: Tinnitus, hearing loss, blurred vision
RESP: Dyspnoea, haemoptysis, bronchospasm, rhinitis, shortness of breath

Contraindications: Hypersensitivity, hypersensitivity to aspirin or other NSAIDs agents; active or suspected peptic ulceration or gastrointestinal haemorrhage; ulcerative colitis, asthma, 3rd trimester of prenancy: avoid rectal administration in inflammatory disease of rectum and peri-anal area

Precautions: Pregnancy, lactation, children, bleeding disorders, GI disorders, cardiac disorders, severe renal disease, severe hepatic disease, hypertension, elderly

Pharmacokinetics:
Period of onset: Peak 1½ hr, half-life 6 hr, metabolised in liver, excreted in urine (metabolites), breast milk, 99% protein bound

Interactions/incompatibilities:
- May increase action of: anticoagulants, phenytoin, sulphonylurea hypoglycaemics
- Decreased effects of: β-blockers, frusemide
- Enhanced toxicity of: methotrexate, cyclosporin, lithium

Clinical assessment:
- Patient at high risk of peptic ulceration or GI bleeding
- Renal and hepatic function if impairment expected

Treatment of overdose:
Gastric lavage, supportive treatment, correct serum electrolytes

NURSING CONSIDERATIONS

Assess:
- Test hearing and eyesight before, during and after treatment

Administer:
- With or after food
- Modified-release, swallow whole

Perform/provide:
- Store suppositories in a cool dry place between 2° and 25°C

Evaluate:
- Response to treatment indicated by decreased pain and joint stiffness, swollen joints and ability to move more easily
- Eye and ear problems: blurred vision, tinnitus may suggest toxicity
- Report any indigestion or black tarry stools

Teach patient/family:
- To inform clinician of blurred vision and tinnitus as these may suggest toxicity
- To avoid driving, operating machinery, etc. if drowsiness or dizziness occur
- To report changes in urinary output, weight gain, oedema, fever and blood in urine as nephrotoxicity may occur
- The drug may not be fully effective until up to a month after start of treatment
- To store medication as above
- To take with food, milk or antacids to avoid gastric upset
- To avoid aspirin and alcohol
- To report any indigestion or black tar-like stools

---

fluspirilene

Redeptin
Func. class.: Antipsychotic, neuroleptic
Chem. class.: Diphenylbutylpiperidine
Legal class.: POM

Action: Dopamine antagonist
Uses: Maintenance treatment in

schizophrenia and related psychoses

Dosage and routes:

• *Adults:* Deep IM injection 2 mg, increased by 2 mg at weekly intervals according to response; usual maintenance dose 2–8 mg weekly, maximum 20 mg weekly

• *Elderly:* A quarter to half the usual starting dose may be required

Available forms include: Injection 2 mg/ml; 1 ml, 3 ml ampoules, 6 ml vials (aqueous suspension)

Side effects/adverse reactions:

CVS: Hypotension, arrhythmias

INTEG: Pain, erythema, swelling, nodules at injection site, pallor, photosensitisation, rashes, sweating

CNS: Extrapyramidal symptoms, tardive dyskinesia, moderate sedative effects, drowsiness, apathy, depression, insomnia, restlessness, agitation, nightmares, blurred vision, headache

GI: Dry mouth, constipation, salivation, jaundice

GU: Difficulty with micturition, impotence

EENT: Nasal congestion

META: Hypothermia, pyrexia, menstrual disturbances, galactorrhoea, gynaecomastia, weight gain

SYST: Neuroleptic malignant syndrome

Contraindications: Coma caused by CNS depressants, hypersensitivity to this drug or other diphenybutylpiperidines, pregnancy, breast-feeding, bone marrow depression

Precautions: Cardiovascular disease, renal or hepatic impairment, parkinsonism, epilepsy, prostatic hypertrophy, elderly, alcoholism, brain damage, lithium therapy

Pharmacokinetics: Duration of action 5–15 days. Maximum plasma concentrations within 4–8 hr after IM injection; half-life 3 weeks, metabolite excreted in urine

Interactions/incompatibilities:

• Reduced effects of: antiepileptics, dopamine agonists (e.g. bromocriptine, levodopa, lysuride, pergolide)

• Enhanced CNS depression with: alcohol, hypnotics, strong analgesics, other CNS depressants

• Possible enhanced toxicity of both drugs: lithium

• Enhanced hypotension with: anaesthetics

• Enhanced antimuscarinic side-effects with: tricyclic antidepressants

Clinical assessment:

• Caution, it masks nausea/vomiting of other conditions

• Monitor renal and hepatic function of impaired

• Monitor for signs of tardive dyskinesia during long-term therapy

Treatment of overdose: Symptomatic treatment, treat extrapyramidal symptoms with antimuscarinics

NURSING CONSIDERATIONS

Assess:

• Baseline BP (lying and standing), pulse, respiration and temperature

Administer:

• By deep IM injection; rotating sites

• Shake well before use

Perform/provide:

• Fluids/boiled sweets for dry mouth

• Local treatment for pain at site

• Safe environment: cot sides, help with mobilisation

• Fibre/fluids for constipation

• Sexual counselling as required

Evaluate:

• Subcutaneous nodules

• Restlessness, agitation, changes in sleep pattern

• Fluid balance

• Sweating, rashes and sore throats

• Fever, hypothermia

- Weight gain
- Mood and mental state

Teach patient/family:

- Warn about side effects such as nightmares, weight gain, blurred vision, sexual problems, menstrual cycle changes and nicturition difficulties
- To report fever, infection and sore throat and rashes
- To avoid the sun and use a sunscreen
- That drug may take several weeks to take effect
- Change position slowly to avoid dizziness
- Avoid hot baths
- May cause drowsiness, if affected do not drive or operate machinery. Take no alcohol or any other medicines unless specifically prescribed

---

flutamide ▼

Drogenil
Func. class.: Antiandrogen
Legal class.: POM

Action: Blocks androgen receptors at target tissues
Uses: Treatment of advanced prostatic carcinoma in which suppression of testosterone effects is indicated
Dosage and routes:

- *Adult:* By mouth 250 mg 3 times a day. Commence 3 days before LHRH analogue if used to prevent 'flare'

Available forms include: Tablets 250 mg
Side effects/adverse reactions:
GI: Nausea, vomiting, diarrhoea, ulcer-like pain, heartburn, liver dysfunction, thirst
CNS: Increased appetite, anorexia, insomnia, tiredness, headache, dizziness, weakness, malaise, blurred vision, anxiety
CV: Oedema, lymphoedema
GU: Gynaecomastia and/or breast tenderness, galactorrhoea, decreased libido, reduced sperm counts
HAEM: Ecchymoses, haemolytic anaemia, macrocytic anaemia
RESP: Chest pain
INTEG: Pruritus, lupus-like syndrome, herpes zoster
Contraindications: Sensitivity to flutamide
Precautions: Cardiac disease, hepatic disease
Pharmacokinetics: Rapid and complete absorption after oral administration, with rapid metabolism to active metabolite. Half-life of both flutamide and major metabolite 5–6 hr
Interactions/incompatibilities:

- Increased effect of warfarin

Clinical assessment:

- Periodic liver function tests
- Monitor concurrent warfarin therapy closely

Treatment of overdose: Forced gastric emptying, supportive care

NURSING CONSIDERATIONS:

Perform/provide:

- All supporting measures for patient with cancer

Evaluate:

- Side effects

Teach patient/family:

- To report side effects and any increasing symptoms

Administer:

- With LHRH analogues as initial treatment to prevent 'flare' from transient testosterone release

fluticasone (inhaled) dipropionate ▼

Flixotide
Func. class.: Corticosteroid
Chem. class.: Synthetic corticosteroid
Legal class.: POM

Action: Reduces inflammation of bronchial mucosa leading to reduced oedema and mucus secretion. At normal therapeutic doses the inhaled preparation lacks systemic side effects
Uses: Prophylaxis of asthma in patients requiring more than occasional use of bronchodilators
Dosage and routes:
• *Adult:* By inhalation of powder 100–1000 mcg twice a day, starting dose chosen according to severity of symptoms and adjusted to the minimum effective dose
• *Child. (4–16 yr):* By inhalation of dry powder: 50–100 mcg twice a day
Available forms include: Dry powder Diskhaler disks containing 50 mcg, 100 mcg, 250 mcg per blister
Side effects/adverse reactions:
EENT: Candidiasis of mouth and throat, hoarse voice, irritation of throat
RESP: Paradoxical bronchospasm, coughing
Contraindications: Hypersensitivity
Precautions: Pregnancy; breast feeding; patient transferring from oral corticosteroids (start inhalation therapy and withdraw oral steroids slowly); unsuitable for relief of acute symptoms, respiratory tract infection; especially active or quiescent tuberculosis
Treatment of overdose: Symptomatic and supportive treatment; consider monitoring adrenal reserve after chronic overdosage; continue treatment at therapeutic dose

NURSING CONSIDERATIONS

Administer:
• Pierce disks immediately before use
Evaluate:
• Therapeutic response
• Side effects
Teach patient/family:
• Correct method of inhaling
• Disks may be kept in Diskhaler but should only be pierced immediately before use
• When inhaled bronchodilators are prescribed, these should be used first
• That rinsing the mouth after use minimises the risk of candidiasis
• About side effects

fluticasone (nasal) propionate

Func. class.: Corticosteroid
Chem. class.: Synthetic corticosteroid
Legal class.: POM

Action: Reduces inflammation of nasal mucosa leading to reduced oedema and mucus secretion. At normal therapeutic doses nasal use lacks systemic side effects
Uses: Prophylaxis and treatment of seasonal allergic rhinitis including hayfever and perennial rhinitis
Dosage and routes:
• *Adult and child over 12 yr:* By nasal spray 100 mcg (2 sprays) into each nostril once a day, increasing to 100 mcg (2 sprays) into each nostril twice a day if needed
• *Child (4–11 yr):* By nasal spray, for seasonal allergic rhinitis only, 50 mcg (1 spray) into each nostril once a day, increasing to 50 mcg (1 spray) into each nostril twice a day if needed

Available forms include: Nasal spray, 50 mcg per spray

Side effects/adverse reactions:

EENT: Dryness and irritation of nose and throat, unpleasant taste and smell, nose bleed, sneezing

Contraindications: Hypersensitivity

Precautions: Pregnancy; lactation; nasal infection; respiratory tract infection (including lung tuberculosis); prolonged use in children; systemic steroid therapy

Treatment of overdose: Symptomatic and supportive treatment; consider monitoring adrenal reserve after chronic overdosage; continue treatment at therapeutic dose

NURSING CONSIDERATIONS

Administer:

- Shake gently before using
- Intranasally only

Evaluate:

- Therapeutic effect
- Side effects

Teach patient/family:

- Correct method of inhalation
- To blow nose before use
- Single doses are best given in the morning
- About side effects
- If sneezing occurs, blow nose and repeat dose

fluvoxamine maleate

Faverin

Func. class.: Antidepressant, serotonin uptake inhibitor

Legal class.: POM

Action: Selectively inhibits re-uptake of central neurotransmitter 5-HT with little effect on noradrenaline

Uses: Depressive illness

Dosage and routes:

- By mouth usually 100–200 mg daily; maximum daily dose 300 mg; doses over 100 mg must be divided

Available forms include: Tablets 50 mg, 100 mg

Side effects/adverse reactions:

GI: Nausea, vomiting, constipation, diarrhoea, raised liver enzyme levels

CNS: Headache, drowsiness, agitation, tremor, convulsions, dizziness, anxiety

CV: Bradycardia, hypotension, ECG changes

Contraindications: History of epilepsy, MAOIs within 2 weeks of starting treatment

Precautions: Renal or hepatic impairment, pregnancy, lactation

Pharmacokinetics: Onset of effect within 2 weeks; half-life is 15 hr, converted in liver to inactive metabolites which are excreted in urine. Completely absorbed orally, 80% protein bound

Interactions/incompatibilities:

- Increased effects of: alcohol
- Potentiation: nicoumalone, warfarin, MAOIs, propranolol, theophylline, phenytoin
- Effects possibly enhanced by: lithium, tryptophan

Clinical assessment:

- ECG if CV side effects occur
- Renal function if impairment suspected
- Liver function if impairment suspected
- Serum levels of oral anticoagulants, phenytoin, theophylline during concomitant therapy

Treatment of overdose: Gastric lavage and activated charcoal; symptomatic treatment

NURSING CONSIDERATIONS

Administer:

- Whole; should not be chewed or crushed
- In the evening
- Avoiding antacids/alkalis

Perform/provide:

- Fibre and fluids for constipation
- Small portions of favourite foods

Evaluate:
• Pulse 4 hrly
• Appetite or nausea
• Fits or neurological events
• Weight, improving sleep pattern, mental state and mood

Teach patient/family:
• To avoid alcohol
• That agitation may increase
• Tablet to be swallowed whole, not chewed
• Not to take indigestion medicines
• Not to drive or operate machinery if drowsy

---

folic acid

Lexpec, many combination products
Func. class.: Vitamin B complex group
Chemical class.: Pteroylglutamic acid
Legal class.: POM, GSL (at doses less than 500 mcg)

Action: Needed for erythropoiesis; increases RBC and platelet formation in megaloblastic anaemias
Uses: Megaloblastic or macrocytic anaemia caused by folic acid deficiency, liver disease, alcoholism, haemolysis
Dosage and routes:
• *Adult:* Initially 5 mg daily for 4 months then 5 mg a day to 5 mg week
• *Child:* Under 1 yr: 500 mcg/kg daily; over 1 yr as adult dose
Prevention of neural tube defect (as oral therapy for the mother) to prevent recurrence:
• By mouth, 5 mg daily until twelfth week of pregnancy
Prevent first occurrence:
• By mouth, 400 mcg daily before conception and during first 12 weeks of pregnancy
Available forms include: Tablets, 100 mcg, 5 mg, syrup 2.5 mg/5 ml. Tablets 400 mcg available as food supplement
Side effects/adverse reactions:
RESP: Bronchospasm
Contraindications: Hypersensitivity, should not be given alone in pernicious anaemia and other B_{12}-deficiency states because of the risk of subacute combined degeneration of the spinal cord; folate deficiency due to dihydrofolate reductase inhibitors
Pharmacokinetics:
Period of onset: Peak ½–1 hr, bound to plasma proteins, excreted in breast milk, methylated in liver, excreted in urine (small amounts)
Clinical assessment:
• Full blood count

NURSING CONSIDERATIONS

Assess:
• Drugs currently taken: alcohol, hydantoins, trimethoprim, these drugs may cause increased folic acid use by body

Evaluate:
• Therapeutic response: increased weight, oriented well-being, absence of fatigue

Teach patient/family:
• Take drug exactly as prescribed
• Notify clinician of side effects, e.g. anorexia, occasionally nausea, abdominal distension and flatulence
• Correct dietary intake
• If suspect pregnancy and not taking supplement start at once and continue until the twelfth week of pregnancy
• If receiving antiepileptic therapy, consult clinician before commencing folic acid supplements

folinic acid

Refolinon, Rescufolin, Calcium Folinate, Calcium Leucovorin, Lederfolin

Func. class.: Vitamin/folic acid antagonist antidote

Chem. class.: Tetrahydrofolic acid derivative

Legal class.: POM

Action: Converted to essential cofactor tetrahydrofolate, circumventing enzyme inhibition by drugs, prevents toxicity during antineoplastic therapy by protecting normal cells. Modifies metabolism of 5-fluorouracil enhancing its potency

Uses: Megaloblastic or macrocytic anaemia caused by folic acid deficiency, overdose of folic acid antagonist, methotrexate toxicity, toxicity caused by pyrimethamine or trimethoprim. Adjunct to 5-fluorouracil treatment of cancer

Dosage and routes:

Megaloblastic anaemia caused by folate deficiency

• *Adult:* By mouth, 10–20 mg once a day

• *Child:* 0.25 mg/kg daily

Prevention of toxicity after therapeutic doses of methotrexate

• *Adult and child:* IM, IV infusion, IV injection up to 120 mg in divided doses over 12–24 hr then 12–15 mg IM or 15 mg by mouth 6-hrly for 48 hr. Prolonged and/or higher doses needed after high doses of methotrexate or when clearance impaired. Begin 8–24 hr after methotrexate infusion started

Prevention of toxicity after methotrexate overdose

• Immediate administration of an equal or greater dose of folinic acid

Potentiation of 5-fluorouracil

• *Adult:* slow IV 25–200 mg/m^2 immediately before 5-fluorouracil

Available forms include: Tablets 15 mg; injection IM/IV 3 mg/ml, 1, 2, 10 ml amps; powder for injection 15, 30, 50, 100, 350 mg (contains 0.7 mmol calcium per vial)

Side effects/adverse reactions:

SYSTEM: Pyrexia

RESP: Wheezing

Contraindications: Pernicious anaemia/megaloblastic anaemia where vitamin B_{12} is deficient

Pharmacokinetics: Not known

Interactions/incompatibilities:

• Nullifies effects of antineoplastic folate antagonists, e.g. methotrexate if given simultaneously

• Increases effect of 5-fluorouracil

Clinical assessment:

• Methotrexate levels during folinic acid rescue after high methotrexate doses or where impaired clearance anticipated

NURSING CONSIDERATIONS

Administer:

• After reconstituting with water for injection by IV or IM injection

• High doses of folinic acid IV injection must be given over at least 3–5 min due to high calcium content

Perform/provide:

• Increase fluid intake if used to treat folic acid inhibitor overdose

Evaluate:

• Therapeutic response: increased weight, oriented well-being, absence of fatigue

• Fluid balance, watch for nausea and vomiting

• Respiratory status, especially wheezing

• Drugs currently taken: alcohol, hydantoins, trimethoprim may cause increased folic acid use by body

Teach patient/family:

• To take drug exactly as prescribed

- To notify clinician of side effects
- To eat vitamin B-rich diet

formestane ▼

Lentaron

Func. class.: Antineoplastic, adrenal steroid inhibitor

Chem. class.: Enzyme inhibitor, androstenedione derivative

Legal class.: POM

Action: Inhibits conversion of androgens to oestrogens in the peripheral tissues

Uses: Treatment of advanced breast cancer in women with natural or artificially induced post-menopausal status

Dosage and routes:

- *Adult:* By IM injection 250 mg every 2 weeks

Available forms include: Powder for preparing suspension for injection 250 mg vials with diluent

Side effects/adverse reactions:

CNS: Lethargy, drowsiness, emotional lability, headache, dizziness

CVS: Leg oedema, thrombophlebitis

EENT: Sore throat

ENDO: Hot flushes

GI: Nausea, vomiting, constipation

GU: Vaginal spotting or bleeding, pelvic cramps, colpitis

INTEG: Local itching, pain, burning, swelling, granuloma, sterile abscess, inflammation, haematoma at the injection site. Rash, pruritis, exanthema, facial hypertrichosis, valopecia

MS: Arthralgia, muscle cramps

SYST: Anaphylaxis

Contraindications: Hypersensitivity; premenopausal endocrine status, pregnancy, breast-feeding

Precautions: Diabetes mellitus (effects on glucose tolerance unknown)

Incompatibilities: Should not be mixed with any other medication for injection

Treatment of overdose: No experience of overdose; give supportive and symptomatic treatment

NURSING CONSIDERATIONS

Assess:

- Baseline vital signs (temperature, pulse, respiration, BP) primarily for underlying illness rather than in connection with use of the drug
- Blood glucose (no studies yet done on use in patients with diabetes mellitus)

Administer:

- IM: into deep muscle (buttock or thigh) finding a new site for every injection (high risk of sterile abscess and haematoma). Injection to be freshly prepared before use but allowed to come to room temperature before use
- Other medications by mouth if possible. Avoid IV, IM, SC routes to prevent infection and bruising
- Anti-emetic 30–60 min before treatment
- All other medication as prescribed, including analgesics, antibiotics, anti-emetics, antispasmodics

Perform/provide:

- Protective isolation if WBC levels are low
- Fluids: increase fluid intake to 2–3 l daily to prevent urate deposits, calculi formation
- Diet: as nutritious as patient will eat, but low in purines (offal, dried beans, peas) to maintain urine alkalinity
- Skincare as appropriate
- Mouthcare: mouth rinsing 3–4 times daily; brush teeth with soft brush or use cotton-tipped appli-

cators for stomatitis; use unwaxed dental floss
• Warm compresses and other suitable treatment at injection site if indicated
• Storage: vials in refrigerator
• All supporting care for patient with breast cancer

Evaluate:
• Therapeutic effect (reduction in size of tumour)
• Side effects

Teach patient/family:
• About the drug
• About side effects and to report these to nurse or clinician
• That any diabetic patient should report any changes in diabetic status promptly

foscarnet sodium ▼

Foscavir
Func. class.: Antiviral
Chem. class.: Inorganic pyrophosphate organic analog
Legal class.: POM

Action: Antiviral activity is produced by selective inhibition at the pyrophosphate binding site on virus-specific DNA polymerases and reverse transcriptases at concentrations that do not affect cellular DNA polymerases

Uses: Treatment of cytomegalovirus retinitis in AIDS patients where ganciclovir is inappropriate

Dosage and routes:
• *Adult:* 20 mg/kg over 30 min by IV infusion, followed by continuous IV infusion of 21–200 mg/kg/day, depending upon renal function (checked every 2 days) for 2–3 weeks

Available forms include: Solution for IV infusion containing foscarnet trisodium hexahydrate 24 mg/ml; 250, 500 ml bottles

Side effects/adverse reactions:
CNS: Seizures, headache, fatigue
CV: Thrombophlebitis if given undiluted by peripheral vein
ELECT: Hypocalcaemia
ENDO: Hypoglycaemia
GI: Nausea, vomiting
GU: Renal impairment/failure
HAEM: Decreased haemoglobin concentrations
INTEG: Rash

Contraindications: Pregnancy; breast-feeding

Precautions: Renal impairment, hypocalcaemia

Interactions:
• Increased risk of renal impairment with IV pentamidine, aminoglycosides, vancomycin, amphotericin, other nephrotoxic drugs
• Increased risk of hypocalcaemia: IV pentamidine

Incompatibilities: IV fluids other than 5% dextrose

Lab. test interferences: N/A

Treatment of overdose: Symptomatic and supportive treatment. Removed by haemodialysis; this may be of benefit in severe overdosage

NURSING CONSIDERATIONS

Assess:
• Baseline vital signs, renal function, urinary pH
• Blood count

Administer:
• With increased fluids before and during drug administration to increase diuresis and minimise renal toxicity
• Undiluted via a central venous line or, after dilution to less than 12 mg/ml, via peripheral vein. Dilute using 5% dextrose only
• Prescribed anti-emetic

Perform/provide:
• 5% dextrose only for infusion (risk of incompatibility with other fluids)
• Monitoring for side effects during therapy

• Warm compresses to injection site if thrombophlebitis occurs

Evaluate:

• Vital signs (raised temperature may indicate infection)

• Renal function every two days

• Therapeutic response

• For all side effects (if severe, drug may be discontinued)

• Fluid balance, urinary output

Teach patient/family:

• That the drug is not a cure but will control symptoms

• About side effects and to report any that occur

• To seek advice from clinician before taking any other medicines (serious drug interactions may occur)

fosfestrol tetrasodium

Honvan

Func. class.: Oestrogen pro-drug

Chem. class.: Salt of the oestrogen stilboestrol

Legal class.: POM

Action: Produces stilboestrol when activated by the enzyme acid phosphatase, producing local cytotoxic effect

Uses: All stages of prostatic carcinoma, including pain due to metastases

Dosage and routes:

• By mouth 100–200 mg 3 times daily, reducing to 100–300 mg daily in divided doses; Slow IV injection 552–1104 mg daily for at least 5 days; maintenance dose 276 mg 1–4 times weekly

Available forms include: Tablets 100 mg; injection 55.2 mg/ml, 5-ml ampoule

Side effects/adverse reactions:

CNS: Dizziness, headache, migraine, depression

CV: Hypertension, thrombophlebitis, oedema, thromboembolism, CVA, pulmonary embolism, myocardial infarction

GI: Nausea, vomiting, diarrhoea, anorexia, pancreatitis, cramps, constipation, increased appetite, increased myopia, astigmatism

GU: Gynaecomastia, testicular atrophy, impotence, feminisation

INTEG: Rash, urticaria, acne, oily skin, seborrhoea, purpura, chloasma

META: Folic acid deficiency, hypercalcaemia, hyperglycaemia

MS: Perineal burning and discomfort, pain in bony metastases

Precautions: Hypertension gallbladder disease, congestive cardiac failure, diabetes, poor cardiac reserve, fluid retention, depression, history of cholestatic jaundice

Clinical assessment:

• Check cardiac functions

• Use only in specialist oncology unit

• Analgesia if given IV for prostatic cancer

• IV administration should be slow, with patient lying supine

• Diuretics if fluid retention present

• Evaluate size of tumour, acid phosphatase, level of side effects

Treatment of overdose: Gastric lavage if swallowed. Supportive treatment paying special attention to electrolytes

NURSING CONSIDERATIONS

Assess:

• Fluid balance, BP and pulse

Administer:

• Orally, with food if required to decrease nausea. Close links to a oncology unit should be maintained

• Intravenously, slowly directly into vein each day, with patient supine. Special handling preparation, administration and disposal of syringe and needle is by trained non-pregnant, staff wearing protective clothing

• Facilities for regular monitoring of clinical, biochemical and haematological effects during and after administration (IV)

Perform/provide:

• Suitable analgesic, antiemetics and diuretics

• Diet suitable to enhance each patient's good health

• Aid with mobility

Evaluate:

• Therapeutic response; destruction of malignant cell, decreased malignant growth, and pain from metastases

• Input and output of fluids, check for retention

• Blood pressure and pulse especially during IV therapy

• Regular urinalysis

• Weigh before initial dose then at regular intervals

• Increased urinary function and patient's well being

• Maintain on lowest dose that will control disease

• Signs of feminising of men, impotence, enlarged breasts, testicular atrophy

• Perineal and bony metastatic pain after IV treatment

Teach patient/family:

• That addition of analgesia is available when required

• To understand body changes may occur, including breasts in men

• To report any body changes; including dizziness, pain, soreness, weight loss or gain, oedema, skin changes, jaundice

framycetin sulphate

Sofradex (with gramicidin and dexamethasone), Soframycin, Sofra-Tulle

Func. class.: Antibiotic
Chem. class.: Aminoglycoside
Legal class.: POM

Action: Impairs bacterial protein synthesis; bactericidal

Uses: Bacterial infection in otitis externa; bacterial skin infections

Dosage and routes:

• Eye drops: Instil 1–2 drops every one or two hours, or more frequently, initially, reducing as infection controlled; eye ointment: apply 2 or 3 times a day; ear drops: 2–3 drops 3 or 4 times a day; ear ointment: apply once or twice a day

• Impregnated dressing: apply directly to infected wound and cover

Available forms include: Eye/eardrops, eye ointment, 0.5%; impregnated paraffin gauze dressing 1%

Side effects/adverse reactions:

EENT: Local sensitivity, ototoxicity

Contraindications: Hypersensitivity to framycetin or other ingredients

Precautions: Perforated eardrum, short term use only or fungal infections may occur, contact lenses, pregnancy, lactation, sensitivity to other aminoglycoside antibiotics

Pharmacokinetics: Significant absorption possible during prolonged use

Clinical assessment:

• Avoid long-term use (fungal infection may occur)

• Systemic antibiotic may be required

• Check sensitivity to framycetin and neomycin

• Culture and sensitivity tests

NURSING CONSIDERATIONS

Assess:

• Check ear drum intact before use

Administer:

• Eye drops may be administered up to every 15–20 min at first

• After obtaining samples for culture and sensitivity

Perform/provide:

• Store in refrigerator (avoid freezing)

• Discard 4 weeks after opening

• Simple comfort e.g. warm cloth

• Ear hygiene

• Hearing tests if ototoxicity occurs

Evaluate:

• Hearing loss

• Discharge from ear

• Improvement in condition

Teach patient/family:

• Ear drop instillation and care of drugs

• Report hearing changes/local reactions

• To finish course

---

frusemide

Lasix, Aluzine, Diuresal, Dryptal, Frumax, Rusyde, many combination products

Func. class.: Loop diuretic

Chem. class.: Sulphonamide derivative

Legal class.: POM

Action: Acts on loop of Henle by increasing excretion of chloride, sodium

Uses: Pulmonary oedema, oedema in congestive cardiac failure, liver disease, renal disease, hypertension

Dosage and routes:

• *Adult:* By mouth 20–80 mg daily in the morning; IM/slow IV 20–50 mg, increased until desired response

• *Child:* By mouth 1–3 mg/kg daily; IM/slow IV 0.5–1.5 mg/kg to maximum of 20 mg daily

Oliguria

• By mouth: initially 250 mg daily increasing by increments of 250 mg every 4–6 hr if necessary to maximum single dose 2 g; IV infusion 0.25–1 g daily, rate not exceeding 4 mg/min

Available forms include: Tablets 20, 40, 500 mg; oral solution 1 mg/ml; injection IM, IV 10 mg/ml, 2 ml, 5 ml and 25 ml ampoules

Side effects/adverse reactions:

GU: Renal failure, glycosuria

ELECT: Hypokalaemia, hypochloraemic alkalosis, hypomagnesaemia, hyperuricaemia, hypocalcaemia, hyponatraemia

CNS: Headache, fatigue, weakness, vertigo, paraesthesia

GI: Nausea, diarrhoea, dry mouth, vomiting, anorexia, cramps, oral, gastric irritations

EENT: Loss of hearing, ear pain, tinnitus, blurred vision

INTEG: Rash, pruritus, purpura, Stevens-Johnson syndrome, sweating, photosensitivity, urticaria

MS: Cramps, gout, stiffness

ENDO: Hyperglycaemia

HAEM: Thrombocytopenia, agranulocytosis, leucopenia, anaemia

CV: Orthostatic hypotension

Contraindications: Hypersensitivity to sulphonamides, anuria, hypovolaemia, electrolyte depletion, precomatose states associated with liver cirrhosis

Precautions: Diabetes mellitus, dehydration, ascites, severe renal disease, pregnancy, lactation, prostatic hypertrophy

Pharmacokinetics:

By mouth: Onset 1 hr, peak 1–2 hr, duration 6–8 hr

IV: Onset 5 min, peak ½ hr, duration 2 hr

Excreted in urine, faeces, excreted in breast milk

Interactions/incompatibilities:

• Increased toxicity: digitalis, aminoglycoside antibiotics, cephalosporins, NSAIDs, antiarrhythmics, vancomycin, corticosteroids, carbenoxolone, cisplatin

• Decreased effects of: antidiabetics, pressor amines, mexiletine, tocainide, lignocaine (as antiarrhythmic)

• Increased action of: antihypertensives especially angiotensin converting enzyme inhibitors, tubocurarine, gallamine lithium, salicylates

• Increased orthostatic hypotension: alcohol, barbiturates, narcotics

• Decreased effect of frusemide: indomethacin and NSAIDs, phenytoin, aspirin, phenobarbitone, carbenoxolone

Clinical assessment:

• Electrolytes; potassium, sodium, chloride; include blood urea nitrogen, blood sugar, full blood count, serum creatinine, serum uric acid

Lab. test interferences:

Interfere: Glucose tolerance test

Treatment of overdose: Lavage if taken orally, monitor electrolytes, administer fluids and electrolytes

NURSING CONSIDERATIONS

Assess:

• Baseline BP, weight and fluid balance

• Initial effect of drug, increase or decrease dose, then reduce where possible to maintenance

• Glucose in urine if patient is diabetic

Administer:

• Orally in the morning to avoid interference with sleep if using drug as a diuretic

• Intravenous injection in emergency only, give slowly directly into vein. If larger doses are then required give by slow infusion and titrate according to response. Maximum dose and rate must be checked.

• IV route preferred to IM

• Potassium replacement if potassium is less than 3.0 mmol/l

• With food, if nausea occurs, absorption may be decreased slightly

Perform/provide:

• Drug increases urinary output; if patient is not able to move quickly ensure toilet facilities nearby

Evaluate:

• Improvement in oedema of feet, legs, sacral area daily if medication is being used in congestive cardiac failure

• Weight, fluid balance daily to determine fluid loss; effect of drug may be decreased if used daily

• Rate, depth, rhythm of respiration, effect of exertion

• BP lying, standing; postural hypotension may occur

• Improvement in CVP 8 hrly

• Signs of metabolic acidosis: drowsiness, restlessness

• Signs of hypokalaemia: postural hypotension, malaise, fatigue, tachycardia, leg cramps, weakness

• Rashes, temperature elevation, pruritis daily

• Confusion, especially in elderly

Teach patient/family:

• To increase fluid intake 2–3 litres daily unless contraindicated

• To rise slowly from lying or sitting position

• To inform clinician if experience muscle cramps, weakness, nausea, dizziness

• Take with food or milk for GI symptoms

• Take early in day to prevent nocturia

gabapentin ▼

Neurontin
Func. class.: Anticonvulsant
Chem. class.: Gamma-aminobutyric acid (GABA) analogue
Legal class.: POM

Action: Mechanism of action is unclear, but different from that of several other drugs that interact with GABA synapses in the CNS. The gabapentin binding site and its function remain to be elucidated
Uses: Adjunctive therapy for the treatment of partial seizures with or without secondary generalisation in patients whose condition is not controlled by or who are intolerant of standard anticonvulsants used alone or in combination
Dosage and routes:
• *Adult:* By mouth; 300 mg on first day of treatment, two 300 mg doses on second day of treatment, three 300 mg doses on third day of treatment. Thereafter the dose can be increased if required using increments of 300 mg per day up to a maximum of 2400 mg daily in 3 equally divided doses
Renal impairment
• By mouth; GFR less than 15 ml/min 300 mg every other day; GFR 15–30 ml/min 300 mg once daily; GFR 30–60 ml/min 300 mg twice daily; GFR 60–90 ml/min 400 mg three times a day
Haemodialysis
• By mouth; 200–300 mg after each 4 hr of dialysis
Available forms include: Capsules, 100, 300, 400 mg
Side effects/adverse reactions:
CNS: Somnolence, dizziness, ataxia, fatigue, headache, tremor, convulsions, amnesia, nervousness
EENT: Nystagmus, diplopia, rhinitis, amblyopia, pharyngitis
GI: Nausea, vomiting, dyspepsia
MS: Dysarthria
RESP: Cough
SYST: Weight gain
Contraindications: Hypersensitivity; breast-feeding
Precautions: Pregnancy; absence seizures or mixed seizures that include absence seizures; if stopping treatment reduce dose gradually over a minimum of one week
Interactions
• Gabapentin absorption is reduced by co-administration of antacids
Treatment of overdose: Symptomatic and supportive treatment; gabapentin can be removed by haemodialysis but this is not normally required except in patients with renal impairment

NURSING CONSIDERATIONS

Assess:
• Weight
Administer:
• By mouth; time between doses in a 3 times a day schedule should not exceed 12 hours
Evaluate:
• Therapeutic effect: reduction in number, severity of seizures
• For side effects, including nausea, vomiting, weight gain
• Excess dosage
Teach patient/family:
• That doses must be taken regularly; not more than 12 hours to elapse between doses
• To check weight regularly
• About other side effects; to report these to nurse or clinician

gallamine triethiodide

Flaxedil
Func. class.: Non-depolarising muscle relaxant
Legal class.: POM

Action: Inhibits transmission of

nerve impulses by competing for cholinergic receptor sites, antagonising action of acetylcholine
Uses: Facilitation of endotracheal intubation, skeletal muscle relaxation during mechanical ventilation, surgery, or general anaesthesia
Dosage and routes:
• *Adult:* IV 80–120 mg then 20–40 mg as required. May be given IM if no suitable vein
• *Child:* IV 1.5 mg/kg
• *Neonate:* 600 mcg/kg
Available forms include: Injection IV 40 mg/ml
Side effects/adverse reactions:
CV: Bradycardia, tachycardia, decreased BP
RESP: Prolonged apnoea, bronchospasm, cyanosis, respiratory depression
EENT: Increased secretions
INTEG: Rash, flushing, pruritus, urticaria
GI: Decreased motility
Contraindications: Hypersensitivity, myasthenia gravis, shock, severe renal impairment (glomerular filtration rate less than 50 ml/min)
Precautions: Pregnancy, cardiac disease, children, electrolyte imbalances, dehydration, respiratory disease, renal disease
Pharmacokinetics:
IV: Onset 2 min, duration 20–60 min; half-life 2 min, 29 min (terminal), excreted in urine, faeces (metabolites)
Interactions/incompatibilities:
• Increased neuromuscular blockade: aminoglycosides, clindamycin, lincomycin, quinidine, local anaesthetics, polymyxin antibiotics, lithium, narcotic analgesics, thiazides, enflurane, isoflurane, halothane, diazepam, nifedipine, verapamil
• Reduced neuromuscular blockade: azathioprine
• Do not mix with barbiturates or pethidine in solution or syringe
Clinical assessment:
• For electrolyte imbalances (potassium, magnesium); may lead to increased action of this drug
• By anaesthetist to determine neuromuscular blockade
Treatment of overdose: Edrophonium or neostigmine, atropine, monitor vital signs; may require mechanical ventilation

NURSING CONSIDERATIONS

Assess:
• History of renal impairment, myasthenia gravis
• Electrolyte levels
• Vital signs (BP, pulse, respirations)
Administer:
• IV: 80–120 mg
• IM: by anaesthetist only if no vein available
• Not to be mixed with barbiturate
• By slow IV over 1–2 min (only by qualified person, usually an anaesthetist)
Perform/provide:
• Flush vein with saline before and after administration
• Reassurance if communication is difficult during recovery from neuromuscular blockade
Evaluate:
• Therapeutic response: level and dose of paralysis
• Vital signs especially tachycardia
• Allergic reactions: rash, fever, respiratory distress, pruritus; drug should be discontinued
Teach patient/family:
• That some muscle weakness present during recovery

ganciclovir

Cymevene
Func. class.: Antiviral
Chem. class.: Synthetic guanine analogue
Legal class.: POM

Action: Phosphorylated to active form within infected cell; inhibits viral DNA replication
Uses: Life-threatening or sight-threatening cytomegalovirus in immunocompromised patients
Dosage and routes: IV infusion over 1 hr, initially 5 mg/kg every 12 hr for 14–21 days; patients at risk of relapse, maintenance dose 6 mg/kg daily for 5 days per week or 5 mg/kg every day. Treatment should be based on individual response and toxicity
Available forms include: IV infusion powder for reconstitution, 500 mg vial
Side effects/adverse reactions:
HAEM: Thrombocytopenia, neutropenia, anaemia, eosinophilia, raised blood urea nitrogen or serum creatinine
GU: Impaired fertility, incontinence, anuria, haematuria
GI: Abdominal pain, bloating, anorexia, constipation, diarrhoea, haemorrhage, melaena
INTEG: Rashes, local reactions at infusion site, alopecia, pruritus
EENT: Sore throat, epistaxis
META: Abnormal liver function tests, acidosis, decreased glucose, potassium and sodium levels
CV: Syncope, hypotension, tachycardia, hypertension, haemorrhage, generalised oedema, arrhythmias, chest pain, cardiac arrest, myocardial infarction, phlebitis, paraesthesia
CNS: Headache, dizziness, anxiety, drowsiness, coma, confusion, hallucinations, ataxia, deafness, retinal detachment
SYSTEM: Sepsis, fever, malaise, facial oedema
MS: Arthralgia, myalgia, muscular twitching
RESP: Asthma, cough, dyspnoea
Contraindications: Pregnancy, breast-feeding within 72 hr of a dose, abnormally low neutrophil counts, hypersensitivity to ganciclovir or acyclovir, neonatal or congenital cytomegalovirus
Precautions: Haematological toxicity, renal impairment, history of exposure to radiation or to drugs toxic to bone marrow, potential carcinogen, vesicant, prevent conception for 90 days after treatment (men and women)
Pharmacokinetics: Half-life 3 hr; eliminated in urine
Interactions/incompatibilities:
- Increase toxicity: cotrimoxazole, pentamidine, dapsone, flucytosine, zidovudine, amphotericin
- Increased risk of seizures when administered with this drug: imipenem-cilastatin

Clinical assessment:
- Renal function; dose adjusted in renal impairment
- Blood counts every 1–2 days for decreasing granulocytes; if Hb is too low, may require blood transfusion or drug to be withheld
- Liver function tests; serum electrolytes

Treatment of overdose: Consider haemodialysis

NURSING CONSIDERATIONS

Administer:
- By infusion over 1 hr, diluted to 10 mg/ml or less. Reduce dose in renal impairment (see data sheet)
- By IV infusion slowly over 1 hr
- Wear gloves and safety goggles when reconstituting solution; toxic and a potential carcinogen

Evaluate:
• For facial oedema and a wide range of side effects
• For changes in physical condition

Teach patient/family:
• Drug is not a cure but will control symptoms
• To notify clinician of sore throat, epistaxis, malaise
• That serious drug interactions could occur if non-prescribed medications are taken
• That other drugs may be necessary to prevent any infections

---

gemeprost

Cervagem
Func. class.: Oxytoxic
Chem. class.: Prostaglandin E analogue
Legal class.: POM

Action: Softens and dilates the cervix, stimulates uterine contractions

Uses: Preparation of cervix prior to trans-cervical termination during first trimester of pregnancy; termination during second trimester

Dosage and routes: Vaginally, first trimester: 1 mg 3 hr before surgery; second trimester therapeutic termination: 1 mg 3-hrly to a maximum of 5 pessaries; repeat 24 hr after first dose if necessary
Use only one course for second trimester intra-uterine death

Available forms include: Pessaries 1 mg

Side effects/adverse reactions:
GU: Vaginal bleeding, uterine pain
GI: Nausea, vomiting, diarrhoea
CNS: Dizziness, headache
CV: Dyspnoea, chest pain, palpitations
MS: Backache, muscle weakness
SYSTEM: Chills, pyrexia
INTEG: Flushing

Contraindications: Hypersensitivity to prostaglandins

Precautions: Cervicitis, vaginitis, cardiovascular insufficiency, obstructive airways disease, raised intraocular pressure

Pharmacokinetics: Duration of effect 12 hr; gastrointestinal side effects and uterine pain greater after 3 hr

NURSING CONSIDERATIONS

Assess:
• Respiratory rate, rhythm; notify clinician of any irregularities
• Vaginal discharge – check for irritation, itchiness
• Pain, type and location

Administer:
• High in posterior fornix of vagina after bladder is emptied
• Anti-emetic/antidiarrhoeal before giving drug if prescribed
• 36–48 hours after oral Mifepristone given for termination

Evaluate:
• For fever, chills; use tepid sponge
• Exclude pregnancy during follow-up

Teach patient/family:
• To remain lying down for 10–15 min after insertion

---

gemfibrozil

Lopid
Func. class.: Hypolipidaemic
Chem. class.: Aryloxisobutyric acid derivative
Legal class.: POM

Action: Decreases serum triglycerides, very low density lipoproteins and low density lipoproteins and increases high density lipoproteins-cholesterol, inhibiting atherosclerosis

Uses: Primary prevention of heart disease in men aged 40–55 with hyperlipidaemia and hyperlipidaemia types IIA, IIB, III, IV and V where diet is insufficient
Dosage and routes:
• *Adult:* By mouth 1200 mg daily in two doses; maximum 1500 mg daily
Available forms include: Capsules 300 mg, tablets 600 mg
Side effects/adverse reactions:
GI: Nausea, vomiting, dyspepsia, diarrhoea, increased liver enzymes, stomatitis, flatulence, hepatomegaly, gastritis
INTEG: Rash, urticaria, pruritus, dry hair and skin, alopecia
HAEM: Leucopenia, anaemia, eosinophilia
CNS: Fatigue, weakness, headache, dizziness
GU: Decreased libido, impotence
MS: Myalgias, arthralgias
Contraindications: Severe hepatic disease, severe renal disease, gallstones, alcoholism, hypersensitivity
Precautions: Peptic ulcer, pregnancy, lactation, monitor serum lipids
Pharmacokinetics:
By mouth: Peak 2–6 hr, plasma protein binding greater than 90%, half-life 6–25 hr, 70% excreted in urine, metabolised in liver
Interactions/incompatibilities:
• May increase effect of suphonylureas used with this drug
• May increase anticoagulant properties of oral anticoagulants
• Decreased effect: rifampicin
Clinical assessment:
• Hepatic function if patient is on long-term therapy
• For signs of vitamin A, D, K deficiency
• Annual eye examination
Treatment of overdose: Symptomatic support

NURSING CONSIDERATIONS

Assess:
• Alcohol intake of patient (should not be used if patient is alcoholic)
• Withdraw drug after 3 months if the response is inadequate
Administer:
• Drug with meals if GI symptoms occur
• After serum lipid and full blood count
Evaluate:
• Bowel pattern daily; increase fibre and water in diet if constipation develops
• Activity levels of patient
Teach patient/family:
• Symptoms of hypothrombinaemia: bleeding mucous membranes, dark tarry stools, petechiae; these symptoms should be reported immediately
• That compliance is needed since toxicity may result if doses are missed
• That other risk factors should be decreased: high fat diet, smoking, absence of exercise
• That non-prescribed preparations should be avoided unless directed by clinician
• Birth control should be practised while on this drug
• Report GU symptoms: decreased libido, impotence, dysuria, proteinuria, oliguria

gentamicin sulphate

Genticin, Cidomycin
Func. class.: Antibiotic
Chem. class.: Aminoglycoside
Legal class.: POM

Action: Interferes with protein synthesis in bacterial cell by binding to ribosomal subunit, causing misreading of genetic code; inaccurate peptide sequence forms in protein chain, causing bacterial death

Uses: Severe systemic infections of CNS, respiratory, GI, urinary tract, bone, skin, soft tissues caused by susceptible strains of Gram-negative organisms and some Gram-positive organisms, including *P. aeruginosa, Proteus* spp, *Klebsiella* spp, *Serratia* spp, *E. coli*, *Enterobacter* spp, *Acinetobacter* spp, *Citrobacter* spp, *Staphylococcus* spp

Dosage and routes:

Severe systemic infections

• *Adult:* IV, IM, IV infusion 2–5 mg/kg daily in divided doses 8 hrly

• *Adult:* Intrathecal 1–5 mg/day with IM 2–4 mg/kg daily in divided doses 8 hrly

• *Child:* Less than 2 weeks 3 mg/kg 12-hrly; 2 weeks–12 yr 2 mg/kg 8-hrly

• Adjust doses in renal impairment

Dental/respiratory procedures/GI/GU surgery (prophylaxis endocarditis)

• *Adult:* IV, IM 120 mg with amoxycillin immediately before induction

• *Child:* IM, IV gentamicin 2 mg/kg with amoxycillin before induction

Available forms include: Injection (as sulphate) IM, IV 10 or 40 mg/ml; intrathecal 5 mg/ml

Side effects/adverse reactions:

GU: Oliguria, renal damage, azotaemia, renal failure

CNS: Confusion, depression, numbness, tremors, convulsions, muscle twitching, neurotoxicity (mostly after intrathecal injection)

EENT: Ototoxicity, visual disturbances

HAEM: Agranulocytosis, thrombocytopenia, leucopenia, anaemia

MS: Neuromuscular blockade, respiratory paralysis

INTEG: Rash, burning, urticaria, photosensitivity, dermatitis

Contraindications: Pregnancy, myasthenia gravis, hypersensitivity

Precautions: Neonates, renal disease, hearing deficits, lactation, elderly

Pharmacokinetics:

IM: Onset rapid, peak 1–2 hr

IV: Onset immediate, peak 1–2 hr. Plasma half-life 1–2 hr; duration 6–8 hr, not metabolised, excreted unchanged in urine

Interactions/incompatibilities:

• Increased ototoxicity, neurotoxicity, nephrotoxicity: other aminoglycosides, amphotericin B, polymyxin, vancomycin, ethacrynic acid, frusemide, mannitol, cisplatin, cephalosporins

• Decreased effects of: parenteral penicillins, neostigmine, pyridostigmine

• Do not mix in solution or syringe: penicillins, amphotericin B, cephalosporins, erythromycin, heparin, sodium bicarbonate, chloramphenicol

• Increased effects: non-depolarising muscle relaxants (e.g. tubocurarine), biphosphonates

Clinical assessment:

• Renal function. Dose adjustment required in impairment

• Serum peak, drawn at 30–60 min after IV infusion or 60 min after IM injection, and trough level drawn just before next dose; dose adjustment required if peak outside range 5–10 mcg/ml or trough above 2 mcg/ml

• Duration of treatment, should not normally exceed 7 days

Treatment of overdose: Haemodialysis, monitor serum levels of drug

NURSING CONSIDERATIONS

Assess:

• Culture and sensitivity to identify infecting organism

• Weight before treatment; calculation of dosage is usually done based on ideal body weight, but may be calculated on actual body weight

• Hearing aids

Administer:
After culture and sensitivity administer appropriate therapy as indicated
• By IV injection over no less than 3 min; if by infusion over no more than 20 min and in no more than 100 ml of solution. Adjust dose according to renal and auditory function; pre-dose (trough) concentrations should be less than 2 mg/l
• IM injection in large muscle mass, rotate injection sites
• Drug in evenly spaced doses to maintain blood level
• Bicarbonate to alkalinise urine if ordered for urinary tract infection, as drug is most active in alkaline environment

Perform/provide:
• Adequate fluids of 2–3 litres daily unless contraindicated to prevent irritation of tubules
• Flush IV line with 0.9% sodium chloride or 5% glucose in distilled water after infusion
• Supervised ambulation, other safety measures for vestibular dysfunction

Evaluate:
• Fluid balance, urinalysis daily for proteinuria, cells, casts; report sudden change in urine output
• Vital signs during infusion, watch for hypotension, change in pulse
• IV site for thrombophlebitis including pain, redness, swelling half hourly: get site changed if necessary
• Urine pH if drug is used for urinary tract infection; urine should be kept alkaline
• Therapeutic effect: absence of fever, draining wounds, negative culture and sensitivity after treatment
• Hearing during and after treatment and/or ringing in ears, vertigo
• Signs of dehydration: high specific gravity, decrease in skin turgor, dry mucous membranes, dark urine
• Overgrowth of infection including increased temperature, malaise, redness, pain, swelling, perineal itching, diarrhoea, stomatitis, change in cough or sputum
• Vestibular dysfunction: nausea, vomiting, dizziness, headache; drug should be discontinued if severe
• Injection sites for redness, swelling, abscesses; use warm compresses at site

Teach patient/family:
• To report headache, dizziness, symptoms of overgrowth of infection, renal impairment
• To report loss of hearing, ringing, roaring in ears or feeling of fullness in head
• About side effects

---

gentamicin sulphate (ophthalmic/otic)

Genticin, Cidomycin, Minims
Func. class.: Antibiotic
Chem. class.: Aminoglycoside
Legal class.: POM

Action: Interferes with protein synthesis in bacterial cell by binding to ribosomal subunit, causing misreading of genetic code; inaccurate peptide sequence forms in protein chain, causing bacterial death

Uses: Infection of external eye, ear

Dosage and routes:
• *Adult and child:* Instil 1 to 3 drops in the eye or 2 to 4 drops in the ear 4–8 hrly; apply ointment to conjunctival sac 2 to 4 times a day

Available forms include: Ointment 0.3%; solution 0.3%

Side effects/adverse reactions:
EENT: Poor corneal wound

healing, temporary visual haze, overgrowth of non-susceptible organisms, irritation, burning, stinging, itching
Contraindications: Hypersensitivity, superinfection
Precautions: Antibiotic hypersensitivity
Interactions/incompatibilities: None known

NURSING CONSIDERATIONS

Administer:
- Eye drops may be instilled every 15–20 min at first, reducing frequency as infection controlled
- After washing hands, cleanse crusts or discharge from eye before application
- Patient may instil drug under nurse's supervision

Evaluate:
- Therapeutic response: absence of redness, inflammation, tearing
- Allergy: itching, lacrimation, redness, swelling

Teach patient/family:
- To use drug exactly as prescribed
- Not to use eye makeup, towels, washcloths, eye medication of others; re-infection may occur
- Each eye should be cleaned completely separately or infection/re-infection to both eyes may occur
- That drug container tip should not be touched to eye
- To report itching, increased redness, burning, stinging, swelling; drug should be discontinued
- That application may cause blurred vision
- Not to wear contact lenses during treatment

gentamicin sulphate (topical)

Cidomycin, Genticin
Func. class.: Antibiotic
Chem. class.: Aminoglycoside
Legal class.: POM

Action: Interferes with protein synthesis in bacterial cell by binding to ribosomal subunit, causing misreading of genetic code; inaccurate peptide sequence forms in protein chain, causing bacterial death
Uses: Skin infections
Dosage and routes:
- *Adult and child:* Topical, rub into affected area 3–4 times daily

Available forms include: Cream, ointment 0.3%
Side effects/adverse reactions:
INTEG: Rash, urticaria, stinging, burning, photosensitivity, pruritus
Contraindications: Hypersensitivity
Precautions: Pregnancy, open, large wounds
Interactions/incompatibilities: None known
Clinical assessment:
- Avoid long-term use, produces skin sensitisation and bacterial resistance
- Consider the need for systemic treatment

NURSING CONSIDERATIONS

Administer:
- Enough medication to cover lesions completely
- After cleansing with soap, water before each application, dry well

Evaluate:
- Allergic reaction: burning, stinging, swelling, redness
- Therapeutic response: decrease in size, number of lesions

Teach patient/family:
- Rub well into skin if not painful
- To apply using gloves
- To avoid use of non-prescribed

creams, ointments, lotions unless directed by clinician
• To wash hands thoroughly before and after each application
• To avoid direct sunlight or wear sunscreen to prevent burns
• Not to exceed stated dose

gestronol hexanoate

Depostat
Func. class.: Depot progestogen
Chem. class.: Progestogen
Legal class.: POM

Action: Arrests endometrial proliferation and reduces prostatic weight
Uses: Endometrial carcinoma, mild benign prostatic hyperplasia when patient is at risk from surgery
Dosage and routes:
Endometrial carcinoma (before hysterectomy and advanced disease) to inhibit metastatic spread before and after surgery
• IM injection 200–400 mg every 5–7 days continue for minimum 12 weeks
For existing metastases, IM injection 200–400 mg every 5–7 days. (Benefit should be seen within 8–12 weeks. Continue as required)
Prostatic hyperplasia
• IM 200 mg weekly, increased to 300–400 mg if no satisfactory response after 3 months
Available forms include: Injection 100 mg/ml, 2 ml ampoule
Side effects/adverse reactions:
GU: Changes in libido, breast tenderness, irregular menstruation inhibition of spermatogenesis
GI: Disturbances
INTEG: Acne, urticaria, jaundice, pain at injection site
META: Weight gain, oedema
RESP: Exacerbation of asthma, cough, dyspnoea
CNS: Exacerbation of migraine, epilepsy
CV: Circulatory irregularities
SYST: Abnormal liver function tests
Contraindications: Undiagnosed vaginal bleeding, mammary carcinoma, pregnancy, history of pemphigoid gestationis, porphyria, severe arterial and coronary heart disease
Precautions: Hepatic or renal disease, hypertension, cardiac disease, diabetes mellitus, lactation, epilepsy, migraine, asthma
Pharmacokinetics: Response in endometrial carcinoma may require 8–12 weeks, in prostatic hyperplasia 3 months
Interactions/incompatibilities:
• Increased plasma concentrations of: cyclosporin
Clinical assessment:
• Prescribe lowest effective dose
• Check liver function periodically in patients with chronic liver disease

NURSING CONSIDERATIONS

Assess:
• Baseline weight and fluid balance
• BP at beginning of treatment and periodically
Administer:
• Titrated dose
• By deep IM injection
• Rotate injection sites
• In one dose daily
Evaluate:
• For hypertension, cardiac symptoms
• Weight and fluid balance
• For any changes in mental state
• Therapeutic response: decreased abnormal bleeding
• Oedema—increase or decrease
Teach patient/family:
• About all aspects of drug usage
• To report suspected pregnancy

• To report any chest pain, vaginal bleeding, oedema, dark urine, clay-coloured stools, headaches, excessive weight gain or GI upsets

glibenclamide

Calabren, Daonil, Diabetamide, Euglucon, Libanil, Malix, Semi-Daonil

Func. class.: Oral hypoglycaemic
Chem. class.: Sulphonylurea
Legal class.: POM

Action: Causes functioning β-cells in pancreas to release insulin, leading to drop in blood glucose levels; may have extrapancreatic action also; not effective if patient lacks functioning β-cells

Uses: Non-insulin dependent diabetes mellitus (type II) not controlled by diet alone

Dosage and routes:

• *Adult:* By mouth 5 mg initially, then increased to desired response; maximum 15 mg daily

• *Elderly:* By mouth 2.5 mg initially, then increased to desired response; maximum 15 mg daily

Available forms include: Tablets 2.5, 5 mg

Side effects/adverse reactions:

META: Weight gain

CNS: Headache, weakness, paraesthesia

GI: Nausea, fullness, heartburn, hepatotoxicity, cholestatic jaundice

HAEM: Leucopenia, thrombocytopenia, agranulocytosis, aplastic anaemia, increased aspartate aminotransferase, alanine aminotransferase, alkaline phosphatase

INTEG: Rash, allergic reactions, pruritus, urticaria, eczema, photosensitivity, erythema

ENDO: Hypoglycaemia, inappropriate ADH secretion with hyponatraemia

Contraindications: Hypersensitivity to sulphonylureas, juvenile or brittle diabetes; diabetic ketoacidosis; coma; severely impaired thyroid, renal, hepatic or adrenocortical function; surgery, breastfeeding; porphyria

Precautions: Elderly, cardiac disease, severe hypoglycaemic reactions, pregnancy

Pharmacokinetics:

By mouth: Completely absorbed by GI route, onset 15–60 min, peak 2–8 hr, duration 10–24 hr; half-life 2–5 hr, metabolised in liver, excreted in urine, faeces (metabolites) 90%–95% is plasma protein bound

Interactions/incompatibilities:

• Effects increased by: MAOIs azapropazone, sulphinpyrazone, phenylbutazone, clofibrate, bezafibrate, salicylates, sulphonamides, chloramphenicol, fenfluramine, tetracyclines, anti-coagulants, β-blockers, alcohol, fluconazole, miconazole

• Antagonised by: corticosteroids, oral contraceptives, thiazide diuretics, thyroid preparations, oestrogens, phenothiazines, rifampicin, frusemide, bumetanide, diazoxide, lithium, nifedipine

Treatment of overdose: Symptomatic treatment of hypoglycaemia with oral glucose or sucrose, or IV glucose, or glucagon 1 mg subcutaneous or IM

NURSING CONSIDERATIONS

Assess:

• Baseline weight

Administer:

• Drug 30 min before meals as a single dose before breakfast

Perform/provide:

• Blood and urine glucose levels during treatment to determine diabetes control

Evaluate:

• Therapeutic response: decrease in polyuria, polydipsia

• Hypoglycaemic/hyperglycaemic reaction that can occur soon after meals

Teach patient/family:

• To use a blood glucose test while on this drug *or* to test urine glucose levels with reagent strip approximately 2 hr after each meal

• The symptoms of hypo/hyperglycaemia, what to do about each

• That drug must be continued on daily basis; explain consequence of discontinuing drug

• To take drug in morning to prevent hypoglycaemic reactions at night

• To avoid non-prescribed medications unless prescribed by a clinician

• That diabetes is a life-long illness, medication will not cure disease

• That all food included in diet plan must be eaten in order to prevent hypoglycaemia

• To carry Diabetic ID card in case of emergency

---

gliclazide

Diamicron

Func. class.: Oral hypoglycaemic
Chem. class.: Sulphonylurea
Legal class.: POM

Action: Increases insulin secretion in diabetes mellitus when some pancreatic β-cell activity is still present; also reduces platelet adhesion and aggregation and increases fibrinolytic activity

Uses: Non-insulin dependent diabetes mellitus (type II) unresponsive to diet alone

Dosage and routes:

• *Adult:* By mouth initially 40–80 mg daily adjusted according to response; up to 160 mg may be given as single dose with breakfast, higher doses should be divided; maximum daily dose 320 mg

Available forms include: Tablets 80 mg

Side effects/adverse reactions:

CNS: Headache
GI: Disturbances, hepatic impairment, liver failure, jaundice
META: Weight gain
HAEM: Thrombocytopenia, agranulocytosis, aplastic anaemia
INTEG: Rash, pruritus, erythema, exfoliative dermatitis

Contraindications: Ketoacidosis, pregnancy, juvenile onset diabetes, surgery, hypersensitivity to sulphonylureas; breast-feeding; porphyria; coma; severe renal or hepatic impairment

Precautions: Elderly, concurrent illness, hepatic or renal impairment

Pharmacokinetics: Well absorbed orally; duration of action at least 12 hr; half-life 10–12 hr; excreted in urine as unchanged drug and metabolite

Interactions/incompatibilities:

• Effects increased by: alcohol, azapropazone, β-blockers, chloramphenicol, clofibrate, cotrimoxazole, MAOIs, miconazole, phenylbutazone, sulphinpyrazone, bezafibrate, fluconazole, tetracyclines, oral anticoagulants

• Antagonised by: rifampicin, bumetanide, corticosteroids, corticotrophin, diazoxide, frusemide, oral contraceptives, thiazides, lithium, nifedipine, corticosteroids, thiazide diuretics, oestrogens, thyroid hormones

Treatment of overdose: Gastric lavage and symptomatic treatment of hypoglycaemia including oral/IV glucose

NURSING CONSIDERATIONS

Assess:

• Baseline weight

Administer:

• Drug 30 min before meals, as a single dose before breakfast or twice daily dose with breakfast and main meal

Perform/provide:

• Blood and urine glucose levels during treatment to determine diabetes control

Evaluate:

• For symptoms of hyper- or hypoglycaemia

• Therapeutic response: decrease in polyuria, polydipsia

Teach patient/family:

• To check blood sugar levels regularly *or* to check and test urine for glucose regularly

• Symptoms of hypoglycaemia/ hyperglycaemia and how to treat

• That drug must be taken regularly as prescribed

• To avoid non-prescribed medication unless approved by clinician

• That diabetes is a life-long illness; medication will not cure the disease

• That a diet should be followed and all food eaten to prevent hypoglycaemia

• To carry a Medic-Alert card

• That some weight gain is possible

---

glipizide

Glibenese, Minodiab

Func. class.: Oral hypoglycaemic

Chem. class.: Sulphonylurea

Legal class.: POM

Action: Causes functioning β-cells in pancreas to release insulin, leading to drop in blood glucose levels; not effective if patient lacks functioning β-cells

Uses: Non-insulin dependent diabetes mellitus (type II) not controlled by diet alone

Dosage and routes:

• *Adult:* By mouth 5 mg initially, then increased to desired response, maximum 40 mg daily. Doses up to 15 mg as a single dose before breakfast, larger doses divided

• *Elderly:* By mouth 2.5–5 mg initially, then increased to desired response

Available forms include: Tablets 2.5, 5 mg

Side effects/adverse reactions:

CNS: Headache, weakness, dizziness, drowsiness

GI: Hepatotoxicity, cholestatic jaundice, nausea, vomiting, diarrhoea, constipation, anorexia, increased aspartate aminotransferase, alanine aminotransferase, alkaline phosphatase

INTEG: Rash, allergic reactions, pruritus, urticaria, eczema, photosensitivity, erythema

ENDO: Hypoglycaemia

META: Weight gain

Contraindications: Hypersensitivity to sulphonylureas; juvenile or brittle diabetes; severe renal, hepatic or thyroid disease; severe trauma, sepsis or surgery, acidosis, pregnancy; breast-feeding; porphyria

Precautions: Elderly, cardiac disease, renal impairment, hepatic impairment

Pharmacokinetics:

By mouth: Completely absorbed by GI route, onset 1–1½ hr, duration 10–24 hr, half-life 2–4 hr, metabolised in liver, excreted in urine, 90%–95% is plasma protein bound

Interactions/incompatibilities:

• Effects increased by: MAOIs, cimetidine, bezafibrate, clofibrate, tetracyclines, cotrimoxazole, salicylates, sulphonamides, chloramphenicol, oral anticoagulants, β-blockers, alcohol, azapropazone, sulphinpyrazone, phenylbutazone, fluconazole, miconazole

• Antagonised by: corticosteroids,

oral contraceptives, thiazide diuretics, thyroid preparations, oestrogens, phenothiazines, rifampicin, frusemide, bumetanide, diazoxide, lithium, nifedipine
Treatment of overdose: Gastric lavage and supportive treatment for hypoglycaemia including oral/IV glucose

NURSING CONSIDERATIONS

Assess:
- Baseline weight

Administer:
- Single daily doses should be taken before breakfast, divided doses should be taken before breakfast and with evening meal

Perform/provide:
- Blood and urine glucose levels during treatment to determine diabetes control

Evaluate:
- Therapeutic response: decrease in polyuria, polydipsia, polyphagia, alertness, absence of dizziness, stable gait
- Hypoglycaemic/hyperglycaemic reaction that can occur soon after meals

Teach patient/family:
- To use blood glucose test while on this drug, *or* to test urine glucose levels with reagent strip approximately 2 hr after each meal
- The symptoms of hypo/hyperglycaemia; what to do about each
- That medication must be continued on daily basis; explain consequence of discontinuing
- To take dose in morning to prevent hypoglycaemic reactions at night
- To avoid non-prescribed medications unless approved by clinician
- That diabetes is a life-long illness; medication will not cure disease
- That all food included in diet plan must be eaten in order to prevent hypoglycaemia
- To carry Diabetic ID card for emergency purposes
- To continue weight control, dietary restrictions, exercise, hygiene

gliquidone

Glurenorm
Func. class.: Oral hypoglycaemic
Chem. class.: Sulphonylurea
Legal class.: POM

Action: Causes functioning β-cells in pancreas to release insulin, leading to drop in blood glucose levels; not effective if patient lacks functioning β-cells
Uses: Non-insulin dependent diabetes mellitus (type II) not controlled by diet alone
Dosage and routes: By mouth initially 15 mg daily before breakfast, adjusted to 45–60 mg daily in 2–3 divided doses; maximum single dose 60 mg; maximum daily dose 180 mg
Available forms include: Tablets 30 mg
Side effects/adverse reactions:
CNS: Headache
GI: Disturbances
META: Weight gain
HAEM: Thrombocytopenia, agranulocytosis, aplastic anaemia
SYSTEM: Sensitivity reactions in first 6–8 weeks of therapy
Contraindications: Ketoacidosis, pregnancy, juvenile onset diabetes, surgery, hypersensitivity to sulphonylureas, severe hepatic or renal impairment; breast-feeding; porphyria
Precautions: Renal impairment, elderly, concurrent illness
Pharmacokinetics: Onset of effect within 1 hour, duration of optimal effect 2–3 hr. Converted in liver to inactive metabolites, half-life 1.4 hr, 95% of dose excreted via bile

Interactions/incompatibilities:
• Effects increased by: alcohol, azapropazone, β-blockers, chloramphenicol, clofibrate, cotrimoxazole, MAOIs, miconazole, phenylbutazone, sulphinpyrazone cimetidine, salicylates, sulphonamides, fluconazole, bezafibrate, clofibrate, oral anticoagulants, tetracyclines
• Antagonised by: rifampicin, oestrogens, thyroid hormones, bumetanide, corticosteroids, corticotrophin, diazoxide, frusemide, oral contraceptives, thiazides, phenothiazines, lithium, nifedipine
• Potentiated by gliquidone: barbiturates, vasopressin, oral anticoagulants
Treatment of overdose:
Gastric lavage and supportive treatment for hypoglycaemia including oral/IV glucose

NURSING CONSIDERATIONS

Assess:
• Baseline weight
Administer:
• Drug 30 min before meals or as a single dose before breakfast
Perform/provide:
• Blood and urine glucose levels during treatment to determine diabetes control
Evaluate:
• Therapeutic response, decrease in polyuria, polydipsia, polyphagia
• Mental status, absence of giddiness, stable gait
• Hypoglycaemic/hyperglycaemic reactions that could occur
Teach patient/family:
• To check urine and test for glucose regularly *or* to check blood sugar levels regularly
• That some weight gain is possible
• Symptoms for hypoglycaemia/hyperglycaemia and how to treat
• That medication must be taken regularly as prescribed
• To avoid non-prescribed drugs unless directed by clinician
• That diabetes is a life-long illness, drug will not cure disease
• That a diet plan should be followed and all food eaten to prevent hypoglycaemia
• To carry a Medic-Alert card in case of emergency

---

glucagon

Func. class.: Hyperglycaemic
Chem. class.: Polypeptide hormone
Legal class.: POM

Action: Increases plasma glucose concentration by mobilising glycogen stores from the liver; reduces intestinal motility
Uses: Acute hypoglycaemia; aid in diagnostic intestinal radiography and endoscopy; symptomatic treatment of β-blocker poisoning (unlicensed indication)
Dosage and routes:
Acute hypoglycaemia
• IM/IV/subcutaneous injection 0.5–1 unit, repeated after 20 min if necessary, followed if no response by intravenous glucose
Radiography
• IM 1–2 units, IV 0.2–2 units
Available forms include: Injection 1 unit vial, 10 unit vial
Side effects/adverse reactions:
GI: Nausea, vomiting, diarrhoea
SYSTEM: Hypersensitivity reactions (rare)
Contraindications: Insulinoma, phaeochromocytoma, glucagonoma
Precautions: Ineffective in chronic hypoglycaemia, starvation, adrenal insufficiency, pregnancy
Pharmacokinetics: Onset of effect on intestine 1 min after IV injection, 5–10 min after IM. Duration of action 10–30 min. Half-life 3–6 min; inactivated in liver, kidney and plasma

Clinical assessment:
• Monitor blood glucose levels in hypoglycaemic patient until stable and asymptomatic
Treatment of overdose: Symptomatic including phentolamine in severe hypertension and potassium in hypokalaemia
NURSING CONSIDERATIONS
Assess:
• Baseline vital signs
Administer:
• Using aseptic technique
Evaluate:
• Therapeutic response: adequate blood and urine glucose, absence of ketones in urine
• Injection sites for redness, swelling
• Monitor vital signs 4-hrly
• Mental status, level of consciousness
Teach patient/family:
• Symptoms of hypoglycaemia
• Importance of taking correct medication and diet
• Supportive care
• To carry a Medic-Alert card if patient is known diabetic

glycerine (glycerol)

Func. class.: Laxative, hyperosmotic
Chem. class.: Trihydric alcohol
Legal class.: GSL

Action: Increases osmotic pressure, draws fluid into colon
Uses: Constipation
Dosage and routes:
• *Adult:* rectal suppository, 4 g
• *Child:* rectal suppository, 2 g
• *Infant:* rectal suppository, 1 g
Available forms include: 1 g, 2 g, 4 g rectal suppository
Contraindications: Hypersensitivity
NURSING CONSIDERATIONS
Assess:
• Bowel pattern
• Cause of constipation; identify whether fluids, or exercise is missing from lifestyle
Administer:
• Moisten with water as necessary for ease of insertion
Perform/provide:
• Storage in cool environment, do not freeze
Evaluate:
• Cramping, rectal bleeding, nausea, vomiting; if these symptoms occur, discontinue use
• Therapeutic response
Teach patient/family:
• Not to use laxatives for long-term therapy; bowel tone will be lost
• That bowel movements do not always occur daily
• Do not use in presence of abdominal pain, nausea, vomiting
• Notify clinician if constipation unrelieved or if symptoms of electrolyte imbalance occur: muscle cramps, pain, weakness, dizziness

glyceryl trinitrate

GTN, Coro-Nitro, Nitrocine, Nitro-Dur, Nitrolingual, Nitrocontin, Suscard, Sustac, Nitronal, Tridil Deponit, Percutol, Transiderm-Nitro, Glytrin
Func. class.: Anti-anginal
Chem. class.: Nitrate
Legal class.: Oral P, Injection POM

Action: Decreases preload, afterload, which is responsible for decreasing left ventricular end diastolic pressure, systemic vascular resistance
Uses: Chronic stable angina pectoris, prophylaxis of angina pain, left ventricular failure
Dosage and routes:
• *Adult:* Sublingual, 0.3–1.0 mg as required

• *Adult:* By mouth, modified-release, 2.6–6.4 mg 2–3 times daily; in severe angina, 10 mg 3 times daily
• *Adult:* Buccal tablets, modified-release, angina, 2 mg as required
• *Adult:* IV infusion 10–200 mcg/min
• *Adult:* Buccal spray, 1–2 doses under the tongue
• *Adult:* Transdermal patches, 1 patch every 24 hr
• *Adult:* Ointment, 0.5–2 inches every 3–4 hours

Available forms include: Sublingual tablets 300 mcg, 500 mcg; tablets, modified-release, 2.6 mg, 6.4 mg, 10 mg; buccal tablets, modified-release, 1 mg, 2 mg, 3 mg, 5 mg; injection 500 mcg/ml, 1 mg/ml, 5 mg/ml; buccal sprays 400 mcg/dose; transdermal patches 2.5 mg/24 hr, 5 mg/24 hr, 10 mg/24 hr, 15 mg/24 hr; ointment 16.64 mg/inch (2%)

Side effects/adverse reactions:
CV: Postural hypotension, tachycardia, collapse, hypotension, palpitations
GI: Nausea, vomiting
INTEG: Pallor, sweating, local irritation and erythema with topical preparations
CNS: Headache, flushing, dizziness, apprehension, restlessness
HAEM: Methaemoglobinaemia

Contraindications: Hypersensitivity to nitrates, raised intracranial pressure, marked anaemia, closed-angle glaucoma, cerebral haemorrhage, acute myocardial infarction, hypovolaemia, severe hypotension

Precautions: Postural hypotension, glaucoma, severe renal or hepatic dysfunction

Pharmacokinetics:
Modified-release: Onset 1 hr, peak 3–4 hr, duration 8–12 hr
By mouth: Onset 15–60 min, peak 1–1½ hr, duration 4–12 hr
Sublingual: Onset 1–3 min, duration 30 min
Transdermal: Onset ½–1 hr, duration 24 hr
IV: Onset immediate, duration variable
Transmucosal: Onset 3 min, duration 10–30 min
Metabolised by liver, excreted in urine

Interactions/incompatibilities:
• Increased effects of this drug: β-blockers, narcotics, tricyclics, diuretics, antihypertensives, major tranquillisers
• Decreased effects: sympathomimetics
• Increased bioavailability of: dihydroergotamine producing coronary vasoconstriction
• Incompatible with PVC infusion systems
• Increased effects of: opiates, anticholinergic effects of tricyclics

Treatment of overdose: Supportive, with bed elevation and vasoconstrictors to maintain blood pressure. IV methylene blue for methaemaglobinaemia. Gastric lavage after oral ingestion

NURSING CONSIDERATIONS

Assess:
• Baseline BP, pulse

Administer:
• IV – give via infusion pump. BP assessed hrly until stable. Sublingual or buccal glyceryl trinitrate is more effective than oral. Topical patch – allow minimum 2 hr break between reapplication of new patch within 24 hr period to avoid developing tolerance

Evaluate:
• BP, pulse, respirations during treatment
• Pain: duration, time started, activity being performed, character
• Tolerance if taken over long period of time
• Headache, lightheadedness, decreased BP, may indicate a need for decreased dosage

Teach patient/family:

• That drug may be taken before stressful activity: exercise, sexual activity
• That sublingual tablet may sting when drug comes in contact with mucous membranes
• To avoid hazardous activities if dizziness occurs
• Stress patient compliance with complete medical regimen
• To make position changes slowly to prevent fainting
• To store sublingual tablets in glass containers with foil-lined cap. Discard remainder after 8 weeks

glycopyrronium bromide

Robinul, combination product
Func. class.: Anticholinergic
Chem. class.: Quaternary ammonium compound
Legal class.: POM

Action: Competes with acetylcholine for muscarinic receptor sites in autonomic nervous system, relaxes intestinal smooth muscle, reduces secretions
Uses: Adjunct to anaesthesia, preventing excessive secretions and bradycardia; to prevent muscarinic effects when using cholinesterase inhibitors to terminate neuromuscular block
Dosage and routes:
• *Adult:* Pre- or intra-operatively 200–400 mcg IV or IM; reversal of non-depolarising block 10–15 mcg/kg with 50 mcg/kg neostigmine, both IV
• *Child:* Pre- or intra-operatively 4–8 mcg/kg IM or IV, maximum 200 mcg; reversal of non-depolarising block 10 mcg/kg with 50 mcg/kg neostigmine, both IV
Available forms include: Injection 200 mcg/ml, 1 ml and 3 ml ampoules
Side effects/adverse reactions:
CNS: Confusion, anxiety, restlessness, irritability, delusions, hallucinations, headache, sedation, depression, incoherence, dizziness
EENT: Blurred vision, photophobia, dilated pupils, difficulty swallowing
CV: Palpitations, tachycardia, postural hypotension
GI: Dryness of mouth, constipation , nausea, vomiting, abdominal distress, paralytic ileus
GU: Hesitancy, retention
Contraindications: Hypersensitivity prostatic hypertrophy, urinary retention, pyloric stenosis, paralytic ileus, closed-angle glaucoma
Precautions: Pregnancy, elderly, lactation, prostatic hypertrophy coronary artery disease, congestive heart failure, arrhythmias, hypertension, thyrotoxicosis, fever, narrow-angle glaucoma, paralytic ileus, pyloric stenosis, myasthenia gravis
Pharmacokinetics:
Subcutaneous/IM: Peak 30–45 min, duration 7 hr
IV: Peak 10–15 min, duration 4 hr
Excreted in urine, bile, faeces (unchanged)
Interactions/incompatibilities:
• Increased anticholinergic effect: alcohol, antihistamines, phenothiazines, amantadine
• Do not mix with diazepam, chloramphenicol, pentobarbitone, dimenhydrinate, methohexitone, thiopentone, pentazocine, sodium bicarbonate in syringe or solution
Treatment of overdose: Administration of IV neostigmine to reverse peripheral anticholinergic effects

NURSING CONSIDERATIONS

Assess:
• Use in patients with cardiac disease
Administer:
• As single bolus intravenously whilst anaesthetised

• Supportive measures during anaesthesia
• Mouth care after
Evaluate:
• Fluid balance; retention commonly causes decreased urinary output
• Increase in sympathetic activity
• Vital signs; observe for tachycardia and palpitations
Teach patient/family:
• That effects include dry mouth and palpitations

gonadorelin HCl

Relefact LH-RH, HRF, Fertiral, combination product
Func. class.: Gonadotrophin
Chem. class.: Synthetic luteinizing hormone-releasing hormone
Legal class.: POM

Action: Causes release of LH and FSH from pituitary gland
Uses: Evaluation of pituitary function; treatment of amenorrhoea and female infertility
Dosage and routes:
• *Adult:* Diagnostic, 100 mcg IV/subcutaneous; therapeutic 10–20 mcg subcutaneous/IV over 1 min every 90 mins for maximum 6 months
Available forms include: Powder for injection subcutaneous, IV 100, 500 mcg/vial; solutions for injection subcutaneous, IV 500 mcg/ml in 2 ml ampoule and 100 mcg/ml in 1 ml ampoule
Side effects/adverse reactions:
CNS: Dizziness, headache, flushing
GI: Nausea
INTEG: Inflammation at injection site
GU: Increased menstrual bleeding
Contraindications: Hypersensitivity, pregnancy, endometrial cyst, polycystic disease of the ovaries
Pharmacokinetics: Excreted by kidneys
Interactions/incompatibilities:
• Increased effects of this drug: levodopa, spironolactone
• Decreased effects of this drug: digoxin, phenothiazines, dopamine antagonists, sex steroids, corticosteroids
• Any interacting drugs will interfere with diagnostic use of this agent

NURSING CONSIDERATIONS
Assess:
• Test result: Levels of FSH and LH are measured and diagnosis is based on comparison with local laboratory normal ranges according to time of menstrual cycle
Administer:
• Pulsatile intravenous infusion may be required (with heparin) for therapeutic use
• Repeated doses may be necessary to elevate pituitary gonadotrophin reserve
Teach patient/family:
• Give advice related to infertility

goserelin

Zoladex
Func. class.: Hormone antagonist
Chem. class.: Gonadotrophin-releasing hormone analogue
Legal class.: POM

Action: Causes initial stimulation of LH release by the pituitary gland followed by a decrease in LH secretion and a reduction in the production of testosterone
Uses: Metastatic prostate cancer, suitable for hormone manipulation
Dosage and routes:
• *Adult:* As implant into anterior abdominal wall 3.6 mg every 28 days

Available forms include: Depot implant 3.6 mg
Side effects/adverse reactions:
GU: During weeks 1–2 of treatment, increased tumour growth may occur causing ureteric obstruction
ENDO: Hot flushes, decrease in libido, rarely gynaecomastia
INTEG: Rashes, bruising at injection site
MS: Initial increase in bone pain due to transient increase in plasma testosterone; tumour growth may cause spinal cord compression
Contraindications:
General: Tumours unresponsive to hormone manipulation, hypersensitivity
Males: Surgical removal of testes
Females: Pregnancy, breast-feeding
Precautions: Disease flare may require treatment with anti-androgen, e.g. cyproterone acetate 300 mg daily, for 3 days before and 3 weeks after starting goserelin

NURSING CONSIDERATIONS

Administer:
- By subcutaneous injection into anterior abdominal wall using applicator provided
- Local anaesthetic may be used

Perform/provide:
- Symptoms should be treated as necessary
- Storage in sealed packet in refrigerator

Evaluate:
- Bone pain; temporary increase may occur and symptoms should be treated
- Signs of spinal cord compression or renal impairment due to ureteric obstruction; these should be reported at once
- Bruising may occur at the injection site

Teach patient/family:
- Possible side effects and the need to report these at once

granisetron

Kytril
Func. class.: Anti-emetic
Chem. class.: Serotonin-antagonist
Legal class.: POM

Action: Antagonises the action of serotonin at receptors in both the CNS and the periphery, interfering with its role in stimulating nausea and vomiting
Uses: Prevention and treatment of nausea and vomiting induced by cytostatic therapy
Dosage and routes:
- *Adult:* IV 3 mg infused over 5 min. Up to two more 3 mg infusions may be given in 24 hr if needed, separated by at least 10 min

Available forms include: Injection IV 1 mg/ml (as hydrochloride)
Side effects/adverse reactions:
CNS: Headache
GI: Constipation, transient increases in liver enzymes
Contraindications: Children
Precautions: Pregnancy, lactation, children
Interactions: N/A
Incompatibilities: N/A
Lab. test interferences: N/A
Treatment of overdose: Supportive and symptomatic treatment

NURSING CONSIDERATIONS

Assess:
- Vital signs (temperature, pulse, respiration, BP); fluid balance
- Blood count including platelets

Administer:
- IV by bolus injection over 5 min diluted to 20 ml using sodium chloride 0.9%, dextrose 5% or dextrose saline

Perform/provide:
- All supportive measures for primary disease (care of skin, mouth, fluid balance; all other medication as prescribed)

• Storage; protect ampoules from direct sunlight

Evaluate:

• Therapeutic response; reduction of nausea and vomiting

• For side effects; headache, constipation

Teach patient/family:

• About the drug and the side effects

• To report any side effects to nurse or clinician

---

griseofulvin

Grisovin, Fulcin

Func. class.: Antifungal

Chem. class.: Penicillium griseofulvum derivative

Legal class.: POM

Action: Arrests fungal cell division at metaphase of development, binds to human keratin making it resistant to disease

Uses: Fungal infections of the skin, scalp, hair and nails when topical treatment is inappropriate or has failed

Dosage and routes:

• *Adult:* By mouth 500–1000 mg daily in single or divided doses

• *Child:* By mouth 10 mg/kg daily

Available forms include: Tablets 125, 500 mg, suspension 125 mg/5 ml

Side effects/adverse reactions:

INTEG: Rash, urticaria, photosensitivity, lichen planus, angioneurotic oedema, exfoliative dermatitis

CNS: Headache, peripheral neuritis, paraesthesias, confusion, dizziness, fatigue, insomnia, psychosis

EENT: Blurred vision, oral candidiasis, taste alterations

GU: Proteinuria

GI: Nausea, vomiting, anorexia, diarrhoea, cramps, dry mouth, flatulence

HAEM: Leucopenia, granulocytopenia, neutropenia

Contraindications: Hypersensitivity, porphyria, severe hepatic disease, lupus erythematosus, pregnancy

Pharmacokinetics: By mouth: Peak 4 hr, half-life 9–24 hr, metabolised in liver, excreted in urine (inactive metabolites), faeces, perspiration

Interactions/incompatibilities:

• Tachycardia: alcohol

• Decreased action of this drug: barbiturates

• Increased effect of: alcohol

• Decreased action of: warfarin, oral anticoagulants, oral contraceptives

Treatment of overdose: Symptomatic treatment only

NURSING CONSIDERATIONS

Assess:

• Fluid balance

• For history of penicillin allergy; may be cross-sensitive to this drug

Administer:

• Take after meals. Give for at least 4 weeks; for nail infections 6 to 12 months treatment may be required. Continue therapy at least 2 weeks after signs of infection resolve

• After meals otherwise absorption is likely to be inadequate

• Until 3 separate cultures are negative for infective organism

Evalute:

• For limited side effects; headaches, nausea, vomiting, photosensitivity

• Therapeutic response

Teach patient/family:

• That long-term therapy may be needed to clear infection (2 weeks to 15 months depending on organism)

• Good hygiene: handwashing

technique, nail care, use of concomitant topical agents if prescribed
• Stress compliance even after symptoms regress
• To use sunscreen or avoid direct sunlight to prevent photosensitivity
• To notify clinician of sore throat, fever, skin rash
• To avoid alcohol (effects enhanced)
• Impairment of driving may occur

guaiphenesin

Many combination products
Func. class.: Expectorant
Legal class.: P, (NHS)

Action: Reported to decrease sputum viscosity which may increase removal of mucus
Uses: Cough
Dosage and routes:
• *Adult:* By mouth 100–400 mg every 4–6 hr in cough mixtures, not to exceed 1.2 g daily
• *Child:* By mouth 12 mg/kg daily in 6 divided doses
Available forms include: Variety of multi-ingredient cough syrups
Side effects/adverse reactions:
CNS: Drowsiness
GI: Nausea, anorexia, vomiting
Contraindications: Hypersensitivity; persistent cough; porphyria
Treatment of overdose: Other ingredients in cough mixtures likely to present more hazard
NURSING CONSIDERATIONS
Perform/provide:
• Increased fluids/room humidification to liquefy secretions
Evaluate:
• Therapeutic response: absence of cough
• Cough: type, frequency, character including sputum
Teach patient/family:
• Avoid driving, other hazardous activities if drowsiness occurs (rare)
• Avoid smoking, smoke-filled room, perfumes, dust, environmental pollutants, cleansers

guanethidine (ophthalmic)

Ismelin, combination products
Func. class.: Anti-hypertensive, ocular; antiglaucoma agent
Chem. class.: Anti-adrenergic agent
Legal class.: POM

Action: Lowers intra-occular pressure, probably by reducing production of aqueous humour and increasing outflow via trabecular network. Interferes with sympathetic neurotransmission
Uses: Treatment of primary open angle or secondary glaucoma; treatment of lid retraction following exopthalmos and endocrine imbalance
Dosage and routes:
Glaucoma
• *Adult:* Instil initially 1 drop twice daily; normal maximum 2 drops twice daily
Lid retraction
• *Adult:* Instil initially 1 drop twice daily for at least 1 week, reducing thereafter to 1 drop daily or on alternate days
Available forms include: Eyedrops 5%, 1% (with adrenaline 0.2%), 3% (with adrenaline 0.5%)
Side effects/adverse reactions:
EENT: Irritation of the eye, conjunctival vasodilation, conjunctival fibrosis with secondary corneal changes, ptosis
CVS: Adrenaline-containing products only: tachycardia, extrasystoles, hypertension

Contraindications: Closed angle glaucoma, hypersensitivity; soft contact lenses
Precautions: Pregnancy, lactation. For adrenaline-containing products only: hypertension, cardiovascular disease, thyrotoxicosis
Pharmacokinetics: Systemic absorption possible
Interactions/incompatibilities:
• Soft contact lenses should not be worn
• Systemic MAOIs may potentiate the effects of adrenaline-containing preparations
Clinical assessment:
• Reduction in intra-occular pressure/improvement in lid retraction
• Use minimum dose to produce therapeutic response
• 6 monthly eye examinations

NURSING CONSIDERATIONS

Assess:
• Use with caution in patients with hypertension, heart disease
Administer:
• One drop into the lower fornix of the appropriate eye
Evaluate:
• BP and pulse
Teach patient/family:
• To report severe smarting and redness of eye
• Do not discontinue use of drug without seeking advice from clinician

guanethidine monosulphate

Ismelin
Func. class.: Antihypertensive
Chem. class.: Anti-adrenergic agent
Legal class.: POM

Action: Inhibits noradrenaline release from postganglionic, adrenergic neurones, depleting noradrenaline stores in adrenergic nerve endings
Uses: Moderate to severe hypertension in conjunction with a diuretic or β-blocker; by injection to control hypertensive crises
Dosage and routes:
• *Adult:* By mouth initially 10 mg daily, increase by 10 mg at weekly intervals; usual daily dose 25–50 mg
• *Adult:* IM 10–20 mg, repeat after 3 hr if necessary
Available forms include: Tablets 10 mg, 25 mg; injection 10 mg/ml
Side effects/adverse reactions:
CV: Orthostatic hypotension, dizziness, bradycardia, congestive cardiac failure, angina, heart block, oedema
CNS: Depression, fatigue, lethargy, paraesthesia, headache
GI: Nausea, vomiting, diarrhoea, constipation, dry mouth, weight gain, anorexia
INTEG: Dermatitis, loss of scalp hair
HAEM: Thrombocytopenia, leucopenia, anaemia
EENT: Nasal congestion, ptosis, blurred vision
GU: Ejaculation failure, impotence, nocturia, retention increased blood urea nitrogen
RESP: Dyspnoea
MS: Muscle weakness
Contraindications: Hypersensitivity, phaeochromocytoma, renal failure, congestive heart failure
Precautions: Renal, cardiac or cerebral insufficiency, pregnancy, lactation, peptic ulcer, asthma
Pharmacokinetics:
By mouth: 50% absorbed, therapeutic level: 1–3 weeks, half-life 5 days, partially metabolised by liver, excreted in urine, breast milk
Interactions/incompatibilities:
• Increased hypotension: diuretics, other antihypertensives, anaesthetics

- Do not use within 14 days of MAOIs: risk hypertensive crisis
- Increased orthostatic hypotension: alcohol
- Decreased hypotensive effect: tricyclic antidepressants, phenothiazines, oral contraceptives, haloperidol, pizotifen
- Sinus bradycardia with digitalis and anti-arrythmics
- Hypersensitivity to: adrenaline, amphetamine, mazindol, phenylpropanolamine and other sympathomimetics

Clinical assessment:

- Renal function studies in renal impairment (blood urea nitrogen, creatinine)

Treatment of overdose:

Lavage, activated charcoal, vasopressors given cautiously, bradycardia treated with atropine

NURSING CONSIDERATIONS

Assess:

- Fluid balance in renal disease patient
- BP

Evaluate:

- BP, pulse, watch for hypotension
- Daily weight—observe for peripheral oedema
- Symptoms of congestive cardiac failure, oedema, dyspnoea

Teach patient/family:

- To avoid driving if drowsiness occurs
- Not to discontinue drug abruptly
- Not to use non-prescribed products unless directed by clinician; cough, cold preparations
- To report bradycardia, dizziness, confusion, depression, fever, sore throat
- That impotence, gynaecomastia may occur, but are reversible
- To rise slowly to sitting or standing position to minimise postural hypotension
- That therapeutic effect may take 2–4 weeks

halofantrine hydrochloride

Halfan

Func. class.: Antimalarial

Legal class.: POM

Action: Exerts a schizonticidal action against the *Plasmodium falciparum* and *Plasmodium vivax* parasites during the erythrocytic stage of their life cycle

Uses: Treatment of uncomplicated chloroguine-resistant malaria caused by *Plasmodium falciparum* and *Plasmodium vivax*

Dosage and routes:

- *Adult and child over 37 kg:* By mouth 1500 mg given as 3 doses of 500 mg at 6-hr intervals
- *Child 32–37 kg:* By mouth 1125 mg given as 3 doses of 375 mg at 6-hr intervals
- *Child 23–31 kg:* By mouth 750 mg given as 3 doses of 250 mg at 6-hr intervals

Available forms include: Tablets 250 mg

Side effects/adverse reactions:

GI: Diarrhoea, abdominal pain, nausea, vomiting, raised liver enzymes

INTEG: Pruritis, rash

Contraindications: Hypersensitivity; breast feeding. Not to be used for prophylaxis

Precautions: Pregnancy; cerebral malaria and other complicated malarial conditions

Interactions: N/A

Incompatibilities: N/A

Lab. test interferences: N/A

Treatment of overdose: Induction of vomiting and/or gastric lavage; symptomatic and supportive treatment

NURSING CONSIDERATIONS

Assess:

- History of malarial episodes

• For possible pregnancy, breast feeding

Administer:

• At regular intervals

Evaluate:

• Therapeutic effect
• Side effects

Teach patient/family:

• Importance of taking tablets as prescribed
• About side effects
• Not to take drug prophylactically
• To avoid becoming pregnant and to report if pregnancy is likely to have occurred

---

haloperidol

Dozic, Haldol, Serenace
Func. class.: Antipsychotic/ neuroleptic; anti-emetic
Chem. class.: Butyrophenone
Legal class.: POM

Action: Depresses cerebral cortex, hypothalamus, limbic system; controls activity and aggression; blocks neurotransmission produced by dopamine at synapse; exhibits strong α-adrenergic, anticholinergic blocking action

Uses: Psychotic disorders including schizophrenia, mania, behavioural or mental problems e.g. aggression, violent or dangerously impulsive behaviour; persistent hiccup, Tourette syndrome, elderly restlessness and agitation, nausea and vomiting, severe anxiety

Dosage and routes:

• *Adult:* By mouth initially 1.5 mg to 20 mg daily in divided doses; may be increased slowly to 100 mg daily and 200 mg daily in severe cases; debilitated or elderly initially half the adult dose. IM: 2–30 mg then 5 mg hrly if necessary (4–8 hrly if satisfactory); anti-emetic, IM 1–2 mg

• *Child:* By mouth initially 25–50 mcg per kg daily, maximum 10 mg daily

• *Adolescents:* Initially as for adults but to a maximum of 30 mg daily and 60 mg in severe cases

For specific indications seek specialist advice

• *Adult:* Depot injection, deep IM, as decanoate, initially 50 mg every 4 weeks; increase at 2-week intervals in increments of 50 mg to 300 mg; repeat every 4 weeks; higher doses may be needed; in elderly, debilitated patients, use 12.5–25 mg every 4 weeks as the initial dose

Available forms include: Tablets 1.5, 5, 10, 20 mg; capsules 0.5 mg; oral liquid 1, 2 mg/ml; oral liquid concentrate 10 mg/ml; injection 5, 10 mg/ml; depot injection 50, 100 mg/ml (as decanoate)

Side effects/adverse reactions:

CNS: Extrapyramidal symptoms: parkinsonism, akathisia, dystonia, rigidity, tremor; tardive dyskinesia, drowsiness, headache, excitement, agitation, insomnia, neuroleptic malignant syndrome (NMS)

INTEG: Pigmentation, photosensitivity, rash, dermatitis

GI: Nausea, appetite loss, dyspepsia, weight loss, dry mouth, constipation

GU: Amenorrhoea, gynaecomastia, impotence, urinary retention

EENT: Blurred vision

CV: Hypotension, ventricular arrhythmias

HAEM: Agranulocytosis, transient leucopenia

ENDO: Galactorrhoea

Contraindications: Hypersensitivity, coma, Parkinson's disease, bone marrow depression, breast-feeding, confusional states, basal ganglia disease

Precautions: Pregnancy, liver disease, renal disease, phaeochromocytoma, epilepsy (or conditions predisposing to epilepsy, e.g. barbiturate, alcohol withdrawal, brain damage), cardiac disease, thyrotoxicosis, convulsions, hypotension.

Pharmacokinetics:

By mouth: Onset erratic, peak 2–6 hr, half-life 24 hr

IM: Onset 15–30 min, peak 15–20 min, half-life 21 hr

IM (Decanoate): Peak 4–11 days, half-life 3 weeks

Metabolised by liver, excreted in urine, bile, crosses placenta, enters breast milk

Interactions/incompatibilities:

- Enhanced sedative effect: alcohol, anxiolytics, hypnotics, sedatives, strong analgesics
- Antagonise action of: adrenaline, other sympathomimetic agents, phenindione
- Increased risk of extrapyramidal symptoms, neurotoxicity: lithium
- Increased metabolism of haloperidol: rifampicin
- Interference with metabolism of: tricyclic antidepressants

Clinical assessment:

- Monitor response and side effects

Treatment of overdose: Gastric lavage or aspiration for oral ingestion, maintain airway, provide artificial ventilation if necessary. For hypotension do not use adrenaline; use a plasma expander and vasopressor agents e.g. noradrenaline

NURSING CONSIDERATIONS

Assess:

- Base line, vital signs, BP standing and lying
- Swallowing of oral medication; check for hoarding or giving of medication to other patients
- Fluid balance
- Urinalysis before and during prolonged therapy

Administer:

- Antimuscarinic agent, to be used if extrapyramidal symptoms occur
- IM depot injection into gluteal muscle

Perform/provide:

- Decreased noise input by dimming lights, avoiding loud noises
- Supervised ambulation until stabilised on medication; do not involve in strenuous exercise programme because fainting is possible; patient should not stand still for long periods of time
- Increased fluids and fibre in diet to prevent constipation
- Sips of water for dry mouth

Evaluate:

- Therapeutic response: decrease in emotional excitement, hallucinations, delusions, paranoia, reorganisation of patterns of thought, speech
- Take pulse and respirations 4 hrly during initial treatment; report drops of 30 mmHg
- Affect, orientation, level of consciousness, reflexes, gait, coordination, sleep pattern disturbances
- Dizziness, faintness, palpitations, tachycardia on rising
- Extrapyramidal symptoms including akathisia (inability to sit still, no pattern to movements, tardive dyskinesia (bizarre movements of jaw, mouth, tongue, extremities), pseudoparkinsonism (rigidity, tremors, pill rolling, shuffling gait)
- Skin turgor daily
- Constipation, urinary retention daily; if these occur, increase bulk, water in diet

Teach patient/family:

- That postural hypotension occurs often, and to rise from sitting or lying position gradually
- To remain lying down after IM

injection for at least 30 min
- To avoid hot baths, hot showers, since hypotension may occur
- To avoid abrupt withdrawal of this drug as relapse may result; drug should be withdrawn slowly
- To avoid non-prescribed preparations (cough, hayfever, cold) unless approved by clinician since serious drug interactions may occur; avoid use with alcohol or CNS depressants, increased drowsiness may occur
- To use a sunscreen during sun exposure to prevent burns
- Regarding compliance with drug regimen
- About extrapyramidal symptoms and necessity for meticulous oral hygiene since oral candidiasis may occur
- To report impaired vision, jaundice, tremors, muscle twitching
- Advise not to drive or operate machinery when treatment started or high doses used until CNS effects known

---

halothane

Fluothane

Func. class.: Anaesthetic, inhalational
Chem. class.: Halogenated hydrocarbon
Legal class.: P

Action: Progressive depression of the central nervous system beginning with the cerebral cortex and spreading to the vital centres in the medulla. Like all anaesthetic agents its precise mode of action is unknown

Uses: Induction and maintenance of anaesthesia for all types of surgery and in patients of all ages

Dosage and routes:

Induction of anaesthesia
- *Adult:* By inhalation via special vaporiser, 2–4% in oxygen or oxygen/nitrous oxide
- *Child:* By inhalation via special vaporiser, 1.5–2% in oxygen or oxygen/nitrous oxide

Maintenance of anaesthesia
- *Adult and child:* By inhalation, 0.5–2%

Available forms include: Bottles, 250 ml

Side effects/adverse reactions:
CNS: Raised CSF pressure
CV: Hypotension (especially during induction), bradycardia, cardiac arrhythmias
GI: Post-operative nausea and vomiting; hepatoxicity including hepatic failure
MISC: Malignant hyperpyrexia

Contraindications: Halothane exposure within the last 3 months; unexplained jaundice or pyrexia after previous exposure to halothane

Precautions: Pregnancy; breast-feeding

Pharmacokinetics: Approximately 80% excreted unchanged via the lungs, remainder metabolised in the liver to trifluoroacetic acid bromide and chloride salts; metabolites excreted renally over approximately 1 week

Interactions
- Increased risk of cardiac arrhythmias with: adrenaline, isoprenaline, other sympathomimetics, levodopa, aminophylline, theophylline, tricyclic antidepressants
- Increased hypotensive effect with: antihypertensives, antipsychotics, β-blockers
- Increased muscle relaxation; non-depolarising muscle relaxants

Incompatibilities:
- Liquid halothane should not be diluted or contaminated with other substances

Treatment of overdose: Cases of

ingestion should be treated symptomatically

NURSING CONSIDERATIONS

Assess:

• Previous anaesthetic history to establish if halothane has been used as an induction agent during last 3 months; if so, warn anaesthetist (risk of halothane hepatitis if used again)

• Family history for evidence of malignant hyperpyrexia

• Vital signs (temperature, pulse, respiration, BP); respiratory function, cardiovascular status

Administer:

• By anaesthetist using calibrated vaporiser with air, oxygen, or nitrous oxide/oxygen mixture as the carrier

Perform/provide:

• Equipment to maintain airway

• Monitoring of cardiovascular system during anaesthesia

• Storage: in bottles stored upright; in locked cupboard. When halothane is transferred to vaporiser this must be locked onto back bar of anaesthetic machine

Evaluate:

• Cardiovascular status during and after anaesthesia

• For side effects including nausea, hypotension, severe hypopyrexia in post-anaesthetic stage

---

heparin

Calciparine, Hep-flush, Heplok Multiparin, Hepsal, Minihep, Minihep Calcium, Monoparin, Monoparin Calcium, Pump-Hep, Unihep, Uniparin, Uniparin Calcium

Func. class.: Anticoagulant

Legal class.: POM

Action: Prevents conversion of fibrinogen to fibrin

Uses: Treatment of arterial and venous thrombosis or embolism, e.g. deep vein thrombosis, myocardial infarction, prevention of post-operative venous thrombosis, extra-corporeal circulation, blood transfusions, coronary thrombosis, pulmonary embolism, thrombophlebitis, fat embolism

Dosage and routes:

Therapeutic use:

• *Adult:* IV 5000 units then continuous infusion (preferred) 1000–2000 units/hr (approximately 14–28 units/kg/hr) or IV 5000–10,000 units every 4 hr; subcutaneous injection, deep vein thrombosis prophylaxis 5000 units 2 hr before surgery then 8–12 hrly until ambulant. Deep vein thrombosis treatment 10,000–20,000 units every 12 hr or 250 units/kg every 12 hr. Consult literature for further doses/indications

Heparin flushes

• 10–100 units in sodium chloride 0.9% every 4–8 hr

Available forms include: Many, IV heparin sodium 1000, 5000, 10,000, 25,000 units/ml. Subcutaneous heparin sodium or calcium 25,000 units/ml. Heparin sodium flushes 10, 100 units/ml (not for therapeutic use)

Side effects/adverse reactions:

INTEG: Alopecia, local irritation at injection site

HAEM: Acute reversible thrombocytopenia, haemorrhage

MISC: Osteoporosis, hypersensitivity

Contraindications: Hypersensitivity, bleeding tendencies, e.g. haemophilia, gastric or duodenal ulcer, severe hypertension, cerebrovascular disorders, thrombocytopenia, bacterial endocarditis, oesophageal varices

Precautions: Surgery of brain, spinal cord, eye or other sites where haemorrhage a risk. Impaired renal or hepatic function.

Preservatives used in heparin preparations have been implicated in adverse effects. Use concentrated solutions if large quantities of heparin to be used. Heparin does not cross the placenta or appear in breast milk

Pharmacokinetics:

IV: Peak 5 min, duration 2–6 hr

Subcutaneous: Onset 20–60 min, duration 8–12 hr. Half-life 1½ hr, excreted in urine

Interactions/incompatibilities:

• Increased action: oral anticoagulants, salicylates, dihydroergotamine, digitalis, steroids, indomethacin, probenecid, dipyridamole

• Many incompatibilities reported with other drugs for parenteral administration e.g. ampicillin sodium, gentamicin, benzylpenicillin sodium, vancomycin hydochloride. Check with manufacturers data sheet and seek advice before administration

Clinical assesment:

• Determine activated partial thromboplastin time and partial prothrombin time daily

• Platelet count should be measured if treatment longer than 5 days. Stop immediately if thrombocytopenia

• Avoid all IM injections that may cause bleeding

Lab. test interferences:

• Inhibition of aminoglycoside estimations

Treatment of overdose:

• Withdraw heparin therapy

• Administer protamine sulphate

NURSING CONSIDERATIONS

Assess:

• Baseline BP

Administer:

• Using aseptic technique when adminestering by subcutaneous or IV routes

• Avoid rubbing of area to prevent bruising

Evaluate:

• Therapeutic response: decrease of deep vein thrombosis, i.e. pain in limb

• BP 4 hrly initially then twice daily

• Observe injection sites for inflammation

• Bleeding gums, petechiae, ecchymosis, black tarry stools, haematuria

• Fever, skin rash, urticaria

• For signs of hypertension

Teach patient/family:

• To avoid non-prescribed preparations that may cause serious drug interactions, e.g. aspirin

• Drug may be witheld during active bleeding (menstruation)

• To use soft-bristle toothbrush or cotton wool to avoid bleeding gums

• To carry a Medic-Alert ID identifying drug taken

• Stress importance of patient compliance with therapy

• On all aspects of adjustments: dosage, route, action, side effects, when to notify clinician

• To report any signs of bleeding: gums, under skin, urine, stools

• To avoid hazardous activities (football, hockey, skiing) or dangerous work

---

hepatitis a vaccine

Havrix ▼

Func. class.: Vaccine, inactivated

Legal class.: POM

Action: Stimulates production of specific antibodies against hepatitis A virus

Uses: Prevention of hepatitis A, especially in those visiting or residing in areas of medium or high endemicity

Dosage and routes:

• *Adult:* By IM injection 720

ELISA units (1 ml) repeated after 2–4 weeks gives immunity for at least 1 yr. In order to obtain more persistent immunity of up to 10 yr a further 720 ELISA units (1 ml) should be given 6–12 months after the initial dose

Note: In patients with severe bleeding tendencies where IM injections are contraindicated, SC injections may be considered

Available forms include: Prefilled, single-dose, syringes 720 ELISA units in 1 ml

Side effects/adverse reactions:
CNS: Malaise, fatigue, headache
GI: Nausea, anorexia, transient elevation of liver enzymes
INTEG: Soreness, erythema and induration at injection site
SYST: Fever

Contraindications: Hypersensitivity (including that to neomycin); severe febrile infections

Precautions: Repeat immunisation may be necessary in haemodialysis patients and those with an impaired immune system; give at a separate site to co-administered vaccines or normal human immunoglobulin; pregnancy; lactation

Interactions:
• Reduced effect with: immunosuppressive agents including high-dose corticosteroids, cytotoxic chemotherapy, azathioprine

Incompatibilities:
• Do not mix with any other vaccine or drug

Treatment of overdose: Overdose unlikely, symptomatic and supportive treatment

Pharmaceutical precautions: Store protected from light and refrigerated at 2°–8°C. Do not freeze

Administration notes for nurses: IM injection should be made into the deltoid and not the gluteal region and at a different site from any co-administered normal human immunoglobulin or other vaccines. Ensure that facilities are available for dealing with anaphylactic reactions

NURSING CONSIDERATIONS

Assess:
• For contra-indications—see above
• For pregnancy. Hepatitis A should only be given in pregnancy if there is a definite risk of infection
• Using blood test for antibodies to hepatitis A (if time allows) for people over 50 years, or with history of jaundice, or who have lived in area of high endemicity

Administer:
• After checking expiry date
• Using pre-filled syringe
• By IM injection into deltoid (not gluteal) muscle and to different site from that used for immunoglobulin if this is given at the same time
• Do not mix with other vaccines or medications
• With adrenalin 1:1000 to hand in case of anaphylaxis

Perform/provide:
• Record name, date, dose, route, site, batch number of vaccine in patient's notes
• Store in refrigerator (2°C–8°C) and protected from light

Evaluate:
• For anaphylactic reaction
• For local/systemic reactions

Teach patient/family:
• About possible side-effects
• Of continued need for high standards of personal, food and water hygiene
• That co-administration of human normal immunoglobulin may affect the duration of protection

hepatitis B vaccine

Engerix B
Func. class.: Vaccine
Legal class.: POM

Action: Provides active immunity to hepatitis B
Uses: Prevention of hepatitis B infection
Dosage and routes:
- *Adult and child over 12 yr:* IM 1 ml, then 1 ml after 1 month, then 1 ml 6 months after initial dose. For more rapid immunisation third dose at 2 months and booster at 12 months

For immune individual booster dose required 3–5 years after initial course
- *Neonates and child under 12:* IM 0.5 ml, then 0.5 ml after 1 month, then 0.5 ml 6 months after initial dose
- *Infants born to HBsAg positive mothers:* 3 doses 0.5 ml, 1st dose at birth with hepatitis B immunoglobulin

Available forms include: IM 20 mcg/ml injection
Side effects/adverse reactions:
INTEG: Soreness at injection site, urticaria, erythema, swelling, rashes, induration
CNS: Headache, dizziness, fever
GI: Nausea, vomiting, abdominal pain
MS: Arthralgia, myalgia
Contraindications: Hypersensitivity, severe febrile infections
Precautions: Renal dialysis, immunocompromised patients, pregnancy (unless definite risk of hepatitis B)
Vaccine may be ineffective if hepatitis B infection is present
Interactions/incompatibilities:
- Do not mix in same syringe as other vaccines or inject at same site

Clinical assessment:
- Prepare for anaphylactic reaction and have injection of adrenaline 1:1000 available

NURSING CONSIDERATIONS
Administer:
- Subcutaneous route may be considered for haemophiliacs (unlicensed route)
- Only with adrenaline 1:1000 on unit to treat laryngospasm
- Administer in deltoid region or antero-lateral aspect of thigh but not gluteal region

Evaluate:
- For skin reactions; rash, induration, urticaria
- For history of allergies, skin conditions (eczema, psoriasis, dermatitis), reactions to vaccinations
- For anaphylaxis: dyspnoea bronchospasm, tachycardia, collapse

Teach patient/family:
- That there could be local effects of soreness and reduces at vaccination site
- That immunity is not immediate, require full course

hetastarch

Hespan
Func. class.: Plasma expander
Chem. class.: Synthetic polymer
Legal class.: POM

Action: Similar to human albumin, which expands plasma volume by colloidal osmotic pressure
Uses: To expand and maintain blood volume in shock due to burns, sepsis, and in blood loss, acute trauma, surgery, etc
Dosage and routes: IV infusion 500–1000 ml, total dose not to exceed 1500 ml a day. Consult specialist information such as data sheet compendium
Available forms include: IV infusion

6% solution in 0.9% sodium chloride

Side effects/adverse reactions:
HAEM: Decreased haematocrit, increased bleeding and coagulation times
INTEG: Urticaria and other skin reactions
RESP: Bronchospasm, wheezing
GI: Vomiting, salivary gland enlargement
SYST: Anaphylaxis
CNS: Headache
EENT: Periorbital oedema
MISC: Fever, muscular pains

Contraindications: Hypersensitivity, use in pregnancy (unless benefits outweigh risks)

Precautions: Renal disease, severe bleeding disorders, congestive cardiac failure, liver disease, children (no information available). Take blood samples for crossmatching before infusion (ideally)

Pharmacokinetics:
IV: Expands blood volume 1–2 times the amount infused, excreted in urine and faeces

Interactions/incompatibilities:
None known

NURSING CONSIDERATIONS

Assess:
- Baseline vital signs including CVP
- Fluid balance

Administer: See dosage and routes

Perform/provide:
- Storage at constant temperature below 25°C; discard unused portions

Evaluate:
- Vital signs: pulse, BP, respiratory rate CVP (5–30 min) observing for signs of fluid overload (hypertension and pulmonary oedema) and allergic reaction
- CVP during infusion
- Urine output every hr
- Clotting studies if a large transfusion given
- Symptoms of allergic reactions
- Tachycardia, hypotension
- For circulatory overload: increased pulse, respirations, shortness of breath, wheezing, chest tightness, chest pain
- For all side effects

hexachlorophane

Dermalex Lotion, Ster-Zac DC Skin Cleanser, Ster-Zac Powder
Func. class.: Antiseptic and disinfectant
Chem. class.: Polychlorinated phenol derivative
Legal class.: Skin cleanser POM, powder P

Action: Inhibits growth of Gram-positive bacteria and to much lesser extent Gram-negative

Uses: Surgical scrub, skin cleanser, neonatal staphylococcal cross-infection prevention, furunculosis, cord stumps of newborn, routine trunk application in midwifery

Dosage and routes:
Skin cleanser cream 3–5 ml to pre-moistened hands and wash for up to 3 min.
Powder, neonatal staphylococcal cross-infection prevention: after cord ligature, dust cord, and axillas, perineum, groin, front of abdomen. Repeat after napkin changes until cord stump drops away and wound heals

Available forms include: Cream cleanser 3%; powder 0.33%, emollient lotion 0.5%

Side effects/adverse reactions:
INTEG: Sensitivity, photosensitivity

Contraindications: Hypersensitivity, burns, badly damaged skin, pregnancy, mucous membranes, vaginally, under occlusive dressings, large areas of skin.

Precautions: Use on premature or low birth-weight infants, reserved for outbreaks of staphylococcal infections in nurseries. To children under 2 yr use on medical advice only

Clinical assessment:

• Monitor skin condition

NURSING CONSIDERATIONS

Administer:

• To body areas only; do not apply to broken skin, face, lips, mouth, eyes, mucous membranes, anus, meata

• Repeated use may lead to systemic absorption

Evaluate:

• Area of body involved; irritation, rash, breaks, dryness, scales

• Effectiveness of wound care

Teach patient/family:

• To report itching, irritation, dizziness, headache, confusion; discontinue drug immediately

hexamine (methenamine) hippurate

Hiprex

Func. class.: Antibiotic, urinary tract

Chem. class.: Hexamine mandelic acid

Legal class.: P

Action: In acid urine it is hydrolysed to formaldehyde which has antimicrobial activity; bacteriostatic

Uses: Treatment and prophylaxis against urinary tract infections caused by a wide range of Gram-positive and Gram-negative organisms including *Escherichia coli, Aerobacter aerogenes, Pseudomonas* spp, some strains of *Proteus* spp

Dosage and routes:

• *Adult:* By mouth 1 g twice a day; may be increased in patients with catheter to 1 g 3 times a day

• *Child 6–12 yr:* 500 mg twice daily

Available forms include: Tablets 1 g

Side effects/adverse reactions:

INTEG: Rash

GI: Nausea, vomiting, diarrhoea and other disturbances

GU: Bladder irritation, painful and frequent micturation, haematuria, proteinuria

Contraindications: Severe dehydration, severe renal impairment, metabolic acidosis

Precautions: Renal insufficiency, pregnancy

Pharmacokinetics:

By mouth: Excreted in urine, half-life 4 hr

Interactions/incompatibilities:

• Insoluble precipitate in urine: (crystalluria): sulphonamides

• Urine alkalinising agents: potassium litrate, acetazolamide

Clinical assessment:

• Culture and sensitivity before treatment, after completion

• Check that urine pH is less than 5.5

• Up to 12 g of vitamin C if needed to acidify urine; cranberry, prune juice may be used

Lab. test interferences: Estimations for catacholamines, 17-hydroxycorticosteroids, oestrogens in urine

Treatment of overdose: Treat vomiting with an anti-emetic, haematuria by drinking copious amounts of water. Treat bladder symptoms by drinking copious amounts of water and 2–3 teaspoonfuls of bicarbonate of soda

NURSING CONSIDERATIONS

Assess:

• Fluid balance, urine pH less than 5.5 is ideal

Administer:

• Tablets may be halved or crushed and taken with milk or fruit juice
• After mid-stream urine or other samples are obtained for culture and sensitivity

Perform/provide:
• Give vitamin C or juices such as cranberry or prune to achieve desired urine activity
• Limited intake of alkaline foods or drugs: milk, dairy products, peanuts, vegetables, alkaline antiacids, sodium bicarbonate

Evaluate:
• Therapeutic response: decreased pain, frequency, urgency, negative culture and sensitivity, absence of infection
• Allergy: fever, flushing, rash, urticaria, pruritus

Teach patient/family:
• Keep urine acidic by eating food that acidifies urine (meats, eggs, fish, gelatin products, prunes, plums, cranberries)
• Fluids must be increased to 3 litres daily to avoid crystallisation in kidneys
• Complete full course of drug therapy; take drug at evenly spaced intervals around clock for best results

---

homatropine hydrobromide (ophthalmic)

Minims
Func. class.: Mydriatic
Chem. class.: Synthetic alkaloid
Legal class.: POM

Action: Blocks response of iris sphincter muscle, muscle of accommodation of ciliary body to cholinergic simulation, resulting in dilatation, paralysis of accommodation

Uses: As a mydriatic and cycloplegic; uveitis

Dosage and routes:
• *Adult and child:* Instil 1 or 2 drops repeat in 5–10 min for refraction; uveitis 1 or 2 drops 2 to 3 times daily

Available forms include: Eyedrops, solution 1%, 2%. Minims 2% and intended as single use

Side effects/adverse reactions:
EENT: Increased intraocular pressure, blurred vision, photophobia, irritation, oedema
INTEG: Contact dermatitis, rash, dry skin
CV: Bradycardia, tachycardia, palpitations, arrhythmias
CNS: Giddiness, ataxia, psychotic reactions
GI: Dry mouth, constipation, abdominal distension

Contraindications: Hypersensitivity, patients allergic to atropine, glaucoma or tendency to glaucoma (e.g. narrow anterior chamber angle), pregnancy, lactation

Precautions: Systemic reactions in young and very old. Due to visual disturbances after use caution patients against driving, etc., until vision is clear

Pharmacokinetics:
INSTIL: Peak ½–1 hr, duration 1–3 days

Interactions/incompatibilities:
Possible enhanced action by other drugs with antimuscarinic properties: some antihistamines, phenothiazines, tricyclic antidepressants, butyrophenones

Treatment of overdose: If systemic toxicity occurs provide supportive treatment
If ingested: emesis or gastric lavage

NURSING CONSIDERATIONS

Perform/provide:
• Cover eye with patch; danger of retinal damage due to excess light entering the eye

Evaluate:

• Monitor patient and report any systemic symptoms to clinician
• Therapeutic response: decrease in inflammation or cycloplegic refraction
• Eye pain, inform clinician, discontinue use

Teach patient/family:
• Teach patient to use clean swabs to wipe eye before and after, using different swabs for each treatment and each eye
• Do not touch dropper to eye
• Wait 5 min to use other drops
• To report change in vision, blurring or loss of sight, trouble breathing, sweating, flushing
• Not to engage in hazardous activities until able to see
• That blurred vision will decrease with repeated use of drug

---

hyaluronidase

Hyalase
Func. class.: Enzyme
Legal class.: POM

Action: Depolymerises the mucopolysaccharide hyaluronic acid which is a component of the 'tissue cement' of tissue space so reducing its viscosity. The tissue is rendered more permeable to injections
Uses: Increased tissue permeability to IM or subcutaneous injections; aids resorption of extravasated blood and excess fluids
Dosage and routes:
• *For tissue permeability:* Subcutaneous or IM injection, 1500 units with other drug or injected in site before drug; by subcutaneous infusion 1500 units before 500–1000 ml infusion
Available forms include: Injection, powder for reconstitution 1500 unit ampoule
Contraindications: Hypersensitivity; use at site of infections or malignancy, bites or stings; by intravenous route; direct application to the cornea

NURSING CONSIDERATIONS

Administer:
• Immediately after mixing since solution is unstable
• Check compatibility before injecting with other drugs

Evaluate:
• Therapeutic response: absence of swelling, pain after hypodermolysis

---

hydralazine hydrochloride

Apresoline
Func. class.: Antihypertensive
Chem. class.: Vasodilator, peripheral
Legal class.: POM

Action: Vasodilatation through relaxation of arteriolar smooth muscle; reduction in blood pressure with reflex increases in cardiac function
Uses: Moderate to severe hypertension in addition to a β-blocker or thiazide diuretic; hypertensive crisis
Dosage and routes:
• *Adult:* By mouth 25 mg twice a day increasing to a maximum of 50 mg twice a day; for higher doses see data sheet compendium
• *Adult:* slow IV injection 5–10 mg over 20 min; repeated if necessary after 20–30 min; IV infusion initially 200–300 mcg/min then maintenance 50–150 mcg/min
Available forms include: Tablets 25 mg, 50 mg; injection 20 mg
Side effects/adverse reactions:
CV: Tachycardia, palpitations, anginal symptoms, flushing, hypotension, oedema, heart failure

GI: Nausea, vomiting, and other disturbances
SYST: Lupus erythematosus-like syndrome
CNS: Headache, peripheral neuritis, dizziness, polyneuritis, paraesthesia
INTEG: Rashes
HAEM: Changes in blood count, anaemia, leucopenia, neutropenia, thrombocytopenia
GU: Proteinuria, haematuria, increased plasma creatinine, renal failure, urinary retention
EENT: Nasal congestion
MISC: Fever

Contraindications: Hypersensitivity to hydralazine or dihydralazine. Idiopathic systemic lupus erythematosus, severe tachycardia, high output heart failure, myocardial insufficiency due to mechanical obstruction, cor pulmonale, dissecting aortic aneurysm, porphyria

Precautions: Pregnancy, breast feeding, renal impairment and hepatic dysfunction—reduce dosage, coronary artery disease, cerebrovascular disease, low parenteral doses, possible over rapid BP reduction. Possible reaction impairment; patients should be warned of possible hazard driving or operating machinery

Pharmacokinetics:
By mouth: Onset 20–30 min, peak 1 hr, duration 2–4 hr
IM: Onset 5–10 min, peak 1 hr, duration 2–4 hr
IV: Onset 5–20 min, peak 10–80 min, duration 2–6 hr
Half-life 2–8 hr, metabolised by liver, less than 10% present in urine

Interactions/incompatibilities:
• Enhanced hypotensive effect: alcohol, anaesthetics, antidepressants, antipsychotics, anxiolytics, hypnotics, β-blockers, calcium channel blockers, diuretics, dopaminergics, muscle relaxants, nitrates, diazoxide
• Additive hypotensive effect: other antihypertensives
• Antagonise hypotensive effect: NSAIDs, corticosteroids, oestragens and combined oral contraceptives, carbenoxolone, use with caution: MAOIs

Clinical assessment:
• Monitor patient for side effects when treatment with hydralazine started

Treatment of overdose: Immediate gastric lavage and supportive measures. Activated charcoal may be used. If hypotension use a pressor agent (not adrenaline which causes tachycardia) to raise BP

NURSING CONSIDERATIONS

Assess:
• Baseline BP

Administer:
• To patient in recumbent position; keep in that position for 1 hr after administration

Perform/provide:
• BP, 5 min for 2 hr, then 1 hrly for 2 hr, then 4 hrly and jugular venous distension 4 hrly if administered parenterally
• Weight daily, fluid balance

Evaluate:
• Oedema in feet, legs daily
• Skin turgor, dryness of mucous membranes for hydration status
• Rales, dyspnoea, orthopnoea
• IV site for extravasation
• Fever, joint pain, tachycardia, palpitations, headache, nausea
• Mental status: affect, mood, behaviour, anxiety; check for personality changes

Teach patient/family:
• To take with food to increase bioavailability
• To avoid non-prescribed preparations unless approved by clinician
• To notify clinician if chest pain, severe fatigue, fever, muscle or joint pain occurs

hydroclorothiazide

HydroSaluric, Esidrex, many combination products
Func. class.: Thiazide diuretic
Chem. class.: Sulphonamide
Legal class.: POM

Action: Inhibits the reabsorption of sodium chloride and water probably at proximal tubules of kidney
Uses: Oedema of various causes e.g. congestive heart failure, renal dysfunction, hepatic conditions, premenstrual tension; hypertension; adjunct to other antihypertensive drugs
Dosage and routes:
• *Adults:* By mouth, oedema 25–100 mg once or twice daily reducing to maintenance of 25–50 mg alternate days; hypertension 25 mg daily increasing if necessary to 100 mg
Available forms include: Tablets 25, 50 mg
Side effects/adverse reactions:
CNS: Paraesthesia, headache, dizziness, vertigo
GI: Gastric irritation, vomiting, jaundice, pancreatitis nausea, anorexia, constipation, diarrhoea, cramps, salivary gland irritation
INTEG: Rash, photosensitivity, purpura
HAEM: Hyperglycaemia, hyperuricaemia, increased cholesterol, neutropenia, thrombocytopenia
ELECT: Hypokalaemia, hypomagnesaemia, hyponatraemia, hypercalcaemia, hypochloraemic alkalosis
CV: Hypotension, orthostatic hypotension
EENT: Yellow vision, blurred vision
GV: Impotence, interstitial nephritis, renal dysfunction, renal failure
SYST: Anaphylactic reactions
Contraindications: Hypersensitivity to thiazides or sulphonamides, severe renal and hepatic impairment, hypercalcaemia, Addison's disease, porphyria, lithium therapy, precoma associated with hepatic cirrhosis
Precautions: Hypokalaemia, renal and hepatic impairment, diabetes, gout, pregnancy, breast feeding, systemic lupus erythematosus
Monitor for signs of electrolyte imbalance
Pharmacokinetics:
By mouth: Onset 2 hr, peak 4 hr, duration 6–12 hr; excreted unchanged by kidneys, enters breast milk
Interactions/incompatibilities:
• Increased toxicity of: non-depolarising muscle relaxants, lithium, cardiac glycosides, tricyclic antidepressants, MAOIs
• Decreased effects of: antidiabetics, sex hormones
• Risk of hypercalcaemia: calcium salts
• Risk of hypokalaemia: corticosteroids, other diuretics, carbenoxolone
• Decreased effect of this drug: NSAIDs
• Electrolytes and renal function
Lab. test interferences:
Tests for parathyroid function
Treatment of overdose: Empty stomach by emesis or lavage, give symptomatic and supportive treatment

NURSING CONSIDERATIONS

Assess:
• Baseline BP, weight and fluid balance
• Rate, depth, rhythm of respiration, effect of exertion
• Glucose in urine if patient is diabetic
Administer:
• In morning to avoid interference with sleep if using drug as a diuretic
• Potassium replacement if potass-

ium is less than 3.0 mmol/litre unless contraindicated
• With food, if nausea occurs, absorption may be decreased slightly
Evaluate:
• Fluid balance daily to determine fluid loss; effect of drug may be decreased if used daily
• Weight daily
• BP lying, standing; postural hypotension may occur
• Improvement in oedema of feet, legs, sacral area daily if medication is being used in heart failure
• Improvement in CVP and BP recordings
• Signs of metabolic acidosis: drowsiness, restlessness
• Signs of hypokalaemia: postural hypotension, malaise, fatigue, tachycardia, leg cramps, weakness
• Rashes, temperature elevation daily
• Confusion, especially in elderly; take safety precautions if needed
Teach patient/family:
• To increase fluid intake 2–3 litres daily unless contraindicated; to rise slowly from lying or sitting position
• To notify clinician of muscle weakness, cramps, nausea, dizziness
• Drug may be taken with food or milk
• That blood sugar may be increased in diabetics
• Take early in day to avoid nocturia

hydrocortisone/ hydrocortisone acetate/ hydrocortisone butyrate

Dioderm, Efcortelan, Mildison, Hydrocortistab, Locoid, Hydrocortisyl, many combination products
Func. class.: Corticosteroid, topical
Chem. class.: Natural non-fluorinated, glucocorticoid
Legal class.: POM; unless in products specifically licensed as P

Action: Possesses antipruritic, anti-inflammatory actions, mildly potent (base and acetate), potent (butyrate)
Uses: Mild inflammatory skin conditions including the following: eczema, contact dermatitis, seborrhoeic dermatitis, intertrigo, insect bites, psoriasis
Dosage and routes:
• *Adult and child:* Apply sparingly 2–3 times a day
Available forms include: Hydrocortisone—ointment 0.5%, 1%, 2.5%; cream 0.1%, 0.125%, 0.5%, 1%, 2.5%; lotion 1%; acetate—cream 0.1%, 0.125%, 0.5%, 1%, 2.5%; butyrate—ointment 0.1%; cream 0.1%; acetate—cream 0.125%, 0.5%, 1%, 2.5% (many others)
Side effects/adverse reactions:
INTEG: Hypopigmentation, subcutaneous atrophy, acne, spread and worsening of untreated infection, striae, allergic contact dermatitis, thinning of skin, increasing hair growth
Contraindications: Hypersensitivity to corticosteroids, fungal, bacterial, or viral infections
Precautions: Pregnancy, lactation, prolonged administration in infants and children, extreme caution in dermatoses of infancy e.g. napkin eruption, use on face
NURSING CONSIDERATIONS

Assess:
• Skin area to be covered
Administer:
• Apply wearing gloves. Wash hands well before and after application
• Only to dermatoses; do not use on weeping, denuded, or infected area
• Only to affected areas; avoid eyes
Perform/provide:
• Cleansing before application of drug
• Treatment for a few days after area has cleared
Evaluate:
• Temperature; if fever develops, drug should be discontinued
• Extent of skin affected and any changes in condition
• Allergic reaction
• Hypopigmentation
• Therapeutic response: absence of severe itching, patches on skin, flaking
Teach patient/family:
• To avoid sunlight on affected area; burns may occur
• Not to use other non-prescribed products unless directed by clinician

hydrocortisone acetate (ophthalmic/otic)

Combination products
Func. class.: Corticosteroid
Chem. class.: Glucocorticoid, short acting
Legal class.: POM

Action: Anti-inflammatory by suppressing various components of the inflammatory reaction
Uses: Inflammation of the eye or ear
Dosage and routes:
• *Adult and child:* Instil 2 to 4 times a day
Available forms include: Ointment 0.5%, eye/ear drops 0.5%
Side effects/adverse reactions:
EENT: Itching, irritation
INTEG: Rash, urticaria
Contraindications: Hypersensitivity, perforated eardrum, bacterial, fungal or viral infection of the eye, corneal ulceration, glaucoma

NURSING CONSIDERATIONS
Administer:
• After removing impacted cerumen by irrigation of ear if necessary
• Drops or ointment directly into inflammed eye/ear
• Without contact of dropper to inflammed area
Perform/provide:
• Suitable analgesics if required
Evaluate:
• Therapeutic response: decreased pain, soreness and inflammation
• For redness, swelling, fever, pain in ear, which indicates infection
Teach patient/family:
• To instil after washing hands well, without touching dropper to ear/eye
• That balance may be impaired and dizziness occur
• Not to drive or operate machinery if dizziness occurs
• That two containers of hydrocortisone are required if both eyes/ears are inflammed. Containers marked 'left' and 'right' to be used only on that corresponding side
• To contact the clinician if redness, swelling, fever, pain in ear occurs

hydrocortisone butyrate

Locoid, combination product
Func. class.: Corticosteroid, topical
Chem. class.: Non-fluorinated corticosteroid, potent
Legal class.: POM

Action: Reduces inflammation
Uses: Severe inflammatory skin disorders, e.g. eczema in patients unresponsive to less potent corticosteroids, psoriasis, etc.
Dosage and routes: Topically, apply thinly 2–4 times a day, reduce as condition responds
Available forms include: Cream, lipocream, ointment, scalp lotion, all 0.1%
Side effects/adverse reactions:
INTEG: Spread and worsening of untreated infection; thinning of the skin; irreversible striae atrophicae; perioral dermatitis; acne at site of application; mild depigmentation and vellus hair; increased hair growth
Contraindications: Untreated bacterial, fungal or viral skin infections
Precautions: Pregnancy and breast feeding (inadequate safety information), long term use, use with occlusion – restrict limited areas, rebound relapses in psoriasis following development of tolerance

NURSING CONSIDERATIONS

Administer:
- To clean, dry skin
- Apply sparingly to affected area only

Evaluate:
- Effect of drug – improving skin rash
- For localised side effects – rash may be worse to begin with, thinning of skin, hair growth
- For systemic reactions (usually only with long term treatment over large skin areas) – hypertension, water and sodium retention, signs of diabetes and adrenal suppression. Notify clinician at once

Teach patient/family:
- To avoid drug contact with eyes
- To apply sparingly to affected areas only
- Not to use for other skin eruptions
- To inform clinician of any side effects
- Check with G.P. before taking any other medications
- Withhold treatment and notify clinician if rash appears worse

hydrocortisone/ hydrocortisone acetate/ hydrocortisone sodium phosphate/ hydrocortisone sodium succinate

Colifoam, Corlan, Efcortelan Soluble, Efcortesol, Hydrocortistab, Hydrocortone, Solu-cortef
Func. class.: Corticosteroid,
Chem. class.: Glucocorticoid, short-acting
Legal class.: POM

Action: Decreases inflammation by suppression of migration of polymorphonuclear leucocytes, fibroblasts, reversal of increased capillary permeability and lysosomal stabilisation
Uses: Severe inflammation including status asthmaticus, acute allergic reactions, anaphylactic drug reactions; shock, acute adrenal insufficiency, joint conditions including tennis elbow, ulcerative colitis, severe erythema multiforme, systemic lupus erythematosus
Dosage and routes:
Adrenal insufficiency/inflammation shock

• *Adult:* IM, IV infusion, slow IV 100–500 mg (succinate or phosphate) repeated 3–4 times in 24 hr as required
• *Child under 1 yr:* IV 25 mg; 1–5 yr: IV 50 mg; 6–12 yr: IV 100 mg repeated 3–4 times in 24 hr as required

Colitis/Proctitis
• *Adult:* By rectum, aerosol: one application nightly for 2–3 weeks then alternate days; suppository: 25 mg night and morning and after a bowel movement

Joints
• *Adult:* Injection intra-articular, peri-articular 5–50 mg (acetate) according to joint; no more than 3 injections in 24 hr
• *Child:* 5–30 mg daily in divided doses

Replacement
• *Adult:* By mouth 20–30 mg daily in divided doses
• *Child:* 10–30 mg in divided doses

Available forms include: Tablets 10, 20 mg; phosphate injection 100 mg/ml; succinate injection 100 mg/vial; acetate injection 25 mg/ml; aerosol 10%; 25 mg suppository

Side effects/adverse reactions:
INTEG: Acne, poor wound healing, bruising, striae, telangiectasia, atrophy
CNS: Depression, psychological dependance, insomnia, euphoria, aggravation of schizophrenia
CV: Thromboembolism, sodium and water retention, hypertension, potassium loss
HAEM: Leucocytosis
MS: Fractures, osteoporosis, proximal myopathy, tendon rupture, avascular osteonecrosis
GI: Nausea, abdominal distension, increased appetite, peptic ulceration with perforation and haemorrhage, dyspepsia, oesophageal ulceration, oesophageal candidiasis, acute pancreatitis
EENT: Increased intra-ocular pressure, glaucoma, exacerbation of ophthalmic viral or fungal disease, exophthalmos, corneal or scleral thinning, papilloedema
ENDO: Growth suppression in children and adolescents, suppression or hypothalomopituitary-adrenal axis, menstrual irregularity and amenorrhoea, weight gain, Cushingoid features, hirsutism, negative nitrogen balance, increased carbohydrate tolerance with increased requirement for antidiabetic therapy
MISC: Recurrence of dormant tuberculosis, opportunist infection

Contraindications: Hypersensitivity, do not inject into tendons, immunisation procedures, systemic infection unless specific anti-infective therapy is employed

Precautions: Pregnancy, lactation, diabetes mellitus, osteoporosis, glaucoma (or family history of glaucoma), peptic ulcer, congestive heart failure, epilepsy, psychosis or severe psychoneuroses, history of tuberculosis, hypertension, previous steroid myopathy, symptoms of infection suppressed, renal insufficiency
See data sheet compendium for further information

Pharmacokinetics:
By mouth: Onset 1–2 hr, peak 1 hr, duration 1–1½ days
IM/IV: Onset 20 min, peak 4–8 hr, duration 1–1½ days
Rectal: Onset 3–5 days
Metabolised by liver, excreted in urine (17-hydroxycorticosteroids, 17-ketosteroids)

Interactions/incompatibilities:
• Decreased action of this drug: barbiturates, carbamazepine, phenytoin, primidone, rifampicin, ephedrine, anticoagulants
• Decreased effects of: Cholecystographic X-ray media, salicylates, anticoagulants, hypoglycaemic

agents, anti-hypertensives, diuretics, anticholinesterases
• Increased risk of hypokalaemia: acetazolamide, loop diuretics, thiazides, carbenoxolone, β_2-sympathomimetics, amphotericin
Clinical assessment:
• Potassium, blood sugar, urine glucose while on long-term therapy; hypokalaemia, hypertension, mental changes, gastric discomfort, hyperglycaemia
• Plasma cortisol levels during long-term therapy (normal level: 138–635 nmol/litre when drawn at 8 a.m.)

NURSING CONSIDERATIONS

Assess:
• Baseline weight and BP
Administer:
• Orally with food or milk to decrease GI symptoms
• Shake suspension (parenteral)
• Titrated dose, use lowest effective dose
• IM injection deeply in large mass, rotate sites, avoid deltoid, use large bore needle
• In one dose in morning to prevent adrenal suppression, avoid subcutaneous administration, damage may be done to tissue
Perform/provide:
• Weight daily or twice weekly if stable
• Assistance with mobility in patient with bone tissue disease to prevent fractures
Evaluate:
• Fluid balance ratio, be alert for decreasing urinary output and increasing oedema
• Therapeutic response: ease of respirations, decreased inflammation
• Infection: increased temperature, WBC, even after withdrawal of medication; drug masks symptoms of infection
• Potassium depletion: paraesthesia, fatigue, nausea, vomiting, depression, polyuria, dysrhythmias, weakness
• Oedema, hypotension, cardiac symptoms
• Mental status: affect, mood, behavioural changes, aggression, weight gain
Teach patient/family:
• That ID as steroid user should be carried
• To notify clinician if therapeutic response decreases; dosage adjustment may be needed
• Not to discontinue this medication abruptly or adrenal crisis can result
• To avoid non-prescribed products: salicylates, alcohol in cough products, cold preparations unless directed by clinician
• Teach patient all aspects of drug use, including Cushingoid symptoms
• Symptoms of adrenal insufficiency: nausea, anorexia, fatigue, dizziness, dyspnoea, weakness, joint pain

---

hydrogen peroxide

Func. class.: Antiseptic and disinfectant
Chem. class.: Oxidising drug
Legal class.: Solution GSL

Action: Bactericidal
Uses: Skin disinfection, wound and ulcer cleaning and deodourising, mouthwash
Dosage and routes:
• *Adult and child:* Solution, use topically as required
Available forms include: Solution 3%, 6%, 27% and 30% (dilute before use)
Side effects/adverse reactions:
INTEG: 'Irritating' burns
EENT: Use as mouthwash – reversible hypertrophy of papillae of tongue

Contraindications: Hypersensitivity, closed wounds
Precautions: Large or deep wounds, normal skin, bleaches fabric and clothing
Pharmacokinetics: Effective to end of bubbling (oxygen release)

NURSING CONSIDERATIONS

Assess:
• Appropriateness of agent as part of wound management/mouth care
• Patient's ability to avoid ingestion by swallowing if used as mouthwash

Administer:
• Only if no evidence that effervescence can enter blood stream (i.e. not in deep wounds) in order to avoid air/gas embolus
• Diluted, as prescribed
• With care, onto sloughing area of wound avoiding healthy tissue where possible
• Irrigate with normal saline after application
• As a diluted mouthwash for stomatitis

Evaluate:
• Effectiveness of wound cleansing by absence of sloughly material and evidence of tissue granulation—change to other non-desloughing agent at such time
• As mouthwash, oral condition improved, again change to a different preparation

Teach patient/family:
• Technique of administration
• Importance of medical review
• Other aspects to influence oral hygiene if appropriate
• To avoid swallowing

hydroxocobalamin (vitamin B_{12})

NHS Neo-Cytamen, Cobalin-H
Func. class.: Fat soluble vitamin
Legal class.: POM

Action: Needed for adequate nerve functioning, protein and carbohydrate metabolism, normal growth, RBC development
Uses: Vitamin B_{12} deficiency, pernicious anaemia, vitamin B_{12} malabsorption syndrome, tobacco amblyopia, Leber's optic atrophy, subacute combined degeneration of the spinal cord

Dosage and routes:
• *Adult and child:* IM 250–1000 mcg at intervals of 2–3 days for 5 doses; maintenance 1 mg every month. See data sheet for further information

Available forms include: Injection 1 mg

Side effects/adverse reactions:
CNS: Dizziness, hot flushes
INTEG: Itching, exanthema, acneform/bullous eruptions
MISC: Anaphylaxis, chills, fever
GI: Nausea

Contraindications: Hypersensitivity, megaloblastic anaemia of pregnancy
Precautions: Give only after establishing diagnosis; investigate folate metabolism if megaloblastic anaemia fails to respond; hypokalaemia
Pharmacokinetics: Stored in liver, kidneys, stomach; 50%–90% excreted in urine, breast milk

Interactions/incompatibilities:
• Decreased effect of this drug: chloramphenicol, oral contraceptives
• Increased absorption: prednisone

Clinical assessment:
• Full blood count for increase in reticulocyte count during first

week of therapy, then increase in RBC and Hb
• Initial therapy: monitor patient for hypersensitivity reactions
Lab. test interferences: B_{12} assays by microbiological techniques invalidated by anti-metabolites and most antibiotics
Treatment of overdose:
Discontinue drug

NURSING CONSIDERATIONS

Assess:
• Potassium levels during beginning treatment
• Full blood count for increased reticulocyte count during 1st week of therapy
Evaluate:
• Therapeutic response: decreased anorexia, dyspnoea on excretion, palpitations, paraesthesia, psychosis, visual disturbances
• Nutritional status: should include good sources of vitamin B_{12}
• For pulmonary oedema, or worsening of congestive cardiac failure in cardiac patients
Teach patient/family:
• That treatment must continue for life if diagnosis is pernicious anaemia
• About taking a well balanced diet
• That itching skin eruptions must be reported to clinician immediately

hydroxychloroquine sulphate

Plaquenil
Func. class.: Antirheumatic
Chem. class.: 4-aminoquinoline derivative
Legal class.: POM

Action: Mode of action in rheumatism uncertain; may modify disease process
Uses: Rheumatoid arthritis, systemic and discoid lupus erythematosus, dermatological conditions sunlight related
Dosage and routes:
Rheumatoid arthritis, systemic lupus erythematosus
(Seek expert advice)
• *Adult:* By mouth initially 400 mg daily in divided doses reduced to 200–400 mg daily maintenance, using minimum effective dose, maximum 6.5 mg/kg daily (ideal body weight *not* actual body weight)
• *Children:* Up to 6.5 mg/kg daily. Discontinue if no improvement in 6 months
Available forms include: Tablets 200 mg
Side effects/adverse reactions:
INTEG: Rashes, pigmentary changes, hair bleaching and loss, pruritus, skin eruptions
CNS: Headache, nervousness, emotional upsets, psychotic episodes
EENT: Visual disturbances, irreversible retinal damage, corneal opacities, photophobia, vertigo, tinnitus, deafness, difficulty focusing
GI: Nausea, vomiting, anorexia, diarrhoea, cramps
HAEM: Thrombocytopenia, agranulocytosis, aplastic anaemia
CV: Hypotension, ECG changes
Contraindications: Hypersensitivity to 4 aminoquinoline compounds, pregnancy, maculopathy
Precautions: Renal and hepatic impairment, porphyria, psoriasis, neurological disorders, severe gastrointestinal disorders, G6PD deficiency, elderly, visual defects, blood disorders. Ophthalmological examination before starting treatment. Possible visual accommodation impairment initially, warn patients against driving or operating machinery

Pharmacokinetics:
By mouth: Peak 1–2 hr, half-life 3–5 days, metabolised in liver, excreted in urine, faeces, breast milk
Interactions/incompatibilities:
• Decreased absorption of this drug: antacids
• Increased plasma concentration of this drug: cimetidine
• Increased plasma concentration of: digoxin
Treatment of overdose: Evacuate stomach by gastric lavage or emesis; further inhibit absorption with charcoal. Administer parenteral diazepam to reverse chloroquine cardiotoxicity. Prepare to give respiratory support and treatment for shock with fluids and if necessary plasma expanders. In severe cases consider using dopamine
NURSING CONSIDERATIONS
Administer:
• With or after meals at same time each day to maintain drug level
Perform/provide:
• Storage injection should be kept in cool environment
Teach patient/family:
• To use sunglasses in bright sunlight to decrease photophobia
• To report hearing, visual problems, fever, fatigue, bruising, bleeding, which may indicate blood dyscrasias
• To take with food to reduce upset stomach and mark bitter taste
• Other side-effects: nausea, diarrhoea, loss of appetite, skin rashes, lightening and thinning of hair
• Skin irritation in sunlight
• Importance of eye testing
• Allow 4 hr between taking indigestion medicine and hydrochloroquine

hydroxyprogesterone hexanoate

Proluton Depot
Func. class.: Progestogen hormone
Legal class.: POM

Action: Replaces progesterone in deficiency to maintain pregnancy
Uses: Habitual abortion associated with progesterone deficiency
Dosage and routes:
• *Adult:* IM 250–500 mg weekly during first half of pregnancy
Available forms include: Injection IM 250, 500 mg ampoules
Side effects/adverse reactions:
CNS: Depression
CV: Oedema
GI: Disturbances, cholestatic jaundice
INTEG: Acne, urticaria, allergic skin rashes
GU: Breast discomfort, gynaecomastia, irregular menstrual cycles, menstrual bleeding
MISC: Weight gain, changes in libido
Contraindications: History of pemphigoid gestationis, existing or previous liver tumours, undiagnosed vaginal bleeding, mammary carcinoma, missed or incomplete abortion, past severe arterial disease or current high risk, porphyria
Precautions: Hypertension, asthma, cardiovascular, renal or hepatic impairment, diabetes mellitus, depression, breast feeding, epilepsy, migraine
Pharmacokinetics:
IM: Half-life 5 min, excreted in urine, faeces, metabolised in liver
Clinical assessment:
• Liver function tests: alanine aminotransferase, aspartate aminotransferase, bilirubin, periodically during long-term therapy

NURSING CONSIDERATIONS

Assess:

- Baseline and fluid balance
- Weight
- BP at beginning of treatment and periodically

Administer:

- Oil solution deeply in large muscle mass (IM), rotate sites
- In one dose in the morning

Evaluate:

- Therapeutic response
- Oedema, hypertension, cardiac symptoms, jaundice
- Mental status: affect, mood, behavioural changes, depression
- Weight gain
- Fluid balance

Teach patient/family:

- All aspects of drug usage, including Cushingoid symptoms
- To report any side effects
- Explain full expected effects of drug

---

hydroxyurea

Hydrea

Func. class.: Antineoplastic

Chem. class.: Synthetic urea analogue

Legal class.: POM

Action: Acts by inhibiting DNA synthesis without interfering with RNA or protein synthesis; incorporates thymidine into DNA, causing direct damage to DNA strands

Uses: Chronic myeloid leukaemia, cancer of the cervix (with radiotherapy)

Dosage and routes:

Doses are highly variable, and dependent on local treatment protocols, concomitant therapy and tumour type; the following dose schedules have been used

- *Adult:* By mouth continuous regimen 20–30 mg/kg daily or intermittent regimen 80 mg/kg every third day

Available forms include: Capsules 500 mg

Side effects/adverse reactions:

HAEM: Leucopenia, anaemia, thrombocytopenia

GI: Nausea, vomiting, anorexia, diarrhoea, stomatitis, constipation, abdominal pain

GU: Increased blood urea nitrogen, uric acid and creatinine, renal function impairment, dysuria

INTEG: Rash, alopecia, erythema

CNS: Headache, drowsiness, dizziness, disorientation, hallucinations, convulsions

Contraindications: Hypersensitivity, marked thrombocytopenia, leucopenia, severe anaemia

Precautions: Renal dysfunction, pregnancy, elderly, increase in myelosuppressive activity with previous or ongoing cytotoxic treatment or radiotherapy. Monitor blood, bone marrow, renal and liver function, uric acid. Correct anaemia before therapy

Pharmacokinetics: Readily absorbed when taken orally, peak level in 2 hr, degraded in liver, excreted in urine, almost totally eliminated in 24 hr; readily crosses blood-brain barrier

Interactions/incompatibilities:

- Increased toxicity: other cytotoxic drugs

Clinical assessment:

- Liver function tests before, during therapy: bilirubin, alkaline phosphatase, aspartate aminotransferase, alanine aminotransferase, lactic dehydrogenase; as needed or monthly
- Other medications by oral route if possible

Treatment of overdose: Gastric lavage, supportive therapy short term. Long term monitor haemopoietic system with blood transfusion if necessary

NURSING CONSIDERATIONS

Administer:

• HANDLING: take safety precautions appropriate to antineoplastic agents
• Following local antineoplastic (cytotoxic) policies
• Anti-emetic 30–60 min before giving drug to prevent vomiting (severe in high doses)
• Transfusion for anaemia
• Antibiotics for prophylaxis of infection if indicated
• Topical or systemic analgesics for pain
• Other medications by oral route if possible

Perform/provide:

• Nutritious diet with iron, vitamin supplements as ordered
• Strict oral hygiene 4 times a day

Evaluate:

• Fluid balance ratio, report fall in urine output to less than 30 ml/hr
• Monitor temperature 4 hrly; fever may indicate beginning infection
• Bleeding: haematuria, bruising or petechiae, mucosa or orifices 8 hrly
• Level of drowsiness which may occur after taking medication
• Buccal cavity 8 hrly for dryness, sores or ulceration, white patches, oral pain, bleeding, dysphagia
• Neurotoxicity: headaches, hallucinations, convulsions, dizziness
• Symptoms indicating severe allergic reaction: rash, urticaria, itching, flushing
• Inflammation of mucosa, breaks in skin
• Food preferences; list likes, dislikes
• Effects of alopecia on body image, discuss feelings about body changes

Teach patient/family:

• To report any complaints, side effects to nurse or clinician
• That hair may be lost during treatment, and wig or hair piece may be available on the NHS; tell patient that new hair may be different in colour, texture
• To avoid foods with citric acid, hot or rough texture if stomatitis is present
• To report stomatitis: any bleeding, white spots, ulcerations in the mouth; tell patient to examine mouth daily, report symptoms
• Contraceptive measures are recommended during therapy
• To drink 2 litres of fluid
• Notify clinician of fever, chills, sore throat, nausea, vomiting, anorexia, diarrhoea, bleeding, bruising; may indicate blood dyscrasias
• About side effects and benefits

hydroxyzine hydrochloride

Atarax

Func. class.: Anxiolytic, antipruritic
Chem. class.: Antihistamine, piperazine group
Legal class.: POM

Action: Depresses subcortical levels of CNS, including limbic system, reticular formation; competitive antagonist at H_1 receptors

Uses: Adjunct in treatment of anxiety, pruritus

Dosage and routes:

Anxiety

• *Adult:* By mouth 50–100 mg 4 times a day

Pruritus

• *Adult:* By mouth 25 mg at night initially and increasing to 25 mg 3 to 4 times daily if required
• *Child:* By mouth, 6 months to 6 yr, 5–15 mg daily increasing to 50 mg daily if necessary in divided doses; over 6 yr, 15–25 mg in-

creasing to 50–100 mg daily if necessary in divided doses
Available forms include: Tablets 10 mg, 25 mg; syrup 10 mg/5 ml
Side effects/adverse reactions:
CNS: Dizziness, drowsiness, confusion, headache, tremor, convulsions, stimulation
GI: Gastrointestinal disturbances, dry mouth
INTEG: Rash, photosensitivity reactions
CV: ECG abnormalities
EENT: Blurred vision
Contraindications: Hypersensitivity, porphyria, early pregnancy
Precautions: Impaired renal function, hepatic disease. May impair mental alertness or physical co-ordination, warn patients against driving or operating machinery if affected
Pharmacokinetics:
By mouth: Onset 15–30 min, duration 4–6 hr, half-life 3 hr
Interactions/incompatibilities:
• Increased CNS depressant effect: alcohol, barbiturates, other anxiolytics, hypnotics
Lab. test interferences:
False increase: estimation of urinary 17-hydroxycorticosteroids
Treatment of overdose: Induction of vomiting in conscious patients and gastric lavage, supportive care. If hypotension, control with intravenous fluids and noradrenaline or metaraminol

NURSING CONSIDERATIONS

Assess:
• Baseline BP (lying, standing), pulse
Administer:
• Crushed if patient is unable to swallow medication whole
• Frequent sips of water for dry mouth
Perform/provide:
• Assistance with mobility during beginning therapy, since drowsiness/dizziness occurs
• Safety measures, including cot sides
• Checking to see oral medication has been swallowed
Evaluate:
• Mental status: mood, alertness, affect
• Physical dependency and withdrawal symptoms: headache, nausea, vomiting, muscle pain, weakness after long-term use
• Increased sedation
Teach patient/family:
• Not to be used for everyday stress or used longer than 4 months
• Avoid non-prescribed preparations (cold, cough, hay fever) unless approved by clinician
• To avoid driving, activities that require alertness
• To avoid alcohol ingestion, or other psychotropic medications
• Not to discontinue medication quickly after long-term use
• To rise slowly or fainting may occur

hyoscine hydrobromide (ophthalmic)

Func. class.: Mydriatic
Chem. class.: Synthetic alkaloid
Legal class.: POM

Action: Blocks response of iris sphincter muscle, muscle of accommodation of ciliary body to cholinergic stimulation, resulting in dilatation, paralysis of accommodation
Uses: Uveitis, iritis, cycloplegic refraction
Dosage and routes:
• *Adult:* Instil 1–2 drops before refraction or 1–2 drops 1–3 times a day for iritis or uveitis
• *Child:* Instil 1 drop before refraction

Available forms include: Eyedrops 0.25%

Side effects/adverse reactions:

EENT: Increased intraocular pressure, blurred vision, photophobia, irritation, oedema

INTEG: Contact dermatitis, rash, dry skin

CV: Bradycardia, tachycardia, palpitations, arrhythmias

CNS: Giddiness, staggering, psychotic reactions

GI: Dry mouth, constipation, abdominal distension

Contraindications: Hypersensitivity, glaucoma or tendency to glaucoma (e.g. narrow anterior chamber angle)

Precautions: Systemic reactions in young and very old, pregnancy, lactation

Pharmacokinetics:

INSTIL: Peak 20–30 min, duration 3–7 days

Interactions/incompatibilities:

- Possible enhanced action by other drugs with antimuscarinic properties: some antihistamines, phenothiazines, tricyclic antidepressants, butyrophenones

Treatment of overdose: If systemic toxicity occurs provide supportive treatment

If ingested: emesis or gastric lavage

NURSING CONSIDERATIONS

Administer:

- Without contact of dropper to eye

Perform/provide:

- Mark container with date of opening and discard weekly if used in hospital ward, but daily if used in outpatients or casualty departments
- In operating theatres previously unopened containers should be used for each patient. Post-operative patient should always use separate contain even in outpatients

Evaluate:

- Therapeutic response: dilation of pupil, paralysis of muscles causing inability to contract pupil, decreased inflammation
- Eye pain, discontinue and inform the clinician

Teach patient/family:

- To install after washing hands well without touching dropper to eye
- To administer correctly never exceed dosage to avoid absorption into whole circulatory system
- To notify clinician if dry mouth, increased pulse, trouble breathing, sweating, flushing occur. Discontinue immediately
- That blurred vision is temporary and will decrease with repeated use
- Not to drive or use machinery until sight has returned to normal
- Wait 5 min before using other drops

---

hyoscine hydrobromide (transdermal)

Scopoderm TTS

Func. class.: Anti-emetic, anticholinergic

Chem. class.: Belladonna alkaloid

Legal class.: POM

Action: Competitive antagonist of acetylcholine and other parasympathomimetic agents. Action in preventing motion sickness in central nervous system unknown

Uses: Prevention of symptoms of motion sickness

Dosage and routes:

- *Adults and child over 10 yr:* Patch applied behind ear 5–6 hr before travel

Available forms include: Self adhesive patch (transdermal drug delivery system). Average drug absorbed over 72 hr 500 mcg

Side effects/adverse reactions:
CNS: Drowsiness, dizziness, restlessness, disorientation, confusion, visual hallucinations, memory and concentration impairment
EENT: Dilated pupils, visual disturbances
GI: Dry mouth
GU: Urine retention
Contraindications: Hypersensitivity, closed-angle glaucoma
Precautions: Pyloric stenosis, bladder outflow obstruction, intestinal obstruction, elderly, impaired hepatic or renal function, pregnancy, lactation, epilepsy
Pharmacokinetics:
Patch: Onset 15–30 min, duration 72 hr
Interactions/incompatibilities:
- Increased antimuscarinic effects with: antidepressants, antihistamines, antipsychotics, use with caution with CNS acting drugs including alcohol

Treatment of overdose: Remove patch; give physostigmine by slow IV injection 1–4 mg (children 0.5 mg). Repeat if necessary. See further information in data sheet compendium
NURSING CONSIDERATIONS
Administer:
- To area behind ear that is not hairy

Teach patient/family:
- Caution patients against driving or operating machinery. Side effects may last up to 24 hr after removing patch
- To wash, dry hands before applying to surface behind ear
- Apply at least 3 hr before traveling
- Change patch every 72 hr
- To wash hands after handling
- To wash application site after removing
- Report blurred vision, severe dizziness, drowsiness occurs; discontinue use
- To read label of all non-prescribed medications; if any hyoscine is found in product, avoid use
- Use only one patch at a time

hyoscine-N-butylbromide/ hyoscine hydrobromide

Buscopan, combination product
Func. class.: Antimuscarinic
Chem. class.: Belladonna alkaloid
Legal class.: POM

Action: Inhibits acetylcholine at receptor sites in autonomic nervous system, which controls secretions, acts on dopamine receptors in CNS, which decrease involuntary movements
Uses: Gastrointestinal antispasmodic, reduction of secretions before surgery, amnesia, motion sickness
Dosage and routes:
Antispasmodic
- *Adult:* By mouth (butylobromide) 20 mg 4 times a day
- *Child 6–12 yr:* 10 mg 3 times a day

Acute spasm
- IV or IV injection (butylbromide) 20 mg repeated after half an hour if necessary

Premedication
- *Adult:* Subcutaneous or IM injection (hydrobromide) 200–600 mcg half an hour to one hour before anaesthesia
- *Child:* 15 mcg per kg.

Usually given with papaveretum
Available forms include: Tablets (butylbromide) 10 mg; injection (butylbromide) 20 mg/ml, 1 ml ampoules; injection (hydrobromide) 400 mcg/ml, 1 ml, 600 mcg/ml, 1 ml
Side effects/adverse reactions:

CNS: Confusion, depression, psychotic reactions
EENT: Blurred vision, photophobia, dilated pupils, difficulty swallowing, increased ocular pressure
CV: Palpitations, bradycardia, tachycardia, arrhythmias
GI: Dry mouth, constipation, abdominal distension
GU: Urine retention
INTEG: Dry skin, rash
Contraindications: Hypersensitivity, prostatic hypertrophy, pyloric stenosis, paralyticileus, urinary retention, closed-angle glaucoma
Precautions: Pregnancy, breast-feeding, cardiac insufficiency, ulcerative colitis, gastro-oesophageal reflux
Pharmacokinetics:
By mouth: Peak 1 hr, duration 6 hr
Subcutaneous/IM: Peak 30–45 min, duration 7 hr
IV: Peak 10–15 min, duration 4 hr
Excreted in urine, bile, faeces (unchanged)
Interactions/incompatibilities:
• Possible enhanced action by other drugs with antimuscarinic properties: some antihistamines, phenothiazines, tricyclic antidepressants, butyrophenones
Treatment of overdose: Orally ingested: emesis or gastric lavage. If systemic toxicity use parasympathetic agents as necessary, e.g. pilocarpine or neostigmine
NURSING CONSIDERATIONS
Assess:
• Baseline fluid balance and pulse
Perform/provide:
• Storage at room temperature in light-resistant containers
• Frequent drinks, mouthwashes to relieve dry mouth
Evaluate:
• Therapeutic response
• Parkinsonism, extrapyramidal symptoms: shuffling gait, muscle rigidity, involuntary movements
• Urinary fluid balance retention
• Constipation; increase fluids, bulk, exercise if this occurs
• For tolerance over long-term therapy; dose may need to be increased or changed
Teach patient/family:
• Not to discontinue this drug abruptly; to taper off over 1 week
• To avoid driving or other hazardous activities; drowsiness may occur
• To avoid non-prescribed medication: cough, cold preparations with alcohol, antihistamines unless advised by clinician

ibuprofen ▼

Apsifen, Arthrofen, Lidifen, Ebufac, Ibular, Isisfen, Ibumed, Rimafen, Motrin, Brufen, Fenbid, Junifen, many other proprietary brands available, combination products
Func. class.: Non-steroidal anti-inflammatory drug
Chem. class.: Propionic acid derivative
Legal class.: POM, but P if labelled for specific dosage and indications

Action: Inhibits prostaglandin synthesis by decreasing enzyme needed for biosynthesis; possesses analgesic, anti-inflammatory, antipyretic properties
Uses: As an analgesic and anti-inflammatory in rheumatoid arthritis, juvenile arthritis, ankylosing spondylitis, osteoarthritis, other musculoskeletal disorders—capsulitis, tendinitis, etc., soft tissue injuries. As an analgesic in dysmenorrhoea, dental pain, migraine, post-operative pain
Dosage and routes:
• *Adult:* 1200–1800 mg daily in 3–4 doses; maximum 2400 mg per

day; usual maintenance 600–1200 mg daily
• Modified-release tablets 1600 mg daily increased in severe cases to 2400 mg daily in 2 divided doses
• Spansules modified-release 300–900 mg every 12 hours
• *Child:* 20 mg/kg daily in divided doses; juvenile arthritis up to 40 mg/kg daily in divided doses. Not recommended for children less than 7 kg

Available forms include: Tablets 200 mg, 400 mg, 600 mg; sustained-release tablets 800 mg; spansules 300 mg; syrup 100 mg/5 ml; granules 600 mg

Side effects/adverse reactions:
GI: Nausea, diarrhoea, gastrointestinal discomfort, bleeding, ulceration, dyspepsia
CNS: Dizziness, headache, nervousness, depression, drowsiness, insomnia
INTEG: Rash, pruritus
GU: Nephrotoxicity, haematuria, oliguria
HAEM: Blood dyscrasias—agranulocytosis, thrombocytopenia
EENT: Tinnitus, blurred vision

Contraindications: Hypersensitivity; hypersensitivity to aspirin or other NSAIDS; active or suspected peptic ulcer or GI haemorrhage; heart failure, 3rd trimester of pregnancy; asthma; severe renal disease; severe hepatic disease

Precautions: Pregnancy, lactation, children, cardiac disorders, bleeding disorders

Pharmacokinetics:
By mouth: Peak 1–2 hr, half-life 2–4 hr, metabolised in liver (inactive metabolites), excreted in urine (inactive metabolites)

Interactions/incompatibilities:
• May increase action of: oral anti-coagulants, thiazide diuretics, lithium

Treatment of overdose: Gastric lavage, correction of plasma electrolytes and symptomatic relief

NURSING CONSIDERATIONS

Administer:
• With or after food or milk
• Mix granules with water
• Swallow sustained- release preparation whole with plenty of water

Evaluate:
• Therapeutic response: decreased pain, stiffness in joints, decreased swelling in joints, ability to move more easily
• For eye, ear problems: blurred vision, tinnitus; may indicate toxicity

Teach patient/family:
• To report any wheeziness or breathlessness, rash, unresolved indigestion or black tarry stools
• To report blurred vision, ringing, roaring in ears; may indicate toxicity
• To avoid driving, other hazardous activities if dizziness, drowsiness occurs
• To report change in urine pattern, increased weight, oedema, increased pain in joints, fever, blood in urine; indicate nephrotoxicity
• That therapeutic effects may take up to 1 month
• To avoid alcohol, salicylates; bleeding may occur

ibuprofen (topical)

Ibugel, Ibuleve Gel, Proflex Cream
Func. class.: Topical non steroidal anti-inflammatory agent
Chem. class.: Propionic acid derivative
Legal class.: P

Action: Inhibits prostaglandin synthesis; possesses analgesic and anti-inflammatory properties

Uses: Topical application to superficial joints affected by osteoarthritis, rheumatic and muscular pain, muscular skeletal injuries, backache and neuralgia

Dosage and routes:

• *Adults:* Topically

Gel: Apply a thin layer to the affected area and massage up to 3 times a day

Cream: Apply 4–10 cm to the affected area and massage 3–4 times a day

Review therapy after a few weeks

Available forms include: Gel 5%, Cream 5%

Side effects/adverse reactions:

INTEG: Erythema and at site of application. Systemic side effects are unlikely

Contraindications: Hypersensitivity or asthma induced by ibuprofen, aspirin or other NSAIDs; children under 14 yr

Precautions: For topical use only; keep away from eyes, lips and mucous membranes; avoid contact with broken skin; pregnancy; lactation; asthma

Pharmacokinetics: Percutaneous absorption of ibuprofen is about 5% that of oral ibuprofen. Maximum systemic concentration after 2 hr approximately 0.64 microgram/ml but higher levels achieved locally

Interactions: Unlikely to occur at low plasma levels achieved

Treatment of overdose: Overdose extremely unlikely from topical use. If ingested orally treat with supportive and symptomatic measures

NURSING CONSIDERATIONS

Assess:

• Hypersensitivity or asthma

Perform/provide:

• Gloves for professional applicant

Administer:

• Massage until absorbed into affected area

Evaluate:

• Clinical response

• Local side effects

Teach patient/family:

• Correct method of application

• Not to apply to broken skin, mucous membranes, lips or near eyes

• To wash hands thoroughly after use

• To discontinue if side effects occur or pregnancy is likely

---

idarubicin HCl

Zavedos

Func. class.: Antineoplastic

Chem. class.: Anthracycline antibiotic

Legal class.: POM

Action: Interferes with DNA topoisomerase II activity, thus causing cell death

Uses: Acute non-lymphocytic leukaemia in adults, for remission induction in untreated patients or relapsed or refactory patients; acute lymphocytic leukaemia as second line treatment in adults and children. May be used in combination chemotherapy regimes

Dosage and routes:

Doses are highly variable, and dependent on local treatment protocols, concomitant therapy and tumour type; the following dose schedules have been used

Acute non-lymphocytic leukaemia

• *Adults:* IV 12 mg/m^2 daily for 3 days with cytarabine or 8 mg/m^2 daily for 5 days as single agent or in combination

Acute lymphocytic leukaemia

• *Adults:* IV 12 mg/m^2 daily for 3 days

• *Child:* IV 10 mg/m^2 daily for 3 days

Available forms include: Injection 5 mg, 10 mg

Side effects/adverse reactions:
GI: Nausea, vomiting, mucositis, oesophagitis, diarrhoea
CV: Cardiac toxicity: congestive heart failure, acute arrhythmias
INTEG: Reversible alopecia, skin rash, irritation
CNS: Fever, chills
HAEM: Severe myelosuppression, elevation of liver enzymes and bilirubin
GU: Red coloured urine

Contraindications: Severe renal and hepatic impairment; uncontrolled infections; breast-feeding; pregnancy should be avoided

Precautions: Pre-existing heart disease and previous therapy with anthracyclines in high cumulative doses are co-factors for increased risk of idarubicin cardiac toxicity. Monitor cardiac function, monitor blood (to include granulocytes, red cells, platelets and uric acid), renal and hepatic function; systemic infection–control prior to therapy, extravasation

Pharmacokinetics:
IV: Half-life 15–18 hr

Interactions/incompatibilities:
- Increased toxicity: other cytotoxic drugs
- Do not mix with heparin or other drugs

Clinical assessment:
- Blood counts, liver function tests
- ECG for cardiotoxity

Treatment of overdose: Supportive treatment for acute myocardial toxicity and myelosupression

NURSING CONSIDERATIONS

Assess:
- Baseline fluid balance prior to therapy and monitor strict fluid balance during therapy
- Careful haematological monitoring is required to check for myelosuppression
- Potentially fatal congestive heart failure, acute life-threatening arrhythmias or other cardiomyopathies may occur during therapy or several weeks after therapy

Administer:
- HANDLING: take safety precautions appropriate to antineoplastic agents
- Following local antineoplastic (cytotoxic) policies
- After reconstituing contents of vial (5 ml of water for 5 mg vial, 10 ml water for 10 mg vial)
- IV: By slow IV injection over 5–10 min into tubing of running infusion of sodium chloride 0.9%
- Do not mix with other drugs
- Taking care to avoid extravasation which can cause severe local tissue necrosis
- Anti-emetic 30–60 min before treatment
- All other medication as prescribed including analgesics, antibiotics, anti-emetics, antispasmodics

Evaluate:
- Liver and kidney function: should be evaluated before and during treatment; uric acid levels should be monitored because of a risk of hyperuricaemia
- Systemic infection: should be controlled before starting therapy
- Extravasation: can cause severe local tissue necrosis

Teach patient/family:
- Idarubicin may give urine a red colour for 1 or 2 days; patients should be advised that this is no cause for alarm

---

idoxuridine

Herpid, Iduridin, Virudox, Idoxene
Func. class.: Antiviral
Chem. class.: Pyrimidine nucleoside
Legal class.: POM

Action: Arrests replication of DNA viruses

Uses: Cutaneous or ocular infection by herpes simplex and other DNA viruses sensitive to idoxuridine

Dosage and routes:

Eye

• *Adult and child:* Apply ointment, 4-hrly. Maximum period of treatment 21 days.

Skin

• *Adult:* Apply 5% solution to lesions 6-hrly for 3–4 days; severe lesions, use 40% solution. Not recommended in children under 12 yr

Available forms include: *Eye:* ointment 0.5%

Skin: solution 5%, 40% in dimethyl sulphoxide

Side effects/adverse reactions:

EENT: Poor corneal wound healing, temporary visual haze, oedema, itching, occlusion of lachrymal puncta

INTEG: Stinging, taste changes, over usage may lead to maceration of skin

Contraindications: Hypersensitivity to idoxaridine or dimethyl sulphoxide, pregnancy, dermographia

Interactions/incompatibilities:

• Do not use boric acid with this drug

NURSING CONSIDERATIONS

Administer:

• Use gloves to avoid re-infecting other areas, especially face, genitalia

• Cleanse crusts or discharge from eye before application

Perform/provide:

• Storage at room temperature. Do not refrigerate

Evaluate:

• Therapeutic response: absence of redness, inflammation, tearing

• Allergy: itching, lacrimation, redness, swelling

Teach patient/family:

• To use drug exactly as prescribed

• Not to use eye makeup, towels, washcloths, eye medication of others; reinfection may occur

• That drug container tip should not be touched to eye

• To report itching, increased redness, burning, stinging, swelling; drug should be discontinued

• That drug may cause blurred vision when ointment is applied

• Skin preparations can damage some synthetic materials e.g. artificial silk, terylene, avoid contact

ifosfamide

Mitoxana

Func. class.: Antineoplastic alkylating agent

Chem. class.: Nitrogen mustard derivative

Legal class.: POM

Action: Alkylates DNA, RNA; inhibits enzymes that allow synthesis in proteins; is also responsible for cross linking DNA strands

Uses: Chronic lymphocytic leukaemia, lymphomas, solid tumours

Dosage and routes:

Ifosfamide must be given with mesna: see manufacturer's data sheet. Doses are highly variable, and dependent on local treatment protocols, concomitant therapy and tumour type; the following dose schedules have been used

• *Adult:* IV 8–10 g/m^2 over 5 days repeated every 2–4 weeks or 5–6 g/m^2 (maximum 10 g) over 24 hr as infusion repeated every 3–4 weeks. Usual number of courses 4, maximum 7 (6 by 24-hr infusion)

Available forms include: Injection 500 mg, 1 g, 2 g

Side effects/adverse reactions:

CV: ECG changes, tachycardia, cardiotoxicity

HAEM: Leucopenia, thrombocytopenia, anaemia

GU: Haemorrhagic cystitis, sterility, haematuria, nephrotoxicity, glycosuria, proteinuria, aminoaciduria, renal rickets
INTEG: Alopecia, dermatitis
GI: Disturbances, diarrhoea, nausea, vomiting, hepatitis
RESP: Fibrosis
CNS: Confusion, lethargy, tonic-clonic spasms, depression of consciousness, motor unrest, emotional lability, disorientation, EEG changes, aggression, echoalia
SYST: Allergy, immunosuppression

Contraindications: Hypersensitivity, bone marrow aplasia, myelosuppression, pregnancy, breast-feeding, active infection including urinary tract infections, renal impairment, acute urothelial toxicity, hepatic impairment

Precautions: Contraception for both partners, elderly, debilitated, diabetes mellitus, evidence of myelosuppression, concomitant radiotherapy or chemotherapy, previous treatment with platinum compounds, nephrectomy

Pharmacokinetics: Converted in liver to active metabolites; excreted in urine

Interactions/incompatibilities:

- Enhanced effects of: Warfarin and other anticoagulants

Clinical assessment:

- Full blood count, differential and platelet count weekly; withhold drug if WBC less than 4000 and platelets less than 75,000
- Pulmonary function tests: chest X-ray before and during treatment
- Renal function tests: blood urea, serum uric acid, urine creatinine clearance
- Liver function tests: bilirubin, aspartate aminotransferase, alanine aminotransferase, lactic dehydrogenase

Treatment of overdose: Recognised with 24 hr, or possibly 48 hr, administer IV mesna
Administer broad spectrum antibiotic, whole blood transfusion as necessary. See data sheet compendium for further information

NURSING CONSIDERATIONS

Assess:

- Food preferences; list likes and dislikes

Administer:

- HANDLING: take safety precautions appropriate to antineoplastic agents
- Following local antineoplastic (cytotoxic) policies
- After ensuring that clinician is aware of blood results
- IV by infusion over 2–24 hours. Can be given by slow IV injection to supine patients after dilution to less than 4%; direct infusion may cause hypotensive reaction
- Other medications by mouth if possible. Avoid IV, IM, SC routes to prevent infection and bruising
- Anti-emetic 30–60 min before treatment and mesna as prescribed
- All other medication as prescribed including analgesics, antibiotics, anti-emetics, antispasmodics

Perform/provide:

- Ensure mesna given as prescribed
- Test all urine for blood (early signs of haemorrhage in cystitis)
- Strict aseptic technique only when indicated. Protective isolation if WBC count is low
- Good skin care
- Physiotherapy and deep breathing exercises
- Increased fluid intake to 2–3 litre/day and strict fluid balance chart
- Sensible diet that can be tolerated

Evaluate:

- For any bleeding (haematuria, gums)

• For dyspnoea, chest pain, unproductive cough
• Effects on body image (i.e. alopecia)
• Abdominal pain, fever, nausea, vomiting, diarrhoea
• Oedema in feet, joint pain
• Symptoms indicating allergic reaction
• Tachypnoea, ECG changes

Teach patient/family:
• Of protective isolation precautions
• To report any complaints or side effects to clinician
• That impotence or amenorrhoea may occur
• To report any changes in breathing or coughing
• To report any change in colour of stool or urine
• To report any bleeding, white spots or ulceration in the mouth. Check daily

imipenem with cilastatin

Primaxin
Func. class.: Antibiotic, broad spectrum
Chem. class.: Thienamycin β-lactam antibiotic with specific enzyme inhibitor
Legal class.: POM

Action: Inhibits bacterial cell wall synthesis; stable to bacterial beta-lactamase and bactericidal. Cilastatin blocks metabolism of imipenem in kidney
Uses: Aerobic, anaerobic Gram-negative or Gram-positive infections
Dosage and routes: Doses are in terms of imipenem
• *Adult:* IV infusion 1–2 g daily in 3–4 divided doses; less sensitive organisms up to 50 mg/kg daily, maximum 4 g daily; IM injection 500–750 mg 12 hrly. Gonococcal urethritis or cervicitis, single dose of 500 mg
• *Child:* over 3 months, IV infusion 60 mg/kg daily in 4 divided doses, maximum 2 g daily
For further dosage information see manufacturer's data sheet
Available forms include: IV infusion powder for reconstitution 250 mg imipenem/250 mg cilastatin, 60 ml vial; 500 mg imipenem/500 mg cilastatin, 120 ml vial. IM injection powder for reconstitution 500 mg imipenem/500 mg cilastatin, 15 ml vial
Side effects/adverse reactions:
GI: Nausea, vomiting, diarrhoea, pseudomembraneous colitis, taste disturbances
CNS: Convulsions, confusion, mental disturbances, myoclonic activity
HAEM: Increased liver enzymes and bilirubin, thrombophlebitis, neutropenia, eosinophilia, thrombocytopenia, positive direct Coombs' test
INTEG: Rash, urticaria, pruritus, erythema, local pain and induration
SYST: Pyrexia, anaphylaxis, abnormal liver function tests
GU: Elevated serum creatinine and blood urea, red discoloration of urine in children, oliguria, anuria, polyuria, acute renal failure
Contraindications: Hypersensitivity to imipenem or cilastatin, lactation, pregnancy (unless risk benefit outweighs risk)
Precautions: Hypersensitivity to penicillins, cephalosporins and other β-lactam antibiotics, history of gastrointestinal disease particularly colitis, renal impairment (reduce dosage), epilepsy and other CNS disorders
Pharmacokinetics: Cilastatin inhibits renal degradation of imi-

penem; excreted in urine largely as unchanged drug

Interactions/incompatibilities:

• Plasma levels of cilastatin increased by: probenecid

Clinical assessment:

• Liver function tests: aspartate aminotransferase, alanine aminotransferase

• Blood studies: Hb, haematocrit, prothrombin time, WBC, RBC

• Renal function tests: urine for blood and protein

• Culture and sensitivity to identify infecting organisms

• Monitor side effects

NURSING CONSIDERATIONS

Assess:

• Fluid balance

• Bowel pattern

• Respiratory state; tightness or wheeziness in chest

Administer:

• If IM, as a suspension prepared by addition of 2 ml of 1% lignocaine solution to 500 mg imipenem, by deep IM injection into a large muscle mass. If IV, as a solution containing 5 mg/ml, by IV infusion over 20–30 minutes for doses up to 500 mg, or 40–60 min for a 1 g dose; infusion rate may be reduced if nausea develops. Adjust dose in renal impairment

• After culture and sensitivity has been taken

• By IV infusion

Perform/provide:

• Equipment for resuscitation in case of severe reaction

• Adequate fluid intake

Evaluate:

• Fluid balance; report any haematuria to clinician

• Mental state for signs of confusion

• Local reaction to injection site

• Any skin eruptions, signs of allergy

• Therapeutic effect; absence of fever

• Bowel pattern

Teach patient/family:

• Culture to be taken when course completed

• To report sore throat/fever—could indicate further infection

• To inform clinician if diarrhoea persists

• To carry a Medic Alert card if allergic to penicillins

---

imipramine hydrochloride

Tofranil

Func. class.: Antidepressant, tricyclic

Chem. class.: Dibenzazepine—tertiary amine

Legal class.: POM

Action: Blocks reuptake of noradrenaline and serotonin into nerve endings, increasing action of noradrenaline and serotonin in nerve cells

Uses: Depression, nocturnal enuresis in children

Dosage and routes:

• *Adult:* By mouth 75 mg daily in divided doses, may increase gradually to 200 mg, up to 150 mg may be given as a single dose at bed time

• *Child:* Nocturnal enuresis by mouth 7 yr: 25 mg at night, 8–11 yr: 25–50 mg at night, over 11 yr 50–75 mg at night, maximum duration 3 months (including gradual withdrawal)

Available forms include: Tablets 10, 25 mg; syrup 25 mg/5 ml

Side effects/adverse reactions:

HAEM: Agranulocytosis, thrombocytopenia, eosinophilia, leucopenia

CNS: Dizziness, drowsiness, confusion, headache, anxiety, tremors, weakness, insomnia, nightmares, increased psychiatric

symptoms, paraesthesia, epileptic seizures
GI: Diarrhoea, dry mouth, nausea, vomiting, paralytic ileus, increased appetite, cramps, epigastric distress, jaundice, hepatitis, stomatitis
GU: Retention, acute renal failure
INTEG: Rash, urticaria, sweating, pruritus, photosensitivity, hair loss
CV: Orthostatic hypotension, ECG changes, tachycardia, hypertension, palpitations
EENT: Blurred vision, tinnitus, mydriasis, glaucoma
ENDO: Weight gain, disturbances of libido, galactorrhoea, hyper- or hypoglycaemia, occasional weight loss
Contraindications: Hypersensitivity to tricyclic antidepressants, recent myocardial infarction, urine retention, narrow angle glaucoma, child under 6 yr, heart block, arrhythmias, severe liver disease, porphyria, mania
Precautions: Suicidal patients, severe depression, increased intraocular pressure, cardiac disease, hepatic disease, hyperthyroidism, electroshock therapy, elective surgery, elderly, pregnancy, convulsive disorders, prostatic hypertrophy
Pharmacokinetics:
By mouth: Steady state 2–5 days; metabolised by liver, excreted in faeces, excreted in breast milk, half-life 6–20 hr
Interactions/incompatibilities:
• Decreased effects of: guanethidine, debrisoquine, clonidine, indirect acting sympathomimetics (ephedrine), antiepileptics
• Increased effects of: direct acting sympathomimetics (adrenaline), alcohol, barbiturates, benzodiazepines, CNS depressants, antihistamines
• Increased concentration by: methylphenidate, neuroleptics, diltiazem, verapamil, cimetidine
• Hyperpyretic crisis, convulsions, hypertensive episode: MAOIs (avoid imipramine for 3 weeks after stopping MAOI)
Clinical assessment:
• Blood studies: full blood count
• Hepatic studies: aspartate aminotransferase, alanine aminotransferase, bilirubin
• ECG for flattening of T wave, bundle branch block, atrioventricular block, dysrhythmias in cardiac patients
Lab. test interferences:
Increase: Serum bilirubin, alkaline phosphatase, blood glucose
Decrease: 5-hydroxyindoleacetic acid, vanillylmandelic acid, urinary catecholamines
Treatment of overdose: ECG monitoring, induce emesis, lavage, activated charcoal, administer anticonvulsant if necessary

NURSING CONSIDERATIONS

Assess:
• Baseline BP (lying, standing), pulse, weight
Administer:
• With food or milk for GI symptoms
• Dosage at bedtime if oversedation occurs during day; may take entire dose at bed time; elderly may not tolerate once daily dosing
• Mouthwashes, or frequent sips of water for dry mouth
Perform/provide:
• Assistance with mobilisation during beginning therapy since drowsiness/dizziness occurs
• Safety measures including cot sides primarily in elderly
Evaluate:
• Take vital signs 4 hrly in patients with cardiovascular disease
• Weight weekly, appetite may increase with drug
• Mental status: mood, alertness,

affect, suicidal tendencies, increase in psychiatric symptoms: depression, panic
• Urinary retention, constipation; constipation is more likely to occur in children; increase fluids, fibre indiet
• Withdrawal symptoms: headache, nausea, vomiting, muscle pain, weakness; do not usually occur unless drug was discontinued abruptly
• Alcohol consumption; if alcohol is consumed, hold dose until morning

Teach patient/family:
• That therapeutic effects may take 2–3 weeks
• Use caution in driving or other activities requiring alertness because of drowsiness, dizziness, blurred vision
• To avoid alcohol ingestion, other CNS depressants
• Not to discontinue medication quickly after long-term use, may cause nausea, headache, malaise
• To wear sunscreen or large hat since photosensitivity occurs

immunoglobulin, human

Sandoglobulin, Gammabulin, Gamimune-N, Endobulin, Kabiglobulin, Venoglobulin
Func. class.: Antibodies, serum
Chem. class.: IgG
Legal class.: POM

Action: Provides passive immunity
Uses: Agammaglobulinaemia, hepatitis A exposure, measles exposure, measles vaccine complications, purpura, rubella exposure, chicken-pox exposure, idiopathic thrombocytopenic purpura, Kawasaki syndrome
Dosage and routes: See specialist literature for advice on doses
Side effects/adverse reactions:
INTEG: Pain at injection site, rash, pruritus
MS: Arthralgia
SYST: Lymphadenopathy, anaphylaxis, fever, chills
CNS: Headache, fatigue, malaise
GI: Abdominal pain, hepatitis
Contraindications: Hypersensitivity
Interactions/incompatibilities:
• Diminished immune response: live virus vaccines (except yellow fever). Do not administer live virus vaccines 3 weeks before or 3 months after this drug

NURSING CONSIDERATIONS

Assess:
• Active or suspected infection
• Weigh before treatment

Administer:
• IM to large muscle site. 3 ml or less in site
• Within six weeks of exposure to hepatitis A
• Repeat doses as directed

Provide:
• Adrenaline 1:1000 and resuscitative equipment nearby
• Store in refrigerator, following manufacturers recommendations

Teach patient/family:
• That passive immunity is temporary

indapamide

Natrilix
Func. class.: Diuretic
Chem. class.: Indoline
Legal class.: POM

Action: Acts on proximal section of distal renal tubule by inhibiting reabsorption of sodium; may act by direct vasodilation caused by blocking of calcium channel
Uses: Hypertension
Dosage and routes:

• *Adult:* By mouth 2.5 mg daily in the morning
Available forms include: Tablets 2.5 mg
Side effects/adverse reactions:
GU: Impotence
ELECT: Metabolic alkalosis, hyperuricaemia, hypokalaemia, hyperglycaemia
CNS: Headache, dizziness, fatigue, weakness, paraesthesia
GI: Nausea, diarrhoea, dry mouth, dyspepsia, anorexia, constipation
EENT: Reversible acute myopia
INTEG: Rash, pruritus, photosensitivity
CV: Orthostatic hypotension
Contraindications: Recent CVA, severe hepatic failure, sulphonamide hypersensitivity
Precautions: Hypokalaemia, dehydration, ascites, hepatic disease, severe renal disease, pregnancy, breast feeding
Pharmacokinetics:
By mouth: Onset 1–2 hr, peak 2 hr, duration up to 36 hr; excreted in urine, faeces, half-life 14–18 hr
Interactions/incompatibilities:
• Increased hypokalaemia: carbenoxolone, diuretics, steroids
• Increased blood levels of: lithium
Clinical assessment:
• Electrolytes: potassium, sodium, include serum urea, serum creatinine
Treatment of overdose: Lavage if taken orally, monitor electrolytes, administer IV fluids
NURSING CONSIDERATIONS
Assess:
• Baseline BP, weight
• Rate, depth, rhythm of respiration, effect of exertion
Administer:
• In morning to avoid interference with sleep
• With food, if nausea occurs, absorption may be decreased slightly
Evaluate:
• Weight daily, fluid balance daily to determine fluid loss; effect of drug may be decreased if used daily
• BP lying, standing; postural hypotension may occur
• Improvement in oedema of feet, legs, sacral area daily if medication is being used in congestive cardiac failure
• Improvement in CVP and BP recordings
• Signs of metabolic alkalosis
• Signs of hyperkalaemia
• Rashes, temperature elevation 6-hrly
• Confusion, especially in elderly; take safety precautions if needed
• Hydration: skin turgor, thirst, dry mucous membranes
Teach patient/family:
• To increase fluid intake 2–3 litres daily unless contraindicated; to rise slowly from lying or sitting position
• Adverse reactions: muscle cramps, weakness, nausea, dizziness
• Take with food or milk for GI symptoms
• Take early in day to prevent nocturia

---

indomethacin

Antracin, Flexin-Continus, Imbrilan, Indocid, Indocid-R, Indomax, Indolar SR, Indomod, Mobilan, Rheumacin LA, Rimacid, Slo-Indo
Func. class.: Non-steroidal anti-inflammatory drug
Chem. class.: Propionic acid derivative
Legal class.: POM

Action: Inhibits prostaglandin synthesis by decreasing enzyme needed for biosynthesis; possesses analgesic, anti-inflammatory, antipyretic properties

Uses: Pain and moderate to severe inflammation in rheumatic disease and other acute musculoskeletal disorders; acute gout, dysmenorrhoea

Dosage and routes:

• *Adult:* By mouth, arthritis 50–200 mg daily in divided doses; dysmenorrhoea, up to 75 mg daily; by rectum, 100 mg once or twice a day; modified-release 75 mg daily, may increase to 75 mg twice a day maximum total daily dose 200 mg

Available forms include: Capsules 25, 50 mg; capsules modified-release 75 mg; tablets modified release 25 mg, 50 mg, 75 mg, suspension 25 mg/5 ml; suppository 100 mg

Side effects/adverse reactions:

GI: Nausea, anorexia, vomiting, diarrhoea, jaundice, cholestatic hepatitis, constipation, flatulence, cramps, dry mouth, ulceration, bleeding

CNS: Dizziness, drowsiness, fatigue, tremors, confusion, insomnia, anxiety, depression, headache

CV: Tachycardia, peripheral oedema, palpitations, dysrhythmias, hypertension, hypotension, chest pain

INTEG: Purpura, rash, pruritus, sweating

GU: Nephrotoxicity, haematuria, proteinuria, interstitial nephritis, nephrotic syndrome

META: Hyperkalaemia, hyperglycaemia

HAEM: Anaemia, inhibition of platelet aggregation

EENT: Tinnitus, hearing loss, eye changes

Contraindications: Hypersensitivity, asthmatic attacks with aspirin or other NSAIDs; active or suspected peptic ulcer or GI haemorrhage; asthma; nasal polyps associated with angioneurotic oedema, history of gastrointestinal lesions; pregnancy; breast-feeding, suppositories in patients with proctitis or rectal bleeding

Precautions: Pregnancy, lactation, children, bleeding disorders, cardiac disorders, hypersensitivity to other NSAIDs psychiatric disorders, epilepsy, parkinsonism, renal or hepatic disorders

Pharmacokinetics:

By mouth: Onset 1–2 hr, peak 3 hr, duration 4–6 hr; metabolised in liver, kidneys, excreted in urine, bile, faeces, excreted in breast milk

Interactions/incompatibilities:

• May increase action of: coumarin, sulphonamides, methotrexate

• Increased toxicity: diflunisal, lithium, potassium-sparing diuretics, angiotensin converting enzyme inhibitors, probenecid

• Reduced efficacy: diuretics, antihypertensives

Clinical assessment:

• Renal function tests, liver, blood studies: serum urea, creatinine, aspartate aminotransferase, alanine aminotransferase, Hb, before treatment, periodically thereafter

• Audiometric, ophthalmic exam before, during, after treatment

NURSING CONSIDERATIONS

Administer:

• With or after food or milk

• Modified-release; swallow whole

• May be taken with an antacid

• Do not mix antacid with indomethacin suspension

Evaluate:

• Therapeutic response: decreased pain, stiffness in joints, decreased swelling in joints, ability to move more easily

• For eye, ear problems: blurred vision, tinnitus; may indicate toxicity

Teach patient/family:

• To report blurred vision, ringing, roaring in ears; may indicate toxicity

• To avoid driving, other hazardous activities if dizziness, drowsiness occurs

• To report change in urine pattern, increased weight, oedema, increased pain in joints, fever, blood in urine; indicate nephrotoxicity

• To report any wheeziness or shortness of breath

• That therapeutic effects may take up to 1 month

• To avoid alcohol, salicylates; bleeding may occur

• To report any related indigestion or black tarry stools (may indicate bleeding)

• Teach patient/relative how to administer suppositories

indoramin

Baratol, Doralese

Func. class.: Antihypertensive

Chem. class.: α-blocker

Legal class.: POM

Action: Decreases peripheral resistance by vasodilatation; reduces urinary outflow obstruction

Uses: Baratol: hypertension, usually in conjunction with β-blocker or thiazide, Doralese: management of urinary outflow obstruction in benign prostatic hypertrophy

Dosage and routes:

Hypertension

• *Adult:* By mouth initially 25 mg twice daily increased by 25–50 mg daily at intervals of 2 weeks; maximum dose 200 mg daily in 2–3 divided doses

Benign prostatic hypertrophy

• *Adult:* By mouth 20 mg twice daily increased by 20 mg increments every 2 weeks to maximum of 100 mg daily in divided doses; elderly, 20 mg at night may be sufficient

Available forms include: Tablets 20 mg, 25 mg, 50 mg

Side effects/adverse reactions:

CNS: Sedation, dizziness, depression, extrapyramidal effects, drowsiness

EENT: Dry mouth, nasal congestion

GU: Failure of ejaculation

META: Weight gain

Contraindications: Established heart failure, concurrent treatment with MAOIs

Precautions: Incipient heart failure, hepatic or renal impairment, pregnancy, lactation, Parkinson's disease, epilepsy, history of depression, elderly (reduce dosage)

Pharmacokinetics: Half-life 5 hr; metabolised in liver and excreted in urine and faeces as metabolites, some of which may be active

Interactions/incompatibilities:

• Do not use concurrently with: MAOIs

Treatment of overdose: Gastric lavage, assisted ventilation and circulatory support, diazepam for convulsions, monitor temperature for hypothermia

NURSING CONSIDERATIONS

Assess:

• Baseline BP and pulse

• Weight and fluid balance

Administer:

• Tablet whole; should not be chewed or crushed

Perform:

• Store in airtight container

Evaluate:

• BP 4-hrly

• Feet and legs daily for oedema

• Skin turgor – dryness of mucous membranes for hydration status

• For dyspnoea and jugular vein distension

Teach patient/family:

• Effects increased by: alcohol

• That fainting occasionally occurs after first dose; do not drive or

operate machinery for 4 hr after first dose
• To report any side effects

influenza virus vaccine, trivalent A & B (surface antigen/split virion)

Fluvirin, Influvac, MFV-ject, Fluzone
Func. class.: Vaccine
Legal class.: POM

Action: Active immunisation against influenza
Uses: Prevention of influenza
Dosage and routes:
• *Adult and child over 13 yr:* IM, deep subcutaneous 0.5 ml in 1 dose
• *Child 4–13 yr:* IM 0.5 ml, repeat in 1 month
• *Child 6 months–3 yr:* IM 0.25 ml, repeat in 1 month (Fluzone)
Available forms include: Injection IM, subcutaneous
Side effects/adverse reactions:
CNS: Fever
INTEG: Urticaria, induration, erythema
SYST: Anaphylaxis, malaise
MS: Myalgia
Contraindications: Hypersensitivity, active infection, chicken or egg allergy
Precautions: Immunosuppression, pregnancy, polymyxin sensitivity

NURSING CONSIDERATIONS

Assess:
• Active or suspected infections
• History of allergies, skin conditions, reactions to vaccines
• History of allergy to chicken, eggs, feathers
Administer:
• Intramuscular or deep subcutaneous after bringing preparation to room temperature
Provide:
• Adrenaline 1:1000 and resuscitative equipment nearby
• Store in light proof container at 2–10°C (check brand used)
Evaluate:
• For anaphylaxis: dyspnoea tachycardia, profuse sweating, collapse
• Redness and soreness at injection site
• Headache, pyrexia, malaise
Teach patient/family:
• That immunity is not long-term

inosine pranobex

Imunovir
Func. class.: Antiviral and immunomodulator
Chem. class.: Inosine with dimepranol and acedoben
Legal class.: POM

Action: Modifies cell-mediated immune mechanisms; mild antiviral action
Uses: Mucocutaneous herpes simplex type I or II, adjunctive treatment of genital warts
Dosage and routes:
Herpes simplex
• By mouth 1 g 4 times daily for 7–14 days
Genital warts
• By mouth 1 g 3 times daily for 14–28 days
Available forms include: Tablets 500 mg
Side effects/adverse reactions:
HAEM: Increased serum uric acid
GU: Increased urinary uric acid
Precautions: History of gout or hyperuricaemia, renal impairment, lactation
Pharmacokinetics: Inosine component converted to uric acid and excreted in urine; remainder metabolised in liver and excreted in urine
Clinical assessment:

• Renal function tests
• Blood serum uric acid

NURSING CONSIDERATIONS

Assess:
• Fluid balance

Evaluate:
• Skin for rashes, urticaria
• Therapeutic response: absence of itchiness, decrease in number and size of lesions

Teach patient/family:
• That drug may be taken orally before infection occurs; should be taken when itching or pain occurs, usually before eruptions
• In genital herpes, sexual partner may also require treatment and/or be at risk from infection
• Advisability of refraining from intimate sexual contact during acute episode of genital herpes
• To report sore throat or fever
• That drug must be taken regularly for the time prescribed to be effective
• To notify clinician of any urinary symptoms

---

insulin zinc suspension

Hypurin Lente, Lentard MC, Human Monotard, Humulin Lente
Func. class.: Antidiabetic
Chem. class.: Insulin, long acting
Legal class.: P

Action: Decreases blood sugar
Uses: Diabetes mellitus (long acting therapy)
Dosage and routes:
• *Adult and child:* Subcutaneous individualised dose; do not give IV
Available forms include: Subcutaneous injection 100 units/ml vials
Side effects/adverse reactions:
CNS: Headache, lethargy, tremors, weakness, fatigue, delirium, sweating
CV: Tachycardia, palpitations
EENT: Blurred vision
GI: Hunger, nausea
META: Hypoglycaemia
INTEG: Flushing, rash, urticaria, warmth, lipodystrophy, erythema, pruritus
SYST: Anaphylaxis
Contraindications: Hypersensitivity, hypoglycaemia
Pharmacokinetics:
Subcutaneous: Onset 4 hr, duration up to 36 hr
Interactions/incompatibilities:
• Increased hypoglycaemia: alcohol, β-blockers, oral hypoglycaemics, MAOIs, octreotide
• Hyperglycaemia: thiazides, thyroid hormones, oral contraceptives, corticosteroids, lithium, diazoxide, loop diuretics
Clinical assessment:
• Fasting blood glucose (3.3–5.6 mmol/litre)
Treatment of overdose: Glucose by mouth if conscious or glucose 50% IV if comatose, glucagon 1 mg IM, subcutaneous, IV

NURSING CONSIDERATIONS

Administer:
• Shake vial before withdrawing dose
• Take care to avoid vascular injection

Perform/provide:
• Store bottle in use at room temperature for less than 1 month; refrigerate all other supply; do not use discoloured or cloudy solution
• Rotation of injection sites: abdomen, thighs, upper arm, buttocks

Evaluate:
• Therapeutic response: decrease in polyuria, polydipsia, alertness
• Hypoglycaemic/hyperglycaemic reaction that can occur

Teach patient/family:
• Dosage, route, mixing instructions, dietary advice, disease process

• Effects of diet and exercise on blood glucose
• To carry dextrasol or lump sugar to treat hypoglycaemia
• That drug does not cure diabetes, but controls symptoms
• That blurred vision occurs, not to change corrective lens until vision is stabilised 1–2 months
• To carry Medic Alert ID as diabetic
• Hypoglycaemia reaction: headache, tremors, fatigue, weakness
• Symptoms of ketoacidosis: nausea, thirst, polyuria, dry mouth, dry flushed skin, acetone breath, drowsiness
• Blood glucose testing; make sure patient is able to determine glucose
• To avoid non-prescribed drugs unless directed by clinician

---

insulin, biphasic isophane

Mixtard 30/70, Actraphane 30/70, Initard 50/50, Humulin M1, Humulin M2, Humulin M3, Humulin M4, Pen Mix 10/90 Penfill, Pen Mix 20/80 Penfill, Pen Mix 30/70 Penfill, Pen Mix 30/70, Pen Mix 40/60 Penfill, Pen Mix 50/50 Penfill, Pur-In Mix 15/85, Pur-In Mix 25–75, Pur-In Mix 50/50

Func. class.: Antidiabetic
Chem. class.: Insulin, intermediate acting
Legal class.: P

Action: Decreases blood sugar
Uses: Diabetes mellitus (intermediate acting therapy)
Dosage and routes:
• *Adult and child:* Subcutaneous individualised dose, do not give IV
Available forms include: Subcutaneous injection 100 units/ml vials, cartridges for injection device and disposable injection devices

Side effects/adverse reactions:
CNS: Headache, lethargy, tremors, weakness, fatigue, delirium, sweating
CV: Tachycardia, palpitations
EENT: Blurred vision
GI: Hunger, nausea
META: Hypoglycaemia
INTEG: Flushing, rash, urticaria, warmth, lipodystrophy, pruritus, erythema
SYST: Anaphylaxis
Contraindications: Hypersensitivity, hypoglycaemia
Pharmacokinetics:
Subcutaneous: Onset 2 hr, peak 4–12 hr, duration up to 24 hr
Interactions/incompatibilities:
• Increased hypoglycaemia: alcohol, β-blockers, oral hypoglycaemics, MAOIs, octreotide
• Hyperglycaemia: thiazides, thyroid hormones, oral contraceptives, corticosteroids, lithium, diazoxide, loop diuretics
Clinical assessment:
• Fasting blood glucose (3.3–5.6 mmol/litre)
Treatment of overdose: Glucose by mouth if conscious or glucose 50% IV if comatose, glucagon 1 mg IM, subcutaneous, IV if glucose not available

NURSING CONSIDERATIONS

Administer:
• Shake vial before withdrawing dose
• Take care to avoid vascular injection
• Not more than 30 min before a meal
Perform/provide:
• Store bottle in use at room temperature for less than 1 month; refrigerate all other supply; do not use discoloured or cloudy solution
• Rotation of injection sites: abdomen, thighs, upper arm, buttocks, keep record of sites
Evaluate:
• Therapeutic response: decrease

in polyuria, polydipsia, alertness
• Hypoglycaemic/hyperglycaemic reaction that can occur

Teach patient/family:
• Dosage, route, mixing instructions, any dietary advice, disease process
• Effect of diet and exercise on blood glucose
• To carry dextrasol or lump sugar to treat hypoglycaemia
• That drug does not cure diabetes, but controls symptoms
• That blurred vision occurs, not to change corrective lens until vision is stabilised 1–2 months
• To carry Medic Alert ID or Diabetic card
• Hypoglycaemia reaction: headache, tremors, fatigue, weakness, sweating, visual disturbances
• Symptoms of ketoacidosis: nausea, thirst, polyuria, dry mouth, dry flushed skin, acetone breath, drowsiness
• Blood glucose testing, make sure patient is able to determine glucose, test urine for ketones if blood sugar is high
• The pregnant patient to use glucose oxidase reagents
• To avoid non-prescribed drugs unless directed by clinician

insulin, isophane

Hypurin Isophane, Insulatard, Humulin I, Protaphane, Protaphane Penfill, Pur-In Isophane

Func. class.: Antidiabetic
Chem. class.: Insulin, intermediate acting
Legal class.: P

Action: Decreases blood sugar
Uses: Diabetes mellitus (intermediate acting therapy)
Dosage and routes:
• *Adult and child:* Subcutaneous individualised dose, do not give IV

Available forms include: Subcutaneous injection 100 units/ml vials, cartridges for injection device

Side effects/adverse reactions:
CNS: Headache, lethargy, tremors, weakness, fatigue, delirium, sweating
CV: Tachycardia, palpitations
EENT: Blurred vision
GI: Hunger, nausea
META: Hypoglycaemia
INTEG: Flushing, rash, urticaria, warmth
SYST: Anaphylaxis

Contraindications: Hypersensitivity, hypoglycaemia

Interactions/incompatibilities:
• Increased hypoglycaemia: alcohol, β-blockers, oral hypoglycaemics, MAOIs, octreotide
• Hyperglycaemia: thiazides, thyroid hormones, oral contraceptives, corticosteroids, lithium, diazoxide, loop diuretics

Pharmacokinetics:
Subcutaneous: Onset 2 hr, peak 4–12 hr, duration up to 24 hr

Clinical assessment:
• Fasting blood glucose (3.3–5.6 mmol/litre)

Treatment of overdose: Glucose by mouth if conscious or glucose 50% IV if comatose, glucagon 1 mg IM, subcutaneous or IV if glucose not convenient

NURSING CONSIDERATIONS

Administer:
• Shake vial before withdrawing dose
• Take care to avoid vascular injection

Perform/provide:
• Store bottle in use at room temperature for less than 1 month; refrigerate all other supply; do not use discoloured or cloudy solution
• Rotation of injection sites: abdomen, thighs, upper arm, buttocks

Evaluate:

• Therapeutic response: decrease in polyuria, polydipsia, polyphagia, clear sensorium, absence of dizziness, stable gait
• Hypoglycaemic/hyperglycaemic reaction that can occur soon after meals

Teach patient/family:
• Dosage, route, mixing instructions, dietary advice
• Effects of diet and exercise on blood glucose
• To carry dextrasol or lump sugar to treat hypoglycaemia
• That drug does not cure diabetes, but controls symptoms
• That blurred vision occurs, not to change corrective lens until vision is stabilised 1–2 months
• To carry Medic Alert or Diabetic Card
• Hypoglycaemia reaction: headache, tremors, fatigue, weakness, sweating, visual disturbances
• Symptoms of ketoacidosis: nausea, thirst, polyuria, dry mouth, dry flushed skin, acetone breath, drowsiness
• Blood glucose testing, make sure patient is able to determine glucose, test urine for ketones if blood sugar is high
• To avoid non-prescribed medicines unless approved by clinician
• To consult clinician in cases of colds/flu as this could necessitate altering dosage

---

insulin, protamine zinc suspension

Hypurin Protamine Zinc
Func. class.: Antidiabetic
Chem. class.: Insulin, long acting
Legal class.: P

Action: Decreases blood sugar
Uses: Diabetes mellitus (long-acting therapy)

Dosage and routes:
• *Adult and child:* Subcutaneous individualised dose, do not give IV

Available forms include: Subcutaneous injection 100 units/ml vials

Side effects/adverse reactions:
CNS: Headache, lethargy, tremors, weakness, fatigue, delirium, sweating
CV: Tachycardia, palpitations
EENT: Blurred vision
GI: Hunger, nausea
META: Hypoglycaemia
INTEG: Flushing, rash, urticaria warmth, lipodystrophy, pruritus, erythema
SYST: Anaphylaxis

Contraindications: Hypersensitivity, hypoglycaemia

Pharmacokinetics:
Subcutaneous: Onset 4–8 hr, peak 14–20 hr, duration 24–36 hr

Interactions/incompatibilities:
• Increased hypoglycaemia: alcohol, β-blockers, oral hypoglycaemics, MAOIs, octreotide
• Hyperglycaemia: thiazides, thyroid hormones, oral contraceptives, corticosteroids, lithium, diazoxide, loop diuretics

Clinical assessment:
• Fasting blood glucose (3.3–5.6 mmol/litre)

Treatment of overdose: Glucose by mouth if conscious or glucose 50% IV if comatose, glucagon 1 mg IM, subcutaneous or IV

NURSING CONSIDERATIONS

Administer:
• Shake vial before withdrawing dose
• Take care to avoid vascular injection

Perform/provide:
• Store bottle in use at room temperature for less than 1 month; refrigerate all other supply; do not use discoloured or cloudy solution
• Rotation of injection sites: abdomen, upper back, thighs,

upper arm, buttocks; keep record of sites

Evaluate:

• Therapeutic response: decrease in polyuria, polydipsia, alertness
• Hypoglycaemic/hyperglycaemic reaction that can occur

Teach patient/family:

• Dosage, route, mixing instructions, if any diet restrictions, disease process
• Effect of diet and exercise on blood glucose
• To carry dextrasol or lump sugar to treat hypoglycaemia
• That drug does not cure diabetes, but controls symptoms
• That blurred vision occurs, not to change corrective lens until vision is stabilised 1–2 months
• To carry Medic Alert ID as diabetic
• Hypoglycaemia reaction: headache, tremors, fatigue, weakness, sweating and visual disturbances
• Symptoms of ketoacidosis: nausea, thirst, polyuria, dry mouth, dry flushed skin, acetone breath, drowsiness
• Blood glucose testing; make sure patient is able to determine glucose
• The pregnant patient to use glucose oxidase reagents
• To avoid non-prescribed drugs unless directed by clinician
• Test urine for ketones if blood sugar is high

---

insulin, soluble (insulin injection, neutral insulin)

Hypurin Neutral, Velosulin, Human Actrapid, Human Actrapid Penfill, Human Velosulin, Humulin S, Pur-In Neutral

Func. class.: Antidiabetic
Chem. class.: Exogenous unmodified insulin, rapid acting
Legal class.: P

Action: Decreases blood sugar, increases blood pyruvate, lactate, decreases phosphate, potassium

Uses: Diabetes mellitus, diabetic ketoacidosis

Dosage and routes:

• *Adult and child:* Subcutaneous, IM, IV injection or IV infusion according to patients' requirements

Available forms include: IV/IM/subcutaneous injection, 100 units/ml vials, cartidges for injection device

Side effects/adverse reactions:

META: Insulin resistance
INTEG: Flushing, rash, urticaria, warmth, lipodystrophy at injection site
SYST: Hypersensitivity

Contraindications: Hypersensitivity, hypoglycaemia

Pharmacokinetics:

Subcutaneous: Onset 30–60 min, peak 2–3 hr, duration 5–7 hr, half-life 4 hr

IV: Onset 10–30 min, peak 30–60 min, duration 1–2 hr, half-life 3–5 min

Metabolised by liver, muscle, kidneys, excreted in urine

Interactions/incompatibilities:

• Increased hypoglycaemia, alcohol, β-blockers, oral hypoglycaemics, clofibrate
• Hyperglycaemia: thiazides, triamterene, phenothiazines, phenytoin, oral contraceptives, lithium

• Mask signs/symptoms of hypoglycaemia: β-blocker
Clinical assessment:
• Fasting glucose test
• Increased doses if tolerance occurs
• Human insulin to those allergic to beef or pork
• IV after diluting with 0.9% sodium chloride injection
Treatment of overdose: 10%–50% glucose by mouth if conscious or IV if comatose, or glucagon 1 mg by subcutaneous injection

NURSING CONSIDERATIONS

Administer:
• Shake vial before withdrawing dose
• Take care to avoid unintentional vascular injection
• Not more than 30 min before a meal
Perform/provide:
• Check blood sugar levels before meals and bedtime
• Storage in a refrigerator between 2°–8°C, do not use discoloured, or cloudy solution
• Rotation of injection sites: abdomen, upper back, thighs, upper arm, buttocks; keep record of sites
Evaluate:
• Therapeutic response: decrease in polyuria, polydipsia, and blood sugar levels within normal range 4–9 mmol/litre
• Hypoglycaemic/hyperglycaemic reaction that can occur soon after meals in newly diagnosed diabetic
Teach patient/family:
• To keep insulin, equipment available at all times
• Dosage, route, mixing instructions, disease process
• To carry glucose sweets, sugar lumps, to treat hypoglycaemia
• Advise insulin action in association with diet and exercise
• That drug does not cure diabetes, but controls symptoms
• If blurred vision occurs, not to change corrective lens until vision is stabilised 1–2 months
• To carry Diabetic or other Medical Identity Card
• Hypoglycaemia reaction: headache, tremors, fatigue, weakness, sweating
• Symptoms of ketoacidosis: nausea, thirst, polyuria, dry mouth, dry, flushed skin, acetone breath, drowsiness
• Home blood glucose monitoring and how to interpret results
• To test urine for ketones if blood sugar is greater than 17
• To avoid non-prescribed drugs unless directed by clinician

insulin, zinc suspension crystalline

Human Ultratard (long acting), Humulin Zn (intermediate acting)
Func. class.: Antidiabetic
Chem. class.: Insulin
Legal class.: P

Action: Decreases blood sugar
Uses: Diabetes mellitus
Dosage and routes:
• *Adult and child:* Subcutaneous individualised dose; do not give IV
Available forms include: Subcutaneous injection 100 units/ml vials
Side effects/adverse reactions:
CNS: Headache, lethargy, tremors, weakness, fatigue, delirium, sweating
CV: Tachycardia, palpitations
EENT: Blurred vision
GI: Hunger, nausea
META: Hypoglycaemia
INTEG: Flushing, rash, urticaria, warmth, lipoatrophy, lipohypertrophy, erythema, pruritus
SYST: Anaphylaxis
Contraindications: Hypersensitivity, hypoglycaemia
Pharmacokinetics:

Subcutaneous: Onset 4–8 hr, peak 16–18 hr, duration 24–36 hr
Interactions/incompatibilities:
• Increased hypoglycaemia: alcohol, β-blockers, oral hypoglycaemics, MAOIs, octreotide
• Hyperglycaemia: thiazides, thyroid hormones, oral contraceptives, corticosteroids, lithium, diazoxide, loop diuretics
Clinical assessment:
• Fasting blood glucose (3.3–5.6 mmol/litre)
Treatment of overdose: Glucose by mouth if conscious or glucose 50% IV if comatose, glucagon 1 mg IM, IV, subcutaneous

NURSING CONSIDERATIONS

Administer:
• Shake vial before withdrawing dose
• Take care to avoid vascular injection
Perform/provide:
• Store bottle in use at room temperature for less than 1 month; refrigerate all other supply; do not use discoloured or cloudy solution
• Rotation of injection sites: abdomen, thighs, upper arm, buttocks
Evaluate:
• Therapeutic response: decrease in polyuria, polydipsia, alertness
• Hypoglycaemic/hyperglycaemic reaction that can occur
Teach patient/family:
• Dosage, route, mixing instructions, dietary advice, disease process
• Effects of diet and exercise on blood glucose
• To carry dextrasol or lump sugar to treat hypoglycaemia
• That drug does not cure diabetes, but controls symptoms
• That blurred vision occurs, not to change corrective lens until vision is stabilised 1–2 months
• To carry Medic Alert ID as diabetic
• Hypoglycaemia reaction: headache, tremors, fatigue, weakness, sweating, visual disturbances
• Symptoms of ketoacidosis: nausea, thirst, polyuria, dry mouth, dry flushed skin, acetone breath, drowsiness
• Blood glucose testing, make sure patient is able to determine glucose test urine for ketones if blood sugar is high
• To avoid non-prescription drugs unless directed by clinician

---

insulin, zinc suspension amorphous

Semitard MC
Func. class.: Antidiabetic
Chem. class.: Insulin, intermediate acting
Legal class.: P

Action: Decreases blood sugar
Uses: Diabetes mellitus (intermediate acting therapy)
Dosage and routes:
• *Adult and child:* Subcutaneous individualised dose; do not give IV
Available forms include: Subcutaneous injection 100 units/ml vials
Side effects/adverse reactions:
CNS: Headache, lethargy, tremors, weakness, fatigue, delirium, sweating
CV: Tachycardia, palpitations
EENT: Blurred vision
GI: Hunger, nausea
META: Hypoglycaemia
INTEG: Flushing, rash, urticaria, warmth, lipoatrophy, lipohypertrophy, erythema, pruritus
SYST: Anaphylaxis
Contraindications: Hypersensitivity, hypoglycaemia
Pharmacokinetics:
Subcutaneous: Onset 2 hr, peak 4–12 hr, duration up to 24 hr
Interactions/incompatibilities:

• Increased hypoglycaemia: alcohol, β-blockers, oral hypoglycaemics, MAOIs, octreotide
• Hyperglycaemia: thiazides, thyroid hormones, oral contraceptives, corticosteroids, lithium, diazoxide, loop diuretics

Clinical assessment:
• Fasting blood glucose (3.3–5.6 mmol/litre)

Treatment of overdose: Glucose by mouth if conscious or glucose 50% IV if comatose, glucagon 1 mg IM, IV, subcutaneous

NURSING CONSIDERATIONS

Administer:
• Shake vial before withdrawing dose
• Take care to avoid vascular injection

Perform/provide:
• Store bottle in use at room temperature for less than 1 month; refrigerate all other supply; do not use discoloured or cloudy solution
• Rotation of injection sites: abdomen, thighs, upper arm, buttocks

Evaluate:
• Therapeutic response: decrease in polyuria, polydipsia, alertness
• Hypoglycaemic/hyperglycaemic reaction that can occur

Teach patient/family:
• Dosage, route, mixing instructions, dietary advice
• Effects of diet and exercise on blood glucose
• To carry dextrasol or lump sugar to treat hypoglycaemia
• That drug does not cure diabetes, but controls symptoms
• That blurred vision occurs, not to change corrective lens until vision is stabilised 1–2 months
• To carry Medic Alert ID as diabetic
• Hypoglycaemia reaction: headache, tremors, fatigue, weakness, sweating, visual disturbances
• Symptoms of ketoacidosis: nausea, thirst, polyuria, dry mouth, dry flushed skin, acetone breath, drowsiness
• Blood glucose testing, make sure patient is able to determine glucose, test urine for ketones if blood sugar is high
• The pregnant patient to use glucose oxidase reagents
• To avoid non-prescribed drugs unless directed by clinician

---

interferons (alpha)

Intron A (interferon alfa-2b), Roferon-A (interferon alfa-N1), Wellferon (interferon alfa-NI)

Func. class.: Cytokine, biological response modifier with antiviral, antitumour and immodulatory actions

Chem. class.: Protein

Legal class.: POM

Action: Alpha-interferons act in a variety of ways that are only poorly understood. They probably act directly against susceptible viruses and tumours as well as stimulating the immune system

Uses: The treatment of a variety of malignancies and viral conditions including: AIDS-related Kaposi's sarcoma, hairy cell leukaemia, chronic myelogenous leukaemia, metastatic renal cell carcinoma, multiple myeloma, chronic active hepatitis B, condyloma acuminata

Dosage and routes:

Note: A variety of dosage schedules are used and different manufacturers make different recommendations for their products. The following schedules are typical

Hairy cell leukaemia
• *Adult:* By subcutaneous/IM injection 3 MU daily for 12–24 weeks, then 3 MU subcutaneous/

IM 3 times a week as maintenance

AIDS-related Kaposi's sarcoma

• *Adult:* By subcutaneous/IM injection 18–36 MU 3 times a week. This may be preceded by an induction phase of daily dosing lasting 10–12 weeks during which the daily dose is gradually escalated to a maximum of 36 MU daily

Chronic myelogenous leukaemia

• *Adult:* By subcutaneous/IM injection 6–9 MU daily; this may be reduced to 6–9 MU on alternate days once complete haematological response has been achieved

Maintenance of remission in multiple myeloma

• *Adult:* By subcutaneous injection 3 MU 3 times a week

Recurrent or metastatic renal carcinoma

• *Adult:* By subcutaneous/IM injection 3 MU daily escalated to a maximum of 36 MU daily over 10–12 weeks; maintenance, 18–36 MU by subcutaneous/IM injection thrice weekly

Chronic active hepatitis B

• *Adult:* By subcutaneous/IM injection 2.5–7.5 MU/M^2 body surface area 3 times a week for 3–6 months

Condyloma acuminata

• *Adult:* By intralesional injection 1.0 MU in 0.1 ml water for injections 3 times a week for 3 weeks. Up to 5 lesions may be treated simultaneously and large lesions may be treated by multiple injections; total weekly interferon dose should not exceed 15 MU

High tumour burden non-Hodgkin's lymphoma (with appropriate chemotherapy)

• *Adult:* By subcutaneous injection 5 MU 3 times a week for 18 months

Available forms include: Powder for preparing IM/subcutaneous injection 3, 4.5, 9, 18 MU vials (interferon alfa-2a); powder for preparing subcutaneous/intralesional injection 3, 5, 10, 30 MU vials (interferon alfa-2b); solution for IM/subcutaneous injection 3, 10 MU vials (interferon alfa-nl)

Side effects/adverse reactions:

CNS: Headache, depression, lethargy, dizziness, vertigo, confusion, seizures, coma, paraesthesia, neuropathy

CV: Hypotension, cardiac arrhythmias, oedema, cyanosis, myocardial infarction, cardiac arrest, cerebrovascular accident

ELECT: Raised serum creatinine and LDH hypocalcaemia, raised serum glucose

ENDO: Thyroid abnormalities

GI: Hepatotoxicity, anorexia, nausea, diarrhoea, vomiting, reactivation of peptic ulcer, gastrointestinal bleeding

HAEM: Leukopenia, neutropenia, thrombocytopenia

INTEG: Psoriasiform rash, injection site reactions, alopecia, dry skin exacerbation of herpes labialis

MS: Myalgia, arthralgia

SYST: Flu-like symptoms including fever

Contraindications: Hypersensitivity; severe cardiac disease; severe renal or hepatic impairment; epilepsy compromised CNS function; chronic hepatitis with advanced decompensated cirrhosis of the liver; chronic hepatitis in patients who are being treated with or who have recently been treated with immunosuppressive agents excluding short term 'steroid withdrawal'

Precautions: History of myocardial infarction and/or cardiac arrhythmia; pregnancy; breastfeeding; mild to moderate renal or hepatic impairment; severe myelosuppression; asthma

Interactions:

• Raised blood levels of: theophyl-

line and, possibly, other drugs metabolised by liver enzymes
• Changes in mental state when given with drugs acting on the CNS
• Enhanced activity and toxicity of: 5-fluorouracil

Treatment of overdose: Symptomatic and supportive treatment

NURSING CONSIDERATIONS

Assess:
• Baseline vital signs (temperature, pulse, respiration, BP), weight, food likes and dislikes
• Full blood count

Administer:
• IM, subcutaneous, intralesionally
• Intralesional injections for condyloma acuminata using a fine (30 gauge) needle. Apply lignocaine gel first if patient is very sensitive
• All other medication as prescribed including anti-emetics, antibiotics and analgesics
• Side effects may be less troublesome if injections are given at night

Perform/provide:
• Good aseptic technique when administering
• Mouthcare: brush teeth with a soft brush or use cotton-tipped applicators for stomatitis; use unwaxed dental floss
• Skincare as appropriate
• Increased fluid intake to 2–3 l daily
• Storage: unused vials in refrigerator; reconstituted powder in a refrigerator at 2–8°C and used within 24 hr

Evaluate:
• Vital signs: raised temperature may indicate infection or be a side effect
• All side effects including yellowing of skin and sclera
• Therapeutic effect: decrease in size of tumour, easier breathing

Teach patient/family:
• About the drug and the side effects
• That fatigue is common and activity may have to be altered
• To avoid becoming pregnant whilst taking the drug
• To report any side effects
• To avoid hazardous tasks as confusion and dizziness may occur
• That impotence may occur during treatment, but is temporary

---

interferon (gamma-1b)

Immukin

Func. class.: Cytokine, biological response modifier
Chem. class.: Protein
Legal class.: POM

Action: Gamma-interferon has a variety of complex effects on the immune system. In chronic granulomatous disease the most important of these is, probably, phagocyte activation

Uses: Adjunctive treatment to antibiotics to reduce the frequency of serious infection in patients with chronic granulomatous disease

Dosage and routes:
• *Adult:* By subcutaneous injection, 50 mcg/m^2 body surface area 3 times a week
• *Child (over 6 months and under 0.5 m^2 body surface area):* by subcutaneous injection, 1.5 mcg/kg 3 times a week

Available forms include: Injection 200 mcg/ml, 0.5 ml vials

Side effects/adverse reactions:
CNS: Headache, fatigue
GI: Nausea, vomiting
INTEG: Rashes, injection-site tenderness
MS: Myalgia, arthralgia
SYST: Fever, chills

Contraindications: Hypersensitivity

Precautions: Pregnancy; breast-feeding; severe hepatic or renal impairment; seizure disorders or compromised central nervous system function; cardiac disease

Interactions:

• CNS side effects exacerbated by: alcohol

• Possibility of enhanced toxicity with: neurotoxic, haemotoxic, cardiotoxic drugs

• Risk of amplified immune response with: heterologous serum protein preparations or immunological preparations (e.g. vaccines) given simultaneously

Treatment of overdose: Symptomatic and supportive

NURSING CONSIDERATIONS

Assess:

• Baseline vital signs (temperature, pulse, respiration, BP), ECG; also weight, food likes and dislikes

• Full blood count

Administer:

• SC: do not shake vial vigorously

• All other medication as prescribed including anti-emetics, antibiotics and analgesics

Perform/provide:

• Good aseptic technique when administering

• Mouth and skin care as appropriate

• Increased fluid intake to 2–3 l/day

• Storage: unused vials in refrigerator, do not freeze; reconstituted powder in a refrigerator at 2–8°C to be used within 24 hours

Evaluate:

• Vital signs including those indicating cardiac problems

• All side effects including influenza-like symptoms and pain at injection site

• Therapeutic effect

Teach patient/family:

• About the drug and the side effects

• To report any side effects to nurse or clinician

ipecacuanha emetic mixture, paediatric

Func. class.: Emetic
Chem. class.: Alkaloids
Legal class.: P

Action: Acts on chemoreceptor trigger zone to induce vomiting, irritates gastric mucosa

Uses: In poisoning to induce vomiting

Dosage and routes:

• *Adult:* By mouth 30 ml, then 200–300 ml water

• *Child 6–18 months:* By mouth 10 ml, then 100–200 ml water

• *Child over 18 months:* By mouth 15 ml, then 100–200 ml water; may repeat dose if needed once after 20 min

Available forms include: Mixture, prepared from ipecacuanha liquid extract

Side effects/adverse reactions:

CNS: Depression, convulsions, coma

GI: Bloody diarrhoea, mucosal damage

RESP: Inhalation of vomitus

CV: Circulatory failure, atrial fibrillation, fatal myocarditis, dysrhythmias

Contraindications: Hypersensitivity; unconscious/semiconscious; depressed gag reflex; poisoning with petroleum or corrosive products; convulsions; low risk of toxicity for ingested product; late presentation

Precautions: Lactation, pregnancy

Pharmacokinetics:

By mouth: Onset 15–30 min

Interactions/incompatibilities:

• Decreased effect of ipecacuanha: activated charcoal

Clinical assessment:
- Type of poisoning; do not administer if petroleum products or caustic substances have been ingested; contact Poisons Centre

NURSING CONSIDERATIONS

Assess:
- Vital signs, BP; check patients with cardiac disease more often

Administer:
- In fully conscious patients only
- Bounce child to increase emetic effect
- Activated charcoal if this drug doesn't work; may begin lavage after 10–15 min

Evaluate:
- Respiratory status before, during, after administration of emetic; check rate, rhythm, character; respiratory depression can occur rapidly with elderly or debilitated patients
- Response—satisfactory quantity of vomit

---

ipratropium bromide

Atrovent, Atrovent Forte, combination product
Func. class.: Antimuscarinic bronchodilator
Chem. class.: Synthetic quaternary ammonium compound
Legal class.: POM

Action: Inhibits interaction of acetylcholine at receptor sites on the bronchial smooth muscle, resulting in bronchodilation
Uses: Bronchodilation in obstructive airways disease
Dosage and routes:
- *Adult:* 2 inhalations (40 mcg) 3–4 times daily, sometimes up to 4 puffs during early treatment
- *Child up to 6 yr:* 1 inhalation 3 times daily; 6–12 yr 1–2 inhalations 3 times daily
- *Adult:* Nebulised 100–500 mcg up to 4 times a day
- *Child:* Nebulised 100–500 mcg up to 3 times a day

Available forms include: Aerosol inhaler 20 mcg/puff, 40 mcg/puff; nebuliser solution 250 mcg, 500 mcg vials
Side effects/adverse reactions:
GI: Constipation
EENT: Dry mouth, blurred vision
Contraindications: Hypersensitivity to this drug or atropine
Precautions: Pregnancy, lactation, glaucoma, prostatic hypertrophy
Pharmacokinetics: Negligible amounts absorbed from the lungs, half-life of swallowed drug 3–4 hr

NURSING CONSIDERATIONS

Assess:
- For bronchoconstriction; if severe, drug may need to be changed

Administer:
- With salbutamol in the same nebuliser if indicated

Perform/provide:
- Frequent drinks, sugarless gum to relieve dry mouth

Evaluate:
- Therapeutic response: ability to breathe adequately—assessed by use of peak flows
- For tolerance over long-term therapy; dose may need to be increased or changed

Teach patient/family:
- Use inhaler/nebuliser according to prescribed number of inhalations/24 hr, or overdose may occur
- It is a preventative treatment rather than for the control of bronchospasm
- How to use inhaler aerosol or nebuliser equipment

isocarboxazid

Marplan
Func. class.: Antidepressant, MAOI
Chem. class.: Hydrazine
Legal class.: POM

Action: Increases concentrations of endogenous adrenaline noradrenaline, serotonin, dopamine in storage sites in CNS by inhibition of monoamine oxidase; increased concentration reduces depression
Uses: Depression
Dosage and routes:
• *Adult:* By mouth initially 30 mg daily in divided doses, if no improvement after 4 weeks 60 mg daily may be tried for no longer than 6 weeks, reduce dose to lowest effective dose when condition improves (usually 10–20 mg)
Available forms include: Tablets 10 mg
Side effects/adverse reactions:
HAEM: Anaemia, purpura, granulocytopenia
CNS: Dizziness, drowsiness, confusion, headache, anxiety, tremors, weakness, hyperreflexia, mania, insomnia, fatigue
GI: Constipation, dry mouth, nausea, vomiting, anorexia, diarrhoea, weight gain
GU: Change in libido, frequency
INTEG: Rash, flushing, increased perspiration, jaundice
CV: Orthostatic hypotension, hypertension, dysrhythmias, hypertensive crisis, peripheral oedema
EENT: Blurred vision
ENDO: SIADH-like syndrome
Contraindications: Hypersensitivity to MAOIs, hepatic impairment, cerebrovascular disease, phaeochromocytoma, porphyria, children
Precautions: Suicidal patients, convulsive disorders, severe depression, schizophrenia, hyperactivity, diabetes mellitus, pregnancy, renal disease, agitation, blood dyscrasias, elderly
Pharmacokinetics:
By mouth: Duration up to 2 weeks; metabolised by liver, excreted by kidneys
Interactions/incompatibilities:
• Increased pressor effects: indirect acting sympathomimetics (ephedrine), amphetamines
• Increased effects of: direct acting sympathomimetics (adrenaline), local anaesthetics, hypoglycaemic agents, antihypertensives, anticholinergic drugs, alcohol, barbiturates, benzodiazepines, CNS depressants, phenothiazines, diuretics
• Hyperpyretic crisis, convulsions, hypertensive episode: tricyclic antidepressants, tyramine-containing foods, amphetamines, phenylpropanolamine, ephedrine, fenfluramine, dopamine, levodopa, pethidine (and possibly other narcotics)
Clinical assessment:
• Blood studies: full blood count, leucocytes, cardiac enzymes if patient is receiving long-term therapy
• Liver function tests: aspartate aminotransferase, alanine aminotransferase, bilirubin, hepatotoxicity may occur
Treatment of overdose: Lavage, activated charcoal, vital signs, diazepam IV for convulsions, phentolamine for severe hypertension, hydrocortisone for severe shock

NURSING CONSIDERATIONS

Assess:
• Baseline BP (lying, standing), pulse
Administer:
• Increased fluids, fibre in diet if constipation, urinary retention occur

• With food or milk for GI symptoms
• Crushed if patient is unable to swallow medication whole
• Dosage at bedtime if over-sedation occurs during day
• Frequent sips of water for dry mouth

Perform/provide:
• Assistance with mobility during beginning therapy since drowsiness/dizziness occurs
• Safety measures including cotsides, with good explanation to patient

Evaluate:
• BP; if systolic drops 20 mmHg notify clinician
• Toxicity: increased headache, palpitation; discontinue drug immediately; prodromal signs of hypertensive crisis
• Mental status: mood, alertness, affect, memory (long, short), increase in pyschiatric symptoms
• Urinary retention, constipation, GI disturbance, oedema
• Weight weekly
• Withdrawal symptoms: headache, nausea, vomiting, muscle pain weakness

Teach patient/family:
• That therapeutic effects may take 1–4 weeks
• To avoid driving or other activities requiring alertness
• To avoid alcohol ingestion, CNS depressants or non-prescribed medications: for colds, hay fever, cough
• Not to discontinue medication quickly after long-term use
• To avoid high tyramine foods: mature cheese, sour cream, beer, wine, pickled products, liver, raisins, bananas, figs, avocados, meat tenderisers, chocolate, yogurt; increased caffeine
• Report headache, palpitation, neck stiffness
• To carry Medical Identity Card detailing drug therapy

isoflurane

Func. class.: Inhalation anaesthetic
Chem. class.: Halogenated ether
Legal class.: P

Action: Produces central nervous system depression and loss of consciousness

Uses: Induction and maintenance of general anaesthesia

Dosage and routes:

Induction
• *Adult and child:* By inhalation from specially calibrated vaporiser 0.5–3.0% in oxygen or nitrous oxide–oxygen. Minimum anaesthetic concentration decreases with advancing age

Maintenance
• *Adult and child:* By inhalation from specially calibrated vaporiser 1–2.5% in nitrous oxide–oxygen; an additional 0.5–1% may be required when given with oxygen alone; caesarean section, 0.5–0.75% in nitrous oxide–oxygen. Minimum anaesthetic concentration decreases with advancing age

Available forms include: Bottles, 100 ml

Side effects/adverse reactions:
CV: Hypotension, tachycardia, cardiac arrhythmias
ELECT: Elevated serum fluoride
GI: Nausea and vomiting during recovery
HAEM: Elevated white blood cell count
MISC: Shivering during recovery
RESP: Respiratory depression

Contraindications: Sensitivity; history of malignant hyperpyrexia following administration

Precautions: Raised intracranial pressure; pregnancy; obstetric anaesthesia

Pharmacokinetics: Readily absorbed on inhalation; mostly excreted unchanged through the

lungs; small amounts are excreted in the urine as inorganic fluoride
Interactions:
• Potentiation of muscle relaxants, especially depolarising agents
• Risk of cardiac arrhythmias with: adrenaline (including, possibly, topical preparations), isoprenaline, levodopa, tricyclic antidepressants, verapamil
• Enhanced hypotensive effect with: antihypertensives, antipsychotics, β-blockers, verapamil

NURSING CONSIDERATIONS
Assess:
• Baseline vital signs (temperature, pulse, respiration, BP)
Administer:
• With adequate concentrations of oxygen to avoid hypoxia
• With all other supporting equipment appropriate for general anaesthesia
Perform/provide:
• Regular monitoring and recording of vital signs
• Storage with bottles tightly closed and in a cool place
Evaluate:
• Effect of drug and any side effects including those occurring during recovery
Teach patient/family:
• About the drug and the side effects, particularly during recovery

---

isoniazid

Rimifon, combination products
Func. class.: Antitubercular
Chem. class.: Isonicotinic acid hydrazide
Legal class.: POM

Action: Interference with bacterial cell metabolism, leading to rupture of cell wall
Uses: Treatment, prophylaxis of tuberculosis in combination with other drugs, tuberculous meningitis
Dosage and routes:
Treatment
• *Adult:* By mouth/IM/IV 300 mg once a day or 15 mg/kg 3 times a week for potentially non-compliant patients
• *Child:* By mouth/IM/IV 10 mg/kg (maximum 300 mg) daily or 15 mg/kg 3 times a week
Tuberculous meningitis
• No generally accepted regimen: consult specialist literature
Prophylaxis
• *Adult:* By mouth 300 mg once daily as single dose for 12 months
• *Child and infants:* By mouth 5–10 mg/kg daily in single or divided doses for 12 months (maximum 300 mg daily)
Available forms include: Tablets 50, 100 mg; injection 25 mg/ml; elixir 50 mg/5 ml
Side effects/adverse reactions:
MS: Peripheral neuropathy
SYST: Systemic lupus erythematosus-like syndrome, hepatitis, hyperglycaemia
INTEG: Dermatitis
CNS: Tremors, convulsions, confusion, psychosis
EENT: Optic neuritis
Contraindications: Hypersensitivity, drug-induced liver disease, porphyria
Precautions: Pregnancy, hepatic disease, epilepsy, alcoholism, lactation, renal disease, diabetic retinopathy, cataracts, ocular defects, child under 13 yr, history of psychosis
Pharmacokinetics:
By mouth: Peak 1–2 hr
IM: Peak 45–60 min
Metabolised in liver, excreted in urine (metabolites), excreted in breast milk
Interactions/incompatibilities:
• Reduced absorption: antacids

• Increased toxicity of: carbamazepine, phenytoin, primidone, ethosuximide, diazepam, theophylline
• Increased CNS toxicity with: cycloserine

Clinical assessment:
• Temperature, if less than 38.5° drug should be reduced
• Liver function tests each week: alanine aminotransferase, aspartate aminotransferase, bilirubin
• Renal status: before, every month, serum urea, creatinine, output, specific gravity, urinalysis
• Resistance to therapy if inadequate therapeutic response

NURSING CONSIDERATIONS

Administer:
• Take half to one hour before meals (improved absorption); dose may require adjustment in hepatic failure. Give concomitant pyridoxine for prophylaxis of peripheral neuropathy
• With meals to decrease GI symptoms
• Anti-emetic if vomiting occurs
• With other antitubercular drugs for effective treatment
• With pyridoxine to reduce risk of peripheral neuropathy

Evaluate:
• Mental status often: affect, mood, behavioural changes; psychosis may occur
• For signs and symptoms of peripheral neuropathy, i.e. tingline or loss of sensation in extremeties
• Hepatic status: decreased appetite, jaundice, dark urine, fatigue

Teach patient/family:
• That compliance with dosage schedule, length is necessary
• That scheduled appointments must be kept or relapse may occur
• Avoid alcohol while taking drug
• Prescribed pyridoxine should also be taken

isoprenaline hydrochloride/ isoprenaline sulphate

Medihaler-Iso, Saventrine, Saventrine IV, Min-I-Jet, combination product
Func. class.: Adrenergic agonist
Chem. class.: Sympathomimetic amine
Legal class.: POM

Action: Causes increased contractility and heart rate by acting on β-receptors in heart, also causes peripheral vasodilatation by acting on β-receptors in blood vessel walls

Uses: Heart block, severe bradycardia, asthma, bronchitis

Dosage and routes:
• By mouth 90 mg–840 g daily in divided doses, ranging from 2-hrly to 8-hrly administration (rarely used)

Asthma, bronchospasm
• *Adult:* Aerosol inhalation 1–3 puffs, may repeat after 30 min, maintenance 1–2 puffs 4–8 times daily

Heart block
• *Adult and child:* Infusion IV 0.5–10 mcg/min

Severe bradycardia
• *Adult and child:* 1–4 mcg/min

Shock
• *Adult and child:* IV 0.5–10 mcg/min, intracardiac 100 mcg in 10 ml water

Available forms include: Aerosol 80, 400 mcg inhalation; tablets 30 mg; injection 20 mcg/ml, 1 mg/ml

Side effects/adverse reactions:
CNS: Tremors, anxiety, headache, dizziness, sweating
CV: Palpitations, tachycardia, hypertension, cardiac arrest
GI: Nausea, diarrhoea

Contraindications: Hypersensitivity to sympathomimetics, acute coronary disease, ventricular fibrillation, tachycardia

Precautions: Pregnancy, cardiac disorders, hyperthyroidism, diabetes mellitus, hypertension

Pharmacokinetics:

Inhalation: Onset rapid; duration 1–2 hr

Metabolised in liver, lungs, GI tract, excreted in urine as unchanged drug and metabolites

Interactions/incompatibilities:

• Increased effects of both drugs: other sympathomimetics

• Increased risk of: arrhythmias with: halothane

Treatment of overdose: Symptomatic care, administer β-blocker (but not in asthmatics), monitor heart rhythm

NURSING CONSIDERATIONS

Assess:

• BP, pulse prior to administration

• Fluid balance; check for urinary retention, frequency, hesitancy

Perform/provide:

• Storage at room temperature, do not use discoloured solutions

• Continuous cardiac monitoring during IV administration, preferably on a cardiac unit if given for arrythmias

• BP ½–1 hrly

• Fluid balance

Evaluate:

• For paraesthesia and coldness of extremities, peripheral blood flow may decrease

• Injection site: tissue sloughing

• Therapeutic response: increased BP and heart rate

• Tachycardias—inform clinician immediately

Teach patient/family:

• Use of inhaler

• To avoid getting aerosol in eyes

• To wash inhaler in warm water and dry daily

isosorbide dinitrate

Sorbitrate, Cedocard, Isoket, Imtack, Isoket Retard, Isordil Tembids, Cedocard IV, Cedocard Retard, Isordil, Soni-slo, Sorbichew, Sorbid SA, Vascardin

Func. class.: Anti-anginal

Chem. class.: Nitrate

Legal class.: P, injection POM

Action: Decreases preload, afterload, which is responsible for decreasing left ventricular end diastolic pressure, systemic vascular resistance

Uses: Chronic stable angina pectoris, prophylaxis of angina pain left ventricular failure

Dosage and routes:

• *Adult:* Sublingual, 5–10 mg

• *Adult:* By mouth, angina, 30–120 mg in divided doses; left ventricular failure, 40–160 mg; maximum 240 mg

• *Adult:* IV infusion 2–10 mg/hr

• *Adult:* Modified-release preparations, 20–120 mg every 12 hour; depends on the preparations, see manufacturer's details

Available forms include: Capsules, modified-release 20 mg, 40 mg; tablets 5 mg, 10 mg, 20 mg, 40 mg; tablets, chewable 5 mg; tablets, modified-release 20 mg, 40 mg; sublingual tablets 5 mg; spray 1.25 mg/dose; IV infusion 1 mg/ml, 0.5 mg/ml

Side effects/adverse reactions:

CV: Postural hypotension, tachycardia

INTEG: Pallor, sweating, rash

CNS: Headache, flushing, dizziness, weakness

Contraindications: Hypersensitivity to nitrates, raised intracranial pressure, marked anaemia, closed-angle glaucoma, cerebral haemorrhage, acute myocardial infarction,

hypovolaemia, severe hypotension
Precautions: Postural hypotension, pregnancy, lactation
Pharmacokinetics:
Modified-release: Duration 6–12 hr
By mouth: Onset 15–30 min, duration 4–6 hr
Sublingual: Onset 2–5 min, duration 1–2 hr
Chewable tablets: Onset 3 min, duration ½–3 hr
Metabolised by liver, excreted in urine as metabolites (80%–100%), which are also active vasodilators
Interactions/incompatibilities:
• Increased effects: β-blockers, narcotics, tricyclics, diuretics, antihypertensives
• Decreased effects: sympathomimetics, anticholinergics (sublingual preps only)

NURSING CONSIDERATIONS

Assess:
• BP ½–1 hrly, pulse in IV use, respirations when beginning therapy
• If used IV to treat heart failure, assess oedema, shortness of breath and fluid balance
Administer:
• With full glass of water on empty stomach (oral tablet)
• Clinician may consider oral administration in the morning and at lunch time to attempt to reduce tolerance (day time angina) and lunch and evening to reduce nocturnal angina
• IV rate is usually titrated to treat unstable angina within the limits of the patient is blood pressure
• IV administration: incompatible with PVC or wide bore IV tubes as the drug is absorbed into the plastic and may be up to 30% less effective
• Ideally administered via 50 ml syringe pump or in a poly fusor or glass container
Evaluate:
• Pain: duration, time started, activity being performed, character
• Headache, lightheadedness, decreased BP; may indicate a need for decreased dosage
Teach patient/family:
• That drug may be taken before stressful activity (exercise, sexual activity)
• That sublingual administration may sting when drug comes in contact with mucous membranes
• To avoid hazardous activities if dizziness occurs
• Stress patient compliance with complete medical regimen
• To make position changes slowly to prevent fainting
• That analgesia (such as paracetamol) may help headaches if taken at the same time as drug (unless otherwise contraindicated)
• Headaches often lessen after the initial first days of treatment
• Inform clinician of any episodes of angina. An ECG may be performed if pain lasts over 20 mins

isotretinoin

Roaccutane
Func. class.: Anti-acne agent, systemic
Chem. class.: Retinoid, vitamin A derivative
Legal class.: POM

Action: Decreases size and activity of sebaceous glands
Uses: Cystic and conglobate acne and severe acne unresponsive to other treatment
Dosage and routes:
• *Adult:* By mouth initially 0.5 mg/kg daily for 4 weeks, continue for 8–12 weeks if improvement is seen; if little response increase to

1 mg/kg daily for 8–12 weeks; if intolerant reduce to 0.1–0.2 mg/kg daily for 8–12 weeks
Available forms include: Capsules 5 mg, 20 mg
Side effects/adverse reactions:
INTEG: Dry skin, pruritus, cheilosis, joint and muscle pain, hair loss, photosensitivity, urticarian bruising, hirsutism, sweating
MS: Myalgia, arthralgia
CV: Chest pain
ENDO: Raised serum triglycerides and cholesterol, hyperglycaemia, hyperuricaemia
GI: Nausea, vomiting, anorexia, increased liver enzymes, jaundice, hepatitis, inflammatory bowel disease
EENT: Eye irritation, conjunctivitis, epistaxis, dry nose, mouth, contact lens intolerance, papilloedema, optic neuritis, cataracts, decreased night vision, photophobia, blurred vision, hearing deficiency
HAEM: Thrombocytopenia, thrombocytosis, neutropaenia, anaemia
CNS: Lethargy, fatigue, headache, drowsiness, benign intracranial hypertension, depression, seizures
Contraindications: Hypersensitivity, hepatic or renal impairment, pregnancy, breast-feeding, inadequate contraception in females, hypervitaminosis A, hyperlipidaemia
Precautions: Diabetes, photosensitivity
Pharmacokinetics:
By mouth: Peak 1–4 hr, half-life 10–20 hr; metabolised in liver, excreted in urine, faeces. Bioavailability is enhanced by taking with meals
Interactions/incompatibilities:
• Additive toxic effects: vitamin A, do not take more than the recommended dietary allowance
• Benign intracranial hypertension: increased risk with tetracyclines
• Increased triglyceride levels: alcohol
Clinical assessment:
• Triglyceride levels, aspartate aminotransferase, alanine aminotransferase, alkaline phosphatase; before, during treatment (monthly)
Treatment of overdose: Gastric lavage, supportive measures

NURSING CONSIDERATIONS

Assess:
• Urinalysis weekly for protein, blood
• Blood glucose in diabetics, periodically
Administer:
• Whole, do not crush; give with meals
Evaluate:
• Therapeutic response: decrease in size and number of lesions
• Area of body involved, what helps or aggravates condition
• Pseudotumour cerebri: headache, vomiting, nausea, visual disturbance; discontinue drug
Teach patient/family:
• To avoid sunlight or wear sunscreen since photosensitivity may occur
• That an increase in acne may occur during initial treatment; decrease in 4–6 weeks
• Not to take vitamin A supplements, to take drug with meals
• Regarding package insert
• Not to crush capsules
• Minimise or eliminate alcohol consumption
• Not to take if pregnancy suspected. Reliable contraceptive measures must be taken in women of childbearing potential for at least 4 weeks before, during and at least 4 weeks after stopping treatment

isoxsuprine HCl

Duvadilan
Func. class.: Myometrial relaxant
Chem. class.: Nylidrin related agent
Legal class.: POM

Action: Adrenergic agonist acts directly on vascular smooth muscle; causes uterine relaxation
Uses: Uncomplicated premature labour
Dosage and routes:
• *Adult:* By intravenous infusion, initially 200–300 mcg/min gradually increased to 500 mcg/min until labour is arrested; subsequently by IM injection, 10 mg every 3 hr for 24 hr, then every 4–6 hr for 48 hr
Available forms include: Injection IM/IV 5 mg/ml
Sides effects/adverse reactions:
CV: Hypotension, tachycardia, palpitations, chest pain
CNS: Dizziness, weakness, tremors, anxiety
GI: Nausea, vomiting, abdominal pain, distention
INTEG: Severe rash, flushing
Contraindications: Hypersensitivity, recent arterial haemorrhage, heart disease, premature detachment of placenta, severe anaemia, infection
Precautions: Tachycardia
Interactions/incompatibilities:
• Increased incidence of tachycardia with atropine

NURSING CONSIDERATIONS
Assess:
• Baseline pulse, BP lying and standing
Evaluate:
• BP lying, standing; orthostatic hypotension is common
• Therapeutic response
• Maternal pulse rate
• Foetal heart rate; may cause hypotension in foetus
• Dilation of cervix
Teach patient/family:
• To report palpitations, flushing if severe
• To avoid changes in temperature; extremities should be kept warm to promote better circulation

ispaghula

Fybogel, Isogel, Metamucil, Regulan
Func. class.: Laxative
Chem. class.: Vegetable fibre
Legal class.: GSL

Action: Increases faecal mass stimulating peristalsis
Uses: Constipation, especially in patients with small, hard stools
Dosage and routes:
• Variable depending upon fibre content of individual products; consult manufacturer's literature
Available forms include: Powder, granules, effervescent granules
Side effects/adverse reactions:
GI: Flatulence, abdominal distension
Contraindications: Intestinal obstruction, colonic atony, faecal impaction
Precautions: Low fluid intake
Pharmacokinetics: Not absorbed from GI tract
Treatment of overdose: Maintain fluid intake; symptomatic treatment

NURSING CONSIDERATIONS
Assess:
• Bowel pattern
• Dietary habits and consumption of fruit, vegetable and fibre
• Fluid intake
Administer:
• With at least one full glass of cold fluid/water
• To be drunk immediately after preparation or 'jelly-like' substance is formed

Perform/provide:
• Adequate fluid intake
Evaluate:
• Therapeutic effect; increased faecal mass; reduction of small hard stools
Teach patient/family:
• How to take the powder or granules (immediately after preparation)
• About possible side effects
• About changing diet and the need to maintain a reasonable fluid intake

itraconazole

Sporanox
Func. class.: Antifungal
Chem. class.: Triazole
Legal class.: POM

Action: Impairs the synthesis of ergosterol in fungal cell membranes
Uses: Vulvovaginal candidiasis, oropharyngeal candidiasis, pityriasis versicolor and other dermatophyte infections
Dosage and routes:
Maximum period of treatment 30 days
Vulvovaginal candidiasis
• *Adult:* By mouth 200 mg twice daily for 1 day
Pityriasis versicolor
• *Adult:* By mouth 200 mg daily for 7 days
Oropharyngeal candidiasis
• *Adult:* By mouth 100 mg daily for 15 days (or 200 mg daily for 15 days in AIDS and neutropenic patients)
Tinea corporis and tinea cruris
• *Adult:* By mouth 100 mg daily for 15 days
Tinea pedis and tinea manuum
• *Adult:* By mouth 100 mg daily for 30 days

Available forms include: Capsules 100 mg
Side effects/adverse reactions:
CNS: Headache
GI: Abdominal pain, nausea, dyspepsia
Contraindications: Pregnancy, contraception must be used during and for 1 month after treatment; hypersensitivity; breast-feeding; history of liver disease
Interactions:
• Reduced blood levels of itraconazole with: rifampicin, phenytoin
• Possible reduction in absorption of itraconazole with: H_2 blockers, antacids

NURSING CONSIDERATIONS

Administer:
• To be taken immediately after meals
• 15–30 min before a meal. When a additional dose is required to control night-time symptoms, the tablet should be taken at bedtime
Teach patient/family:
• Not to take non-prescribed antacids (reduce absorption)
• History of liver disease, liver toxicity with other drug therapy, lactation

kanamycin sulphate

Kannasyn
Func. class.: Antibiotic
Chem. class.: Aminoglycoside
Legal class.: POM

Action: Interferes with protein synthesis in bacterial cell by binding to ribosomal subunit, causing inaccurate peptide sequence to form in protein chain, causing bacterial death
Uses: Serious infections due to susceptible Gram-negative organisms which have proved resistant

to other antibiotics; also certain staphylococcal infections due to multi-resistant strains and gonorrhoea

Dosage and routes:

Severe systemic infections

• *Adult and child:* IV infusion 15–30 mg/kg daily in 2–3 doses

• *Adult:* IM acute infections 1 g daily in 2–4 doses maximum 6 days (not more than 10 g total dose), chronic infection, 3–4 g a week on alternate days, maximum 50 g total dose

• *Child:* IM acute infections 15 mg/kg daily in 2–4 doses for not more than 6 days

Available forms include: Injection IM, IV 1 g powder

Side effects/adverse reactions:

GU: Haematuria, renal damage, azootaemia, renal failure, nephrotoxicity

EENT: Ototoxicity, deafness, vestibular damage

INTEG: Rash, burning, urticaria, local intolerance and haematoma at IM injection site, photosensitivity, dermatitis

Contraindications: Hypersensitivity, pregnancy, lactation

Precautions: Neonates, myasthenia gravis, hearing deficits, renal disease

Pharmacokinetics:

IM: Onset rapid, peak 1 hr

IV: Onset immediate, peak 1–2 hr

Plasma half-life 3 hr; not metabolised, excreted unchanged in urine

Interactions/incompatibilities:

• Increased ototoxicity, neurotoxicity, nephrotoxicity: other aminoglycosides, amphotericin B, polymyxin, vancomycin, ethacrynic acid, frusemide, mannitol, cisplatin, cephalosporins

Clinical assessment:

• Weight before treatment; calculation of dosage is usually done based on ideal body weight, but may be calculated on actual body weight

• Serum peak, drawn at 30–60 min after IV infusion or 60 min after IM injection; trough level drawn just before next dose; peak levels should be less than 30 mcg/ml; trough levels should be less than 10 mcg/ml

• Renal impairment by measuring creatinine clearance, blood urea nitrogen, serum creatinine; adjust doses according to blood levels

• Deafness by audiometric testing, ringing, roaring in ears, vertigo; assess hearing before, during, after treatment

• Culture and sensitivity before starting treatment to identify infecting organism

• Vestibular dysfunction: nausea, vomiting, dizziness, headache; drug should be discontinued if severe

Treatment of overdose: Haemodialysis or peritoneal dialysis, monitor serum levels of drug

NURSING CONSIDERATIONS

Assess:

• Culture and sensitivity before treatment

• Weight before treatment

• Regular blood level studies, to monitor serum peak

Administer:

• Preferably IM, as solution containing 250 mg/ml; if IV, then as solution containing 2.5 mg/ml by slow infusion at rate of 3–4 ml/min. Adjust dosage according to renal and auditory function; predose (trough) concentrations should be less than 10 mg/litre

• IM injection in large muscle mass, rotate injection sites

• Drug in evenly spaced doses to maintain blood level

• Bicarbonate to alkalinise urine if ordered in treating urinary tract infection, as drug is most active in alkaline environment

• Intravenously: slow infusion at 3–4 ml/min (2.5 mg/ml). Close observation during infusion
• Blood level studies, repeated 30–60 min after infusion

Perform/provide:

• Adequate fluids of 2–3 litres daily unless contraindicated to prevent irritation of tubules
• Supervised mobilisation, other safety measures with vestibular dysfunction

Evaluate:

• Therapeutic effect: absence of inflammation, redness, fever, draining wounds, lesions
• Input and output of fluids; report haematuria and signs of renal impairment. Special care and treatment for patients with known renal disease
• Urinalysis if drug used for urinary tract infection
• Vestibular damage, tinnitus followed by affected hearing
• Overgrowth of infection: increased temperature, malaise, redness, pain, swelling, perineal itching, diarrhoea, stomatitis, change in cough, sputum
• Injection sites for redness, swelling, rash, haematoma, usually transient
• Effects of any other drug therapy

Teach patient/family:

• To report headaches, tinnitus loss of hearing immediately
• Not to drive or use machinery if dizziness occurs
• To report sore throat, fever malaise, pain, change in cough, sputum and urine indicate superimposed infection

---

kaolin, pectin

Kaopectate
Func. class.: Antidiarrhoeal
Chem. class.: Hydrated aluminium silicate
Legal class.: GSL

Action: Increases solidity of stool
Uses: Diarrhoea
Dosage and routes:

• *Adult:* By mouth 10–30 ml 4-hrly
• *Child 1–5 yr:* By mouth 10 ml 4-hrly
• *Child 1 yr:* By mouth 5 ml 4-hrly

Available forms include: Suspension Kaolin 1.03 g/5 ml
Side effects/adverse reactions: None known
Contraindications: Intestinal obstruction
Interactions/incompatibilities: May reduce absorption of other drugs from GI tract

NURSING CONSIDERATIONS

Assess:

• Stool consistency and frequency
• Dehydration (especially children)

Administer:

• For 48 hr only
• Shake suspension before use
• Increased fluids or oral rehydration solutions

Evaluate:

• Therapeutic response: decreased diarrhoea
• Bowel pattern before; for rebound constipation
• Dehydration in children

Teach patient/family:

• Not to exceed recommended dose
• To shake well before administration

ketamine hydrochloride

Ketalar
Func. class.: Anaesthetic, general
Chem. class.: Phencyclidine derivative
Legal class.: POM

Action: Acts on limbic system, cortex to provide anaesthesia
Uses: Short anaesthesia for diagnostic/surgical procedures; induction agent
Dosage and routes:
• *Adult and child:* Pre-op: IV 2 mg/kg, IM 10 mg/kg
• Induction: IV 1–4.5 mg/kg IM 6.5–13 mg/kg
• Maintenance: ½-full induction dose as required, if used with other anaesthetics, dose may be reduced
Available forms include: Injection IM, IV 10 mg/ml (20 ml), 50 mg/ml (10 ml), 100 mg/ml (5 ml)
Side effects/adverse reactions:
CNS: Hallucinations, confusion, delirium, tremors, polyneuropathy, fasciculations, pseudo-convulsions
CV: Increased B/P, hypotension, bradycardia, increased pulse, arrhythmia
EENT: Diplopia, salivation, small increase in intraocular pressure, nystagmus
INTEG: Rash, pain at injection site
RESP: Apnoea, respiratory depression, laryngospasm
Contraindications: Hypersensitivity, CVA, increased intracranial pressure, severe hypertension, cardiac decompensation, pre-eclampsia, eclampsia
Precautions: Pregnancy, seizure disorders, psychiatric disorders, alcoholism
Pharmacokinetics:
IV: Peak 30 sec, duration 5–10 min
IM: Peak 3–4 min, duration 12–25 min
Interactions/incompatibilities:
• Increased action of this drug: narcotics, barbiturates
• Do not mix with barbiturates in solution or syringe, chemically incompatible

NURSING CONSIDERATIONS

Administer:
• Only with emergency trolley, resuscitation equipment nearby
• IV slowly over 60 seconds
• Narcotic, or diazepam to control recovery symptoms
Perform/provide:
• Quiet environment for recovery to decrease psychotic symptoms
Evaluate:
• Therapeutic response: maintenance of anaesthesia
• Vital signs every 10 min during IV administration, half hrly after IM dose
• Hallucinations, delusions, separation from environment
• Extrapyramidal reactions: dystonia, motor restlessness
• Increasing heart rate or decreasing BP, notify clinician at once

ketoconazole

Nizoral
Func. class.: Antifungal
Chem. class.: Imidazole derivative
Legal class.: POM

Action: Alters cell membranes and interferes with fungal enzyme systems
Uses: Systemic candidiasis, chronic mucocandidiasis, severe candiduria, coccidioidomycosis, histoplasmosis, paracoccidioidomycosis, chronic unresponsive vaginal candidiasis, fungal infections of the skin or fingernails which have not responded to other treatment, prophylaxis of mycotic

infections in the immunosuppressed

Dosage and routes:

• *Adult:* By mouth 200 mg once daily usually for 14 days may increase to 400 mg once daily if needed

• *Child:* By mouth 50–100 mg once daily (3 mg/kg daily)

Chronic vaginal candidiasis

• *Adult:* By mouth, 400 mg once daily for 5 days

Prophylaxis or maintenance for mycoses

By mouth, 200 mg once daily

Dermatophyte infections

Topical, apply cream 2% once or twice daily

Seborrhoeic dermatitis, dandruff

Topical, apply shampoo 2% twice weekly for 2 to 4 weeks, reduce to once every 1 to 2 weeks for prophylaxis

Available forms include: Tablets 200 mg; suspension 100 mg/5 ml; cream 2%; shampoo 2%

Side effects/adverse reactions:

GU: Gynaecomastia

INTEG: Pruritus, rash, dermatitis, purpura, urticaria

CNS: Headache

SYST: Anaphylaxis, angio-oedema

GI: Nausea, vomiting, diarrhoea, cramps, abdominal pain, constipation, flatulence, hepatotoxicity

HAEM: Thrombocytopenia

Contraindications: Hypersensitivity, pregnancy, hepatic disease

Pharmacokinetics:

By mouth: Peak 1–2 hr, half-life 8 hr, metabolised in liver, excreted mainly in bile, faeces, some in urine; requires acid pH for absorption, distributed poorly to CSF, highly protein bound

Interactions/incompatibilities:

• Hepatotoxicity: other hepatotoxic drugs

• Increased concentration of cyclosporin, phenytoin

• Decreased ketoconazole action: antacids, H_2-receptor antagonists (anticholinergics, antihistamines), rifampicin, phenytoin

• Increased anticoagulant effect: coumarin anticoagulants

• Decreased concentration of: rifampicin

Clinical assessment:

• Liver studies (alanine aminotransferase, aspartate aminotransferase, bilirubin) if on long-term therapy

NURSING CONSIDERATIONS

Assess:

• Temperature, blood pressure, pulse and respiration

• Fluid balance

Administer:

• Take with food

• In the presence of acid products only; do not use alkaline products or antacids within 2 hr of drug; may give coffee, tea, acidic fruit juices

• With food to decrease GI symptoms

Evaluate:

• Therapeutic response: decreased fever, malaise, rash, negative culture and sensitivity for infecting organism

• For allergic reaction: rash, photosensitivity, urticaria, dermatitis

• For hepatotoxicity: nausea, vomiting, jaundice, clay-coloured stools, fatigue

Teach patient/family:

• That long-term therapy may be needed to clear infection (1 week–6 months depending on infection)

• To avoid antacids, non-prescribed drugs, alkaline products

• Stress patient compliance with drug regimen

• To notify clinician if GI symptoms, signs of liver dysfunction (fatigue, nausea, anorexia, vomiting, dark urine, pale stools)

ketoprofen

Orudis, Alrheumat, Oruvail
Func. class.: Non-steroidal anti-inflammatory drug
Chem. class.: Propionic acid derivative
Legal class.: POM

Action: Inhibits prostaglandin synthesis by decreasing enzyme needed for biosynthesis; possesses analgesic, anti-inflammatory, antipyretic properties

Uses: Rheumatoid arthritis, osteoarthritis, ankylosing spondylitis, acute articular and periarticular disorders, fibrositis, cervical spondylitis, low back pain, painful musculoskeletal conditions, dysmenorrhoea (not suppositories), acute gout, control of pain and inflammation following orthopaedic surgery

Dosage and routes:

- *Adult:* By mouth 100–200 mg daily in divided doses; modified-release 100–200 mg daily, rectal 100 mg at night, IM 50–100 mg 4 hrly to a maximum of 200 mg in 24 hr. IM treatment should not exceed 3 days

Available forms include: Capsules 50 mg, 100 mg; capsules modified-release 100 mg, 200 mg; suppository 100 mg, IM injection 100 mg/2 ml

Side effects/adverse reactions:

GI: Nausea, anorexia, vomiting, diarrhoea, jaundice, cholestatic hepatitis, constipation, flatulence, cramps, dry mouth, peptic ulcer, indigestion

CNS: Dizziness, drowsiness, fatigue, tremors, confusion, insomnia, anxiety, depression, vertigo, headache

CV: Tachycardia, peripheral oedema, palpitations, dysrhythmias, anaphylaxis

INTEG: Purpura, rash, pruritus, sweating

GU: Nephrotoxicity: dysuria, haematuria, oliguria, azotaemia

HAEM: Thrombocytopenia

EENT: Tinnitus, hearing loss, blurred vision

RESP: Bronchospasm

Contraindications: Hypersensitivity; hypersensitivity to aspirin or other NSAIDs; active or suspected peptic ulcer or GI haemorrhage, history of recurrent peptic ulcer; severe renal dysfunction; asthma; 3rd trimester of pregnancy. Suppositories should not be used in recent proctitis or haemorrhoids.

Precautions: Pregnancy, lactation, children, bleeding disorders, GI disorders, cardiac disorders, renal disease, hepatic disease, asthma, allergic disorders

Pharmacokinetics:

By mouth: Peak ½–1 hr, half-life 2–3 hr, modified-release: peak 6–8 hr, half-life 8 hr metabolised in liver, excreted in urine (metabolites), and faeces

Interactions/incompatibilities:

- May increase action of: coumarins, sulphonamides, methotrexate
- Excretion delayed by: probenicid

NURSING CONSIDERATIONS

Administer:

- With or after food

Evaluate:

- Therapeutic response: decreased pain, stiffness in joints, decreased swelling in joints, ability to move more easily
- For eye, ear problems: blurred vision, tinnitus; may indicate toxicity

Teach patient/family:

- To report blurred vision, ringing, roaring in ears; may indicate toxicity
- To report change in urine pattern, increased weight, oedema,

increased pain in joints, fever, blood in urine; indicate nephrotoxicity
• To report unresolved indigestion or black tarry stools
• To avoid driving, other hazardous activities if dizziness, drowsiness occurs
• That therapeutic effects may take up to 1 month

ketoprofen (topical)

Oruvail Gel
Func. class.: Topical non steroidal anti-inflammatory agent
Chem. class.: Propionic acid derivative
Legal class.: POM

Action: Inhibits prostaglandin synthesis; possesses analgesic and anti-inflammatory properties
Uses: Relief of acute painful musculoskeletal conditions caused by trauma
Dosage and routes:
• Apply to affected area 2–3 times a day and massage
• Usual recommended dose 15 g per day
• Use for up to 7 days
Side effects/adverse reactions:
INTEG: Pruritis and erythema at site of application. Systemic side effects are unlikely
Contraindications: Hypersensitivity; asthma induced by ketoprofen, aspirin or NSAIDs; asthma; exudative dermatoses; eczema; sores; infected lesions; broken skin; children
Precautions: Severe renal impairment; for topical use only. Keep away from eyes, lips and mucous membranes. Avoid contact with broken skin; pregnancy; lactation
Pharmacokinetics: Percutaneous absorption of ketoprofen is about 5% that of oral absorption
Interactions: Unlikely as systemic levels are low
Treatment of overdose: Unlikely from topical use, if large quantities are ingested treatment would be supportive and symptomatic

NURSING CONSIDERATIONS

Assess:
• Hypersensitivity or asthma
Perform/provide:
• Gloves for professional applicant
Administer:
• By massaging well into the affected area
Evaluate:
• Clinical effect
• Any side effects
Teach patient/family:
• Correct method of application including replacement of cap after use
• Not to apply to broken skin, mucous membranes, lips or near eyes
• To wash hands thoroughly after application
• To store in a cool place
• To discontinue if side effects occur or pregnancy is likely
• Not to use for longer than 7 days

ketorolac trometamol ▼

Toradol
Func. class.: NSAIDs
Chem. class.: Trometamol salt
Legal class.: POM

Action: Inhibits prostaglandin synthesis by action on the cyclo-oxygenase enzyme system
Uses: Pain associated with surgical procedures, e.g. main abdominal or dental surgery
Dosage and routes:
• *Adult:* By IM/IV injection, 10 mg initially, then 10–30 mg every 4–6 hr as required. May be used every 2 hr in post-operative

period, maximum 90 mg per day; elderly 60 mg per day; duration of treatment maximum 2 days

• *Adult:* By mouth, 10 mg every 4–6 hr, maximum 40 mg daily. Duration of treatment maximum 7 days. Elderly 10 mg every 6–8 hr

• *Children under 16:* Not recommended

Available forms include: Injection 30 mg in 1 ml, tablets 10 mg

Side effects/adverse reactions:

GI: Discomfort, nausea, haemorrhage, dyspepsia, diarrhoea, constipation, pain, flatulence, fullness, melaena, peptic ulcer, rectal bleeding, stomatitis, vomiting perforation, abnormal liver function, dry mouth

CNS: Drowsiness, dizziness, headache, myalgia, convulsions, abnormal thinking and dreams, hallucinations, sweating, insomnia, vertigo, paraesthesia, asthenia

EENT: Abnormal vision, abnormal taste, tinnitus, hearing loss

INTEG: Pruritis, urticaria, pain at injection site, Lyell's syndrome, Stevens-Johnson syndrome, exfoliative dermatitis, macropapular rash

RESP: Pulmonary oedema, asthma, dyspnoea.

HAEM: Thrombocytopenia

CV: Hypertension, purpura, oedema, bradycardia

GU: Acute renal failure, flank pain with or without haematuria, frequency, oliguria, raised blood urea

MISC: Hypersensitivity reactions including anaphylaxis, hypotension, bronchospasm

Contraindications: Active peptic ulcer on history of peptic ulcer; coagulation disorders; hypersensitivity; patients with allergic reactions to aspirin any other drugs inhibiting prostaglandin synthesis; patients on lithium therapy; pregnancy; breast-feeding; obstetric analgesia; hypovolaemia; moderate on severe renal impairment; history of asthma; patients on anticoagulants

Precautions: Elderly; use with other NSAIDs; renal disease; impaired renal and liver function; bronchial asthma, allergic disease; children under 16; complete or partial syndrome of nasal polyps; angio-oedema; bronchospasm

Pharmacokinetics: 99% protein bound; plasma half life 5–7 hr; primary excretion via urine

Interactions:

• May increase action of: oral anticoagulants, lithium, thiazide diuretics

• Decreases action of frusemide

• Increased toxicity: methotrexate

• Increased plasma level and half life of drug with probenecid

Incompatibilities: Precipitation with morphine sulphate, petmidine hydrochloride, promethazine hydrochloride or hydroxyzine hydrochloride when mixed in a small volume

Treatment of overdose: supportive measures

NURSING CONSIDERATIONS

Assess:

• Baseline vital signs

• Level of pain

Administer:

• IM or by mouth after ensuring that other medication is compatible

Evaluate:

• Therapeutic effect (relief of pain)

• Side effects, including postoperative haemorrhage and pain at injection site

Teach patient/family:

• That prescribed dose must not be exceeded

• About side effects and to report any of these to the nurse or clinician

• Not to take OTC medicines without professional advice

ketotifen

Zatiden
Func. class.: Anti-asthmatic/anti-allergic agents
Chem. class.: Thiophenone
Legal class.: POM

Action: Thought to prevent release of pharmacological mediators of bronchospasm by stabilising mast-cell membranes, also shows properties of antihistamines
Uses: Prophylaxis of asthma, relief of allergy including rhinitis and conjunctivitis
Dosage and routes:
• *Adult:* By mouth 1–2 mg twice daily with food
• *Child over 2 yr:* By mouth 1 mg twice daily with food
Initial treatment in readily sedated patients: 0.5–1 mg at night for first few days
Available forms include: Tablets 1 mg; capsules 1 mg; elixir 1 mg/5 ml
Side effects/adverse reactions:
CNS: Sedation, dizziness
EENT: Dry mouth
Contraindications: Should not be taken with oral antidiabetic drugs; pregnancy; breast-feeding
Precautions: Warn patient of drowsiness effect, alcohol. Continue any pre-existing anti-asthma treatment for at least 2 weeks after starting ketotifen
Interactions/incompatibilities:
• Reversible thrombocytopenia with: oral antidiabetics
• Enhanced sedative effect with: alcohol, other antimuscarinic drugs
Treatment of overdose: Elimination of drug by gastric lavage or emesis is recommended. General supportive treatment
NURSING CONSIDERATIONS:
Administer:
• With food
Perform/provide:
• Mouthwashes to relieve dry mouth
• Frequent rest periods to reduce drowsiness
Evaluate:
• Therapeutic effects or respiratory status
Teach patient/family:
• Not to drive or operate machinery
• To continue all other anti-asthma treatment for at least 2 weeks
• To continue regular usage as prescribed

labetalol hydrochloride

Trandate, Labrocol
Func. class.: Antihypertensive
Chem. class.: β-blocker, α-blocker, non-selective
Legal class.: POM

Action: Produces falls in BP without reflex tachycardia or significant reduction in heart rate through mixture of α-blocking, β-blocking effects; elevated plasma renins are reduced
Uses: Mild-severe hypertension, hypertensive crisis, controlled hypotension during surgery
Dosage and routes:
Hypertension
• *Adult:* By mouth 100 mg twice a day, increased by 100 mg twice a day at intervals of 14 days to maximum of 800 mg daily, further increases to a maximum of 2.4 g daily should be split into 3–4 daily doses. More rapid dose escalation

in severe hypertension possible in hospital

Hypertensive crisis

• *Adult:* IV injection, 50 mg over 1 min, may repeat after 5 min, not to exceed 200 mg total dose

• *Adult:* IV infusion, 2 mg/min; usual range 50–200 mg

Hypertension of pregnancy

• *Adult:* IV infusion, 20 mg/hr doubled every 30 min if needed, usual maximum 160 mg/hr

Following myocardial infarction

• *IV infusion*, 15 mg/hr gradually increased to maximum 120 mg/hr

Available forms include: Tablets 50, 100 mg, 200 mg, 400 mg; injection 5 mg/ml

Side effects/adverse reactions:

CV: Orthostatic hypotension, bradycardia, atrioventricular block, ankle oedema

CNS: Dizziness, mental changes, drowsiness, fatigue, headache, depression, tremor, nightmares, paraesthesia, lethargy

GI: Nausea, vomiting, diarrhoea, liver damage, epigastric pain

INTEG: Rash, urticaria, pruritus, sweating, lichenoid rash

EENT: Tinnitus, visual changes, burning eyes, nasal congestion

GU: Impotence, dysuria, ejaculatory failure, retention

RESP: Bronchospasm, dyspnoea

SYST: Allergic reactions: angio-edema, lupus-like syndrome, fever

Contraindications: Uncontrolled heart failure, second or third degree heart block, cardiogenic shock, bradycardia (less than 50 beats/min), history of asthma or obstructive airways disease, metabolic acidosis

Precautions: Pregnancy, lactation, diabetes mellitus, hyperthyroidism, chronic obstructive airways disease, well compensated heart failure

Pharmacokinetics:

By mouth: Well absorbed, extensive first-pass metabolism, peak plasma levels 1–2 hr

IV: Peak 5 min

Half-life 2–8 hr, metabolised by liver (metabolites inactive), excreted in urine, bile, excreted in breast milk

Interactions/incompatibilities:

• Increased hypotension: diuretics, other antihypertensives, halothane and other anaesthetics, cimetidine

• Decreased effects: sympathomimetics, theophylline

• Increased risk of hypoglycaemia: insulin, oral hypoglycaemics

• Increased risk of cardiotoxicity: amiodarone, diltiazem, nifedipine, verapamil, cardiac glycosides

• Increased risk of tremor with: tricyclic antidepressants

Lab. test interferences:

False increase: urinary catecholamines

Treatment of overdose: Lavage, IV atropine for bradycardia, nebulised β_2-agonist for bronchospasm; cardiac glycoside, O_2, diuretic for cardiac failure; noradrenaline for circulatory collapse. Keep patient supine, legs raised

NURSING CONSIDERATIONS

Assess:

• Baseline vital signs

Administer:

• By mouth, before meals, tablet may be crushed or swallowed whole

• Notify clinician of any significant changes in BP and pulse after oral administration

• Consider cardiac monitoring during IV administration

• BP and pulse every 15 min for 1 hr during IV administration

• IV, keep patient on bed rest for 3–6 hrs

Perform/provide:

• Storage in dry area at room temperature, do not freeze

Evaluate:

• Therapeutic response: decreased BP after 1–2 weeks
• Fluid balance, weight daily
• BP, pulse 4 hrly; note rate, rhythm, quality
• Signs of heart failure: evaluate daily for increased weight, ankle oedema, shortness of breath

Teach patient/family:
• Not to discontinue drug unless instructed by doctor
• Not to use non-prescribed drugs containing α-adrenergic stimulants (nasal decongestants, cold preparations) unless directed by clinician
• To report dizziness, confusion, depression, fever and impotence to the doctor
• To avoid hazardous activities if dizziness is present
• To report: difficult breathing, especially on exertion or when lying down, night cough, swelling of extremities
• Rise slowly to sitting or standing position to minimise postural hypotension

---

lactitol ▼

Func. class.: Laxative
Chem. class.: Disaccharide
Legal class.: POM

Action: Increases osmotic pressure in colon and stool water content after degradation to short chain organic acids by colonic bacteria. Reduces formation and absorption of ammonia in colon

Uses: Constipation, hepatic encephalopathy

Dosage and routes:

Constipation
• *Adult:* By mouth; initially 20 g daily as a single dose with morning or evening meal, subsequently adjusted to produce one stool daily
• *Child 1–6 yr:* By mouth, 2.5–5 g once daily
• *Child 6–12 yr:* By mouth, 5–10 g once daily
• *Child 12–16 yr:* By mouth, 10–20 g once daily

Hepatic encephalopathy
• *Adult and child:* By mouth, 500–700 mg/kg bodyweight daily in 3 divided doses with meals, subsequently adjusted to produce 2 soft stools daily

Available forms include: Sachets 10 g

Side effects/adverse reactions:
ELECT: Electrolyte disturbances following prolonged, excessive use
GI: Abdominal discomfort; flatulence; cramps; sensation of fullness; nausea; borborygmi; anal pruritus; vomiting

Contraindications: Intestinal obstruction; unexplained abdominal pain or bleeding, galactosaemia

Precautions: Fluid or electrolyte imbalances

Pharmacokinetics: Minimal systemic absorption metabolised by colonic bacteria

Interactions:
• Reduced effectiveness in hepatic encephalopathy (but not in constipation) given with: antacids, neomycin
• Increased risk of hypokalaemia with: amphotericin B, carbenoxolone, corticosteroids, thiazide diuretics

Treatment of overdose: Symptomatic and supportive

NURSING CONSIDERATIONS

Assess:
• Bowel habit (frequency, type of stool, straining)
• Fluid intake
• Life-style including amount of exercise, diet

Administer:
• By mouth; mixed with hot or cold beverage, cereal or pudding. Dose adjusted to produce one stool daily

• Via naso-gastric tube; a 40% solution can be prepared as follows: add 200 g lactitol to 200 ml hot distilled water, stirring continuously. When dissolved, dilute to a final volume of 500 ml with cold distilled water

Perform/provide:

• Plenty of fluids
• Appropriate diet

Evaluate:

• Therapeutic effect (may take 2–3 days before effect takes place)
• For side effects (mostly affecting GI tract)
• Fluid balance

Teach patient/family:

• To adjust doses to give one stool daily
• About the side effects
• That lactitol must be taken regularly; NOT suitable for occasional use
• About other methods for reducing constipation (diet, fluids, exercise)

---

lactulose

NHS Duphalac
Func. class.: Laxative
Chem. class.: Disaccharide
Legal class.: P (only prescribable generically on NHS)

Action: Increases osmotic pressure within colon after bacterial degradation, stimulates peristalsis. Prevents formation and absorption of ammonia in colon

Uses: Constipation, hepatic encephalopathy/coma

Dosage and routes:

Constipation

• *Adult:* By mouth 15 ml twice daily adjusted to patient needs
• *Child under 1 yr:* By mouth 2.5 ml twice a day; 1–5 yr; 5 ml twice a day; 6–12 yr; 10 ml twice a day. Reduce dose gradually according to needs

Regular dosing essential—takes up to 48 hr to work

Encephalopathy

• *Adult:* By mouth 30–50 ml 3 times a day, adjusted to produce 2–3 soft stools daily

Available forms include: Oral solution 3.35 g/5 ml

Side effects/adverse reactions:

GI: Nausea, vomiting, cramps, diarrhoea, flatulence

MISC: Electrolyte imbalances if used excessively

Contraindications: Hypersensitivity; galactosaemia; intestinal obstruction

Precautions: Lactose intolerance

Pharmacokinetics: Metabolised in intestine

NURSING CONSIDERATIONS

Assess:

• Fluid balance
• Cause of constipation; identify whether fluids, bulk, or exercise is missing from diet or lifestyle

Administer:

• May be taken with water or fruit juice
• May be taken with meals to decrease any GI side effects

Perform/provide:

• Increase fluids to 2 litres daily

Evaluate:

• Therapeutic response
• Cramping, rectal bleeding, nausea, vomiting; if these symptoms occur, drug should be discontinued
• Clearing of confusion, lethargy, restlessness, irritability

Teach patient/family:

• That instant relief should not be expected
• That medication takes up to 48 hr to take effect
• Not to use laxatives for long-term therapy; bowel tone will be lost
• About changes in diet and lifestyle to relieve constipation

lamotrigine ▼

Lamictal
Func. class.: Anticonvulsant
Chem. class.: Phenyltriazine compound
Legal class.: POM

Action: Possibly inhibits release of glutamate (neurotransmitter) by acting at voltage-sensitive channels to stabilise neuronal membranes
Uses: Partial seizures and secondary generalised tonic-colonic seizures as an adjunct where control not satisfactory with other anti-epileptic drugs
Dosage and routes:
• *Adult and child over 12 yr:* By mouth, 50 mg initially twice daily for 2 weeks, usual maintenance 200–400 mg daily in two divided doses
• Patients taking sodium valproate 50 mg initially daily for 2 weeks, usual maintenance 100–200 mg daily in two divided doses
Available forms include: Tablets 25 mg, 50 mg, 100 mg
Side effects/adverse reactions:
INTEG: Rashes, angioedema, Stevens–Johnson syndrome.
EENT: Diplopia, blurred vision
CNS: Dizziness, drowsiness, headache, unsteadiness, tiredness, irritability, aggression
GI: Disturbances
Contraindications: Hypersensitivity, impaired hepatic or renal function
Precautions: Monitor closely, especially in first month of treatment (including hepatic, renal, and clotting parameters) if unexplained rash, fever, influenza-like symptoms or worsening of seizure control develop; adjunct treatment with other anti-epileptics; relationship (not established) with rapidly progressive illness with status epilepticus, multi-organ dysfunction, disseminated intravascular coagulation and death; avoid abrupt withdrawal; breast-feeding; pregnancy
Pharmacokinetics: Metabolised in liver, renal excretion
Interactions:
• Possible enhanced toxicity: concurrent administration of two or more antiepileptics
• Enhanced metabolism: drugs which induce drug metabolising enzymes e.g. phenytoin, carbamazepine, barbiturates
• Reduced metabolism: sodium valproate
Treatment of overdose: Supportive therapy, gastric lavage if indicated

NURSING CONSIDERATIONS
Assess:
• Current epileptic status of patient
• Baseline vital signs plus blood clotting time and renal and hepatic function
Perform/provide:
• Close monitoring for side effects particularly in the first month of treatment
Evaluate:
• Therapeutic effects (reduction in number and severity of seizures)
Teach patient/family:
• About the drug and the side effects, particularly in the first month of treatment
• To report regularly to nurse or clinician and immediately if any side effects occur
• Not to discontinue the drug suddenly

lanatoside C

Cedilanid
Func. class.: Antidysthythmic, cardiac glycoside
Chem. class.: Digitalis preparation
Legal class.: POM

Action: Acts by influx of calcium

ions from extracellular to intracellular cytoplasm; increases cardiac contractility and cardiac output

Uses: Congestive heart failure, atrial fibrillation, atrial flutter, atrial tachycardia

Dosage and routes:

• *Adult:* By mouth slow digitalisation 1.5–2 mg daily for 3–5 days; maintenance 0.25–1 mg daily

• *Child:* Seek specialist advice

Available forms include: Tablets 250 mcg

Side effects/adverse reactions:

CV: Arrhythmias, heart block, bradycardia

CNS: Headache, drowsiness, apathy, confusion, fatigue, depression, hallucinations

GI: Anorexia, nausea, vomiting, abdominal pain, diarrhoea

INTEG: Pruritus, urticaria, macular rashes

EENT: Blurred vision, yellow green halos, photophobia, diplopia

ENDO: Gynaecomastia

Contraindications: Complete atrioventricular block and 2nd degree atrioventricular block (especially 2:1), excessive sinus bradycardia, supraventricular arrythmias caused by Wolff-Parkinson-White syndrome

Precautions: Recent myocardial infarction; hypothyroidism; elderly patients (reduce dose), pregnancy, electrolyte disturbance (especially hypokalaemia), renal insufficiency

Pharmacokinetics: Poorly absorbed from GI tract, 20% of dose inactivated daily. Duration of action is 3–6 days. Mostly converted to digoxin and excreted in urine

Interactions/incompatibilities:

• Drugs increasing risk of hypokalaemia and lanatoside toxicity: diuretics, amphotericin B, corticosteroids, lithium, carbenoxolone

• Increased lanatoside blood levels: quinidine, verapamil, diltiazem, nicardipine, amiodarone, possibly other calcium antagonists, prazosin, erythromycin, tetracyclines, quinine

• Decreased lanatoside blood levels: anticholinergics, neomycin, sulphasalazine, certain cytotoxics, cholestyramine, colestipol

• Increased risk of cardiotoxicity: β-blockers, verapamil, suxamethonium, IV calcium

Clinical assessment

• Renal function tests: urea, creatinine before treatment; if change/toxicity suspected

• Serum electrolytes especially potassium before treatment; if change/toxicity suspected

• Monitor plasma levels of digoxin (therapeutic level 1.5–3.0 mcg/litre) once therapy stabilised; if toxicity suspected

Treatment of overdose: Gastric lavage if ingestion recent, correct any hypokalaemia, treat arrhythmias with non-cardiac glycoside drugs, consider administration of digoxin specific antibody fragments, monitor ECG continuously

NURSING CONSIDERATIONS

Assess:

• Baseline vital signs

• Apical pulse for 1 min before each dose: if greater than 60, take again in 1 hr; if greater than 60, call clinician and withold drug

• Fluid balance, weight daily

Administer:

• Orally using the lowest effective dose

• Potassium supplements if prescribed for potassium levels less than 3.0 mmol/litre

Evaluate:

• Visual changes headache

• Cardiac status, apical pulse, character, rate, rhythm

• Therapeutic response, decreased weight, oedema, pulse, respiration and increased urine output

Teach patient/family:

• Not to discontinue drug abruptly
• To report symptoms of toxicity, oedema
• To only take other medication on clinician's advice
• To take own pulse and contact clinician if it falls below 60
• Not to take antacid at the same time

levobunolol hydrochloride (ophthalmic)

Betagan
Func. class.: Antihypertensive, ocular; antiglaucoma agent
Chem. class.: Non-selective β-blocker
Legal class.: POM

Action: Non-selective β-adrenergic agent
Uses: Reduction of intra-ocular pressure in chronic open-angle glaucoma and ocular hypertension
Dosage and routes:
• *Adult:* One drop in the affected eye(s) once or twice a day
Available forms include: Eyedrops 0.5%
Side effects/adverse reactions:
EENT: Transient burning or stinging on instillation, blepharoconjunctivitis and iridocyclitis
CV: Bradycardia, hypotension
INTEG: Urticaria, pruritus
RESP: Dyspnoea, asthma
CNS: Headache, lethargy, transient ataxia, dizziness
Contraindications: Asthma, history of obstructive airways disease, bradycardia, heart block, heart failure
Precautions: Pregnancy, breast-feeding
Pharmacokinetics: Onset of action within 1 hr, peak 2–8 hr, duration 24 hr. Significant systemic absorption possible; metabolised in liver, excreted in urine, half-life 6–7 hr
Interactions/incompatibilities:
• Should be used with caution in patients on oral β-blocking drugs (additive effects)

Assess:
• History of asthma, bronchospasm or wheeziness
• Diabetic status
Administer:
• With appropriate support in case of bronchospasm
Evaluate:
• For side effects including transitory dryness of eyes
Teach patient/family:
• Should not be used in patients wearing hydrophilic (soft) contact lenses
• Full clinical response may take several weeks

levodopa

Brocadopa, Larodopa
Func. class.: Antiparkinsonian agent
Chem. class.: Phenylalanine derivative
Legal class.: POM

Action: Decarboxylation to dopamine, which increases dopamine levels in brain
Uses: Parkinsonism
Dosage and routes:
• *Adult:* By mouth 125–500 mg daily divided 2 to 5 times a day with meals, may increase by 0.5–1 g every 3–7 days, depending upon response, not normally to exceed 8 g daily. Non-hospitalised patients may require slower dose elevation and smaller dosage increments
Available forms include: Capsules 125, 250, 500 mg; tablets 500 mg
Side effects/adverse reactions:

HAEM: Haemolytic anaemia, transient leucopenia/thrombocytopenia
CNS: Choreiform involuntary movements, fatigue, headache, anxiety, twitching, numbness, weakness, confusion, agitation, insomnia, nightmares, psychosis, hallucination, hypomania, depression, dizziness, peripheral neuropathy
GI: Nausea, vomiting, anorexia, abdominal distress, bitter taste, transient rises in liver enzymes, GI bleeding
INTEG: Sweating, alopecia, flushing
CV: Orthostatic hypotension, tachycardia, hypertension, palpitation, arrhythmias
MISC: Reddish colouration of urine and other body fluids
Contraindications: Concurrent use of MAOIs (except selegiline), hypersensitivity, narrow-angle glaucoma, history of or active malignant melanoma, psychosis, drug-induced parkinsonism
Precautions: Renal disease, cardiovascular disease, hepatic disease, peptic ulcer, diabetes, pregnancy
Pharmacokinetics:
By mouth: Peak 1–3 hr, metabolised in gut, liver, kidney, excreted in urine (metabolites), plasma half-life 45–65 min
Interactions/incompatibilities:
• Hypertensive crisis: MAOIs (except selegiline) or within 21 days of stopping
• Dysrhythmias: cyclopropane, halogenated hydrocarbon anaesthetics
• Increased effects of: guanethidine, methyldopa, other antihypertensives
• Decreased effects of: antipsychotics
• Effects of levodopa reduced by: benzodiazepines, pyridoxine, iron, metoclopramide

Clinical assessment:
• Adjust dosage depending on patient response
• Hepatic, haematological, renal, cardiovascular, psychiatric surveillance during prolonged therapy
• Prescribe domperidone for nausea
Lab. test interferences:
False positive: Urine ketones, urine glucose
False negative: Urine glucose (glucose oxidase)
Treatment of overdose: Gastric lavage, ECG monitoring, supportive treatment

NURSING CONSIDERATIONS

Administer:
• Drug to be given until patient is starved (before surgery)
• With meals; limit protein taken with drug
Perform/provide:
• Assistance with ambulation, during beginning or therapy
• Testing for diabetes mellitus, acromegaly if on long-term therapy
Evaluate:
• Mental status: affect, mood, behavioural changes, depression
• Assess suicidal tendencies
• Therapeutic response: decrease in involuntary movements, increased, increase mood
Teach patient/family:
• To change positions slowly to prevent orthostatic hypotension
• To report side effects: twitching, eye spasms; indicate overdose
• To use drug exactly as prescribed; if drug is discontinued abruptly, parkinsonian crisis may occur
• That urine, sweat may darken
• To avoid vitamin B_6 preparations, and vitamin-fortified foods containing B_6; these foods can reverse effects of levodopa

lignocaine and prilocaine (topical)

Emla

Func. class.: Anaesthetic, topical, local

Chem. class.: Aminoacyl amide

Legal class.: POM

Action: Inhibits conduction of nerve impulses from sensory nerves

Uses: Topical anaesthetic for skin anaesthesia, and genital mucosa to facilitate removal of warts in adults

Dosage and routes:

Skin

Adult and child over 1 year: Minor topical procedures 2 g Emla for minimum 60 mins, maximum 5 hr; larger areas, 1.5–3 g/10 cm^2 minimum 2 hr, maximum 5 hr

Genital mucosa

Adult: Up to 10 g for 5–10 min prior to procedure

Available forms include: Cream 5%

Side effects/adverse reactions:

EENT: Swelling, burning, stinging, tissue necrosis, irritation

INTEG: Rash, urticaria, oedema

HAEM: Prilocaine has been known to cause methaemoglobinaemia when given parenterally

Contraindications: Hypersensitivity, secondary bacterial infections, infants

Precautions: Sepsis of affected area, pregnancy

Pharmacokinetics:

Topical: Peak 2–5 min, duration ½–1 hr

NURSING CONSIDERATIONS

Administer:

• For surface anaesthesia, not to wounds, or mucous membranes (except genital warts in adults) or atopic dermatitis

• Using spatula provided

• Thickly, under occlusive dressing at least 1 hr before venepuncture (except for infants)

• 5–10 min before removal of genital warts

• Avoiding use near eyes or in middle ear

Perform/provide:

• Storage at room temperature in tight container

Evaluate:

• For therapeutic response

• For redness, swelling

Teach patient/family:

• Not to apply cream to mucous membrane (except for genital warts in adults)

lignocaine hydrochloride

Xylocard, Min-I-Jet lignocaine, Select-A-Jet lignocaine

Func. class.: Anti-arrhythmic (Class Ib)

Chem. class.: Aminoacyl amide

Legal class.: POM

Action: Increases electrical stimulation threshold of ventrical, HIS Purkinje system, by stabilising cardiac membrane

Uses: Ventricular tachycardia, extrasystole, and arrhythmias especially after myocardial infarction

Dosage and routes:

• *Adult:* Slow IV injection 50–100 mg over 2 min, repeated once or twice after 5–10 min intervals if necessary, not to exceed 300 mg in 1 hr; follow by IV infusion 2–4 mg/min

Available forms include: Injection 10 mg, 20 mg/ml; injection for dilution 1 g, 2 g equivalent to 200 mg/ml lignocaine; infusion solution 1 mg/ml, 2 mg/ml

Side effects/adverse reactions:

CNS: Headache, dizziness, drowsiness, paraesthesia, tremor, convulsions, unconsciousness

EENT: Tinnitus, blurred vision
CV: Hypotension, bradycardia, heart block, cardiac arrest
RESP: Dyspnoea, respiratory depression
Contraindications: Hypersensitivity to amides, atrioventricular block, other severe cardiac conduction disturbances and decompensation not dependant on treatable tachyarrhythmias, porphyria
Precautions: Renal disease, liver disease, congestive cardiac failure, hypokalaemia; solutions containing 200 mg/ml are for dilution before use
Pharmacokinetics:
IV: Onset 2 min, duration 20 min
Half-life 8 min, 1–2 hr (terminal), metabolised in liver, excreted in urine
Interactions/incompatibilities:
• Increased effects of lignocaine: cimetidine, phenytoin, propranolol, quinidine and other antiarrhythmics
Clinical assessment:
• ECG
Treatment of overdose: Supportive symptomatic care; temporary pacing may be required for atrioventricular block

NURSING CONSIDERATIONS

Assess:
• BP, pulse, ECG
Administer:
• Intravenously: bolus injection over 2 min directly into vein; effects can be observed within minutes, if necessary injection can be repeated at 5–10 min intervals once or twice
• Infusion at a rate of about 2–4 mg/min
Evaluate:
• Hypotension and bradycardia; may lead to cardiac arrest
• Cardiac rate, respiration: rate, rhythm, character, continuously
• Respiratory status: rate, rhythm, sound, watch for respiratory depression
• CNS effects: dizziness, confusion, loss of consciousness, paraesthaesia, convulsions; drug should be discontinued
• Lung fields, bilateral rales may occur in congestive cardiac failure patient
• Increased respiration, increased pulse; drug should be discontinued

lignocaine HCl (local)

Lignostab, Xylocaine, Lignostab A
Func. class.: Anaesthetic, local
Chem. class.: Aminoacyl amide
Legal class.: POM

Action: Inhibits nerve impulses from sensory nerves by stabilising neuronal membrane
Uses: Peripheral nerve block, infiltration anaesthesia, caudal, epidural, spinal anaesthesia, dental procedures
Dosage and routes:
Varies depending on route of anaesthesia; by injection usual maximum 200 mg given alone or 500 mg when given with adrenaline
Available forms include: Injection 0.5% 1%, 1.5%, 2%, injection with adrenaline 0.5%, 1%, 2%
Side effects/adverse reactions:
CNS: Anxiety, dizziness, convulsions, loss of consciousness, drowsiness, tremors
CV: Myocardial depression, cardiac arrest, dysrhythmias, bradycardia, hypotension
EENT: Blurred vision, tinnitus
INTEG: Rash, urticaria, allergic reactions, oedema
RESP: Respiratory arrest, anaphylaxis
Contraindications: Hypersensitivity, hypovolaemia, heartblock, porphyria

Precautions: Elderly, debilitated, epilepsy, impaired cardiac conduction, impaired respiratory function, impaired hepatic function, bradycardia, pregnancy; facilities for resuscitation should be available; solutions containing adrenaline should not be used in appendages (vasoconstriction may impair blood supply)

Pharmacokinetics:
Onset 4–17 min, duration 3–6 hr; metabolised by liver, excreted in urine (metabolites)

Interactions/incompatibilities:
- Possibly increased systemic effects of lignocaine: cimetidine anti-arrhythmics, propranolol
- Possible interaction with adrenaline containing solutions: general anaesthetics, MAOIs, tricyclic anti-depressants

Treatment of overdose: Supportive symptomatic care

NURSING CONSIDERATIONS

Assess:
- For pre-existing local infection (anaesthesia may be ineffective)
- BP, pulse respiration

Administer:
- As appropriate for procedure to be undertaken. Wide range of uses e.g. subcutaneous for sutures, spinal infiltration
- Smallest dose producing required effect

Perform/provide:
- Resuscitation equipment
- Discard part-used units

Evaluate:
- Therapeutic response: anaesthetic level for procedure
- Allergic reactions; rash urticaria, oedema
- Foetal heart during labour
- Any changes in patient's speech, level of consciousness, complaints of dizziness during therapy
- Patient continuously during major use

Teach patient/family
- To seek medical help if dizziness, convulsions, drowsiness, breathing difficulties occur (up to 6 hr after therapy)

lignocaine/lignocaine HCl (topical)

Xylocaine

Func. class.: Topical anaesthetic
Chem. class.: Aminoacyl amide
Legal class.: P

Action: Inhibits nerve impulses from sensory nerves, by stabilising neuronal membrane

Uses: Surface anaesthesia of skin, mucous membranes during examination, catheterisation, intubation or endoscopy; minor burns and abrasions of skin; local symptomatic relief of pain

Dosage and routes:
- *Adult:* Instilled into urethra up to 40 ml gel; topical application, up to 35 g ointment in 24 hr, or up to 7.5 ml topical solution or 20 activations of topical spray as a single dose

Available forms include: Gel 2% (hydrochloride); ointment 5%; metered spray 10% (10 mg/activation); topical solution 4% (hydrochloride)

Side effects/adverse reactions:
INTEG: Allergy, sensitisation
MISC: Systemic effects (CNS stimulation, CV depression) due to excessive absorption

Contraindications: Hypersensitivity

Precautions: Pregnancy, application to large areas or to denuded skin or in sepsis (risk of systemic absorption)

NURSING CONSIDERATIONS

Assess:
- For pre-existing infection (anaesthetic may be ineffective)

Administer:
- Using sterile dressing technique
- Topically to area for surface anaesthesia using gloves, swab, nozzle or spray
- Instil into urethra through nozzle applicator before catheterisation
- To dirty skin abrasions (children's knees and hands) before scrubbing clean

Evaluate:
- Therapeutic response: absence of local pain, decreased sensitivity during examination and catheterisation
- Allergy: sensitisation, redness swelling

Teach patient/family:
- How to apply
- Not to use on large areas or excessively as absorption into whole circulatory system occurs
- To report any signs of sensitivity

---

lindane (gamma benzene hexachloride)

Quellada
Func. class.: Parasiticide
Chem. class.: Chlorinated hydrocarbon (synthetic)
Legal class.: P

Action: Stimulates nervous system of arthropods, resulting in seizures, death of organism
Uses: Scabies, lice (body/head/pubic), nits
Dosage and routes:
Scabies
- Apply to skin surfaces excluding face and scalp, wash off after 24 hr; reapply after 7 days if needed

Lice
- Apply shampoo to dry hair, leave for 4 min, add water to form lather, rinse, towel dry and comb

Available forms include: Lotion 1%; shampoo 1%
Side effects/adverse reactions:
INTEG: Irritation
CNS: Tremors, convulsions, stimulation, dizziness (ingestion or systemic absorption)
Contraindications: Hypersensitivity, pregnancy, children under 6 months; patients with known seizure disorders, broken or infected skin, low body weight
Precautions: Avoid contact with eyes and mucous membranes; no more than 2 applications/course
Pharmacokinetics: Stored in body fat, metabolised in liver, excreted in urine, faeces
Interactions/incompatibilities:
- Simultaneous application of creams, ointments, or oils may enhance absorption

NURSING CONSIDERATIONS

Assess:
- Signs of infection: scabies between toes and fingers, tracking, blisters, irritation
- Lice, nits, itching inflamed skin patches

Administer:
- To body areas, scalp only; do not apply to broken skin, face, lips, mouth, eyes, any mucous membrane, anus, or meatus
- Not more than twice in any one week or infestation
- Topical corticosteroids as ordered to decrease contact dermatitis
- Lotions of menthol or phenol to control itching
- Prescribed antibiotics if infection present

Perform/provide:
- Isolation until areas on skin, scalp have cleared and treatment is completed
- Removal of nits by using a fine-tooth comb rinsed in vinegar after treatment

Evaluate:

• Area of body involved, including crusts, nits, brownish trails on skin, itching papules in skin folds
Teach patient/family:
• To wash all inhabitants' clothing, using insecticide; preventive treatment may be required of all persons living in same house, using lotion or shampoo to decrease spread of infection
• That itching may continue for 4–6 weeks
• That drug must be reapplied if accidently washed off or treatment will be ineffective
• Do not apply to face
• Treat sexual contact simultaneously

---

liothyronine sodium (T_3)

Tri-iodothyronine injection, Tertroxin
Func. class.: Thyroid hormone
Chem. class.: Levoisomer of triiodothyronine
Legal class.: POM

Action: Increases metabolic rates, increases cardiac output, O_2 consumption, body temperature, blood volume, growth, development at cellular level
Uses: Severe hypothyroid states
Dosage and routes:
• *Adult:* By mouth 10–20 mcg daily increased gradually to 60 mcg daily in divided doses
• *Child:* Adult dose reduced in proportion to body weight
• *Elderly:* Initial dose 5 mcg daily, increased gradually as necessary
Hypothyroid coma
• IV 5–20 mcg by slow injection repeated every 4–12 hr if necessary, or IV 50 mcg initially then 25 mcg every 8 hrs reducing to 25 mcg twice daily
Available forms include: Tablets 20 mcg, injection 20 mcg

Side effects/adverse reactions:
INTEG: Sweating, flushing
CNS: Restlessness, excitability, tremors, headache
CV: Tachycardia, palpitations, angina, arrhythmias, heart failure (overdose)
GI: Vomiting, diarrhoea
MISC: Weight loss, heat intolerance
MS: Muscle cramp, weakness
Precautions: Cardiovascular disorders, elderly, adrenal insufficiency (give corticosteroids first)
Pharmacokinetics:
By mouth: Peak 12–48 hr, half-life 1–2 days
Interactions/incompatibilities:
• Decreased absorption of liothyronine: colestipol, cholestyramine
• Increased effects of: anticoagulants, tricyclic antidepressants
Clinical assessment:
• Thyroid function tests
NURSING CONSIDERATIONS
Assess:
• BP, pulse before each dose
• Fluid balance
Administer:
• In morning if possible as a single dose to decrease sleeplessness
• At same time each day to maintain drug level
Perform/provide:
• Removal of medication 4 weeks before radioactive iodine uptake test
Evaluate:
• Therapeutic response: absence of depression
• Increased weight loss, diuresis, pulse, appetite
• Absence of constipation, peripheral oedema, cold intolerance, pale, cool dry skin, brittle nails, alopecia, coarse hair, menorrhagia, night blindness, paraesthesia, syncope, stupor, coma, carotenaemia skin, rosy cheeks
• Increased nervousness, excit-

ability, irritability, which may indicate too high dose of medication, usually after 1–3 weeks of treatment
• Cardiac status: angina, palpitation, chest pain, change in vital signs–seek medical advice
Teach patient/family:
• Hair loss will occur in child, but is temporary
• Report excitability, irritability, anxiety, which indicates overdose
• That hypothyroid child will show almost immediate behaviour/personality change
• That treatment drug is not to be taken to reduce weight
• To avoid non-prescribed medication containing iodine, read labels
• To avoid iodine in food; salt-iodinized, soya beans, tofu, turnips, some seafood, some breads

liquid paraffin

Petrolagar, combination product
Func. class.: Laxative
Chem. class.: Petroleum hydrocarbon
Legal class.: P

Action: Eases passage of stool by lubricating and softening
Uses: Constipation
Dosage and routes:
• *Adult:* By mouth 10–30 ml at night when required or 10 ml morning and night
Available forms include: Emulsion
Side effects/adverse reactions:
GI: Nausea, anal seepage of paraffin and consequent irritation
RESP: Lipoid pneumonia
MISC: Granulomatous reactions caused by absorption (especially from emulsion)
Contraindications: Hypersensitivity, children under 3 yr; abdominal pain; nausea/vomiting; prolonged use
Pharmacokinetics: Excreted in faeces
Interactions/incompatibilities:
• May decrease absorption of: fat-soluble vitamins

NURSING CONSIDERATIONS

Administer:
• Alone for better absorption; not within 1 hr of other drugs or within 1 hr of antacids, milk or cimetidine
• Shake before use
Evaluate:
• Therapeutic response: decrease in constipation
• Cause of constipation; identify whether fluids, bulk, or exercise is missing from patient's diet and lifestyle
• Nausea, vomiting; if these symptoms occur, drug should be discontinued
Teach patient/family:
• Not to use laxatives for long-term therapy; bowel tone will be lost
• That normal bowel movements do not always occur daily
• Not to use in presence of abdominal pain, nausea, vomiting
• Notify clinician if constipation unrelieved or if symptoms of electrolyte imbalance occur: muscle cramps, pain, weakness, dizziness
• Avoid prolonged use

lisinopril

Zestril, Carace, combination products
Func. class.: Antihypertensive
Chem. class.: Angiotensin converting enzyme (ACE) inhibitor
Legal class.: POM

Action: Inhibits angiotensin converting enzyme, preventing conversion of angiotensin I to angiotensin II

Uses: Hypertension, congestive heart failure

Dosage and routes:

Diuretics should be stopped if possible for 2–3 days before starting treatment to minimise the risk of a rapid fall in blood pressure and hypotension

Hypertension

• *Adult:* By mouth initially 2.5 mg daily; maintenance 10–20 mg daily, maximum 40 mg daily

Congestive heart failure

• *Adult:* Initially 2.5 mg daily under hospital supervision, adjusted according to response within the range 5–20 mg daily

Available forms include: Tablets 2.5, 5, 10, 20 mg

Side effects/adverse reactions:

CVS: Hypotension, chest pain, palpitations

GI: Nausea, diarrhoea

GU: Renal insufficiency, impotence

INTEG: Rash, angioedema

CNS: Dizziness, headache, fatigue, asthenia

RESP: Cough, possible airways obstruction due to angioedema

Contraindications: Hypersensitivity, pregnancy, breast-feeding, aortic stenosis or outflow obstruction, renovascular disease, porphyria

Precautions: Lactation, renal disease, peripheral vascular or cerebrovascular disease, ischaemic heart disease, congestive heart failure, volume depletion

Pharmacokinetics: Peak 6–8 hr, excreted unchanged in urine

Interactions/incompatibilities:

• Increased hypotensive effect: diuretics, other antihypertensives, alcohol, anaesthetics, antidepressants, anxiolytics, baclofen, levodopa, phenothiazines

• Decreased hypotensive effects when used with: NSAIDs, carbenoxolone, corticosteroids, oestrogens, oral contraceptives

• Increased potassium levels: potassium salt substitutes, potassium-sparing diuretics, potassium supplements

• Possibly increased toxicity: NSAIDs, lithium

Clinical assessment:

• Assess renal function before and during therapy

Treatment of overdose: Supportive symptomatic care

NURSING CONSIDERATIONS

Assess:

• Establish baseline fluid balance and assessment of renal function and electrolytes

Administer:

• Preferably at night to avoid possible postural hypotension

• Under medical supervision at start of treatment

Evaluate:

• Blood pressure and pulse 4 hrly when established drug dosage

• Hrly observations on instigation of drug; marked hypotension may occur

• For postural hypotension

• Hypertensive control to gauge maintenance dose

• Daily weight (often given with diuretictherapy)

• Control of symptoms of congestive cardiac failure—oedema dyspnoea and productive cough

Perform/provide:

• Bed rest at start of drug therapy

• Safe environment if postural hypotension occurs

Teach patient/family:

• Seek medical advice if symptoms recur

• To avoid sudden ceasation of therapy

• Possible side-effect—care on rising/standing up; headaches, fatigue are common

• General advice to manage symptoms of cardiac failure

lithium carbonate

Camcolit, Liskonum, Phasal, Priadel
Func. class.: Antimania agent
Chem. class.: Alkali metal ion salt
Legal class.: POM

Action: May alter sodium, potassium ion transport across cell membrane biogenic amines of noradrenaline, serotonin in CNS areas involved in emotional responses
Uses: Mania, prevention of manic depressive illness or recurrent depression
Dosage and routes:
Doses should be adjusted to achieve therapeutic plasma concentrations, avoiding overdosage and toxic plasma concentrations; measure initially weekly, then monthly, and every 2 months thereafter; therapeutic plasma concentration of lithium ion 0.4–1.0 mmol/litre; concentrations at the higher end for control of acute symptoms, at the lower end for prophylaxis and for the elderly; restabilisation and monitoring is essential is a formulation is changed because of wide variations in bioavailability
• *Adult:* By mouth initially 0.4–1.2 g daily, initially in divided doses; single doses may be used after stabilisation; modified-release preparations may be used
Available forms include: Tablets 250 mg; tablets modified-release 200 mg, 300 mg, 400 mg, 450 mg
Side effects/adverse reactions:
CNS: Headache, drowsiness, dizziness, tremors, ataxia, cognitive impairment, slurred speech, incoordination, hyperreflexia, psychosis, confusion, stupor, memory loss, clonic movements; convulsions, coma (severe overdosage)
GI: Anorexia, nausea, vomiting, diarrhoea
GU: Polyuria, polydipsia, oedema, renal impairment (long-term)
CV: Hypotension, ECG changes, arrhythmias, circulatory collapse
INTEG: Acne, rash, exacerbation of psoriasis
HAEM: Leucocytosis
EENT: Tinnitus, blurred vision
ENDO: Hypothyroidism, hyperparathyroidism
MS: Muscle weakness
MISC: Weight gain, antinuclear antibody formation
Contraindications: Renal impairment, heart disease, sodium imbalance, dehydration, Addison's disease, debilitated patients
Precautions: Elderly, pregnancy, breast feeding, myasthenia, disturbances of salt/fluid balance (e.g. vomiting, diarrhoea, excessive sweating), surgery
• Different preparations vary in bioavailability: a change in preparation requires monitoring and stabilisation as for initiation of therapy
Pharmacokinetics:
By mouth: Onset rapid, peak ½–4 hr, half-life 7–36 hr depending on age; crosses blood-brain barrier, excreted in urine, enters breast milk, well absorbed by oral method
Interactions/incompatibilities:
• Increased plasma lithium concentration: NSAIDs, angiotensin converting enzyme inhibitors, diuretics, tetracycline
• Decreased plasma-lithium concentration: sodium bicarbonate, acetazolamide, aminophylline
• Increased toxicity: antidepressants, anti-epileptics, diltiazem, methyldopa, metoclopramide, metronidazole, sumatriptan, verapamil
• Possibly decreased effects of: antidiabetics, diuretics, neostigmine, pyridostigmine
• Possibly increased effects of: muscle relaxants

Clinical assessment:
• Monitor plasma lithium weekly initially and for one month after stable dosage achieved, then every 1–3 months
• Monitor cardiac, renal, and thyroid function periodically
Treatment of overdose: Supportive symptomatic care; forced diuresis with an osmotic diuretic or sodium lactate or bicarbonate infusion, or dialysis for severe intoxication

NURSING CONSIDERATIONS

Assess:
• Baseline weight
• Sodium intake; decreased sodium intake with decreased fluid intake may lead to lithium retention; increased sodium and fluids may be decrease lithium retention

Administer:
• The same formulation each time; bioavailability changes between formulation
• Modified-release tablets whole, not to be crushed or chewed; may be broken in half if required

Evaluate:
• Observe for CNS changes
• Signs of oedema

Teach patient/family:
• Symptoms of minor toxicity: vomiting, diarrhoea, poor coordination, fine motor tremors, weakness, lassitude; major toxicity: coarse tremors, severe thirst, tinnitus, dilute urine
• Action, dosage, side effects; when to notify clinician
• To monitor urine specific gravity
• That contraception is necessary since lithium may harm fetus
• Not to operate machinery until lithium levels are stable
• Maintain adequate fluid intake avoid dietary changes

lofepramine

Gamanil
Func. class.: Antidepressant
Chem. class.: Tricyclic
Legal class.: POM

Action: Block reuptake of biogenic amines from nerve endings in CNS; action in depression not fully understood
Uses: Depressive illness
Dosage and routes:
• *Adult:* By mouth, 140–210 mg daily in divided doses
Available forms include: Tablets, 70 mg (as hydrochloride)
Side effects/adverse reactions:
HAEM: Agranulocytosis, leucopenia, eosinophilia, purpura, thrombocytopenia
CNS: Headache, agitation, paraesthesia, tremor, confusion, hypomania, convulsions, dizziness, drowsiness
META: Blood sugar and weight changes
GI: Nausea, dry mouth, constipation
GU: Difficulty with micturition, changes in sexual function
INTEG: Sweating, rashes
CV: Postural hypotension, tachycardia, syncope
Contraindications: Hypersensitivity, recent myocardial infarction, arrhythmias, heart block, mania, porphyria, pregnancy and breast-feeding (unless compelling medical reason), severe renal or hepatic impairment
Precautions: Diabetes, cardiac disease, epilepsy, renal or hepatic impairment, thyroid disease, psychoses, urinary retention; avoid abrupt cessation of therapy; caution in anaesthesia, narrow angle glaucoma, prostatic hypertrophy, elderly
Pharmacokinetics: Absorbed from

GI tract, extensively demethylated during first pass metabolism in liver to primary metabolite desipramine

Interactions/incompatibilities:
- Concurrent administration with or within 2 weeks of cessation of treatment with MAOIs should be avoided
- Increased toxicity: alcohol, anaesthetic agents, antihypertensives, antihistamines, antimuscarinics, anxiolytics, diuretics, oral contraceptives, phenothiazines, sympathomimetics
- Increased effects of lofepramine: cimetidine, diltiazem, disulfiram, verapamil
- Decreased effects of lofepramine: antiepileptics, oral contraceptives
- Decreased effects of: adrenergic neurone blockers, antiepileptics, clonidine, sublingual nitrates

Treatment of overdose: Supportive symptomatic care

NURSING CONSIDERATIONS

Assess:
- All drugs patient is on for compatibility
- Pulse and blood pressure

Administer:
- Orally as directed
- Laxatives if necessary

Perform/provide:
- Store at room temperature in own packaging to protect from light and moisture
- Frequent drinks to prevent a dry mouth
- Diet high in fibre to alleviate constipation

Evaluate:
- Therapeutic response; decreased depression
- Most side effects are mild and transient, agitation, dizziness, postual hypotention, tachycardic sweating

Teach patient/family:
- To take high fibre/bulk diet
- That alcohol should be avoided
- That therapeutic effect may take up to 2 weeks
- Not to discontinue medication without medical advice. Drug should be tapered off slowly
- To take other medication only if directed by clinician. The effect of lofepramine is increased and decreased by several drugs and also effect other drugs

---

Iodoxamide (ophthalmic) ▼

Alomide

Func. class.: Anti-inflammatory
Chem. class.: Dioxamic acid derivative
Legal class.: POM

Action: Similar to sodium cromoglycate and thought to stabilise mast cells preventing release of histamine and other inflammatory mediators

Uses: Non-infective allergic conjunctivitis

Dosage and routes:
- *Adult and child over 4 yr:* 1 or 2 drops 4 times daily

Available forms include: Eye drops 0.1%

Side effects/adverse reactions:
EENT: Discomfort, burning, stinging, itching, tearing

Contraindications: Hypersensitivity to drug or formulation components (benzalkonium chloride, disodium edetate)

Precautions: Pregnancy; nursing mothers

Incompatibilities: Contact lenses

Treatment of overdose: Use running water to flush from eye. Ingestion, consider emesis.

NURSING CONSIDERATIONS

Assess:
- Ability of patient (or carer) to instil eye drops

Evaluate:
• Therapeutic effect
Teach patient/family:
• How to instil drops
• About the side effects and to report any of these
• That contact lenses must not be worn

lofexidine hydrochloride ▼

Britlofex
Chem. class.: Imidazoline derivative
Legal class.: POM

Action: Centrally acting to produce reduction in sympathetic tone
Uses: Symptomatic relief in opioid withdrawal
Dosage and routes:
• By mouth, initially 200 mcg twice daily, increasing if necessary by increments of 200–400 mcg per day to a maximum of 2.4 mg per day. If no opioid use, duration of treatment 7–10 days (longer if necessary); withdraw treatment over at least 2–4 days
Available forms include: Tablets 200 mcg
Side effects/adverse reactions:
CNS: Drowsiness
EENT: Dry mouth, throat and nose
CV: Hypotension, bradycardia, rebound hypertension (on withdrawal)
Contraindications: Hypersensitivity to imidazoline derivatives
Precautions: Pregnancy, breast-feeding, severe coronary insufficiency, recent myocardial infarction, cerebrovascular disease, marked bradycardia, chronic renal failure, renal impairment, history of depression
Interactions:
• Enhanced sedative effect: alcohol, anxiolytics, hypnotics
Treatment of overdose: Supportive measures; gastric lavage if necessary

NURSING CONSIDERATIONS

Assess:
• Degree of likely cooperation from patient
Administer:
• As prescribed but withdraw over 2–4 days
Evaluate:
• Therapeutic effect of drug
• For side effects
Teach patient/family:
• About the drug and possible side effects
• Not to discontinue the drug suddenly
• To avoid hazardous activity (driving, using heavy machinery); drug may induce drowsiness
• Not to take alcohol

lomustine

CCNU
Func. class.: Antineoplastic alkylating agent
Chem. class.: Nitrosourea
Legal class.: POM

Action: Alkylates DNA, RNA; inhibits enzymes that allow synthesis of amino acids in proteins; also responsible for cross-linking DNA strands
Uses: Hodgkin's disease resistant to conventional therapy, other lymphomas, melanomas, multiple myeloma; brain, lung, bladder, kidney, gastrointestinal tract, breast, cervix tumours
Dosage and routes:
Doses are highly variable, and dependent on local treatment protocols, concomitant therapy and

tumour type; the following dose schedules have been used

• *Adult:* By mouth 120–130 mg/m^2 as a single dose every 6 weeks. Do not give repeat dose unless WBC is above 4000/mm^3, platelet count above 100,000/mm^3

• *Children:* Only under exceptional circumstances and expert supervision. Dose as for adults

Available forms include: Capsules 10 mg, 40 mg

Side effects/adverse reactions:

HAEM: Thrombocytopenia, leucopenia, anaemia, possibility of permanent marrow damage with prolonged use

GI: Nausea, vomiting, anorexia, stomatitis, raised liver enzymes

INTEG: Loss of scalp hair

CNS: Confusion, lethargy

Contraindications: Hypersensitivity, severe bone marrow depression, pregnancy, breast feeding, failure to respond to other nitrosoureas

Precautions: Radiation therapy

Pharmacokinetics: Metabolised in liver, excreted in urine; half-life 16–48 hr, 50% protein bound, crosses blood-brain barrier, appears in breast milk. Maximal bone marrow depression 4–6 weeks post dose, may last several weeks

Interactions/incompatibilities:

• Increased metabolism of this drug: phenobarbitone

Clinical assessment:

• Full blood count, differential, platelet count weekly; withhold drug if WBC is below 4000 or platelet count is below 100,000

• Liver function tests before, and monthly during therapy

Treatment of overdose: Supportive, no specific antidote. Blood products or filgrastim for marrow suppression

NURSING CONSIDERATIONS

Assess:

• Baseline temperature

• Fluid balance

Administer:

• HANDLING: take safety precautions appropriate to antineoplastic agents

• Following local antineoplastic (cytotoxic) policies

• After ensuring that clinician is aware of blood results

• By mouth; capsules to be swallowed whole

• Other medications by mouth if possible. Avoid IV, IM, SC routes to prevent infection and bruising

• Anti-emetic 30–60 min before treatment

• All other medication as prescribed including analgesics, antibiotics, anti-emetics, antispasmodics

Perform/provide:

• Strict medical asepsis, protective isolation if WBC levels are low

• Special skin care

• Increase fluid intake to 2–3 litres daily to prevent urate deposits, calculi formation

• Strict oral hygiene

Evaluate:

• Bleeding: haematuria, bruising or petechiae, mucosa or orifices 8 hrly

• Dyspnoea, rales, unproductive cough, chest pain, tachypnoea

• Food preferences; list likes, dislikes

• Inflammation of mucosa, breaks in skin

• Buccal cavity 8 hrly for dryness, sores or ulceration, white patches, oral pain, bleeding, dysphagia

• Symptoms indicating severe allergic reaction: rash, pruritus, urticaria, purpuric skin lesions, itching, flushing

Teach patient/family:

• Of protective isolation precautions if indicated

• To report any complaints or side effects to nurse or clinician

• To report any changes in breathing or coughing
• To avoid foods with citric acid, hot or rough texture
• To report any bleeding, white spots or ulcerations in mouth to clinician; tell patient to examine mouth daily

loperamide HCl

Amet, Diocalm Ultra, Imodium
Func. class.: Antidiarrhoeal
Chem. class.: Piperidine derivative
Legal class.: P, POM

Action: Direct action on intestinal muscles to decrease GI peristalsis
Uses: Diarrhoea
Dosage and routes:
Acute diarrhoea
• *Adult:* By mouth 4 mg, then 2 mg after each loose stool, not to exceed 16 mg daily for up to 5 days
• *Child 4 to 8 yr:* By mouth 1 mg 4 times daily for up to 3 days
• *Child 9–12 yr:* By mouth 2 mg 4 times a day for up to 5 days
Chronic diarrhoea
• *Adult:* By mouth 4–8 mg daily in divided doses initially, adjust according to response
Available forms include: Capsules 2 mg; liquid 1 mg/5 ml
Side effects/adverse reactions:
CNS: Dizziness, drowsiness, fatigue
GI: Abdominal cramps, dry mouth, bloating, ileus
INTEG: Rash, urticaria
Contraindications: Hypersensitivity; severe ulcerative colitis; pseudomembranous colitis; abdominal distension; ileus; constipation; children under 4 yr
Precautions: Pregnancy, lactation, children, liver disease, dehydration, dysentery
Pharmacokinetics:
By mouth: Onset ½–1 hr, duration 4–5 hr, half-life 7–14 hr; metabolised in liver, excreted in faeces as unchanged drug, small amount in urine
Clinical assessment:
• Electrolytes if on long-term therapy (K, Na, Cl)
NURSING CONSIDERATIONS
Assess:
• Fluid balance
• Diet
• Discontinue if acute diarrhoea persists longer than 5 days in adults and 3 days in a child, and seek further medical advise. Seek advice earlier if necessary
Perform/provide:
• Store a dilution of syrup for up to 2 weeks at 20°C
• Diet that does not cause increased peristalsis or irritation. Especially in chronic, long-term use
Evaluate:
• Therapeutic response; decreased diarrhoea
• Input and output of fluid especially in children. Observe for dehydration
• Bowel patterns before; rebound constipation
• Dehydration, especially children and elderly
• Potentially more serious condition—continuous diarrhoea, abdominal cramps distention
• Side effects urticaria, rash
Teach patient/family:
• That overuse will cause constipation
• To seek medical advice if children appear 'ill'
• To wash, dry gently and use a suitable cream on sore bottoms

Ioprazolam NHS dormonoct

Func. class.: Hypnotic
Chem. class.: Benzodiazepine
Legal class.: CD (Sch 4) POM

Action: Depresses CNS with sedative effect

Uses: Short-term treatment of insomnia

Dosage and routes:

• *Adult:* By mouth, 1 mg at bedtime; may be increased to 1.5–2 mg in severe insomnia; maximum dose in elderly or debilitated patients, 0.5–1 mg

Available forms include: Tablets, 1 mg

Side effects/adverse reactions:

CNS: Drowsiness, headaches, dizziness, and lightheadness the following day; ataxia, confusion, especially in elderly; amnesia; dependence; rarely excitement, depression, aggression

GI: Nausea, jaundice

GU: Urinary retention, changes in libido

INTEG: Rash

HAEM: Blood dyscrasias

CV: Hypotension

EENT: Blurred vision

Contraindications: Acute pulmonary insufficiency, respiratory depression, phobic or obsessional states, chronic psychosis, porphyria, hypersensitivity to benzodiazepines

Precautions: History of alcohol or drug abuse or personality disorder; cerebrovascular disease, renal or hepatic impairment; pregnancy, lactation; reduce dose in elderly or debilitated patients; avoid prolonged use and abrupt withdrawal

Pharmacokinetics: Absorbed from GI, metabolised to desmethyldiazepam, half-life reported as 7 to 15 hr

Interactions/incompatibilities:

• Enhanced CNS effects: alcohol, anaesthetics, opioid analgesics, antidepressants, antihistamines, α-blockers, antipsychotics, baclofen, cimetidine

• Possibly enhanced effects of: antihypertensives

• Possibly reduced effects of: levodopa

NURSING CONSIDERATIONS

Assess:

• Pulse and blood pressure

• All drugs patient is taking for compatibility (elderly often hoard drugs)

Administer:

• Orally at bedtime

Evaluate:

• Therapeutic response; decreased insomia

• Side effects, particularly drowsiness, dizziness, headache, ataxia, nausea the following morning

• For suicidal tendencies which may be released in depressed patients

• Drug dependency if used long term

Teach patient/family:

• That treatment is for a few weeks only

• Not to take alcohol

• To take other medication only if directed by clinician (enhances effect of several drugs and alcohol)

• Not to discontinue medication without medical advice. Drug should be tapered off slowly

• To avoid driving or use of machinery if drowsiness or dizziness occurs

• Not to sleep during the day

• That suitable physical activity may enhance sleep pattern

• Not to drink coffee, take or do anything at night to interfere with sleep

loratidine

Clarityn
Func. class.: Antihistamine, H_1-receptor antagonist
Chem. class.: Ethylpiperidine derivative
Legal class.: POM

Action: Decreases allergic response by antagonising the action of histamine at H_1-receptor sites in the eyes, respiratory tract, GI tract and skin
Uses: Relief of symptoms associated with seasonal allergic rhinitis and allergic skin conditions such as idiopathic urticaria in adults and children and chronic perennial allergic rhinitis in adults
Dosage and routes:
• *Adult and child over 30 kg bodyweight:* By mouth, 10 mg once daily
• *Child 2–12 yr under 30 kg bodyweight:* By mouth, 5 mg once daily
Available forms include: Tablets, 10 mg; syrup 5 mg/ml
Side effects/adverse reactions:
CNS: Fatigue, headache
GI: Nausea
Contraindications: Hypersensitivity; pregnancy; breast-feeding
Pharmacokinetics: Rapidly absorbed after oral administration, peak plasma concentrations reached in about 1 hr; extensively metabolised to active metabolites, excreted in urine and faeces; elimination half-lives of loratidine and active metabolite 12 and 18 hr respectively
Lab. test interferences: Reduced response to allergens during skin testing for allergy—discontinue treatment 4 days prior to testing
Treatment of overdose: Induce vomiting even if emesis has occurred spontaneously (preferably using ipecacuanha) and administer activated charcoal; if emesis fails or is contraindicated perform gastric lavage; thereafter provide symptomatic and supportive treatment
NURSING CONSIDERATIONS:
Assess:
• Advise prescribing clinicians *re* previous adverse reactions to antihistamines and/or respiratory disease
Administer:
• With meals if GI symptoms occur. Be aware of possible decreased absorption
Perform/provide:
• Sips of water, frequent mouthwashes to alleviate dry mouth
Evaluate:
• Therapeutic response: absence of running or congested nose
• For signs of fatigue, headaches and nausea during therapy
• For signs of hypersensitivity/allergy, e.g. rash, pruritus, photosensitivity
• Adverse response: discontinue treatment if serious reactions occur
Teach patient/family:
• Avoid in breast-feeding mothers/during pregnancy
• All aspects of drug use and notify clinician immediately if adverse reactions occur
• To avoid driving or other hazardous activities if drowsiness occurs

lorazepam

~~NHS~~ Ativan
Func. class.: Hypnotic, anxiolytic, anti-epileptic, premedicant
Chem. class.: Benzodiazepine
Legal class.: CD (Sch 4) POM

Action: Depresses subcortical levels of CNS, including limbic system and reticular formation
Uses: Anxiety, insomnia in

psychiatric or organic disorders, premedication, status epilepticus

Dosage and routes:

Anxiety

• *Adult:* By mouth 1–4 mg daily in divided doses; elderly, debilitated, half adult dose

• *Adult:* IM or slow IV injection, acute panic attacks, 25–30 mcg/kg; repeat every 6 hr if required

Insomnia

• *Adult:* By mouth 1–2 mg at bedtime

Premedication

• *Adult:* By mouth 2–3 mg the night before procedure, then 2–4 mg 1–2 hr before procedure; slow IV 50 mcg/kg 30–45 min before procedure; IM 50 mcg/kg 1–1.5 hr before procedure

Status epilepticus

• *Adult:* IV 4 mg

• *Child:* IV 2 mg

Available forms include: Injection 4 mg/ml; tablets 1 mg, 2.5 mg

Side effects/adverse reactions:

CNS: Dizziness, drowsiness, confusion, headache, hangover, restlessness, ataxia, depression, sleep disturbances, hallucinations

GI: Nausea, vomiting

INTEG: Rash

CV: Hypertension, hypotension

EENT: Blurred vision, diplopia

HAEM: Blood dyscrasias

Contraindications: CNS depression, coma, reporter depression, sleep apnoea

Precautions: History of alcohol or drug abuse or personality disorder; cerebrovascular disease, renal or hepatic impairment; pregnancy; lactation; reduce dose in elderly or debilitated patients; avoid prolonged use and abrupt withdrawal

Pharmacokinetics:

By mouth: Peak 1–3 hr, duration 3–6 hr, metabolised by liver, excreted by kidneys, breast milk, half-life 12 hr

Interactions/incompatibilities:

• Enhanced CNS effects: alcohol, anaesthetics, opioid analgesics, antidepressants, antihistamines, α-blockers, antipsychotics, baclofen, cimetidine

• Possibly enhanced effects of: antihypertensives

• Possibly reduced effects of: levodopa

NURSING CONSIDERATIONS

Assess:

• Weight

Administer:

• Orally

• Intramuscular injection after diluting with equal volume of sodium chloride 0.9% or water for injection

• IM or slow IV only when oral route is not available

• IV slowly into a large vein

• At recommended times when used as premedication

Perform/provide:

• Store injections in refrigerator 0–4°C protect from light

• Assist with mobility

• Safety measures; e.g. side rails

Evaluate:

• Drug dependency if used long term

• Blood pressure and pulse, also respiration if IM or IV administration

Teach patient/family:

• That treatment should be for short-term use only

• To take other medication only if directed by clinician (enhances effect of several drugs and alcohol)

• Not to take alcohol

• Not to discontinue medication without medical advice. Drug should be tapered off slowly

• To avoid driving or hazardous activities if dizziness or drowsiness occurs

• That suitable physical activity may aid sleep

• To seek psychiatric help if necessary

lormetazepam

Func. class.: Hypnotic
Chem. class.: Benzodiazepine
Legal class.: CD (Sch 4) POM

Action: Depresses CNS with sedative effect

Uses: Short treatment of insomnia

Dosage and routes:

• *Adult:* By mouth, 0.5–1.5 mg at bedtime; reduce dose to 0.5 mg in elderly patients

Available forms include: Tablets, 0.5, 1 mg

Side effects/adverse reactions:

CNS: Drowsiness, headache, dizziness and lightheadness the following day; ataxia, confusion, especially in elderly; amnesia; dependence; rarely excitement, aggression or uncovering suicidal tendencies

GI: Nausea, jaundice

GU: Urinary retention, changes in libido

CVS: Hypotension

INTEG: Rash

HAEM: Blood dyscrasias

EENT: Blurred vision

Contraindications: Acute pulmonary insufficiency, hypersensitivity to benzodiazepines, myasthenia gravis, respiratory depression, phobic or obsessional states, chronic psychosis, porphyria

Precautions: History of alcohol or drug abuse or personality disorder; cerebrovascular disease, renal or hepatic impairment; pregnancy, lactation; reduce dose in elderly or debilitated patients; avoid prolonged use and abrupt withdrawal

Pharmacokinetics: Rapidly absorbed from GI tract, metabolised to inactive glucuronide, half-life reported as 11 hr

Interactions/incompatibilities:

• Enhanced CNS effects: alcohol, anaesthetics, opioid analgesics, antidepressants, antihistamines, α-blockers, antipsychotics, baclofen, cimetidine

• Possibly enhanced effects of: antihypertensives

• Possibly reduced effects of: levodopa

NURSING CONSIDERATIONS

Assess:

• Pulse and blood pressure

• All drugs patient is taking for compatibility (elderly often hoard drugs)

Administer:

• Orally at bedtime

Evaluate:

• Therapeutic response

• Side effects, particularly drowsiness, headache, ataxia, nausea the following morning

• For suicidal tendencies which may be released in depressed patients

• Drug dependency if used long term

Teach patient/family:

• That treatment is for a few weeks only

• Avoid alcohol

• To take other medication only if by clinician. Enhanced effect of several drugs and alcohol

• To avoid driving or use of machinery if drowsiness or dizziness occurs

• Not to discontinue medication without medical advice. Drug should be tapered off slightly

• Not to sleep during the day

• That suitable physical activity may enhance sleep pattern

• Not to drink coffee, take or do anything at night that may interfere with sleep

loxapine

Loxapac
Func. class.: Antipsychotic/neuroleptic
Chem. class.: Dibenzoxazepine
Legal class.: POM

Uses: Treatment of acute and chronic psychotic states
Dosage and routes:
• *Adult:* By mouth initially 20–50 mg daily in 2 divided doses, then increased over 7–10 days to 60–100 mg daily in 2 to 4 doses, until control achieved. Maximum 250 mg daily. Maintenance doses should be adjusted to the needs of the patient
Available forms include: Capsules 10, 25, 50 mg (as succinate)
Side effects/adverse reactions:
CNS: Dizziness, drowsiness, faintness, headache, staggering gait, muscle twitching, weakness, paraesthesia, confusional states, extrapyramidal reactions, akathisia, tardive dyskinesia, neuroleptic malignant syndrome
INTEG: Dermatitis, oedema, pruritus, seborrhoea, flushing
CV: Tachycardia, hypotension, hypertension, syncope
GI: Nausea, vomiting, constipation
EENT: Dry mouth, nasal congestion, blurred vision (anticholinergic effects)
RESP: Dyspnoea
MISC: Weight gain or loss, ptosis, hyperpyrexia, abnormal thirst
Contraindications: Comatose or semi-comatose patients, bone marrow depression, severe drug-induced depressed states, hypersensitivity, children, porphyria
Precautions: Convulsive disorders, cardiovascular disease, pregnancy, glaucoma, urinary retention; anti-emetic effect of this drug may mask signs of overdosage of toxic drugs and obscure conditions such as intestinal obstruction, brain tumour
Interactions/incompatibilities:
• Increased anticholinergic effect: anticholinergic antiparkinsonian agents, other anticholinergic drugs (tricyclic antidepressants, antihistamines, other antipsychotics)
• Increased CNS depression: alcohol, anxiolytics and hypnotics, opioid analgesics
• Possibly increased effects of: antihypertensives
• Possibly decreased effects of: anti-epileptics
Treatment of overdose: Gastric lavage and general supportive measures
NURSING CONSIDERATIONS:
Administer:
• Ensuring dose is swallowed
Evaluate:
• Therapeutic effect
• For anti-emetic effect masking other conditions
• For extra pyramidal symptoms
Teach/patient/family:
• About side effects including extra-pyramidal symptoms and skin reaction
• Of need to take medication as prescribed (doses may be adjusted)

lypressin

Syntopressin
Func. class.: Pituitary hormone
Chem. class.: Lysine vasopressin
Legal class.: POM

Action: Promotes reabsorption of water by action on renal tubular epithelium, smooth muscles causing constriction with a vasopressor effect
Uses: Pituitary diabetes insipidus
Dosage and routes:
• *Adult:* Intranasally 2.5–10 units

into one or both nostrils 3–7 times daily
Available forms include: Nasal spray 50 units/ml
Side effects/adverse reactions:
EENT: Nasal irritation, congestion, mucosal ulceration
GI: Nausea, abdominal pain, urge to defaecate
CV: Increased BP
Contraindications: Coronary heart disease, anaesthesia with halothane or cyclopropane
Precautions: Pregnancy, arteriosclerosis, peripheral vascular disease, hypertension, epilepsy, heart failure, asthma, migraine, renal failure
Pharmacokinetics:
Intranasal: Onset 1 hr duration 3–8 hr, half-life 15 min: metabolised in liver, kidneys, excreted in urine
Interactions/incompatibilities:
• Possibly enhanced effect of lypressin: carbamazepine, chlorpromamide, clofibrate
• Possibly decreased effect of lypressin: lithium

NURSING CONSIDERATIONS

Assess:
• Baseline weight
• Fluid balance

Evaluate:
• Therapeutic response: absence of severe thirst, decreased urine output, osmolality
• Weight daily, check for oedema in extremities, if water retention is severe, diuretic may be prescribed
• Water intoxication: lethargy, behavioural changes, disorientation, neuromuscular excitability

Teach patient/family:
• To clear nasal passages before using drug, not to inhale spray
• Use nasal spray within one month of opening
• To carry drug at all times
• All aspects of drug: action, side effects, dose, when to notify clinician

lysuride maleate ▼

Revanil
Func. class.: Dopamine agonist
Chem. class.: Ergot alkaloid derivative
Legal class.: POM

Action: Direct stimulation of surviving dopamine receptor
Uses: Parkinsonism
Dosage and routes:
• *Adult:* By mouth initially 200 mcg with food at bedtime, gradually increasing at weekly intervals by 200 mcg daily to a maximum of 5 mg daily in three divided doses
Available forms include: Tablets 200 mcg
Side effects/adverse reactions:
CV: Hypotension, Raynaud's syndrome
GI: Nausea, vomiting, abdominal pain, constipation
CNS: Dizziness, headache, drowsiness, lethargy, malaise, psychotic reactions, hallucinations
INTEG: Transient exanthemata
Contraindications: Severe disturbances of peripheral circulation, coronary insufficiency, porphyria
Precautions: Pituitary tumour, pregnancy, history of psychosis
Interactions/incompatibilities
• Possibly reduced effects of both drugs: antipsychotics

NURSING CONSIDERATIONS

Assess:
• Blood pressure before, during and after treatment

Administer:
• Orally following the dosage regime for suitable gradual introduction
• Commence at bedtime and increase dosage until equal day and night time dosages are established
• With food to prevent nausea and vomiting

Evaluate:
• Therapeutic response: decreased dyskinesia, slow movement and excressive salivation
Teach patient/family:
• To stand up slowly to prevent postural hypotension
• That alcohol should not be taken, decreases effect of lysuride maleate
• Not to drive or operate machinery if dizziness occurs
• It may be necessary to use additional contraception if oral contraception is used or if female is of child bearing age

magaldrate (aluminum magnesium complex)

Dynese
Func. class.: Antacid
Chem. class.: Aluminium/magnesium hydroxide
Legal class.: GSL

Action: Neutralises gastric acidity
Uses: Antacid
Dosage and routes:
• *Adult:* By mouth 800–1600 mg (5–10 ml) after meals and at bedtime
• *Child 6–12 years:* By mouth: 400–800 mg (2.5–5 ml) after meals, at bedtime
Available forms include: Suspension 800 mg/5 ml
Side effects/adverse reactions:
GI: Constipation, diarrhoea
META: Hypermagnesaemia
Contraindications: Hypersensitivity; hypophosphataemia; renal failure; GI obstruction; porphyria; hypermagnesaemia
Precautions: Renal disease
Pharmacokinetics:
By mouth: Duration 60 min, little absorption, excreted in urine
Interactions/incompatibilities:
• Decreased absorption of: iron salts, phenothiazines, phenytoin, tetracyclines, 4-quinolone antibiotics, rifampicin, isoniazid, pivampicillin, azithromycin, itraconazole, ketoconazole, dipyridamole, bisphosphonates, penicillamine

NURSING CONSIDERATIONS
Administer:
• After or between meals
• Shake suspension before use
• Laxatives or stool softeners if constipation occurs
Evaluate:
• Therapeutic response: absence of pain, decreased acidity
• Constipation: increase bulk in diet if needed
Teach patient/family:
• The need to eat small regular meals to reduce acidity

magnesium carbonate

Func. class.: Antacid
Chem. class.: Magnesium salt
Legal class.: GSL (some combinations P or POM) many proprietories NHS

Action: Neutralises gastric acidity
Uses: Hyperacidity, constipation
Dosage and routes:
Antacid
• *Adult:* By mouth 250–500 mg after meals and at bedtime or as required
Laxative
• *Adult:* By mouth 2–5 g
Available forms include: Suspensions, combined preparations
Side effects/adverse reactions:
GI: Diarrhoea, flatulence, cramps, belching
META: Hypermagnesaemia
Contraindications: Hypersensitivity; hypophosphataemia; renal failure; intestinal obstruction; hypermagnesaemia

Precautions: Severe renal disease, diarrhoea
Pharmacokinetics:
By mouth: Little absorption, excreted in urine
Interaction/incompatibilities:
• Decreased absorption of: iron salts, phenothiazines, phenytoin, tetracyclines, 4-quinolone antibiotics, rifampicin, isoniazid, pivampicillin, azithromycin, itraconazole, ketoconazole, dipyridamole, bisphosphonates, penicillamine

NURSING CONSIDERATIONS

Assess:
• Dietary habits
Administer:
• Shake suspension before use
• Give in water
• Magnesium carbonate mixture should be freshly prepared
Evaluate:
• Attacks of diarrhoea. (Aluminium hydroxide may be prescribed instead)
• Therapeutic response: absence of pain, decreased acidity, decreased constipation
Teach patient/family:
• Not to change antacids unless directed by clinician
• To increase bulk in diet to aid constipation
• Store in tightly covered container

magnesium hydroxide/ oxide

Milk of Magnesia, many combination products
Func. class.: Antacid
Chem. class.: Magnesium salt
Legal class: GSL

Action: Neutralises gastric acidity
Uses: Antacid, laxative
Dosage and routes:
• *Adult:* By mouth 250 mg–1 g after meals and at bedtime or as required
Laxative
• *Adult:* By mouth 2–4 g
Available forms include: Mixture 550 mg/10 ml
Side effects/adverse reactions:
GI: Diarrhoea
META: Hypermagnesaemia
Contraindications: Hypersensitivity; hypophosphataemia; renal failure; intestinal obstruction; hypermagnesaemia
Precautions: Severe renal disease, diarrhoea
Pharmacokinetics:
By mouth: Little absorption, excreted in urine
Interactions/incompatibilities:
• Decreased absorption of: iron salts, phenothiazines, phenytoin, tetracyclines, 4-quinolone antibiotics, rifampicin, isoniazid, pivampicillin, azithromycin, itraconazole, ketoconazole, dipyridamole, bisphosphonates, penicillamine

NURSING CONSIDERATIONS

Assess:
• Cause of acidity or constipation
Administer:
• After meals and at bedtime
• Shake mixture before use
• Aluminium antacids if diarrhoea occurs
Evaluate:
• Therapeutic response: absence of pain, decreased acidity
• Decreased constipation, characteristics of stools
Teach patient/family:
• Not to change antacids unless directed by clinician
• Not to take at the same time as antibiotics
• About dietary causes

magnesium salts

Citramag, Epsom Salts, Magnesium Sulphate, Magnesium Hydroxide Mixture, Milk of Magnesia, many combination products
Func. class.: Laxative, osmotic
Legal class.: GSL

Action: Increases osmotic pressure, draws fluid into colon
Uses: Constipation, bowel preparation before surgery or examination
Dosage and routes:
• *Adult:*
For bowel preparation:
By mouth (Magnesium Sulphate), 5–10 g in a tumblerful of water before breakfast—acts in 2–4 hours; by mouth (Magnesium Citrate), 17.7 g as effervescent powder in 200 ml water about 8.00 pm on evening prior to procedure
• *Child:* By mouth (Magnesium Citrate) over 10 yr, half adult dose; 5–9 yr, one third adult dose
For constipation:
• *Adult:* By mouth, 25 to 50 ml (Magnesium Hydroxide Mixture)
Available forms include: Powder (Magnesium Sulphate), effervescent powder (Magnesium Citrate), suspension (Magnesium Hydroxide)
Side effects/adverse reactions:
GI: Gastrointestinal irritation, colic
META: Electrolyte, fluid imbalances
Contraindications: Acute gastrointestinal conditions
Precautions: Renal impairment (risk of hypermagnesaemia and systemic magnesium toxicity)

NURSING CONSIDERATIONS

Assess:
• Cause of constipation; identify whether fluids, bulk or exercise is missing from diet and lifestyle
• Fluid balance; check for decrease in urinary output
Administer:
• With a full glass of water
• Shake mixtures before use
• Effervescent powder should be made in 200 ml hot water and allowed to stand for 2 hours before taking
Evaluate:
• Therapeutic response: decreased constipation
• Cramping, rectal bleeding, nausea, vomiting; if these symptoms occur, drug should be discontinued
• Magnesium toxicity: thirst, confusion, decrease in reflexes
Teach patient/family:
• Not to use laxatives for long-term therapy; bowel tone will be lost
• About changes in diet and lifestyle

magnesium trisilicate

Func. class.: Antacid
Chem. class.: Magnesium salt
Legal class.: GSL

Action: Neutralises gastric acidity
Uses: Dyspepsia
Dosage and routes:
• *Adult:* By mouth 10 ml of mixture, 1–2 tablets (chewed) or 1–5 g of powder 3 times a day, with water
Available forms include: Powder, mixture, tablets, (all compound preparations)
Side effects/adverse reactions:
GI: Diarrhoea
Contraindications: Hypersensitivity to this drug; hypophosphataemia; renal failure; hypermagnesaemia
Precautions: Severe renal disease
Pharmacokinetics:
By mouth: Little absorption

Interactions/incompatibilities:
• Decreased absorption of: tetracyclines, 4-quinolones, isoniazid, rifampicin, biphosphonates chloroquine, hydroxychloroquine, penicillamine, anticholinergics, chlordiazepoxide, cimetidine, corticosteroids, oral iron salts, phenothiazines, phenytoin, fat-soluble vitamins, itraconazole, ketoconazole, fosinopril

NURSING CONSIDERATIONS

Administer:
• Given on an empty stomach, effect lasts for about 40 min. If given 1 hr after meals, effects last for approximately 2 hr
• Tablets to be chewed
• Shake mixture before use
• Give mixture in water
• Mix powder in water before taking
• Mixture should be recently prepared

Evaluate:
• Therapeutic response: absence of pain, decreased acidity
• Observe for loose stools. Change to aluminium antacid if diarrhoea occurs

Teach patient/family:
• Not to use non-prescribed antacids unless directed by clinician

malathion

Derbac-M, Prioderm, Suleo-M
Func. class.: Parasiticide
Chem. class.: Organophosphorous compound
Legal class.: P

Action: Inhibits the enzyme cholinesterase in lice and mites resulting in a build up of the neurotransmitter acetylcholine, which results in interference with neuromuscular transmission, paralysis and death

Uses: Eradication of head, pubic and crab lice and scabies; also used as agricultural pesticide. Not for routine prophylactic use

Dosage and routes:

Treatment of head lice
• *Adult and child:* By single (most products) or multiple (Prioderm Cream Shampoo) topical application, following the manufacturer's instructions for individual products. Contact time required varies: 5 min (Prioderm Cream Shampoo); 2 hr (Prioderm Lotion); 12 hr (Derbac-M and Suleo-M lotions)

Treatment of pubic lice
• *Adult:* By topical application (Prioderm Cream Shampoo), two five minute applications separated by rinse, following manufacturer's instructions

Treatment of crab lice
• *Adult and child:* By single topical application (Derbac-M) to the whole body except the non-hairy areas above the neck; wash off after a contact time of at least 1 hr, preferably overnight

Treatment of scabies:
• *Adult and child:*
By single topical application (Derbac-M and Prioderm Lotion) to the body surfaces from the neck down (when treating children under 2 yr with Derbac-M a thin application should also be made to the scalp and face avoiding eyes and mouth), washing off after a contact time of 12 hr (Prioderm Lotion) or 24 hr (Derbac-M)

Available forms include: Alcoholic lotion 0.5%; non-alcoholic lotion 0.5%; cream shampoo 1.0%

Side effects/adverse reactions:
INTEG: Skin irritation
MISC: May affect permed, coloured or bleached hair
RESP: Isopropyl alcohol in some products may cause wheezing in asthmatics

Contraindications: Hypersensitivity
Precautions: Children under 6 months of age should only be treated under medical supervision; not intended for regular use – it should not be used more than once a week for 3 weeks at a time; pregnancy; breast-feeding
Pharmacokinetics: Little absorption when used correctly
Treatment of overdose: Gastric lavage, symptomatic and supportive care, atropine and pralidoxime may be required to counteract cholinesterase inhibition. Some preparations are alcohol-based and will result in alcohol intoxication as well as malathion toxicity

NURSING CONSIDERATIONS

Assess:
• Signs of infection: scabies between toes and fingers, tracking, blisters, irritation
• Signs of head and pubic lice

Administer:
• Wearing protective rubber or plastic gloves if handling malathion regularly
• Keeping away from mouth and eyes
• Allowing lotions to dry naturally; do not apply heat
• Leaving on for recommended period of time

Perform/provide:
• Isolation until treatment completed and areas on skin and scalp have cleared
• Removal of nits by using a fine-tooth comb; rinse in vinegar after treatment

Evaluate:
• Scabies – area of body involved, including crusts, nits, brownish trails on skin, itching papules in skin folds
• Eradication of head and pubic lice, scabies

Teach patient/family:
• When treating scabies to pay particular attention to applying lotion to skin folds, finger and toe-webs and underneath nails
• To wash clothing of all residents using insecticide: preventative treatment may be required for all persons living in same house, using lotion or shampoo to decrease spread of infection
• Sexual contacts should be treated simultaneously
• Not to wash treated area before recommended contact time has elapsed
• Not to use alcohol-based solutions near sources of ignition
• That itching may continue for 4–6 weeks in cases of scabies
• Lotion/shampoo may affect permed, coloured or bleached hair
• May cause wheezing in asthmatics
• May cause skin irritation
• To seek medical advice if accidentally swallowed

---

mannitol

Min-I-Jet Mannitol
Func. class.: Osmotic diuretic
Chem. class.: Hexahydric alcohol
Legal class.: POM

Action: Acts by increasing osmolarity of glomerular filtrate, which raises osmotic pressure of fluid in renal tubules; there is a decrease in reabsorption of water, increase in urinary output
Uses: To promote systemic diuresis in cerebral oedema, decrease intraocular pressure, improve renal function in acute renal failure
Dosage and routes:
Oliguria, treatment, renal failure
• *Adult:* IV, 1–2 test doses of 200 mg/kg (50 ml of 25%) over 3–5 min, then 50–100 g daily (maximum 200 g daily) adjusted to maintain urine flow of 30–50 ml/hr

Intraocular pressure/intracranial pressure
• *Adult:* IV 1.5–2 g/kg of a 15%–25% solution over ½–1 hr
• *Children:* 1–2 g/kg of a 15–25% solution over ½–1 hr
Available forms include: Injection IV 10%, 20%; Min-I-Jet 25%
Side effects/adverse reactions:
GU: Marked diuresis, acute renal failure
CNS: Dizziness, headache, convulsions
GI: Nausea, vomiting, dry mouth, thirst
CV: Oedema, thrombophlebitis, hypotension, hypertension, tachycardia, angina-like chest pains, fever, chills
RESP: Pulmonary oedema
ELECT: Fluid and electrolyte imbalances, acidosis, dehydration
EENT: Blurred vision, decreased intra-ocular pressure
Contraindications: Hypersensitivity, anuria, severe pulmonary congestion, severe dehydration metabolic oedema
Precautions: Dehydration, pregnancy, severe renal disease (test dose of 200 mg/kg body-weight may be required), lactation
Pharmacokinetics:
IV: Onset 30–60 min for diuresis, ½–1 hr for intra-ocular pressure, 25 min for cerebrospinal fluid; duration 2–3 hr for diuresis, 4–6 hr for intra-ocular pressure, 3–8 hr for cerebrospinal fluid; excreted in urine
Interactions/incompatibilities:
• Incompatible with whole blood, in solution or syringe with any other drug or solution
Clinical assessment:
• Electrolytes: potassium, sodium, chloride; include blood urea nitrogen, full blood count, serum creatinine, blood pH, arterial blood gases
Treatment of overdose: Discontinue infusion, correct fluid, electrolyte imbalances, haemodialysis

NURSING CONSIDERATIONS

Assess:
• Rate, depth, rhythm of respiration, effect of exertion
Administer:
• IV in 15%–25% solutions slowly do not mix with blood in transfusion apparatus use in-line filter for solutions of 20–25%
Perform/provide:
• Storage at 20–30°C, storage below 20°C may cause deposition of crystals, if necessary, redissolve crystals by heating to 60°C, cool to blood heat before use
Evaluate:
• Improvement in oedema of feet, legs, sacral area daily if medication is being used in congestive cardiac failure
• Weight, fluid balance daily to determine fluid loss; effect of drug may be decreased if used daily
• BP lying, standing, postural hypotension may occur
• Improvement in CVP 8 hrly
• Signs of metabolic acidosis: drowsiness, restlessness
• Signs of hypokalaemia: postural hypotension, malaise, fatigue, tachycardia, leg cramps, weakness
• Rashes, temperature elevation daily
• Confusion, especially in elderly; take safety precautions if needed
• Hydration including skin turgor, thirst, dry mucous membranes
Teach patient/family:
• To increase fluid intake 2–3 litres daily unless contraindicated; to rise slowly from lying or sitting position

maprotiline HCl

Ludiomil
Func. class.: Antidepressant
Chem. class.: Tetracyclic
Legal class.: POM

Action: Blocks reuptake of noradrenaline into nerve endings, increasing action of noradrenaline on nerve cells

Uses: Depression, especially where sedation is required. Use in children not recommended

Dosage and routes:

• *Adults:* By mouth, initially 25–75 mg daily in 3 divided doses or as a single dose at night. Increasing at intervals of 1–2 weeks to a maximum of 150 mg daily

• *Elderly:* By mouth, initially 30 mg daily in 3 divided doses or as a single dose at night, increasing at intervals of 1–2 weeks to a maximum of 75 mg daily

Available forms include: Tablets 10, 25, 50, 75 mg

Side effects/adverse reactions:

HAEM: Agranulocytosis, eosinophilia, leucopenia

CNS: Dizziness, drowsiness, confusion (in elderly), headache, anxiety, tremors, stimulation, weakness, behavioural disturbances (in children), nightmares, insomnia, hypomania, extrapyramidal symptoms (in elderly) (e.g. tremor, akathisia, myoclonus), ataxia, dysarthria, paraesthesia, increased psychiatric symptoms, convulsions

GI: Dry mouth, nausea, vomiting, paralytic ileus, increased appetite, weight gain, cramps, epigastric distress, jaundice, stomatitis, taste disturbance, constipation

META: Hyperglycaemia, breast enlargement, galactorrhoea

GU: Urinary retention, difficulty with micturition, acute renal failure, interference with sexual function

INTEG: Rash, urticaria, sweating, pruritus, photosensitivity, angioedema, purpura, oedema, alopecia

CV: Postural hypotension, arrhythmias, tachycardia, syncope, hypertension, palpitations, atrioventricular block

EENT: Blurred vision, tinnitus, mydriasis

Contraindications: Hypersensitivity, recent myocardial infarction, convulsive disorders, prostatic hypertrophy, urinary retention, should not be given concurrently or within 2 weeks of therapy with MAOIs, heart block, mania, narrow-angle glaucoma, severe renal or liver disease, porphyria

Precautions: Suicidal patients, cardiac disease, hyperthyroidism, concurrent treatment for hypothyroidism, electroconvulsive therapy, elective surgery, pregnancy, elderly

Pharmacokinetics:

By mouth: Onset 15–30 min, peak 8 hr, duration up to 3 weeks, steady state 6–10 days; metabolised by liver, excreted by kidneys, in faeces, half-life 27–58 hr (mean 43 hr)

Interactions/incompatibilities:

• Decreased effects of: guanethidine, clonidine

• Increased effects of: direct acting sympathomimetics, alcohol, barbiturates, benzodiazepines, CNS depressants, antihistamines, antihypertensives, phenytoin

• Hyperpyretic crisis, convulsions, hypertensive episode: MAOIs within 14 days

• Plasma levels increased by: neuroleptics and methylphenidate cimetidine

• Increased risk of arrhythmias and hyportension with anaesthesia

Clinical assessment:

• Blood studies: White blood cell count, leucocytes, differential, cardiac enzymes if patient is receiving long-term therapy

• Hepatic studies: aspartate aminotransferase, alanine aminotransferase, bilirubin, creatinine if impairment expected

• ECG for flattening of T wave, bundle branch block. Atrioventricular block, dysrhythmias in cardiac patients

Lab. test interferences:

Increase: Serum bilirubin, blood glucose, alkaline phosphatase

False increase: Urinary catecholamines

Decrease: Vanillylmandelic acid, 5-hydroxyindoleacetic acid

Treatment of overdose: ECG monitoring, induce emesis, lavage, activated charcoal, administer anticonvulsant. IV diazepam if convulsions occur. Treat hypotension and circulatory collapse with a plasma expander, reduced myocardial function with dopamine/dobutamine, correct metabolic acidosis

NURSING CONSIDERATIONS

Assess:

• Baseline BP, pulse and weight

Administer:

• Increased fluids and fibre in diet if urinary retention and/or constipation occur

• With food or milk for GI symptoms

• Dosage at bedtime if oversedation occurs during day; patient may take entire dose at bedtime; elderly may not tolerate once daily dosing

• Chewing gum, boiled sweets or frequent sips of water for dry mouth

• Take with fruit juice, water, or milk to disguise taste

Perform/provide:

• Assistance with ambulation during beginning therapy since drowsiness/dizziness occurs

• Safety measures including siderails primarily in elderly

• Checking to see oral medication swallowed

Evaluate:

• Pulse 4 hrly BP (lying, standing) if systolic BP drops 20 mmHg withhold drug, notify clinician; take vital signs 4 hrly in patients with cardiovascular disease

• Weight weekly; appetite may increase with drug

• Extrapyramidal symptoms primarily in elderly: rigidity, dystonia, motor restlessness

• Mental status: mood, alertness affect, suicidal tendencies, increase in psychiatric symptoms: depression, panic

• Urinary retention, constipation; constipation is more likely to occur in children

• Withdrawal symptoms: headache, nausea, vomiting, insomnia restlessness; do not usually occur unless drug was discontinued abruptly

• Alcohol consumption; if alcohol is consumed, withhold dose until morning

Teach patient/family:

• That therapeutic effects may take 2–3 weeks

• Caution in driving or other activities requiring alertness because of drowsiness, dizziness, blurred vision

• To avoid alcohol, other CNS depressants

• Not to discontinue medication quickly after long-term use, may cause nausea, headache, insomnia

• To take precautions since photosensitivity can occur

mebendazole

Vermox, Ovex
Func. class.: Anthelmintic
Chem. class.: Benzimidazole derivative
Legal class.: POM/P

Action: Inhibits glucose, nutrient uptake, degeneration of cytoplasmic microtubules in the cell; interferes with absorption, secretory function
Uses: Pinworms, roundworms, hookworms, whipworms, threadworms
Dosage and routes:
Threadworm
• *Adult and child over 2 yr:* By mouth 100 mg as a single dose. If re-infection occurs, give a second dose after 2 weeks.
Hookworm, roundworm, whipworm
• By mouth 100 mg twice a day for 3 days
Available forms include: Tablets, chewable 100 mg; syrup 100 mg/5 ml
Side effects/adverse reactions:
CNS: Dizziness, fever
GI: Transient diarrhoea, abdominal pain
Contraindications: Hypersensitivity, pregnancy
Pharmacokinetics:
By mouth: Peak ½–7 hr, excreted in faeces primarily (metabolites), small amount in urine (unchanged), highly bound to plasma proteins
Interactions/incompatibilities: None known
Treatment of overdose: Gastric lavage
NURSING CONSIDERATIONS
Assess:
• Stools during entire treatment; specimens must be sent to laboratory while still warm
Administer:
• May be crushed, chewed if unable to swallow whole
• By mouth after meals to avoid GI symptoms since absorption is not altered by food
• Second course after 3 weeks if needed; usually recommended
Evaluate:
• For therapeutic response: expulsion of worms and 3 negative stool cultures after completion of treatment
• For allergic reaction: rash (rare)
• For diarrhoea during expulsion of worms; prevent contamination with faeces
• For infection in other family members since transmission from person to person is common
Teach patient/family:
• Proper hygiene after bowel movement including handwashing technique; tell patient to avoid putting fingers in mouth
• That infected person should sleep alone
• To change bed linen daily, wash self and clothing in hot water
• To clean toilet daily with disinfectant
• Need for compliance with dosage schedule, duration of treatment
• To wear shoes
• To wash all fruits and vegetables well before eating

mebeverine HCl

Colofac, Colven, Fomac
Func. class.: Antispasmodic
Chem. class.: Butyl veratrate derivative
Legal class.: POM

Action: Relaxes intestinal smooth muscle, without affecting motility
Uses: Gastrointestinal disease characterised by smooth muscle spasm, irritable bowel syndrome

Dosage and routes:
• *Adults and children over 10:* By mouth 1 tablet or 15 ml liquid 3 times daily, 20 min before food
• *Adult and children over 12:* Granules: By mouth one sachet twice a day, half an hour before meals, increasing to 3 times a day if necessary.
Available forms include: Tablets 135 mg; liquid 50 mg/5 ml; granules 135 mg (with ispaghula)
Side effects/adverse reactions: None serious
Contraindications: All preparations: paralytic ileus; porphyria; children less than 10 yr. Sachets: intestinal obstruction or colonic atomy, contain 6.1 mmol of sodium and are therefore contraindicated in severe renal and cardiovascular disease
Precautions: Paralytic ileus, pregnancy, porphyria

NURSING CONSIDERATIONS

Administer:
• Mix granules in 250 ml of cold water and take immediately, swallow carefully and do not take immediately before going to bed
• Shake liquid before use
• 20–30 min before food

Perform/provide:
• Increased fluids, fibre in diet, exercise to decrease constipation

Evaluate:
• Therapeutic response, absence of abdominal pain—nausea
• Decrease in constipation

Teach patient/family:
• That tablets should be swallowed, not chewed
• That bowel actions do not occur daily
• That tablets should not be taken if there is severe pain or vomiting

---

medroxyprogesterone acetate

Depo-Provera, Farlutal, Provera
Func. class.: Progestogen
Chem. class.: Progesterone derivative
Legal class.: POM

Action: Inhibits secretion of pituitary gonadotrophins, which prevents follicular maturation and ovulation, stimulates growth of mammary tissue, antineoplastic action against endometrial renal and breast cancer
Uses: Uterine bleeding (abnormal), secondary amenorrhoea, endometriosis, endometrial, prostate, renal cancer, postmenopausal, breast cancer, contraception

Dosage and routes:

Contraception
• By deep IM, 150 mg during first 5 days menstrual cycle or before 6th week post partum, repeat every 3 months

Secondary amenorrhoea
• *Adult:* By mouth 2.5–10 mg for 5–10 days from 16th day of menstrual cycle for 3 consecutive cycles

Breast cancer
• *Adult:* By mouth 400–1500 mg daily, increasing to 2000 mg daily. IM initially 500 mg–1000 mg daily for 28 days, then 500 mg twice weekly for as long as response satisfactory

Endometriosis
• *Adult:* By mouth 10 mg 3 times a day starting from the first day of menstrual cycle for 90 days. Deep IM injection 50 mg once a week or 100 mg every 2 weeks for 6 months or more

Prostatic cancer
• *Adult:* By mouth 100–500 mg daily. IM initially 500 mg twice

weekly, maintenance 500 mg once a week

Endometrial/renal cancer

• *Adult:* By mouth 100–500 mg daily. IM 400–1000 mg weekly. Dose may be increased to 1000 mg daily. Once disease is stabilised maintenance may be as little as 400 mg each month

Dysfunctional uterine bleeding

• *Adult:* By mouth 2.5–10 mg daily for 5–10 days starting on 16th day of menstrual cycle for 2 cycles. IM 50 mg weekly

Available forms include: Tablets 5, 10, 100, 200, 250, 400 and 500 mg; oral suspension 80 mg in 1 ml; injection: 50, 150, 200 mg/ml

Side effects/adverse reactions:

CNS: Dizziness, migraine headache, nervousness, insomnia, depression, fatigue

CV: Thrombophlebitis, oedema, thromboembolism, stroke, pulmonary embolism, myocardial infarction

GI: Nausea, vomiting, anorexia, cramps, increased weight, cholestatic jaundice

EENT: Diplopia, acute impairement of vision

GU: Amenorrhoea, cervical erosion, breakthrough bleeding, dysmenorrhoea, vaginal candidiasis, breast changes, galactorrhoea, gynaecomastia, testicular atropy, impotence, endometriosis, spontaneous abortion, transient infertility (up to 2 yr following continuous treatment)

INTEG: Rash, urticaria, acne, hirsutism, alopecia, oily skin, seborrhoea, purpura, melasma, photosensitivity, angioneurotic oedema

SYST: Anaphylaxis, hyperpyrexia, back pain

META: Hyperglycaemia, hypercalcaemia

Contraindications: Pregnancy, hypersensitivity, thromboembolic disorders, reproductive cancer, genital bleeding (abnormal, undiagnosed), hepatic disease, missed abortion, hypercalcaemia linked with boney metastases

Precautions: Lactation, puerperium, hypertension, asthma, blood dyscrasias, gallbladder disease, hypercalcaemia, congestive cardiac failure, diabetes mellitus, bone disease, depression, migraine headache, convulsive disorders, renal disease, family history of cancer of breast or reproductive tract, undiagnosed abnormal uterine bleeding hormone dependent tumours

Pharmacokinetics:

By mouth: Plasma half-life 2 days, steady state reacted in 10 days, excreted in urine and faeces, metabolised in liver

Interactions/incompatibilities:

None known

Clinical assessment:

• Titrated dose, use lowest effective dose

Lab. test interferences: Gonadotrophin levels, plasma progesterone, testosterone (male), oestrogen (female), cortisol levels, urinary pregnanediol levels, glucose tolerance and metyrapone tests

NURSING CONSIDERATIONS

Assess:

• Baseline BP and fluid balance

Administer:

• Shake vigorously to disperse IM injection

• Solution deeply in large muscle mass (IM), rotate sites

• In one dose in morning

• With food or milk to decrease GI symptoms with oral dose

Evaluate:

• BP periodically

• Fluid balance; be alert for decreasing urinary output; increasing oedema

• Therapeutic response: decreased abnormal uterine bleeding, ab-

sence of amenorrhoea
• Oedema, hypertension, cardiac symptoms, jaundice
• Mental status: affect, mood, behavioural changes, depression
• Hypercalcaemia

Teach patient/family:
• Counsel patient on long-term nature of product if used as contraceptive
• To avoid sunlight or use sunscreen; photosensitivity can occur
• All aspects of drug usage, including Cushingoid symptoms
• To report breast lumps, vaginal bleeding, oedema, jaundice, dark urine, clay-coloured stools, dyspnoea, headache, blurred vision, abdominal pain, numbness or stiffness in legs, chest pain; male to report impotence or gynaecomastia
• To report suspected pregnancy

---

mefenamic acid

Ponstan
Func. class.: Non-steroidal anti-inflammatory drug
Chem. class.: Anthranilic acid derivative
Legal class.: POM

Action: Inhibits prostaglandin synthesis by inhibiting an enzyme needed for biosynthesis; possesses analgesic, anti-inflammatory, antipyretic properties

Uses: Mild to moderate pain, osteoarthritis, rheumatoid arthritis pyrexia, primary dysmenorrhoea, menorrhagia due to dysfunctional cause

Dosage and routes:
• *Adult and child more than 12 yr:* By mouth 500 mg, 3 times a day
• *Child less than 12 yr:* By mouth, infants over 6 months, 25 mg/kg daily in divided doses, or 6 months–1 yr, 50 mg 8 hrly, 2 yr–4 yr 100 mg 8 hrly, 5 yr–8 yr 150 mg 8 hrly, 9 yr–12 yr 200 mg 8 hrly

Discontinue treatment in children after 7 days (except Still's disease)

Available forms include: Capsules 250 mg; dispersible tablets 250 mg; suspension 50 mg/ml; tablets 500 mg

Side effects/adverse reactions:
GI: Nausea, anorexia, vomiting, diarrhoea leading to proctocolitis (discontinue), jaundice, cholestatic hepatitis, discomfort, dyspepsia, peptic ulcer
CNS: Dizziness, drowsiness
INTEG: Rash (discontinue)
GU: Nephrotoxicity: glomerulonephritis, dysuria, haematuria, oliguria, uraemia, renal failure (elderly)
HAEM: Thrombocytopenia, haemolytic anaemia
EENT: Tinnitus, hearing loss, blurred vision
RESP: Bronchospasm

Contraindications: Hypersensitivity; hypersensitivity to aspirin or other NSAIDS; 3rd trimester of pregnancy; asthma; severe renal disease, severe hepatic disease, inflammatory bowel disease; active or suspected peptic ulcer or GI haemorrhage; porphyria

Precautions: Pregnancy, lactation, children, bleeding disorders, GI disorders, cardiac disorders, hypersensitivity to other NSAIDs, renal disease, concurrent use with other plasma protein binding drugs, elderly especially with dehydration or renal disease

Pharmacokinetics:
By mouth: Peak 2 hr, half-life 3–3½ hr; metabolised in liver, excreted in urine (metabolites), excreted in breast milk. Highly bound to plasma proteins

Interactions/incompatibilities:
• May increase action of:

coumarin anticoagulants, phenytoin, sulphonamides
• May antagonise: antihypertensives due to fluid retention
Clinical assessment:
• Renal, liver, blood studies: blood urea nitrogen, creatinine, aspartate aminotransferase, alanine aminotransferase, Hb before treatment, periodically thereafter if problems anticipated
• Audiometric, ophthalmic exam during, treatment if problems develop
Treatment of overdose: Gastric lavage and activated charcoal, intensive supportive measures

NURSING CONSIDERATIONS

Administer:
• With or after food
• Dispersible tablets in water
Evaluate:
• Therapeutic response: decreased pain, stiffness, swelling in joints, ability to move more easily
• For eye, ear problems: blurred vision, tinnitus (may indicate toxicity)
Teach patient/family:
• To report blurred vision, or ringing, roaring in ears (may indicate toxicity)
• To avoid driving or other hazardous activities if dizziness or drowsiness occurs
• To report change in urine pattern, weight increase, oedema, pain increase in joints, fever, blood in urine (indicates nephrotoxicity)
• That therapeutic effects may take up to 1 month
• To take with food or milk
• To report any indigestion or black tarry stools

mefloquine ▼

Lariam
Func. class.: Antimalarial
Chem. class.: Quinine derivative
Legal class.: POM

Action: Is thought to work by damaging the malarial plasmodium membrane
Uses: Therapy and prophylaxis of malaria. The drug is especially indicated for therapy of *Plasmodium falciparum* malaria in which the pathogen has become resistant to other antimalarial agents. Mefloquine prophylaxis is particularly recommended for travellers to malarious regions in which multiple resistant *P. falciparum* strains occur
Dosage and routes:
Malaria prophylaxis
(for brief stays 1–3 weeks)
• *Adult and children over 45 kg:* By mouth 250 mg once weekly
• *Children:* By mouth under 15 kg weight, not recommended; 15–19 kg, one quarter adult dose; 20–30 kg, half adult dose; 31–45 kg three-quarter adult dose
• Dose should be taken once a week, always on the same day beginning one week before departure and continued for 4 weeks after leaving malarious area
For prolonged stays (more than 3 weeks): As above for first 4 weeks then take further doses at 2-week intervals. First dose 1 week before arriving in endemic area
Malaria treatment
• *Non-immune adults and children 45–60 kg:* By mouth, 3 tablets followed by 2 tablets after 6–8 hr
• *Non-immune adults and children over 60 kg:* By mouth 3 tablets followed by 2 tablets after 6–8 hr and 1 tablet after a further 6–8 hr
• *Semi-immune patients living in*

malarious areas 45–60 kg: By mouth a single dose of 3 tablets
• *Semi-immune patients living in malaria areas over 60 kg:* By mouth 3 tablets, followed by 1 tablet after 6–8 hr
• *Children under 45 kg irrespective of immune status*: By mouth a single dose of 25 mg/kg
Available forms include: Tablets 250 mg mefloquine (as hydrochloride)
Side effects/adverse reactions:
Mainly at higher doses
CNS: Dizziness, disturbed sense of balance, loss of appetite, headache, feeling of weakness, rare cases of depression, confusion, anxiety, hallucinations and paranoid reactions. In prophylaxis—occasional reports of psychological changes. If noticed the drug must be discontinued
GI: Nausea, vomiting, diarrhoea, abdominal pain, elevation of transaminases (rare)
CV: Bradycardia
INTEG: Rash, pruritus
Contraindications: Prophylactic use in pregnancy, breast-feeding, renal insufficiency, severe impairment of liver function, or in patients with a history of psychiatric disturbances or convulsions
Precautions: Women of child-bearing potential should take reliable contraceptive precautions during use and for 3 months after the last dose
Pharmacokinetics:
By mouth: peak plasma level is reached within 2–12 hr. Average half-life is 21 days and excretion is primarily in bile and faeces
Interactions: Avoid concurrent use of quinine due to increased incidence of convulsions except in severe cases where 1–2 days of IV quinine may be necessary followed by mefloquine. Possible increased risk of bradycardia with β-blockers, digoxin, some calcium channel blockers

NURSING CONSIDERATIONS
Assess:
• Baseline observations. BP, temperature, pulse, respiration
Administer:
• Take with meals; swallow whole with plenty of liquid
Perform/provide:
• Observe for side-effects
Evaluate:
• Fluid balance, watch for nausea, vomiting, diarrhoea
• Vital signs: bradycardia may occur
• Psychological status
Teach patient/family:
• Driving and similar tasks requiring fine coordination are not recommended during and 2 weeks after malaria treatment. Caution with regard to driving in prophylactic use
• If psychological changes occur when mefloquine is used for prophylaxis the drug must be stopped
• Give advice on contraception for women of child-bearing potential
• To take medication on same day of every week when taking for prophylaxis

---

megestrol acetate

Megace
Func. class.: Antineoplastic
Chem. class.: Progestogen
Legal class.: POM

Action: Affects endometrium by antiluteinising effect; this is thought to bring about cell death
Uses: Hormone dependent, breast, endometrial cancer
Dosage and routes:
Breast cancer
• *Adult:* 160 mg daily as a single dose or in divided doses
Endmetrial cancer

• *Adult:* By mouth 40–320 mg daily in divided doses
Available forms include: Tablets 40, 160 mg
Side effects/adverse reactions:
GI: Nausea, vomiting, diarrhoea, abdominal cramps, increased appetite
GU: Gynaecomastia, fluid retention, hypercalcaemia, changes in libido
INTEG: Alopecia, rash, pruritus, urticaria, acne, weight gain
CNS: Mood swings, carpal tunnel syndrome
HAEM: Thrombophlebitis
Contraindications: Hypersensitivity, pregnancy, undiagnosed vaginal bleeding, missed abortion, previous severe arterial disease, prophyria, thromboembolic disorders
Precautions: Thrombophlebitis, diabetes, lactation, hypertension, hepatic, cardiac and renal disease
Interactions/incompatibilities: None known
Clinical assessment:
• Pulmonary function tests, chest X-ray films before, during therapy; chest film should be obtained every 2 weeks during treatment
• Serum calcium

NURSING CONSIDERATIONS

Assess:
• Vital signs, fluid balance before treatment is commenced
Administer:
• Antacid before oral agent, give drug after evening meal, before bedtime
• Anti-emetic 30–60 min before giving drug to prevent vomiting
• Antispasmodics as prescribed
Perform/provide:
• Increase fluid intake to 2–3 litres daily to prevent dehydration
• Nutritious diet with iron, vitamin supplements as ordered
• Limitation of calcium (dairy products)
Evaluate:
• Vital signs 4 hrly
• Dyspnoea, râles, unproductive cough, chest pain, tachypnoea, fatigue, increased pulse, pallor, lethargy
• Food preferences; list likes, dislikes
• Effects of alopecia on body image; discuss feelings about body changes
• Fluid balance
• Oedema in feet, joints, hands, ankles; oliguria
• Symptoms indicating severe allergic reaction; rash, pruritus, urticaria, purpuric skin lesions, itching, flushing
• Frequency of stools, characteristics: cramping, acidosis, signs of dehydration (rapid respirations, poor skin turgor, decreased urine output, dry skin, restlessness, weakness)
• Mood swings
• Nausea, vomiting, diarrhoea constipation, weakness, loss of muscle tone
Teach patient/family:
• To report any complaints or side effects to nurse or clinician
• That (for women) gynaecomastia can occur; reversible after discontinuing treatment

melphalan

Alkeran
Func. class.: Antineoplastic alkylating agent
Chem. class.: Nitrogen mustard
Legal class.: POM

Action: Alkylates DNA, RNA; inhibits enzymes that allow synthesis of amino acids in proteins; also responsible for cross-linking DNA strands
Uses: Multiple myeloma, advanced breast cancer, soft tissue sarcoma,

malignant melanoma, polycythaemia vera, advanced ovarian adenocarcinoma

Dosage and routes:

Doses are highly variable, and dependent on local treatment protocols, concomitant therapy, and tumour type; the following dose schedules have been used

Multiple myeloma

• *Adult:* By mouth 0.15 mg/kg body weight daily in divided doses for 4 days with 40 mg prednisolone a day for 4 days. Repeat at intervals of 6 weeks for 12 months

Ovarian adenocarcinoma

• *Adult:* By mouth 0.2 mg/kg daily in 3 divided doses for 5 days. Repeat every 4–8 weeks provided the bone marrow has recovered

• *Adult:* IV infusion 1 mg/kg every 4 weeks

Advanced breast carcinoma

• *Adult:* By mouth 0.15 mg/kg daily or 6 mg/m^2 body surface area for 5 days. Repeat every 6 weeks

Malignant melanoma and soft tissue sarcoma

• Seek specialist's advice; given by regional perfusion

Polycythaemia vera

• *Adult:* To induce remission, by mouth 6–10 mg daily for 5–7 days. For maintenance, by mouth 2–6 mg weekly

Available forms include: Tablets 2 mg, 5 mg; injection 50 mg

Side effects/adverse reactions:

HAEM: Thrombocytopenia, neutropenia, haemolytic anaemia, leucopenia, leukaemia

GI: Nausea, vomiting, stomatitis, diarrhoea

GU: Amenorrhoea, hyperuricaemia

INTEG: Rash, urticaria, alopecia

RESP: Pulmonary fibrosis

Contraindications: Hypersensitivity

Precautions: Lactation, pregnancy, radiation therapy, bone marrow depression, concurrent cytotoxic therapy, renal impairment (in moderate–severe disease reduce dose and adjust according to response)

Pharmacokinetics:

Oral absorption maybe variable. Metabolised in liver, excreted in urine, half-life 1½ hr, highly bound to plasma proteins

Interactions/incompatibilities:

• Increased toxicity: antineoplastics, radiation, cyclosporin. Avoid concurrent use of nalidixic acid

• Unstable in IV infusion fluids but may be given in sodium chloride 0.9%, at room temperature within 2 hr of reconstitution. Do not use dextrose

Clinical assessment:

• Full blood count, differential, platelet count weekly; withhold drug if WBC is less than 2000/mm^3 or platelet count is less than 75,000/mm^3. Other institutions may have own guidelines

• Renal function studies: blood urea nitrogen, serum uric acid, urine creatinine clearance before, during therapy

• Liver function tests before, during therapy (bilirubin, aspartate aminotransferase, alanine aminotransferase, lactic dehydrogenase) as needed or monthly

Treatment of overdose: Supportive; monitor blood counts, give infusion products, filgrastin as appropriate

NURSING CONSIDERATIONS

Assess:

• Baseline vital signs including fluid balance

Administer:

• HANDLING: take safety precautions appropriate to antineoplastic agents

• Following local antineoplastic (cytotoxic) policies

• After ensuring that clinician is aware of blood results

• Regional perfusion for malignant melanoma and soft tissue sarcoma

• IV: by infusion over 2 hours; by injection into tubing of fast-running infusion
• Using sodium chloride 0.9% for dilution or infusion. Dextrose solutions must not be used
• By mouth; tablets should be swallowed whole
• Other medications by mouth if possible. Avoid IV, IM, SC routes to prevent infection and bruising
• Anti-emetic 30–60 min before treatment
• All other medication as prescribed including analgesics, antibiotics, anti-emetics, antispasmodics

Perform/provide:
• Strict medical asepsis, protective isolation if WBC levels are low
• Strict fluid balance chart
• Increase fluid intake to 2–3 litres a day to prevent urate deposits, calculi formation
• Rinsing of mouth 3 or 4 times a day with water and prescribed mouthwashes to prevent ulceration and infection; brushing of teeth 2 or 3 times a day with soft brush or cotton tipped applicators for stomatitis; use unwaxed dental floss
• Warm compresses at injection site for inflammation, if indicated

Evaluate:
• Fluid balance; report fall in urine output of 30 ml/hr
• Bleeding: haematuria, bruising, petechiae due to thrombocytopenia mucosa or orifices 8 hrly
• IV site for extravasation and pain; if leakage stop infusion
• Food preferences; list likes, dislikes
• Yellowing of skin, sclera, dark urine, clay-coloured stools, itchy skin, abdominal pain, fever, diarrhoea
• Inflammation of mucosa, breaks in skin
• Buccal cavity 8 hrly for dryness, due to stomatitis and potential fungal infections, sores, ulceration, white patches, oral pain, bleeding, dysphagia
• Symptoms indicating severe allergic reaction: rash, pruritus, urticaria, purpuric skin lesions, itching, flushing

Teach patient/family:
• Of protective isolation precautions due to neutropenia
• To report any complaints or side effects to nurse or clinician
• That sterility, amenorrhoea can occur; reversible after discontinuing treatment
• That hair may be lost during treatment; a wig or hairpiece is available on NHS prescription; new hair may be different in colour, texture
• Good mouthcare and to report any bleeding, white spots, or ulcerations in mouth to clinician; tell patient to examine mouth daily

meningococcal vaccine BP (groups A & C polysaccharides)

AC VAX, Mengivac (A + C)
Func. class.: Vaccine
Legal class.: POM

Action: Active immunisation
Uses: Immunisation against meningococcal meningitis caused by group A and group C meningococci
Dosage and routes:
• *Adults and children aged 2 months and over:* Deep subcutaneous injection 0.5 ml of reconstituted vaccine
Available forms include: Subcutaneous injection 50 mcg of group A polysaccharide and 50 mcg of group C polysaccharide in 0.5 ml
Side effects/adverse reactions:

INTEG: Erythema, slight induration and tenderness or pain at the site of injection
CNS: Febrile reactions, chills
Contraindications: Hypersensitivity, febrile conditions
Precautions: If administered to patients on immunosuppressive therapy, the vaccine may not induce an effective response. It should not be given in pregnancy unless there is a definite risk from groups A and C meningococcal disease. The Menigivac brand is not recommended in children under 18 months (except in an epidemic) because of an alleged transient response to serogroup C and increased incidence of side effects

NURSING CONSIDERATIONS

Assess:
• Infection; vaccination must be delayed if acute infection

Administer:
• The vaccine must not be given intravenously under any circumstances
• The vaccine should be reconstituted with the diluent supplied by adding the entire contents of the diluent vial to the vaccine vial. As with all vaccinations a solution of 1:1000 adrenaline should be available for injection should an anaphylactic reaction occur; additionally follow local protocols

Perform/provide:
• Store between 2°C and 8°C. The reconstituted vaccine should be used immediately, and certainly within 1 hr

Teach patient/family:
• That low grade fever, irritability and fatigue may occasionally occur in the first 72 hr following vaccination

menotrophin

Pergonal, Humegon
Func. class.: Gonadotrophin
Chem. class.: Human follicle stimulating hormone (FSH); human luteinising hormone (LH)
Legal class.: POM

Action: In women increases follicular growth, maturation; in men, when given with HCG, stimulates spermatogenesis
Uses: Infertility in amenorrhoeic anovulatory women, women undergoing *in vitro* fertilisation, hypogonadotrophic hypogonadism in men
Dosage and routes:
Amenorrhoeic anovulatory women
• By IM injection, either a total of 3–5 ampoules given as 3 equal doses on alternate days, followed by up to 10,000 units of HCG 1 week after first injection or; by IM injection 1–2 ampoules each day, followed by up to 10,000 units HCG 24–48 hr after last injection. Both regimens should be adjusted at weekly intervals to gain best response
In vitro fertilisation and associated techniques
• 100 mg of clomiphene by mouth on days 2–6 followed by IM injection of 2–3 ampoules of menotrophin starting on day 5. Adjust dose according to response. A dose of up to 10,000 units of HCG is administered 24–48 hr after the last menotrophin injection or; by IM injection 2–3 ampoules of menotrophin daily from day 2–3 of cycle. Adjust dose according to response. A dose of up to 10,000 HCH is administered 24–48 hr after the last menotrophin injection
Hypogonadotrophic hypogonadism in men
• By IM injection 1 ampoule 3

times a week, with 2000 units HCG twice a week for at least 4 months
Available forms include: Powder for injection 75 units FSH/75 units LH, 150 units FSH/150 units LH
Side effects/adverse reactions:
CNS: Fever
CV: Hypovolaemia
GI: Nausea, vomiting, diarrhoea, abdominal pain and distension
GU: Ovarian enlargement, ovarian hyperstimulation, multiple births, ascites, pleural effusion
INTEG: Joint pain
Contraindications: Hypothyroidism, adrenal deficiency, hyperprolactinaemia, pituitary tumour unless these conditions have been treated. Ovarian dysgenesis, absent uterus, premature menopause
Treatment of overdose: The acute toxicity of menotrophin has been shown to be very low. However, too high a dosage for more than one day may lead to hyperstimulation of the ovaries

NURSING CONSIDERATIONS

Assess:
- Weight on alternate days

Administer:
- After reconstituting with 1–2 ml sterile saline injection; use immediately

Evaluate:
- Rapid weight gain
- Ovarian enlargement, abdominal distention/pain; report symptoms immediately

Teach patient/family:
- That multiple births are possible, pregnancy usually occurs in 4–6 weeks after start of treatment
- To keep appointment during treatment every other day for 2 weeks
- That daily intercourse is necessary from day preceding administration of gonadotrophin until ovulation occurs

meptazinol

Meptid
Func. class.: Narcotic analgesic
Chem. class.: Partial opiod agonist
Legal class.: POM

Action: Acts on opiod receptors in CNS, stimulation of mu or kappa receptors produces analgesic effects
Uses: Moderate to severe pain, including postoperative pain, obstetric pain, renal colic
Dosage and routes:
- *Adults:* By mouth, 200 mg 3–6 hrly; IM injection, 75–100 mg 2–4 hrly, but for obstetric analgesia, 100–150 mg (approximately 2 mg/kg) 2–4 hrly
- Slow IV injection, 50–100 mg 2–4 hrly

Available forms include: Tablets, 200 mg; injection, 100 mg (as hydrochloride)/ml
Side effects/adverse reactions:
CNS: Drowsiness, alteration of pupillary responses, dizziness, headache
GI: Nausea, vertigo, vomiting, dyspepsia, abdominal pain, diarrhoea
GU: Diarrhoea
INTEG: Pain and tissue at injection site, sweating
SYST: Tolerance, dependence
Contraindications: Hypersensitivity
Precautions: Myocardial infarction, pregnancy (other than labour), severe respiratory depression, asthma, hepatic or renal impairment, head injury, elevated intracranial pressure
Pharmacokinetics: Onset within 15 min, duration of action 2 to 7 hr. Tablets subject to first pass hepatic metabolism and metabolites are excreted in the urine.
Interactions/incompatibilities:
- Delays absorption of: mexiletine

may potentiate other CNS depressants
• Injection, should not be mixed with other drugs in the same syringe or infusion

Treatment of overdose:
• Resuscitate if necessary
• Gastric lavage if taken orally
• Naloxone if respiratory depression is evident
• Supportive therapy

NURSING CONSIDERATIONS

Assess:
• Pain and appropriate analgesia

Administer:
• An anti-emetic if vomiting occurs
• Do not mix injection in same syringe as other drugs
• If given intravenously, flush system with saline before and after administration

Evaluate:
• For side effects – nausea, vomiting, diarrhoea, constipation, sweating, abdominal pain, dyspepsia, rash, drowsiness
• For withdrawal symptoms when drug is stopped
• Therapeutic effect – diminished pain

Teach patient/family:
• Dizziness may occur so avoid any task requiring alertness (e.g. driving) until sure they are not affected
• Check with clinician before taking any other drugs

mercaptopurine (6-MP)

Puri-Nethol
Func. class.: Antineoplastic, antimetabolite
Chem. class.: Purine analogue
Legal class.: POM

Action: Inhibits purine metabolism by blocking inosinic acid conversion to adenine, which is responsible for DNA, RNA synthesis

Uses: Chronic granulocytic leukaemia, acute lymphoblastic leukaemia, acute myelogenous leukaemia

Dosage and routes:
Doses are highly variable, and dependent on local treatment protocols, concomitant therapy and tumour type; the following dose schedules have been used
• *Adult and child:* By mouth 2.5 mg/kg daily. Adjusted to the needs of the individual patient. Reduce dose if renal or hepatic function is reduced

Available forms include: Tablets 50 mg

Side effects/adverse reactions:
CNS: Fever, headache, weakness
HAEM: Thrombocytopenia, leucopenia, myelosuppression, anaemia
GI: Nausea, vomiting, anorexia, oral ulceration, hepatotoxicity (with high doses), jaundice
GU: Renal failure, hyperuricaemia, hyperuricosuria
INTEG: Rash

Precautions: Patients with prior drug resistance, leucopenia, thrombocytopenia, anaemia, pregnancy. Renal or hepatic disease

Pharmacokinetics: Incompletely absorbed when taken orally, metabolised in liver, excreted in urine

Interactions/incompatibilities:
• Increased toxicity: radiation or other antineoplastics
• Potentiated by: allopurinol (quarter mercaptopurine dose)
• Effects of warfarin reduced by mercaptopurine

Clinical assessment:
• Full blood count, differential, platelet count weekly; withhold drug if WBC is less than 3500 or platelet count is less than 100,000; drug should be discontinued
• Renal function studies: blood urea nitrogen, serum uric acid,

urine creatinine clearance, electrolytes before, during therapy
• Liver function tests before, during therapy: bilirubin, alkaline phosphatase, aspartate aminotransferase, alanine aminotransferase, weekly during beginning therapy

Treatment of overdose: Supportive measures and blood transfusion if required

NURSING CONSIDERATIONS

Administer:
• HANDLING: take safety precautions appropriate to antineoplastic agents
• Following local antineoplastic (cytotoxic) policies
• After ensuring that clinician is aware of blood results
• By mouth; tablets should not be crushed. Avoid inhaling/ingesting dust when breaking tablets. Give after evening meal but before bedtime and preceded by antacid
• Other medications by mouth if possible. Avoid IV, IM, SC routes to prevent infection and bruising
• Anti-emetic 30–60 min before treatment
• All other medication as prescribed including analgesics, antibiotics, anti-emetics, antispasmodics

Perform/provide:
• Increase fluid intake to 2–3 litres daily to prevent urate deposits, calculi formation, unless contraindicated
• Observe for signs of stomatitis and encourage oral hygiene four times a day

Evaluate:
• Monitor temperature 4 hrly, when indicated; fever may indicate beginning infection
• Effects of alopecia on body image; discuss feelings about body changes
• Inflammation of mucosa, breaks in skin
• Buccal cavity 8 hrly for dryness, sores, ulceration, white patches, oral pain, bleeding, dysphagia
• Symptoms indicating severe allergic reaction: rash, urticaria, itching, flushing

Teach patient/family:
• To report any complaints, side effects to nurse or clinician
• To avoid foods with citric acid, hot or rough texture if stomatitis is present
• To report stomatitis: any bleeding, white spots, ulcerations in mouth; tell patient to examine mouth daily, report symptoms
• Teach good oral hygiene
• Contraceptive measures are recommended during therapy
• To drink 10–12 glasses of fluid daily
• Notify clinician of fever, chills, sore throat, nausea, vomiting, anorexia, diarrhoea, bleeding, bruising, which may indicate blood dyscrasias

---

mesalazine

Asacol, Pentasa, Salofalk
Func. class.: Anti-inflammatory
Chem. class.: Aminosalicylate
Legal class.: POM

Action: May diminish inflammation by inhibiting prostaglandin production in colon

Uses: Maintenance or remission of ulcerative colitis

Dosage and routes:

Acute disease
• *Adult:* By mouth 2400 mg daily in divided doses
• Rectally 750–1500 mg daily in divided doses (last dose at bedtime) or a 1 g enema once daily at night

Maintenance
• *Adult:* By mouth 1200–2400 mg daily in divided doses

• Rectally 750–1500 mg daily in divided doses as above

Available forms include: Tablets 250 mg, 400 mg; enema 1 g/ 100 ml; suppositories 250 mg, 500 mg

Side effects/adverse reactions:

GI: Cramps, gas, nausea, diarrhoea, abdominal pain, pancreatitis, exacerbation of colitis, hepatitis

CNS: Headache

HAEM: Leucopenia, neutropenia, thrombocytopenia

GU: Nephritis, nephrotic syndrome, renal failure

Contraindications: Hypersensitivity to salicylates; severe renal impairment; (glomerular filtration rate less than 20 ml/min); children under 2 yr

Precautions: Renal disease, pregnancy, lactation, children, elderly

Pharmacokinetics:

Absorbed from colon; excreted rapidly by the kidney mainly as metabolite

NURSING CONSIDERATIONS

Administer:

• Swallow tablets whole

• Do not take indigestion medicines with enteric coated tablets

Evaluate:

• Response to treatment: absence of pain, bleeding from the gastrointestinal tract and decrease in diarrhoea

• Signs of gastrointestinal irritation indicated by cramp, flatulence, nausea, diarrhoea, rectal discomfort. If severe the drug must be discontinued

Teach patient/family:

• To inform clinician of gastrointestinal symptoms

• Advice on diet

mesna

Uromitexan

Func. class.: Urothelial antitoxicity agent

Chem. class.: Sulphydryl containing compound

Legal class.: POM

Action: Reacts with acrolein (metabolite of cyclophosphamide and ifosamide) in urinary tract to reduce urothelial toxicity

Uses: In conjunction with cyclophosphamide or ifosfamide to prevent urothelial toxicity

Dosage and routes:

• When cytotoxic given as IV bolus: 20% of cytotoxic dose w/w given simultaneously over 15–30 min then repeat after 4 and 8 hr. Dose can be increased to 4 doses of 40% w/w of cytotoxic dose given at 3 hrly intervals (larger dose recommended in children, previous urothelial toxicity, pelvic irradiation)

• When ifosfamide is given as 24 hr infusion, give an initial 20% w/w of cytotoxic dose as an IV bolus then 100% w/w of cytotoxic dose over 24 hr, then a further 60% w/w of cytotoxic dose over 12 hr (or for the last 12 hr, 3 doses of 20% w/w of cytotoxic dose given at 28, 32 and 36 hr)

• By mouth, 40% w/w of cytotoxic dose is given with the infusion or as it stops and repeated after 4 and 8 hr

Available forms include: Injection 100 mg/ml, 4 ml, 10 ml ampoules

Side effects/adverse reactions:

(Difficult to distinguish from cytotoxic therapy)

CNS: Headache, depression, irritability

GI: Nausea, vomiting, colic, diarrhoea

SYST: Fatigue, limb pains
INTEG: Rash
Contraindications: None known
Pharmacokinetics: Excreted in urine, inactivates toxic metabolite of cyclophosphamide or ifosfamide
Clinical assessment:
• Full blood count, differential, platelet count weekly
• Renal function tests, blood urea, electrolytes
Lab. test interferences: Mesna causes a false positive for urinary ketones test, producing a red-violet colour which fades rapidly on addition of glacial acetic acid

NURSING CONSIDERATIONS

Administer:
• Orally, drug should be taken immediately the ampoule is opened, in a soft drink (orange juice)
• Anti-emetic 30–60 mins before drug
• Slow IV infusion using appropriate size needle
Perform/provide:
• Reconstituted solution should be destroyed after 24 hr
• Plenty of fluids in diet—fluid intake 2–3 litres daily
• Frequent mouthwashes
Evaluate:
• Fluid balance, test urine for blood and protein. Report fall in urine output below 30 ml/hr
• Raised temperature; may indicate infection
• For any bleeding, haematuria; report to clinician
• For oedema in feet, joint pain, abdominal pain
• For all side effects
Teach patient/family:
• Of protective isolation precaution
• To report any complaints of side effects
• To report any bleeding
• To report any urinary symptoms

mesterolone

Pro-Viron
Func. class.: Male sex hormone
Chem. class.: Synthetic androgen
Legal class.: POM

Action: Supplements endogenous androgen production
Uses: Androgen deficiency, male infertility
Dosage and routes:
Androgen deficiency
• By mouth 25 mg 3–4 times daily for several months; maintenance dose 50–75 mg daily in divided doses
Male infertility
• 100 mg daily for several months
Available forms include: Tablets 25 mg
Side effects/adverse reactions:
GU: Prostatism in elderly, priapism
META: Oedema, weight gain
GI: Benign and in rare cases malignant liver tumours leading to isolated cases of life threatening intra-abdominal haemorrhage
Contraindications: Prostatic carcinoma, previous or existing liver tumours, breast cancer in men, hypercalcaemia, nephrosis
Clinical assessment:
• Liver function tests, aspartate aminotransferase, alanine aminotransferase, bilirubin
Treatment of overdose: There have been no reports of ill effects from overdosage and treatment is generally unnecessary

NURSING CONSIDERATIONS

Assess:
• Baseline weight and BP
Perform/provide:
• Diet with increased protein; decrease salt if oedema occurs
• Regular examination of prostate during treatment
Evaluate:

• Regular examination of the prostate during treatment is advised.
• Weight gain; notify clinician if gain is greater than 2.5 kg
• For oedema and hypertension
• Mental status—behavioural pattern
• For signs of impotence, testicular atrophy in males
• For symptoms of hypoglycaemia, lethargy, GI upsets
• Therapeutic response; may take several months

Teach patient/family:
• Drug needs to be combined with good diet, rest and exercise
• To notify clinician if therapeutic response decreases
• Teach patient all aspects of drug, including change in sex characteristics

---

metaraminol tartrate

Aramine
Func. class.: Adrenergic agonist
Chem. class.: Substituted β-phenylethylamine, sympathomimetic
Legal class.: POM

Action: Both direct and indirect effects on sympathetic nerve terminals; inhibits GI, smooth muscle and vascular smooth muscle supplying skeletal muscle; cardiac excitatory effects; increases heart rate and force of heart muscle contraction
Uses: Acute hypotension
Dosage and routes:
Hypotension
• *Adult:* IV Infusion: 15–100 mg in 500 ml Dextrose 5% or sodium chloride 0.9%. Adjust rate according to response every 10 min
Grave emergency
• *Adult:* IV bolus 0.5–5 mg, then IV infusion of 15–100 mg/500 ml solution, adjusting dose every 10 min
Available forms include: Injection IV, 10 mg/ml
Side effects/adverse reactions:
CV: Palpitations, sinus or ventricular tachycardia, hypotension, ectopic beats, angina, circulatory collapse
INTEG: Necrosis, tissue sloughing with extravasation, abscess
RESP: Respiratory collapse, pulmonary oedema
Contraindications: Hypersensitivity, myocardial infarction, pregnancy
Precautions: Pregnancy, lactation, cardiac disease, history of malaria, treatment with digoxin, arterial embolism, peripheral vascular disease, hypertension, thyroid disease, diabetes mellitus, cirrhosis, concurrent use with cyclopropane or halothane anaesthesia
Pharmacokinetics:
IV: Onset 1–2 min duration 20 min–1 hr
Interactions/incompatibilities:
• Dysrhythmias: general anaesthetics
• Decreased action of this drug: other β-blockers
• Increased BP: oxytocics
• Increased pressor effect: tricyclic antidepressant, MAOIs
• Incompatible with alkaline solutions: sodium bicarbonate
• Concurrent use with cyclopropane or halothone unless clinical circumstance demands
Treatment of overdose: Administer an α-blocker, then noradrenaline for severe hypotension

NURSING CONSIDERATIONS

Assess:
• Baseline vital signs
• Fluid balance

Administer:
• Parenteral IV dose slowly, after diluting with 500 ml of dextrose 5% or 0.9% sodium chloride

• Plasma expanders for hypovolaemia if ordered

Perform/provide:

• Keep drug refrigerated
• Do not use discoloured solutions
• Continuous monitoring of vital signs (preferably with patient in ICU)

Evaluate:

• ECG during administration continuously, if BP increases, drug is decreased
• BP and pulse every 5 min after parenteral route
• CVP during infusion if possible
• For paraesthesia and coldness of extremities, peripheral blood flow may decrease
• Injection site for tissue sloughing
• Therapeutic response: increased BP with stabilisation

Teach patient/family:

• Reason for drug administration

metformin HCl

Glucophage, Orabet
Func. class.: Oral hypoglycaemic agent
Chem. class.: Biguanide
Legal class.: POM

Action: Uptake of glucose from gastrointestinal tract delayed; increases peripheral utilization of glucose; decreases gluconeogenesis

Uses: Non-insulin dependent diabetes; as an adjuvant in insulin dependent diabetic patients who are poorly controlled

Dosage and routes:

• By mouth 500 mg 8-hrly or 850 mg 12-hrly with or after food; maximum dose 3 g daily in divided doses

Available forms include: Tablets 500, 850 mg

Side effects/adverse reactions:

GI: Anorexia, nausea, vomiting, decreased absorption of vitamin B_{12}, diarrhoea
METAB: Lactic acidosis

Contraindications: Lactic acidosis or conditions associated with lactic acidosis such as hypoxaemia, pulmonary insufficiency, alcoholism; renal or hepatic impairment; cardiac failure or recent myocardial infarction; severe infection or trauma, dehydration, pregnancy; breast-feeding; children, hypersensitivity, diabetic coma and ketoacidosis

Pharmacokinetics: Control may be achieved after several days but full effects may not be seen for up to 2 weeks. Excreted unchanged in urine

Interactions/incompatibilities:

• Enhanced hypoglycaemic effect: alcohol, β-blockers, MAOIs, bezafibrate, clofibrate, cimetidine, lithium
• Antagonise hypoglycaemic effect: diazoxide, corticosteroids, diuretics, oral contraceptives

Clinical assessment:

• Monitor for hyperglycaemia or hypoglycaemia
• Monitor renal function, estimate B_{12} levels annually.

Treatment of overdose: Supportive measures with particular attention to correct metabolic disturbances and fluid loss

NURSING CONSIDERATIONS

Administer:

• With or after food

Evaluate:

• For signs of hyperglycaemic reaction
• Therapeutic response; decrease in polyuria, polydipsia, polyphagia

Teach patient/family:

• To check blood sugar regularly whilst taking the drug OR
• To check urine for sugar
• The symptoms of hyperglycaemia and how to respond to this

• That the drug should be taken regularly as prescribed
• To avoid non-prescribed medications unless approved by a clinician
• That diabetes is a life-long illness and that drug will not cure disease
• To carry a Medic Alert card for emergency purposes

methadone HCl

Physeptone
Func. class.: Narcotic analgesic
Chem. class.: Synthetic opioid
Legal class.: CD (Sch 2) POM

Action: Inhibits ascending pain pathways in CNS, increases pain threshold, alters pain perception
Uses: Severe pain, narcotic withdrawal
Dosage and routes:
Pain
• *Adult:* By mouth, subcutaneous, IM, 5–10 mg 6–8 hrly and adjusted depending on response
Narcotic withdrawal
• *Adult:* By mouth doses in range 15–20 mg (higher in some patients to 40 mg) daily and reduce gradually
Available forms include: Injection subcutaneous, IM 10 mg/ml; tablets 5 mg; linctus 2 mg/5 ml; mixture 1 mg/ml
Side effects/adverse reactions:
CNS: Drowsiness, dizziness, euphoria, confusion, changes of mood, hallucinations
GI: Nausea, vomiting, constipation
GU: Difficulty with micturition, dysuria
INTEG: Urticaria, pruritus, flushing
EENT: Miosis
CV: Hypotension, bradycardia, palpitations
RESP: Respiratory depression
Contraindications: Hypersensitivity, respiratory depression, obstructive airways disease, obstetric use, concurrent administration with MAOIs or within 2 weeks of their discontinuation, raised intracranial pressure, head injuries
Precautions: Addiction, pregnancy, breast feeding, hepatic disease, asthma, obstructive bowel disorders, hypotension, hypothyroidism, myasthenia gravis; reduce dosage in renal impairment, elderly, debilitated
Pharmacokinetics:
By mouth: Onset 30–60 min, duration 6–8 hr
Subcutaneous/IM: Onset 10–20 min, peak 1 hr, duration 6–8 hr, cumulative 22–48 hr
Metabolised by liver, excreted by kidneys, excreted in breast milk, half-life 15–25 hr
Interactions/incompatibilities:
• Effects may be increased with other CNS depressants: alcohol, narcotics, sedative/hypnotics, antipsychotics, skeletal muscle relaxants
• Concurrent use of MAOIs
Treatment of overdose: Naloxone IV repeated every 5–10 min; elimination rate by kidney increased by acidification of urine.
N.B: lavage, dialysis and CNS stimulation are contraindicated

NURSING CONSIDERATIONS

Assess:
• Pain levels
• Vital signs
Administer:
• With anti-emetic if nausea, vomiting occur
Perform/provide:
• Storage according to CD regulations and local procedures
• Assistance with mobility
Evaluate:

- Therapeutic response: decrease in pain
- Fluid balance check for decreasing output; may indicate urinary retention
- CNS changes: dizziness, drowsiness, hallucinations, euphoria, level of consciousness, pupil reaction
- Allergic reactions: rash, urticaria
- Respiratory dysfunction: respiratory depression, character, rate, rhythm; notify clinician if respirations are less than 12/min
- Need for pain medication, physical dependence

Teach patient/family:

- To report any symptoms of CNS changes, allergic reactions
- That physical dependency may result when used for extended periods of time
- Withdrawal symptoms may occur: nausea, vomiting, cramps, fever, faintness, anorexia
- To report increase in pain
- Abstain from narcotic drug abuse whilst undergoing methadone withdrawal regimen

methicillin sodium

Celbenin

Func. class.: Antibiotic, broad-spectrum

Chem. class.: Penicillinase resistant penicillin

Legal class.: POM

Action: Interferes with cell wall replication of susceptible organisms; osmotically unstable cell wall swells, bursts from osmotic pressure

Uses: Infections caused by β-lactamase producing staphylococci

Dosage and routes:

- *Adult:* IM or IV injection (over 3–4 min) 1 g 4–6 hrly; may also be given by IV infusion. Dosage may be increased in severe infections
- *Child under 2 yr:* Quarter adult dose; 2–10 yr half adult dose
- May be administered by other routes in conjunction with systemic therapy

Available forms include: Powder for injection 1 g

Side effects/adverse reactions:

HAEM: Bone marrow depression, leucopenia, agranulocytosis, anaemia, increased bleeding time, defective platelet function

GI: Upsets including diarrhoea and nausea, glossitis

MISC: Allergic reactions, anaphylatic shock

Contraindications: Penicillin hypersensitivity

Precautions: Pregnancy, lactation, history of allergy, renal impairment

Pharmacokinetics:

IM: Peak ½–1 hr, duration 4 hr

IV: Peak 15 min, duration 2 hr

Metabolised in liver, excreted in urine, bile, breast milk

Interactions/incompatibilities:

- Reduced excretion of methicillin: probenecid

Clinical assessment:

- Renal studies: urinalysis, protein, blood
- Culture and sensitivity before drug therapy; drug may be taken as soon as culture is taken
- Scratch test to assess allergy; usually done when penicillin is only drug of choice

Treatment of overdose: Symptomatic treatment in the unlikely event

NURSING CONSIDERATIONS

Assess:

- Bowel pattern
- Any patient with compromised renal system since drug is excreted

slowly in poor renal system function; toxicity may occur rapidly

Administer:

- If given IV, 1 g should be dissolved in 20 ml water for injections, and given over 3–4 min, or added to IV infusion
- Drug after culture and sensitivity has been completed

Perform/provide:

- Adequate fluid intake 2 litres daily during diarrhoea episodes

Evaluate:

- Therapeutic effectiveness: absence of fever, draining wounds
- Bowel pattern before, during treatment
- Fluid balance; report haematuria, oliguria since penicillin in high doses is nephrotoxic
- Monitor for skin rash and report if seen. Treatment should be stopped
- Respiratory status: rate, character, wheezing, tightness in chest
- Allergies before initiation of treatment, reaction of each medication; highlight allergies on Nursing Care Plan

Teach patient/family:

- Culture may be taken after completed course of medication
- To report sore throat, fever, fatigue; could indicate superimposed infection
- To wear or carry Medic Alert identify if allergic to penicillins
- To notify nurse or clinician of diarrhoea

---

methixene hydrochloride

Tremonil

Func. class.: Anticholinergic, antiparkinsonian agent

Chem. class.: Synthetic tertiary amine

Legal class.: POM

Action: Corrects central relative cholinergic excess thought to occur in parkinsonism as a result of dopamine deficiency

Uses: Parkinsonism, drug-induced extrapyramidal symptoms, senile tremor

Dosage and routes:

- By mouth 2.5 mg 3 times daily increased gradually; maintenance dose 15–60 mg daily in divided doses, 15–30 mg daily in divided doses for elderly

Available forms include: Tablets 5 mg

Side effects/adverse reactions:

CNS: Dizziness, nervousness, excitability, confusion, psychiatric disturbances

CV: Tachycardia

GU: Urinary retention

GI: Disturbances, dry mouth, constipation

EENT: Transient visual disturbances

Contraindications: Prostatic hypertrophy, urinary retention, narrow angle glaucoma, cardiac arrythmias, intestinal hypotonia, alcoholism, myasthenia gravis, intoxication with analgesics, hypnotics, psychotropics, alcohol, pyloric stenosis, paralytic ileus

Precautions: Hepatic or renal impairment, cardiovascular disease, initial autonomic disturbances, avoid sudden discontinuation of drug, drug liable to abuse

Pharmacokinetics: Absorbed from GI tract, excreted in urine partly unchanged and partly as isomeric sulphoxides or their metabolites

Interactions/incompatibilities:

- Increased antimuscarinic effects: drugs with antimuscarinic properties including disopyramide, anti-depressants, antihistamines, phenothiazines, amantadine, domperidone, metoclopramide

Treatment of overdose: Gastric lavage and supportive measures, giving fluids freely. Peripheral symptoms may be relieved by neostigmine

NURSING CONSIDERATIONS

Administer:

• With or after meals to prevent GI upsets

• At bedtime to avoid daytime drowsiness in patient with parkinsonism

Perform/provide:

• Frequent fluids, mouthwashes to relieve dry mouth

Evaluate:

• For extrapyramidial symptoms, shuffling gait, muscle rigidity, involuntary movements

• Fluid balance: retention commonly causes decreased urinary output

• For urinary hesitancy, retention

• For constipation—increase fluids, bulk, exercise

• For tolerance over long-term therapy—dose may need to be changed

• Mental status: affect, mood, CNS depression; if mental symptoms worsen during initial treatment, inform clinician

Teach patient/family:

• Not to discontinue drug abruptly

• To avoid driving or other hazardous activities; drowsiness may occur

• To avoid non-prescribed medications, alcohol, antihistamines, unless approved by clinician

---

methocarbamol

Robaxin 750, Robaxin Injectable, combination product

Func. class.: Skeletal muscle relaxant

Chem. class.: Carbamate derivative

Legal class.: POM

Action: CNS depressant; action may be from sedative effects; precise mechanism of action is unknown

Uses: Pain due to spasm in musculoskeletal conditions or trauma, tetanus management

Dosage and routes:

• *Adult:* By mouth 1.5 g 4 times daily but may be effective in reduced dosage, 750 mg 3 times daily

• *Elderly:* Half adult dose or less

• *Adult:* IV injection or infusion 1–3 g daily for maximum of 3 days (maximum dose 3 g/day)

• *Elderly:* Maximum dose 1.5 g/day

Available forms include: Tablets 750 mg; injection IV 1 g/10 ml

Side effects/adverse reactions:

CNS: Dizziness, drowsiness, tremor, lassitude, light-headedness, restlessness, anxiety, confusion, convulsions, vertigo, headache, syncope

GI: Nausea, vomiting, metallic taste

INTEG: Allergic rash, urticaria, flushing

EENT: Blurred vision

CV: Hypotension, bradycardia, angioedema

SYST: Anaphylaxis

Contraindications: Hypersensitivity, coma or pre-coma states; brain damage, epilepsy; myaesthenia gravis, use in children, pregnancy, breast-feeding, injection should be avoided in renal impairment

Precautions: Renal disease, hepatic disease. May cause drowsiness—warn patients not to drive or operate machinery until affects known

Pharmacokinetics:

By mouth: Onset ½ hr, peak 1–2 hr, half-life 1–2 hr, metabolised in liver, excreted in urine (unchanged)

Interactions/incompatibilities:

• Increased CNS depression: alcohol, barbiturates
• Potentiation of effects: anorectics, antimuscarinics, some psychotropic agents

Clinical assessment:
• Monitor response and side effects

Lab. test interferences:
False positive: possibly in test for raised 5-hydroxyindoleacetic acid

Treatment of overdose: Gastric lavage with supportive measures; continue for 24 hr

NURSING CONSIDERATIONS

Administer:
• IV: by slow injection, or infusion at maximum of 300 mg/min, 1 g to be diluted to no more than 250 ml with glucose 5% or sodium chloride 0.9%
• By mouth with meals for GI symptoms

Evaluate:
• Therapeutic response: decreased pain, spasticity (short-term acting drug)
• Allergic reactions: rash, fever, respiratory distress
• Severe weakness, numbness in extremities
• Psychological dependency: increased need for medication, more frequent requests for medication, increased pain
• CNS depression: dizziness, drowsiness, psychiatric symptoms

Teach patient/family:
• Not to discontinue medication quickly; insomnia, nausea, headache, spasticity, tachycardia will occur; drug should be tapered off over 1–2 weeks
• Not to take with alcohol, other CNS depressants
• To avoid changes to lifestyle whilst taking this drug
• To avoid hazardous activities if drowsiness, dizziness occurs; avoid driving operating machinery
• To avoid using non-prescribed drugs: cough preparations, antihistamines, unless directed by clinician

---

methohexitone sodium

Brietal Sodium
Func. class.: Anaesthetic, general
Chem. class.: Barbiturate
Legal class.: POM

Action: Acts in reticular-activating system to produce anaesthesia

Uses: Rapid very short acting anaesthetic agent for induction and maintenance of anaesthesia in short procedures, used with other agents for more prolonged anaesthesia

Dosage and routes:

Induction
• *Adult:* IV 1% solution, 50–120 mg given at a rate of 10 mg in 5 seconds according to response
• *Child:* 1 mg/kg

Maintenance
• *IV:* 20–40 mg every 4–7 min of a 1% solution

Available forms include: Injection IV 100, 500 mg powder for reconstitution

Side effects/adverse reactions:
RESP: Transitory apnoea, respiratory depression, respiratory arrest, bronchospasm, sneezing, cough
CNS: Headache, persistent drowsiness
CV: Circulatory depression, cardiac arrest, hypotension, tachycardia
GI: Salivation, nausea, hiccup
INTEG: Shivering, thrombophlebitis, pain at injection site
MS: Skeletal muscle hyperactivity
MISC: Acute allergic reactions

Contraindications: Hypersensitivity to barbiturates, porphyria, epilepsy, status asthmaticus

Precautions: Cardiovascular disease, renal disease, liver disease, impaired respiratory function, impaired endocrine function, debilitated patients. Pregnancy, lactation, labour and delivery, severe anaemia, extreme obesity

Pharmacokinetics:

IV: Onset 30–40 sec; half-life 11.5 hr

Interactions/incompatibilities:

• Increased action: CNS depressants

• Decreased action: coumarin anticoagulants, endogenous steroids

• Increased occurrence of abnormal muscle movements: cyclizine, some phenothiazines

• Not to be mixed with acid solutions including: atropine sulphate, tubocurarine, succinylcholine

• Do not mix with solutions containing bacteriostats

• Do not allow contact with silicon treated components of syringes, etc.

Clinical assessment:

• Monitor and report level of anaesthesia during post-operative period

Treatment of overdose: Life-support measures as required

NURSING CONSIDERATIONS

Assess:

• Baseline vital signs

• Level of orientation before administration

Administer:

• Slowly, after preparation with sodium chloride solution of 0.9% or 5% dextrose as a 1% solution of methohexitone

• With resuscitative equipment nearby

• IV slowly only under direction of anaesthetist

Evaluate:

• Extravasation, if it occurs use nitroprusside or chloroprocaine to decrease pain, increase circulation

• Dysrhythmias or myocardial depression

• Level of respiratory excitability immediately after administration

• Vital signs for dysrhythmias, myocardial depression or hypotension

methotrexate

Methotrexate (Lederle), Maxtrex

Func. class.: Antineoplastic antimetabolite

Chem. class.: Folic acid antagonist

Legal class.: POM

Action: Inhibits dihydrofolate reductase that reduces folic acid, which is needed for nucleic acid synthesis in reproducing cells

Uses: Choriocarcinoma and other trophoblastic tumours, childhood acute lymphoblastic leukaemia, meningeal leukaemia in children, non-Hodgkin's lymphoma, breast cancer, osteogenic sarcoma, bronchogenic sarcoma, head and neck cancer, bladder carcinoma, psoriasis

Dosage and route:

Cancer chemotherapy

Doses are highly variable, and dependent on local treatment protocols, concomitant therapy and tumour type

Psoriasis

• *Adult:* By mouth 10–25 mg weekly

Available forms include: Tablets 2.5 mg, 10 mg; injection (as sodium salt) 2.5 mg/ml, 25 mg/ml, 100 mg/ml

Side effects/adverse reactions:

HAEM: Bone marrow depression, leucopenia, thrombocytopenia, anaemia

GI: Nausea, vomiting, diarrhoea, ulcerative stomatitis, hepatic cirrhosis, acute liver atrophy, intestinal perforation, haemorrhagic enteritis

GU: Renal failure, severe nephropathy, suppression of ovarian and testicular function
INTEG: Rash, alopecia, photosensitivity, vasculitis, ulceration
EENT: Blurred vision
CNS: Headache, drowsiness, ataxia, transient paresis, dementia, major convulsions

Contraindications: Serious Leucopenia, thrombocytopenia, anaemia, severe renal or hepatic impairment, pregnancy, breast-feeding, porphyria

Precautions: Lactation, haematological depression, renal impairment, ulceration of gastrointestinal tract, diarrhoea, debility, very young elderly.

Pharmacokinetics:
By mouth: Readily absorbed when taken orally, peak 1–4 hr
IV/IM: Peak ½–2 hr
Not metabolised, excreted in urine (unchanged), crosses blood-brain barrier, 50% plasma protein bound

Interactions/incompatibilities:
• Increased toxicity: aspirin and other salicylates, sulphonamides, diuretics, hypoglycaemic agents, diphenylhydantoin, chloramphenicol, tetracyclines, NSAIDs, cotrimoxazole, trimethoprim, phenytoin, tetretinate, probenecid
• Concurrent administration of: live vaccines
• Decreased effects of this drug: folic acid supplements

Clinical assessment:
• Full blood count prior to treatment and 10 days post treatment. Do not give next dose whilst patient neutropenic
• Renal function studies before/during treatment when impairment suspected or high dose therapy being given
• Liver function tests before and during therapy if severe impairment anticipated; liver biopsy should be done before start of therapy (psoriasis patients)
• Sodium bicarbonate to maintain urine pH above 7 during excretion phase after medium-high dose (greater than 100 mg/m^2 approximately) therapy

Treatment of overdose: IM, IV or orally calcium leucovorin at a dose equal or higher than overdose and administered within 1 hr, further doses if required
Supporting therapy of blood transfusion and renal dialysis if necessary

NURSING CONSIDERATIONS

Assess:
• Baseline vital signs

Administer:
• HANDLING: take safety precautions appropriate to antineoplastic agents
• Following local antineoplastic (cytotoxic) policies
• After ensuring that clinician is aware of blood results
• May be given IV, or as a prolonged IV infusion, or IM, or by mouth; also intra-arterially, or as intrathecal or intraventricular injection. Reconstituted and diluted solutions stable for 24 hours
• Should not be mixed with other IV drugs
• Antacid before oral agent; give tablets with food at the end of evening meal and before bedtime
• Anti-emetic 30–60 min before treatment
• Other medications by mouth if possible. Avoid IV, IM, SC routes to prevent infection and bruising
• All other medication as prescribed including analgesics, antibiotics, anti-emetics, antispasmodics

Perform/provide:
• Strict medical asepsis and protective isolation if WBC levels are low
• Liquid diet: carbonated beverage, dry toast, plain biscuits may

be added when patient is not nauseated or vomiting
• Increased fluid intake to 2–3 litres daily to prevent urate deposits, calculi formation, unless contraindicated
• Diet low in purines: avoid offal meats (kidney, liver), dried beans, peas to maintain alkaline urine
• Rinsing of mouth 3 or 4 times a day with water, hydrogen peroxide; brushing of teeth 2 or 3 times a day with soft brush or cotton-tipped applicators for stomatitis; use unwaxed dental floss
• Nutritious diet with iron, vitamin supplements

Evaluate:
• Fluid balance; report fall in urine output to less than 30 ml/hr
• Bleeding: haematuria, bruising or petechiae, mucosa or orifices 8 hrly
• Food preferences; list likes, dislikes
• Effects of alopecia on body image; discuss feelings about body changes
• Hepatotoxicity: yellowing of skin, sclera, dark urine, clay-coloured stools, pruritus, abdominal pain, fever, diarrhoea
• Buccal cavity 8 hrly for dryness, sores, ulceration, white patches, oral pain, bleeding, dysphagia
• Symptoms indicating severe allergic reaction: rash, urticaria, itching, flushing

Teach patient/family:
• Why protective isolation precautions are needed
• To report any complaints, side effects to nurse or clinician: black tarry stools, chills, fever, sore throat, bleeding, bruising, cough, shortness of breath, dark or bloody urine
• That hair may be lost during treatment and wig or hairpiece is available on NHS prescription; tell patient that new hair may be different in colour, texture (alopecia is rare)
• To avoid foods with citric acid, hot or rough texture if stomatitis is present
• To report stomatitis: any bleeding, white spots, ulcerations in mouth; tell patient to examine mouth daily, report symptoms to nurse
• Contraceptive measures are recommended during therapy for at least 8 weeks following cessation of therapy
• To drink 10–12 glasses of fluid daily
• To avoid alcohol, salicylates
• Importance of regular blood tests

---

methotrimeprazine

Nozinan
Func. class.: Sedative anti-emetic
Chem. class.: Aliphatic propylamine-phenothiazine derivative
Legal class.: POM

Action: Depresses cerebral cortex, hypothalamus, limbic system; blocks neurotransmission produced by dopamine at synapse; exhibits strong α-adrenergic, anticholinergic blocking action

Uses: Terminal care-severe pain (with restlessness, distress, or vomiting), sedation, schizophrenia

Dosage and routes:

Terminal illness
• *Adult:* By mouth 12.5–50 mg orally 4–8 hrly; IM injection 12.5–25 mg; IV injection 12.5–25 mg (after dilution with equal volume of sodium chloride 0.9%) every 6–8 hr (severe agitation up to 50 mg); continuous subcutaneous infusion 25–200 mg daily diluted with sodium chloride 0.9% via a syringe driver

Schizophrenia
• *Adult:* By mouth (Ambulant) 25–50 mg daily orally in 3 divided doses and increased as necessary. Bed-patients 100–200 mg daily orally in 3 divided doses increased as necessary to 1 g daily
Available forms include: Injection (hydrochloride) 25 mg/ml, tablets (maleate) 25 mg
Side effects/adverse reactions:
HAEM: Agranulocytosis, leucopenia, haemolytic anaemia, jaundice
CNS: Weakness, drowsiness, apathy, nightmares, insomnia, depression, agitation, extrapyramidal symptoms
GI: Dry mouth, constipation
INTEG: Sensitisation, rashes
EENT: Nasal congestion, blurred vision
CV: Hypotension, tachycardia, arrhythmias, ECG changes
Contraindications: Hypersensitivity, pregnancy (safety not established), coma caused by CNS depressants, bone-marrow depression, phaeochromocytoma
Precautions: Postural hypotension (especially patients over 50 and elderly), children (maximum daily dose 40 mg, average for 10 yr old 15–20 mg daily), cardiac, renal and hepatic disease
Pharmacokinetics:
By mouth: Onset 20–30 min, peak 1–2 hr, duration 4 hr; metabolised by liver, excreted by kidneys and in faeces, excreted in breast milk
Interactions/incompatibilities:
• Increased sedation: alcohol, anxiolytics, hypnotics
• Enhanced hypotensive effect: anaesthetics, antihypertensives, calcium-channel blockers
• Avoid simultaneous administration of prochlorperazine and desferrioxamine
Treatment of overdose: Gastric lavage if within 6 hr, give activated charcoal, supportive care. See data sheet for further information
NURSING CONSIDERATIONS
Assess:
• Baseline vital signs
Administer:
• IV injection and subcutaneous infusion as indication under dosage and routes, above
Perform/provide:
• Bedrest for several hours after injection if orthostatic hypotension occurs
• Safety measure: siderails, nightlight, callbell within easy reach
• Assistance with ambulation for 6 hr after injection
Evaluate:
• Decreasing BP with increased pulse that may occur 10–30 min after injection
• Effect on uterine contractions, foetal heart tones if using for labour
• Therapeutic response: decrease in pain, grimacing, absence of change in vital signs, ability to cough and breathe deeply after surgery
• For extra-pyramidal signs
Teach patient/family:
• Drug may impair mental alertness or physical co-ordination, warn patients against driving or operating machinery if affected

---

methoxamine hydrochloride

Vasoxine
Func. class.: Adrenergic agonist
Chem. class.: Sympathomimetic amine
Legal class.: POM

Action: Constricts peripheral blood vessels causing transient rise in BP

Uses: Hypotension in anaesthesia
Dosage and routes:
• *Adults:* IM injection 5–20 mg, slow IV injection 5–10 mg at rate of 1 mg/min
• *Child:* IM injection 250 mcg/kg body weight, IV injection 80 mcg/kg body weight
Available forms include: Injection 20 mg/ml, 1 ml ampoule
Side effects/adverse reactions:
CV: Hypertension, bradycardia
GI: Projectile vomiting
CNS: Headache
INTEG: Feeling cold, other skin sensations
GU: Desire to micturate
MISC: Sensation of fullness in neck and chest
Contraindications: Severe coronary or cardiovascular disease, pre-existent severe hypertension
Precautions: Hyperthyroidism, pregnancy, second dose to be injected only when first has ceased to act, make repeated arterial pressure measurements
Pharmacokinetics: Acts 1 or 2 min after IV injection and about 15–20 min after IM injection, in the latter case duration of action is 1½ hr
Interactions/incompatibilities:
• Increased response to drug: MAOIs, tricyclic antidepressants, β–blockers, other sympathomimetic agents, some appetite suppressants and amphetamine-like psychostimulants
Treatment of overdose: Administer phentolamine 5 mg IV if blood pressure does not return to normal after an appropriate time; repeat as necessary
NURSING CONSIDERATIONS
Assess:
• Baseline vital signs
Administer:
• Parenteral (IV) dose slowly according to manufacturers' instructions
Evaluate:
• Fluid balance—notify clinician if output less than 30 ml/hr
• ECG during administration; if BP increases, drug is decreased
• BP and pulse every 5 min after parenteral route
• CVP during infusion if possible
• For paraesthesiae and coldness of extremities, peripheral blood flow may decrease
• Therapeutic response: increased BP with stabilisation
Teach patient/family:
• The reason for drug administration

methyclothiazide

Enduron
Func. class.: Thiazide diuretic
Chem. class.: Sulphonamide derivative
Legal class.: POM

Action: Acts on distal tubule by increasing excretion of water, sodium, chloride, potassium
Uses: Oedema, hypertension
Dosage and routes:
• *Adult:* By mouth 2.5–5 mg daily, if necessary increased to 10 mg daily
Available forms include: Tablets 5 mg
Side effects/adverse reactions:
GU: Glycosuria, impotence
CNS: Dizziness, headache, weakness, paraesthesia
GI: Nausea, vomiting, anorexia, constipation, diarrhoea, pancreatitis
HAEM: Increased plasma cholesterol thrombocytopenia, agranulocytosis, aplastic anaemia, leucopenia, neutropenia
INTEG: Purpura, rash, photosensitivity
CV: Hypotension

ELECT: Hyperglycaemia, hyperuricaemia, hypokalaemia, hypomagnesaemia, hyponatraemia, hypercalcaemia, hypochloraemic alkalosis

Contraindications: Hypersensitivity to thiazides or sulphonamides, severe renal or hepatic disease, Addison's disease, hypercalcaemia, lithium therapy, porphyria

Precautions: May cause hypokalaemia, renal and hepatic impairment, pregnancy, lactation, diabetes, gout, electrolyte imbalance in elderly. May precipitate pancreatitis

Pharmacokinetics:

By mouth: Onset 2 hr, peak 6 hr, duration greater than 24 hr; excreted unchanged by kidneys, enters breast milk

Interactions/incompatibilities:

- Increased toxicity of: lithium, digitalis
- Decreased effects of: antidiabetics
- Decreased absorption of thiazides: cholestyramine, colestipol
- Risk of hypercalcaemia: calcium salts
- Increased risk of hypokalaemia: corticosteroids

Clinical assessment:

- Electrolytes; potassium, sodium, chloride, calcium
- Blood lipid analysis

Treatment of overdose: Recent ingestion: gastric lavage or emesis, supportive measures

NURSING CONSIDERATIONS

Assess:

- Baseline vital signs including BP standing/lying
- Weight
- Rate, depth, rhythm of respiration, effect of exertion
- Glucose in urine if patient is diabetic

Administer:

- In morning to avoid interference with sleep if using drug as a diuretic
- With food, if nausea occurs, absorption may be decreased slightly

Perform/provide:

- Daily blood sugar estimations
- Daily weighing, fluid balance

Evaluate:

- BP lying, standing, postural hypotension may occur early in use
- Improvement in oedema of feet, legs, sacral area daily if medication is being used in congestive cardiac failure
- Improvement in CVP 8 hrly
- Signs of metabolic acidosis: drowsiness, restlessness
- Signs of hypokalaemia: postural hypotension, malaise, fatigue, tachycardia, leg cramps, weakness
- Rashes, temperature elevation daily
- Confusion, especially in elderly; take safety precautions if needed

Teach patient/family:

- To increase fluid intake 2–3 litres daily unless contraindicated. To rise slowly from lying or sitting position
- To notify clinician of muscle weakness, cramps, nausea, dizziness
- Drug may be taken with food or milk
- That blood sugar may be increased in diabetics, urine or blood should be tested daily
- Take early in day to avoid nocturia

---

methylcellulose

Celevac

Func. class.: Laxative, bulk

Chem. class.: Hydrophilic, semisynthetic cellulose derivative

Legal class.: GSL

Action: Attracts water, expands in

intestine to increase peristalsis; also absorbs excess water in stool; decreases diarrhoea

Uses: Constipation, colostomy/ ileostomy control, diverticular disease, diarrhoea, appetite control

Dosage and routes:

- *Adult:* By mouth 3–6 tablets twice a day; for constipation take with at least 300 ml water; for colostomy/ileostomy control and diarrhoea take with a minimum of liquid and avoid liquids 30 min before and after each dose
- For appetite control, 3 tablets 30 min before meals with 300 ml warm water, repeated between meals if necessary

Available forms include: Tablets 500 mg

Side effects/adverse reactions:

GI: Flatulence, abdominal distension, intestinal obstruction

Contraindications: Intestinal obstruction, faecal impaction, hypersensitivity, colonic atony, dehydration

Precautions: Diarrhoea due to a pathological cause, e.g. infective bowel disease

Pharmacokinetics:

By mouth: Onset 12–24 hr, peak 1–3 days

Treatment of overdose: Gastric lavage if necessary; rectal washout if obstruction develops

NURSING CONSIDERATIONS

Assess:

- Cause of constipation; identify whether fluids, bulk, or exercise is missing from lifestyle
- Fluid balance to identify fluid loss

Administer:

- Take care when swallowing as swells in water
- Alone for better absorption (especially colostomy/ileostomy); do not take within 1 hr of other drugs or within 1 hr of antacids, milk, or cimetidine
- In morning or early evening (oral dose); should not be taken before going to bed
- 1–2 litres of fluid daily if used as laxative or appetite suppressant

Evaluate:

- Therapeutic response: decrease in constipation
- Cramping, rectal bleeding, nausea, vomiting; if these symptoms occur, drug should be discontinued

Teach patient/family:

- That normal bowel movements do not always occur daily
- Not to use if abdominal pain, nausea, vomiting occur
- Notify clinician if constipation unrelieved or if symptoms of electrolyte imbalance occur: muscle cramps, pain, weakness, dizziness
- That preparations swell in contact with liquid; carefully swallow with water and do not take immediately before going to bed
- About diet

---

methyldopa/ methyldopate hydrochloride

Aldomet, Dopamet, combination product

Func. class.: Antihypertensive

Chem. class.: Centrally acting α agonist

Legal class.: POM

Action: Stimulates central α-adrenergic receptors or acts as false transmitter, resulting in reduction of arterial pressure

Uses: Hypertension in conjunction with a diuretic; hypotensive crisis

Dosage and route:

- *Adult:* By mouth 250 mg 2 or 3 times daily, then adjusted every

2 days as required, maximum daily dose 3 g daily; IV injection or infusion 250−500 mg 6 hrly; not to exceed 1 g 6 hrly

• *Child:* By mouth 10 mg/kg daily is 2−4 divided doses; maximum daily dose 65 mg/kg or 3 g, whichever less; IV injection or infusion 20−40 mg/kg daily in divided doses every 6 hr; maximum daily dose 65 mg/kg or 3 g, whichever less

• *Elderly:* By mouth 125 mg twice a day initially, adjusted as required; maximum daily dose 2 g

Available forms include: Tablets (methyldopa) 125, 250, 500 mg; oral suspension (methyldopa) 250 mg/5 ml; injection (methyldopate HCl) 50 mg/ml

Side effects/adverse reactions:

GI: Nausea, vomiting, diarrhoea, constipation, hepatic dysfunction, distension, flatus, colitis, dry mouth, pancreatitis, sore or black tongue, sialadenitis, liver disorders

CV: Bradycardia, myocarditis, orthostatic hypotension, angina, oedema, weight gain, prolonged carotid sinus

CNS: Sedation, weakness, dizziness, headache, depression, psychosis, parkinsonism, paraesthesia, bell's palsy, involuntary choreoathetotic movement, impaired mental acuity, nightmares

INTEG: Eczema, lichenoid eruption, toxic epidermal necrolysis

GU: Decreased libido, impotence, failure to ejaculate

MISC: Allergic reactions

HAEM: Positive Coombs' test, bone marrow depression, leucopenia, thrombocytopenia, haemolytic anaemia, granulocytopenia

EENT: Nasal congestion

Contraindications: Hypersensitivity, active hepatic disease, depression, phaeochromocytoma, porphyria

Precautions: Pregnancy, lactation, Coombs' test, renal disease (reduce initial dose), severe cardiac disease

Pharmacokinetics:

By mouth: Peak 2−4 hr, duration 12−24 hr

IV: Peak 2 hr, duration 10−16 hr

Metabolised by liver, excreted in urine

Interactions/incompatibilities:

• Reduced antihypertensive effect with: phenothiazines, sympathomimetics, tricyclic antidepressants, MAOIs, NSAIDs, corticosteroids, oestrogens and combined oral contraceptives

• Enhanced hypotensive effect: anaesthetics, alcohol, other antihypertensives, antipsychotics, anxiolytics, hypnotics, β-blockers, calcium channel blockers, levodopa, nitrates

• Increased lithium toxicity

Clinical assessment:

• Blood counts

• Renal studies: protein, blood urea nitrogen, creatinine, watch for increased levels, may indicate nephrotic syndrome

• Baselines in renal, liver function tests before therapy begins

• Potassium levels, although hyperkalaemia rarely occurs

Lab. test interferences:

Positive direct Coombs' test in up to 20% of patients. Urinary uric acid measurement by phosphotungstate method, serum creatinine by alkaline picrate method, aspartate aminotransferase (SGOT) by colourimetric method, estimation of urinary catacholamines by fluorescent measurements

Treatment of overdose: Gastric lavage or emesis. Symptomatic treatment. Drug is dialysable

NURSING CONSIDERATIONS

Assess:

• BP prior to treatment as baseline

Evaluate:

- Therapeutic response: decrease in BP
- Allergic reaction: rash, fever, pruritus, urticaria; refer to medical staff if any reactions occur
- Symptoms of congestive cardiac failure: oedema, dyspnoea, BP
- Renal symptoms: polyuria, oliguria, frequency

Teach patient/family:

- To take 1 hr before meals
- Not to discontinue drug abruptly or withdrawal symptoms may occur: anxiety, increased BP, headache, insomnia, increased pulse, tremors, nausea, sweating
- Not to use non-prescribed (cough, cold, allergy) products unless directed by clinician
- Stress compliance with medication regime even if feeling better
- To rise slowly to sitting or standing position to minimise risk of postural hypotension
- Notify clinician if mouth sores, sore throat, fever, swelling of hands or feet, irregular heartbeat or chest pain, oedema occur
- Excessive perspiration, dehydration, vomiting and diarrhoea may lead to fall in BP; consult clinician if these occur
- Dizziness, fainting, lightheadedness may occur during first few days of therapy
- May cause skin rash or impaired perspiration

---

methylphenobarbitone

Prominal
Func. class.: Anticonvulsant
Chem. class.: Barbiturate
Legal class.: CD (Sch 3) POM

Action: Depresses the activity of the CNS

Uses: Generalised tonic-clonic (grand mal) seizures, partial (focal) seizures

Dosage and routes:

- *Adult:* By mouth 100–400 mg daily; dose increased every 2–3 weeks according to response; up to 600 mg daily may be needed
- *Child:* By mouth 5–15 mg/kg daily; doses increased every 2–3 weeks according to response

Available forms include: Tablets 30 mg, 60 mg, 200 mg

Side effects/adverse reactions:

HAEM: Megaloblastic anaemia, hypoprothrombinaemia (neonates exposed to drug)
CNS: Drowsiness, ataxia, lethargy, mental depression, paradoxical excitement, confusion, restlessness, dependence
INTEG: Maculopapular rash, photosensitivity, fixed drug eruptions, exfoliative dermatitis, erythema multiform, toxic epidermal necrolysis
CV: Hypotension
RESP: Respiratory depression
GU: Acute interstitial nephritis
MISC: Arthritis, hepatitis
GI: Stomatitis

Contraindications: Severe respiratory depression, porphyria

Precautions: Impaired renal or hepatic function, respiratory depression, pregnancy, lactation

Pharmacokinetics:

By mouth: Onset 20–60 min, duration 6–8 hr
Metabolised by liver, excreted by kidneys, half-life 34 hr

Interactions/incompatibilities:

- Increased effects: CNS depressants, other anti-epileptics
- Reduced effects of: disopyramide, quinidine, chloramphenicol, metronidazole, nicoumalone, warfarin, tricyclic antidepressants, griseofulvin, calcium channel blockers, digitoxin, corticosteroids, cyclosporin, oral contraceptives, theophylline, thyroxine

Treatment of overdose: Recent ingestion (4 hr): gastric lavage and aspiration; supportive therapy with attention particularly to cardiovascular, respiratory and renal function, and electrolyte balance

NURSING CONSIDERATIONS

Evaluate:

- Mental status: mood, alertness, affect, memory (long, short)
- Respiratory depression: respiration less than 10/min, shallow
- Blood dyscrasias: fever, sore throat, bruising, rash, jaundice

Teach patient/family:

- All aspects of drug usage: action, side effects, dose, when to notify clinician
- To avoid alcohol

Teach patient/family:

- Drug may cause drowsiness, caution against driving on operating machinery if affected

---

methylprednisolone, methylprednisolone acetate, methylprednisolone sodium succinate

Medrone, Solu-Medrone, Depo-Medrone

Func. class.: Corticosteroid
Chem. class.: Glucocorticoid
Legal class.: POM

Action: Decreases inflammation by suppression of migration of polymorphonuclear leucocytes, fibroblasts, reversal of increased capillary permeability and lysosomal stabilisation

Uses: Suppression of severe inflammatory and allergic disorders including severe erythema multiform, anaphylaxis, bronchial asthma, ulcerative colitis, etc.; cerebral oedema, shock

Dosage and routes:

- *Adult:* By mouth, usual range 2–40 mg in 3 or 4 equally divided doses
- *Child:* By mouth, dose is based on clinical response
- *Adults and child:* IM injection/slow IV injection or infusion, doses in range initially 10 mg to 500 mg; graft rejection by IV infusion up to 1 g daily up to 3 days
- By deep IM injection, 40–120 mg, repeated every 2–3 weeks if required
- For specific indication seek further information in the BNF and manufacturer's data sheet

Available forms include: Tablets 2, 4, 16 mg; injection IV (sodium succinate) 40 mg, 125 mg, 500 mg, 1 g, 2 g; depot injection IM (acetate) 40 mg/ml ampoules 1 ml, 2 ml, 3 ml

Side effects/adverse reactions: Consult BNF and data sheet compendium for further information

INTEG: Acne, poor wound healing, bruising, striae
CNS: Depression, mood changes, euphoria, insomnia, convulsions, dependance
CV: Cardiovascular collapse (rapid administration), embolism, hypertension, congestive heart failure
HAEM: Leucocytosis
METAB: Primary and secondary adrenal insufficiency
MS: Fractures, osteoporosis, proximal myopathy, avascular osteonecrosis, tendon rupture
GI: Nausea, increased appetite, dyspepsia, peptic ulceration, abdominal distension, haemorrhage, pancreatitis, oesophageal ulceration and candidiasis
EENT: Increased intra-ocular pressure, glaucoma, exacerbation of viral disease

Contraindications: Hypersensitivity, systemic fungal infections, immunisation procedures

Precautions: Pregnancy, lactation, children, masking of signs of infection, tuberculosis, non-specific ulcerative colitis, prolonged use, hypokalaemia, osteoporosis, increased susceptibility to infections, diabetes, glaucoma, epilepsy, chronic psychotic reactions, congestive cardiac failure, myasthenia gravis, renal insufficiency, thrombophlebitis, hypertension, active or latent peptic ulcer, diverticulitis, ocular herpes simplex, fresh intestinal anastomoses,
Doses must be reduced slowly

Pharmacokinetics:
By mouth: Peak 1–2 hr
IM: Peak 4–8 days

Interactions/incompatibilities:
- Decreased effect of this drug: rifampicin, carbamazepine, phenobarbitone, phenytoin, primidone
- Decreased effects of: antidiabetics, antihypertensions, diuretics
- Increased risk of hypokalaemia with: acetazolamide, loop diuretics, thiazides, carbenoxolone

Clinical assessment:
- Potassium, blood sugar, urine glucose while on long-term therapy; hypokalaemia and hyperglycaemia
- Plasma cortisol levels during long-term therapy (normal level: 138–635 nmol/litre when drawn at 8 a.m.
- Titrated dose, use lowest effective dose

Lab. test interferences:
False negative: Skin allergy tests

NURSING CONSIDERATIONS

Assess:
- Baseline weight, BP, pulse, fluid balance

Administer:
- Tablets with food or milk to decrease GI symptoms
- Suspension; after shaking (parenteral)
- Depot IM injection deeply in large mass, rotate sites, avoid deltoid, sub-cutaneous route, use 19G needle

Perform/provide:
- Assistance with ambulation in patient with bone tissue disease to prevent fractures

Evaluate:
- Fluid balance, be alert for decreasing urinary output and increasing oedema
- Therapeutic response: ease of respirations, decreased inflammation
- Weight gain daily; notify if weekly gain is greater than 2.5 kg
- Infection: increased temperature, WBC, even after withdrawal of medication; drug masks symptoms of infection
- Potassium depletion: paraesthesia, fatigue, nausea, vomiting, depression, polyuria, dysrhythmias, weakness
- Hypotension, cardiac symptoms, chest pain
- Mental status: affect, mood, behavioural changes, aggression

Teach patient/family:
- That steroid card must be carried at all times
- To notify clinician of any side effects or if therapeutic response decreases; dosage adjustment may be needed
- Not to discontinue this medication abruptly or adrenal crisis can result
- To avoid non-prescribed drugs: salicylates, alcohol in cough products, cold preparations unless directed by clinician
- Teach patient all aspects of drug use, including Cushingoid symptoms
- Symptoms of adrenal insufficiency: nausea, anorexia, fatigue, dizziness, dyspnoea, weakness, joint pain

methysergide maleate

Deseril
Func. class.: Antimigraine agent
Chem. class: Ergot derivative
Legal class.: POM

Action: Potent serotonin antagonist in CNS; potentiates the effects of vasoconstrictor stimuli and inhibits pain-facilitating and permeability-increasing actions of serotonin
Uses: Prophylactic treatment of cluster headache, other vascular headaches, migraine, diarrhoea in Carcinoid syndrome
Dosage and routes:
• *Adult:* By mouth 1 mg at bedtime increased over 2 weeks to 1 or 2 mg 2 to 3 times daily
Carcinoid syndrome
• *Adult:* By mouth 12–20 mg daily
Available forms include: Tablets 1 mg
Side effects/adverse reactions:
CNS: Dizziness, insomnia, psychic reactions, drowsiness, euphoria, confusion, ataxia, weakness, hallucinations
GI: Nausea, vomiting, heartburn, abdominal discomfort
MS: Leg cramps, joint and muscle pains
INTEG: Rashes, loss of scalp hair, eruptions
MISC: Retroperitoneal fibrosis, fibrosis in other areas
CV: Postural hypotension, tachycardia, vascular reactions including arterial spasm
Contraindications: Collagen disease, pregnancy, breast-feeding, peripheral vascular disorders, pulmonary and cardiovascular disease, urinary tract disorders, cachetic or septic conditions, cellulitis, severe hypertension, impaired hepatic or renal function
Precautions: History of peptic ulceration, abrupt withdrawal, regular clinical supervision, concomitant use of ergotamine
Pharmacokinetics:
By mouth: Half-life 10 hr, metabolised by liver, excreted in urine (metabolites/unchanged drug)
Interactions/incompatibilities:
• Enhanced vasoconstriction: vasoconstrictors or vasopressors
Treatment of overdose: Aspiration or gastric lavage, supportive measures. See further information in data sheet compendium
NURSING CONSIDERATIONS
Assess:
• Baseline weight
Administer:
• Use requires hospital supervision
• At beginning of headache, dose must be titrated to patient response
• Give with or after food to avoid GI symptoms
• Continuous therapy should not exceed 6 months. Drug-free period of 1 month required before recommencing
Perform/provide:
• Storage in dark area; do not use discoloured solutions
• Quiet, calm environment with decreased stimulation for noise, bright light, or excessive talking
Evaluate:
• Weight daily, check for peripheral oedema in feet, legs
• Withdraw treatment for reassessment after 6 months
• Therapeutic response: decrease in frequency, severity of headache
• For stress level, activity, recreation, coping mechanisms of patient
• Neurological status: level of consciousness, blurring vision, nausea, vomiting, tingling in extremities that occur preceding headache
Teach patient/family:
• Not to use non-prescribed drugs,

serious drug interactions may occur
- To maintain dose at approved level, not to increase even if drug does not relieve headache
- To report side effects: increased vasoconstriction starting with cold extremities, then paraesthesia, weakness
- That an increase in headaches may occur when this drug is discontinued after long-term use
- Report at once: dyspnoea, paraesthesia, urinary problems, pain in abdomen, chest, back, legs

metipranolol (ophthalmic)

Minims Metipranolol
Func. class.: Antihypertensive, ocular
Chem. class.: Non-selective β-blocker
Legal class.: POM

Action: Reduces intra-ocular pressure, probably by reducing the rate of production of aqueous humour
Uses: Primary open-angle glaucoma, secondary glaucoma
Dosage and routes:
- *Adults:* Instil one drop twice daily; initially 0.1%, 0.3% if control not achieved

Available forms include: Eye drops, unit-dose (preservative-free), 0.1%, 0.3%
Side effects/adverse reactions:
EENT: Eye irritation—burning, stinging, blurred vision, transitory dry eyes, allergic blepharojunctivitis, superficial keratitis, anterior uveitis
CV: Bradycardia, hypotension
RESP: Bronchospasm, dyspnoea, respiratory failure
CNS: Weakness, fatigue, headache, ataxia
INTEG: Rash, oedema
Contraindications: Asthma, history of obstructive airways disease, bradycardia, heart block, heart failure
Precautions: Breast feeding, patients wearing soft contact lenses, diabetic control monitored, cardiac disease
Interactions/incompatibilities:
Additive effect: other β-blockers—oral administration
Treatment of overdose: Flush immediately with water or saline
NURSING CONSIDERATIONS
Teach patient/family:
- To report change in vision, with blurring or loss of sight
- Method of instillation; not to touch dropper to eye
- That long-term therapy could be required
- That blurred vision will decrease with continued use of the drug

metoclopramide

Maxolon, Gastrobid, Gastromax, Gastroflux, Parmid, Metramid, Primperan, combination products
Func. class.: Anti-emetic
Chem. class.: Central dopamine receptor antagonist
Legal class.: POM

Action: Enhances response of tissue to acetylcholine in upper GI tract, which causes contraction of gastric muscle, relaxes pyloric, duodenal segments, increases peristalsis. Selective action on the chemoreceptor trigger zone by inhibiting central dopamine receptors. Decreases sensitivity of visceral afferent nerves to the vomiting centre
Uses: Digestive disorders, relief of symptoms of heatburn, sickness, dyspepsia, flatulence, milk regurgitation and pain associated

with gastro-duodenal dysfunction; nausea and vomiting associated with gastrointestinal disorders, treatment with cytotoxics or radiotherapy, migraine; post-operative conditions such as gastric hypotonia, diagnostic procedures

Dosage and routes:

Nausea/vomiting

• *Adult:* By mouth IV/IM 10 mg (5 mg in young adults 15–19 yr) 3 times a day
• *Child:* By mouth IV/IM
• *Up to 1 yr:* 1 mg twice a day
• *1–2 yr:* 1 mg 2 or 3 times a day
• *3–5 yr:* 2 mg 2 or 3 times a day
• *6–9 yr:* 2.5 mg 3 times a day
• *10–14 yr:* 5 mg 3 times a day. Do not exceed 0.5 mg/kg

Delayed gastric emptying

• *Adult:* By mouth 10 mg 30 min before meals for 2–8 weeks

Acute migraine

• *Adult:* By mouth/IM 10 mg at onset of attack

Gastroesophageal reflux

• *Adult:* By mouth 10–15 mg 4 times a day 30 min before meals

Nausea vomiting—(cytotoxics)

• *Adult:* Intermittent IV, up to 2 mg/kg in at least 50 ml infusion over at least 15 mins starting 30 mins before chemotherapy and may be repeated every 2 hours for up to 5 doses in 24 hours. (Max. in 24 hours 10 mg/kg)
• Continuous IV infusion. Seek specialist advice

Radiological examination

• *Adult:* IM/IV 10–20 mg 5–10 min prior to exam (young adult 10 mg)
• *Child:* IV/IM
• Up to 3 yrs 1 mg
• 3–5 yr 2 mg
• 5–9 yr 2.5 mg
• 9–14 yr 5 mg

Available forms include: Tablets 10 mg; syrup 5 mg/5 ml; injection IV 5 mg/ml; tablets modified-release 15 mg; capsules modified-release 30 mg. Paediatric liquid 1 mg/ml

Side effects/adverse reactions:

CNS: Drowsiness, restlessness, depression, extrapyramidal reactions of dystonic type, tardive dyskinesia
MS: Increased muscle tone
GI: Diarrhoea, constipation
GU: Galactorrhoea or related disorders, hyperprolactinaemia
CV: Hypotension

Contraindications: Hypersensitivity to metoclopramide; first trimester of pregnancy; patients under 20 except for intractable vomiting of known cause, e.g. radiotherapy and cytotoxic therapy; pre-medication for surgical procedures; porphyria

Precautions: Renal or hepatic impairment (reduce dose), pregnancy, lactation, hypertensive response in phaeochromocytoma, masking of underlying disorder e.g. cerebral irritation, do not use for 3–4 days after gastrointestinal surgery

Pharmacokinetics:

IV: Onset 1–3 min, duration 1–2 hr
By mouth: Onset ½–1 hr, duration 1–2 hr
IM: Onset 10–15 min, duration 1–2 hr
Metabolised by liver, excreted in urine, half-life 4 hr

Interactions/incompatibilities:

• Increased absorption (and enhanced effect) of: aspirin, paracetamol
• Decreased action of this drug: opioid analgesics, antimuscarinics
• Increased risk of extrapyramidal effects: ranwolfia alkaloids, antipsychotics, lithium, tetrabenazine
• Increased sedation: CNS depressants
• Antagonism of hypoprolac-

tinaemic effect of bromocriptine
• Increased plasma level: levodopa
Lab. test interferences:
Increase: Prolactin
Treatment of overdose: Gastric lavage with supportive measures; dystonic symptoms, treat in severe cases with anticholinergic drugs

NURSING CONSIDERATIONS
Administer:
• By mouth ½–1 hr before meals for better absorption
• IV infusion and injection slowly
• IV infusion may be given in 0.9% sodium chloride, 5% glucose, glucose/sodium chloride, compound sodium lactate
• Injection over 1–2 min
• IV preparations can be mixed with morphine/diamorphine and some cytotoxics under certain conditions: consult data sheet
Perform/provide:
• Frequent sips of water for dryness mouth
• Discard open ampoules
• Measure paediatric doses accurately with pipette
Evaluate:
• Therapeutic response: absence of nausea, vomiting, anorexia, fullness; extrapyramidal effect
• For side effects
• GI complaints: nausea, vomiting, anorexia, constipation
Teach patient/family:
• Avoid driving or other hazardous activities until patient is stabilised on this medication
• Avoid alcohol or other CNS depressants that will enhance sedating properties of this drug
• Accurate dosage
• Report side effects especially extrapyramidal side effects

metolazone

Metenix 5, Xuret
Func. class.: Diuretic
Chem. class.: Thiazide-like; quinazoline derivative
Legal class.: POM

Action: Acts on distal tubule by increasing excretion of water, sodium, chloride, potassium
Uses: Mild and moderate hypertension cardiac, renal and hepatic oedema, ascites or toxaemia of pregnancy
Dosage and routes:
Oedema
• *Adult:* By mouth 5–10 mg daily, as single dose. Maximum 80 mg/24 h
Hypertension
• *Adult:* By mouth 5 mg daily as a single morning dose for 3–4 weaks then maintenance 5 mg on alternate days
Available forms include: Tablets 5, 10 mg. 500 mcg available only as Xuret brand
Side effects/adverse reactions:
GU: Uraemia, glycosuria
CNS: Anxiety, headache, dizziness, fatigue, weakness
GI: Nausea, vomiting, anorexia, abdominal discomfort, cramps, pancreatitis
INTEG: Rash, urticaria, fever, chills
META: Latent diabetes, hyperuricaemia, azotaemia. Rarely clinical gout
HAEM: Leucopenia
CV: Orthostatic hypotension, tachycardia, chest pain
ELECT: Hypokalaemia, hypercalcaemia, hyponataemia, hypochloraemia, hypomagnasemia on prolonged use
Contraindications: Hypersensitivity to metolazone, anuria,

electrolyte deficiency states, coma or precomatose states associated with liver cirrhosis

Precautions: Hypokalaemia, diabetes, gout, pregnancy, breast feeding, renal and hepatic impairment

Pharmacokinetics:

By mouth: Onset 1 hr, peak 2 hr, duration 12–24 hr; excreted unchanged by kidneys, enters breast milk, half-life 8 hr

Interactions/incompatibilities:

• Increased toxicity of: cardiac glycosides
• Increased risk of hypokalaemia: corticosteroids
• Decreased effects of: antidiabetics, insulin
• Decreased doses of non-diuretic antihypertensive agents may be needed
• Profound diuresis with: loop diuretics

Clinical assessment:

• Electrolytes: potassium, sodium, chloride; include blood urea nitrogen, blood sugar, serum creatinine

Treatment of overdose: Danger of dehydration and electrolyte depletion. Treatment should be aimed at fluid replacement and correction of electrolyte imbalance

NURSING CONSIDERATIONS

Assess:

• Baseline weight, fluid balance
• Rate, depth, rhythm of respiration, effect of exertion
• Glucose in urine if patient is diabetic

Administer:

• In morning to avoid interference with sleep if using drug as a diuretic
• Potassium replacement if potassium is less than 3.0 mmol/litre, unless contraindicated
• With food if nausea occurs; absorption may be decreased slightly

Evaluate:

• Weight, fluid balance daily to determine fluid loss; effect of drug may be decreased if used daily
• BP lying, standing; postural hypotension may occur
• Improvement in oedema of feet, legs, sacral area daily if medication is being used in congestive cardiac failure
• Improvement in CVP and BP recordings
• Signs of metabolic acidosis: drowsiness, restlessness
• Signs of hypokalaemia: postural hypotension, malaise, fatigue, tachycardia, leg cramps, weakness
• Rashes, temperature elevation daily
• Confusion, especially in elderly; take safety precautions if needed

Teach patient/family:

• To increase fluid intake 2–3 litres daily unless contraindicated. To rise slowly from lying or sitting position
• To notify clinician of muscle weakness, cramps, nausea, dizziness, loss of appetite
• Drug may be taken with food or milk
• That blood sugar may be increased in diabetics
• Take early in day to avoid nocturia

metoprolol tartrate

Betaloc, Arbralene, Betaloc SA, Mepranix Lopresor SR, Lopresor, combination products

Func. class.: Antihypertensive anti-arrhythmic, anti-anginal, anti-migraine agent

Chem. class.: Cardioselective β-blocker

Legal class.: POM

Action: Produces falls in BP without reflex tachycardia or significant reduction in heart rate through

β-blocking effects; elevated plasma renins are reduced; blocks β_2-adrenergic receptors in bronchial, vascular smooth muscle only at high doses (decreases rate of sino-atrial node)

Uses: Mild to moderate hypertension, acute myocardial infarction to reduce cardiovascular mortality, angina pectoris, adjunct in treatment of hyperthyroidism, prophylaxis of migraine, cardiac arrhythmias

Dosage and routes:

Hypertension

• *Adult:* Initial dose 100 mg; maintenance 100–200 mg in 1–2 doses

Angina

• *Adult:* By mouth 50–100 mg 2 or 3 times a day

Arrhythmias

• *Adult:* By mouth 50 mg 2 or 3 times a day up to 300 mg daily in divided doses

• *Adult:* IV injection up to 5 mg at 1–2 mg/min; repeat after 5 min if required; total dose 10–15 mg

Following acute phase of myocardial infarction (within 12 hr)

• *Adult:* IV injection 5 mg every 2 min, maximum 15 mg; then by mouth after 15 min, 50 mg every 6 hr, and then maintenance 200 mg daily in divided doses

Hyperthyroidism

• *Adult:* By mouth 50 mg 4 times daily

Migraine prophylaxis

• *Adult:* By mouth 100–200 mg in divided doses daily

Available forms include: Tablets 50 mg, 100 mg; tablets modified-release 200 mg; injection 1 mg/ml

Side effects/adverse reactions:

CV: Bradycardia, postural hypotension, heart failure, palpitations, cardiac arrhythmias, Raynaud's phenomenon, peripheral oedema and precordial pain. Isolated reports of cardiac conduction abnormalities, gangrene in patients with pre-existing severe peripheral circulating disorders

CNS: Sleep disturbances, dizziness, paraesthesia, personality changes, depression, anxiety, headaches, fatigue, lassitude

GI: Nausea, vomiting, abdominal pain, diarrhoea, constipation, dry mouth, abnormal liver function tests

INTEG: Rash, alopecia, urticaria, increased sweating, photosensitivity

HAEM: Thrombocytopenia

EENT: Dry irritated eyes, conjunctivities, vision disturbance, tinnitus

RESP: Bronchospasm, dyspnoea, wheezing, rhinitis

META: Weight gain, muscle cramps

Contraindications: Bronchospasm, asthma, history of obstructive airways disease, metabolic acidosis, sinus bradycardia, partial heart block, uncontrolled congestive heart failure

Precautions: May aggravate bradycardia, peripheral arterial circulatory disorders and anaphylactic shock. Should be withdrawn gradually over 10 days, diminishing doses to 25 mg a day for the last 6 days, patients should be monitored. Reversible obstructive airways disease. Labile and insulin dependant diabetes; hypoglycaemic therapy may need alteration. Bioavailability may be increased in liver cirrhosis. α-blocker should be given concomitantly in phaeochromocytoma. Pregnancy, lactation. Warn anaesthetist if patient on β-blocker therapy. Diabetes mellitus

Pharmacokinetics:

By mouth: Peak 1.5–2 hr, duration 13–19 hr; half-life 3–4 hr, metabolised in liver (metabolites), exhibits genetic polymorphism, i.e. fast and poor metabolisers, excreted in urine, enters breast milk, no significant β-blocking effects in the neonate if mother on normal doses

Interactions/incompatibilities:

- Increased blood pressure with: adrenaline
- Increased hypotension, bradycardia: reserpine, hydralazine, methyldopa, prazosin, anticholinergics
- Should not be given with: verapamil
- Decreased antihypertensive effects: indomethacin, sympathomimetics
- Increased hypoglycaemic effects: insulin
- Decreased bronchodilatation: theophyllines

Clinical assessment:

- ECG, directly when giving IV during initial treatment
- Reduced dosage in hepatic dysfunction
- IV, keep patient recumbent for 3 hr

Treatment of overdose: Lavage, IV atropine for bradycardia, IV theophylline for bronchospasm, digitalis, O_2, diuretic for cardiac failure, haemodialysis, hypotension administer vasopressor (dopamine or dobutamine)

NURSING CONSIDERATIONS

Assess:

- Baseline weight
- BP, pulse note rate, rhythm, quality
- Respiratory rate – note any wheeze

Administer:

- By mouth before meals or bedtime; tablet may be crushed or swallowed whole

Perform/provide:

- Regular peak flow readings if any previous chest disease or the patient complains of tight, wheezy chest

Evaluate:

- Therapeutic response: decreased BP after 1–2 weeks
- Weight increase
- May affect libido and/or potency
- For signs of heart failure, such as ankle oedema

Teach patient/family:

- Take with or immediately after meals
- Not to discontinue drug abruptly, taper over 2 weeks, may cause precipitate angina
- Not to use non-prescribed drugs containing α-adrenergic stimulants, (nasal decongestants, cold preparations) unless directed by clinician
- To report bradycardia, dizziness, confusion, depression, fever, sore throat, shortness of breath to clinician
- To take pulse at home, advise when to notify clinician
- To avoid alcohol, smoking
- Limit sodium intake
- To comply with weight control, dietary adjustments, modified exercise programme
- To avoid hazardous activities if dizziness is present
- To report symptoms of congestive cardiac failure: difficult breathing, especially on exertion or when lying down, night cough, swelling of extremities
- Take medication at bedtime to maintain effect of orthostatic hypotension
- Wear support hose to minimise effects of orthostatic hypotension

metronidazole (topical gel)

Metrogel, Metrotop
Func. class.: Antibiotic
Chem. class.: Nitroimidazole derivative
Legal class.: POM

Action: Direct-acting amoebocide/ trichomonacide binds, degrades DNA in organism
Uses: De-odorisation of fungating malodorous tumours (acting against anaerobic bacteria associated with odour); acute inflammatory exacerbations of acne rosacea
Dosage and routes:
• Topically, malodorous tumours; to clean wound apply liberally 1 to 2 times daily; cavities, pack with paraffin gauze smeared with gel 1 to 2 times daily. Acne rosacea, apply thinly 2 times daily for 8 to 9 weeks
Available forms include: 0.75% and 0.8%
Side effects/adverse reactions:
Not reported with topical use but in systemic use of metronidazole:
CNS: Headache, dizziness, ataxia, drowsiness, peripheral neuropathy, uncoordination
EENT: Dry mouth, unpleasant taste, furry tongue
GI: Nausea, vomiting, gastrointestinal disturbance
GU: Darkening of urine
HAEM: Leucopenia
INTEG: Rash, pruritis, urticaria
Contraindications: Hypersensitivity
Precautions: No evidence of significant absorption from topical use but if so:
Peripheral neuropathy with prolonged use; metabolites retained in renal failure – significance unknown; pregnancy
Interactions:
• Disulfiram-like reaction: alcohol may increase action: warfarin
• Increased toxicity: lithium
• Decreased action of this drug: phenobarbitone
Treatment of overdose: Gastric lavage, dialysis

NURSING CONSIDERATIONS

Perform/provide:
• Good wound dressing technique and non-adherent dressing
• Other support and techniques to improve quality of life for the patient, including other methods of controlling smell
Evaluate:
• Therapeutic effect (reduction in smell)
• For side effects – only likely in long-term systemic use
Teach patient/family:
• Wound dressing technique and method of using Metronidazole
• About possible side effects
• All other supportive measures

metronidazole/ metronidazole HCl

Elyzol, Flagyl S, Flagyl, Flagyl Compak, Metrolyl, Vaginyl, Zadstat
Func. class.: Antibiotic, antiprotozoal
Chem. class.: Nitroimidazole derivative
Legal class.: POM

Action: Direct-acting amoebicide/ trichomonacide binds, degrades DNA inside, outside organism. High activity against anaerobic bacteria and protozoa
Uses: Intestinal and extraintestinal amoebiasis, including symptomless cyst passers, amoebic abscess, trichomoniasis, prevention and treatment of bacterial vaginitis, bacterial anaerobic infections, giardiasis, acute ulcerative gingi-

vitis, acute dental infections, e.g. ulcers and pressure sores

Dosage and routes:

Anaerobic infections (usually treated for 7 days)

• *Adult:* By mouth 800 mg initially then 400 mg 8 hrly (e.g. ulcers and pressure sores 400 mg 8 hrly); by rectum 1 g 8 hrly for 3 days, then 1 g 12 hrly; by IV infusion 500 mg 8 hrly

• *Child:* Any route 7.5 mg/kg 8 hrly

Bacterial vaginosis

• By mouth 400 mg twice daily for 7 days, or 2 g as single dose

Acute ulcerative gingivitis

• *Adult:* By mouth 200 g 8 hrly for 3 days

• *Child:* 1–3 yr 50 mg 8 hrly for 3 days, 3–7 yr 100 mg 12 hrly, 7–10 yr 100 mg 8 hrly

Acute dental infections

• By mouth 200 mg 8 hrly for 3–7 days

Surgical prophylaxis

• *Adult:* By mouth 400 mg 8 hrly during 24 hr before surgery followed by postoperative IV or rectal administration until able to take tablets; IV 500 mg, shortly before surgery, repeat 8 hrly, start oral therapy 400 mg 8 hrly as soon as feasible; rectal 1 g 8 hrly

• *Child:* By mouth, IV 7.5 mg/kg 8 hrly; rectal 250–500 mg 8 hrly

Trichomoniasis

• By mouth 200 mg 8 hrly or 400 mg 12 hrly for 7 days or 800 mg in morning and 1200 mg at night for 2 days or 2 g as single dose

• *Child:* 7–10 yr 100 mg 8 hrly for 7 days, 3–7 yr 100 mg 12 hrly for 7 days, 1–3 yr 50 mg 8 hrly for 7 days

Protozoal infections

See specialist texts

Available forms include: Tablets 200, 400 mg; film coated tablets 200, 400 mg; IV infusion 5 mg/ml; IV injection 5 mg/ml; suppositories 500 mg, 1 g; suspension 200 mg/(as benzoate)/5 ml

Side effects/adverse reactions:

HAEM: Leucopenia, anaphylaxis

INTEG: Rash, pruritus, urticaria

CNS: Headache, dizziness, ataxia, drowsiness, peripheral neuropathy, incoordination, transient epileptiform seizures

EENT: Dry mouth, unpleasant taste, furry tongue, angioedema

GI: Nausea, vomiting, gastrointestinal disturbance

GU: Darkening of urine

Contraindications: Hypersensitivity

Precautions: Persistent gonococci infection after trichomonal treatment, metabolites retained in renal failure, significance unknown; both active drug and metabolites removed by dialysis. Dose reduction not required in renal failure. No routine dose reduction required in patients undergoing intermittent peritoneal dialysis or continuous ambulatory peritoneal dialysis. Impairment or clearance in hepatic disease. Dose reduction to one third given once daily to patients with hepatic encephalopathy. Active disease of the CNS other than brain abscess

Pharmacokinetics:

By mouth: Peak 20 min–3 hr, half-life 5–11 hr, excreted mainly in urine as metabolites

Interactions/incompatibilities:

• Disulfiram-like reaction: alcohol

• May increase action: warfarin

• May increase plasma level of: lithium. Lithium treatment should be tapered or withdrawn before concomitant treatment

• Psychosis: disulfiram

• Decreased action of this drug: phenobarbitone

Clinical assessment:

• Regular clinical and laboratory monitoring if drug given for more than 10 days

• Plasma concentration of lithium, creatinine and electrolytes should be monitored in patients given metronidazole and lithium together

Lab. test interferences:

Decrease: Aspartate aminotransferase alanine aminotransferase

NURSING CONSIDERATIONS

Assess:

• Fluid balance, stools for number, frequency, character

Administer:

• By mouth, tablets should be swallowed whole with plenty of water during or after a meal; suspension should be taken at least 1 hr before meals. IV, as solution containing 5 mg/ml, by infusion at a rate of about 5 ml/min

• Suspension should be taken at least an hour before food

• Tablets, after meals, to avoid GI symptoms, metallic taste

• Other routes as indicated in pharmacological section

Evaluate:

• Stools during entire treatment; should be clear at end of therapy, for 1 yr before patient is considered cured (amoebiasis)

• Neurotoxicity: peripheral neuropathy, seizures, dizziness, incoordination, pruritus, joint pains; may be discontinued

• Ophthalmic examination during, after therapy; visual problems occur often

• Allergic reaction: fever, rash, itching, chills; drug should be discontinued if these occur

• Superimposed infection: fever, monilial growth, fatigue, malaise

• Renal and reproductive dysfunction: dysuria, polyuria, impotence, dyspareunia, decreased libido

Teach patient/family:

• Urine may turn dark reddish brown

• Proper hygiene after bowel movements: hand-washing technique

• Need for compliance with dosage schedule, duration of treatment

• To use condoms if treatment for trichomoniasis or cross contamination may occur

• Treatment of both partners is necessary

• To avoid alcohol (because disulfiram-like reaction will occur) even with the smallest amounts of alcohol

---

metyrapone

Metopirone

Func. class.: Cortisol inhibitor

Legal class.: POM

Action: Inhibits biosynthesis of cortisol (and to a lesser extent aldosterone) production leading to increased production of ACTH

Uses: Assessment of anterior pituitary function; Cushing's syndrome; resistant oedema due to increased aldosterone secretion in cirrhosis, nephrosis, congestive cardiac failure

Dosage and routes:

Assessment of pituitary function

• *Adult:* By mouth 750 mg 4-hrly for 6 doses

• *Child:* By mouth 15 mg/kg 4-hrly for 6 doses; minimum single dose 250 mg

Management of Cushing's syndrome

• *Adult:* By mouth: 250 mg–6 g daily tailored to cortisol production; use only under specialist advice

Oedema

• *Adult:* By mouth: 2.5–4.5 g daily in divided doses (with glucocorticoids)

Available forms include: Capsules 250 mg

Side effects/adverse reactions:

CNS: Dizziness, headache
CV: Hypotension
GI: Nausea, vomiting
INTEG: Allergic reactions

Contraindications: Pregnancy, lactation, hypersensitivity, adrenocortical insufficiency

Precautions: Patients with liver cirrhosis may show delayed response to metyrapone because of liver damage delaying cortisol metabolism. In thyroid hypofunction, urinary steroid levels may rise very slowly or not at all in response to metyrapone

Pharmacokinetics: Rapidly absorbed and eliminated from plasma. Peak plasma levels occur after 1 hr, following a dose of 750 mg, plasma levels average 3.7 mcg/ml decreasing to a mean value of 0.5 mcg/ml after 4 hr. Half-life is 20–26 min

Lab. test interferences: Anticonvulsants, antidepressants, neuroleptics, hormones affecting the hypothalamo-pituitary axis and antithyroid agents may affect the metyrapone diagnostic test

Treatment of overdose: Gastric lavage, forced emesis. Administer a large dose of hydrocortisone together with IV sodium chloride 0.9% and glucose. Repeat as necessary according to patient's clinical condition

NURSING CONSIDERATIONS

Assess:
• Baseline weight and BP

Administer:
• With meals and/or milk to prevent GI symptoms

Perform/provide:
• Fluid balance; weight daily

Evaluate:
• Standing/sitting BP to detect postural hypotension following treatment
• Additional symptom support as fatigue, heart failure, muscle weakness, may all be established resulting from disease

Teach patient/family:
• That capsules should be taken with milk or after food
• To change position slowly to prevent hypotension
• To use contraceptives to prevent pregnancy
• That therapeutic effect may take 2 months
• To avoid hazardous activity if dizziness occurs
• Supplemental information concerning management of Cushing's Syndrome symptoms

---

mexiletine hydrochloride

Mexitil
Func. class.: Anti-arrhythmic (Class Ib)
Chem. class.: Lignocaine analogue
Legal class.: POM

Action: Depresses maximum rate of depolarisation with little or no modification of resting potentials or duration of action potentials

Uses: Ventricular tachycardia, ventricular dysrhythmias during cardiac surgery, myocardial infarction or ischaemic heart disease. Ventricular arrhythmias indured by digitalis and other drugs. *Not* of proven value in arrhythmias in pre-excitation syndromes

Dosage and routes:
• *Adult:* By mouth, loading dose 400 mg (600 mg if opioids administered); maintenance after 2 hr, 200–250 mg 3–4 times a day; usual daily dose 600–800 mg in divided doses
• *Adult:* By mouth, modified-release capsules, 1 twice daily
• *Adult:* IV injection 100–250 mg at 25 mg/min; then IV infusion 250 mg (0.1% solution) over 1 hr,

then 150 mg/hr for 2 hr, then 500 mcg/min

Available forms include: Capsules 50 mg, 200 mg; modified-release capsules 360 mg; injection 25 mg/ml

Side effects/adverse reactions: Mainly related to blood concentration

CNS: Headache, dizziness, lightheadedness, drowsiness, confusion, dizziness, incoordination, dysarthria, ataxia, tremor, paraesthesia, convulsions, psychiatric disorder

EENT: Blurred vision, nystagmus, diplopia

GI: Nausea, vomiting, indigestion, constipation, diarrhoea, abdominal pain, dry mouth, unpleasant taste, hiccups, jaundice

CV: Hypotension, bradycardia, atrial fibrillation, palpitation, conduction defects, exacerbation of arrhythmias and torsade de pointes

MS: Arthralgia

INTEG: Rash

SYST: Fever

HAEM: Thrombocytopenia, appearance of positive but symptomless antinuclear factor titres

Contraindications: Hypersensitivity, cardiogenic shock, high degree atrioventricular block unless a pacemaker is *in situ*

Precautions: Pregnancy, lactation, myocardial infarction results in prolonged absorption half-life mexiletine. Plasma elimination half-life prolonged in moderate to severe hepatic disease and where creatinine clearance in less than 10 ml/min

Pharmacokinetics:

By mouth: Peak 1 hr; half-life 12 hr, metabolised by liver, excreted by kidneys, small proportion of unchanged drug

Interactions/incompatibilities:

• Oral therapy: drugs which delay absorption rate e.g. opiates may reduce peak plasma concentration. Rate of absorption but not bioavailability may be delayed

• Drugs inducing hepatic mixed function oxidase system may lower levels of plasma mexiletine

• Drugs acidifying or alkálinising the urine may enhance or reduce rate of drug elimination

• Concomitant IV therapy with other local anaesthetic type agents e.g. lignocaine/procanamaide is not recommended. This has not been seen as a problem with oral mexiletine

Clinical assessment:

• ECG and BP monitoring should be carried out during treatment

• Blood levels (therapeutic level 0.75 mcg/ml)

• Electrolytes potassium, sodium, chloride

Treatment of overdose: Gastric lavage where appropriate. Transfer to intensive/coronary care unit for cardiopulmonary support. Arrhythmias: treat appropriately. Diazepan may be useful for convulsions

NURSING CONSIDERATIONS

Assess:

• Baseline vital signs

• Fluid balance, ECG

Administer:

• IV infusion rate using infusion pump, run at less than 4 mg/min

Perform/provide:

• Continuous cardiac monitoring during intravenous administration, preferably in a coronary care/cardiac unit

Evaluate:

• Malignant hyperthermia: tachypnoea, tachycardia, changes in BP, increased temperature

• BP continuously for fluctuations

• Cardiac rate, respiration: rate, rhythm, character, continuously

• Respiratory status: rate, rhythm, watch for respiratory depression

• CNS effects: dizziness, confusion, psychosis, paraesthesia, convulsions; inform medical staff if these occur

• Record any arrhythmias to medical staff. Infusions may need to be discontinued immediately if arrhythmias are life threatening

Teach patient/family:

• To take medication as prescribed

• That medication is a treatment rather than a cure

• Mexiletine can cause hiccups indigestion and dry mouth

---

mianserin hydrochloride

Bolvidon, Norval

Func. class.: Antidepressant

Chem. class.: Tetracyclic

Legal class.: POM

Action: Blocks presynaptic α-adrenoceptors and increases turnover of brain noradrenaline

Uses: Depressive illness, particularly where sedation is required

Dosage and routes:

• *Adult:* By mouth, initially 30–40 mg daily, in divided doses or preferably as single dose at bedtime, increased gradually as necessary; maximum initial dose in elderly 30 mg; usual dose range 30–90 mg

Available forms include: Tablets 10, 20, 30 mg

Side effects/adverse reactions:

HAEM: Agranulocytosis, leucopenia, eosinophilia, purpura, aplastic anaemia, thrombocytopenia, jaundice

CNS: Sedation, blurred vision, confusion, hypomania, convulsions, dizziness, tremor, behavioural disturbances

GI: Nausea, dry mouth, constipation

INTEG: Sweating, rashes, breast disorders

CV: Arrhythmias, postural hypotension, oedema

MS: Arthritis, arthralgia, polyarthropathy

SYST: Influenza-like syndrome

Contraindications: Recent myocardial infarction or heart block

Precautions: Diabetes, cardiac disease, epilepsy, pregnancy, hepatic impairment, symptoms of prostatic hypertrophy; psychoses, urinary retention; avoid abrupt cessation of therapy; caution in anaesthesia, elderly, suicidal patients, renal disease, narrow angle glaucoma

Pharmacokinetics: Readily absorbed. Bioavailability reduced to 70% by first pass hepatic metabolism. Metabolised to desmethylmianserin and 8-hydroxymianserin which are active. Excreted in urine as metabolites either free or conjugated. Same also in faeces. Biphasic half-life, duration of terminal phase in 6–39 hr. Effect may not be seen for 2–4 weeks

Interactions/incompatibilities:

• Hypertensive crises: MAOIs

• Increased effect: alcohol

• Possible side effects: phenytoin (monitor plasma levels), antihypertensives (monitor BP), anticoagulants (monitor prothrombin time)

Clinical assessment:

• Blood tests: Full blood count, every 4 weeks during first 3 months of treatment. Monitor and if fever, sore throat or other signs of infection develop, stop treatment. Obtain full blood count

• ECG for flattening of T-wave, bundle branch block, atrioventricular block, dysrhythmias in cardiac patients

Treatment of overdose: Empty stomach by lavage. Treat symptomatically

NURSING CONSIDERATIONS

Assess:

• BP (lying, standing), pulse

- Weight

Administer:

- With food or milk for GI symptoms
- Dosage at bedtime if over-sedation occurs during the day. May take entire dose at bedtime, elderly may not tolerate more than once a day dosing
- Add to fruit juice, water or milk to disguise taste

Perform/provide:

- Check to see oral medication swallowed
- Mouthwashes or frequent sips of water for dry mouth
- Increased fluids, fibre in diet if constipation, urinary retention occur
- Assistance with walking during beginning of therapy since drowsiness/dizziness occurs
- Safety measures, including cot sides, primarily in elderly; reason for using such measures should be fully explained to patient

Evaluate:

- BP (lying, standing) and pulse 4-hrly; if systolic BP drops 20 mmHg withhold drug and notify clinician
- Vital signs 4-hrly in patients with cardiovascular disease
- Weight gain; appetite may increase with drug
- Mental status, alertness, affect, sleeping pattern, drowsiness, dizziness
- For signs of physical dependence: withdrawal symptoms; nausea, vomiting, headache, muscle pain, weakness after long-term use
- For urinary retention, constipation; more likely to occur in younger people
- For alcohol consumption; if alcohol is consumed, hold dose until morning
- For signs of suicidal tendencies
- Therapeutic response, decreased anxiety, restlessness, sleeplessness

Teach patient/family:

- That therapeutic effects may take 2–4 weeks
- To avoid driving, activities that require alertness, since drowsiness may occur
- To avoid alcohol or other psychotropic medications
- Not to discontinue medication quickly after long-term use

---

miconazole

Daktarin

Func. class.: Antifungal

Chem. class.: Imidazole

Legal class.: POM; 15 g oral gel P

Action: Interferes with fungal DNA replication

Uses: Coccidioidomycosis, candidiasis, cryptococcosis, blastomycosis, paracoccidioides, chronic mucocutaneous candidiasis, systemic fungal intertain and of ovophorynx, gastrointestinal tract and suprainfections due to Gram-positive bacteria. IV used for severe infections only

Dosage and routes:

- *Adult:* IV infusion in 250–500 ml fluid 600 mg 8 hrly, adjusted as required
- *Child:* IV infusion up to 40 mg/kg daily, maximum 15 mg/kg in one infusion
- *Adult:* By mouth, 2% gel 5–10 ml 6 hrly tablets 250 mg 6 hrly for 10 days or up to 2 days after symptoms clear
- *Child:* By mouth, under 2 yr gel 2.5 ml twice a day; 2–6 yr 5 ml twice a day; over 6 yr 5 ml 4 times a day

Available forms include: Injection 10 mg/ml; tablets 250 mg; oral gel 2%

Side effects/adverse reactions:

CV: Tachycardia, dysrhythmias (rapid IV)
INTEG: Pruritus, rash, fever, flushing, anaphylaxis, urticaria, phlebitis
CNS: Drowsiness, headache
GI: Nausea, vomiting, anorexia, diarrhoea, cramps
HAEM: Decreased haematocrit, thrombocytopenia, hyperlipidaemia

Contraindications: Hypersensitivity, due to polyethoxylated castor oil in IV preparation

Precautions: Rapid IV may cause arrhythmias

Pharmacokinetics:
IV: Terminal half-life 24 hr, metabolised in liver to inactive metabolites, excreted in urine, 50% of oral dose may be excreted unchanged in faeces. Over 90% protein binding

Interactions/incompatibilities:
• Increased action of: anticoagulants anti-epileptics, hypoglycaemic drugs
• Antagonism of *in vitro* miconazole activity by: amphotericin

Clinical assessment:
• Cardiac system: BP, pulse, ECG; watch for increasing pulse, cardiac dysrhythmias; drug should be discontinued if these occur
• Blood studies: haemoglobin, haematocrit, serum sodium, lipids

Treatment of overdose: Tablets: gastric lavage, followed by a purgative and supportive treatment

NURSING CONSIDERATIONS
Administer:
• Infusion must be diluted with 0.9% sodium chloride or 5% dextrose and given by slow infusion over at least 30 min. For oral infections gel or tablets should be retained in the mouth as long as possible
• After culture and sensitivity is obtained to identify causative organism
• Anti-emetic for nausea and vomiting as ordered
• After test dose of 200 mg is given; watch for allergic reactions
• IV after diluting with dextrose 5% 0.9% sodium chloride if hyponatraemia has occurred

Evaluate:
• For phlebitis, pruritus; may need IV antihistamine; continue unless reaction is severe
• Allergic reaction after test dose; have adrenaline available
• Therapeutic response: decreased fever, malaise, rash, negative culture and sensitivity for infecting organism

Teach patient/family:
• That long-term therapy may be required to clear infection (1 week–1 month)
• Proper hygiene: handwashing techniques, nail care
• Avoid contact with eyes, nose

---

miconazole nitrate

Daktarin, Gyno-Daktarin, combination product
Func. class.: Antifungal
Chem. class.: Imidazole derivative
Legal class.: POM

Action: Interferes with fungal DNA replication

Uses: *Tinea pedis*, *tinea cruris*, *tinea corporis*, *tinea versicolor*, vaginal or vulvae *Candida albicans* and superinfection due to susceptible Gram-positive bacteria, intertigo, candida nappy rash, paronychia, erythrasma, fungal infection of the outer ear, nail infections, fungal skin infections

Dosage and routes:
Cream 2%
• *Adult and child:* Apply twice daily continuing for 10 days after lesions have healed; nail infections, apply daily under occlusive dressing

Powder

• *Adult and child:* Apply twice daily to skin lesions, separately or with cream, may also be dusted on clothing in contact with affected area

Not recommended for nail and hair infections

Intravaginal

• *Adult:* Cream 2%: insert two 5 g applicatorfuls nightly for 7 nights, use cream topically to anogenital area twice daily

• *Adult:* Pessary 100 mg: insert 2 pessaries for 7 nights

• *Adult:* Tampons 100 mg: insert 1 tampon night and morning for 5 days

• *Adult:* Ovule 1.2 g: insert 1 ovule at night as single dose

Available forms include: Cream 2%; vaginal tampon 100 mg; powder 2%; spray powder 0.16%; vaginal cream 2%; pessary 100 mg; vaginal ovule 1200 mg

Side effects/adverse reactions:

GU: Vulvovaginal burning, itching

Contraindications: Hypersensitivity

Precautions: Child less than 2 yr, pregnancy

Interactions/incompatibilities:

• Vaginal contraceptive diaphragms

Treatment of overdose: Appropriate method of gastric emptying may be used

NURSING CONSIDERATIONS

Administer:

• After cleansing with soap, water before each application, dry well

• 1 filled applicator or 1 tablet/ovule deep-intravaginally each night; 1 tampon to be inserted night and morning for 5 days as directed

• Enough medication to cover lesions completely

• Powder/spray can be used in socks/clothing in contact with affected areas

Evaluate:

• Allergic reaction: burning, stinging, swelling, redness

• Therapeutic response: decrease in size, number of lesions

Teach patient/family:

• To avoid use of non-prescribed creams, ointments, lotions unless directed by data

• To wash hands before, after each application

• To avoid contact with eyes

• That intravaginal preparations damage latex condoms and diaphragms

• That cream should be applied daily to the partner's penis to prevent re-infection in vaginal, vulval infection

midazolam

Hypnovel

Func. class.: Anaesthetic induction agent, sedative

Chem. class.: Benzodiazepine, short-acting

Legal class.: POM

Action: Depresses subcortical levels in CNS; may act on limbic system, reticular formation; may potentiate aminobutyric acid (GABA) by binding to specific benzodiazepine receptors

Uses: Induction of general anaesthesia, sedation for diagnostic endoscopic procedures, intubation, dental surgery

Dosage and routes:

Intravenous sedation

• *Adults:* Slow IV injection over 30 seconds 2 mg followed after 2 min by increments of 0.5–1 mg if necessary. Usual range 2.5–7.5 mg

• *Elderly:* Slow IV injection over 30 seconds initially 1–1.5 mg followed after 30 seconds by increments of 0.5–1 mg if necessary. Usual range 1–2 mg

If opiates are being used for analgesia reduce initial doses

Premedication before surgery

• *Adults:* IM injection 70–100 mcg/kg 30–60 min preoperatively. Usual dose is 5 mg

• *Elderly:* IM injection as above but 2.5 mg may be adequate

Induction of anaesthesia

• *Adults:* Slow IV injection, following opiate pre-medication 200 mcg/kg. Increase to 300 mcg/kg if no pre-medication has been given

• *Elderly:* Slow IV injection, following opiate pre-medication 100 mcg/kg. Increase to 200 mcg/kg if no pre-medication has been given

• *Child over 7 yr:* Slow IV injection 150 mcg/kg

Available forms include: Injection 2.5 mg/ml, 5 mg/ml (as hydrochloride)

Side effects/adverse reactions:

CNS: Retrograde amnesia, euphoria, confusion, headache, anxiety, insomnia, slurred speech, paraesthesia, disinhibition

RESP: Respiratory depression

CV: Hypotension, reduced cardiac output, stroke volume, systemic vascular resistance

EENT: Vertigo, visual disturbances

GI: Nausea, vomiting, increased salivation

INTEG: Pain, swelling at injection site, thrombophlebitis

Contraindications: 3rd trimester of pregnancy, hypersensitivity to benzodiazepines, respiratory depression, acute pulmonary insufficiency

Precautions: Impaired renal or hepatic function, elderly, myasthenia gravis, 1st and 2nd trimester of pregnancy, lactation, concurrent CNS depressants pulmonary insufficiency, personality disorders

Pharmacokinetics:

IM: Onset 15 min, peak ½–1 hr

IV: Onset 3–5 min, onset of anaesthesia 1½–2½ min, protein binding 97%, half-life 2 hr, metabolised in liver, metabolites excreted in urine, crosses placenta, blood–brain barrier

Interactions/incompatibilities:

• Prolonged respiratory depression: other CNS depressants, alcohol, barbiturates

• Increased hypnotic effect: fentanyl, narcotic agonists, analgesics, droperidol

NURSING CONSIDERATIONS

Assess:

• Vital signs

• Baseline level of consciousness

Administer:

• IM or IV at onset of anaesthesia (duration 1½–2½ min) or as continuous infusion

Perform/provide:

• Respiratory ventilation equipment if required

Evaluate:

• Degree of respiratory depression due to muscle relaxation

• Response to administration of induction agent/sedative

• Ensure patient is sedated as well as paralysed

• Ensure patient remains on bed resting until drug effects have worn off

• Injection site for signs of inflammation

Teach patient/family:

• To avoid driving and other activities requiring mental alertness until drowsiness and weakness subside

• If receiving drug by continuous infusion, some muscle weakness may be experienced

mifepristone ▼

Mifegyne
Func. class.: Oxytoxic
Chem. class.: Prostaglandin analogue
Legal class.: POM. Supplied *only* to NHS hospitals and premises approved under the Abortion Act 1967

Action: Mifepristone is an anti-progestational agent
Uses: Termination of intra-uterine pregnancy of up to 63 days gestation, in conjunction with administration of a prostaglandin analogue
Dosage and routes:
• 600 mg orally, followed 36–48 hr later by gemeprost 1 mg vaginally (unless abortion already completed)
• Should be administered in the presence of the clinician
Available forms include: tablets, 200 mg
Side effects/adverse reactions:
GI: Nausea, vomiting
INTEG: Vaginal bleeding, malaise, faintness, rashes, uterine pain after gemeprost administration
Side effects may also be caused by gemeprost
Contraindications: Desired pregnancy, pregnancy exceeding 64 days, gestation; suspected ectopic pregnancy; chronic adrenal failure; long-term corticosteroid therapy, haemorrhagic disorders and anti-coagulant therapy; smokers over 35 years of age; porphyria; known allergy to mifepristone
Precautions: Asthma and chronic obstructive airways disease; cardiovascular disease or risk factors; not recommended in renal or hepatic failure. If patient has prosthetic heart valves or history of infective endocarditis, then appropriate prophylactic antibiotics should be administered. Follow-up at 8 to 12 days to confirm efficacy. Oral contraception initiated 3–9 days after mifepristone administration
Pharmacokinetics: Well absorbed orally; peak plasma levels after 1.5 hr; half-life is approx. 24 hr; it is excreted in the bile
Interactions: Non-steroidal inflammatory drugs, should not be administered for at least 8–12 days after mifepristone dose
Lab. test interferences: Plasma adrenocorticotrophic hormone (ACTH) and plasma cortisol levels may be elevated by mifepristone
Treatment of overdose: Treatment of adrenal failure may be needed

NURSING CONSIDERATIONS

Assess:
• Psychological suitability for this method of termination
• Patient's level of knowledge, understanding and acceptance of termination by this method
• Patient's understanding that treatment, once begun, must be completed, and cannot be stopped
• That if vomiting begins within 2 hr of administration, suction evacuation may be necessary
• Smoking habits
• Baseline vital signs (temperature, pulse, respiration, BP)
Administer:
• By mouth, with or without food, but with fluids; followed 36–48 hr later by gemeprost vaginally (unless abortion is complete)
• After clinician has completed HSA 4 form
• In presence of clinician on named-only basis
Perform/provide:
• Storage: in locked cupboard
• Clinician to complete post-marketing surveillance form
• Contact number (for patient not

in hospital or clinic) if there are problems

Evaluate:

• Vital signs

• Therapeutic effect; loss of products of conception

• Side effects: pain, excessive vaginal blood loss. If vomiting occurs within two hours of taking dose, inform clinician and prepare patient for suction evacuation

• Psychological state: aggression, depression, grief

Teach patient/family:

• About side effects and to report any promptly to nurse or clinician

• That suction evacuation may be necessary if side effects (vomiting) occur

• To complete treatment as agreed and prescribed

• To avoid any of the following: aspirin and NSAID drugs, cigarettes and alcohol until after follow-up visit

milrinone

Primacor

Func. class.: Cardiac inotropic agent

Chem. Class.: Phosphodiesterase inhibitor

Legal class.: POM

Action: Selective inhibitor of peak III phosphodiesterase isoenzyme in cardiac and vascular muscle. Positive inotrope and vasodilator with little chronotropic activity; also improves left ventricular diastolic relaxation

Uses: Short-term treatment of severe congestive heart failure unresponsive to conventional maintenance therapy

Dosage and routes:

• *Adult:* Slow IV injection 50 mcg/kg followed by maintenance IV infusion titrated between 0.375–0.75 mcg/kg/min to a maximum haemodynamic effect 12 hr following surgery, 48–72 hr following congestive heart failure; total dose should not exceed 1.13 mg/kg daily

Available forms include: Injection 1 mg/ml (as lactate)

Side effects/adverse reactions:

CNS: Headache, tremor

CV: Supraventricular and ventricular arrhythmias, hypotension, angina

META: Hypokalaemia, thrombocytopenia

Contraindications: Hypersensitivity

Precautions: Following myocardial infarction, obstructive aortic or pulmonary vascular disease, hypertrophic subaortic stenosis, uncontrolled atrial flutter or fibrillation, hypotension, reduced cardiac filling pressures (e.g. patients on diuretics), hypokalaemia, renal impairment, pregnancy, breast-feeding

Pharmacokinetics: In congestive heart failure volume of distribution is approximately 0.4 litre/kg, half-life is approximately 2.3 hr and clearance is 0.13 litre/kg/hr. Milrinone is approximately 70% bound to plasma proteins and primarily excreted in the urine

Interactions/incompatibilities:

• Precipitation occurs if parenteral milrinone is mixed with: frusemide, bumetanide, sodium bicarbonate

NURSING CONSIDERATIONS:

Assess:

• Baseline vital signs including fluid balance

Administer:

• By slow IV infusion, consult manufacturer's data sheet

Perform/provide:

• Continuous monitoring preferably on intensive therapy unit or coronary care unit

Evaluate:
• Therapeutic response
• The usual period is 48 to 72 hr, but some patients have been maintained for up to 5 days
• Cardiovascular parameters, electrolytes and renal function should be monitored closely during the infusion

minocycline HCl

Minocin, Minocin MR
Func. class.: Antibiotic, broad spectrum
Chem. class.: Tetracycline
Legal class.: POM

Action: Inhibits protein synthesis, phosphorylation in micro-organisms by binding to 30S ribosomal sub-units, reversibly binding to 50S ribosomal subunits
Uses: Syphilis, gonorrhoea, lymphogranuloma venereum, staphylococci meningococcal carriers
Dosage and routes:
Routine use
• *Adult and child over 12 yr:* By mouth 100 mg 12 hrly
Gonorrhoea
• *Adult:* By mouth a single dose of 200 mg followed by 100 mg every 12 hr for at least 4 days in males. Females may require prolonged treatment
Acne
• *Adult:* By mouth 50 mg twice a day, modified release capsule 100 mg daily
Prophylaxis of asymptomatic meningococcal carriers
• *Adult:* By mouth 100 mg twice daily for 5 days followed by rifampicin
Available forms include: Tablets 50, 100 mg, modified release capsule 100 mg
Side effects/adverse reactions:
CNS: Headache, dizziness and vertigo, raised intracranial pressure
HAEM: Eosinophilia, neutropenia, thrombocytopenia, haemolytic anaemia
EENT: Decreased calcification of deciduous teeth
GI: Nausea, vomiting, diarrhoea, pseudomembranous colitis
CV: Pericarditis
INTEG: Rash, urticaria, photosensitivity, increased pigmentation, exfoliative dermatitis, pruritus
SYST: Angioneurotic oedema, Stevens-Johnson syndrome, anaphylaxis
Contraindications: Hypersensitivity to tetracyclines, children under 12 yr, systemic lupus erythematosus, complete renal failure
Precautions: Renal disease, hepatic disease, lactation, pregnancy
Pharmacokinetics:
By mouth: Half-life 11–17 hr; excreted in faeces, excreted in breast milk, 55%–88% protein bound
Interactions/incompatibilities:
• Decreased effect of this drug; antacids, large amounts of dairy products, alkali products, (less significant than other tetracyclines), iron, calcium, magnesium salts, sucralfate, bismute chelate
• Increased effect: anticoagulants
• Decreased effect: penicillins
• Nephrotoxicity: methoxyflurane
Clinical assessment:
• Blood studies: prothrombin time, full blood count, aspartate aminotransferase, alanine aminotransferase, blood urea nitrogen, creatinine

NURSING CONSIDERATIONS

Assess:
• Culture and sensitivity before treatment
• Bowel pattern
• Fluid balance

Administer:
• Not to be taken with iron preparations or antacids
• Orally; dose and length of treatment appropriate for disease, e.g. Gonorrhoea, bolus; streptococcal infection, 10 days
• Not suitable for young children

Evaluate:
• Therapeutic response, absence of fever, lesions, redness, inflammation
• Negative culture and sensitivity
• Effect of any other drug therapy, e.g. increased action of anticoagulants
• Decreased drug action due to antacids
• Side effects nausea, diarrhoea, dizziness vertigo, rash, urticaria, photosensitivity overgrowth resistant glossitis, stomatitis vaginitis

Teach patient/family:
• To avoid large amounts of dairy products – decrease drug effect
• To take at evenly spaced intervals, always to complete course
• Report sore throat, fever, malaise, pain, could indicate superimposed infection
• Do not take alcohol
• Not to drive or use machinery if dizziness occurs during treatment
• To eat regular small amount of yoghurt if stomatitis occurs (small, white ulcers on mucous membrane)

---

minoxidil

Loniten, Regaine
Func. class.: Antihypertensive
Chem. class.: Vasodilator – peripheral
Legal class.: POM

Action: Directly relaxes arteriolar smooth muscle, causing vasodilatation

Uses: Severe hypertension not responsive to other therapy; topically to treat alopecia

Dosage and routes:

Hypertension
• *Adult and child over 12 yr:* By mouth initially 5 mg daily in single or divided doses, increasing to 10 mg daily then by 10 mg every 3 days if necessary. Maximum daily dose 100 mg; elderly, initial dose 2.5 mg in patients over 65 years of age
• *Child under 12 yr:* Initially 0.2 mg/kg daily in single or divided doses; increasing by 0.1–0.2 mg/kg every 3 days if necessary. Maximum daily dose 1.0 mg/kg

Available forms include: Tablets 2.5 mg, 5 mg, 10 mg

Side effects/adverse reactions:
CV: Severe rebound hypertension, tachycardia, angina, increased T wave, congestive cardiac failure, pulmonary oedema, sodium, water retention, peripheral, oedema
CNS: Dizziness, headache
GI: Nausea, vomiting
GU: Gynaecomastia, breast tenderness, increased blood urea nitrogen and creatinine
INTEG: Rash, hypertrichosis

Contraindications: Hypersensitivity, phaeochromocytoma, porphyria

Precautions: Pregnancy, lactation, children, renal disease, congestive cardiac failure, elderly, pericardial effusion

Pharmacokinetics:
By mouth: Onset 30 min, peak 2–3 hr, duration 75 hr; half-life 4.2 hr, metabolised in liver, metabolites, excreted in urine, faeces.

Interactions/incompatibilities:
• Concurrent use with quanethidine may cause orthostatic hypotension

Clinical assessments:
• Electrolytes: potassium, sodium chloride, CO_2
• Renal function studies: cate-

cholamines, blood urea nitrogen, creatinine
• Hepatic function studies: aspartate aminotransferase, alanine aminotransferase, alkaline phosphatase
Treatment of overdose: Administer sodium chloride 0.9%. Phenylephrine, angiotensin II, vasopressor, dopamine may reverse hypotension may be used if inadequate perfusion of a vital organ is evident

NURSING CONSIDERATIONS

Assess:
• Fluid balance
• Baseline weight
• Weigh before and during treatment
• Blood pressure and pulse ECG before and during treatment

Administer:
• Topically to scalp for alopecia
• Orally with food, following the dosage regimen for suitable gradual introduction until optimum blood pressure control is achieved
• With a diuretic to control salt and water retention; with a beta adrenergic blocking agent

Evaluate:
• Therapeutic decreased and controlled blood pressure
• Increased hair growth for alopecia
• ECG alterations. Most changes are transient (increased T wave)
• Angina, peripheral oedema, increased heart rate
• Growth of body hair
• Input and output of fluids, check for fluid retention—oedema
• Report weight gains of 1.5 kg or more weekly
• Nausea and dizziness
• Breast tenderness, rash

Teach patient/family:
• That increased body hair will reverse when treatment finished
• Not to discontinue medication without medical advice. Drug should be tapered off slowly
• To avoid driving or hazardous activity if dizziness occurs
• To report pitting oedema, dizziness, weight gain more than 2.2 kg, shortness of breath, bruising or bleeding

---

misoprostol

Cytotec, combination product
Func. class.: Antiulcer and gastroprotective agent
Chem. class.: Prostaglandin E_1 analogue
Legal class.: POM

Action: Inhibits gastric acid secretion, protects gastroduodenal mucosa; increases bicarbonate, mucus production
Uses: Prophylaxis and healing of gastric and duodenal ulcers including those induced by NSAIDs
Dosage and routes:
• *Adult:* Healing, 800 mcg daily in 2–4 divided doses for 4–8 weeks
• Prophylaxis of NSAID induced ulceration 400–800 mcg daily in 2–4 divided doses
Available forms include: Tablets 200 mcg
Side effects/adverse reactions:
GI: Diarrhoea, nausea, vomiting flatulence, dyspepsia, abdominal pain
GU: Menorrhagia, abnormal vaginal bleeding
CNS: Dizziness
SYST: Rashes
Contraindications: Hypersensitivity; pregnancy; breast-feeding; women of child-bearing age unless effective contraceptive measures are ensured
Precautions: Cerebrovascular disease, hypertension, coronary artery disease, severe peripheral vascular disease

Pharmacokinetics:
By mouth: Peak 30 min, half-life is 20–40 min, plasma steady state achieved within 2 days, excreted in urine
Treatment of overdose: General supportive measures
NURSING CONSIDERATIONS
Assess:
• Fluid balance, blood urea nitrogen, creatinine
Administer:
• With breakfast or main meals and at bedtime
Evaluate:
• Response to treatment indicated by absence of pain and gastrointestinal symptoms
Teach patient/family:
• Black pepper, caffeine, alcohol, spices and very hot or cold food are best avoided
• Not to take non-prescription medicines for coughs and colds, antacids and aspirin
• Pregnancy should be avoided while taking drug as it can cause miscarriage. If pregnancy is suspected the drug should be discontinued and the clinician informed
• Advise appropriate contraceptive methods

---

mitomycin

Mitomycin-C, Kyowa
Func. class.: Antineoplastic, antibiotic
Legal class.: POM

Action: Inhibits DNA synthesis, primarily; appears to cause cross-linking of DNA
Uses: Pancreas, breast, stomach cancer; adenocarcinoma of lung; skin, bladder, rectal and other cancers
Dosage and routes:
Doses are highly variable, and dependent on local treatment protocols, concomitant therapy and tumour type; the following dose schedules have been used
• *Adult:* IV 5–10 mg/m^2 every 3–6 weeks; bladder instillation in bladder cancer, 10–40 mg in 20–40 ml water 1–3 times a week for 10–20 doses; doses of 4–10 mg administered to a similar schedule have been used to prevent recurrent bladder tumours
Available forms include: Injection 2 mg, 10 mg, 20 mg
Side effects/adverse reactions:
HAEM: Thrombocytopenia, leucopenia, anaemia, toxicity cumulative
GI: Nausea, vomiting, anorexia, stomatitis, hepatotoxicity, diarrhoea
GU: Renal failure, oedema, fibrosis of bladder following instillation
INTEG: Rash, alopecia, severe necrosis following extravasation
RESP: Fibrosis, pulmonary infiltrate, dyspnoea
CNS: Fever, paraesthesia
EENT: Blurred vision
Contraindications: Hypersensitivity, pregnancy, breast-feeding
Precautions: Renal disease, bone marrow depression
Pharmacokinetics:
IV: Half-life approximately 17 min, metabolised in liver, 10% excreted in urine (unchanged). Blood count nadir around 4 weeks post treatment
Interactions/incompatibilities:
• Increased toxicity: other antineoplastics or radiation
Clinical assessment:
• Full blood count, differential, platelet count prior to treatment and at nadir; withhold drug if patient excessively myelosuppressed
• Renal function studies: before, during therapy

• Liver function tests before, during therapy

Treatment of overdose: Supportive, no specific antidote, blood products or filgrastim for marrow suppression

NURSING CONSIDERATIONS

Administer:

• HANDLING: take safety precautions appropriate to antineoplastic agents

• Following local antineoplastic (cytotoxic) policies

• After ensuring that clinician is aware of blood results

• IV; preferably into tubing of fast-running sodium chloride infusion

• By installation into bladder

• Other medications by mouth if possible. Avoid IV, IM, SC routes to prevent infection and bruising

• Anti-emetic 30–60 min before treatment

• All other medication as prescribed including analgesics, antibiotics, anti-emetics, antispasmodics

Perform/provide:

• Strict medical asepsis, protective isolation if WBC levels are low

• Strict oral hygiene 4 times a day

• Warm compresses at injection site for inflammation; check for extravasation

Evaluate:

• Bleeding: haematuria, bruising, petechiae, mucosa or orifices 8 hrly

• Dyspnoea, rales, unproductive cough, chest pain, tachypnola fatigue, increaed pulse, pallor, lethargy

• Food preferences; list likes, dislikes

• Effects of alopecia on body image; discuss feelings about body changes

• Oedema in feet, joint, stomach pain, shaking

• Inflammation of mucosa, breaks in skin

• Buccal cavity 8 hrly for dryness, sores, ulceration, white patches, oral pain, bleeding, dysphagia

• Local irritation, pain, burning at injection site

• GI symptoms: frequency of stools, cramping

• Acidosis, signs of dehydration: rapid respirations, poor skin turgor, decreased urine output, dry skin, restlessness, weakness

Teach patient/family:

• Why protective isolation precautions are necessary

• To report any complaints, side effects to nurse or clinician

• That hair may be lost during treatment and wig or hairpiece is available on NHS; tell patient that new hair may be different in colour, texture

• To avoid foods with citric acid, hot or rough texture

• To report any bleeding, white spots, ulcerations in mouth; tell patient to examine mouth daily

---

mitozantrone

Novantrone

Func. class.: Antineoplastic

Chem. class.: Synthetic anthracenedione derivative

Legal class.: POM

Action: Binds to DNA, cytocidal effect on both proliferating and nonproliferating cells suggesting lack of cell cycle phase specificity

Uses: Acute non-lymphocytic leukaemia (adult), advanced breast cancer, non-Hodgkin's lymphoma, palliation of non-resectable primary hepatocellular carcinoma

Dosage and routes:

Doses are highly variable, and dependent on local treatment protocols, concomitant therapy and tumour type; the following dose schedules have been used

• *Adult:* Breast cancer, non-Hodgkin's lymphoma, hepatoma: single agent, IV 12–14 mg/m^2 repeated at 21-day intervals; adjusted according to WBC and platelet count; combination therapy, reduce dose by 2–4 mg/m^2 according to regimen. Acute non-lymphocytic leukaemia relapse, IV 12 mg/m^2 daily on 5 consecutive days as single agent, or IV 10–12 mg/m^2 on 2–3 consecutive days with cytarabine

Available forms include: Injection 2 mg/ml (as hydrochloride)

Side effects/adverse reactions:

GI: Nausea, vomiting, diarrhoea, anorexia, mucositis, hepatotoxicity, gastrointestinal bleeding

HAEM: Thrombocytopenia, leucopenia, anaemia

INTEG: Rash, necrosis at injection site, dermatitis, thrombophlebitis at injection site, alopecia

CV: congestive cardiac failure, cardiomyopathy, dysrhythmias

MISC: Fever

RESP: Dyspnoea

EENT: Transient blue colouration of sclerae

CNS: Fatigue, weakness

GU: Transient blue-green coloration of urine, amenorrhoea

Contraindications: Hypersensitivity, pregnancy, breast-feeding

Precautions: Myelosuppression, cardiac disease, children, renal, severe hepatic disease

Pharmacokinetics: Highly bound to plasma proteins, metabolised in liver, excreted via renal, hepatobiliary systems; elimination half-life 5–18 days. WBC nadir 10 days post-dosing

Interactions/incompatibilities:

• Do not mix with: heparin, precipitate will form

• Increased bone marrow depression given with: other cytotoxics, radiotherapy

Clinical assessment:

• Perform full blood count, differential WBC pre-treatment and 10 days post-treatment

• Regular assessment of cardiac function in patients with pre-existing cardiac disease or after cumulative dose greater than 160 mg/m^2

Treatment of overdose: Supportive, no specific antidote, blood products or filgrastim for marrow suppression

NURSING CONSIDERATION

Administer:

• HANDLING: take safety precautions appropriate to antineoplastic agents

• Following local antineoplastic (cytotoxic) policies

• After ensuring that clinician is aware of blood results

• IV: Following dilution to at least 50 ml of infusion; over at least 3 min, preferably into tubing of a fast-running sodium chloride 0.9% infusion

• Other medications by mouth if possible. Avoid IV, IM, SC routes to prevent infection and bruising

• Anti-emetic 30–60 min before treatment

• All other medication as prescribed including analgesics, antibiotics, anti-emetics, antispasmodics

Perform/provide:

• Care to avoid contact of mitozantrone with the skin, mucous membranes, or eyes

• Strict oral hygiene 4 times a day

Evaluate:

• Bleeding e.g. haematuria, melaena, bruising and petechiae. Observe mucosal surfaces for bleeding 8 hrly

• Be aware of food preferences

• Observe for signs of jaundice e.g. yellowing of skin and sclera, dark urine, clay-coloured stools, itching, abdominal pain, fever, diarrhoea

• Acidosis and signs of dehydration indicated by heightened respiratory rate, poor skin elasticity, decreased urinary output, restlessness or weakness

Teach patient/family:

• Mitozantrone may impart a blue-green coloration to the urine for 24 hr after administration

• Blue coloration of the sclerae may be seen very rarely and is reversible

• Patients and their partners should be advised to avoid conception for at least 1–6 months after cessation of therapy

• All side effects must be reported to clinician or nurse

• Hot foods and those which are coarse or contain citric acid are best avoided

• To report bleeding, mouth ulceration and white patches (indicative of *Candida*) to the clinician or nurse at once. The patient should examine his/her mouth at least once a day

---

moclobemide ▼

Manerix

Func. class.: Antidepressant

Chem. class.: Reversible inhibitor of the enzyme monoamine oxidase A (RIMA)

Legal class.: POM

Action: Reversibly inhibits monoamine oxidase, showing preferential action against type A of the enzyme which metabolises noradrenaline and serotonin resulting in increased brain concentrations of these neurotransmitters

Uses: Severe depression

Dosage and routes:

• *Adult:* By mouth, initially 300 mg daily in divided doses, reduced to 150 mg daily or increased to max. 600 mg daily depending on severity of condition and individual response

Hepatic impairment: When hepatic drug metabolism is severely inhibited by disease or drugs which inhibit microsomal mono-oxygenase activity (e.g. cimetidine) normal plasma levels are achieved using doses one-third to half those usually employed

Available forms include: Tablets 150 mg

Side effects/adverse reactions:

CNS: Sleep disturbance, dizziness, headache, confusion

GI: Nausea, elevated hepatic enzymes

Contraindications: Hypersensitivity; phaeochromocytoma; patients receiving treatment with tricyclic or serotonin reuptake inhibitory antidepressants – a washout period equal to 4–5 half lives of the drug and of any active metabolites should elapse before starting meclobemide; patients receiving pethidine or codeine

Precautions: Pregnancy; lactation; diets rich in tyramine; patients whose predominant clinical feature is excitation or agitation; bipolar disorders; schizophrenia; schizo-affective disorders; thyrotoxicosis

Pharmacokinetics: Completely absorbed after oral administration, with 20% first-pass metabolism in the liver; peak plasma concentrations reached within one hr of dosage; almost completely metabolised in liver to inactive metabolites, excreted in urine; elimination half-life 1–2 hr

Interactions:

• CNS toxicity, hypertensive crisis: Tricyclic and serotonin reuptake inhibitory antidepressants – a period equal to 4–5 half lives of the drug or of any active metabolites should elapse between stopping these and starting

meclobemide, but tricyclics can start as soon as meclobemide is stopped; pethidine, codeine, sympathomimetics including those found in proprietary cold remedies
• Potentiation of: Ibuprofen, opiates – use particular caution with morphine, fentanyl
• Potentiation of meclobemide: Cimetidine-halve meclobemide dose

Treatment of overdose: Experience limited; symptomatic and supportive treatment

Pharmaceutical precautions: N/A

NURSING CONSIDERATIONS

Assess:
• Baseline BP
• Mental status
• If patient is not taking any other medication, particularly Ibuprofen or opiates

Administer:
• By mouth at the end of a meal

Perform/provide:
• Increased fluid for dry mouth and if constipation occurs

Evaluate:
• Therapeutic effect; lessening of depression
• Side effects, particularly changes in sleep pattern, dizziness, confusion, headache
• Changes in BP

Teach patient/family:
• That dose should be taken at the end of a meal
• About dietary restrictions (MAOIs). Not to eat cheese, pickled herrings or broad bean pods, or take Bovril, Oxo, Marmite or any similar extract. Reasons why these are prohibited
• Not to take any other medicines including remedies for colds, coughs, pain, without advice from clinician or pharmacist
• To abstain from alcohol
• To carry their MAOI card always
• To report any side effects to nurse or clinician but not to discontinue taking medication without advice

molgramostim (Granulocyte macrophage-colony stimulating factor; GM-CSF) ▼

Leucomax

Func. class.: Haematopoietic growth factor
Chem. class.: Protein
Legal class.: POM

Action: Stimulates the production and maturation of neutrophils and macrophages from pluripotent haematopoietic stem cells in the bone marrow

Uses: As an adjunctive treatment to cytotoxic chemotherapy, bone marrow transplantation and ganciclovir treatment, reducing the severity and duration of neutropenia

Dosage and routes:

After cytotoxic chemotherapy
• By SC injection 60,000–110,000 U/kg body weight daily, starting at least 24 hr after chemotherapy, continued until absolute neutrophil count is in the desired range

After bone-marrow transplantation
• By IV infusion 110,000 U/kg bodyweight daily, starting day after transplantation, continued until absolute neutrophil count is in the desired range; max. duration of treatment 30 days

Adjunct to ganciclovir treatment
• By SC injection 60,000 U/kg body weight daily for 5 days, dosage then adjusted to maintain absolute neutrophil count and white blood cell count in the desired range

Note: Variations on these dosage regimens are commonly used in specialist centres to make most cost effective use of this expensive drug
Available forms include: Injection 1.67 million, 3.33 million, 7.77 million U (150, 300, 700 mcg)
Side effects/adverse reactions:
CNS: Asthenia, fatigue, headache, paraesthesia, confusion, convulsions, intracranial hypertension
CV: Peripheral oedema, cardiac failure, capillary leak syndrome, cerebrovascular disorders, hypotension, cardiac arrhythmias, pericarditis, pericardial effusion, syncope
EENT: Stomatitis
GI: Nausea, diarrhoea, vomiting, anorexia, abdominal pain
INTEG: Rash, injection site reactions, increased sweating, pruritus
MISC: Non-specific chest pain
MS: Musculoskeletal pain
RESP: Dyspnoea, pleural effusion, pulmonary oedema
SYST: Fever, rigors, anaphylaxis
Contraindications: Hypersensitivity, myeloid malignancies
Precautions: Pulmonary disease; history of autoimmune disease; pregnancy; breast-feeding; patients under 18 yr of age
Pharmacokinetics: Elimination half-life 1–2 hr following IV administration, 2–3 hr following SC administration
Interactions: Increased myelosuppression given within 24 hr of cytotoxic chemotherapy
Incompatibilities: Some infusion sets, e.g. Port-A-Cath; should not be mixed with any other drug
Treatment of overdose: Symptomatic and supportive

NURSING CONSIDERATIONS

Assess:
- Vital signs (temperature, pulse, respiration, BP), fluid balance
- Full blood count including platelets

Administer:
- IV infusion (started not less than 24 hr after antineoplastic chemotherapy)
- SC injection
- If dilution is required 5% dextrose should be used. If diluted to a final concentration of less than 200,000 U (2 mcg), 1 ml human serum albumin should first be added to a final concentration of 2 mg/ml to prevent drug absorption on to infusion apparatus

Perform/provide:
- Platelet count twice weekly
- Storage in a refrigerator or at room temperature for a single period of up to 7 days
- All supportive measures for primary disease

Evaluate:
- Therapeutic effect, reduction/ absence of infection
- Side effects, including enhanced myelosuppression, musculoskeletal pain, tumour growth
- Urinary output (dysuria occurs occasionally)

Teach patient/family:
- About the drug and its side effects
- To report any side effects promptly to the nurse or clinician
- Technique for administration (if being carried out by patient or family member)
- To store the drug in a refrigerator

morphine sulphate

MST Continus SRM-Rhotard, Oramorph, Sevredol, combination products
Func. class.: Narcotic analgesic
Chem. class.: Opioid
Legal class.: CD (Sch 2) POM

Action: Inhibits ascending pain

pathways in CNS, increases pain threshold, alters pain perception. Acts of CNS opiate receptors
Uses: Severe pain
Dosage and routes:
Acute pain
• *Adult:* Subcutaneous/IM 4–15 mg 4 hrly as needed; By mouth 30–60 mg 4 hrly as needed; modified-release 8–12 hrly; rectal 30–60 mg 4 hrly as needed; slow IV half to quarter IM dose
• *Child:* Subcutaneous or IM injection; up to 1 month 150 mcg/kg, 1–12 months 200 mcg/kg, 1–5 yr 2.5–5 mg, 6–12 yr 5–10 mg. Doses should be repeated 4 hrly
Myocardial infarction
• Slow IV 10 mg followed by 5–10 mg if required (rate 2 mg/min)
Acute pulmonary oedema
• Slow IV 5–10 mg
Chronic pain
• *Adult:* By mouth, subcutaneous/IM injection 5–20 mg 4 hrly; rectally, 15–30 mg 4 hrly
• Modified-release tablets: By mouth, take previous daily oral morphine requirement, divide by two and give this dose 12 hrly. Alternatively in adults start with 30 mg twice daily and increase with increments of 25–50%
Available forms include: Injection subcutaneous, IM, IV 10, 15, 30 mg/ml; oral solution 10 mg/5 ml, 100 mg/5 ml, 8.4 mg/ml; oral tablets 10, 20 mg; rectal suppository 15, 30 mg; modified-release tablets 10, 30, 60, 100, 200 mg
Side effects/adverse reactions:
CNS: Drowsiness, confusion, hallucinations, sedation, euphoria, alteration of pupillary responses
GI: Nausea, vomiting, anorexia, constipation, cramps, dry mouth
SYST: Tolerance, dependence
INTEG: Urticaria, flushing, pruritus, sweating, pain at site of injection
EENT: Miosis
GU: Retention
CV: Palpitations, bradycardia, hypotension
RESP: Respiratory depression, cough suppression
META: Hypothermia
Contraindications: Hypersensitivity, respiratory depression, head injury, raised intracranial pressure, within 21 days of taking MAOIs
Precautions: Addictive personality, pregnancy, lactation, myocardial infarction (acute), severe heart disease, respiratory depression, hepatic disease, renal disease, obstructive airways disease, elderly (dosage reduction), hypothyroidism
Pharmacokinetics:
By mouth: Onset variable, peak variable, duration variable
Subcutaneous: Onset 15–30 min, peak 50–90 min
IV: Peak 20 min
Metabolised by liver, excreted by kidneys, excreted in breast milk, half-life 2½–3 hr
Interactions/incompatibilities:
• Effects may be increased with: other CNS depressants, alcohol, narcotics, sedative/hypnotics, antipsychotics, skeletal muscle relaxants, cimetidine
• Absorption of mexiletine may be delayed by opiates and cisapride action may be antagonised
Treatment of overdose: Naloxone 0.4–2 mg IV at 2 to 3 min intervals up to 10 mg, O_2, IV fluids, vasopressors; Gastric lavage

NURSING CONSIDERATIONS

Assess:
• When pain is beginning to return; determine dosage interval by patient response
Administer:
• With anti-emetic if nausea, vomiting occur
Perform/provide:
• Assistance with ambulation

• Safety measures: siderails, night light, call bell within easy reach
• Fluids and fibre if constipated

Evaluate:
• Therapeutic response: decrease in pain
• Fluid balance, check for decreasing output; may indicate urinary retention
• CNS changes: drowsiness, hallucinations, euphoria, level of consciousness, pupil reaction
• Allergic reactions: urticaria
• Respirations: respiratory depression, character, rate, rhythm; notify clinician if respirations are less than 12/min
• Need for additional analgesia, physical dependence

Teach patient/family:
• To report any symptoms of CNS changes, allergic reactions
• That dependency may result if dose taken is more than that needed to relieve pain
• Withdrawal symptoms may occur if high dose reduce too quickly: nausea, vomiting, cramps, fever, faintness, anorexia
• Importance of secure storage for controlled drug—social implications, risk to adults and children

mupirocin

Bactroban, Bactroban Nasal
Func. class.: Antibiotic, topical
Chem. class.: Pseudomonic acid
Legal class.: POM

Action: Inhibits bacterial protein synthesis by binding to specific protein complex, shows no cross resistance to most antibiotics

Uses: Bacterial skin infection, elimination of nasal carriage of *Staphylococcus aureus* including methicillin-resistant *Staphylococcus aureus* (MRSA)

Dosage and routes:
• Apply small amount to affected area 3 times a day for up to 10 days. Intranasal apply to anterior part of each nostril 2–3 times daily for 5–7 days. Gently press sides of nose together to spread ointment

Available forms include: Ointment 2% (20 mg/g); nasal ointment 2%

Side effects/adverse reactions:
INTEG: Burning, stinging, itching

Contraindications: Hypersensitivity to mupirocin, polyethylene glycols

Precautions: Pregnancy, lactation, moderate to severe renal impairment

NURSING CONSIDERATIONS

Assess:
• Affected area for persistent infection (indicated by increase in size of the lesions or an increase in their number)

Administer:
• After samples have been sent for culture and sensitivity
• Cover with gauze after application if indicated

Perform/provide:
• In presence of MRSA, patient should be barrier nursed with strict hygiene control of staff to avoid further spread of infection
• Regular swabs to determine evidence of continuing infection
• Follow local policy for MRSA infection
• Wash hands after applying ointment and wear gloves
• In hospital children should be nursed in isolation (2–5 days)

Evaluate:
• Response to treatment: reduction in size and number of lesions

Teach patient/family:
• Hands must be washed after applying ointment
• Child's fingernails must be trimmed to prevent scratching
• Irritation and worsening of con-

dition must be reported to clinician or health visitor

mustine hydrochloride

Func. class.: Antineoplastic alkylating agent
Chem. class.: Nitrogen mustard
Legal class.: POM

Action: Alkylates DNA, RNA; also responsible for cross-linking DNA strands
Uses: Principally Hodgkin's disease. Occasionally other cancers; topically in mycosis fungoides
Dosage and routes:
Doses are highly variable, and dependent on local treatment protocols, concomitant therapy and tumour type; the following dose schedules have been used
• *Adult:* IV 0.4 mg/kg as a single dose or 0.1 mg/kg as a course of 4 daily injections. Reconstituted in sodium chloride 0.9% or water for injections. Topical (in mycosis fungoides) as a 0.02% solution in sodium chloride 0.9%
Available forms include: Injection 10 mg
Side effects/adverse reactions:
After injection
EENT: Tinnitus, hearing loss
HAEM: Thrombocytopenia, leucopenia, agranulocytosis, anaemia
GI: Nausea, vomiting, diarrhoea, stomatitis, weight loss
CNS: Headache, dizziness, drowsiness
INTEG: Alopecia, pruritus
GU: Amenorrhoea, reduced spermatogenesis
SYST: Fever
After topical use
INTEG: Contact dermatitis, rash, alopecia
Contraindications: Pregnancy, severe leucopenia, thrombocytopenia or anaemia and coexistent or suspected granuloma, breastfeeding
Precautions: Vesicant, only ever give systemically by IV injection, avoid extravasation. If extravasation occurs seek specialist advice
• Irrritant to skin and mucous membranes, accidental contamination requires irrigation or washing with large amounts of water—seek medical advice
Pharmacokinetics: Metabolised in liver, excreted in urine. Disappears from blood in 10 min
Interactions/incompatibilities:
• Increased toxicity: antineoplastics, radiation
• Rapidly unstable in alkaline solution
Clinical assessment:
• Full blood count, differential, before treatment and at nadir 10 days post-treatment. Withhold treatment if WBC below limits set in the treatment unit
• Anti-emetic 30–60 min before giving drug to prevent vomiting
Treatment of overdose: Sodium thiosulphate infusion 64 mg per mg mustine will neutralise mustine if given *immediately* afterwards, otherwise treatment is supportive

NURSING CONSIDERATIONS

Assess:
• Baseline temperature and fluid balance
Administer:
• HANDLING: take safety precautions appropriate to antineoplastic agents. Vesicant; irritant to skin and mucous membranes. Accidental contamination requires irrigation or washing with copious amounts of water. Seek specialist advice if contamination occurs
• Following local antineoplastic (cytotoxic) policies
• After ensuring that clinician is aware of blood results
• Vesicant: only ever give system-

atically by IV injection; preferably into tubing of fast-running sodium chloride 0.9% infusion
• Topically to lesions, avoiding normal and broken skin, eyes, mucous membranes
• Other medications by mouth if possible. Avoid IV, IM, SC routes to prevent injection and bruising
• Anti-emetic 30–60 min before treatment
• All other medication as prescribed including analgesics, antibiotics, anti-emetics, antispasmodics

Perform/provide:
• Trained personnel should reconstitute drug in designated area
• Strict medical asepsis, protective isolation if WBC levels are low
• Special skin care
• Increase fluid intake to 2–3 litres daily to prevent urate deposits, calculi formation
• Strict oral hygiene 4 times a day with prescribed mouthwashes
• Warm compresses at injection site for inflammation

Evaluate:
• Bleeding: haematuria, bruising or petechiae, mucosa or orifices 8 hrly
• For extravasation; infusion should be stopped if local pain experienced
• Food preferences; list likes, dislikes
• Yellowing of skin, sclera, dark urine, clay-coloured stools, itchy skin, abdominal pain, fever, diarrhoea
• Effects of alopecia on body image; discuss feelings about body changes
• Inflammation of mucosa, breaks in skin
• Buccal cavity 8 hrly for dryness, sores, ulceration, white patches, oral pain, bleeding, dysphagia
• Local irritation, pain, burning, discoloration at injection site
• Symptoms indicating severe allergic reaction: rash, pruritus, urticaria, purpuric skin lesions, itching, flushing

Teach patient/family:
• Of protective isolation precautions
• To report any complaints or side effects to nurse or clinician
• That sterility, amenorrhoea can occur; reversible after discontinuing treatment
• That hair may be lost during treatment; a wig or hairpiece is available on NHS prescription; new hair may be different in colour, texture
• To avoid foods with citric acid, hot or rough texture
• To report any bleeding, white spots, or ulcerations in mouth to clinician; tell patient to examine mouth daily

nabilone

Cesamet
Func. class.: Anti-emetic
Chem. class.: Synthetic cannibinoid
Legal class.: POM

Action: Inhibition of vomiting control mechanism in the medulla oblongata

Uses: Nausea and vomiting caused by cytotoxic drugs, unresponsive to conventional anti-emetics

Dosage and routes:
• *Adult over 18 yr:* By mouth, 1 mg twice daily, increased if necessary to 2 mg twice daily, throughout each cycle of cytotoxic therapy and, if necessary, for 48 hr after last dose of each cycle; maximum 6 mg daily
• First dose taken the night before initiation of cytotoxic therapy, 2nd

dose 1–3 hr before the first dose of cytotoxic drug
Available forms includes: Capsules 1 mg (hospital only)
Side effects/adverse reactions:
CNS: Drowsiness, confusion, disorientation, euphoria, psychosis, depression, hallucinations, lapses in concentration, decreased coordination, headache, blurred vision, tremors
CV: Postural hypotension, tachycardia
GI: Dry mouth, decreased appetite, abdominal cramps
Contraindications: Known allergy to cannabinoid agents, nausea and vomiting causes from any cause other than cancer chemotherapy
Precautions: History of psychosis, pregnancy, lactation, elderly, heart disease, hypotension
Pharmacokinetics: Absorbed from the GI tract, undergoes metabolism possible to active metabolite, excreted predominately by biliary route. Half-life is 2 hr
Interactions/incompatibilities:
• Increased effects of: CNS depressants, including alcohol and narcotic analgesics
Treatment of overdose: Symptomatic and supportive therapy. Anticipate psychotic episodes, including hallucinations and anxiety reactions. Consider administration of a neuroleptic agent or activated charcoal to decrease absorption from GI tract
• Maintain airway
• Maintain body temperature
• Assess conscious state

NURSING CONSIDERATIONS

Assess:
• Baseline BP: lying and standing
• Pulse
Administer:
• See under dose
• For 48 hr after end of chemotherapy if necessary
Perform/provide:
• Boiled sweets, frequent sips of water for dry mouth
Evaluate:
• For neurological side effects including drowsiness, confusion, disorientation: may require assistance with ambulation
• Therapeutic effect: reduction of nausea and vomiting
• For postural hypotension and tachycardia
Teach patient/family:
• Rise slowly as fainting may occur
• Not to perform potentially hazardous tasks since mental and physical abilities may be impaired
• Avoid alcohol
• Deep breathing to assist in control of nausea

---

nabumetone

Relifex
Func. class.: Non-steroidal anti-inflammatory drug
Chem. class.: Butanone
Legal class.: POM

Action: Prostaglandin synthesis inhibitor. Has both analgesic and anti-inflammatory effects
Uses: Osteoarthritis, rheumatoid arthritis
Dosage and routes:
• By mouth 1 g at night; in severe conditions 0.5–1 g in morning as well, elderly patients 0.5–1 g daily
Available forms include: Tablets 500 mg; suspension 500 mg in 5 ml
Side effects/adverse reactions:
GI: Nausea, diarrhoea, constipation, dyspepsia, flatulence, abdominal pain
CNS: Headache, dizziness, vertigo, sedation
INTEG: Rashes, pruritus
Contraindications: Active or suspected peptic ulceration or GI

haemorrhage; severe hepatic impairment; hypersensitivity; hypersensitivity to aspirin or other NSAIDS; pregnancy; breast-feeding; asthma

Precautions: Elderly patients, history of peptic ulceration, allergic disorders, asthma, renal impairment, aspirin hypersensitivity

Pharmacokinetics: Absorbed from GI tract and rapidly metabolised in liver to principal active metabolite, 6-methoxy-2-naphthylacetic acid, which has a plasma half-life of 12–36 hr

Interactions/incompatibilities:

• Increased risk of side effects: anticoagulants, antihypertensives, anticonvulsants, sulphonylurea hypoglycaemics, cardiac glycosides, diuretics

Clinical assessment:

• Renal function tests: blood urea, creatinine, before treatment and periodically thereafter if problem anticipated

Treatment of overdose: No specific antidote. Treatment with gastric lavage, activated charcoal using up to 60 g orally in divided doses

NURSING CONSIDERATIONS

Administer:

• With or after food

• Swallow whole

Evaluate:

• Therapeutic response: decreased pain, stiffness, swelling in joints, ability to move more easily

Teach patient/family:

• To avoid driving or other hazardous activities if dizziness or drowsiness occurs

• To report change in urine pattern, weight increase, oedema, pain increase in joints, fever, blood in urine (indicates nephrotoxicity)

• That therapeutic effects may take up to 1 month

• To take with food or milk

• To report any indigestion or black tarry stools

nadolol

Corgard, combination product

Func. class.: Antihypertensive, anti-anginal, anti-arrhythmic, anti-migraine agent, antithyroid agent

Chem. class.: Non-selective β-blocker

Legal class.: POM

Action: Long-acting, nonselective β-adrenergic receptor blocking agent; mechanism is similar to propranolol

Uses: Chronic stable angina pectoris, mild to moderate hypertension prophylaxis of migraine, arrhythmias, thyrotoxicosis

Dosage and routes:

Angina

• *Adult:* By mouth 40 mg daily increased at weekly intervals to 160 mg daily

Hypertension

• *Adult:* By mouth 80 mg daily increased at weekly intervals to maximum 240 mg daily

Arrhythmias

• *Adult:* By mouth 40 mg daily increased to 160 mg daily; reduce to 40 mg daily if bradycardia occurs

Migraine prophylaxis

• *Adult:* By mouth 40 mg daily increased at weekly intervals; usually 80–160 mg daily

Hyperthyroidism (adjunct)

• *Adult:* By mouth 80–160 mg daily

Available forms include: Tablets 40 mg, 80 mg

Side effects/adverse reactions:

RESP: Respiratory dysfunction

CV: Bradycardia, hypotension

CNS: Fatigue, lightheadedness, paraesthesia, depression, insomnia

GI: Nausea, vomiting, diarrhoea, colitis, constipation, cramps, dry mouth

INTEG: Rash, pruritus, fever, cold extremities, alopecia

Contraindications: Bronchospasm, asthma, history of obstructive airways disease, metabolic acidosis, sinus bradycardia, partial heart block, uncontrolled congestive heart failure
Precautions: Diabetes mellitus, pregnancy, renal disease, lactation, congestive cardiac failure, hyperthyroidism, chronic obstructive airways disease, angina, hepatic disease
Pharmacokinetics:
By mouth: Onset variable, peak 3–4 hr, duration 17–24 hr; half-life 16–20 hr, not metabolised, excreted in urine (unchanged), bile, breast milk
Interactions/incompatibilities:
• Increased effects: alcohol, anaesthetics, anti-arrhythmics, antidiabetics, antihypertensives, calcium channel blockers, cardiac glycosides, corticosteroids, diuretics
• Decreased effects: analgesics, sympathomimetics, MAOIs
Clinical assessment:
• Fluid balance; creatinine clearance if kidney damage is diagnosed
Treatment of overdose: Excessive bradycardia treated with atropine; if no response isoprenaline given with caution. Cardiac failure with digitalisation and diuretics. Glucagon may be useful. Hypotension managed with adrenaline. Bronchospasm counteracted with isoprenaline and aminophylline. May be removed from circulation by haemodialysis

NURSING CONSIDERATIONS
Assess:
• Baseline vital signs
Evaluate:
• Therapeutic response (dependant on dose)
• Reduction in hypertension
• Relief of angina
• Reduced arrhythmias
• Respiratory status, may cause bronchospasm
• Heart rate – bradycardia, heart block
• Observe for increased cardiac failure (oedema, weight gain, dyspnoea)
• Reduced doses required with renal failure
• Control of migraine
• Relief from thyrotoxic symptoms
Teach patient/family:
• May cause cold extremities, fatigue, sleep disturbances

---

naftidrofuryl oxalate

Praxilene, Praxilene Forte
Func. class.: Vasodilator
Legal class.: POM

Action: Potent spasmolytic; exerts a direct effect on intracellular metabolism increasing ATP levels and decreasing lactic acid levels in ischaemic conditions
Uses: Cerebral and peripheral vascular disease, intermittent claudication, night cramps, Raynaud's syndrome
Dosage and routes:
Cerebral vascular disease
• By mouth 100 mg 3 times daily
Peripheral vascular disease
• By mouth 100–200 mg 3 times daily; IV or intra-arterial infusion 200 mg in 250–500 ml of dextrose 5% or sodium chloride 0.9% over at least 90 min twice daily
Available forms include: Capsules 100 mg; injection 20 mg/ml, 10 ml ampoule
Side effects/adverse reactions:
GU: Nausea, epigastric pain
INTEG: Rash
Contraindications: Parenteral administration in atrioventricular block, bolus injection, hypersensitivity
Precautions: Pregnancy, lactation,

severe cardiac insufficiency, renal, hepatic disease
Interactions: β-Blockers, antiarrhythmic drugs, incompatible with solutions containing calcium ions
Treatment of overdose: Depression of cardiac conduction may require isoprenaline, convulsions may be managed by diazepam

NURSING CONSIDERATIONS

Assess:
- Baseline BP and pulse

Administer:
- With meals to reduce GI upsets
- Do not give IV dose as a bolus

Evaluate:
- Therapeutic response: increased temperature in extremities, orientation, long- and short-term memory
- BP, pulse during treatment until stable
- Record BP lying and standing—postural hypotension is common

Teach patient/family:
- That medication may need to be taken continuously, therapeutic response may not be seen for 2–3 months
- That it is necessary to stop smoking to prevent excessive vasoconstriction
- Dizziness may occur
- To make positional changes slowly, or fainting may occur
- To discontinue drug, notify clinician if rash develops
- To report palpitations, flushing if severe
- To avoid changes in temperature; extremities should be kept warm to promote better circulation

nalbuphine hydrochloride

Nubain
Func. class.: Narcotic analgesic
Chem. class.: Partial opiate agonist
Legal class.: POM

Action: Inhibits ascending pain pathways in CNS, increases pain threshold, alters pain perception
Uses: Moderate to severe pain, peri-operative analgesia
Dosage and routes:
- *Adult:* Subcutaneous/IM/IV 10–20 mg every 3–6 hr as required
- *Child:* Up to 300 mcg/kg repeated once or twice as necessary

Myocardial infarction, suspected
- *Adult:* Slow IV 10–20 mg repeated after 30 min if necessary

Premedication
- *Adult:* Subcutaneous/IM/IV 100–200 mcg/kg

Induction
- *Adult:* IV 0.3–1 mg/kg over 10–15 min

Intra-operative analgesia
- *Adult:* IV 250–500 mcg/kg at 30 min intervals

Available forms include: Injection subcutaneous, IM, IV 10 mg/ml 1 ml, 2 ml
Side effects/adverse reactions:
CNS: Dizziness, confusion, headache, sedation, speech difficulty
GI: Nausea, vomiting
INTEG: Urticaria, flushing
EENT: Blurred vision
CV: Tachycardia, bradycardia, change in BP
RESP: Respiratory depression
Contraindications: Hypersensitivity, addiction (opioid), head injury, increased intracranial pressure
Precautions: Addictive personality, pregnancy, lactation, respiratory depression, hepatic disease, renal disease, asthma
Pharmacokinetics:

Subcutaneous/IM/IV: Duration 3–6 hr; metabolised by liver, excreted by kidneys, half-life 5 hr

Interactions/incompatibilities:

• Effects may be increased with other CNS depressants: alcohol, narcotics, sedative/hypnotics, antipsychotics

Treatment of overdose: Naloxone IV, O_2, IV fluids, vasopressors

NURSING CONSIDERATIONS

Assess:

• Baseline vital signs, pupil size and reaction

• Fluid balance

• When pain is beginning to return; determine dosage interval by patient response

Administer:

• With anti-emetic if nausea, vomiting occur

Perform/provide:

• Storage in CD cupboard

• Assistance with ambulation

• Safety measures: siderails, night light, call-bell within easy reach

Evaluate:

• Therapeutic response: decrease in pain

• CNS changes: drowsiness, hallucinations, euphoria, level of consciousness, pupil reaction

• Allergic reactions: rash, urticaria

• Respirations: respiratory depression, character, rate, rhythm; notify clinician if respirations are less than 12/min

• Therapeutic response

Teach patient/family:

• To report any symptoms of CNS changes, allergic reactions

• That physical dependency may result when used for extended periods of time

• Withdrawal symptoms may occur: nausea, vomiting, cramps, fever, faintness, anorexia

• Importance of safe storage; risk to children

nalidixic acid

Negram, Mictral, Uriben

Func. class.: Antibiotic, urinary tract

Chem. class.: 4-Quinolone

Legal class.: POM

Action: Appears to inhibit DNA polymerisation, primary target being single-stranded DNA precursors in late stages of chromosomal replication

Uses: Urinary tract infections

Dosage and routes:

• *Adult:* By mouth 1 g 4 times a day for 7 days reduced to 500 mg every 6 hr in long-term treatment. Granules, 660 mg in water 3 times daily for 3 days

• *Child over 3 months:* By mouth 50 mg/kg daily in 4 divided doses; 30 mg/kg daily for long-term treatment

Available forms include: Tablets 500 mg; suspension 300 mg/5 ml, granules 660 mg/4.1 g sachet

Side effects/adverse reactions:

INTEG: Pruritus, rash, urticaria, photosensitivity, angioedema, arthralgia

CNS: Dizziness, headache, drowsiness, convulsions, weakness

GI: Nausea, vomiting, abdominal pain, diarrhoea

EENT: Sensitivity to light, blurred vision, change in colour perception

Contraindications: Hypersensitivity, infants less than 3 months, history of convulsive disorders, porphyria

Precautions: Elderly, renal disease, hepatic disease, G6PD deficiency

Pharmacokinetics:

By mouth: Peak 1–2 hr, metabolised in liver, excreted in urine (unchanged conjugates)

Interactions/incompatibilities:

• Increased effects of: oral anti-

coagulants
• Decreased effects of: antacids, iron supplements
Clinical assessment:
• Blood count for patients on chronic therapy
• Renal, hepatic function
Lab. test interferences:
False positive: Urinary glucose
False increase: 17-hydroxycorticosteroids, vanillylmandelic acid
NURSING CONSIDERATIONS
Assess:
• Fluid balance
Administer:
• Granules should be dissolved in water. Adjust dose in patients with creatinine clearance below 20 ml/min to half standard dosage
• After mid-stream urine is obtained for culture and sensitivity
Perform/provide:
• 2 litre fluid daily ensures that urinary pH is greater than 5.5
• Limited intake of alkaline foods, drugs: milk, dairy products, peanuts, vegetables, alkaline antacids, sodium bicarbonate
• Protect drug from freezing
Evaluate:
• CNS symptoms: insomnia, vertigo, headache, drowsiness, convulsions
• Allergy: fever, flushing, rash, urticaria, pruritus
• For photosensitivity
Teach patient/family:
• That photosensitivity occurs; that patient should avoid sunlight or use sunscreen to prevent burns
• Instruct patient to protect suspension from freezing, shake well before taking
• May cause drowsiness; advise patient not to drive or operate machinery while on medication and to seek help for walking if affected
• Instruct patients with diabetes that Clinitest may prove false positive for glucose

naloxone HCl

Narcan, Narcan Neonatal, Min-I-Jet
Func. class.: Narcotic antagonist
Chem. class.: Thebaine derivative
Legal class.: POM

Action: Competes with opioids at opioid receptor sites
Uses: Opioid-induced respiratory depression including pentazocine, dextropropoxyphene
Dosage and routes:
Opioid-induced respiratory depression
• *Adult:* IV/subcutaneous/IM 0.8–2 mg; repeat every 2–3 min, if required to maximum 10 mg (IV route faster onset)
• *Child:* 100 mcg/kg; then 100 mcg/kg if no response
Postoperative respiratory depression
• *Adult:* IV 0.1–0.2 mg every 2 min as required. Further doses by IM injection after 1–2 hr if required
• *Child:* IV 10 mcg/kg, then 0.1 mg/kg if no response. If IV route not possible may be given by IM or subcutaneous route in divided doses
• *Neonate:* IV/subcutaneous/IM 10 mcg/kg repeated every 2–3 min or 200 mcg (60 mcg/kg) IM at birth (onset on action slower)
Available forms include: Injection IV, IM, subcutaneous 20 mcg/ml, 0.4 mg/ml, 1 mg/ml
Side effects/adverse reactions:
GI: Nausea, vomiting
Contraindications: Hypersensitivity
Precautions: Pregnancy, opiate dependence (may precipitate acute withdrawal symptoms), cardiac irritability
Pharmacokinetics:
Metabolised by liver, excreted by kidneys, excreted in breast milk, half-life 1–3½ hr
NURSING CONSIDERATIONS

Assess:
• Baseline vital signs and neurological status
• Level of consciousness and respiratory rate to determine whether complete or partial reversal of opiate is required

Administer:
• IV, IM or subcutaneously
• Can be diluted in 0.9% sodium chloride or in 5% dextrose

Evaluate:
• Signs of withdrawal in drug-dependent individuals
• Therapeutic effect
• Cardiac status: tachycardia, hypertension
• Respiratory dysfunction: respiratory depression, character, rate, rhythm; if respirations are less than 10/min, respiratory stimulant should be administered

nandrolone decanoate/ nandrolone phenylpropionate

Deca-Durabolin, Deca-Durabolin 100, Durabolin

Func. class.: Androgenic anabolic steroid
Chem. class.: Halogenated testosterone derivative
Legal class.: POM

Action: Increases weight by building body tissue, increases potassium, phosphorus, chloride, nitrogen levels, increases bone development

Uses: Osteoporosis in postmenopausal women; aplastic anaemia

Dosage and routes:

Post-menopausal women
• Deep IM 50 mg every 3 weeks (decanoate). Deep IM 50 mg weekly (phenylpropionate)

Aplastic anaemia
• Deep IM 50–150 mg weekly (decanoate)

Anaemia of CRF
• Males, deep IM injection 200 mg weekly (decanoate)
• Females, deep IM injection 100 mg weekly (decanoate)

Anaemia due to cytotoxic chemotherapy
• Deep IM injection 200 mg weekly; to start at least 2 weeks prior to chemotherapy, then continue until blood count returned to normal

Available forms include: Phenylpropionate injection IM 25, 50 mg/ml; decanoate injection IM 25, 50, 100 mg/m (Deca-Durabolin 100)

Side effects/adverse reactions:
INTEG: Acneiform lesions, oily hair, acne vulgaris, hirsutism
MS: Premature epiphyseal closure
GU: Amenorrhoea, increased libido, inhibition of spermatogenesis, sodium and water retention, decreased breast size, clitoral hypertrophy
GI: Occasionally abnormal liver function tests
EENT: Voice deepening, hoarseness
ENDO: Abnormal glucose tolerance test

Contraindications: Known or suspected carcinoma of the prostate or mammary carcinoma in the male

Precautions: Diabetes mellitus, CV disease, liver dysfunction, skeletal metastases, renal dysfunction, hypertension, epilepsy, migraine

Pharmacokinetics:
IM: Metabolised in liver, excreted in urine, excreted in the breast milk

Interactions/incompatibilities:
• Increased effects of: oral antidiabetics
• Increased prothrombin urine:

anticoagulants
• Decreased effects of: insulin
Clinical assessment:
• Electrolytes: potassium, sodium, chloride calcium; cholesterol
• Liver function studies: alanine aminotransferase, aspartate aminotransferase, bilirubin

NURSING CONSIDERATIONS

Assess:
• Baseline weight, and BP
Administer:
• By deep IM injection
Perform/provide:
• Diet with increased calories, protein; decrease sodium if oedema occurs
Evaluate:
• Weight daily, notify clinician if weekly weight gain is greater than 2.5 kg
• Fluid balance; be alert for decreasing urinary output, increasing oedema
• Growth rate in children since growth rate may be uneven (linear/bone growth) when used for extended periods of time
• Therapeutic response: increased appetite, increased stamina
• Oedema, hypertension, cardiac symptoms, jaundice
• Mental status: affect, mood, behavioural changes, aggression
• Signs of masculinisation in female: increased libido, deepening of voice (sometimes irreversible), male: gynaecomastia, impotence, testicular atrophy
• Hypoglycaemia in diabetics; since oral anticoagulant action is decreased
• Acne, hirsutism
Teach patient/family:
• Drug needs to be combined with complete health plan: diet, rest, exercise
• To notify clinician if therapeutic response decreases
• Not to discontinue medication abruptly
• All aspects of drug usage; drug can be abused by athletes
• Females to report menstrual irregularities
• That long-term use may be necessary

naproxen/naproxen sodium

Naprosyn Nycopren, Synflex, Pranoxen, Continus, Arthrosin, Prosaid, Arthroxen, Rheuflex, Laraflex, Valrox, combination product
Func. class.: Non-steroidal anti-inflammatory drug
Chem. class.: Propionic acid derivative
Legal class.: POM

Action: Inhibits prostaglandin synthesis by decreasing an enzyme needed for biosynthesis; possesses analgesic, anti-inflammatory, antipyretic properties
Uses: Mild to moderate pain, osteoarthritis, rheumatoid arthritis (including juvenile arthritis), acute gout, other musculoskeletal disorders
Dosage and routes:
250 mg naproxen is equivalent to 275 mg naproxen sodium
• *Adult:* By mouth 500 mg–1 g daily in 2 divided doses, or 1 g once daily (base); Rectal route 500 mg at bedtime; if necessary another 500 mg in the morning
Available forms include: Tablets 250 mg, 275 mg, 375 mg, 500 mg, granules 500 mg/sachet, suspension 125 mg/5 ml, suppositories 500 mg tablets modified-release 375 mg, 500 mg
Side effects/adverse reactions:
GI: Nausea, vomiting, cholestatic jaundice; ulcerative stomatitis, peptic ulcer, colitis, bleeding
CNS: Insomnia, headache, in-

ability to concentrate, vertigo
CV: Peripheral oedema
INTEG: Purpura, rash, pruritus, sweating, vasculitis
GU: Nephrotoxicity: haematuria
HAEM: Blood dyscrasias
EENT: Tinnitus, hearing loss, blurred vision

Contraindications: Hypersensitivity, hypersensitivity to aspirin or other NSAIDS; asthma; severe renal disease; severe hepatic disease, active or suspected peptic ulcer or GI bleed; 3rd trimester of pregnancy

Precautions: Pregnancy, lactation, children, bleeding disorders, GI disorders, cardiac disorders, hypersensitivity to other NSAIDs

Pharmacokinetics:
By mouth: Peak 2 hr, half-life 3–3½ hr; metabolised in liver, excreted in urine (metabolites), excreted in breast milk

Interactions/incompatibilities:
- May increase action of: coumarin, phenytoin, sulphonamides when used with this drug
- Decreased antihypertensive effect of: propranolol and other β-blockers
- Increased blood levels of: lithium
- Increased levels of this drug: probenecid
- Enhanced toxicity of: methotrexate

Clinical assessment:
- Renal, liver, blood studies: blood urea nitrogen, creatinine, aspartate aminotransferase, alanine aminotransferase, Hb before treatment, periodically thereafter if problems anticipated

Lab. test intereferences:
Discontinue therapy 48 hr prior to adrenal function tests. May affect tests for urinary 5-hydroxyindoleacetic acid

Treatment of overdose: Gastric lavage and supportive measures; administer activated charcoal; haemodialysis may be appropriate in a patient with renal failure

NURSING CONSIDERATIONS

Administer:
- With or after food
- Mix granules in water and take immediately
- Swallow modified-release or enteric coated tablets whole not chewed
- Do not take indigestion mixtures at the same time as enteric coated tablets

Evaluate:
- Therapeutic response: decreased pain, stiffness, swelling in joints, ability to move more easily
- For eye, ear problems: blurred vision, tinnitus (may indicate toxicity)

Teach patient/family:
- To report blurred vision, ringing, roaring in ears (may indicate toxicity)
- To avoid driving or other hazardous activities if dizziness or drowsiness occurs
- To report change in urine pattern, weight increase, oedema, pain increase in joints, fever, blood in urine (indicates nephrotoxicity)
- That therapeutic effects may take up to 1 month
- To take with food or milk
- To report indigestion or black tarry stools

---

nedocromil sodium

Tilade
Func. class.: Anti-asthmatic
Chem. class.: Quinoline
Legal class.: POM

Action: Thought to prevent release of pharmacological mediators of bronchospasm by stabilising mast-cell membranes

Uses: Prophylaxis of reversible obstructive airways disease

Dosage and routes:

• *Adult:* Inhale 2 puffs (4 mg) twice daily increased to 2 puffs 6 hrly if necessary

Available forms include: Aerosol inhalation, 2 mg/dose

Side effects/adverse reactions:

CNS: Headache

GI: Nausea

EENT: Bitter taste in mouth

Contraindications: Children under 12 yr; known hypersensitivity

Precautions: Pregnancy, lactation

Pharmacokinetics: After inhalation nedocromil is deposited in the lungs, absorbed and excreted unchanged in bile and urine. Drug deposited in oropharynx is swallowed and poorly absorbed from GI tract. Drug does not accumulate on long term dosing and is not retained in any tissues

NURSING CONSIDERATIONS

Administer:

• By inhalation

Perform/provide:

• Gargle, sip of water to decrease irritation in throat

Evaluate:

• Respiratory status, respiratory rate, rhythm characteristics, cough, wheezing, dyspnoea

Teach patient/family:

• To clear mucus before using

• Proper inhalation technique: exhale, use inhaler, inhale deeply, remove, hold breath, exhale, repeat until all of the drug is inhaled

• That therapeutic effect may take up to 4 weeks

• Regular use is necessary

• Not effective during asthma attack

nefopam hydrochloride

Acupan

Func. class.: Analgesic

Chem. class.: Benzoxazocine

Legal class.: POM

Action: Not established

Uses: Relief of acute and chronic pain

Dosage and routes:

• By mouth initially 60 mg 3 times daily adjusted according to response; usual range 30–90 mg 3 times daily; elderly: half adult initial dose

• IM injection 20 mg 6-hrly

Available forms include: Tablets 30 mg; injection 20 mg/ml, 1 ml ampoule

Side effects/adverse reactions:

CNS: Nervousness, insomnia, drowsiness, blurred vision, headache

GI: Nausea, dry mouth, vomiting

CV: Tachycardia

INTEG: Sweating

GU: Urinary retention, may colour urine pink

Contraindications: Convulsive disorders, myocardial infarction, patients receiving MAOIs

Precautions: Renal or liver disease, glaucoma, urinary retention. Administer IM injection with patient lying down. Reduced dosage for elderly

Pharmacokinetics: Onset of effect after IM injection is 15–20 min, peak effect within 1½ hr. 60 mg oral is equivalent to 20 mg IM

Interactions:

• Tricyclic antidepressants, MAOIs

Tests/investigations: Renal and liver function tests if impairment suspected

Treatment of overdose: Gastric lavage and supportive measures. Administer activated charcoal

NURSING CONSIDERATIONS

Assess:

• Location, duration and severity of pain

Administer:

• With food to decrease GI symptoms

Perform/provide:

• Mouthwashes to relieve mouth dryness

Evaluate:

• Therapeutic response: decreased pain, stiffness, swelling in joints, ability to move more easily

• For eye, ear problems: blurred vision, tinnitus (may indicate toxicity)

• Urinary output

Teach patient/family:

• To report blurred vision, ringing, roaring in ears (may indicate toxicity)

• To avoid driving or other hazardous activities if dizziness or drowsiness occurs

• To report change in urine pattern, weight increase, oedema, pain increase in joints, fever, blood in urine (indicates nephrotoxicity)

• That therapeutic effects may take up to 1 month

---

neomycin sulphate

Mycifradin, Nivemycin

Func. class.: Antibiotic

Chem. class.: Aminoglycoside

Legal class.: POM

Action: Interferes with protein synthesis in bacterial cell by binding to ribosomal subunit causing inaccurate peptide sequence to form in protein chain, causing bacterial death

Uses: Hepatic coma. Pre-operatively to sterilise bowel

Dosage and routes: By mouth

Pre-operative bowel sterilisation

• *Adult:* 1 g every 1 hr for 4 doses, then 4 hrly for 2 or 3 days

• *Child more than 12 yr:* 1 g 4 hrly for 2–3 days

• *Child 6–12 yr:* 250–500 mg 4 hrly for 2–3 days

• *Child 1–5 yr*: 200–400 mg 4 hrly for 2–3 days

Hepatic coma

• *Adults:* 4–12 g daily in divided doses for 5–7 days

• *Child*: 50–100 mg/kg daily in divided doses

Available forms include: Tablets 500 mg; elixir 100 mg/5 ml

Side effects/adverse reactions:

GU: Nephrotoxicity

CNS: Confusion, nystagmus, paraesthesia, disorientation

EENT: Ototoxicity

HAEM: Haemolytic anaemia, blood dyscrasias

GI: Nausea, vomiting, diarrhoea, increased salivation, stomatitis, increased alanine aminotransferase, aspartate aminotransferase, bilirubin

CV: Hypotension, myocarditis

INTEG: Dermatitis, pruritus, drug fever, anaphylaxis

Contraindications: Bowel obstruction, hypersensitivity, children under 1 yr

Precautions: Neonates, hepatic coma (minimum period of administration), renal disease, pregnancy, hearing deficits, lactation, neuromuscular disorders

Pharmacokinetics: Only about 3% absorbed orally, but accumulation to toxic levels can occur especially in renal impairment. Excreted unchanged by kidneys, half-life 2 hr

Interactions/incompatibilities:

• Increased ototoxicity, neurotoxicity, nephrotoxicity: other aminoglycosides, amphotericin B, polymyxin, vancomycin, cyclosporin, cisplatin, cephalosporins, loop diuretics

• Increased effects: non-depolari-

sing muscle relaxants, oral anti-coagulants when given with oral neomycin
• Decreased effects of: oral digoxin, oral penicillin, oral contraceptives when given with oral neomycin
Treatment of overdose: Monitor renal and auditory function—if impaired dialysis indicated

NURSING CONSIDERATIONS

Assess:
• Weight before treatment; calculation of dosage is usually done based on ideal body weight, but may be calculated on actual body weight

Administer:
• After specimens taken for culture and sensitivity
• For oral use only (too toxic for parenteral use)

Perform/provide:
• Adequate fluids of 2–3 litres daily unless contraindicated to prevent irritation of tubules
• Supervised ambulation, other safety measures for patients with vestibular dysfunction

Evaluate:
• Fluid balance, urinalysis daily for proteinuria, cells, casts; report sudden change in urine output
• Urine pH if drug is used for urinary tract infection; urine should be kept alkaline
• When given in hepatic coma, or as pre-operative bowel preparation ensure that bowel motions take place
• Therapeutic effect: absence of fever, draining wounds, negative culture and sensitivity after treatment
• Renal impairment by securing urine for creatinine clearance testing, blood urea nitrogen, serum creatinine; lower dosage should be given in renal impairment (creatinine clearance less than 80 ml/min)
• Deafness by audiometric testing, ringing, roaring in ears, vertigo; assess hearing before, during, after treatment
• Dehydration: high specific gravity, decrease in skin turgor, dry mucous membranes, dark urine
• Vestibular dysfunction: nausea, vomiting, dizziness, headache; drug should be discontinued if severe

Teach patient/family:
• To report headache, dizziness, symptoms of overgrowth of infection, renal impairment
• To report loss of hearing, ringing, roaring in ears or a feeling of fullness in head

neomycin sulphate (ophthalmic/otic)

Minims, Neomycin sulphate, many combination products
Func. class.: Antibiotic
Chemical class.: Aminoglycoside
Legal class.: POM

Action: Inhibits protein synthesis in susceptible micro-organisms
Uses: Eye/ear infection (external)
Dosage and routes:
• *Adult and child:* Instil 2–4 drops 3 or 4 times a day into affected eye or ear. Eye ointment apply to eye one or more times daily
Available forms include: Single use Minims eye drops 0.5%, 0.5 ml. Many combination preparations of ear/eye drops/ointment
Side effects/adverse reactions:
EENT: Itching, irritation in ear/eye
INTEG: Rash
Contraindications: Hypersensitivity
Precautions: Perforated eardrum, glaucoma, short-term use only or resistant infections may occur; contact lenses, pregnancy

NURSING CONSIDERATIONS
Evaluate:
• Therapeutic response: decreased pain, reduced inflammation of the eye
• For redness, swelling, fever, pain in ear/eye, which indicates superimposed infection
Teach patient/family:
• Method of instillation using aseptic technique, including not touching dropper to ear/eye
• That dizziness may occur after instillation into ears

neomycin sulphate (topical)

Many combination products
Func. class.: Antibiotic
Chemical class.: Aminoglycoside
Legal class.: POM

Action: Interferes with bacterial protein synthesis
Uses: Skin infections
Dosage and routes:
• *Adult and child:* Topical apply to affected area 2 or 3 times a day
Available forms include: Combinations in cream, ointment, dusting powder, powder spray, spray application
Side effects/adverse reactions:
INTEG: Rash, urticaria, scaling, redness
Contraindications: Hypersensitivity, large areas, deafness, avoid prolonged usage, broken skin
Precautions: Pregnancy, lactation
Interactions/incompatibilities: None known
NURSING CONSIDERATIONS
Administer:
• After cleansing with soap and water before each application, dry well
• Enough medication to cover lesions completely
• Treatment should not be repeated for at least 3 months. Do not cover with occlusive dressings
Evaluate:
• Allergic reaction: burning, stinging, swelling, redness
• Therapeutic response: decrease in size, number of lesions
Teach patient/family:
• To wash hands before, after each application
• To apply using gloves to prevent further infection
• To avoid use of non-prescribed creams, ointments, lotions unless directed by clinician

neostigmine bromide/ neostigmine methylsulphate

Prostigmin, combination product
Func. class.: Anticholinesterase, cholinergic
Chem. class.: Quaternary compound
Legal class.: POM

Action: Inhibits destruction of acetylcholine, which increases concentration at sites where acetylcholine is released; this facilitates transmission of impulses across myoneural junction
Uses: Myasthenia gravis, neuromuscular blocking agent antagonist, bladder distention, paralytic ileus
Dosage and routes:
Myasthenia gravis
• *Adult:* By mouth 15–30 mg at intervals throughout the day. Total daily dose usually 5–20 tablets (higher doses may be needed); IM/subcutaneous injection 1–2.5 mg at intervals throughout the day, usual daily dose 5–20 mg

• *Child up to 6 yr:* By mouth, initially 7.5 mg
• *Child 6–12 yr:* By mouth initially 15 mg, usual total daily dose 15–90 mg
• *Child:* IM/subcutaneous injection 200–500 mcg as required
• *Neonate:* By mouth initially 1–2 mg then titrate to patient needs usually 1–5 mg every 4 hr, half an hour before feeds; IM/subcutaneous injection initially 0.1 mg then titrate to patient needs usually 50–250 mcg every 4 hr

Tubocurarine antagonist
• *Adult:* Slow IV over 1 min 0.05–0.07 mg/kg, may repeat if required, give 0.02–0.03 mg/kg atropine with or before this drug

Other indications
• *Adult:* IM/subcutaneous injection 0.5–2.5 mg or 1–2 tablets orally 4–6 hrly depending on condition
• *Child:* 2.5–15 mg orally or IM/subcutaneous injection 0.125–1 mg 4–6 hrly depending on condition

Approximate equivalent of different routes: 0.5 mg IV = 1–1.5 mg IM or subcutaneous = 15 mg orally

Available forms include: Tablets (bromide) 15 mg; injection (methylsulphate) 0.5 mg/ml, 2.5 mg/ml

Side effects/adverse reactions:
GI: Nausea, diarrhoea, vomiting, cramps, increased salivation

Contraindications: Gastrointestinal or urinary obstruction; hypersensitivity to drug or bromide in case of tablets

Precautions: Seizure disorders, bronchial asthma, coronary occlusion, vagotonia, peptic ulcer, bradycardia, parkinsonism, hypotension

Pharmacokinetics:
By mouth: Onset 2–4 hr, duration 2½–4 hr
IM/IV/subcutaneous: Onset 10–30 min, duration 2½–4 hr
Metabolised in liver, excreted in urine

Interactions/incompatibilities:
• Decreased action of: gallamine, metocurine, pancuronium, tubocurarine, atropine
• Increased action of: decamethonium, suxamethonium
• Decreased action of this drug: aminoglycosides, anaesthetics, β-blockers, lithium, procainamide, quinidine

Treatment of overdose: Artificial ventilation initiated if respiratory depression is severe. Atropine IV 1–2 mg antidote to muscarinic effects

NURSING CONSIDERATIONS

Assess:
• Baseline vital signs

Administer:
• On empty stomach for better absorption but with milk to avoid GI symptoms
• Give IV very slowly
• Always have atropine available when giving by injections
• Smaller doses required after thymectomy
• Dose titration to give best results with least toxicity
• May be given with atropine to minimise muscarinic effects

Perform/provide:
• Storage at room temperature

Evaluate:
• Therapeutic response: increased muscle strength, hand grasp, improved gait, absence of laboured breathing (if severe)
• Vital signs, respiration 4 hrly; more frequently if given to reverse anaesthetic paralysis
• Fluid balance; check for urinary retention or incontinence
• Bradycardia, hypotension, bronchospasm, headache, dizziness, convulsions, respiratory depression; drug should be discontinued if toxicity occurs

Teach patient/family:
• That drug is not a cure, it only relieves symptoms
• All aspects of drug: action, side effects, dose, when to notify clinician
• To wear Medic Alert ID specifying Myasthenia Gravis and drugs

---

netilmicin sulphate

Netillin
Func. class.: Antibiotic
Chem. class.: Aminoglycoside
Legal class.: POM

Action: Interferes with protein synthesis in bacterial cell by binding to ribosomal subunit, causing inaccurate peptide sequence to form in protein chain, causing bacterial death
Uses: Severe systemic infections of CNS, respiratory, GI, urinary tract, bone, skin, soft tissues, bacteraemia, septicaemia caused by *P. aeruginosa, E. coli, Enterobacter, Acinetobacter, Providencia, Citrobacter, Staphylococcus* spp, *K. pneumoniae, P. mirabilis, Serratia* spp plus all Gram-negative infections resistant to gentamicin
Dosage and routes:
Normal renal function
• *Adult and child over 12 yr:* IM/IV 4–6 mg/kg daily as a single daily dose or in divided doses 8–12 hrly, severe infections up to 7.5 mg/kg daily in divided doses every 8 hr
• *Child and infants 6 weeks–12 yr:* IM/IV 6.0–7.5 mg/kg daily in divided doses 8–12 hrly
• *Neonate over 1 week:* IM/IV 7.5–9.0 mg/kg daily in divided doses 8 hrly
• *Neonates under 1 week:* IM/IV 6 mg/kg daily in divided doses 12 hrly
• Adjust dose in renal impairment and according to blood drug level
Available forms include: Injection IM, IV 10, 50, 100 mg/ml
Side effects/adverse reactions:
GU: Adverse renal effects, generally mild in nature
CNS: Dizziness, headache, paraesthesia, vertigo
EENT: Ototoxicity, deafness, visual disturbances, tinnitus, roaring in the ears
GI: Vomiting, malaise, diarrhoea
CV: Hypotension, myocarditis, tachycardia
INTEG: Rash
Contraindications: Hypersensitivity
Precautions: Neonates, renal disease, pregnancy, children less than 12 yr, lactation, myasthenia gravis, hearing deficit
Pharmacokinetics:
IM: Onset rapid, peak 1–2 hr
IV: Onset immediate, peak 1–2 hr
Plasma half-life 2–3 hr, not metabolised, excreted unchanged in urine
Interactions/incompatibilities:
• Increased ototoxicity, neurotoxicity, nephrotoxicity: other aminoglycosides, amphotericin B, polymyxin, vancomycin, frusemide, mannitol, cisplatin, cephalosporins
• Do not mix in solution or syringe: carbenicillin, ticarcillin, amphotericin B, cephalothin, erythromycin, heparin
• Increased effects: non-depolarising muscle relaxants
Clinical assessment:
• Serum peak, drawn at 60 min after IV infusion or 60 min after IM injection (peak 5–12 mg/litre); trough level drawn just before next dose (trough less than 2 mg/litre). Higher peak acceptable in once daily dosing
Lab. test interferences:
Increase: Blood sugar, alkaline phosphatase, aspartate aminotransferase, alanine aminotransferase, prothrombin time

Decrease: Hb, WBC, platelets
Treatment of overdose: Haemodialysis, monitor serum levels of drug

NURSING CONSIDERATIONS

Assess:
- Baseline vital signs
- Weight before treatment; calculation of dosage is usually done based on ideal body weight, but may be calculated on actual body weight
- Fluid balance
- Ensure "peak and trough" levels are seen before administering second 24 hr prescribed regime

Administer:
- Preferably IM, but if necessary IV bolus over 3–5 min or IV infusion in 50–200 ml of fluid over half to 2 hr. Adjust dosage according to renal and auditory function; pre-dose (trough) concentrations should be less than 2 mg/l
- After samples have been sent for culture and sensitivity
- IM injection in large muscle mass, rotate injection sites
- IV as 3–5 min bolus or, more safely as an infusion over 30 min
- Drug in evenly spaced doses to maintain blood level

Perform/provide:
- Adequate fluids of 2–3 litre daily unless contraindicated to prevent irritation of tubules
- Flushing of IV line with sodium chloride 0.9% or dextrose 5% after infusion
- Supervised mobilisation, other safety measures for patients with vestibular dysfunction

Evaluate:
- Vital signs during infusion, watch for hypotension, change in pulse
- IV site for thrombophlebitis including pain, redness, swelling every 30 min, change site if needed; apply warm compresses to discontinued site
- Therapeutic effect: absence of fever, draining wounds, negative culture and sensitivity after treatment
- Daily fluid balance, urinalysis for proteinuria, cells, casts; report sudden change in urinary output
- Dehydration: high specific gravity, decrease in skin turgor, dry mucous membranes, dark urine
- Renal impairment by securing urine for creatinine clearance testing, blood urea nitrogen, serum creatinine; a lower dosage should be given in renal impairment (creatinine clearance less than 100 ml/min)
- Deafness by audiometric testing, ringing, roaring in ears, vertigo; assess hearing before, during, after treatment
- Secondary infection: increased temperature, malaise, redness, pain, swelling, perineal itching, diarrhoea, stomatitis, change in cough or sputum
- Vestibular dysfunction: nausea, vomiting, dizziness, headache; drug should be discontinued if severe

Teach patient/family:
- To report headache, dizziness, symptoms of overgrowth of infection, renal impairment
- To report loss of hearing, ringing, roaring in ears or feeling of fullness in head

---

nicardipine hydrochloride

Cardene, Cardene SR
Func. class.: Antihypertensive, anti-anginal
Chem. class.: Dihydropyridine calcium-channel blockers
Legal class.: POM

Action: Inhibits calcium ion influx across cell membrane during cardiac depolarisation; produces relaxation of coronary vascular smooth muscle, peripheral vascular smooth muscle

Uses: Chronic stable angina pectoris, mild to moderate hypertension

Dosage and routes:

Angina

• *Adult:* By mouth initially 20 mg 3 times a day (range 60–120 mg daily)

Hypertension

• *Adult:* By mouth 20 mg 3 times a day initially (range 60–120 mg daily); if controlled on 20–30 mg 3 times daily can be given 30–40 mg twice daily; modified-release, initially 30 mg twice daily, usual dose 45 mg twice daily, range 30–60 mg twice daily

Available forms include: Capsules 20 mg, 30 mg; capsules, modified-release 30 mg, 45 mg

Side effects/adverse reactions:

CV: Dysrythmia, oedema, atrioventricular block, ventricular tachycardia, hypotension, palpitations, myocardial infarction, intracranial haemorrhage

GI: Nausea, vomiting, diarrhoea, gastric upset, constipation, hepatitis, salivation

GU: Polyuria, acute renal failure

INTEG: Rash, pruritus, urticaria

CNS: Headache, drowsiness, dizziness, depression, paraesthesia, somnolence

Contraindications: Hypersensitivity to dihydropyridines, cardiogenic shock

Precautions: Congestive cardiac failure, hypotension, hepatic impairment, children, renal disease, elderly

Pharmacokinetics:

By mouth: Onset 10 min, peak 1–2 hr, half-life 2–5 hr; metabolised by liver, excreted in urine (98% as metabolites)

Interactions/incompatibilities:

• Increased effects of: digitalis, neuromuscular blocking agents, cyclosporin

• Increased effects of nicardipine: cimetidine

Lab. test interferences:

Transient elevation of liver function tests, glucose, serum bilirubin, blood urea nitrogen and creatinine. Triiodothyronine, thyroxine and TSH may also be affected abnormally

NURSING CONSIDERATIONS

Assess:

• Baseline vital signs, ECG

Evaluate:

• Response to treatment: decrease in pain from angina, fall in blood pressure

• Cardiac function: blood pressure, pulse, respirations, ECG daily

• For side effects

Teach patient/family:

• To avoid non-prescription medicines unless directed by clinician

• Emphasise the importance of every aspect of treatment: diet, exercise, reduction in stress and smoking as well as taking drug

• Clinician must be informed of palpitations, shortness of breath, swollen feet and hands, pronounced dizziness, constipation, nausea

---

niclosamide

Yomesan

Func. class.: Anthelmintic

Chem. class.: Salicylamilide derivative

Legal class.: P

Action: Inhibits synthesis in mitochondria; leads to destruction in intestine where worm may be digested, removed in faeces; not effective for ova or larval stage

Uses: Regular, dwarf tapeworms
Dosage and routes:
Taenia solium
• *Adult:* By mouth 2 g as a single dose after a light breakfast, followed by a purgative after 2 hr
• *Child up to 2 yr:* By mouth 500 mg
• *Child 2–6 yr:* By mouth 1 g
T. saginata and Diphyllobothrium latum
• As for *T. solium*, but half the dose may be taken after breakfast and the remainder 1 hr later followed by a purgative after a further 2 hr
Hymenolepsis nana
• *Adult:* 2 g on first day, then 1 g daily for 6 days
• *Child up to 2 yr:* By mouth quarter adult dose
• *Child 2–6 yr:* By mouth half adult dose
Available forms include: Tablets, chewable 500 mg
Side effects/adverse reactions:
INTEG: Pruritus
CNS: Dizziness
GI: Nausea, vomiting, abdominal pain
Contraindications: Hypersensitivity
Precautions: Child under 2 yr, pregnancy, lactation
Treatment of overdose: Enemas, laxatives; do not induce vomiting

NURSING CONSIDERATIONS

Assess:
• Stools during entire treatment, 1, 3 months after treatment; specimens must be sent to laboratory while still warm. Gloves must be worn when handling any stools
Administer:
• May be crushed and washed down with water, mixed with water if unable to swallow whole
• Laxatives if constipated; not necessary for drug to work, but will assist expulsion of worm
• After breakfast, tablet must be chewed, and then swallowed
Perform/provide:
• Storage in original packaging
Evaluate:
• Therapeutic response; expulsion of worms, 3 negative stool cultures after completion of treatment
• For allergic reaction: rash
• For diarrhoea during expulsion of worms
• For infection in other family members since infection from person to person is common
Teach patient/family:
• Proper hygiene after bowel movement including handwashing technique; tell patient to avoid putting fingers in mouth
• That infected person should sleep alone
• That bed linen should be changed daily and washed in hot water
• Bed clothes should not be shaken
• To clean toilet daily with disinfectant
• Need for compliance with dosage schedule, duration of treatment
• To drink fruit juice to remove mucous that intestinal tapeworms burrow in, aids in expulsion of worms (dwarf tapeworms only)
• To avoid alcohol
• To wash all fresh fruit and vegetables

nicotinamide

Func. class.: Vitamin B group
Chem. class.: Pyridine derivative
Legal class.: GSL

Action: Necessary for conversion of fats, protein, carbohydrates by oxidation reduction. Deficiency causes pellagra
Uses: Prophylactic, vitamin B deficiency
Dosage and routes:

Prophylactic

• *Adult:* By mouth 15–30 mg daily

Vitamin B deficiency

• *Adult:* By mouth usually 60–120 mg, but up to 920 mg daily by IV infusion (as high potency vitamins B and C injection) in Wernicke's encephalopathy and Korsakoff's psychosis

Available forms include: Tablets 50 mg; many combination products tablets, capsules, injections

Side effects/adverse reactions: Unlikely in therapeutic doses, though anaphylactic reactions possible with vitamins B and C injection IV

Contraindications: Hypersensitivity

Pharmacokinetics: Well absorbed orally, metabolised in liver, small amounts excreted unchanged in urine

Treatment of overdose: Unlikely to be of clinical significance

NURSING CONSIDERATIONS

Assess:

• Baseline vital signs

• Ability of patient to manage own medication

Administer:

• IV, slowly (over 10 min); IM into large muscle mass; when oral intake is inadequate or impossible orally

Perform/provide:

• Equipment and drugs to deal with anaphylaxis

Evaluate:

• For allergic reactions during or shortly after IV or IM administration

• That tablets are taken

• Therapeutic response

Teach patient/family:

• Reason for medication

• Other supporting mechanisms (in chronic alcoholism)

nicotine

NHS Nicorette, Nicorette Plus Nicotinelle TTS Nicabate

Func. class.: Smoking deterrant

Chem. class.: Cholinergic

Legal class.: POM/P (depending upon strength)

Action: Increase catecholamine release from adrenal medulla by stimulating receptors in CNS

Uses: Nicotine substitution as an aid to smoking cessation

Dosage and routes:

Chewing gum

• *Adult:* 1 piece 2 mg or 4 mg chewed for ½ hr as required to abstain from smoking, maximum 15 4-mg pieces daily; withdraw gradually after 3 months

Transdermal patches

Nicabate

• *Adult:* Smoking more than 10 cigarettes daily, initially 21 mg patch applied to skin and replaced every 24 hr for 4–6 weeks, then 14 mg patch for 2–4 weeks, then 7 mg patch for 2–4 weeks; individual smoking fewer than 10 cigarettes daily or with cardiovascular disease or weighing less than 45 kg, initially 14 mg patch daily for 4–6 weeks, then 7 mg patch daily for a further 2–4 weeks

Nicorette

• *Adult:* Initially 15 mg patch applied to skin for 16 hr in every 24 hr for 8 weeks, then 10 mg patch for 16 hr daily for 2 weeks, then 5 mg patch for 16 hr daily for 2 weeks

Nicotinell TTS

• *Adult:* Smoking more than 20 cigarettes daily, initially '30' patch applied to skin and replaced every 24 hr, withdraw gradually by changing to lower strength patch every 3–4 weeks; individuals smoking fewer than 20 cigarettes

daily start with '20' patch
Available forms include: Chewing gum 2, 4 mg (as resin complex); Transdermal patches 5, 10, 15 mg/16 hr and 7, 14, 21 mg/24 hr
Side effects/adverse reactions:
EENT: Jaw ache, irritation in buccal cavity, excessive salivation
CNS: Dizziness, headache
GI: Nausea, indigestion
INTEG: At site of patch, skin reactions have included erythema, pruritus, blisters, burning/pinching sensations
MISC: Hiccup
Contraindications: Hypersensitivity, pregnancy, breast-feeding
Precautions: Gastritis, peptic ulcer, angina, coronary artery disease
Pharmacokinetics: Metabolised in liver, excreted in urine, half-life 2–3 hr, all available nicotine is released from gum after 30 min chewing. Patch: 1–2 hr for nicotine passage into plasma. Plateau plasma concentrations at 8–10 hr after application
Treatment of overdose: Gastric lavage with wide bore tube, activated charcoal, supportive care

NURSING CONSIDERATIONS

Assess:
• Number of cigarettes smoked and dependence
• Local skin reaction due to patch application
Administer:
• Gum: Ensure that patient understands that gum should be chewed slowly
• Patches: Should be applied to dry, non-hairy skin on trunk or upper arm; application sites should be rotated; 16-hour patches should be removed at night
Evaluate:
• Adverse reaction: irritation of buccal cavity, dislike of taste, jaw ache
• Therapeutic response: decrease in urge to smoke, decreased need for gum after 3–6 months
Teach patient/family:
• To chew gum slowly for 30 min to promote buccal absorption of the drug; do not chew over 45 min
• Not to exceed the recommended dose
• To begin drug withdrawal after 3 months use; not to exceed 6 months
• All aspects of drug; give package insert to patient
• That gum will not stick to dentures, dental appliances
• That gum is as toxic as cigarette; it is to be used only as an aid to smoking cessation
• Not to use during pregnancy; birth defects may occur

nicotinic acid

Func. class.: Hypolipidaemic
Chem. class.: Pyridine derivative
Legal class.: P

Action: B vitamin with actions of nicotinamide, though seldom used in deficiency because of side effects; high doses decrease serum lipids
Uses: Hyperlipidaemias, has also been used in peripheral vascular disease
Dosage and routes:
Adjunct in hyperlipidaemia
• *Adult:* By mouth 300–600 mg daily in 3 divided doses after meals, may be increased to 6 g daily over 2–4 weeks
Available forms include: Tablets 50 mg; many combination products
Side effects/adverse reactions:
CNS: Headache, dizziness, faintness
GI: Nausea, vomiting, anorexia, flatulence, jaundice, diarrhoea, peptic ulcer, abdominal cramps

GU: Hyperuricaemia, glycosuria
CV: Postural hypotension, pounding in head
EENT: Blurred vision, ptosis
INTEG: Flushing, dry skin, rash, hyperpigmentation, pruritus
SYST: Sensation of heat
METAB: Decreased glucose tolerance
Contraindications: Hypersensitivity, pregnancy, lactation
Precautions: Glaucoma, cardiovascular disease, diabetes mellitus, gout, history of peptic ulceration, impaired liver function
Pharmacokinetics:
By mouth: Peak 30–70 min, half-life 45 min, metabolised in liver, 30% excreted unchanged in urine (more after high doses)

NURSING CONSIDERATIONS

Assess:
• Blood glucose before and during treatment

Administer:
• With meals for GI symptoms
• If CNS and INTEG side effects severe, take low initial doses with meals or take aspirin 300 mg 30 min before the dose

Evaluate:
• Therapeutic response: decreased lipids, warm extremities, absence of numbness in extremities
• Nutritional status
• Liver dysfunction: clay coloured stools, itching, dark urine, jaundice
• CNS symptoms: headache, paraesthesias, blurred vision

Teach patient/family:
• To remain recumbent if postural hypotension occurs
• To abstain from alcohol if drug is prescribed for hyperlipidaemia
• To avoid sunlight if skin lesions are present
• To take a diet rich in liver, yeast, legumes, lean poultry, offal

nicoumalone

Sinthrome
Func. class.: Anticoagulant
Chem. class.: Coumarin
Legal class.: POM

Action: Interferes with blood clotting. Antagonises effects of vitamin K-dependent coagulation factors
Uses: Deep vein thrombosis, pulmonary embolism, transient ischaemic attacks, prophylaxis of embolism with prosthetic heart valves, rheumatic
Dosage and routes:
• *Adult:* By mouth 8–12 mg on day 1; 4–8 mg on day 2; maintenance dose usually 1–8 mg daily
Available forms include: Tablets 1 mg, 4 mg
Side effects/adverse reactions:
CNS: Fever
GI: Loss of appetite, nausea, vomiting
HAEM: Haemorrhage
INTEG: Reversible alopecia, dermatitis, urticaria, haemorrhagic skin necrosis
Contraindications: Severe hypertension, pericarditis, pericardial effusion, subacute endocarditis, severe hepatic or renal disease, increased fibrinolytic activity, following surgery on lung, prostate and uterus, peptic ulcer, pregnancy, hypersensitivity, haemorrhagic diathesis, blood dyscrasias, pre- and post-surgery on CNS or eyes, haemorrhage in GI, urogenital or respiratory tracts and cardiovascular system
Precautions: Hepatic or renal disease, lactation (give infant vitamin K), thyrotoxicosis, tumours, infection, inflammation, severe heart failure, elderly, other IM injections

Pharmacokinetics: Rapidly absorbed, at least 60% of dose is available systemically. Peak plasma concentration after 1–3 hr. Over 98% bound to plasma protein. Extensively metabolised, in liver and excreted in faeces and urine. Plasma half-life is 8–11 hr

Interactions/incompatibilities:

• May be inhibited by: aminoglutethimide, barbiturates, carbamazepine, dichloralphenazone, griseofulvin, oral contraceptives, phenytoin, primidone, rifampicin, vitamin K, cholestyramine, thiazide diuretics

• May be potentiated by: alcohol, allopurinol, amiodarone, anabolic steroids, androgens, anti-arrhythmics, azapropazone, aztreonam, bezafibrate, cephamandole, chloral hydrate, chloramphenicol, cimetidine, clofibrate, co-trimoxazole, danazol, azithromycin, ciprofloxacin, dextropropoxyphene, enoximone, diflunisal, disulfiram, erythromycin, ethacrynic acid, glucagon, heparin, fluvoxamine, ifosfamide, oral hypoglycaemics paroxetine, omeprazole, flurbiprofen, fluconazole, itraconazole, gemfibrozil, ketoconazole, latamoxef, mefenamic acid, metronidazole, miconazole, nalidixic acid, neomycin, norfloxacin, flutamide, influenza vaccine, phenylbutazone, phenytoin, piroxicam, quinidine, propafenone, proguanil, simvastatin, rowachol, sulindac, sulphinpyrazone, sulphonamides, tamoxifen, tetracyclines, thyroxine, tolmetin, trimethoprim

• Increased prothrombin time: broad-spectrum antibiotics

• Increased risk of bleeding due to antiplatelet effect: aspirin, dipyridamole

Clinical assessment:

• Blood tests (Hb, platelets, occult blood in stools) 3 monthly

• Prothrombin time daily until stabilised

Lab. test interferences:

Increase: Triiodothyronine uptake

Decrease: Uric acid

Treatment of overdose: If patient's thromboplastin time was normal at time of overdosage, reduce drug absorption by emesis or gastric lavage combined with activated charcoal or fast-acting laxative. Vitamin K may antagonise nicoumalone in 3–5 hr. Moderate haemorrhage: give vitamin K by mouth 2–5 mg, severe cases require 1–10 mg by very slow IV injection. In life-threatening haemorrhage give fresh frozen plasma or whole blood

NURSING CONSIDERATIONS

Assess:

• BP

Administer:

• At the same time each day to maintain steady blood levels

• Alone—do not give with food

• Avoid all IM injections that may cause bleeding

Evaluate:

• For signs of hypertension

• Therapeutic response: decrease in deep vein thrombosis

• Any signs of bleeding, e.g. black stools, haematuria

Teach patient/family:

• To take drug at same time every day

• To avoid non-prescribed medications unless directed by clinician

• Urine may be discoloured

• To report any signs of bleeding to the clinician

nifedipine

Adalat, Adalat Retard, Adalat LA, Adalat IC, Corceten, Nifensar XL, Angiopine, Calcilat, combination products
Func. class.: Antihypertensive, antianginal
Chem. class.: Dihydropyridine calcium-channel blocker
Legal class.: POM

Action: Inhibits calcium ion flux across cell membranes relaxing arterial smooth muscle both in the coronary and peripheral circulation
Uses: Prophylaxis and treatment of angina, treatment of Raynaud's phenomenon, and hypertension
Dosage and routes:
Angina
• *Adult:* By mouth initially 10 mg 3 times daily; maintenance 5–20 mg 3 times daily; for immediate effect, capsule may be bitten, liquid retained or swallowed
Hypertension
• *Adult:* By mouth, modified-release, usual dose 10–40 mg
Coronary vasospasm
• *Adult:* By coronary catheter, 100–200 mcg over 90–120 seconds; maximum 6 dose of 200 mcg over 3 hr
Raynaud's phenomenon
• *Adult:* By mouth initially 10 mg 3 times daily; maintenance 5–20 mg 3 times daily
Available forms include: Capsules 5 mg, 10 mg; tablets modified-release 10 mg, 20 mg, 30 mg, 60 mg; capsules modified-release 10 mg, 20 mg; coronary injection 100 mcg/ml
Side effects/adverse reactions:
CV: Oedema, tachycardia, hypotension, palpitations, ischaemic pain
GI: Nausea, gastric upset, gingival hyperplasia
INTEG: Rash, pruritus, flushing
CNS: Headache, fatigue, drowsiness, dizziness, anxiety, depression, paraesthesia
Contraindications: Hypersensitivity to dihydropyridines, cardiogenic shock
Precautions: Congestive cardiac failure, hypotension, hypovolaemia, hepatic impairment, children, renal disease, diabetes mellitus, pregnancy
Pharmacokinetics:
By mouth: Capsules onset 10 min, peak 30 min, tablets duration 6–12 hr, half-life 4 hr; 90% protein bound, metabolised by liver, excreted in urine (98% as metabolites)
Interactions/incompatibilities:
• Effects of nifedipine may be potentiated by: cimetidine
• Increased effects of: hypoglycaemia, levodopa, quinidine
• Decreased effects: noradrenaline, isoprenaline, digitoxin
Treatment of overdose: Gastric lavage and charcoal instillation have been used. Calcium gluconate may be helpful with IV atropine for bradycardia

NURSING CONSIDERATIONS

Assess:
• Baseline vital signs and ECG; blood sugar (glucose) levels
Administer:
• Sublingually; break capsule
Perform/provide:
• Ensure capsule breaks and content is absorbed in the mouth
Evaluate:
• Therapeutic response: decreased anginal pain
• Improvement in temperature of digits
Teach patient/family:
• How to take pulse before taking drug; record or graph should be kept

• To avoid hazardous activities until stabilised on drug or dizziness is no longer a problem
• To limit caffeine consumption (coffee, tea, chocolate)
• To avoid non-prescribed drugs unless directed by clinician
• Stress patient compliance to all areas of medical regimen, diet, exercise, stress reduction, drug therapy
• To report side effects; headaches, dizziness, paraesthesia

---

nimodipine

Nimotop
Func. class.: Cerebral vasodilator
Chem. class.: Calcium channel blocker
Legal class.: POM

Action: Interferes with inward displacement of calcium ions through the slow channels of active smooth muscle cell membranes resulting in relaxation
Uses: Treatment and prevention of ischaemic neurological deficits caused by arterial spasm following subarachnoid haemorrhage
Dosage and routes:
Prophylactic
• *Adult:* By mouth, 60 mg 4-hrly for 21 days
Therapeutic
• *Adult:* IV infusion via central catheter; initially 1 mg/hr (5 ml/hr neat solution), increased after 2 hr to 2 mg/hr (10 mg/hr neat solution), provided no severe decrease in BP has occurred; in patients with unstable BP or weighing less than 70 kg initially 500 mcg/hr. Treatment to start as soon as possible and continue for 5–14 days; if surgery performed while treatment is in progress, continue for at least 5 days after
Available forms include: IV infusion, 200 mcg/ml; tablets 30 mg
Side effects/adverse reactions:
CV: Hypotension, variation in heart rate
CNS: Headache
GI: Disturbances, nausea, transient increase in liver enzymes during infusion
SYST: Feeling of warmth
INTEG: Flushing
Precautions: Cerebral oedema, raised intracranial pressure, impaired renal function, pregnancy
Pharmacokinetics: 50% absorbed orally, extensive first-pass metabolism. Metabolised in liver, plasma half-life 1–6 hr; 95% protein bound
Interactions/incompatibilities:
• Nimodipine potentiates: other hypotensives, avoid co-administration with calcium channel blockers/β-blockers if possible
• Increased risk of nephrotoxicity with: nephrotoxic drugs
• Incompatible with: PVC infusion materials
Clinical assessment:
• BP
• Renal function in patients with impairment or on nephrotoxic drugs
Treatment of overdose: Gastric lavage and activated charcoal after oral ingestion/stop IV infusion. Monitor BP, give dopamine or noradrenaline if very low

NURSING CONSIDERATIONS

Assess:
• Baseline vital signs and weight (if possible)
Administer:
• By intravenous infusion via central catheter using a controlled delivery pump
• Use Y-connection to dilute infusion solution during administration
• Orally in tablet form
Evaluate:

• Therapeutic response
• Vital signs

Perform/provide:

• Full neurological observations
• Use of PVC apparatus should be avoided

nitrazepam

Mogadon, Remnos, Somnite, Unisomnia

Func. class.: Sedative hypnotic
Chem. class.: Benzodiazepine
Legal class.: CD (Sch. 4), POM (only prescribable generically on NHS)

Action: Depresses CNS with sedative and hypnotic effects

Uses: Short-term treatment of insomnia

Dosage and routes:

• *Adult:* By mouth, 5–10 mg at bedtime
• *Elderly or debilitated:* By mouth, 2.5–5 mg at bedtime

Available forms include: Tablets, 5 mg; oral suspension, 2.5 mg/5 ml; capsules, 5 mg

Side effects/adverse reactions:

CNS: Drowsiness, and lightheadedness the following day; ataxia and confusion, especially in the elderly; dependence, rebound insomnia on withdrawal; headache; vertigo, changes in libido, paradoxical excitement and aggression
CV: Hypotension
GI: GI upsets, jaundice
GU: Urinary retention
HAEM: Dyscrasia
INTEG: Rash

Contraindications: Hypersensitivity; respiratory depression; acute pulmonary insufficiency; phobic or obsessional states; chronic psychosis; porphyria

Precautions: Respiratory disease; muscle weakness; history of drug abuse; marked personality disorder; pregnancy; breast-feeding; hepatic impairment; renal impairment; elderly or debilitated patients; prolonged use; abrupt withdrawal after prolonged use; bereavement or loss (may inhibit psychological adjustment)

Pharmacokinetics: Well absorbed following oral administration, peak plasma levels within 2 hr of administration; metabolised in the liver to inactive metabolites; excreted in urine; elimination half-life 24 hr

Interactions:

• Enhanced sedative effect with: alcohol, anaesthetics, opioid analgesics, isoniazid, cimetidine, antidepressants, antihistamines, alpha-blockers, antipsychotics, lofexidine, baclofen, nabilone
• Reduced anticonvulsant action of: clonazepam
• Increased CNS side-effects given with: anticonvulsants, especially barbiturates and phenytoin

Treatment of overdose: Gastric lavage if performed promptly; supportive treatment; flumazenil may be used to antagonise

NURSING CONSIDERATIONS

Assess:

• The need for hypnotic prior to administration if prescribed PRN

Administer:

• Short term treatment for insomnia
• Tablets at bedtime, lower dose in elderly or debilitated
• Avoiding in respiratory disease/disorder

Perform/provide:

• Storage protected from the light

Evaluate:

• Therapeutic response: ability to sleep at night
• Mental status, confusion; excitement, aggression
• Dependence
• Drowsiness, lightheadedness the following day

- BP as may cause hypotension
- Jaundice
- Urinary output as can cause urinary retention
- Respiratory status

Teach patient/family:

- To avoid activities (i.e. driving) requiring alert status until stabilized
- To avoid: alcohol ingestion; opiod analgesics; antidepressants; as these can enhance sedative effect
- Alternative measures to improve sleep

---

nitrofurantoin

Furandantin, Macrodantin
Func. class.: Antibiotic
Chem. class.: Nitrofuran derivative
Legal class.: POM

Action: Unclear but may involve interference with a number of bacterial enzymes

Uses: Urinary tract infection, pyelitis

Dosage and routes:

Acute infection

- *Adults:* By mouth 50 mg 4 times a day for 7 days, increased to 100 mg 4 times a day in severe infection
- *Child over 3 months:* By mouth 3 mg/kg daily in 4 divided doses for 7 days

Surgical prophylaxis

- *Adults:* By mouth 50 mg 4 times a day on the day of procedure and for another 3 days

Long-term suppressive treatment

- *Adults:* By mouth 50–100 mg daily
- *Child over 3 months:* By mouth 1 mg/kg daily as a single dose

Available forms include: Capsules 50, 100 mg; tablets 50, 100 mg; suspension 25 mg/5ml

Side effects/adverse reactions:

INTEG: Pruritus, rash, urticaria, angioedema, alopecia, erythema multiforme, exfoliative dermatitis, arthralgia

CNS: Dizziness, headache, drowsiness, vertigo, nystagmus, asthenia

RESP: Acute and subacute pulmonary reactions (fever, chills, cough, chest pain, dyspnoea, pulmonary infiltration and consolidation, pleural effusion), chronic pulmonary reactions (malaise, dyspnoea on exertion, cough, altered pulmonary function

HAEM: Agranulocytosis, leucopenia, granulocylopenia, haemolytic anaemia, anaemia, thrombocytopenia, megaloblastic anaemia, eosinophilia, aplastic anaemia

GI: Nausea, vomiting, abdominal pain, diarrhoea, cholestatic jaundice, chronic active hepatitis, pancreatitis

Contraindications: Hypersensitivity, severe renal disease (creatinine clearance less than 60 ml/min), infants under 3 months, pregnancy at term, G6PD deficiency

Precautions: Pregnancy, lactation, G6PD deficiency, anaemia, diabetes mellitus, electrolyte imbalance, vitamin B_{12} or folate deficiency, pulmonary disease, hepatic impairment, neurological disorders, allergic diathesis

Interactions:

- Effects of nitrofurantoin increased by: probenecid
- Effects of nitrofurantoin antagonised by: nalidixic acid, quinolones
- Absorption of nitrofurantoin decreased by: magnesium trisilicate

Treatment of overdose: Induction of emesis or gastric lavage, maintain a high fluid intake. Nitrofurantoin can be haemodialysed

NURSING CONSIDERATIONS

Assess:
• Fluid balance, urine pH less than 5.5 is ideal for urinary tract infection
Administer:
• To be taken with or after food
• After clean-catch urine is obtained for culture and sensitivity
• As two daily doses if urine output is high or if patient has diabetes (medical decision)
• 2 litres fluid in 24 hr
Perform provide:
• Limited intake of alkaline foods or drugs: milk, dairy products, peanuts, vegetables, alkaline antacids, sodium bicarbonate
Evaluate:
• CNS symptoms: insomnia, vertigo, headache, drowsiness, convulsions
• Allergy: fever, flushing, rash, urticaria, pruritus
Teach patient/family:
• Take medication with food to decrease GI irritation
• Instruct patient to protect suspension from freezing and shake well before taking
• May cause drowsiness; instruct patient to seek aid in walking and other activities; advise patient not to drive or operate machinery while on medication
• Instruct patients with diabetes that Clinitest may prove false-positive for glucose; Clinistix or Labstix should be used
• Urine may be coloured dark yellow or brown whilst receiving drug

---

nizatidine

Axid
Func. class.: H_2-receptor antagonist
Chem. class.: Substituted thiazole
Legal class.: POM

Action: Blocks H_2 receptors thereby reducing gastric acid output
Uses: Benign gastric and duodenal ulceration, prevention of duodenal ulcer recurrence, symptomatic relief of gastro-oesophageal reflux
Dosage and routes:
Gastric and duodenal ulcer disease
• *Adult:* By mouth 300 mg at night or 150 mg twice daily for 4–8 weeks; maintenance 150 mg at night for up to 1 yr
Gastro-oesophageal reflux
• *Adult:* By mouth, 150–300 mg twice daily for up to 12 weeks
Available forms include: Capsules 150 mg, 300 mg
Side effects/adverse reactions:
CNS: Headache, somnolence, confusion, abnormal dreams
ENDO: Gynaecomastia
HAEM: Thrombocytopenia, eosinophilia
INTEG: Pruritus, sweating, urticaria, exfoliative dermatitis
MS: Myalgia
RESP: Bronchospasm, laryngeal oedema
METAB: Hyperuricaemia
GI: Elevated liver enzymes, hepatitis, jaundice, nausea
Contraindications: Hypersensitivity
Precautions: Renal or hepatic impairment (reduce dose in renal impairment), pregnancy, lactation
Pharmacokinetics: Partially metabolised by the liver and principally excreted by the kidney, plasma half-life 1.5 hr, 70% absorbed orally, small amount (0.1% of plasma concentration) enters breast milk, 35% bound to plasma proteins
Clinical assessment:
• Renal function tests: if impairment anticipated
Treatment of overdose: Symptomatic and supportive therapy is recommended. Activated charcoal, emesis or lavage may reduce absorption

NURSING CONSIDERATIONS

Assess:
• Gastric pH (greater than 5 should be maintained)
• Fluid balance

Administer:
• With meals for prolonged drug effect
• Antacids 1 hr before or 1 hr after drug

Evaluate:
• Mental status, confusion, dizziness, depression, anxiety, weakness, tremors, psychosis, diarrhoea, jaundice, report immediately
• For GI symptoms; nausea, vomiting, diarrhoea, cramps

Teach patient/family:
• That occasionally gynaecomastia, impotence may occur but are reversible
• Avoid driving or other hazardous activities until patient is stabilised
• To avoid black pepper, caffeine, alcohol, harsh spices, extremes in temperature of food
• To avoid non-prescribed preparations; aspirin, cough, cold preparations

---

noradrenaline acid tartrate

Levophed Levophed Special
Func. class.: Adrenergic agonist
Chem. class.: Sympathomimetic amine
Legal class.: POM

Action: Causes increased contractility and heart rate by acting on β-receptors in heart; also, acts on α-receptors, causing vasoconstriction in blood vessels; when larger doses are administered, causes vasodilatation in renal, intracerebral, coronary blood vessels
Uses: Acute hypotension
Dosage and routes:
• *Adult:* IV infusion 8–12 mcg/min titrated to BP
Levophed special
• *Adult:* Rapid IV or intracardiac injection 0.5–0.75 ml
Available forms include: Injection IV 200 mcg, 2 mg/ml
Side effects/adverse reactions:
CNS: Headache
CV: Palpitations, tachycardia, hypertension, ectopic beats, angina
GI: Nausea, vomiting
INTEG: Necrosis, tissue sloughing with extravasation, gangrene
Contraindications: Hypersensitivity, ventricular fibrillation, tachydysrhythmias, phaeochromocytoma
Precautions: Pregnancy, lactation, arterial embolism, peripheral vascular disease
Pharmacokinetics:
IV: Onset 1–2 min, metabolised in liver, excreted in urine (inactive metabolites)
Interactions/incompatibilities:
• Do not use within 2 weeks of MAOIs or hypertensive crisis may result
• Dysrhythmias: general anaesthetics, cardiac sensitising agents
• Decreased action of this drug: other β-blockers
• Increased BP: oxytocics
• Increased pressor effect: tricyclic antidepressant, MAOIs
• Incompatible with alkaline solutions: sodium bicarbonate, frusemide injection, phenytoin
Clinical assessment:
• ECG during administration continuously, if BP increases, drug is decreased
• CVP during infusion if possible
Administer:
• Plasma expanders for hypovolaemia
• Using 2 bottle set up so drug may be discontinued while IV is still running
Treatment of overdose: Admin-

ister phentolamine with care

NURSING CONSIDERATIONS

Assess:

- Baseline vital signs and ECG
- Fluid balance

Perform/provide:

- Dilute with dextrose 5% if necessary in preference to other infusion solutions
- Storage of reconstituted solution if refrigerated for no longer than 24 hr
- Do not use discoloured solutions
- Protect from light
- Continuous monitoring of vital signs (patient preferably in ICU)

Evaluate:

- For paraesthesia and coldness of extremities, peripheral blood flow may decrease: doppler monitoring
- Injection site: tissue sloughing; if this occurs, administer phentolamine mixed with normal saline
- Therapeutic response: increased BP with stabilisation

Teach patient/family:

- Reason for drug administration

---

norethisterone acetate/ enanthate

Micronor, Noristerat, Primolut-N, Utovlan, Noriday, Menzon, SH420, many combination products

Func. class.: Progestogen

Chem. class.: Progesterone derivative

Legal class.: POM

Action: Inhibits secretion of pituitary gonadotrophin, which prevents follicular maturation and ovulation

Uses: Menorrhagia, premenstrual syndrome, amenorrhea, endometriosis, progestogen-only contraception, also component of several oestrogen/progestogen oral contraceptives, inoperable breast cancer

Dosage and routes:

Menorrhagia, premenstrual tension

- *Adult*: By mouth 5 mg 2–3 times daily from the 19th–26th day of the cycle

Dysmenorrhoea

- *Adult:* By mouth 5 mg 3 times daily for 20 days, starting from the 5th day of the cycle for 3–4 cycles

Dysfunctional uterine bleeding

- *Adult:* By mouth 5 mg 3 times daily for 10 days

Prophylaxis

- 5 mg twice daily on the 19th to 26th days of cycle

Progestogen-only contraception

- *Adult:* By mouth 350 mcg (1 tablet) daily continuously. IM injection 200 mg within the first 5 days of menstrual cycle. Effects last for 8 weeks and injection may be repeated once

Endometriosis

- *Adult:* By mouth initially 10 mg daily commencing on 5th day of cycle, increasing to 30 mg daily if spotting occurs. After bleeding has stopped, the initial dose is usually adequate. Duration of treatment, 4–6 months

Inoperable breast cancer

- *Adult:* By mouth 10 mg (as acetate) 3 times a day for 6 weeks, then increase to 20 mg 3 times a day if necessary

Available forms include: Tablets 350 mcg, 5 mg; tablets 10 mg (as acetate), injection 200 mg/ml (as enanthate)

Side effects/adverse reactions:

CNS: Dizziness, headache, migraine, depression, fatigue, exacerbation of epilepsy

CV: Hypotension, thrombophlebitis, oedema, thromboembolism, stroke, pulmonary embolism, myocardial infarction

GI: Nausea, vomiting, anorexia,

cramps, weight gain, cholestatic jaundice
EENT: Diplopia
GU: Amenorrhoea, cervical erosion, breakthrough bleeding, dysmenorrhoea, vaginal candidiasis, breast changes, (gynaecomastia, testicular atrophy, impotence), endometriosis, chloasma, spontaneous abortion
INTEG: Hirsutism, acne, photosensitivity
META: Hyperglycaemia, malignant and benign hepatic tumours, hypercholesterolaemia
Contraindications: Breast cancer, or hormone dependant neoplasia, hypersensitivity, thrombophlebitis, thromboembolic disorders, reproductive cancer, genital bleeding (abnormal, undiagnosed), pregnancy, history of idiopathic jaundice, severe pruritus or herpes gestationis during pregnancy, Dubin–Johnson or Rotor syndromes
Precautions: Lactation, hypertension, asthma, congestive cardiac failure, myocardial infarction, diabetes mellitus, bone disease, depression, migraine headache, convulsive disorders, hepatic disease, renal disease, family history of breast or reproductive tract cancer, amenorrhoea, fluid retention
Pharmacokinetics:
By mouth: Duration 24 hr, excreted in urine, faeces, metabolised in liver
Interactions/incompatibilities:
• Efficacy of norethisterone may be reduced by: rifampicin, barbiturates, phenytoin, ampicillin, tetracycline, griseofulvin

NURSING CONSIDERATIONS

Assess:
• Baseline weight
• BP at beginning of treatment and periodically thereafter
Administer:
• Titrated dose, use lowest effective dose
• Solution deeply in large muscle mass (IM), rotate sites
• In one dose in morning
• With food or milk to decrease GI symptoms
Evaluate:
• Therapeutic response: decreased abnormal uterine bleeding, absence of amenorrhea
• For potential side-effects regularly
Teach patient/family:
• To avoid sunlight or use sunscreen, photosensitivity can occur
• All aspects of drug usage, including cushingoid symptoms
• To report side-effects, e.g. breast lumps, vaginal bleeding, oedema, jaundice, dark urine, clay-coloured stools, dyspnoea, headache, blurred vision, abdominal pain, numbness or stiffness in legs, chest pain; male to report impotence or gynaecomastia
• To report suspected pregnancy promptly

---

norfloxacin (ophthalmic.) ▼

Noroxin
Func. class.: Broad spectrum antibiotic
Chem. class.: Fluoroquinolone
Legal class.: POM

Action: Inhibits bacterial deoxyribonucleic acid synthesis, bactericidal
Uses: Topical treatment of external ocular infections including conjunctivitis, keratoconjunctivitis
Dosage and routes:
• *Adult and Child:* Instil one or two drops into affected eye 4 times a day. Severe infections, instil

drops every 2 hr during waking hours for first day of therapy.
Available forms include: Eyedrops 0.3%, 5 ml
Side effects/adverse reactions:
EENT: local burning or smarting, conjunctival hyperaemia, chemosis, photophobia.
GI: Bitter taste after instillation
Contraindications: Hypersensitivity
Precautions: Breast-feeding; pregnancy
Treatment of overdose: Flush eye thoroughly with water

NURSING CONSIDERATIONS

Assess:
- Ability of patient (or carer) to instil drops

Administer:
- After culture and sensitivity tests
- After cleaning the eye(s)
- As prescribed

Evaluate:
- Therapeutic effect: reduction in pain, swelling and obvious signs of infection
- For side effects

Teach patient/family:
- How to instil drops
- About side effects and to report any to nurse or clinician
- About hygiene related to eye infection; not to share face flannels, towels; not to touch or rub the eyes
- Not to use eye drops if wearing hydrophilic (soft) contact lenses

norfloxacin ▼

Utinor
Func. class.: Broad spectrum antibiotic
Chem. class.: Fluoroquinolone
Legal class.: POM

Action: Inhibits bacterial deoxyribonucleic acid synthesis, bactericidal
Uses: Treatment of urinary tract infections
Dosage and routes:
- *Orally:* Need not be taken on an empty stomach

Uncomplicated lower urinary tract infections
- 400 mg twice daily for 3 days

Urinary tract infections
- 400 mg twice daily for 7 days

Chronic relapsing urinary tract infection
- 400 mg twice daily for up to 12 weeks (reduced to 400 mg once daily after 4 weeks if adequate suppression achieved)

Available forms include: Tablets, 400 mg
Side effects/adverse reactions:
CNS: Headache, dizziness, sleep disturbances, depression, anxiety/nervousness, irritability, euphoria, disorientation, hallucination, epiphoria, confusion
GI: Nausea, heartburn, abdominal pain/cramps, diarrhoea, anorexia, pseudomembranous colitis, pancreatitis
INTEG: Rash, photosensitivity, Stevens-Johnson syndrome, toxic epidermal necrolysis, exfoliative dermatitis, erythema multiforme, pruritus
MS: Tinnitus, hypersensitivity: anaphylaxis, interstitial nephritis, angioedema, vasculitis, urticaria, arthritis, myalgia and arthralgia, abnormal liver function tests, blood disorders (eosinophilia, leucopenia, neutropenia, thrombocytopenia)
Contraindications: Hypersensitivity to norfloxacin or any quinolone antibiotic. Tablets are contraindicated in prepubertal children and growing adolescents
Precautions: History of convulsions. Use in pregnancy and lactation not recommended. Renal impairment (reduce dose)
Pharmacokinetics: Peak plasma levels after 1–2 hr; half-life

4 hr, excreted in urine and bile as active drug and metabolites
Interactions:
• Decreased absorption: antacids, iron sucralfate (administer two hrs apart).
• Increased risk of convulsions with non-steroidal anti-inflammatories
• Effect of oral anticoagulants increased
• Increased cyclosporin nephrotoxicity due to elevated blood levels
• Increased theophylline levels with norfloxacin
Treatment of overdose: Gastric lavage following oral ingestion

NURSING CONSIDERATIONS

Assess:
• Vital signs (temperature, pulse, respiration, BP)
• Fluid intake
• Age of patient (contraindicated in growing adolescents)
Administer:
• After culture and sensitivity tests, urine test
• May be taken with or without food, but with full glass of water
Perform/provide:
• Fluids 2–3 l daily, unless contraindicated
Evaluate:
• Therapeutic effect: reduction in fever; pain; frequency of micturition
• For side effects; wide variety affecting several systems
• Fluid intake and balance
Teach patient/family:
• That tablets must be taken as prescribed and the full course finished
• About side effects and to report any of these to nurse or clinician
• To take 2–3 l of clear fluids daily
• Not to be taken with antacids or iron preparations (reduced absorption)

norgestrel (levonorgestrel)

Cyclo-Progynova, Prempack C (all with oestrodiol)
Func. class.: Progestogen
Chem. class.: Progesterone derivative
Legal class.: POM

Action: Inhibits secretion of pituitary gonadotrophins, which prevents follicular maturation and ovulation
Uses: In combined preparations for menopausal symptoms
Dosage and routes:
• *Adult:* By mouth 1 tablet daily for 10 days of cycle (as combination product)
Side effects/adverse reactions:
CNS: Dizziness, headache, migraine, depression, fatigue, anxiety
CV: Hypotension, thrombophlebitis, oedema, thromboembolism, stroke, pulmonary embolism, myocardial infarction, cardiac symptoms
GI: Nausea, vomiting, anorexia, cramps, increased weight and appetite, cholestatic jaundice, dyspepsia
Available forms include: Tablets 500 mcg (with 1 mg or 2 mg oestradiol), 150 mcg (with 0.625 mg or 1.25 mg oestrogens, conjugated).
EENT: Diplopia
GU: Amenorrhoea, cervical erosion, breakthrough bleeding, dysmenorrhoea, vaginal candidiasis, breast changes, endometriosis, spontaneous abortion, altered libido
INTEG: Rash, acne, hirsutism, photosensitivity, leg pain and swelling
META: Hyperglycaemia
Contraindications: Breast cancer, hypersensitivity, thromboembolic

disorders, hormone dependent cancer, genital bleeding (abnormal, undiagnosed), cerebral haemorrhage, pregnancy, severe hepatic disease, liver tumour, history of idiopathic jaundice or pruritus in pregnancy, Dubin–Johnson or Rotor syndrome, sickle-cell anaemia, congenital disturbance of lipid metabolism, history of herpes gestationis, endometriosis, severe diabetes with vascular changes
Precautions: Lactation, hypertension, asthma, blood dyscrasias, gallbladder disease, congestive cardiac failure diabetes mellitus, bone disease, depression, migraine headache, convulsive disorders, hepatic disease, renal disease, family history of breast or porphyria, otosclerosis, reproductive tract cancer, multiple sclerosis, epilepsy, thyrotoxicosis
Pharmacokinetics:
By mouth: Duration 24 hr, excreted in urine and faeces, metabolised in liver
Clinical assessment:
• Liver function studies, aspartate aminotransferase, alanine aminotransferase, bilirubin, periodically during long-term therapy
• Use lowest effective dose
NURSING CONSIDERATIONS
Assess:
• Baseline BP, weight
Evaluate:
• Weight gain
• Alterations in BP
• Therapeutic response: decreased abnormal uterine bleeding, resumption of menses
• Oedema, hypertension, cardiac symptoms, jaundice
• Mental status: anxiety levels, mood, behavioural changes, depression
• Hypercalcaemia
Teach patient/family:
• Photosensitivity can occur rarely
• All aspects of drug usage, including Cushingoid symptoms
• To report side effects
• To report suspected pregnancy
• To monitor blood sugar, if diabetic
• Importance of taking tablets as prescribed

---

nortriptyline

Aventyl, Allegron, combination products
Func. class.: Antidepressant, tricyclic
Chem. class.: Dibenzocycloheptene—secondary amine
Legal class.: POM

Action: Blocks reuptake of noradrenaline, serotonin into nerve endings, increasing action of noradrenaline, serotonin in nerve cells
Uses: Endogenous depression, nocturnal enuresis
Dosage and routes:
• *Adult:* By mouth, initially 20–40 mg (elderly 30 mg) daily, increased gradually; maximum 100 mg daily
Nocturnal enuresis
• *Child:* By mouth 6–7 yr (20–25 kg) 10 mg at night, 8–11 yr (25–35 kg) 10–20 mg at night, over 11 yr (35–54 kg) 25–35 mg at night. Treatment should be for a maximum of 3 months
Available forms include: Capsules 10, 25 mg; tablets 10, 25 mg
Side effects/adverse reactions:
HAEM: Agranulocytosis, thrombocytopenia, eosinophilia, leucopenia, purpura
CNS: Dizziness, drowsiness, confusion, headache, anxiety, hallucinations, disorientation, delusions, restlessness, agitation, panic, hypomania, tremors, stimulation, weakness, insomnia, nightmares, extrapyramidal symptoms

(elderly), increased psychiatric symptoms, numbness, tingling, paraesthesia of extremeties, ataxia, peripheral neuropathy, seizures, EEG changes
GI: Constipation, dry mouth, nausea, vomiting, paralytic ileus, taste disturbance, weight gain or loss, parotid swelling, increased appetite, cramps, epigastric distress, jaundice, hepatitis, stomatitis, gingivitis, black tongue
GU: Retention, acute renal failure, urinary frequency, nocturia
INTEG: Rash, urticaria, sweating, pruritus, photosensitivity
CV: Orthostatic hypotension, ECG changes, tachycardia, hypertension, myocardial infarction, arrhythmias, heart block, stroke
EENT: Blurred vision, tinnitus, mydriasis
META: Breast enlargement, galactorrhoea, altered libido, altered blood glucose levels, inappropriate secretion of antidiuretic hormone
Contraindications: Hypersensitivity to tricyclic antidepressants, heart block, cardiac arrhythmias, recent myocardial infarction, convulsive disorders, severe liver disease, mania, children under 6 yr, breast-feeding, porphyria
Precautions: Suicidal patients, schizophrenia, severe depression, increased intra-ocular pressure, narrow-angle glaucoma, urinary retention, cardiac disease, hepatic disease, hyperthyroidism, electroshock therapy, elective surgery, pregnancy, cardiovascular disease, epilepsy
Pharmacokinetics:
By mouth: Steady state 4–19 days; metabolised by liver, excreted by kidneys, excreted in breast milk, half-life 18–28 hr
Interactions/incompatibilities:
• Decreased effects of: guanethidine, clonidine
• Increased effects of: direct acting sympathomimetics, adrenaline, alcohol, barbiturates, benzodiazepines, CNS depressants
• Hyperpyretic crisis, convulsions, hypertensive episode: MAOIs or within 2 weeks of their administration
• Effects of nortriptyline may be reduced by: barbiturates
• Effects of nortriptyline may be potentiated by: cimetidine, fluoxetine
Treatment of overdose: ECG and electrolyte monitoring, induce emesis, lavage, activated charcoal, administer anti-arrhythmics or anticonvulsants if necessary

NURSING CONSIDERATIONS

Assess:
• BP (lying, standing), pulse
• Vital signs 4-hrly in patients with cardiovascular disease
• Weight
• Mental status; mood, affect, depression, panic
Administer:
• Increased fluids, bulk in diet if constipation, urinary retention occur
• With food or milk for GI symptoms
• A single dose or divided doses for depression
• Dosage at bedtime if oversedation occurs during day; may take entire dose at bedtime; elderly may not tolerate once day dosing
• Mouthwashes, or frequent sips of water for dry mouth
• Mix with fruit juice, water, or milk to disguise taste
Perform/provide:
• BP; if systolic drops 20 mmHg inform clinician and withhold drug
• Assistance with ambulation during beginning therapy since drowsiness/dizziness occurs
• Safety measures including siderails primarily in elderly
• Checking to see oral medication swallowed

Evaluate:
• Extrapyramidal symptoms primarily in elderly: rigidity, dystonia, motor restlessness alertness
• Mental status: mood, affect, suicidal tendencies, increase in psychiatric symptoms: depression, panic
• Urinary retention, constipation; constipation is more likely to occur in children
• Withdrawal symptoms: headache, nausea, vomiting, muscle pain, weakness; do not usually occur unless drug was discontinued abruptly
• Alcohol consumption; if alcohol is consumed, hold dose until morning

Teach patient/family:
• That therapeutic effects may take 2–3 weeks
• Use caution in driving or other activities requiring alertness because of drowsiness, dizziness, blurred vision
• To avoid alcohol other CNS depressants
• Not to discontinue medication quickly after long-term use, may cause nausea, headache, malaise
• To wear sunscreen or large hat since photosensitivity occurs

noxythiolin

Noxyflex S
Func. class.: Antibacterial/ Antifungal
Chem. class.: Thiourea derivative
Legal class.: POM

Action: Destroys most fungal and bacterial pathogens partly by slow release of formaldehyde into solution

Uses: Bladder infections, peritonitis, treatment of other infected body cavities

Dosage and routes:
Refer to manufacturer's data sheet for further details of dosage routes and methods of administration

Bladder infections
• Instil 100 ml of 2.5% solution twice daily (2–3 times weekly for prophylaxis)

Intraperitoneal use
• Instil 200 ml of 2.5% solution prior to closure or 500 ml of 1% solution via a catheter over 12 hrs, continued for 3–7 days post-operatively
• Should not exceed a daily dose of 10 g for accumulative installations or continuous irrigation regimens

Available forms include: Powder for reconstitution 2.5 g in 20-ml vial

Side effects/adverse reactions:
GU: Burning sensation on application to bladder

Precautions: Requires aseptic technique during preparation, not a substitute for appropriate systemic antibacterial/antifungal therapy

NURSING CONSIDERATIONS

Assess:
• Fluid balance, odour and concentration of urine
• Temperature daily

Administer:
• Dissolve in an appropriate volume of water for injections or 0.9% sodium chloride, using aseptic technique to produce a 1 or 2.5% solution; warm to 37°C before instillation
• After samples have been sent for culture and sensitivity
• Reconstituted solution into bladder only using aseptic technique
• Local anaesthetic may be desirable for certain procedures

Evaluate:
• For bladder irritation: frequency of micturation, urinary output

• For decrease in fever

Teach patient/family:

• The importance of using an aseptic technique

• The importance of fluid intake—2 litre/day

• To report any haematuria, or burning sensation in bladder

nystatin (oral)

Nystan, Nystatin-Dome

Func. class.: Antifungal

Chem. class.: Amphoteric polyene macrolide

Legal class.: POM

Action: Binds to sterols in cell membrane of fungi, allowing intracellular components to leak

Uses: Oral, intestinal infections caused by *Candida* spp

Dosage and routes:

Oral infection

• *Adult, children:* 100,000 units as suspension or pastille 4 times a day after meals

GI infection

• *Adult:* By mouth 500,000–1,000,000 units 4 times a day

• *Child:* By mouth 100,000 units 4 times a day

Available forms include: Tablets 500,000 units; pastilles 100,000 units; suspension 100,000 units/ml

Side effects/adverse reactions:

GI: Nausea, vomiting, diarrhoea

Contraindications: Hypersensitivity

Pharmacokinetics:

By mouth: Negligible absorption, excreted in faeces

Treatment of overdose: Absorption negligible, no systemic toxicity

NURSING CONSIDERATIONS

Administer:

• After samples have been sent for culture and sensitivity

• Oral suspension dose by placing ½ in each cheek, retain for as long as possible, then swallow

• Topical dose after cleansing area; mouth may be swabbed

• For oral infection the suspension should be kept in contact with affected areas as long as possible

Evaluate:

• For allergic reaction: rash, urticaria; drug may need to be discontinued

• For predisposing factors, antibiotic therapy, pregnancy, diabetes mellitus

Teach patient/family:

• That long-term therapy may be required to clear infection; to complete entire course of medication

• Good oral hygiene

nystatin (topical)

Nystan, many combination products

Func. class.: Antifungal

Chem. class.: Amphoteric polyene macrolide

Legal class.: POM

Action: Binds sterols in fungal cell membrane, which increases permeability, causing leaking of cell contents

Uses: Cutaneous and vulvovaginal candidiasis

Dosage and routes:

Topical

• *Adult and child:* Topical apply to affected area 2–4 times a day continuing at least 7 days after lesions heal

Vaginal

• Vaginally 100,000–200,000 units as pessaries or vaginal cream each night for at least 14 nights. Apply gel or cream to anogenital area 2–4 times a day for vulval infection

Available forms include: Cream, gel, ointment (all 100,000 units/g); vaginal pessaries 100,000 units; vaginal cream 100,000 units/application

Side effects/adverse reactions:
INTEG: Rash, urticaria, stinging, burning
Contraindications: Hypersensitivity
Precautions: Pregnancy
Interactions/incompatibilities:
• Vaginal cream damages condoms and contraceptive diaphragms

NURSING CONSIDERATIONS
Administer:
• After samples have been taken for culture and sensitivity
• After cleansing with soap, water before each application, dry well
• Enough medication to cover lesions completely
• Vaginal tablets by inserting high into vagina
• In vaginal candidiasis, treat partner concurrently to avoid re-infection

Evaluate:
• Allergic reaction: burning, stinging, swelling, redness
• Therapeutic response: decrease in size, number of lesions, decreased itching, white patches on vulvae

Teach patient/family:
• Wash hands before, after each application
• To avoid use of non-prescribed creams, ointments, lotions in area of treatment unless directed by clinician
• To apply with glove to prevent further infection
• Avoid sexual contact during treatment of vaginal infection to minimise re-infection
• That relief from itching should occur after 24–72 hr

octreotide

Sandostatin
Func. class.: Somatostatin analogue
Chem. class.: Peptide
Legal class.: POM

Action: Inhibits secretion of peptides of the gastroenteropancreatic endocrine system and of growth hormone. Synthetic analogue of somatostatin with a longer duration of action

Uses: Relief of symptoms associated with gastroenteropancreatic endocrine tumours, carcinoid tumours with features of the carcinoid syndrome, VIPomas, and glucagonomas

Dosage and routes:
Gastroenteropancreatic endocrine tumours
• *Adult:* Subcutaneous initially 50 mcg once or twice daily gradually increased up to 200 mcg 3 times a day if needed. Exceptionally, higher doses may be required. Maintenance doses are variable

Acromegaly
• Subcutaneous 100–200 mcg 3 times daily

Available forms include: Injection subcutaneous octreotide (as acetate) 50 mcg/ml, 100 mcg/ml, 500 mcg/ml, 1 ml ampoules; 200 mcg/ml, 5 ml vial

Side effects/adverse reactions:
GI: Anorexia, nausea, vomiting, abdominal pain, diarrhoea, steatorrhoea, bloating, flatulence, formation of gallstones, liver enzyme abnormalities, hepatitis
INTEG: Pain, stinging, burning at injection site with redness and swelling
ENDO: Impaired postprandial glucose tolerance, rarely persistent hyperglycaemia

Contraindications: Hypersensitivity, pregnancy, breast-feeding
Precautions: Sudden escape of gastroenteropancreatic endocrine tumours from symptomatic control may occur infrequently. Diabetics may show reduced hypoglycaemic requirements, increased depth and duration of hypoglycaemia in insulinoma
Pharmacokinetics: Metabolised in the liver. Plasma half-life 90–120 min
Interactions/incompatibilities:
• Alters requirements for insulin/oral hypoglycaemics in diabetics
Clinical assessment:
• Monitor hypoglycaemic control closely in diabetics
• Ultrasonic examination of the gall bladder is recommended prior to and at 6–12 month intervals during therapy
• Monitor thyroid function during long-term therapy

NURSING CONSIDERATIONS

Assess:
• Thyroid function during long term therapy
• Gall bladder by ultra sonic examination before and six monthly during therapy
• Electrolytes
• Input and output of fluids
• Blood sugar levels
• Weight
Administer:
• If rapid response needed, initial dose given by IV injection diluted to 10–50% with sodium chloride 0.9%
• Subcutaneously following the dosage regimen for suitable gradual introduction
• Injections should be given with solution at room temp
• Avoid multiple injections at short intervals at the same site
• In carcinoid tumour, discontinue if there is no beneficial effect within 1 week
Perform/provide:
• For prolonged storage ampoules should be stored between 2 and 8°C. For day-to-day use store at room temperature for up to 2 weeks
Evaluate:
• Therapeutic response, improved symptoms, quality of life, electrolyte abnormalities; reduced excretions and diarrhoea
• Weight gain
• Fluctuation of blood glucose
• Local skin reactions pain, stinging, redness and swelling
• Flatulence, bloating, signs of jaundice
Teach patient/family:
• That insulin or oral hypoglycaemic drugs may be reduced for diabetics
• That drug needs to be combined with complete health plan: diet, rest exercise
• To notify clinician if it is any yellowing in skin, clay coloured stool, dark urine

oestradiol/oestradiol valerate

Estraderm TTS, Climaval Progynova, Hormonin, Zumenon, Vagifem
Func. class.: Oestrogen
Chem. class.: Nonsteroidal synthetic oestrogen
Legal class.: POM

Action: Necessary for adequate functioning of female reproductive system; affects release of pituitary gonadotropins, inhibits ovulation, adequate calcium use in bone structures
Uses: Menopause, primary amenorrhoea, atrophic vaginitis
Dosage and routes:
Menopause/hypogonadism/casttration/ovarian failure

• *Adult:* By mouth 1 mg daily for 3 weeks of each cycle. Increase to 2 mg daily if necessary
• *Adult:* Implant 25–100 mg every 4–8 months with cyclical progesteron on 10–13 days of each cycle if uterus intact
• Transderm patch, menopausal symptoms (not oestoporosis prophylaxis) initially one 50 mcg patch applied twice a week. Adjust dose according to response. Maximum dose 100 mcg daily, Progestrogen essential (unless hysterectomy) on last 12 days of cycle
• Vaginal tablets; 1 tablet inserted daily for 2 weeks, then reduce to one twice weekly. Discontinue after 3 months to assess need

Available forms include: Tablets 1, 2 mg; implants 25, 50, 100 mg; patch 25, 50, 100 mcg, vaginal tablet, 25 mcg

Side effects/adverse reactions:
CNS: Dizziness, headache, migraine, depression, vertigo
CV: Thrombophlebitis, oedema, thromboembolism, stroke, pulmonary embolism, myocardial infarction, hypertension, palpitations
GI: Nausea, vomiting, diarrhoea, anorexia, pancreatitis, cramps, dyspepsia, flatulence, constipation, increased appetite, abdominal pain, increased weight, cholestatic jaundice
EENT: Contact lens intolerance, increased myopia, astigmatism
GU: Amenorrhoea, cervical erosion, breakthrough bleeding, dysmenorrhoea, vaginal candidiasis, breast changes
INTEG: Rash, urticaria, acne, chloasma, hirsutism, melasma, erythema nodosum
META: Hyperglycaemia, sodium and water retention

Contraindications: Breast cancer, hyperlipoproteinaemia, thromboembolic disorders, oestrogen-dependent neoplasms, cholestatic jaundice, history of jaundice or herpes gestationis, pregnancy, Dubin–Johnson syndrome, Rotor syndrome, moderate-to-severe sickle cell anaemia, genital bleeding (abnormal, undiagnosed), pregnancy porphyria, congestive cardiac failure, severe hepatic disease or renal disease, endometriosis, uterine fibromyomata

Precautions: Asthma, blood dyscrasias, gallbladder disease, diabetes mellitus, bone disease, multiple sclerosis, depression, migraine headache, severe varicose veins, chloasma, convulsive disorders, family history of cancer of breast or reproductive tract, hypertension, cholelithiasis

Pharmacokinetics:
By mouth: Degraded in liver, excreted in urine
Transdermal: Onset 4 hr, duration up to 4 days

Interactions/incompatibilities:
• Decreased action of: anticoagulants, oral hypoglycaemics and insulins
• Toxicity: tricyclic antidepressants
• Decreased action of this drug: anticonvulsants, barbiturates, phenylbutazone, rifampicin
• Increased action of: corticosteroids

Clinical assessment:
• Liver function studies, including aspartate aminotransferase, alanine aminotransferase, bilirubin, alkaline phosphatase

Lab. test interferences:
Increase: Thyroxine, thyroxine-binding globulin (TBG)
Decrease: Triiodothyronine resin uptake test

NURSING CONSIDERATIONS

Assess:

• Baseline weight and BP before therapy and regularly during the course

Administer:

• Titrated dose, use lowest effective dose

• Implant should be inserted subcutaneously into an area where there is little or no movement or blood supply, e.g. buttock, lower abdominal wall

• Insert implant using a trocar and cannular under local anaesthetic; could insert in wound at time of laparotomy

• With food or milk to decrease GI symptoms (oral)

• Patch to be applied to clean, dry, unbroken skin on trunk below waistline; not to be applied on or near breasts

• Insert vaginal tablets using disposable applicator

Evaluate:

• Urinary glucose in patient with diabetes, increased urine glucose may occur

• Weight daily, notify clinician of weekly weight gain greater than 2.5 kg; if increase, diuretic may be ordered

• BP 4 hrly watch for increase caused by water and sodium retention

• For decreasing urinary output and increasing oedema

• Therapeutic response: absence of breast engorgement, reversal of menopausal symptoms

• Oedema, hypertension, cardiac symptoms, jaundice

• Mental status: affect, mood, behavioural changes, aggression

Teach patient/family:

• Weight weekly, report gain greater than 2.5 kg

• Warn contact lense wearers that vision may alter slightly; allow time to settle before seeking opticians advice

• Avoid sunlight or wear sunscreen; burns may occur

• Patch should be removed after 3–4 days and replaced with fresh patch on slightly different site

oestriol

Ovestin, combination products

Func. class.: Oestrogen

Chem. class.: Female sex hormone

Legal class.: POM

Action: Enables female reproductive system to function adequately; affects release of pituitary gonadotrophins; inhibits ovulation

Uses: GU symptoms associated with oestrogen deficiency states; infertility associated with poor cervical penetration

Dosage and routes:

GU symptoms

• *Adult:* By mouth, 0.5–3 mg daily as single dose for up to 1 month then 0.5–1 mg daily until epithelial integrity is restored (short term use only)

Infertility

• *Adult:* By mouth, 0.25–1 mg daily as single dose on days 6–15 of menstrual cycle (with regular monitoring)

Available forms include: Tablets 0.25 mg (250 mcg)

Side effects/adverse reactions:

HAEM: Changes in liver function

CNS: Depression, headache

GU: Endometrial carcinoma in postmenopausal women treated with unopposed oestrogen therapy. For patients with intact uterus, progestogen should be administered cyclically. Withdrawal bleeding (rarely)

GI: Nausea, vomiting

META: Weight gain, breast ten-

derness and enlargement, sodium retention with oedema
INTEG: Jaundice, chloasma, rashes
Contraindications: Oestrogen-dependent carcinoma, history of thromboembolism, hepatic impairment, sickle-cell anaemia, undiagnosed vaginal bleeding, pregnancy, severe hypertension
Precautions: Diabetes mellitus, epilepsy, hypertension, migraine, cardiac or renal disease, history of jaundice, wearing of contact lenses, lactation. Prolonged treatment, endometriosis, fibrocystic mastopathy, hyperlipoproteinaemia, history of herpes gestationis, porphyria
Pharmacokinetics: Oestriol is short acting, due to short nuclear retention time in the target tissues, its low affinity for plasma protein and rapid metabolic clearance
Interactions/incompatibilities:
• Decreased effect: concurrent administration of liver enzyme inducing agents, e.g. rifampicin, barbiturates, carbamazepine, phenytoin
Treatment of overdose: Symptomatic treatment only
NURSING CONSIDERATIONS
Assess:
• Baseline BP, weight, urinalysis (in diabetics)
Administer:
• Titrated dose
• With food or milk to avoid GI symptoms
Evaluate:
• Therapeutic response, absence of breast enlargement, reversal of menopause
• Mental changes—mood and behavioural patterns
• Oedema, hypertension, cardiac symptoms, jaundice, hyperglycaemia
• Fluid balance; observe urinary output and increasing oedema
• Glucose in urine; may increase in diabetic patients
Teach patient/family:
• To weigh weekly, report gain more than 2.5 kg
• To report breast lumps, vaginal bleeding, oedema, GI upsets, abdominal pain or numbness in joints

oestrogens, conjugated

Premarin, combination product
Func. class.: Oestrogen
Chem. class.: Equine and synthetic oestrogens
Legal class.: POM

Action: Oestrogens needed for adequate functioning of female reproductive system; it affects release of pituitary gonadotropins, inhibits ovulation, adequate calcium use in bone structures
Uses: Oestrogen replacement therapy in menopausal and postmenopausal women. Menopause, breast cancer, prostatic cancer, primary ovarian failure, osteoporosis, atrophic vaginitis, Kraurosis vulvae. Unopposed oestrogen therapy in women following hysterectomy. In patients with intact uterus cyclical progestogen must be administered
Dosage and routes:
Menopause
• *Adult:* By mouth 0.625–1.25 mg daily 3 weeks on, 1 week off for each cycle maintaining on lowest effective dose
Prostatic cancer
• *Adult:* By mouth 1.25–2.5 mg three times a day
Breast cancer
• *Adult:* By mouth 10 mg 3 times a day for 3 months or longer; palliative, for women who are at least 5 years post menopause

Primary ovarian failure/ osteoporosis
• *Adult:* By mouth 0.25–1.25 mg daily 3 weeks on, 1 week off
Atrophic vaginitis
• By mouth 0.625–1.25 cyclically daily; vaginal cream 1–2 g daily 3 weeks on, 1 week off
Available forms include: Tablets 0.625, 1.25, 2.5 mg; cream 0.625 mg/g
Side effects/adverse reactions:
CNS: Dizziness, headache, migraine, depression
CV: Hypotension, thrombophlebitis, oedema, thromboembolism, stroke, pulmonary embolism, myocardial infarction
GI: Nausea, vomiting, diarrhoea, anorexia, pancreatitis, cramps, constipation, increased appetite, increased weight, cholestatic jaundice
EENT: Contact lens intolerance, increased myopia, astigmatism
GU: Amenorrhoea, cervical erosion, breakthrough bleeding, dysmenorrhoea, vaginal candidiasis, breast changes, gynaecomastia, testicular atrophy, impotence
INTEG: Rash, urticaria, acne, hirsutism, alopecia, oily skin, seborrhoea, purpura, melasma
META: Folic acid deficiency, hypercalcaemia, hyperglycaemia, alters lipid profile in postmenopausal women
Contraindications: Thromboembolic disorders, oestrogen-dependent neoplasm, genital bleeding (abnormal, undiagnosed), pregnancy, active thromboembolic disease, acute liver disease severe cardiac, renal disease, Rotor Syndrome, Dubin-Johnson syndrome, symptomatic endometrious, fibromyomalae
Precautions: Hypertension, asthma, blood dyscrasias, gallbladder disease, congestive cardiac failure, diabetes mellitus, bone disease, depression, migraine headache, convulsive disorders, hepatic disease, renal disease, family history of cancer of breast or reproductive tract, long term treatment should be accompanied by administration of a progestogen
Pharmacokinetics:
By mouth, IV/IM: Degraded in liver, excreted in urine, excreted in breast milk
Interactions/incompatibilities:
• Decreased action of: anticoagulants, oral hypoglycaemics
• Toxicity: tricyclic antidepressants
• Decreased action of this drug: anticonvulsants, barbiturates, phenylbutazone, rifampicin
• Increased action of: corticosteroids
Clinical assessment:
• Liver function studies including aspartate aminotransferase alanine aminotransferase, bilirubin, alkaline phosphatase

NURSING CONSIDERATIONS

Assess:
• Baseline BP, weight, urinalysis (in diabetics)
Administer:
• Titrated dose, use lowest effective dose
• With food or milk to decrease GI symptoms by mouth
Evaluate:
• BP 4 hrly; watch for increase caused by water and sodium retention
• Fluid balance, be alert for decreasing urinary output and increasing oedema
• Therapeutic response: absence of breast engorgement, reversal of menopausal symptoms, or decrease in tumour size in prostatic cancer
• Oedema, hypertension, cardiac symptoms, jaundice, hypercalcaemia

• Mental status: affect, mood, behavioral changes, aggression
Teach patient/family:
• Weigh weekly, report gain greater than 2.5 kg
• Report any breakthrough bleeding, amenorrhoea; gynaecomastia, testicular atrophy (male)

ofloxacin ▼

Tarivid
Func. class.: Broad spectrum antibiotic
Chem. class.: Fluoroquinolone
Legal class.: POM

Action: Inhibits bacterial deoxyribonucleic acid synthesis; bactericidal
Uses: Urinary tract infections—upper and lower tract infections; infections of the lower respiratory tract; sexually transmitted diseases including uncomplicated urethral and cervical gonorrhoea, non gonococcal urethritis, cervicitis
Dosage and routes:
Lower urinary tract infections
• *Adult:* By mouth, 200–400 mg daily as a morning dose
Upper urinary tract infections
• *Adult:* By mouth, 200–400 mg daily increasing to 400 mg twice daily if necessary
Lower respiratory tract infections
• *Adult:* By mouth, 400 mg daily increasing to 400 mg twice daily if necessary
Uncomplicated urethral and cervical gonorrhoea
• A single oral dose of 400 mg
Non gonococcal urethritis and Cervicitis:
• By mouth, 400 mg daily
Complicated urinary tract infections
• IV 200 mg daily administered over at least 30 min
Lower respiratory tract infections
• IV 200 mg twice daily administered over at least 30 min
Septicaemia
• IV 200 mg twice daily administered over at least 30 min increasing to 400 mg twice daily in severe complicated infections
Impaired renal function
• Following a normal initial dose the dosage should be reduced in patients with renal impairment; for acute infection usually a course of treatment lasting 7 to 10 days is sufficient
Available forms include:
Ofloxacin tablets, 200 mg and 400 mg; ofloxacin hydrochloride 2 mg/ml; for IV infusion 50 ml, 100 ml
Side effects/adverse reactions:
CNS: Headaches, dizziness, sleep disturbance, nightmares, unsteady gait and tremor, disturbed taste and smell including neurological complications such as convulsions, hallucinations, restlessness, agitation, confusion and psychotic episodes
CV: Reduced blood pressure with IV infusion (rare); tachycardia
EENT: Disturbed vision
GI: Abdominal pain, anorexia, nausea, vomiting, diarrhoea
INTEG: Thrombophlebitis; pain and reddening at site of infusion
HAEM: Blood dyscrasia
MS: Pain in joints and muscles, weakness
SYST: Hypersensitivity: facial oedema, swelling of tongue, oedema of glottis, fever
Contraindications: Avoid in patients with known hypersensitivity to fluoroquinolone antibiotics or in epileptic patients and patients with pre-existing CNS lesions involving a lowered convulsion threshold. Ofloxacin should be avoided in children or growing adolescents or pregnant

or lactating women. Patients with known G6PD deficiency may be predisposed to haemolytic reactions

Precautions: Patients receiving treatment with ofloxacin should avoid exposure to strong sunlight and avoid UV rays. Since there have been occasional reports of somnolence, impairment of skills, dizziness and visual disturbance, patients should know how they react to ofloxacin before driving or operating machinery. These effects may be enhanced by alcohol

Pharmacokinetics: Ofloxacin is well absorbed from the gastrointestinal tract, 81–94% following oral administration. Peak plasma levels reached approx. one hr post oral ingestion. Half-life is 3.5–5.5 hr increasing to 10–50 hr in anuria. Ofloxacin is predominantly excreted 90% unchanged in urine

Interactions:
- Increased serum levels of ofloxacin: probenecid
- Reduced oral absorption: milk, antacids

Lab. test interferences: Altered liver function tests

Treatment of overdose: Treatment of overdose should be symptomatic. Gastric lavage following oral ingestion

NURSING CONSIDERATIONS

Assess:
- Vital signs (temperature, pulse, respiration, BP); fluid balance, urine test
- For known sensitivities
- History of previous psychiatric or epileptic episodes

Administer:
- After culture and sensitivity tests
- IV infusion: immediately after bottle has been opened and contents diluted with 0.9% sodium chloride for infusion and glucose 5% infusion; administer over at least 30 min and use alone
- By mouth, with or without food, but with a full glass of water

Perform/provide:
- Fluids: 2–3 l daily (for oral preparation) unless contraindicated
- Monitoring of BP during IV infusion
- Storage: IV ofloxacine protected from light

Evaluate:
- Therapeutic effect; control of infection
- For side effects: hypotension, pain at site of infusion

Teach patient/family:
- That tablets must be taken as prescribed and the full course finished
- About side effects and to report any of these to nurse or clinician
- To take 2–3 l of clear fluids daily
- Not to be taken with antacids or iron preparations (reduced absorption)
- That patients should avoid exposure to strong sunlight or use high factor sun cream if exposure is unavoidable
- To avoid hazardous tasks, including driving, if any dizziness occurs

---

ofloxacin (ophthalmic) ▼

Exocin

Func. class.: Broad spectrum antibiotic

Chem. class.: Fluoroquinolone

Legal class.: POM

Action: Inhibits bacterial deoxyribonucleic acid synthesis; bactericidal

Uses: Topical treatment of external ocular infection including conjunctivitis, keratoconjunctivitis

Dosage and routes:

• *Adult and Child:* Instil one or two drops in the affected eye(s) every 2 to 4 hr for first 2 days and then four times daily for up to 10 days treatment
Available forms include: Eyedrops (0.3%) 5 ml
Side effects/adverse reactions:
EENT: Ocular irritation: burning, stinging, redness, itching, photophobia
CNS: Dizziness, headache
GI: Nausea
Contraindications: Hypersensitivity
Precautions: Resistance to therapy; breast-feeding; pregnancy
Pharmacokinetics: Maximum serum ofloxacin concentrations are achieved after 10 days of topical administration
Treatment of overdose: Flush eye thoroughly with water
NURSING CONSIDERATIONS
Assess:
• Ability of patient (or carer) to instil drops
Administer:
• After culture and sensitivity tests
• After clearing the eye(s)
• As prescribed
Evaluate:
• Therapeutic effect; reduction in pain, swelling, obvious signs of infection
• For side-effects
Teach patient/family:
• How to instil drops
• About side-effects and to report any to nurse or clinician
• About hygiene related to eye infection; not to share face flannels, towels; not to rub or touch the eyes

olsalazine

Dipentum
Func. class.: Anti-inflammatory
Chem. class.: Salicylate derivative
Legal class.: POM

Action: Olsalazine is converted in the colon to 5-aminosalicylic acid which acts topically on the colonic mucosa
Uses: Treatment and maintenance of remission in acute mild ulcerative colitis
Dosage and routes:
Acute mild disease
• *Adult:* By mouth initially 1 g daily in divided doses increased up to a maximum of 3 g daily over 1 week. A single dose should not exceed 1 g
Remission maintenance
• *Adult and elderly:* By mouth 500 mg twice a day
Available forms include: Capsules 250 mg
Side effects/adverse reactions:
GI: Diarrhoea, abdominal cramps, nausea, dyspepsia, reversible pancreatitis
INTEG: Rash
CNS: Headache
MS: Arthralgia
Contraindications: Hypersensitivity to salicylates, significant renal impairment
Pharmacokinetics: The systemic absorption of olsalazine is minimal
Treatment of overdose: Minimal systemic absorption, no specific antidote, treatment supportive
NURSING CONSIDERATIONS
Assess:
• Nutritional status, dietary habits
Administer:
• With or just after food
Evaluate:
• Therapeutic effect
• For side effects; diarrhoea and GI disturbance, rashes arthralgia

Teach patient/family:
• Importance of maintenance dose
• About diet, stress alleviation
• To report side effects

omeprazole

Losec
Func. class.: Proton pump inhibitor, anti ulcer
Chem. class.: Benzimidazole
Legal class.: POM

Action: Specific inhibitor of the gastric proton pump (H^+, K^+, ATPase) in the parietal cell, producing dose-dependent inhibition of acid secretion by binding to the enzyme and reducing gastric acid secretion
Uses: Treatment of oesophageal reflux disease; duodenal and benign gastric ulcers; including those complicating NSAID therapy; Zollinger–Ellison syndrome
Dosage and routes:
Reflux oesophagitis
• *Adult:* By mouth, 20 mg once daily up to max. 40 mg daily. For patients not fully healed after 4 weeks a further 4–8 weeks treatment may be required
Duodenal and benign gastric ulcers
• *Adult:* By mouth, 20 mg daily up to max. 40 mg daily for 4 weeks. Patients with benign gastric ulcers may require 8 weeks. Long term therapy is not currently recommended
Zollinger Ellison syndrome
• *Adult:* By mouth, initially 60 mg once daily up to 120 mg daily according to response. For doses above 80 mg daily, the total dose should be divided and given twice daily
Available forms include: Capsules, 20 mg

Side effects/adverse reactions:
CNS: Headache, dizziness, lightheadedness and feeling faint, somnolence, insomnia and vertigo. Reversible mental confusion, agitation, depression and hallucinations have occurred in severely ill patients
GI: Constipation, diarrhoea, nausea, vomiting, flatulence and abdominal pain. Stomatitis and candidiasis have been reported in isolated cases; liver dysfunction; hepatitis; jaundice
HAEM: Blood dyscrasia
MS: Arthritic and myalgic symptoms
SYST: Malaise, fever, peripheral oedema, sweating
Contraindications: Pregnancy and breast-feeding; when gastric ulcer is suspected, the possibility of malignancy should be excluded before treatment with omeprazole is instituted, as treatment may alleviate symptoms and delay diagnosis
Precautions: Dosage adjustment may be necessary with impaired hepatic function. Severe liver disease: max. dose 20 mg daily
Pharmacokinetics: Oral dosing of omeprazole 20 mg produces inhibition of gastric acid secretion within 1–2 hr of the first dose. The maximum effect is achieved within 4 days of starting treatment after which the degree of acid inhibition remains constant. The mean decrease in pentagastrin stimulated peak acid output 24 hr after dosing with omeprazole is about 70%. The inhibition of acid secretion is not directly related to the plasma concentration of omeprazole at a given time
Interactions:
• Delayed elimination of: diazepam, phenytoin and warfarin
• Increased plasma levels of: digoxin

Treatment of overdose: Symptomatic and supportive therapy should be provided as necessary. Single doses of up to 160 mg have been given without adverse effect

NURSING CONSIDERATIONS

Assess:

• Digoxin levels in elderly patients already taking digoxin

Administer:

• By mouth; capsules to be swallowed whole, not chewed

Perform/provide:

• Storage: in dry area (omeprazole is sensitive to moisture)

Evaluate:

• Therapeutic effect: reduction of pain in oesophagus and upper GI tract

Teach patient/family:

• To take the dose as prescribed

• About side effects and to report any of these to nurse or clinician

• About changes in diet (reduction of fibre, fruit and vegetable if diarrhoea occurs; increase if constipation occurs)

• Not to undertake hazardous activity, including driving, if dizziness occurs

---

ondansetron ▼

Zofran

Func. class.: Anti-emetic

Chem. class.: Serotonin-antagonist, methylcarbazolone derivative

Legal class.: POM

Action: Antagonises the action of serotonin at receptors in both the CNS and the periphery, interfering with its role in stimulating nausea and vomiting

Uses: Prevention and treatment of postoperative nausea and vomiting and nausea and vomiting precipitated by radiotherapy and chemotherapy

Dosage and routes:

Emetogenic chemotherapy and radiotherapy

• *Adult:* Moderately emetogenic chemotherapy or radiotherapy, by mouth 8 mg 1–2 hr before treatment or, slowly, IV 8 mg immediately before treatment, then, by mouth 8 mg every 12 hr for up to 5 days. Severely emetogenic chemotherapy, slowly IV 8 mg immediately before treatment, followed by 8 mg at intervals of 2–4 hr for 2 further doses (or followed by 1 mg/hr by continuous IV infusion for up to 24 hr) then 8 mg by mouth every 12 hr for up to 5 days. Alternatively, by IV infusion 32 mg over 15 min immediately before treatment, then, by mouth 8 mg every 12 hr for up to 5 days.

• *Child:* By slow IV injection or infusion over 15 min, 5 mg/m^2 body surface area immediately before chemotherapy then, by mouth 4 mg every 12 hr for up to 5 days

Hepatic impairment Total daily dose should not exceed 8 mg in patients with moderate or severe impairment

Postoperative nausea and vomiting

•*Adult:* By mouth 8 mg given 4 hr before anaesthesia followed by 2 further doses at intervals of 8 hr, or, slowly, IV 4 mg at induction of anaesthesia

Hepatic impairment Total daily dose should not exceed 8 mg in patients with moderate or severe impairment

Available forms include: Tablets 4, 8 mg (as hydrochloride dihydrate); injection IV 2 mg/ml (as hydrochloride dihydrate) 2, 4 ml ampoules

Side effects/adverse reactions:

CNS: Headache

GI: Constipation, transient increases in liver enzymes

MISC: Sensation of warmth or flushing of face/epigastrium
SYST: Anaphylaxis
Contraindications: Hypersensitivity
Precautions: Pregnancy, breast feeding, hepatic impairment
Treatment of overdose: Supportive and symptomatic treatment

NURSING CONSIDERATIONS

Assess:
- Vital signs (temperature, pulse, respiration, BP), fluid balance
- Full blood count including platelets

Administer:
- IV: by slow injection immediately before chemo- or radiotherapy
- By mouth 1–2 hours before chemo- or radiotherapy

Perform/provide:
- All supportive measures for primary disease (care of skin, mouth, fluid balance, all other medication as prescribed)
- Storage; protect ampoules from direct sunlight

Evaluate:
- Therapeutic response, reduction or lessening of nausea and vomiting
- For side effects; headache, constipation

Teach patient/family:
- About the drug and the side effects
- To report any side effects to nurse or clinician

oral contraceptives, combined

Mercilon, Loestrin, Marvelon, Conova, Femodene, Minulet, Microgynon, Ovranette, Eugynon, Ovran, Brevinor, Ovysmen, Neocon, Norimin, Cilest, Norinyl, Ortho-Novin
Phased: Triadene, Tri-Minulet, Logynon, Trinordiol, BiNovum, Synphase, TriNovum
Func. class.: Hormone
Chem. class.: Oestrogen/progestogen combinations
Legal class.: POM

Action: Prevents ovulation by suppressing follicle stimulating, luteinizing hormone
Uses: To prevent pregnancy, endometriosis, hypermenorrhoea
Dosage and routes:
- *Adult:* By mouth 1 tablet daily starting on day 1 of menstrual cycle

21 tablet packs
- 1 tablet daily for 21 days followed by a 7 day gap

28 tablet packs
- 1 tablet daily continuously

Triphasic/Biphasic
- 1 tablet daily as shown on package insert

Available forms include: Tablets, many combinations
Side effects/adverse reactions:
GI: Nausea, vomiting, cramps, diarrhoea, bloating, constipation, change in appetite, cholestatic jaundice, weight gain, impairment of liver function, hepatic tumours
INTEG: Chloasma, melasma, acne, rash, urticaria, erythema, pruritus, hirsutism, photosensitivity
CV: Increased BP, thromboembolic conditions, fluid retention, oedema

ENDO: Decreased glucose tolerance
GU: Breakthrough bleeding, amenorrhoea, spotting, dysmenorrhoea, galactorrhoea, endocervical hyperplasia, vaginitis, cystitis-like syndrome, breast change, changes in libido
CNS: Depression, fatigue, dizziness, nervousness, anxiety, headache
EENT: Retinal thrombosis
HAEM: Increased fibrinogen, clotting factor

Contraindications: Pregnancy, lactation, reproductive cancer, history of thromboembolic disease, recurrent jaundice, porphyria, undiagnosed vaginal bleeding, history of pruritus of pregnancy or herpes gestationis, deterioration of otosclerosis, thrombophlebitis, myocardial infarction, hepatic tumours, hepatic disease, coronary artery disease, women over 40 yr, hyperlipidaemia, severe or focal migraine, Dubin-Johnson and Rotor syndrome, mammary, endometrial or oestrogen dependent tumours

Precautions: Depression, hypertension, renal disease, seizure disorders, lupus erythematosus, multiple sclerosis, rheumatic disease, migraine headache, amenorrhoea, irregular menses, breast cancer (fibrocystic), gallbladder disease

Pharmacokinetics: Degraded in liver, excreted in urine

Interactions/incompatibilities:

- Decreased effectiveness of oral contraceptives: ampicillin, tetracycline, rifampicin, analgesics, carbamazepine, phenobarbitone, phenytoin, primidone, antihistamines, griseofulvin
- Decreased action of: oral anticoagulants, antidepressants, oral hypoglycaemics and insulins, antihypertensives
- Increased clotting: aminocaproic acid
- Increased plasma concentrations of: cyclosporin, theophylline

Clinical assessment:

- Glucose, thyroid function, liver function tests

Lab. test interferences:

Increase: Thyroid binding globulin, protein bound iodine, thyroxine, platelet aggregability, protein bound iodine
Decrease: Triiodothyronine, antithrombin

NURSING CONSIDERATIONS

Evaluate:

- Therapeutic response: absence of pregnancy, endometriosis, menorrhagia
- Reproductive changes: change in breasts, tumours, positive PAP smear; drug should be discontinued if changes occur

Teach patient/family:

- Detection of clots using Homan's sign (dorsiflexion of foot causing pain in calf)
- To use sunscreen or avoid sunlight; photosensitivity can occur
- To take at same time each day to ensure equal drug level
- To report GI symptoms that occur after 4 months
- To use another birth control method during 1st week of oral contraceptive use
- To take another tablet as soon as possible if one is missed. If this is more than 12 hr late contraception may not work. Continue taking tablets but use additional precautions for 7 days. If these 7 days run beyond the end of the pack, start the new pack immediately the current one is finished
- That after drug is discontinued, pregnancy may not occur for several months
- To report abdominal pain, change in vision, shortness of breath, change in menstrual flow,

spotting, breakthrough bleeding, breast lumps, swelling
• That continuing medical care is needed: PAP smear and gynaecologic examinations 6 monthly

orciprenaline sulphate (inhaled)

Alupent
Func. class.: Bronchodilator
Chem. class.: Synthetic sympathomimetic amine
Legal class.: POM

Action: Relaxes bronchial smooth muscle by direct action on β-adrenergic receptors
Uses: Bronchial asthma, bronchospasm
Dosage and routes:
• *Adult:* Inhalation, 1–2 puffs, may repeat if necessary after not less than 30 min, not to exceed 12 puffs daily
• *Child up to 6 yr:* 1 puff up to 4 times daily; 6–12 yr 1–2 puffs up to 4 times daily
• *Adult:* By mouth 20 mg 6–8 hrly
• *Child:* By mouth, up to 1 yr 5–10 mg 3 times daily; 1–3 yr 5–10 mg 4 times daily; 3–12 yr 40–60 mg daily in divided doses
Available forms include: Tablets, 20 mg; aerosol 750 mcg/metered inhalation; syrup 10 mg/5 ml;
Side effects/adverse reactions:
CNS: Tremors, anxiety, insomnia, headache, dizziness, stimulation
CV: Palpitations, tachycardia, hypertension, cardiac arrest
GI: Nausea
Contraindications: Hypersensitivity to sympathomimetics; thyrotoxicosis
Precautions: Pregnancy, cardiac disorders, diabetes mellitus, prostatic hypertrophy, hyperthyroidism, hypertension, elderly, MAOIs. Due to risk of arrhythmias and other side effects, more selective β_2-adrenoreceptor stimulants are preferred for routine therapy
Interactions/incompatibilities:
• Increased effects of both drugs: other sympathomimetics
• Decreased action: β-blockers
Clinical assessment:
• Respiratory function: vital capacity, forced expiratory volume, arterial blood gases
• Monitor serum potassium particularly if administered with xanthines

NURSING CONSIDERATIONS

Administer:
• Shake inhaler before use
• Using correct inhaler technique
• Wait for 1 min between puffs
• 2 hr before bedtime to avoid sleeplessness (tablets and syrup)
Evaluate:
• Therapeutic response: absence of dyspnoea, wheezing
• Tolerance over long-term therapy, dose may need to be increased or changed
Teach patient/family:
• Not to use non-prescribed drug, extra stimulation may occur
• Inhaler technique and advise on maximum number of inhalations in 24 hr
• Review package insert with patient
• To avoid getting aerosol in eyes
• To wash inhaler in warm water and dry daily
• On all aspects of drug; avoid smoking, smoke-filled rooms

orphenadrine citrate/hydrochloride

Norflex, Biorphien, Disipal
Func. class.: Skeletal muscle relaxant, central acting
Chem. class.: Tertiary amine
Legal class.: POM

Action: Acts centrally on skeletal muscle to relax, inhibit muscle spasm
Uses: Parkinsonism short term relief of muscle spasm
Dosage and routes:
Parkinson's disease
• *Adult:* By mouth 150 mg daily in divided doses. Increase by 25–50 mg daily every 2–3 days if necessary. Maximum dosage is 400 mg daily
Short term relief of muscle spasm
• *Adult:* IM or IV injection 60 mg (given over 5 min if IV). Repeat after 12 hr
Available forms include: Tablets 50 mg, injection 30 mg/ml (citrate); solution 25 mg, 5 ml
Side effects/adverse reactions:
HAEM: Aplastic anaemia
CNS: Dizziness, weakness, fatigue, drowsiness, headache, disorientation, insomnia, stimulation, euphoria, hallucination, agitation, nervousness
EENT: Nasal congestion, blurred vision, increased intra-ocular pressure
CV: Hypotension, tachycardia
GI: Nausea, vomiting, constipation, dry mouth, numbness of the tongue and mouth, difficulty with micturition
GU: Urinary frequency, hesitancy
INTEG: Rash, pruritus, urticaria
Contraindications: Hypersensitivity, closed-angle glaucoma, GI obstruction, myasthenia gravis, stenosing peptic ulcer, urinary retention, breast-feeding, children under 12 yr, acute pulmonary insufficiency, prostatic hypertrophy, tardive dyskinesia
Precautions: Pregnancy, cardiac disease, chronic pulmonary insufficiency, elderly, tachycardia, hypertension, liver or kidney dysfunction
Interactions/incompatibilities:
• Increased CNS effects: coproxamol
Clinical assessment:
• Blood studies: full blood count, WBC, differential, blood dyscrasias may occur (rare)
Lab. test interference: Elevated triiodothyronine (Sephadex method)
Treatment of overdose: Gastric lavage, emetic and high enema. Cholinergic agents such as carbachol may be useful

NURSING CONSIDERATIONS

Assess:
• Blood studies before and periodically in long-term use. Check for anaemia and dyscrasis
Administer:
• Intravenous injection directly into vein over 5 min. Further doses at 12 hr intervals
• Intramuscular or intravenous injection
• Orally with meals if nausea occurs. Increase dosage at recommended rate until optimum response with minimum side effects
Perform/provide:
• Help with mobility
• Frequent drink to prevent dry mouth
Evaluate:
• Therapeutic response: decreased rigidity, spasms
• Input and output of fluids, retention, frequency, hesitancy
• Side effects: nausea, dry mouth, numb tongue and mouth, visual disturbances, dizziness, micturition difficulties are usually tran-

sient or controlled by slight reduction in dosage
• Blood; plastic anaemia, rash, dyscrasis-rare

Teach patient/family:
• Not to discontinue medication without medical advice. Drug should be tapered off slowly
• To take other medication only if directed by clinician
• That alcohol should not be taken nor CNS depressants
• To avoid driving or use of machinery until therapy established

oxazepam

Func. class.: Anxiolytic
Chem. class.: Benzodiazepine
Legal class.: CD (Sch 4) POM

Action: Depresses subcortical levels of CNS, including limbic system and reticular formation
Uses: Anxiety (short-term use), alcohol withdrawal
Dosage and routes:
Anxiety
• *Adult:* By mouth 15–30 mg 3 or 4 times a day
• *Elderly, debilitated:* By mouth 10–20 mg 3 or 4 times a day
Insomnia
• *Adult:* By mouth 15–25 mg at bedtime; maximum 50 mg
Available forms include: Tablets 10 mg, 15 mg
Side effects/adverse reactions:
CNS: Dizziness, drowsiness, confusion, headache, anxiety, excitement, disorientation amnesia, ataxia, vertigo, syncope, lethargy, tremors, stimulation, fatigue, depression, insomnia, hallucinations, suicidal tendency, paradoxical aggression
GI: Constipation, dry mouth, nausea, vomiting, anorexia, diarrhoea, increased liver enzymes, jaundice
GU: Altered libido, urinary retention
HAEM: Blood dyscrasias, leucopenia
INTEG: Rash, dermatitis, itching
CV: Hypotension, oedema
EENT: Blurred vision
Contraindications: CNS depression, coma, respiratory depression, sleep apnoea
Precautions: Elderly, debilitated, hepatic disease, renal disease, history of alcoholism or drug abuse, personality disorders, chronic pulmonary insufficiency, concurrent CNS depressants including alcohol, general anaesthesia, opiates, MAOIs, antidepressants
Pharmacokinetics:
By mouth: Peak 2–4 hr, metabolised by liver, excreted by kidneys, half-life 6–8 hr
Interactions/incompatibilities:
• Increased effects of this drug: CNS depressants, alcohol, cimetidine, disulfiram, omeprazole
• Increased effects of: alcohol, general anaesthetics, opioid analgesics, MAOIs, antihypertensives
Clinical assessment:
• Blood studies: Full blood count during long-term therapy, blood dyscrasias have occurred rarely
• Liver function tests; aspartate aminotransferase, alanine aminotransferase, bilirubin, creatinine, lactic dehydrogenase, alkaline phosphatase
Treatment of overdose: Lavage, vital signs, supportive care

NURSING CONSIDERATIONS

Assess:
• Baseline pulse; BP
Administer:
• Crushed if patient is unable to swallow medication whole
Perform/provide:
• Frequent sips of water for dry mouth
Evaluate:

• Pulse, BP for first 24 hr of treatment
• Lying and standing BP if indicated
• Therapeutic response: decreased anxiety, restlessness, insomnia
• Mental status: mood, alertness, affect, sleeping pattern, drowsiness, dizziness
• Physical dependency, withdrawal symptoms: headache, nausea, vomiting, muscle pain, weakness after long-term use
• Suicidal tendencies

Teach patient/family:
• That drug may be taken with food
• Not to be used for everyday stress or used longer than 4 months, unless directed by clinician
• Avoid non-prescribed preparations (cough, cold, hay fever) unless approved by physician
• To avoid driving, activities that require alertness, since drowsiness may occur
• To avoid alcohol or other psychotropic medications unless prescribed by clinician
• Not to discontinue medication abruptly after long-term use
• To stand up slowly or fainting may occur
• That drowsiness might worsen at beginning of treatment

oxidized cellulose

Oxycel, Surgicel
Func. class.: Haemostatic
Chem. class.: Cellulose product
Legal class.: GSL

Action: Forms gel acting as physical barrier to bleeding
Uses: Haemostasis in surgery, epistaxis
Dosage and routes:
• *Adult and child:* Topical, apply using sterile technique as needed, remove after bleeding stops, if possible, or leave in place if not
Available forms include: Knitted fabric, gauze or lint
Side effects/adverse reactions:
EENT: Sneezing and burning when used in the nose
INTEG: Burning, stinging at site of application
CNS: Headache when used in the nose
MISC: Inhibits epithelialisation
Contraindications: Hypersensitivity, large artery haemorrhage, oozing surfaces, implantation or packing in bone surgery, infected wounds
Interactions/incompatibilities:
• Application after silver nitrate or other escharotics inhibits absorption
• Inactivates thrombin

NURSING CONSIDERATIONS

Administer:
• Using sterile technique
• Dry, use only amount needed to control bleeding
• Loosely, remove excess before closure in surgery; irrigate first, then remove using sterile technique

Evaluate:
• Allergy: fever, rash, itching, burning, stinging
• Bleeding: mucous membranes, epistaxis, ecchymosis, petechiae, haematuria, haematemesis

Teach patient/family:
• To report any signs of bleeding: gums, under skin, urine, stools, emesis

oxprenolol hydrochloride

Apsolox, Slow-Trasicor, Oxyprenix SR, Trasicor, combination product
Func. class.: Antihypertensive, anti-anginal, anti-arrhythmic
Chem. class.: Non-selective β-blocker blocker, non cardio-selective
Legal class.: POM

Action: Decreases preload, after-load, which is responsible for decreasing left ventricular end diastolic pressure, systemic vascular resistance

Uses: Angina, arrhythmias, hypertension, anxiety-induced tachycardia, hypertrophic obstructive cardiomyopathy, thyrotoxicosis

Dosage and routes:

Angina

• *Adult:* By mouth, 40–160 mg 3 times daily

Arrhythmias, hypertrophic obstructive cardiomyopathy

• *Adults:* By mouth, initially 20–40 mg 3 times daily, increased as required, maximum dose 480 mg daily; modified-release, 160 mg daily increasing to 320–480 mg daily if required

Hypertension

• *Adult:* By mouth, initially 80 mg twice daily; increased at weekly intervals as needed; maximum 480 mg daily; modified-release, 160 mg once daily, increased to twice daily if required; maximum 480 mg

Anxiety symptoms

• *Adults:* By mouth 40 mg twice daily; increase to a maximum of 160 mg daily

Available forms include: Tablets 20 mg, 40 mg, 80 mg, 160 mg; tablets, modified-release 160 mg

Side effects/adverse reactions:

CNS: Dizziness, drowsiness, headache, insomnia, excitability
CV: Heart failure, bradycardia, atrioventricular conduction disorders, peripheral vasoconstriction, hypotension
EENT: Visual disturbances, keratoconjuctivitis, dry eyes
GI: Disturbances, dry mouth
GU: Loss of libido
RESP: Bronchospasm, dyspnoea
HAEM: Thrombocytopenia
INTEG: Cold extremities, rash

Interactions/incompatibilities:

• Effects of oxprenolol may be enhanced by: other antihypertensives, calcium antagonists, anti-arrhythmics, cimetidine, fluvoxamine, mefloquine, digoxin, diuretics
• Oxprenolol, may potentiate: alcohol, analgesia, antihistamines, tricyclic antidepressants, anti-arrhythmics of the quinidine type and amiodarone, insulin, oral anti-diabetic agents, chlorpromazine
• Effects of oxprenolol may be reduced by: indomethacin, rifampicin, corticosteroids, thyroxine, carbenoxolone, xamoterol
• Oxprenolol may reduce effects of: neostigmine, pyridostigmine, xamoterol
• Severe hypertension may occur with concurrent use of: sympathomimetics such as adrenaline, noradrenaline and also in cough and cold remedies

Contraindications: Bronchospasm, asthma, history of obstructive airways disease, metabolic acidosis, sinus bradycardia, partial heart block, uncontrolled congestive heart failure

Precautions: Pregnancy, lactation, hepatic or renal impairment, avoid abrupt withdrawal in angina, chronic bronchitis, hypoglycaemia, insulin dependent or labile diabetes, thyrotoxic crisis, peripheral vascular disorders, uncontrolled cardiac failure, pulse rate less than 50 beats/min, alcoholism diabetic acidosis, emphysema, Raynaud's disease, phaeochromocytoma (unless treated with a α-adrenergic blocker)

Pharmacokinetics:
Almost completely absorbed from GI tract, subject to considerable first pass metabolism. Peak levels occur after 1–2 hr. Metabolised the liver and excreted in urine

Clinical assessment:
• Perform creatinine clearance if kidney damage is diagnosed

Lab. test interferences:
Increase: Serum potassium, serum uric acid, alanine aminotransferase, aspartate aminotransferase alkaline phosphatase, lactic dehydrogenase
Decrease: Blood glucose

Treatment of overdose: For sinus bradycardia and hypotension 10.5–2 mg atropine by slow 1V infusion followed by isoprenaline of 25 mcg IV if necessary. In cardiogenic shock 5–10 mg glucagon IV may be helpful. Salbutamol by inhalation or 4 mcg/kg slow IV injection can be given for bronchospasm

NURSING CONSIDERATIONS

Assess:
• Baseline BP, pulse, respirations and weight
• Fluid balance
• Pain: duration, time started, activity being performed

Administer:
• With full glass of water on empty stomach

Evaluate:
• Observe for postural hypotension
• Tolerance, if taken over a long period of time
• Therapeutic response, degree of palpitations, breathlessness, anxiety levels
• BP, heart and respiratory rates

Teach patient/family:
• That dose must be taken with a glass of water
• That drug should be taken before stressful activity or exercise
• That if taken sublingually, mucous membranes may sting
• To avoid hazardous activities if dizziness occurs
• Stress patient compliance with complete medical regime
• To make positional changes slowly to prevent fainting

---

oxybutynin hydrochloride

Cystrin, Ditropan ▼
Func. class.: Antispasmodic, anticholinergic
Legal class.: POM

Action: Direct antispasmodic action on smooth muscle of the bladder detrusor and anticholinergic action blocking the muscarinic effects of acetylcholine on smooth muscle. Cause relaxation of the detrusor muscle of the bladder and for patients with an unstable bladder, increase bladder capacity reducing the incidence of spontaneous contractions of the detrusor muscle

Uses: Urinary incontinence, urgency and frequency in the unstable bladder, whether due to neurogenic bladder disorders (detrusor hyperreflexia) in conditions such as multiple sclerosis and spina bifida or to idiopathic detrusor instability (motor urge incontinence). Nocturnal enuresis in children

Dosage and routes:
• *Adult:* By mouth, 5 mg two or three times daily increasing as clinically required to a maximum of 20 mg daily in divided doses
• *Elderly:* By mouth, initially 2.5 to 3 mg twice daily, titrating dose according to response
• *Children over 5 yr of age:*

Neurogenic bladder instability: By mouth, 5 mg twice a day increasing to three times a day to obtain a clinical response provided side effects are tolerated
Nocturnal Enuresis: By mouth, 5 mg two or three times a day, the last dose being administered before bedtime
Available forms include: Tablets 2.5 mg, 3 mg, 5 mg; elixir 2.5 mg in 5 ml
Side effects/adverse reactions: The most frequently reported side effects (>1%) to oxybutynin are:
CNS: Headache, dizziness, drowsiness, blurred vision
CV: Arrhythmias, facial flushing
GI: Dry mouth, constipation, nausea, abdominal discomfort, diarrhoea
GU: Urinary retention, difficulty in micturition
INTEG: Dry skin
Contraindications: Achalasia; obstruction of the bladder or gastrointestinal tract including intestinal atony, toxic megacolon; severe ulcerative colitis; myasthenia gravis, glaucoma; breast feeding; prostatic hypertrophy; pyloric stenosis; renal impairment; cardiac disease
Precautions: Elderly and in patients with autonomic neuropathy, hepatic or renal disease. The symptoms of hyperthyroidism, coronary artery disease, congestive cardiac failure, cardiac arrhythmias, tachycardias and prostatic hypertrophy may be aggravated following administration of oxybutynin
Interactions: Increased antimuscarinic effects: anticholinergics, phenolthiazines, butyrophenones, amantidine, tricyclic antidepressants
Treatment of overdose: Immediate gastric lavage after oral ingestion. Slow injection of 1.0 to 2.0 mg physostigmine salicylate repeated as necessary up to a total of 5 mg. Contact Poisons Information Service for specialist advice. Fever should be treated symptomatically with tepid sponging or ice packs. In pronounced restlessness or excitation, 10 mg diazepam by IV injection should be administered. Tachycardia may be treated with intravenous injection of propranolol and urinary retention managed by catheterisation. If paralysis of respiratory muscles occurs, mechanical ventilation will be required

NURSING CONSIDERATIONS

Assess:
- Bladder management, fluid balance, urine test
- Age and physical state (frailty) of patient

Administer:
- By mouth; titrated dose

Evaluate:
- Therapeutic response; reduction in incontinence, urgency, frequency; control of enuresis
- For side effects

Teach patient/family:
- About side effects of oxybutynin
- Other techniques for bladder management; reduction of fluids before bedtime, manual bladder expression
- About side effects and to report any of these to nurse or clinician. Many side effects can be controlled or eliminated by reducing the dose.

oxycodone pectinate

Func. class.: Narcotic analgesic
Chem. class.: Opioid, semisynthetic derivative
Legal class.: CD (Sch 2) POM

Action: Inhibits ascending pain pathways in CNS, increases pain threshold, alters pain perception
Uses: Moderate-to-severe pain in terminal illness

Dosage and routes:
• *Adult:* Rectally 30–60 mg every 6–8 hr
Available forms include: Suppositories 30 mg (special order from Boots)
Side effects/adverse reaction:
CNS: Drowsiness, dizziness, confusion, sedation, euphoria
GI: Nausea, vomiting, anorexia, constipation, cramps
GU: Dysuria
INTEG: Rash, urticaria, flushing, diaphoresis, pruritus
EENT: Tinnitus, blurred vision, miosis, diplopia, dry mouth
CV: Palpitations, bradycardia, orthostatic hypotension
RESP: Respiratory depression
SYST: Hypothermia
Contraindications: Hypersensitivity
Precautions: Addictive personality, pregnancy, lactation, increased intracranial pressure, respiratory depression, hepatic disease, renal disease, hyperthyroidism, prostatic hypertrophy, myxoedema, adrenocortical insufficiency
Pharmacokinetics: Well absorbed from GI tract, metabolised in liver excreted in urine as metabolite and unchanged
Interactions/incompatibilities:
• Increased CNS depression with: alcohol, sedative/hypnotics, antipsychotics, skeletal muscle relaxants, other CNS depressants
• Serious hypertensive/hypotensive reactions with CNS excitation/depression with: MAOIs
• Antagonism of GI effects of: cisapride, metoclopramide, domperidone
Treatment of overdose: Naloxone IV, symptomatic treatment
NURSING CONSIDERATIONS
Assess:
• Pain levels
• Fluid balance
Administer:
• With anti-emetic if nausea, vomiting occur
Perform/provide:
• Storage in CD cupboard
• All supportive measures
• Assistance with ambulation
• Safety measures: cot sides, night light, callbell within easy reach
Evaluate:
• Therapeutic response: decrease in pain
• CNS changes: dizziness, drowsiness, hallucinations, euphoria, level of consciousness, pupil reaction
• GI symptoms including constipation
• Respiratory rate and character
• Need for pain medication, physical dependence, other supportive care
Teach patient/family:
• To report any gross changes
• Withdrawal symptoms may occur; nausea, vomiting, cramps, fever, faintness, anorexia
• How to insert suppositories
• The need for secure storage

oxymetholone

Anapolon 50
Func. class.: Androgenic anabolic steroid
Chem. class.: Testosterone derivative
Legal class.: POM

Action: Increases weight by building body tissue, increases potassium, phosphorus, chloride, and nitrogen levels, increases bone development, stimulates erythropoiesis
Uses: Aplastic anaemia
Dosage and routes:
• *Adult:* By mouth 2–5 mg/kg daily, titrated to patient response, for at least 3 months. Maintain dose for further 3 months after

initial response. Gradual dose reduction under expert supervision should then be performed watching for signs of relapse

Available forms include: Tablets 50 mg

Side effects/adverse reactions:

INTEG: Acne, alopecia, hirsutism

CNS: Excitation, insomnia

MS: Cramps, premature skeletal maturation in children

CV: Congestive heart failure, oedema

GU: Amenorrhoea, vaginitis, virilisation, decreased libido, decreased breast size, clitoral enlargement, testicular atrophy, gynaecomastia

GI: Nausea, vomiting, diarrhoea, cholestatic jaundice

ENDO: Abnormal glucose tolerance test

Contraindications: Severe renal disease, porphyria, severe hepatic disease, hypersensitivity, pregnancy, lactation, hypercalcaemia, carcinoma of breast or prostrate in males, nephrosis or nephrotic phase of nephritis, porphyria

Precautions: Diabetes mellitus, cardiac, renal, or hepatic disease, prostatic hypertrophy, myocardial infarction, epilepsy, hypertension, migraine

Pharmacokinetics:

By mouth: Metabolised in liver, excreted in urine, excreted in breast milk

Interactions/incompatibilities:

- Adjustments in insulin, oral antidiabetic dosage
- Increased prothrombin time: anticoagulants
- Oedema: ACTH, adrenal steroids

Clinical assessment:

- Electrolytes: potassium, sodium, chloride, calcium; cholesterol
- Liver function studies: aspartate aminotransferase, alanine aminotransferase, bilirubin

Lab. test interferences:

Glucose tolerance, thyroid function

NURSING CONSIDERATIONS

Administer:

- With food to reduce GI symptoms
- Titrated dose, use lowest effective dose

Perform/provide:

- Diet with increased calories and protein; decrease sodium if oedema occurs

NB. That drug is one of abuse by athletes

Evaluate:

- Weight daily, notify clinician if weekly weight gain is greater than 2.5 kg
- BP 4 hrly
- Fluid balance oedema, be alert for decreasing urinary output, increasing oedema
- Growth rate in children since growth rate may be uneven (linear/bone growth) when used for extended period; premature closure of epiphyses in children
- Oedema, hypertension, cardiac symptoms, jaundice
- Mental status: affect, mood, behavioural changes, aggression
- Signs of masculinisation in female: increased libido, deepening of voice, breast tissue, enlarged clitoris, menstrual irregularities; male: gynaecomastia, impotence, testicular atrophy
- Hypercalcaemia: lethargy, polyuria, polydipsia, nausea, vomiting, constipation; drug may need to be decreased
- Hypoglycaemia in diabetics, since oral anticoagulant action is decreased

Teach patient/family:

- Drug needs to be combined with complete health plan: diet, rest, exercise
- To notify clinician if therapeutic response decreases

• Not to discontinue this medication abruptly
• Teach patient all aspects of drug usage, including changes in sex characteristics
• Women to report menstrual irregularities
• That 1–3 month course is necessary for response in breast cancer
• That drug can be abused

oxyphenbutazone (ophthalmic)

Tanderil
Func. class.: Non-steroidal anti-inflammatory drug
Chem. class.: Pyrazolone derivative
Legal class.: POM

Action: Inhibits prostaglandin synthesis by inhibiting an enzyme needed for biosynthesis; possesses analgesic, anti-inflammatory, antipyretic properties
Uses: Local treatment of ocular inflammation
Dosage and routes:
• *Adult:* Apply to inner surface of lower eyelid, 2–5 times a day
Available forms include: Eye ointment 10%
Side effects/adverse reactions:
EENT: Oedema of eyelid, redness of conjunctiva
Contraindications: Hypersensitivity, pregnancy, lactation, infants under 6 months of age
Precautions: Glaucoma
NURSING CONSIDERATIONS
Administer:
• Use aseptic technique
• Use within 1 month of opening tube
Evaluate:
• For eye, ear problems; blurred vision, tinnitus (may indicate toxicity)
Teach patient/family:
• To report blurred vision, or ringing, roaring in ears (may indicate toxicity)

oxytetracycline HCl

Berkmycen, Imperacin, Unimycin, Terramycin
Func. class.: Antibiotic broad spectrum
Chem. class.: Tetracycline
Legal class.: POM

Action: Inhibits protein synthesis, phosphorylation in micro-organisms by binding to 30S ribosomal subunits, reversibly binding to 50S ribosomal subunits
Uses: Syphilis, gonorrhoea, Lyme disease, leptospirosis, infections due to *Brucella*, *Chlamydia*, *Mycoplasma* and *Rickettsiae* spp, other sensitive bacterial infections, exacerbations of chronic bronchitis, acne vulgaris
Dosage and routes:
• *Adult:* By mouth 250–500 mg 6 hrly
Acne
• *Adult:* By mouth 250 mg 3 times a day for 1–4 weeks then 250 mg twice a day
Available forms include: Tablets 250 mg; capsules 250 mg; mixture 125 mg/5 ml
Side effects/adverse reactions:
CNS: Raised intracranial pressure, headache
HAEM: Neutropenia, thrombocytopenia, haemolytic anaemia
EENT: Discolouration and enamel defects in developing teeth, oral candidiasis
GI: Nausea, vomiting, hepatotoxicity, stomatitis, pseudomembranous colitis
CV: Pericarditis
GU: Increased blood urea nitro-

gen, polyuria, polydipsia, renal failure
INTEG: Rash, photosensitivity, exfoliative dermatitis
Contraindications: Hypersensitivity to tetracyclines, children under 12 yr, pregnancy, porphyria, chronic renal failure
Precautions: Hepatic disease, lactation, pregnancy
Pharmacokinetics:
By mouth: Peak 2–4 hr, half-life 6–9 hr; excreted in urine, bile, faeces, 10%–40% protein bound
Interactions/incompatibilities:
- Impaired oxytetracycline absorption: antacids, sodium bicarbonate, dairy products, iron products, alkali products
- Increased effect: anticoagulants
- Decreased effect: penicillins
- Nephrotoxicity: methoxyflurane

Lab. test interferences:
False positive: Urine glucose with Clinistix
False increase: Urinary catecholamines

NURSING CONSIDERATIONS

Assess:
- Fluid balance
- Bowel patterns

Administer:
- By mouth an hour before food or on an empty stomach; not to be taken with milk, iron preparations, or antacids
- After specimens have been sent for culture and sensitivity
- 2 hr before or after laxative or ferrous products, 3 hr after antacid
- Not to children under 8

Evaluate:
- Therapeutic response: decreased temperature, absence of lesions, negative culture and sensitivity
- Allergic reactions: rash, itching, pruritus, angioneurotic oedema
- Nausea, vomiting, diarrhoea; administer anti-emetic, antacids as ordered
- Overgrowth of infection: increased temperature, malaise, redness, pain, swelling, drainage, perineal itching, diarrhoea, changes in cough or sputum

Teach patient/family:
- To avoid sun exposure since burns may occur; sunscreen does not seem to decrease photosensitivity
- If diabetic to avoid use of Clinistix, Diastix, for urine glucose testing
- That all prescribed medication must be taken unless advised otherwise by clinician
- To avoid milk products for a few hours before and after taking tablets

---

oxytocin, synthetic

Syntocinon, Syntometrine, (combination product)
Func. class.: Oxytocic
Chem. class.: Synthetic Hormone
Legal class.: POM

Action: Directly acts on myofibrils producing uterine contraction, breast stimulation
Uses: Stimulation of labour, induction; missed or incomplete abortion; postpartum bleeding
Dosage and routes:
Stimulation of labour
- *Adult:* IV infusion, as solution containing 1 unit/l in glucose 5% or other suitable diluent, 1 to 3 milliunits/min increase gradually until contractions occur every 2 to 5 min; rate should not exceed 12 milliunits/min

Incomplete abortion
- *Adult:* IV infusion, as solution containing 10 to 20 units/500 ml of glucose 5% or other suitable diluent, 10 to 30 drops/min, increased in strength by 10–20 units/500 ml every hour; should not exceed 100 units/500 ml

Third stage of labour (routine)
• IM injection of syntometrine 1 ml with or after delivery of shoulders
Post-partum haemorrhage
• IV infusion 10–20 units/500 ml after delivery of shoulders (high-risk cases with atonic uterus).
Available forms include: Injection IV 2 units/2 ml, 5 units/ml, 10 units/ml and 50 units/5 ml
Side effects/adverse reactions:
CNS: Headache, lethargy, coma, and convulsions (water intoxication)
GI: Nausea, vomiting
CV: Hypertension, subarachnoid, haemorrhage
GU: Uterine rupture, uterine spasm
MISC: Fetal asphyxia, neonatal jaundice
Contraindications: Hypersensitivity, severe toxaemia, cephalopelvic disproportion, hypertonic uterine inertia, mechanical obstruction to delivery, failed trial labour, fetal distress, placenta praevia, predisposition to amniotic fluid embolism or uterine rupture
Precautions: Hypertension, multiple pregnancy, high parity, abnormal presentation, previous Caesarean section
Pharmacokinetics:
IV: Onset 1 min, duration 30 min, half-life 12–17 min
Interactions/incompatibilities:
• May cause hypertension when used with vasopressors
NURSING CONSIDERATIONS
Assess:
• Baseline vital signs for mother and baby (if appropriate)
Administer:
• Do not administer through same line as blood/plasma
• By IV infusion keeping volume low
• With resuscitation equipment and drugs at hand
• With continuous monitoring
Evaluate:
• Fluid balance
• Contraction, fetal heart trace, BP, pulse, respiration
• BP, pulse; watch for changes that may indicate haemorrhage
• Respiratory rate, rhythm, depth; notify clinician of abnormalities
• Length, duration of contraction; report contractions lasting over 1 min or absence of contractions
Teach patient/family:
• To report increased blood loss, abdominal cramps, increased temperature or foul-smelling lochia

pamidronate disodium 

Aredia
Func. class.: Parathyroid agent (calcium regulator)
Chem. class.: Bisphosphonate
Legal class.: POM

Action: Potent inhibitor of bone resorption, exact mechanism of action not yet established
Uses: Tumour-induced hypercalcaemia
Dosage and routes:
• *Adult:* Slow IV infusion, 15 to 90 mg, according to plasma calcium concentration as single infusion or in divided doses over 2–4 days
Consult data sheet for calculating dosage regimen (seek expert advice)
Available forms include: IV infusion concentrate 15 mg/5 ml; 30 mg/vial with 10 ml solvent
Side effects/adverse reactions:
CNS: Convulsions (due to electrolyte disturbances)
HAEM: Transient lymphocytopenia
SYST: Mild transient rise in body temperature

Contraindications: Hypersensitivity
Precautions: Pregnancy, renal insufficiency
NURSING CONSIDERATIONS
Administer:
- After appropriate parenteral/oral rehydration
- Dilute ampoule contents in a calcium free infusion solution to a maximum 30 mg/250 ml and infuse slowly depending on concentration
- Dosage is determined by the patient's initial calcium level
- Total dosage may be given as a single infusion or in divided doses

Evaluate:
- Serum calcium levels start to decrease 24 to 28 hr after drug administration and maximum lowering can be expected after 4 to 5 days. If normocalcaemia is not achieved within this period, a further dose may be given
- Duration of response varies. Treatment can be repeated when hypercalcaemia recurs
- Do not give as a bolus injection since severe local reactions and thrombophlebitis may occur.
- Transient asymptomatic hypocalcaemia is not uncommon; symptomatic hypocalcaemia is rare
- In patients with severe renal insufficiency, it is recommended that the chosen dose be administered as multiple doses

Perform/provide:
- Store ampoules in a refrigerator
- Do not store the diluted infusion
- Do not mix with calcium containing infusion solutions

pancreatin

Creon, Nutrizym, Pancrease, Pancrex, Pancrex V
Func. class.: Digestant
Chem. class.: Pancreatic enzyme concentrate—porcine
Legal class.: P or GSL

Action: Pancreatic enzyme needed for proper pancreatic functioning
Uses: Exocrine pancreatic secretion insufficiency in cystic fibrosis, pancreatectomy, total gastrectomy, chronic pancreatitis
Dosage and routes:
- *Adults and children:* By mouth adjust according to size, number and consistency of stool, so that patient thrives; extra allowance may be required for snacks between meals

Available forms include: Tablets, capsules, granules and powder, providing varying amounts of protease, lipase and amylase activity, doses providing 160 to 3300 units of protease activity, 5000 to 56,000 units lipase activity, 3300 to 60,000 units amylase activity available
Side effects/adverse reactions:
GI: Anal soreness
GU: Hyperuricosuria, hyperuricaemia
INTEG: Rash, hypersensitivity
EENT: Buccal soreness
Contraindications: Hypersensitivity to pig protein; early stages of acute pancreatitis
Interactions/incompatibilities:
- Concurrent antacids may dissolve enteric coatings

NURSING CONSIDERATIONS
Assess:
- For allergy to pork

Administer:
- If not enteric coated 30–45 min after antacid or cimetidine; decreased pH inactivates drug
- Mixed with food (contents

of capsules, granules, powder) or swallowed whole (capsules, tablets)
• Low-fat diet to decrease GI symptoms
• With or immediately before or after food
• If mixed with food or liquids eat within an hour. Do not chew contents of capsules
• Do not mix with very hot food or liquids
• Do not retain in the mouth

Evaluate:
• Therapeutic effect; dose may be adjusted freely depending on stools

Teach patient/family:
• All aspects of enzyme including side effects

pancuronium bromide

Pavulon
Func. class.: Non-depolarising muscle relaxant
Chem. class.: Synthetic curariform
Legal class.: POM

Action: Inhibits transmission of nerve impulses by binding with cholinergic receptor sites, antagonizing action of acetylcholine
Uses: Facilitation of endotracheal intubation, skeletal muscle relaxation during mechanical ventilation, surgery, or general anaesthesia
Dosage and routes:
• *Adult surgery:* IV 50–80 mcg/kg or 80–100 mcg/kg. Incremental doses: 10–20 mcg/kg
• *Child surgery:* Initial dose 60–100 mcg/kg. Incremental doses, 10–20 mcg/kg
• *Neonatal surgery:* IV 30–40 mcg/kg. As neonates are sensitive incremental doses should be adjusted according to initial response
• *Intensive care adults:* IV 60 mcg/kg every 1½ hr or even less frequently
• Doses should be reduced if given after suxamethonium

Available forms include: Injection IV 2 mg/ml
Side effects/adverse reactions:
CV: Tachycardia, increased, decreased BP
RESP: Prolonged apnoea, bronchospasm (rare)
EENT: Increased secretions
MS: Weakness due to prolonged skeletal muscle relaxation
Contraindications: Hypersensitivity, use before suxamethonium
Precautions: Pregnancy, reduced dose in renal disease, altered circulation time, hypothermia, electrolyte imbalances, dehydration, neuromuscular disease, respiratory disease, liver disease, carcinomatosis, myasthenia gravis
Pharmacokinetics:
IV: Onset 30–45 sec, peak 1½–5 min; metabolised (small amounts), excreted in urine (unchanged), duration 45–60 mins
Interactions/incompatibilities:
• Increased neuromuscular blockade: general anaesthetics, narcotic analgesics, diazepam, other muscle relaxants; also aminoglycosides, some polypeptide antibiotics (azlocillin, clindomycin, lincomycin, mezlocillin, polymyxins), β-blockers, diuretics, glyceryl trinitrate, lithium, magnesium salts (parenteral), MAOIs, metronidazole, nifedipine, phenytoin, qúinidine, verapamil
• Decreased effect: proprandol, neostigmine, pyridostigmine, endrophonium, noradrenaline, adrenaline, potassium, sodium, or calcium chloride, heparin, azathioprine, theophylline, previous corticosteroid therapy
• Arrhythmias: tricyclic antidepressants

Administer:

• Using nerve stimulator by anaesthetist to determine neuromuscular blockade

• Anticholinesterase to reverse neuromuscular blockade

• By qualified persons, usually an anaesthetist

Treatment of overdose: Endrophonium or neostigmine, atropine, monitor vital signs; maintain mechanical ventilation until spontaneous breathing restored

NURSING CONSIDERATIONS

Assess:

• Baseline vital signs (BP, pulse, respirations, airway)

Perform/provide:

• Reassurance if communication is difficult during recovery from neuromuscular blockade

Administer:

• As IV bolus or by continous infusion under direction of anaesthetist

• Always preceded by sedation

Evaluate:

• Therapeutic response: paralysis of jaw, eyelid, head, neck, rest of body

• Recovery: decreased paralysis of face, diaphragm, leg, arm, rest of body

• Allergic reactions: rash, fever, respiratory distress, pruritus; drug should be discontinued

• Vital signs

• Fluid balance, retention

• Degree of respiratory depression due to muscle relaxation

• Ensure that patient is sedated as well as paralysed

• Use nerve stimulator to determine degree of neuromuscular block

Teach patient/family:

• Discuss effects of the drug with patient

• Reassure that sedation precedes paralysis

papaveretum

Omnopon (mixed opium alkaloids), Papaveretum

Func. class.: Narcotic analgesic

Chem. class.: Hydrochlorides of opium alkaloids containing morphine, codeine, noscapine and papaverine. *Note* Omnopon preparations do not contain noscapine

Legal class.: CD (Sch 2) POM

Action: Exerts marked narcotic effect on CNS and on the periphery as an antispasmodic

Uses: Pre-operative sedation, analgesia during and after surgery, relief of severe chronic pain

Dosage and routes:

Acute pain

• *Adult:* Subcutaneous, IM injection, 10–20 mg (according to weight), slow IV injection 2.5–10 mg, repeated 4 hrly if necessary

• *Infant up to 1 month:* 150 mcg/kg

• *Infant 1–12 months:* 200 mcg/kg

• *Child 1–12 yr:* 200–300 mcg/kg; when given IV, dose is generally quarter to half corresponding subcutaneous/IM dose

Pre-operative sedation

• *Adult:* Subcutaneous, IM injection, 10–20 mg, 45–60 min before anaesthesia

• *Child:* Single doses as above

Available forms include: Injection, 10 mg/ml, 20 mg/ml, 20 mg with hyoscine hydrobromide 400 mcg/ml

Side effects/adverse reactions:

RESP: Respiratory depression, cough suppression, pulmonary oedema (overdosage)

CNS: Drowsiness, alteration of pupillary responses, hallucinations, mood changes, dependence, confusion, neonatal convulsions

CV: Bradycardia, palpitations, postural hypotension
GI: Nausea, vomiting, reduced motility, constipation, dry mouth
GU: Urinary retention
INTEG: Urticaria, pruritus
SYSTEM: Hypothermia

Contraindications: Respiratory depression, head injury, raised intracranial pressure, obstructive airways disease, coma, hypersensitivity, treatment with MAOIs in last 2 weeks. Noscapine in papaveretum containing preparations is contraindicated in women of child-bearing potential

Precautions: History of drug abuse, acute alcoholism, convulsive disorders, respiratory insufficiency; dosage may need to be reduced for elderly or debilitated patients. Pregnancy, lactation, severe renal or hepatic impairment, biliary tract disorders, hypothyroidism, adrenocortical insufficiency, shock, prostatic hypertrophy, supraventricular tachycardia

Interactions/incompatibilities:
- Actions may be potentiated by other CNS depressants, such as anaesthetic agents, alcohol. MAOIs, phenothiazines

Treatment of overdose: Signs are similar to overdosage with morphine. Supportive care. Administer naloxone for reversal

NURSING CONSIDERATIONS

Assess:
- Respiratory rate BP
- Fluid balance
- Pain control and appropriateness of analgesia

Administer:
- Before the patient is in severe pain for the best effect
- With anti-emetic if nausea, vomiting, occur

Perform/provide:
- Storage in CDA cupboard (hospital)

Evaluate:
- Therapeutic response; decrease in pains
- Respiratory rate and depth for signs of respiratory depression
- Pulse, BP for signs of cardiovascular depression
- Other side effects—nausea, vomiting, constipation, urinary retention
- Dependence on drug. Increased dose may be indicated

Teach patient/family:
- Avoid alcohol whilst taking drug
- Advise patient not to mobilise unaided
- Check with clinician before taking other medications
- Need for secure storage

---

paracetamol

Alvedon, Calpol, Disprol, Panadol, Salzone, Cupanol, many combination products

Func. class.: Non-opioid analgesic
Chem. class.: Nonsalicylate, para aminophenol derivative
Legal class.: P, GSL

Action: Inhibition of prostaglandin synthesis; antipyretic action results from inhibition of hypothalamic heat-regulating centre

Uses: Mild to moderate pain or fever

Dosage and routes:
- *Adult and child over 12 yr:* By mouth 0.5–1 g 4–6 hrly, maximum 4 g in 24 hr
- *Child 2 months:* 60 mg for post-immunisation pyroxia only
- *Child 3 months–1yr:* By mouth 60–120 mg
- *1–5 yr:* By mouth, 120–250 mg; rectal, 125–250 mg
- *6–12 yr:* By mouth 250–500 mg. Doses given 4–6 hrly, maximum 4 doses in 24 hr

• *Child 1–5 yr:* By rectum 125–250 mg up to 4 times daily
Available forms include: Tablets 500 mg, elixir (oral solution) 120 mg/5 ml, mixture (oral suspension) 120 mg/5 ml, 250 mg/5 ml, suppositories 125 mg
Side effects/adverse reactions:
HAEM: Blood dyscrasias (rare)
GI: Overdosage may produce nausea, vomiting, abdominal pain; delayed, progressive, hepatotoxicity leading to death
GU: Papillary necrosis (long-term use), nephrotoxicity (overdosage)
INTEG: Rash, urticaria
Contraindications: Hypersensitivity
Precautions: Hepatic disease, renal disease, chronic alcoholism
Pharmacokinetics:
By mouth: Onset 10–30 min, peak ½–2 hr, duration 4–6 hr. Metabolised by liver, excreted by kidneys, half-life 1–4 hr
Interactions/incompatibilities:
• Increased effects of: anticoagulants, chloramphenicol
• Increased risk of neutropenia: zidovudine
• Decreased effects of this drug: cholestyramine, oral contraceptives, narcotics, anticholinergics, anticonvulsants
• Increased effect of this drug: metoclopramide
• Increased toxicity: barbiturates, alcohol, rifampicin, anticonvulsants
Treatment of overdose: Gastric lavage, administer prompt IV acetylcysteine or oral methionine; further treatment based on plasma paracetamol concentrations 4 hr or more after ingestion. Antidotes are generally ineffective more than 15 hr after overdose

NURSING CONSIDERATIONS
Assess:
• Fluid balance; decreasing output may indicate renal failure (long-term therapy)
Evaluate:
• Therapeutic response: absence of pain, fever
• For rash, blood disorders, acute pancreatitis
• Renal dysfunction: decreased urine output
Teach patient/family:
• Not to exceed recommended dosage; acute poisoning may result
• To read label on other non-prescribed medicines; many contain paracetamol

paraldehyde

Func. class.: Anticonvulsant
Chem. class.: Cyclic ether
Legal class.: POM

Action: CNS depressant; exact mechanism of action is unknown
Uses: Refractory seizures, status epilepticus
Dosage and routes:
• *Adult:* Deep IM 5–10 ml; maximum 20 ml
• *Adult:* IV infusion, 4–5 ml
• *Adult:* By rectum (solution) 5–10 ml
• *Child:* Deep IM or by rectum (solution), up to 3 months, 0.5 ml; 3–6 months, 1 ml; 6–12 months, 1.5 ml; 1–2 yr 2 ml; 3–5 yr, 3–4 ml; 5–12 yr, 5–6 ml
Available forms include: Injection 5 ml, 10 ml paraldehyde
Side effects/adverse reactions:
CNS: Drowsiness
GI: Foul breath, local irritation, hepatotoxicity (overdosage)
GU: Nephrotoxicity (overdosage)
INTEG: Rash
CV: Hypotension, collapse
MISC: Pain, sterile abscess after IM injection
RESP: Pulmonary oedema, pulmonary haemorrhage
Contraindications: Hypersensitivity; rectally in colitis

Precautions: Asthma, hepatic disease, pulmonary disease; avoid contact with rubber and plastic (use glass syringe) injection near sciatic or other nerves may cause nerve damage

Interactions/incompatibilities:

• Enhanced effect of paraldehyde: alcohol, CNS depressants, general anaesthetics, disulfiram

NURSING CONSIDERATIONS

Assess:

• Baseline vital signs including temperature

Administer:

• Deep IM maximum volume 5 ml at one site

• IV infusion in sodium chloride 0.9% at a concentration of 0.4%; only in specialist centres where intensive care facilities are available

• By rectal route as an enema with a 10% solution in sodium chloride 0.9%

Perform/provide:

• Ventilation of room (drug is excreted via lungs)

Evaluate:

• Mental status: mood, alertness, affect, memory (long, short)

• Respiratory dysfunction; respiratory depression, character, rate, rhythm; hold drug if respirations are more than 12/min or if pupils are dilated

Teach patient/family:

• That physical dependency may result when used for extended periods of time

• To avoid driving, other activities that require alertness

• Not to discontinue medication quickly after long-term use, taper over several weeks

• Dangers of misuse

paroxetine ▼

Seroxat

Func. class.: Anti-depressant

Chem. class.: Serotonin (5HT) reuptake inhibitor

Legal class.: POM

Action: Selectively inhibits reuptake of the central neurotransmitter serotonin with little effect on noradrenaline

Uses: Depressive illness, including that accompanied by anxiety

Dosage and routes:

• *Adult:* By mouth initially 20 mg once daily in the morning increased if necessary to maximum 50 mg once daily

• *Elderly:* By mouth initially 20 mg once daily in the morning; maximum 40 mg once daily

Available forms include: Tablets 20, 30 mg

Side effects/adverse reactions:

CNS: Somnolence, tremor, asthenia, insomnia

EENT: Dry mouth

ELECT: Hyponatraemia

GI: Nausea

GU: Sexual dysfunction

INTEG: Sweating

Contraindications: Hypersensitivity; MAOIs within 14 days of starting treatment

Precautions: Pregnancy; breast feeding; history of mania epilepsy; electroconvulsive therapy; cardiac disease

Interactions:

• Risk of toxicity with MAOIs—do not give paroxetine with, or for 14 days after MAOIs; do not give MAOIs for at least 14 days after stopping paroxetine

• Effects of oral anticoagulants enhanced

• Risk of CNS toxicity with: lithium, sumatriptan, tryptophan

• Reduced plasma levels of paroxetine and increased side effects with: phenytoin and possibly other anticonvulsants

Treatment of overdose: Gastric lavage and activated charcoal to reduce absorption; symptomatic and supportive treatment

NURSING CONSIDERATIONS

Assess:

- Sleeping pattern

Administer:

- Tablets with food

Evaluate:

- Therapeutic response

Teach patient/family:

- To take tablets with food
- Need for compliance with regime
- Not to take alcohol, or with MAOIs

---

penicillamine

Distamine, Pendramine

Func. class.: Antirheumatic

Chem. class.: Chelating agent

Legal class.: POM

Action: A chelating agent which aids the elimination from the body of certain heavy metal ions by forming stable soluble complexes which can be excreted via kidney

Uses: Severe active or progressive rheumatoid arthritis, cystinuria, chronic active hepatitis, Wilson's disease, copper or lead poisoning

Dosage and routes: By mouth

Rheumatoid arthritis

Seek expert advice

- *Adult:* By mouth initial dose 125–250 mg daily before food, for 1 month, then increase dose by this amount every 4–12 weeks until remission occurs. Usual maintenance dosage 500–750 mg daily, but up to a maximum of 1.5 g may be required
- *Elderly:* By mouth initial dose 50–125 mg increased in similar increments at a minimum of 4 week intervals to maximum 1 g daily
- *Child:* By mouth initial dose 50 mg daily before food, for 1 month, then increase dose at 4 week intervals to maintenance dose of 15–20 mg/kg daily

Drug to be discontinued if no improvement within 1 year

Wilson's disease

- *Adults:* By mouth 1.5–2 g daily in divided doses before food, reduced to 0.75–1 g daily once disease is controlled. Do not continue dose of 2 g daily for more than 1 yr
- *Elderly:* By mouth 20 mg/kg/day in divided doses before food
- *Child:* By mouth up to 20 mg/kg/day in divided doses. Minimum 500 mg/day

Cystinuria: dissolution of stones

- *Adults:* By mouth 1–3 g daily in divided doses 30 min before food—urine cystine levels of not more than 200 mg/l should be maintained

Prevention of cystine stones:

- *Adult:* By mouth 0.5–1 g at bedtime. Maintain fluid intake above 3 litres daily
- *Elderly and children:* By mouth no dosage range established, use the minimum dose to maintain urinary cystine level below 200 mg/l

Lead poisoning

- *Adults:* By mouth 1–2 g daily in divided doses before meals until total daily urinary lead is less than 0.5 mg daily
- *Elderly and child:* By mouth 20 mg/kg daily in divided doses before meals

Chronic active hepatitis

- *Adults:* By mouth (Maintenance only after disease controlled with corticosteriods)—500 mg daily in divided doses before meals increasing to 1.25 g daily over 3 months. Monitor disease status with periodic liver function tests

Available forms include: Tablets 50, 125, 250 mg

Side effects/adverse reactions:

HAEM: Agranulocytosis, severe thrombocytopenia, leucopenia

GI: Nausea, anorexia, taste loss, mouth ulcers

GU: Proteinuria, nephrotic syndrome, haematuria (rare)

INTEG: Rashes, pruritus, epidermolysis bullosa, increased skin friability, Stevens-Johnson syndrome, pemphigus

MS: Muscle weakness, joint pain

SYSTEM: Fever, myasthenia, lupus erythematosus

Contraindications: Hypersensitivity, lupus erythematosus, agranulocytosis, thrombocytopenia

Precautions: Renal impairment, pregnancy, portal hypertension; withdraw if platelets or WBC count low

Pharmacokinetics: Absorbed from GI tract, peak concentration in 1 hr. Rapidly excreted in urine, traces in plasma after 48 hr due to protein binding

Interactions/incompatibilities:

- Concomitant nephrotoxic or myelosuppressant drugs such as gold, antimalarials, cytotoxics and immunosuppressants
- Phenylbutazone, iron salts should not be given within 2 hr of penicillamine

Clinical assessment:

- Attempt dose reduction if remission is achieved in treatment of rheumatoid arthritis
- Full blood count weekly or two weekly in first 8 weeks of therapy and after each increase in dose, or monthly during maintenance
- Periodic liver function tests in chronic active hepatitis
- Urinalysis weekly initially and after each dosage increase, monthly during maintenance

NURSING CONSIDERATIONS

Administer:

- Take with water
- 1 hr before food or at bedtime for maximum absorption
- Do not give iron or other heavy metals or antacids within 2 hr

Evaluate:

- Urine—test weekly for proteinuria and haematuria
- Withhold drug and inform clinician if haematuria presents
- Urine measurement for signs of renal failure
- For signs of side effects—nausea and vomiting, anorexia, fever, rash, loss of taste. Treat these as appropriate
- Patient's response to drug—any improvement in condition

Teach patient/family:

- That improvement in their condition may not occur for 6–12 weeks
- To check with clinician before taking any other medication
- Serious side effects—any which occur must be reported at once
- May experience metallic taste which will disappear
- If rashes, nausea, loss of appetite, mouth ulcers occur these should be reported
- Teach patient to test own urine (if appropriate) for protein or have regular testing via the clinician
- To carry penicillamine record card
- Importance of 4 weekly blood testing
- The difference between penicillamine and penicillin
- Need to drink 3 litres daily

pentaerythritol tetranitrate

Cardiacap, Mycardol
Func. class.: Vasodilator, coronary
Chem. class.: Nitrate
Legal class.: P

Action: Decreases vascular resistance and venous return, thus decreasing left ventricular work
Uses: Chronic stable angina pectoris, prophylaxis of angina pain as an adjunct to glyceryl trinitrate
Dosage and routes:
• *Adult:* By mouth 60 mg 3 to 4 times a day before meals SUS REL 30 mg every 12 hr
Available forms include: Capsules modified release 30 mg; tablets 30 mg
Side effects/adverse reactions:
CV: Postural hypotension, tachycardia, syncope, cyanosis, methaemoglobinaemia
GI: Nausea, vomiting
INTEG: Pallor, sweating, rash
CNS: Headache, flushing, dizziness, lethargy, drowsiness
Contraindications: Hypersensitivity to this drug or other nitrates, anaemia, increased intracranial pressure due to head trauma or cerebral haemorrhage, acute myocardial infarction
Precautions: Pregnancy, closed-angle glaucoma, hypotension
Pharmacokinetics:
By mouth: Onset 20–60 min, peak 4–8 hr
Modified release: Duration 12 hr. Metabolised by liver, excreted in faeces and urine
Interactions/incompatibilities:
• Increased effects: alcohol, β-blockers, narcotics, tricyclics antidepressants, diuretics, antihypertensives, general anaesthetics
• Decreased effects: sympathomimetics, acetylcholine, histamine

NURSING CONSIDERATIONS
Assess:
• BP, pulse, respirations before beginning therapy
Administer:
• Orally before meals
Evaluate:
• Therapeutic response, stabilizing of angina pectoris
• Effect of any other drug therapy
• Pain—duration, character, activity being performed
• Headache, lethargy and nausea, if at commencement of treatment should be transient
• Side effects: toxicity—cyanosis, syncope, methaemoglobin-aernia, rash, servere headache fall in blood pressure, dizziness, palpitation
Perform/provide:
• Suitable physical activity to encourage healthier living
Teach patient/family:
• To give up smoking and encourage a healthy diet and physical activity
• To avoid driving and hazardous activities if dizziness occurs
• Not to drink alcohol
• To take other medication only if directed by clinician
• To report palpitations or vomiting immediately

pentamidine isethionate

Pentacarinat
Func. class.: Antiprotozoal
Chem. class.: Aromatic diamidine derivative
Legal class.: POM

Action: Interferes with DNA/RNA synthesis in protozoa

Uses: *Pneumocystis carinii* infections; visceral leishmaniasis, cutaneous leishmaniasis, trypanosomiasis

Dosage and routes:

Pneumocystis carinii

• *Adult and child:* Slow IV infusion/deep IM injection 4 mg/kg daily for 2 weeks

• Inhalation, 600 mg daily via a suitable nebuliser system; for prophylaxis, 300 mg every 4 weeks

Visceral leishmaniasis

• Deep IM 3–4 mg/kg alternate days to maximum total of 10 injections. Repeat if required

Cutaneous leishmaniasis

• Deep IM 3–4 mg/kg, once or twice weekly

Trypanosomiasis

• Deep IM/slow IV infusion 4 mg/kg daily or alternate days to total of 7–10 injections

Available forms include: Injection 300 mg/vial; nebuliser solution 300 mg/bottle

Side effects/adverse reactions:

CV: Hypotension, cardiac arrhythmias, ventricular tachycardia, hypertension, syncope, flushing

HAEM: Anaemia, leucopenia, thrombocytopenia

INTEG: Sterile abscess, pain at injection site (IM); pruritus, urticaria, rash

GU: Acute renal failure, azotaemia

GI: Nausea, vomiting, taste disturbances, hepatic impairment, acute pancreatitis

CNS: Disorientation, hallucinations, dizziness

META: Hyperkalaemia, hypocalcaemia, hypoglycaemia, hyperglycaemia

RESP: Cough, bronchospasm, or pneumothorax (inhalation route)

Precautions: Blood dyscrasias, hepatic disease, renal disease (reduce dose), hyperglycaemia, hypoglycaemia, hypertension, hypotension, pregnancy, lactation

Pharmacokinetics: Elimination half-life about 6 hr (IV), 9 hr (IM); accumulates in liver, kidney. Small amounts excreted unchanged in urine. Half-life in lung fluid prolonged; about 5% of inhaled dose absorbed

Clinical assessment:

• Blood studies, fasting blood glucose (daily during therapy and periodically afterwards); full blood count, platelets (daily); serum calcium (weekly); serum electrolytes (daily)

• ECG for cardiac dysrhythmias

• Liver function tests: aspartate aminotransferase, alanine aminotransferase bilirubin, alkaline phosphatase

• Renal studies daily: urinalysis, blood urea nitrogen, creatinine

NURSING CONSIDERATIONS

Assess:

• Bowel pattern

• Fluid balance

• Allergies before treatment, reaction of each medication; place allergies on nursing care plan; notify all people giving drugs

Administer:

• Avoid bolus intravenous injection if possible; if IV is necessary give slowly. IM injection should be deep, preferably into the buttock. Patients should receive the drug lying down if given parenterally, under BP monitoring

• Inhaled bronchodilators prior to nebulised solution

Perform/provide:

• Storage in refrigerator for reconstituted solution

Evaluate:

• Therapeutic response: decreased temperature, ability to breathe

• BP during administration and at intervals during treatment

• Bowel pattern during treatment
• Sterile abscess, pain at injection site
• Respiratory status: rate, character, wheezing, dyspnoea
• Fluid balance; report haematuria, oliguria
• Any patient with compromised renal system; drug is excreted slowly in poor renal system function; toxicity may occur rapidly
• Dizziness, confusion, hallucination

Teach patient/family:

• To report sore throat, fever, fatigue, could indicate superimposed infection

---

pentazocine

Fortral

Func. class.: Narcotic analgesic
Chem. class.: Synthetic benzomorphan
Legal class.: CD (Sch 3) POM

Action: Inhibits ascending pain pathways in CNS, increases pain threshold, alters pain perception

Uses: Moderate to severe pain

Dosage and routes:

• *Adult:* By mouth, pentazocine HCl 50–100 mg 3–4 hrly as needed; IV/IM/subcutaneous injection, pentazocine 30–60 mg (as lactate) 3–4 hrly as needed, dose not to exceed 1 mg/kg (subcutaneous, IM) or 0.5 mg/kg (IV); rectal, pentazocine 50 mg (as lactate) up to 4 times daily
• *Child 1–6 yr:* IM/subcutaneous injection, pentazocine (as lactate) 1 mg/kg; IV, pentazocine (as lactate) 0.5 mg/kg
• *Child 6–12 yr:* By mouth, pentazocine HCl 25 mg 3–4 hrly as needed; IM/subcutaneous injection, pentazocine (as lactate) 1 mg/kg; IV, pentazocine (as lactate) 0.5 mg/kg

Available forms include: Injection, pentazocine (as lactate) 30 mg/ml; suppositories, pentazocine (as lactate) 50 mg; capsules, pentazocine HCl 50 mg; tablets, pentazocine HCl 25 mg

Side effects/adverse reactions:

CNS: Drowsiness, sleep disturbances, dizziness, confusion, headache, hallucinations, sedation, paraesthesia, mood changes, raised intracranial pressure, convulsions, coma (overdosage), dependence
GI: Nausea, vomiting, dry mouth, constipation
GU: Urinary retention, biliary spasm
INTEG: Sweating, flushing, pruritus, local damage at injection site
EENT: Visual disturbances
CV: Tachycardia, hypotension, transient hypertension
RESP: Respiratory depression

Contraindications: Hypersensitivity, dependence (narcotic), respiratory depression, raised intracranial pressure, head injury, hypertension, heart failure, porphyria

Precautions: Pregnancy, lactation, myocardial infarction (acute), hepatic disease, renal disease, phaeochromocytoma, hypothyroidism, adrenocortical insufficiency, prostatic hypertrophy, inflammatory or obstructive bowel disease

Pharmacokinetics:

By mouth, about 50% available, peak 1–3 hr
Subcutaneous/IM: Onset 15–30 min, peak 1–2 hr, duration 2–4 hr
IV: Onset 2–3 min, duration 4–6 hr
Metabolised by liver, excreted by kidneys

Interactions/incompatibilities:
- Effects may be increased with other CNS depressants: alcohol, anaesthetics, sedative/hypnotics, antipsychotics
- Enhanced clearance in smokers (decreased effect)
- May decrease effects of other opioids (weak antagonist properties)
- Interacts with MAOIs (enhanced toxicity)

Treatment of overdose: Naloxone, gastric lavage, supportive care including anticonvulsants as required

NURSING CONSIDERATIONS

Assess:
- Fluid balance
- Respiratory function
- Pain control and appropriateness of analgesia

Administer:
- With anti-emetic if nausea, vomiting occur

Perform/provide:
- Storage in CD cupboard (hospital)
- Assistance with ambulation, only after dose has taken effect in case of dizziness
- Safety measures: cot sides, night light, callbell within easy reach as necessary

Evaluate:
- Therapeutic response: decrease in pain
- CNS changes: dizziness, drowsiness, hallucinations, euphoria, level of consciousness, pupil reaction
- Decrease in urinary output: may indicate urinary retention
- Allergic reactions: rash, urticaria
- Respiratory dysfunction: respiratory depression, character, rate, rhythm; notify clinician if respirations are less than 12/min
- Need for pain medication, physical dependence

Teach patient/family:
- To report any symptoms of CNS changes, allergic reactions
- That physical dependency may result when used for extended periods of time
- Avoid potentially hazardous tasks until certain that dizziness does not occur
- Measures to reduce risk of constipation
- Withdrawal symptoms may occur: nausea, vomiting, cramps, fever, faintness, anorexia if drug is suddenly stopped after a long period
- Not to exceed prescribed dosage without consulting clinician

---

pergolide ▼

Celance

Func. class.: Dopamine agonist
Chem. class.: Ergot alkaloid derivative
Legal class.: POM

Action: Direct stimulation of D_1 and D_2 dopamine receptors

Uses: Adjunctive to levodopa in the treatment of parkinsonism

Dosage and routes:
- *Adult:* By mouth 50 mcg daily for 2 days, increased by 100–150 mcg every third day over next 12 days, further increases of 250 mcg every third day until optimal therapeutic response achieved; usual maintenance 3 mg daily; usually administered in divided doses 3 times per day

Available forms include: Tablets 50, 250, 1000 mcg (as mesylate)

Side effects/adverse reactions:

CNS: Dyskinesia, hallucinations, somnolence, insomnia, confusion
CV: Hypotension, arrhythmias
EENT: Diplopia, rhinitis
GI: Nausea, dyspepsia, constipation, diarrhoea
MISC: Pain

RESP: Dyspnoea

Contraindications: Hypersensitivity to this drug or other ergot derivatives

Precautions: Arrhythmias; cardiac disease; history of confusion or hallucinations; dyskinesia; pregnancy; breast feeding; increase dosage and withdraw drug gradually

Interactions:

- Antagonism of and by: antipsychotics
- Risk of hypotension with: antihypertensives
- Possible potentiation of: oral anticoagulants

Treatment of overdose: Gastric lavage and/or activated charcoal to reduce absorption; symptomatic and supportive treatment including cardiac monitoring

NURSING CONSIDERATIONS

Assess:

- Baseline BP

Administer:

- With particular attention to variations in dosage

Evaluate:

- Therapeutic response
- Side-effects including hypotension

Teach patient/family:

- Reasons for varying amounts of drug
- Importance of compliance with regime
- About side effects
- To report any side effects to nurse or clinician
- Not to drive or use heavy machinery particularly during early stages of taking this medication. May affect performance of skilled tasks

pericyazine

Neulactil

Func. class.: Antipsychotic/neuroleptic

Chem. class.: Phenothiazine

Legal class.: POM

Action: Depresses cerebral cortex, hypothalamus, limbic system, which controls aggression; blocks neurotransmission produced by dopamine at synapse; exhibits strong α-adrenergic, anticholinergic blocking action

Uses: Behavioural disturbances, schizophrenia and related psychotic disorders, short-term adjunctive treatment of severe anxiety, psychomotor agitation

Dosage and routes:

- *Adult:* By mouth short-term anxiety, agitation, behaviour disorders, 15–30 mg (elderly 5–10 mg) daily (anxiety, agitation); give in 2 unequal doses, taking the larger at bedtime; adjust according to response
- By mouth, schizophrenia, other psychoses, 75 mg daily in divided doses; increase by 25 mg at weekly intervals; usual maintenance dose up to 300 mg daily
- *Child:* By mouth, severe behaviour/mental disorders, initially 0.5 mg daily for child weighing 10 kg; increased by 1 mg for each additional 5 kg body weight up to maximum 10 mg daily; maintenance dose not to exceed twice initial dose

Available forms include: Tablets 2.5, 10, 25 mg; syrup 10 mg/5 ml

Side effects/adverse reactions:

CNS: Extrapyramidal symptoms, tardive dyskinesia, sedation, drowsiness, apathy, nightmares, insomnia, depression, agitation

CV: Arrhythmias, hypotension, ECG changes

HAEM: Agranulocytosis, leucopenia, haemolytic anaemia
GU: Difficulty with micturition, menstrual disturbances, impotence
ENDO: Galactorrhoea, gynaecomastia, weight gain
SYST: Neuroleptic malignant syndrome
INTEG: Pallor, photosensitisation, contact sensitization, rashes
EENT: Dry mouth, nasal congestion, blurred vision, corneal and lens opacities
GI: Constipation, jaundice
Contraindications: Coma caused by CNS depressants, bone marrow depression, hypersensitivity
Precautions: Cardiovascular or cerebrovascular disease, respiratory disease, parkinsonism, epilepsy, phaeochromocytoma, renal or hepatic impairment, history of jaundice or leucopenia, myasthenia gravis, hypothyroidism, elderly patients, pregnancy, lactation, prostatic hypertrophy
Pharmacokinetics: None known
Interactions/incompatibilities:
• Effects may be increased with other CNS depressants: alcohol, sedative/hypnotics
• Increased antimuscarinic effect, possibly reduced antipsychotic effect with other antimuscarinic drugs
• Decreased absorption with antacids, antiparkinsonian agents, lithium
• Decreased effect of amphetamines, levodopa, clonidine, guanethidine, adrenaline, oral hypoglycaemics
• Possible encephalopathy with desferrioxamine
Clinical assessment:
• Periodic eye, skin examinations on long-term therapy
Treatment of overdose:
• Lavage, supportive care
Lab. test interferences:
False positive: Pregnancy tests

NURSING CONSIDERATIONS
Assess:
• Fluid balance
Administer:
• Antimuscarinic antiparkinsonian agent may be prescribed if extrapyramidal symptoms appear
Perform/provide:
• Urinalysis before and during prolonged therapy
• Supervised ambulation, until stabilised on medication, do not involve in strenuous exercise programme because fainting is possible; patient should not stand still for long periods of time
• Increased fluids to prevent constipation
• Sips of water, mouthwashes for dry mouth
Evaluate:
• For dizziness, faintness, palpitations, tachycardia on rising
• For extrapyramidal symptoms including akathisia (inability to sit still, no pattern to movement), tardive dyskinesia (bizarre movements of jaw, mouth, tongue, extremities), pseudoparkinsonism (rigidity, tremors, pill rolling, shuffling gait)
• For constipation, urinary retention daily; if these occur, increase bulk, water in diet
• Affect, orientation, level of consciousness, reflexes, gait, coordination, sleep pattern; report any disturbances to clinician
• Therapeutic response: decrease in emotional excitement, hallucinations, delusions, paranoia, reorganisation of patterns of thought, speech
Teach patient/family:
• That orthostatic hypotension occurs frequently, and to rise from sitting or lying position gradually
• To remain lying down after IM injection for at least 30 min
• To avoid hot baths, hot showers since hypotension may occur

• To avoid abrupt withdrawal of this drug, drugs should be withdrawn slowly
• To avoid non-prescribed medication (cough, hayfever, cold) unless approved by clinician, since serious drug interactions may occur; avoid use with alcohol or CNS depressants, increased drowsiness may occur
• To use sunscreen during sun exposure to prevent burns
• Importance of compliance with drug regimen
• To report sore throat, malaise, fever, bleeding, mouth sores; if these occur, full blood count should be done and drug discontinued

perindopril

Conversyl
Func. class.: Antihypertensive
Chem. class.: Angiotensin-converting enzyme inhibitor
Legal class.: POM

Action: Inhibits the conversion of angiotensin I to vasoconstrictive angiotensin II and reduces degradation of vasodilatory bradykinin
Uses: Essential hypertension where standard therapy is ineffective or inappropriate; adjunct in heart failure
Dosage and routes:
Diuretics should be stopped if possible for 2–3 days before starting treatment to minimise the risk of a rapid fall in blood pressure and hypotension
Hypertension
• *Adult:* By mouth, initially, 2 mg daily increasing to maintenance dose of 4 to 8 mg daily
Congestive heart failure
• *Adult:* By mouth, initially 2 mg in the morning, under close hospital supervision, increase if necessary to usual maintenance dose of 4 mg
Available forms include: Tablets 2 mg, 4 mg
Side effects/adverse reactions:
HAEM: Decreases in haemoglobin, red cells and platelets
CV: Hypotension (with initial doses, especially with concurrent diuretics)
CNS: Fatigue, asthenia, malaise, headache, mood and sleep disturbances
GU: Proteinuria, increased blood urea and creatinine
RESP: Cough
GI: Taste impairment, epigastric discomfort, nausea, abdominal pain
INTEG: Skin rashes, pruritus, flushing, angioneurotic oedema
Contraindications: Hypersensitivity, pregnancy, breast-feeding, aortic stenosis or outflow obstruction, renovascular disease, porphyria
Precautions: Renal insufficiency (reduce dose), peripheral vascular disease, atherosclerosis
Pharmacokinetics: Perindopril acts through its active metabolite perindoprilat, the other metabolites being inactive
Interactions/incompatibilities
• Increased hypotensive effect: diuretics and other antihypertensives, neuroleptics, tricyclic antidepressants, anaesthetics
• Increased plasma concentrations of: lithium, potassium
Clinical assessment:
• The doses should be titrated against blood pressure to achieve optimum control
• It is recommended that diuretic therapy is discontinued 3 days before starting treatment, if required, the diuretic should be reintroduced at the lowest dose

• Potassium sparing diuretics should be avoided or used with extreme caution
• Assess renal function before and during treatment where appropriate
• Combination of potassium supplements or potassium sparing diuretics with perindopril is not recommended
• The dose should be taken before a meal

NURSING CONSIDERATIONS

Assess:
• Renal and liver function tests before therapy and occasionally during treatment

Evaluate:
• Pulse and blood pressure regularly until therapeutic response obtained; lower blood pressure
• Oedema in feet and legs
• Input and output of fluids check for fluid retention
• Effect of any other medication
• Hypotension
• Symptoms of congestive cardiac failure

Teach patient/family:
• To take other medication only if directed by clinician
• To report oedema
• To avoid driving or use of machinery until therapy establish
• To report oliguria and any other renal changes

---

permethrin

Lyclear
Func. class.: Parasiticide
Chem. class.: Synthetic pyrethroid
Legal class.: P

Action: Induces sensory hyperexcitability, uncoordination, prostration and death in lice and mites

Uses: Eradication of head lice and scabies

Dosage and routes:

Head lice
• *Adult and child over 6 months of age:* By topical application of hair lotion after shampooing hair with a normal shampoo; leave on hair for 10 min then rinse

Scabies
• *Adult (and child over 2 yr of age):* By topical application of skin cream to the skin of the whole body excluding the head; leave on for at least 8 hr before washing
• *Child (2 months–2 years of age):* By topical application of skin cream to the skin of the whole body including the face, neck, scalp and ears; leave on for at least 8 hr before washing

Available forms include: Hair lotion 1%, skin cream 5%

Side effects/adverse reactions:
INTEG: Irritation of skin or scalp

Contraindications: Hypersensitivity

Precautions: Children under 6 months of age treated with shampoo and children under 2 yr of age and elderly patients treated with skin cream should be treated under medical supervision; pregnancy; breast-feeding

Pharmacokinetics: Only about 1% absorbed percutaneously even after whole body administration; rapidly metabolised and excreted in urine

Treatment of overdose: No experience of toxicity; ingestion of whole bottle of lotion or tube of cream unlikely to cause overt toxicity; lotion may cause alcohol intoxication in a small child which could be prevented by gastric lavage within 2 hr of ingestion

NURSING CONSIDERATIONS

Assess:
• Signs of scabies between toes and fingers, tracking, blisters,

irritation; area of body involved, including crusts, nits, brownish trails on skin, itching papules in skin folds
• Signs of head lice

Administer:
• Wearing protective plastic or rubber gloves if handling permethrin regularly
• Keeping away from mouth and eyes
• Ensuring very young children do not lick it off

Perform/provide:
• Isolation until treatment completed and areas on skin and scalp have cleared
• Removal of nits by using a fine-tooth comb, rinsed in vinegar after treatment

Evaluate:
• Eradication of head lice, scabies

Teach patient/family:
• When treating scabies to pay particular attention when applying lotion to skin folds, finger and toe-webs and underneath nails
• To wash clothing of all residents using insecticide. Preventative treatment may be required for all persons living in same house, using lotion or shampoo to decrease spread of infection
• That sexual contacts should be treated simultaneously
• Not to wash treated area before recommended contact time has elapsed

perphenazine

Fentazin

Func. class.: Antipsychotic/neuroleptic, anti-emetic
Chem. class.: Phenothiazine
Legal class.: POM

Action: Depresses cerebral cortex, hypothalamus, limbic system, which control activity, aggression; blocks neurotransmission produced by dopamine at synapse; exhibits strong α-adrenergic, anticholinergic blocking action; as antiemetic inhibits medullary chemoreceptor trigger zone

Uses: Psychotic disorders, schizophrenia, short-term adjunctive treatment of severe anxiety, psychomotor agitation, nausea, vomiting

Dosage and routes:

Nausea and vomiting
• *Adult:* By mouth initially 4 mg 3 times daily adjusted according to response to a maximum of 24 mg daily
• *Elderly:* By mouth, quarter to half usual adult dose

Psychoses
• *Adult:* By mouth 4 mg 3 times a day; maximum 24 mg daily; elderly, half adult dose

Available forms include: Tablets 2, 4 mg

Side effects/adverse reactions:
CNS: Extrapyramidal symptoms especially dystonia, tardive dyskinesia; seizures, headache, drowsiness, confusion, sedation, agitation, insomnia, paradoxical excitement
HAEM: Anaemia, leucopenia, agranulocytosis
INTEG: Rash, photosensitivity
EENT: Blurred vision, dry mouth, nasal congestion, corneal and lens opacities, retinopathy
GI: Constipation, jaundice
GU: Urinary retention, impotence, amenorrhoea
CV: Orthostatic hypotension, arrhythmias, ECG changes (prolongation of QT interval and T-wave changes), tachycardia
ENDO: Galactorrhoea, gynaecomastia, weight gain
SYST: Neuroleptic malignant syndrome, hypothermia

Contraindications: Hypersensi-

tivity, blood dyscrasias, coma, child below 14 yr, bone marrow depression

Precautions: Pregnancy, lactation, renal failure, hypothyroidism, hepatic disease, arrhythmias, cardiac failure, coronary artery disease, severe respiratory disease, epilepsy, Parkinson's disease, myasthenia gravis, personal or family history of closed-angle glaucoma, phaeochromocytoma, prostatic hypertrophy, elderly patients, especially during extreme climatic conditions

Pharmacokinetics:

By mouth: Onset erratic, peak 2–4 hr

IM: Onset 10 min, peak 1–2 hr, duration 6 hr, occasionally 12–24 hr

Metabolised by liver, excreted in urine, enters breast milk

Interactions/incompatibilities:

• Oversedation: other CNS depressants such as alcohol, analgesics, sedative/hypnotics

• Decreased absorption: antacids, tea, coffee (concurrent administration)

• Decreased effects of: lithium, levodopa, anticonvulsants, oral hypoglycaemics, adrenaline and other sympathomimetics, guanethidine, clonidine

• Increased effects of: quinidine, diazoxide, neuromuscular blockers, corticosteroids, digoxin

• Increased anticholinergic effects: anticholinergics

Lab. test interferences:

False positive: Pregnancy tests

Treatment of overdose: Lavage, supportive care

NURSING CONSIDERATIONS

Assess:

• Fluid balance

Administer:

• Orally, dose titrated to patient's requirements

Perform/provide:

• Urinalysis before and during prolonged therapy

• Supervised ambulation until stabilised on medication; do not involve in strenuous exercise programme because fainting is possible; patient should not stand still for long periods of time

• Increased fluids to prevent constipation

• Sips of water for dry mouth

Evaluate:

• Therapeutic response: decrease in emotional excitement, hallucinations, delusions, paranoia, reorganisation of patterns of thought, speech

• Affect, orientation, level of consciousness, reflexes, gait, coordination, sleep pattern disturbances

• Dizziness, faintness, palpitations, tachycardia on rising

• Extrapyramidal symptoms including motor restlessness (inability to sit still, no pattern to movements), tardive dyskinesia (bizarre movements of jaw, mouth, tongue, extremities), pseudoparkinsonism (rigidity, tremors, pill rolling, shuffling gait)

• Constipation, urinary retention daily; if these occur, increase bulk, water in diet

Teach patient/family:

• That postural hypotension occurs frequently, and to rise from sitting or lying position gradually

• To remain lying down after IM injection for at least 30 min

• To avoid hot showers, or baths since hypotension may occur

• To avoid abrupt withdrawal of this drug, drugs should be withdrawn slowly

• To avoid non-prescribed preparations (cough, hayfever, cold) unless approved by clinician since serious drug interactions may occur; avoid use with alcohol or CNS

depressants, increased drowsiness may occur
- To use a sunscreen during sun exposure to prevent burns
- Importance of compliance with drug regimen
- About necessity for meticulous oral hygiene since oral candidiasis may occur
- To report sore throat, malaise, fever, bleeding, mouth sores; if these occur, full blood count should be drawn and drug discontinued

pethidine HCl

Pethidine-Roche, combination product
Func. class.: Narcotic analgesic
Chem. class.: Opioid, phenylpiperidine derivative
Legal class.: CD (Sch 2) POM

Action: Inhibits ascending pain pathways in CNS, increases pain threshold, alters pain perception
Uses: Moderate to severe pain, peri-operative analgesia, obstetric analgesia
Dosage and routes:
Pain
- *Adult:* By mouth 50–150 mg every 4 hr as needed; subcutaneous/IM 25–100 mg every 4 hr as needed; slow IV 25–50 mg every 4 hr as needed
- *Child:* By mouth/subcutaneous/IM 0.5–2 mg/kg every 4 hr as needed

Peri-operatively
- *Adult:* IM 25–100 mg 1 hr before surgery, IV 10–25 mg as needed (adjunct to nitrous oxide/oxygen)
- *Child:* IM 0.5–2 mg/kg 1 hr before surgery

Obstetric analgesia
- Subcutaneous/IM 50–100 mg, repeat after 1–3 hr as needed, maximum 400 mg in 24 hr

Available forms include: Injection 10 mg/ml, 50 mg/ml; tablets 50 mg
Side effects/adverse reactions:
CNS: Drowsiness, dizziness, confusion, headache, sedation, CNS stimulation, mood changes, convulsions, coma (overdosage), raised intracranial pressure, dependence
GI: Nausea, vomiting, dry mouth, constipation
GU: Urinary retention, biliary spasm
INTEG: Sweating, flushing, pruritus, local reaction at injection site
EENT: Visual disturbances
CV: Palpitations, bradycardia, hypotension
RESP: Respiratory depression
Contraindications: Hypersensitivity, coma, severe renal impairment, obstructive airways disease
Precautions: Dependence, pregnancy, lactation, head injury or increased intracranial pressure, adrenocortical insufficiency, biliary tract disorders, shock, respiratory depression, hepatic disease, renal disease, neonates, premature babies, hypothyroidism, prostatic hypertrophy, supraventricular tachycardia, elderly or debilitated, cancer, sickle cell disease
Pharmacokinetics:
By mouth: Onset 15 min, peak 1 hr, duration 2–4 hr
Subcutaneous/IM: Onset 10 min, peak 1 hr, duration 2–4 hr
IV: Onset 5 min, duration 2 hr
Metabolised by liver (to active/inactive metabolites), excreted by kidneys, excreted in breast milk
Interactions/incompatibilities:
- Effects may be increased with other CNS depressants: alcohol, anaesthetics, narcotics, sedative/hypnotics, antipsychotics
- Interacts with MAOIs (enhanced toxicity)

Treatment of overdose: Naloxone,

gastric lavage, supportive care including anticonvulsants as required

NURSING CONSIDERATIONS

Assess:

• Respiratory rate, BP

• Pain control and appropriateness of analgesia

Administer:

• With anti-emetic if nausea, vomiting occur

Perform/provide:

• Storage in CD cupboard (hospital)

Evaluate:

• Therapeutic response: decrease in pain

• CNS changes: dizziness, drowsiness, hallucinations, level of consciousness, pupil reaction

• Allergic reactions: rash, urticaria

• Respiratory dysfunction: respiratory depression

• Side effects—nausea, vomiting, constipation urinary retention

• Need for pain medication, physical dependence, tolerance

Teach patient/family:

• To report any symptoms of CNS changes, allergic reactions

• Advise patient not to mobilise unsupervised

• Need for secure storage

phenazocine hydrobromide

Narphen

Func. class.: Narcotic analgesic

Chem. class.: Synthetic benzomorphan

Legal class.: CD (Sch 2) POM

Action: Inhibits ascending pain pathways in CNS, increases pain threshold, alters pain perception; considered to be less sedating than morphine

Uses: Severe pain

Dosage and routes:

• By mouth or sublingually, 5 mg 4–6 hrly when necessary; maximum single dose, 20 mg

Available forms include: Tablets 5 mg

Side effects/adverse reactions:

RESP: Respiratory depression, cough suppression

CV: Hypotension

CNS: Drowsiness, dizziness, dependence

GI: Nausea, reduced motility, constipation, vomiting, dry mouth

GU: Urinary retention

INTEG: Pruritus, sweating

Contraindications: Hypotension, myxoedema, respiratory depression, obstructive airways disease, coma, convulsive disorders, delirium tremens, alcoholism

Precautions: Labour (may cause neonatal respiratory depression), history of drug abuse, renal impairment, head injury, raised intracranial pressure; dosage may need to be reduced for elderly patients, in hepatic disease, or hypothyroidism

Pharmacokinetics: Onset within 20 min, duration 5–6 hr

Interactions/incompatibilities:

• MAOIs (increased toxicity)

• Enhanced effect with narcotic analgesics, sedatives/hypnotics, anaesthetics

Treatment of overdose: Naloxone, supportive care

NURSING CONSIDERATIONS

Assess:

• Pain control and effectiveness of analgesia

• Respiratory function, baseline

• Blood pressure baseline

• Urinary output

Administer:

• Sublingually as prescribed

• With anti-emetic if indicated

Perform/provide:

• Safe environment (potent analgesic). Patient not to mobilise until

drug has taken effect as dizziness may occur
- Storage in CD cupboard (hospital)

Evaluate:
- CNS and respiratory function as drug is a respiratory depressant
- BP
- Urinary output for retention
- Effectiveness of pain control
- Tolerance and/or dependence

Teach patient/family:
- Not to exceed the prescribed dose without medical advice
- To report signs of CNS disturbance
- To avoid potentially hazardous tasks until drug has taken effect without dizziness occurring
- That physical dependence may result if taken for long periods and then stopped suddenly
- Need for safe storage

phenelizine

Nardil
Func. class.: Antidepressant (MAOI)
Chem. class.: Hydrazine
Legal class.: POM

Action: Increases concentrations of endogenous adrenaline, noradrenaline, serotonin, dopamine in storage sites in CNS by inhibition of monoamine oxidase; increased concentration reduces depression

Uses: Depression, especially where phobic symptoms are present, when uncontrolled by other means

Dosage and routes:
- *Adult:* By mouth 15 mg 3 times daily, may increase to 15 mg 4 times daily if necessary (up to 30 mg 3 times daily in hospital), reduced to lowest possible maintenance dose once response occurs

Available forms include: Tablets phenelzine 15 mg (as sulphate)

Side effects/adverse reactions:
HAEM: Blood dyscrasias
CNS: Dizziness, drowsiness, peripheral neuropathy, paraesthesia, headache, anxiety, tremors, weakness, euphoria, mania, insomnia, fatigue, convulsions
GI: Constipation, dry mouth, nausea, vomiting, increased appetite, weight gain, jaundice
GU: Micturition difficulty, impotence, delayed ejaculation
INTEG: Rash, sweating, purpura
CV: Orthostatic hypotension, arrhythmias, hypertensive crisis (interaction with drugs or food)
EENT: Blurred vision

Contraindications: Hypersensitivity to MAOIs, hepatic impairment, cerebrovascular disease, phaeochromocytoma, porphyria or serotonin uptake inhibitors

Precautions: Suicidal patients, epilepsy, cardiovascular disease, blood dyscrasias, renal disease, diabetes mellitus, pregnancy, elderly or agitated patients

Pharmacokinetics: Metabolised by liver, excreted by kidneys

Interactions/incompatibilities:
- Increased pressor effects (hypertensive crisis): indirect acting sympathomimetics, dopamine, levodopa, amphetamines, anoectics, tyramine-containing foods
- Increased effects of: alcohol, barbiturates and other hypnotics, antimuscarinics, diuretics, antihypertensives, hypoglycaemics
- Hypotension, convulsions: tricyclic antidepressants, pethidine and other opioid analgesics (administer in reduced dose initially)

Treatment of overdose: Lavage, symptomatic care (IV fluids, hydrocortisone for hypotension, phentolamine for hypertension, chlorpromazine for restlessness)

NURSING CONSIDERATIONS

Assess:
• Baseline BP
Administer:
• Increased fluids, bulk in diet if constipation, urinary retention occur
• With food or milk or GI symptoms
• Dosage at bedtime if oversedation occurs during day
• Frequent sips of water for dry mouth
Perform/provide:
• Assistance with ambulation during beginning therapy since drowsiness/dizziness occurs
• Check patient compliance
Evaluate:
• BP (lying, standing), pulse; if systolic BP drops 20 mmHg notify clinician
• Toxicity: increased headache, palpitation, discontinue drug immediately; prodromal signs of hypertensive crisis
• Mental status: mood, alertness, affect, memory (long, short); increase in psychiatric symptoms
• Urinary retention, constipation, oedema, take weight weekly
• Withdrawal symptoms: headache, nausea, vomiting, muscle pain, weakness
Teach patient/family:
• That therapeutic effects may take 1–4 weeks
• To avoid driving or other activities requiring alertness
• Give patient MAOI warning card to be carried at all times
• To avoid alcohol ingestion, CNS depressants or non-prescribed drugs: cold, weight, hay fever, cough syrup
• Not to discontinue medication quickly after long-term use
• To avoid high tyramine foods: cheese, sour cream, beer, wine, pickled products, liver, raisins, bananas, figs, avocados, meat tenderisers, chocolate, yoghurt; bovril, caffeine containing products, oxo, marmite, broad beans, heavy red wines
• Report headache, palpitation, neck stiffness

phenobarbitone

Gardenal Sodium
Func. class.: Anticonvulsant
Chem. class.: Barbiturate
Legal class.: CD (Sch 3) POM

Action: Decreases impulse transmission, increases seizure threshold at cerebral cortex level
Uses: All forms of epilepsy (except absence seizures), status epilepticus, febrile seizures in children
Dosage and routes:
Phenobarbitone and phenobarbitone sodium are therapeutically equivalent and given in the same doses
Epilepsy
• *Adult:* By mouth 60–180 mg at bedtime
• *Adult:* IM or IV 50–200; repeat after 6 hr if required; maximum 600 mg daily
• *Child:* By mouth 8 mg/kg daily
Status epilepticus
• *Adult:* IV maximum rate 100 mg/min, maximum dose 15 mg/kg
Available forms include: Phenobarbitone: tablets 15 mg, 30 mg, 60 mg, 100 mg; elixir 15 mg/5 ml. Phenobarbitone sodium: tablets 30 mg, 60 mg; injection 200 mg/ml (other strengths available)
Side effects/adverse reactions:
HAEM: Folate deficiency, megaloblastic anaemia
CNS: Paradoxical stimulation drowsiness, sedation, lethargy, hangover, dependence, coma (overdosage)
GI: Nausea, vomiting
INTEG: Rash, urticaria, Stevens-

Johnson syndrome, angioneurotic oedema, local pain at injection site
RESP: Respiratory depression (overdosage)
Contraindications: Severe respiratory depression, porphyria
Pharmacokinetics:
By mouth: Onset 20–60 min, peak 8–12 hr, duration 6–10 hr, metabolised by liver, excreted by kidneys, excreted in breast milk, half-life 53–118 hr
Interactions/incompatibilities:
- Increased effects: CNS depressants, alcohol, chloramphenicol, valproic acid
- Decreased effects: antidepressants, antipsychotic agents
- Enhances hepatic metabolism and may decrease effects of: anticoagulants, tricyclic antidepressants, calcium channel blockers, corticosteroids, chloramphenicol, cyclosporin, oral contraceptives, griseofulvin, metronidazole, phenytoin

Clinical assessment:
- Therapeutic level 10–40 mg/litre

Treatment of overdose: Supportive care

NURSING CONSIDERATIONS

Assess:
- Mental status

Administer:
- IV diluted 1 in 10 with water for injection
- IV in status epilepticus in specialist centres only where intensive care facilities are available; patients should not have recently received phenobarbitone or primidone

Perform/provide:
- Regular assessment of respiratory status

Evaluate:
- Control of seizures
- Mental status: mood, alertness affect, memory (long, short)
- Respiratory depression
- Blood dyscrasias: fever, sore throat, bruising, rash, jaundice

Teach patient/family:
- All aspects of drug administration: action, dose, route, when to notify clinician
- Not to withdraw medication abruptly

phenoperidine HCl

Operidine
Func. class.: Narcotic analgesic
Chem. class.: Opioid phenylpiperidine derivative
Legal class.: CD (Sch 2) POM

Action: Inhibits ascending pain pathways in CNS, increases pain threshold, alters pain perception
Uses: Enhancement of anaesthetics, analgesia during surgery; as respiratory depressant in prolonged assisted respiration
Dosage and routes:
With spontaneous respiration
- *Adult:* IV injection up to 1 mg, then 0.5 mg every 40–60 min as required
- *Child:* IV injection 30–50 mcg/kg

With assisted ventilation
- *Adult:* IV injection 2–5 mg, then 1 mg as required
- *Child:* IV injection 100–150 mcg/kg

Available forms include: Injection 1 mg/ml
Side effects/adverse reactions:
RESP: Respiratory depression, cough suppression
CNS: Drowsiness
CV: Bradycardia
EENT: Visual disturbances
GI: Nausea, vomiting, reduced motility, constipation, jaundice
GU: Urinary retention
MS: Rigidity
SYST: Reduced tolerance, dependence

Contraindications: Hypersensitivity, obstructive airways disease, respiratory depression (if not ventilating mechanically)

Precautions: Hypothyroidism, hepatic impairment, dependence, pregnancy, renal disease, biliary tract disorders, adrenocortical insufficiency, shock, prostatic hypertrophy, supraventricular tachycardia, head injury, raised intraneonates, premature infants, elderly or debilitated patients

Pharmacokinetics: Metabolised in liver, excreted in urine

Interactions/incompatibilities:

- MAOIs (enhanced toxicity)
- Effects may be enhanced with other CNS depressants: alcohol, anaesthetics, narcotics, sedative/hypnotics, antipsychotics

Treatment of overdose: Naloxone, supportive care

NURSING CONSIDERATIONS

Assess:

- Baseline vital signs, pupil size and reaction
- Fluid balance
- When pain is starting to return

Administer:

- With anti-emetic if nausea or vomiting occurs

Perform/provide:

- Storage in CD cupboard
- Assistance with walking; drowsiness, dizziness may occur
- Safety measures including cot-sides if necessary

Evaluate:

- For CNS changes
- For respiratory changes; depression, rate, rhythm; notify clinician if respirations are under 12/min
- Therapeutic response; dependency

Teach patient/family:

- About all aspects of the drug
- That physical dependence may occur if drug is used for an extended period
- That withdrawal symptoms could occur if drug is discontinued abruptly
- Not to drive or engage in other hazardous activities if drowsiness/dizziness occur
- Secure storage

phenothrin

Full Marks

Func. class.: Parasiticide

Chem. class.: Synthetic pyrethroid

Legal class.: P

Action: Induces sensory hyperexcitability, uncoordination, prostration and death in lice

Uses: Eradication of head and pubic lice

Dosage and routes:

Head and pubic lice

- *Adult and child:* Topically by single application of alcoholic lotion left on hair for 2 hr

Available forms include: Alcohol-based lotion 0.2%

Side effects/adverse reactions:

INTEG: Alcohol-based lotion may cause skin irritation in people with eczema

MISC: May affect permed, coloured or bleached hair

RESP: Alcohol-based lotion may cause wheezing in asthmatics

Contraindications: Hypersensitivity

Precautions: Children under 6 months should only be treated under medical supervision

Pharmacokinetics: Little absorption when used correctly

Treatment of overdose: Empty stomach of contents and provide symptomatic and supportive care

NURSING CONSIDERATIONS

Assess:

- For signs of head and pubic lice

Administer:

- Wearing protective rubber or

plastic gloves if using phenothrin regularly
• Keeping away from eyes
• Allowing lotion to dry naturally – do not apply heat
• Leaving on for recommended period of time
Perform/provide:
• Isolation until treatment completed
• Removal of lice by using a fine toothed comb rinsed in vinegar after the treatment
Evaluate:
• Eradication of head and/or pubic lice
Teach patient/family:
• To wash clothing of all residents. Preventative treatment may be required for all persons living in the same house
• To treat sexual contacts simultaneously
• That it may cause skin irritation in people with eczema
• That it may cause wheezing in asthmatics
• That it may affect bleached, coloured or permed hair
• To seek medical advice if accidentally swallowed
• Alcohol-based lotion is flammable – do not use near sources of ignition
• Not to wash treated area before recommended contact time has elapsed

---

phenoxybenzamine hydrochloride

Dibenyline
Func. class.: Antihypertensive
Chem. class.: α-Adrenergic blocker
Legal class.: POM

Action: α-Adrenergic blocker, which binds to α-adrenergic receptors, dilating peripheral blood vessels, lowers peripheral resistance, lowers blood pressure
Uses: Phaeochromocytoma
Dosage and routes:
• *Adult:* By mouth 10 mg daily, increase by 10 mg daily; usual range 1–2 mg/kg daily in 2 doses
Phaeochromocytoma hypertensive crisis and adjunct in severe shock
• *Adult:* IV infusion 1 mg/kg daily in 200 ml sodium chloride 0.9% over at least 2 hr; do not repeat within 24 hr
Available forms include: Capsules 10 mg, injection 50 mg/ml (hospital only)
Side effects/adverse reactions:
GI: Dry mouth, nausea, vomiting, diarrhoea
CV: Postural hypotension, tachycardia
CNS: Dizziness, drowsiness, sedation, lassitude
GU: Inhibition of ejaculation
EENT: Nasal congestion, miosis
Contraindications: Hypersensitivity, history of cerebrovascular accident, 3–4 weeks after myocardial infarction, porphyria
Precautions: Severe heart disease, congestive heart failure, cerebrovascular disease, renal damage, respiratory infection, elderly, pregnancy
Pharmacokinetics:
By mouth: Onset 2 hr, peak 4–6 hr, duration 3–4 days; half-life 24 hr, metabolised in liver, excreted in urine, bile
Interactions/incompatibilities:
• Hypotensive response: adrenaline, antihypertensives
Treatment of overdose: Supportive care (IV saline, noradrenaline, elevate legs)
NURSING CONSIDERATIONS
Assess:
• Weight before initial dose
• Pulse, blood pressure lying and

standing before and regularly during treatment

Administer:

- IV infusion with intensive care facilities available
- Avoid contamination of hands with injection solution due to risk of contact sensitivity
- Orally following dosage regime for suitable gradual introduction, until control of hypertension or postural hypotension occurs
- With food or milk if GI symptoms occur

Perform/provide:

- Frequent drinks to prevent a dry mouth

Evaluate:

- Effect of any other therapy
- Therapeutic response: decreased BP, increased peripheral pulses
- Nausea, vomiting, diarrhoea, dry mouth
- Postural hypotension, tachycardia
- Dizziness

Teach patient/family:

- Avoid alcohol
- To report dizziness, palpitations, fainting
- To change position slowly or fainting may occur
- To take drug exactly as prescribed
- To avoid driving and hazardous activities until treatment established
- To only take other medication if directed by clinician
- To give up smoking and encourage or healthy diet

phenoxymethylpenicillin potassium (Penicillin V)

Apsin VK, Distaquaine VK, Stabillin VK, V-Cil-K

Func. class.: Antibiotic, broad-spectrum

Chem. class.: Penicillin

Legal class.: POM

Action: Interferes with cell wall replication of susceptible organisms; osmotically unstable cell wall swells, bursts from osmotic pressure

Uses: Mild to moderate streptococcal, pneumococcal, staphylococcal, spirochaetal and other bacterial infections due to susceptible organisms; prophylaxis of rheumatic fever

Dosage and routes:

- *Adult:* By mouth 250–500 mg every 6 hr at least 30 min before meals
- *Child 6–12 yr:* By mouth 250 mg 6 hrly before meals
- *Child 1–5 yr:* 125 mg 6 hrly before meals
- *Child up to 1 yr:* 62.5 mg 6 hrly before meals

Prophylaxis of rheumatic fever

- By mouth, 250 mg twice daily

Available forms include: Capsules 250 mg; tablets 250 mg; powder for oral suspension 62.5, 125, 250 mg/5 ml

Side effects/adverse reactions:

GI: Nausea, vomiting, diarrhoea, abdominal pain, glossitis

META: Hyperkalaemia

SYST: Hypersensitivity (anaphylaxis, rashes, urticaria, serum sickness, chills, fever, oedema, arthralgia, eosinophilia, angioedema)

MISC: Infection (overgrowth) with resistant organisms

Contraindications: Hypersensitivity to penicillins; severe acute

infection (absorption may be inadequate), meningococcal or gonococcal infection
Precautions: History of significant allergies and/or asthma, impaired renal function
Pharmacokinetics:
By mouth: Absorption variable, incomplete; peak 30–60 min, duration 6–8 hr, half-life 30 min, metabolised in liver, excreted in urine
Interactions/incompatibilities:
• Decreased antimicrobial effectiveness of this drug: bacteriostatic agents such as tetracyclines, erythromycin; chloroquine, guar gum (decreased absorption)
• Increased penicillin concentrations when used with: probenecid
Clinical assessment:
• Culture organism and assess sensitivity before drug therapy; drug may be taken once culture sample is taken
• Consider patch test to assess allergy, if penicillin is only drug of choice
Lab. test interferences:
Decrease: Uric acid
False positive: Urine glucose, urine protein
Treatment of overdose: Activated charcoal plus sorbitol, symptomatic supportive care

NURSING CONSIDERATIONS

Assess:
• Bowel pattern
• Fluid balance
• Allergy status, history of allergies (asthma, hay fever)
• Any patient with compromised renal system since drug is excreted slowly in poor renal system function; toxicity may occur rapidly
Administer:
• To be taken at least 30 min before food
• On an empty stomach for best absorption
• After culture and sensitivity has been completed
Perform/provide:
• Adequate fluid intake (2 litres/day) during diarrhoea episodes
• Refrigerate after reconstituting oral elixir
Evaluate:
• Therapeutic effectiveness: absence of fever, draining wounds
• Bowel pattern before and during treatment
• Fluid balance; report haematuria, oliguria since penicillin in high doses is nephrotoxic
• Skin eruptions after administration of penicillin to 1 week after discontinuing drug
• Respiratory status: rate, character, wheezing, tightness in chest
• Allergies before initiation of treatment, reaction of each medication; highlight allergies on nursing care plan
Teach patient/family:
• Aspects of drug therapy, including need to complete entire course of medication to ensure organism death (10–14 days); culture may be taken after completed course
• To report sore throat, fever, fatigue; could indicate superimposed infection
• To wear or carry ID if allergic to penicillins
• To notify nurse of diarrhoea stools

phentermine

Duromine, Ionamin
Func. class.: Appetite suppressant
Chem. class.: Sympathomimetic
Legal class.: CD (Sch 3) POM

Action: Increases release of noradrenaline, dopamine in CNS reduces appetite
Uses: Severe obesity

Dosage and routes:

• *Adult:* By mouth 15–30 mg daily before breakfast

Available forms include: Capsules, modified-release, 15 mg, 30 mg

Side effects/adverse reactions:

CNS: Hyperactivity, insomnia, restlessness, dizziness, nervousness

GI: Nausea, dry mouth, constipation, unpleasant taste, vomiting

GU: Impotence, change in libido, urinary frequency

CV: Palpitations, tachycardia, hypertension

INTEG: Urticaria, facial oedema

MISC: Risk of dependence

Contraindications: Hypersensitivity, hyperthyroidism, hypertension, glaucoma, severe cardiovascular disease, peptic ulcer, epilepsy, prostatic hypertrophy, depression, pregnancy, breastfeeding, children, elderly, unstable personality, history of psychiatric illness or drug abuse, porphyria

Precautions: Anxiety, cardiovascular disease, pregnancy, diabetes mellitus

Pharmacokinetics:

Modified-release capsules: Duration 10–14 hr; metabolised by liver, excreted by kidneys

Interactions/incompatibilities:

• Risk of hypertensive crisis when given within 14 days of MAOIs

• Decrease effect of: antihypertensives

• Hypoglycaemic treatment may require adjustment in diabetics

• Diminished effect of sedatives

Clinical assessment:

• Discontinue if weight gain not achieved

Treatment of overdose: Gastric lavage or emesis if ingestion within last 4 hr, activated charcoal, supportive treatment including diazepam for sedation if needed. Forced acid diuresis possible

NURSING CONSIDERATIONS

Assess:

• Vital signs, BP (drug may reverse antihypertensives). Check patients with cardiac disease more often

• Height and growth rate in children; growth rate may be decreased

Administer:

• At least 6 hr before sleeping; 1 hr before breakfast

• For obesity only if patient is on weight reduction programme including dietary changes, exercise; patient will develop tolerance, and loss of weight will not occur without additional methods

• Limit therapy to 4–8 weeks

• Frequent sips of water for dry mouth

Perform/provide:

• Check to see oral medication has been swallowed

Evaluate:

• Mental status: mood, alertness, affect, stimulation, insomnia, aggressiveness

• For symptoms of abuse

• Physical dependency: should not be used for extended periods of time; dose should be discontinued gradually

• Withdrawal symptoms: headache, nausea, vomiting, muscle pain, weakness

• Drug tolerance after long-term use

Teach patient/family:

• Drug should not be increased if tolerance develops

• To decrease caffeine consumption (coffee, tea, cola, chocolate), which may increase irritability, stimulation

• Avoid non-prescribed preparations unless approved by clinician

• To taper off drug over several weeks, or depression, increased sleeping, lethargy may ensue

• To avoid alcohol ingestion

• To avoid hazardous activities

including driving until patient is stabilised on medication
- To get needed rest; patients will feel more tired at end of day
- That drug is one of abuse

phentolamine mesylate

Rogitine
Func. class.: Antihypertensive
Chem. class.: α-Blocker
Legal class.: POM

Action: α-Adrenergic blocker, binds to α-adrenergic receptors, dilating peripheral blood vessels, lowering peripheral resistances, lowering blood pressure
Uses: Cardiogenic shock, paroxysmal, hypertension, diagnostic test for phaeochromocytoma
Dosage and routes:
Cardiogenic shock
- *Adult:* IV infusion 5–6 mg over 10–30 min at 0.2–2.0 mg/min; may be increased to 5 mg/min in the first min; reduce infusion rate if BP falls below 100 mmHg

Paroxysmal hypertension
- *Adult:* IV/IM injection 5–10 mg once, repeat as required. Prior to surgical removal of phaeochromocytoma, administer 2 hr prior to surgery and repeat as necessary
- *Child:* IV injection 1–5 mg during surgery for removal of phaeochromocytoma

Diagnostic test for phaeochromocytoma
- *Adult:* Establish basal BP then IV 5 mg; positive response is seen as a rapid fall in BP with quick return to basal levels; maximum depressor effect occurs within 2 mins
- *Child:* IV injection 1 mg, test as for adults

Available forms include: Injection 10 mg/ml

Side effects/adverse reactions:
GI: Dry mouth, nausea, vomiting, diarrhoea, abdominal pain
CV: Hypotension, tachycardia, angina, arrhythmias, myocardial infarction
CNS: Dizziness, weakness, anxiety
EENT: Nasal congestion
INTEG: Flushing, sweating
Contraindications: Hypersensitivity, hypotension, angina, myocardial infarction, coronary artery disease
Precautions: Pregnancy, severe hypotension, lactation, myocardial infarction, coronary insufficiency, angina
Pharmacokinetics:
IV: Peak 2 min, duration 10–15 min
IM: Peak 15–20 min, duration 3–4 hr
Metabolised in liver, excreted in urine, plasma half life 19 min
Interactions/incompatibilities:
- May increase effects of antihypertensives
- Not to be mixed in solution or syringe with any drug

Clinical assessment:
- Monitor blood pressure

Treatment of overdose: Discontinue drug. Effects can be attenuated with noradrenaline if necessary

NURSING CONSIDERATIONS

Assess:
- Baseline vital signs including B/P lying, standing

Administer:
- Frequent mouth washes for dry mouth
- After having vasopressor nearby
- After discontinuing all medication for 24 hr if using for diagnostic purpose

Evaluate:
- Postural hypotension
- Cardiac system: pulse, ECG, B/P (lying, standing) 4 hourly
- Dryness of mucous membrane

• Oedema in feet, legs daily

Teach patient/family:

• That bedrest is required during treatment, and for 1 hr after

phenylbutazone

Butacote

Func. class.: Non-steroidal anti-inflammatory drug

Chem. class.: Pyrazolone derivative

Legal class: POM

Action: Inhibits prostaglandin synthesis by decreasing an enzyme needed for biosynthesis; possesses analgesic, anti-inflammatory antipyretic properties

Uses: Ankylosing spondylitis (hospitals only)

Dosage and routes:

• *Adult:* 200 mg 2 or 3 times a day for 2 days, then reduce to the minimum effective, usually 100 mg, 2 or 3 times a day; keep duration of treatment as short as possible. Not for children under 14 yr

Available forms include: Tablets 100 mg

Side effects/adverse reactions:

GI: Nausea, dyspepsia, ulcerative stomatitis, vomiting, hepatitis, peptic ulcer, epigastric pain, bleeding

CNS: Headache

CV: Peripheral oedema due to sodium retention

INTEG: Purpura, rash, pruritus, Stevens-Johnson syndrome

GU: Nephritis

HAEM: Agranulocytosis, aplastic anaemia, thrombocytopenia, leucopenia

EENT: Blurred vision

META: Goitre

RESP: Acute pulmonary syndrome (rare)

Contraindications: Thyroid disease; history of peptic ulceration; GI haemorrhage, blood dyscrasias, Sjögren's syndrome, asthma, hypersensitivity to pyrazolones, aspirin or other NSAIDs; bleeding disorders, severe cardiac disease, severe renal disease; severe hepatic disease; last trimester of pregnancy; porphyria; children under 14 yrs; breast-feeding

Precautions: Lactation, children, history of dyspepsia, elderly (reduce dose), hypersensitivity to other NSAIDs, pregnancy

Pharmacokinetics:

By mouth: Peak 2 hr, half-life 3–3½ hr; metabolised in liver, excreted in urine (metabolites), excreted in breast milk

Interactions/incompatibilities:

• May increase action of anticoagulants, antidiabetics, phenytoin, sulphonamides, methotrexate, lithium

• Reduced action of this drug: with concurrent hepatic microsomal enzyme inducers, e.g. rifampicin, phenobarbitone

Clinical assessment:

• Renal, liver, blood studies: serum urea, creatinine, aspartate aminotransferase, alanine aminotransferase, Hb, before treatment, periodically thereafter

• If decrease in leucocyte and/or platelets or haematocrit observed, drug should be withdrawn

Treatment of overdose: Evacuation of the stomach and activated charcoal. If necessary, haemofiltration and supportive therapy

NURSING CONSIDERATIONS

Administer:

• With or after food

• Swallow whole with water

• Do not take indigestion mixtures at the same time

Evaluate:

• Therapeutic response: decreased pain, stiffness, swelling in joints, ability to move more easily

• For eye, ear problems: blurred vision, tinnitus (may indicate toxicity)
• Persistent indigestion

Teach patient/family:

• To report blurred vision or ringing, roaring in ears (may indicate toxicity)
• To avoid driving or other hazardous activities if dizziness or drowsiness occurs
• To report persistent indigestion or black tarry stools
• To take with food or milk
• To report change in urine pattern, weight increase, oedema, pain increase in joints, fever, blood in urine (indicates nephrotoxicity)
• To report bruising, fever, sore throat, rash, mouth ulceration
• That therapeutic effects may take up to 1 month

---

phenylephrine hydrochloride

Func. class.: Adrenergic, direct acting
Chem. class.: Substituted phenylethylamine, Sympathomimetic
Legal class.: POM

Action: Selective (α1) receptor agonist causing contraction of blood vessels

Uses: Acute hypotension

Dosage and routes:

Hypotension

• *Adult:* Subcutaneous, IM 2–5 mg, IV 0.1–0.5 mg, may repeat after at least 15 min if necessary. Continuous IV infusion 30–60 mcg/minute according to response

Available forms include: Injection, IV, Subcutaneous, IM, 1% (10 mg/ml)

Side effects/adverse reactions:

CNS: Headache
CV: Palpitations, tachycardia, ectopic beats, angina, hypertension, reflex bradycardia
GI: Nausea, vomiting
INTEG: Necrosis, tissue, sloughing with extravasation, gangrene, skin tingling

Contraindications: Hypersensitivity, ventricular fibrillation, tachydysrhythmias, phaeochromocytoma, myocardial infarction, pregnancy, severe hypertension, hyperthyroidism

Precautions: Lactation, arterial embolism, peripheral vascular disease, angina pectoris, diabetes mellitus closed angle glaucoma

Pharmacokinetics:

IV: Duration 20–30 min
IM, subcutaneous: Duration 45–60 min

Interactions/incompatibilities:

• Reversal of effects of antihypertensives with potentially serious consequences
• Do not use within 2 weeks of MAOIs or hypertensive crisis may result
• Increased risk of cardiac arrhythmias when given with inhalation anaesthetics, quinidine, cardiac glycosides
• Decreased action of this drug: α-blockers
• Increased pressor effect when given with: tricyclic antidepressant
• Incompatible with alkaline solutions, e.g. sodium bicarbonate

Clinical assessment:

• ECG during administration continuously; if BP increases, drug is decreased
• CVP during infusion if possible

Treatment of overdose: Administer a phentolamine with care

NURSING CONSIDERATIONS

Assess:

• Baseline vital signs, CVP, ECG

Administer:

• Plasma expanders for hypovolemia

• IV directly into vein, wait 15 min to repeat if necessary
• IV by infusion, 500 ml of dextrose 5% or sodium chloride 0.9% at 30–60 mcg per minute, according to response

Evaluate:
• Input and output of fluids, check output hourly
• E.C.G continuously during administration; if blood pressure increases, drug is decreased
• Blood pressure and pulse at 5 min intervals after administration
• CVP during infusion
• Patients medication
• Side effects, palpitation, ectopic beats, tachycardia, angina hypertension, reflex bradycardia, nausea, vomiting
• Injection site: tissue sloughing, if this occurs administer phentolamine mixed with 0.9% sodium chloride
• For therapeutic response: increase BP with stabilization

Teach patient/family:
• The reason for drug administration
• To report pain, loss of sensation at injection site immediately

---

phenylephrine HCl (ophthalmic)

Minims, Isopto Frin
Func. class.: Mydriatic
Legal class.: P

Action: Blocks response of iris sphincter muscle, muscle of accommodation of ciliary body to cholinergic stimulation, resulting in dilation of pupil, paralysis of accommodation, causes vasoconstriction

Uses: Mydriasis, posterior synechia, redness due to minor eye irritation

Dosage and routes:

Mydriatic prior to examination
• *Adult:* Instil 1 drop of 10% solution
• *Elderly, child:* Instil 1 drop of 2.5% solution

Therapeutic mydriasis
• *Adult:* Instil 1 drop of 10% solution as necessary

Redness due to minor irritation
• *Adult and child:* 1 drop 0.12% solution up to 4 times a day

Available forms include: Solution 0.12, 2.5, 10%

Side effects/adverse reactions:
CV: Palpitations, tachycardia, hypertension, myocardial infarction
RESP: Bronchospasm
EENT: Blurred vision, stinging, photophobia

Contraindications: Hypersensitivity to sympathomimetic amines, narrow-angle glaucoma, dysrhythmias, cardiogenic shock

Precautions: Elderly, hypertension, diabetes mellitus, cerebral arteriosclerosis, pregnancy, contact lenses

Pharmacokinetics: Onset 1 hr, peak 4–8 hr, duration 12–24 hr

Interactions/incompatibilities:
• Reversal of effects of antihypertensives with potentially serious consequences
• Increased pressor effects when given with: tricyclic antidepressants
• May interact with systemic MAOIs, increasing risk of hypertensive reactions
• Increased risk of cardiac arrhythmias when given with: inhalation anaesthetics, quinidine, cardiac glycosides

Clinical assessment:
• Tonometer readings during long-term treatment
• Risk of systemic side-effects and

drug interactions much smaller with 0.12% drops

Treatment of overdose: Supportive, injection of α-blocker e.g. phentolamine 5–10 mg IV may be useful

NURSING CONSIDERATIONS

Assess:

- BP, pulse, respirations

Evaluate:

- Allergic reaction: itching, oedema of eyelids, eye discharge; drug should be discontinued

Teach patient/family:

- To report pain or loss of sight, trouble breathing, sweating, flushing
- Method of instillation: into lower conjunctival sac. Keep eye closed for approx 1 min; use cotton wool ball to mop up excess, discourage rubbing the eye; do not touch dropper to eye

phenytoin

Epanutin, Pentran

Func. class.: Anticonvulsant

Chem. class.: Hydantoin

Legal class.: POM

Action: Inhibits spread of seizure activity in brain

Uses: All types of epilepsy except absence seizures, trigeminal neuralgia, arrhythmias

Dosage and routes:

Epilepsy, trigeminal neuralgia

- *Adult:* By mouth 150–300 mg (3–4 mg/kg) daily in single or two divided doses; increase according to plasma concentrations at weekly intervals; usual range 300–400 mg daily; maximum 600 mg daily
- *Child:* By mouth 5–8 mg/kg daily in a single or two divided doses

Status epilepticus

- *Adult:* Slow IV, loading dose, 15 mg/kg; maintenance 100 mg every 6 hr
- *Neonate:* Slow IV, loading dose 15–20 mg/kg

Arrhythmias

- *Adult:* Slow IV 3.5–5 mg/kg; repeat once if required

Available forms include: Phenytoin: tablets, chewable, 50 mg; suspension 30 mg/5 ml. Phenytoin sodium: tablets 50 mg, 100 mg; capsules 25 mg, 50 mg, 100 mg, 300 mg; injection 50 mg/ml

Side effects/adverse reactions:

HAEM: Agranulocytosis, leucopenia, aplastic anaemia, lymphadenopathy, megaloblastic anaemia

CNS: Drowsiness, dizziness, insomnia, paraesthesias, aggression, headache, nystagmus, slurred speech, dyskinesias, ataxia

HAEM: Lymphadenopathy

GI: Nausea, vomiting, constipation, anorexia, weight loss, hepatitis, jaundice

GU: Nephritis, albuminuria, Peyronie's disease

INTEG: Rash, exfoliative dermatitis, hirsutism, gingival hyperplasmia acne

CV: Atrial and ventricular arrhythmias after IV use

MS: Muscle twitching, polyarthropathy

EENT: Blurred vision

ELECT: Hypocalcaemia

Contraindications: Hypersensitivity, porphyria; IV: sinus bradycardia, sino-atrial block, atrioventricular block, Stokes-Adams syndrome

Precautions: Allergies, hepatic disease, serious renal disease, pregnancy

Pharmacokinetics:

By mouth: Absorption by mouth slow but nearly complete. Half life variable, about 22 hr, metabolised by liver, excreted by kidneys. About 90% protein bound, therapeutic plasma range 10–20 mg/litre

Interactions/incompatibilities:

- Decreased effects of phenytoin: alcohol (chronic use), antacids, rifampicin, folic acid, carbamazepine, sucralfate, tricyclic antidepressants, neuroleptics
- Increased effects of phenytoin: chloramphenicol, disulfiram, sulphonamides, cimetidine, phenylbutazone, isoniazid, dicoumarol, sulphinpyrazone, omeprazole, imidazole anti-fungals, amiodarone
- Increased or decreased effects of phenytoin: phenobarbitone, sodium valproate
- Effects increased or decreased by phenytoin: sodium valproate, phenytoin, warfarin
- Decreased effect of: corticosteroids, dicoumarol, doxycycline, oral contraceptives, quinidine, vitamin D, cyclosporin, disopyramide, mexiletine
- Do not mix injection with any other drug or infusion solution; risk of crystallisation

Clinical assessment:

- Serum phenytoin levels to adjust dosage initially and if problems develop

Treatment of overdose: Empty stomach if ingested in last 4 hr, then supportive measures

NURSING CONSIDERATIONS

Assess:

- Baseline vital signs, including ECG if given for cardiac arrhythmia
- Body weight
- Frequency of seizures

Administer:

- Oral formulations with or after food
- Differences in bioavailability between tablets and capsules may be clinically insignificant; however, care should be taken when changing formulations
- Suspension of phenytoin 90 mg/15 ml may be approximately equivalent to 100 mg tablets or capsules; however, care should be taken when changing formulations
- Chewable tablets should be sucked or chewed; these contain phenytoin and therefore care should be taken when changing to tablets or capsules of phenytoin sodium
- IV slowly with BP and ECG monitoring at a maximum rate of 50 mg/min
- IV slowly in neonates at 1–3 mg/kg/min
- IV with care; solutions are alkaline and irritant; use large vein, large gauge needle or IV catheter; flush with sodium chloride 0.9% after administration
- IV infusion causes precipitation, not recommended
- IM injection gives erratic absorption, not recommended

Evaluate:

- Mental status: mood, alertness, effects, memory (long, short)
- Respiratory depression
- Blood dyscrasias: fever, sore throat, bruising, rash, jaundice
- Therapeutic response: reduction in number and severity of seizures
- Local inflammation at injection site
- Monitor ECG continuously during IV administration

Teach patient/family:

- All aspects of drug administration: route, action, dose, when to notify clinician
- Seek advice about ability to drive. Patient should be seizure free for 2 yr, or if subject to attacks only while asleep, have established a 3 yr period of asleep attacks without awake attacks
- Patients affected by drowsiness should not drive or operate machinery
- To carry a Medical alert Card detailing medication
- About side effects

phosphates (rectal)

Carbalax (Beogex), Fletchers' Phosphate Enema
Func. class.: Osmotic laxative
Chem. class.: Phosphate
Legal class.: P

Action: Increases water absorption in colon by osmotic action
Uses: Constipation, bowel evacuation prior to abdominal procedures and surgery
Dosage and routes:
• *Adult:* 1 enema (128 ml), as required. 1 suppository, inserted 30 min before evacuation required
• *Children over 3 yr:* Enema only, reduced volume according to body weight
Available forms include: Enemas, 128 ml suppositories 1.72 g
Side effects/adverse reactions:
GI: Nausea, cramps, diarrhoea, anal irritation (with prolonged use)
META: Electrolyte, fluid imbalances
Contraindications: Hypersensitivity; abdominal pain; nausea/vomiting; appendicitis; inflammatory or ulcerative bowel conditions; increased colonic absorption capacity; acute gastrointestinal conditions; children under 3 yr
Precautions: Intestinal obstruction
Pharmacokinetics: Excreted in faeces
Interactions/incompatibilities: None known
Clinical assessment:
• Electrolyte balance should be maintained during extend use
NURSING CONSIDERATIONS
Assess:
• Fluid balance to identify fluid loss
• Cause of constipation
Administer:
• At room temperature or warmed in warm water before use
• With patient lying on his/her left side
• Moisten suppository with water before use
• Carefully so as not to use undue force in administration of enema
Evaluate:
• Therapeutic response
• Cramping, rectal bleeding, nausea, vomiting; seek medical advice if these occur
Teach patient/family:
• That normal bowel movements do not always occur daily
• That shortage of fluids, fibre and lack of exercise contribute to constipation
• Not to use laxatives for long-term therapy; bowel tone will be lost
• Do not use in presence of abdominal pain, nausea, vomiting
• Notify clinician if constipation unrelieved or if symptoms of electrolyte imbalance occur: muscle cramps, pain, weakness, dizziness
• That necrosis of bowel can occur with overuse

physostigmine sulphate (ophthalmic)

Func. class.: Antiglaucoma agent
Chem. class.: Cholinesterase inhibitor
Legal class.: POM

Action: Increases concentration of acetylcholine at cholinergic transmission sites, thus causing prolonged, exaggerated action; induces miosis, spasm of accommodation, fall in intraocular pressure by opening up drainage channels, aiding in aqueous humour drainage
Uses: Used in treatment of chronic simple glaucoma, usually with pilocarpine

Dosage and routes:
• *Adult, child:* Instil 1–2 drops of a 0.25% or 0.5% solution into conjunctival sac 2–6 times a day according to response
Available forms include: Drops 0.25%, 0.5%
Side effects/adverse reactions:
CNS: Convulsions, headache
CV: Hypotension, bradycardia, irregular pulse
GI: Nausea, vomiting, abdominal cramps
RESP: Bronchospasm, dyspnoea, pulmonary oedema
EENT: Blurred vision, conjunctivitis, allergic reactions, rhinorrhoea, salivation, brow pain, lacrimation, twitching of eyelids
Contraindications: Inflammatory disease of iris or ciliary body, soft contact lenses
Precautions: Epilepsy, parkinsonism, bradycardia, hypertension, obstructive airway disease
Clinical assessment:
• Awareness of possibility of systemic side effects

NURSING CONSIDERATIONS

Administer:
• Topically to conjunctival sac
• Only clear solutions, never pink or brown
Teach patient/family:
• To report change in vision, blurring or loss of sight, trouble breathing, sweating, flushing
• Method of instillation, not to touch dropper to eye
• That long-term therapy may be required
• That blurred vision will decrease with repeated use of drug
• That drug may be prescribed for bedtime use to prevent nocturnal rise in ocular tension
• That maximal effect of topical application is reached in 30 min, may last 12–36 hr
• To observe eyes for irritation, development of cataracts

phytomenadione (vitamin K_1)

Konakion
Func. class.: Fat-soluble vitamin
Legal class.: POM

Action: Needed for adequate blood clotting (Factors II, VII, IX, X)
Uses: Actual or threatened haemorrhage associated with low blood prothrombin, Factor VII. Coumarin anticoagulant overdose. Prevention/treatment of neonatal haemorrhage
Dosage and routes:
• *Adult:* ***As an antidote to anticoagulant drugs***
• *Potentially fatal and severe haemorrhage:* IV 10–20 mg repeated if prothrombin time 3 hr post-dose shows inadequate response, maximum 40 mg in 24 hr, should be accompanied by whole blood/clotting factors
• *Less severe haemorrhage:* By mouth/IM 10 mg repeated if prothrombin level 8-12 hr post-dose shows inadequate response. Maximum 40 mg in 24 hr
• *Dangerously lowered prothrombin without haemorrhage:* By mouth 5–10 mg as a single dose
• ***Other indications:*** 10–20 mg as required
• *Elderly:* Use dose towards bottom end of dose range
• *Children:* By mouth/IM/IV 5–10 mg
• *Neonates:* Prophylactic: IM 1 mg; therapeutic: IM 1 mg repeated 8 hrly if required
Available forms include: Tablets, chewable 10 mg, injection IV, IM 1 mg in 0.5 ml, 10 mg in 1 ml
Side effects/adverse reactions:
SYST: Anaphylactoid reactions after too rapid IV injection
INTEG: Rash, urticaria. Local cu-

taneous changes after repeated IM injection

Contraindications: Hypersensitivity

Precautions:

- Should only be given IV in life-threatening situations
- IV injections must be very slow
- Pregnancy

Pharmacokinetics: Onset of action up to 12 hr, duration several days–weeks

Interactions/incompatibilities:

- Decreased absorption of this drug: cholestyramine, mineral oil
- Decreased action of: oral anti-coagulants
- Do not dilute injection

Clinical assessment:

- Prothrombin time during treatment

NURSING CONSIDERATIONS

Administer:

- IV: only in cases of severe haemorrhage or critical illness with hepatic dysfunction
- By slow infusion over 30 min
- Do not dilute injection in aqueous diluent

Evaluate:

- Therapeutic response: decreased bleeding tendencies, prothrombin time, clotting time

Perform/provide:

- Monitor ECG if given by infusion

Teach patient/family:

- Not to take other supplements, unless directed by clinician

---

pilocarpine hydrochloride/nitrate (ophthalmic)

Isopto Carpine, Sno-pilo, Ocusert, Minims Pilocarpine Nitrate

Func. class.: Antiglaucoma agent
Chem. class.: Cholinergic agonist
Legal class.: POM

Action: Directly acts on cholinergic receptor sites, induces miosis, spasm of accommodation, fall in intraocular pressure by opening up drainage channels causing outflow of aqueous humour

Uses: Treatment of chronic simple glaucoma and, prior to surgery treatment of acute (closed angle) glaucoma. Also used to produce miosis to counter effects of mydriatic and cycloplegic eye drops. Primary glaucoma, early stages of wide-angle glaucoma (less useful in advanced stages), chronic open-angle glaucoma, acute narrow-angle glaucoma before emergency surgery; also used to neutralise mydriatics used during eye exam; may be used alternately with mydriatics to break adhesions between iris and lens

Dosage and routes:

- *Adult:* Instil 1–2 drops up to 4 times a day; strength of drops and frequency adjusted to response; Ocusert 20/40 in conjunctival sac of eye once a week at bedtime

Available forms include: Eye drops 0.5%, 1%, 2%, 3%, 4%; modified-release intraocular delivery systems, Ocusert Pilo-20, Pilo-40

Side effects/adverse reactions:

CV: Hypertension, tachycardia
RESP: Bronchospasm
GI: Nausea, vomiting, abdominal cramps, diarrhoea
EENT: Blurred vision, brow ache, twitching of eyelids, eye pain with change in focus, hypersalivation, lens changes, retinal detachment

Contraindications: Acute iritis, anterior uveitis, soft contact lenses, hypersensitivity

Precautions: Bronchial asthma, hypertension, pregnancy, breast feeding

Interactions/incompatibilities:

- Ocusert products may increase systemic absorption of autonomic drugs, e.g. adrenaline from the eye

NURSING CONSIDERATIONS

Administer:
- Topically to conjunctival sac

Perform/provide:
- Protect solution from light
- Store Ocusert systems between 2° and 8°C
- Atropine should be readily available as antidote

Teach patient/family:
- To report change in vision, blurring or loss of sight, trouble breathing, sweating, flushing
- To store in fridge
- Not to touch dropper to eye
- That long-term therapy may be required
- That blurred vision will decrease with repeated use of drug
- To discontinue use if local hypersensitivity reaction occurs
- That acuity in dim light will be reduced

pimozide

Orap

Func. class.: Antipsychotic/ neuroleptic
Chem. class.: Diphenylbutylpiperidine
Legal class.: POM

Action: Depresses cerebral cortex, hypothalamus, and limbic system, which control activity, aggression; blocks neurotransmission produced by dopamine at synapse by blocking CNS dopamine receptors

Uses: Acute and chronic schizophrenia, other psychoses, mania and hypomania

Dosage and routes:

Schizophrenia
- *Adult and child over 12 yr:* In acute phase by mouth 10 mg daily increased gradually, if needed, maximum 20 mg daily
- Prevention of relapse 2–20 mg daily

Monosymptomatic hypochondria, other paranoid states
- *Adult:* By mouth, 4 mg daily increased gradually, if needed to 16 mg daily

Mania, hypomania, psychomotor agitation
- *Adult:* By mouth 10 mg daily, increased gradually, if needed, maximum 20 mg daily
- *Elderly:* Half normal starting dose

Available forms include: Tablets 2, 4, 10 mg

Side effects/adverse reactions:

CNS: Extrapyramidal symptoms: pseudoparkinsonism, akathisia, dystonia; tardive dyskinesia, drowsiness, headache, seizures, anxiety, loss of libido, respiratory depression
INTEG: Rash
EENT: Blurred vision, cataracts
GI: Dry mouth, nausea, vomiting, anorexia, constipation, diarrhoea, dyspepsia
GU: Impotence, amenorrhoea, gynaecomastia
CV: Orthostatic hypotension, hypertension, cardiac arrest, ECG changes, tachycardia
MISC: Neuroleptic malignant syndrome

Contraindications: History of cardiac arrhythmias, congenital prolongation of QT interval, severe CNS depression, bone marrow depression, coma caused by CNS depressants, breast-feeding

Precautions: Pregnancy, epilepsy, parkinsonism, lactation, hepatic disease, cardiac disease, renal disease, alcohol withdrawal, brain damage, electrolyte disturbances

Pharmacokinetics:
By mouth: 50% absorbed, peak 6–8 hr, metabolised by liver, excreted in urine, half-life 50–55 hr

Interactions/incompatibilities:
- Decreased convulsive threshold: anticonvulsants

• Increased CNS depression: analgesics, sedatives, anxiolytics, alcohol
• Reduced effect of: bromocriptine, lysuride, pergolide, levodopa
• Increased cardiotoxicity with: phenothiazines, tricyclics, antidysrhythmics, other cardioactive drugs

Clinical assessment:
• Review need for treatment in those developing arrhythmias/ ECG changes
• Those taking anticonvulsants for increased seizure activity

Treatment of overdose: Lavage if orally ingested; provide an airway; monitor ECG; *do not induce vomiting*; procyclidine treatment if extrapyramidal side effects severe; observe for at least 4 days

NURSING CONSIDERATIONS

Assess:
• Swallowing of oral medication; check for hoarding or giving of medication to other patients
• Fluid balance
• Baseline BP
• Urinalysis is recommended before and during prolonged therapy

Administer:
• Procyclidine agent, after securing order from clinician to be used if extrapyramidal systems occur

Perform/provide:
• ECG before starting treatment and at regular intervals if daily dose greater than 16 mg
• Supervised walking until stabilised on medication; do not involve in strenuous exercise programme because fainting is possible; patient should not stand still for long periods of time
• Increased fluids to prevent constipation
• Sips of water, mouthwashes or dry mouth

Evaluate:
• BP standing and lying; also pulse, respirations 4 hrly during initial treatment; report drops of 30 mmHg from baseline
• Dizziness, faintness, palpitations, tachycardia on rising
• Extrapyramidal symptoms including akathisia (inability to sit still, no pattern to movements), tardive dyskinesia (bizarre movements of the jaw, mouth, tongue, extremities), pseudoparkinsonism (rigidity, tremors, pill rolling, shuffling gait)
• Skin turgor daily
• Constipation, urinary retention daily; if these occur increase bulk, water in diet

Teach patient/family:
• That tardive dyskinesia may develop with chronic use
• Not to exceed prescribed dose
• That postural hypotension may occur and to rise from sitting or lying position gradually
• To avoid hot baths or showers, since hypotension may occur
• To avoid abrupt withdrawal of this drug; drugs should be withdrawn slowly
• To avoid non-prescribed preparations (cough, hayfever, cold) unless approved by clinicians since serious drug interactions may occur; avoid use with alcohol or CNS depressants, increased drowsiness may occur
• To avoid hazardous activities if drowsiness or dizziness occurs
• Importance of compliance with drug regimen
• About necessity for meticulous oral hygiene since oral candidiasis may occur
• To report impaired vision, jaundice, tremors, muscle twitching

pindolol

Visken, combination product
Func. class.: Antihypertensive, anti-anginal
Chem. class.: Non-selective β-blocker
Legal class.: POM

Action: Competitively blocks stimulation of β-adrenergic receptor within vascular smooth muscle causing vasodilation and reduction in blood pressure. Cardiac β-blockade prevents excessive stimulation with increase in myocardial oxygen demand. Intrinsic sympathomimetic activity minimises myocardial depression
Uses: Mild to moderate hypertension, angina pectoris
Dosage and routes:
Hypertension
• *Adult:* By mouth, initially 5 mg 2–3 times daily or 15 mg once daily; increase at weekly intervals, maximum 45 mg daily
Angina
• *Adult:* By mouth 2.5–5 mg 3 times daily
Available forms include: Tablets 5 mg, 15 mg
Side effects/adverse reactions:
CV: Hypotension, bradycardia, congestive heart failure, oedema, chest pain, palpitation, claudication, tachycardia, cold extremities, AV block
CNS: Insomnia, dizziness, hallucinations, anxiety, fatigue, depression, headaches
GI: Nausea, vomiting, ischaemic colitis, diarrhoea, abdominal pain
INTEG: Rash, alopecia, pruritus, fever
HAEM: Agranulocytosis
EENT: Visual changes, dry burning eyes
RESP: Bronchospasm, dyspnoea
MS: Muscle fatigue

Contraindications: Bronchospasm, asthma, history of obstructive airways disease, metabolic acidosis, sinus bradycardia, partial heart block, uncontrolled congestive heart failure
Precautions: Major surgery, pregnancy, lactation, diabetes mellitus, renal disease, thyroid disease, chronic obstructive air-ways disease, well compensated heart failure, coronary artery disease; do not give without α-blocker in phaeochromocytoma
Pharmacokinetics:
By mouth: Almost completely absorbed; peak 2–4 hr; half-life 3–4 hr, excreted 30%–45% unchanged, 60%–65% is metabolised by liver, excreted in breast milk
Interactions/incompatibilities:
• Increased hypotension, bradycardia: reserpine, hydralazine, methyldopa, prazosin, nifedipine, verapamil, other antihypertensives
• Hypertensive reactions when given with: adrenaline, noradrenaline, sympathomimetics
• Increased hypoglycaemic effect: of antidiabetics (and masking of warning signs)
• Risk of heart block/failure with: diltiazem, nifedipine, verapamil amiodarone
• Increased myocardial depression: halothane, cyclopropane, trichloroethylene, ether, chloroform
Clinical assessment:
• Baseline renal, liver function tests before therapy begins if significant impairment suspected
Treatment of overdose: Lavage, IV atropine for bradycardia, IV theophylline for bronchospasm, digitalis, O_2, diuretic for cardiac failure, haemodialysis, hypotension; administer vasopressor (isoprenaline)

NURSING CONSIDERATIONS

Assess:

• Fluid balance, weight
• Apical/radial pulse before administration; notify clinician of any significant changes

Administer:
• Orally, before meals, at bedtime, tablet may be crushed or swallowed whole
• Reduced dosage in renal dysfunction

Perform/provide:
• Storage in dry area at room temperature

Evaluate:
• Therapeutic response: decreased BP after 1–2 weeks
• BP, pulse 4 hrly, note rate, rhythm, quality
• Peripheral oedema
• Weight daily

Teach patient/family:
• Take with or immediately after meals
• Not to discontinue drug abruptly, taper over 2 weeks may cause precipitate angina
• Not to use non-prescribed products containing α-adrenergic stimulants (nasal decongestants, non-prescribed cold preparations)
• To report bradycardia, dizziness, confusion, depression, fever, sore throat, shortness of breath to clinician
• To take pulse at home, advise when to notify clinician
• To avoid alcohol, smoking, sodium intake
• The importance of weight control, dietary adjustments, modified exercise programme
• To avoid hazardous activities if dizziness is present
• To report symptoms of congestive cardiac failure: difficult breathing, especially on exertion or when lying down, night cough, swelling of extremities

piperacillin sodium

Pipril

Func. class.: Antibiotic, antipseudomonal
Chem. class.: Ureidopenicillin
Legal class.: POM

Action: Bactericidal antibiotic, interferes with cell wall replication of susceptible organisms

Uses: Treatment of severe local/systemic infection where parenteral therapy is indicated. Surgical prophylaxis, effective against Gram-positive cocci (*S. aureus, S. pyogenes, S. viridans, S. faecalis, S. bovis, S. pneumoniae*); Gram-negative cocci (*N. gonorrhoeae, N. meningitidis*); anaerobes, (*C. perfringens, C. tetani, Bacteroides, Peptococcus* spp); Gram-negative bacilli (*E. coli, Klebsiella* spp, *P. mirabilis, P. vulgaris, P. rehgesii, Enterobacter* spp, *Citrobacter* spp, *P. aeruginosa, Serratia* spp, *Acinetobacter* spp, *H. influenza*). *Not* effective against β-lactamase-producing *Staphylococcus* spp

Dosage and routes:

Systemic infections
• *Adult and child:* IM/IV 100–300 mg/kg in divided doses 6–8 hrly. Maximum single IM dose 2 g (0.5 g in children)
• *Neonates and infants:* IM/IV 100–300 mg/kg daily in 2 divided doses

Prophylaxis of surgical infections
• *Adult:* IV/IM 2 g just before procedure, repeated at least twice at 4 or 6 hr intervals

Acute gonorrhoea
• *Adult*: IM 2 g single dose

Available forms include: Injection IM, IV 1, 2 g; IV infusion 4 g

Side effects/adverse reactions:
HAEM: Increased bleeding time, bone marrow depression

GI: Nausea, vomiting, diarrhoea, raised liver enzymes, abdominal pain, glossitis, colitis, cholestatic jaundice
GU: Haematuria, vaginitis, moniliasis, glomerulonephritis
CNS: Lethargy, twitching, coma, convulsions
SYST: Anaphylaxis
INTEG: Rash, pruritus, rarely exfoliative dermatitis
MISC: Thrombophlebitis and pain at injection site
Contraindications: Hypersensitivity to penicillins
Precautions: Pregnancy, hypersensitivity to cephalosporins, lactation, infectious mononucleosis, renal insufficiency (modify dose)
Pharmacokinetics:
IM: Peak 30–50 min
Half-life 0.7–1.33 hr, excreted in urine, bile, breast milk largely unchanged
Interactions/incompatibilities:
• Decreased antimicrobial effect of this drug: cefoxitin
• Increased penicillin concentrations: aspirin, probenecid
• Synergistic with aminoglycoside antibiotics (but incompatible *in vitro*)

piperazine citrate
piperazine phosphate

Pripsen, Expelix
Func. class.: Anthelmintic
Legal class.: P

Action: Causes paralysis in worm, leading to expulsion
Uses: Pinworm, roundworm, threadworm
Dosage and routes (Recommendations vary with product):
Threadworm
• *Adult:* Pripsen sachets: By mouth, one sachet, repeated after 14 days
• Elixir 750 mg/5 ml: By mouth, 3 × 5 ml daily for 7 days, repeated after 7 days if necessary
• *Child:* Pripsen sachets: By mouth, as a single dose, repeated after 14 days, 3 months–1 year, ⅓ sachet; 1–6 yr, ⅔ sachet; over 6 yr, 1 sachet.
• Elixir 750 mg/5 ml: By mouth, dose given daily for 7 days and repeated after 7 days if necessary, under 2 yr, 0.3 to 0.5 ml per kg, 2–3 years 5 ml, 4–6 years 7.5 ml, 7–12 years 10 ml
Roundworm
• *Adult:* Pripsen sachets: By mouth, one sachet, repeated after 14 days. Repeat at monthly intervals for up to 3 months if reinfection risk
• Elixir 750 mg/5 ml: By mouth, 30 ml as a single dose, repeated after 14 days
• *Child:* Pripsen sachets: By mouth, as a single dose, repeated after 14 days, 3 months–1 year, ⅓ sachet; 1–6 yr, ⅔ sachet; over 6 yr, 1 sachet
• Elixir 750 mg/5 ml: By mouth as a single dose, repeated after 14 days, under 1 year 0.8 ml per kg, 1–3 years 10 ml, 4–5 years 15 ml, 6–8 years 20 ml, 9–12 years 25 ml
Available forms include: Elixir 750 mg (hydrate)/5 ml; oral granules 4 g (with senna)/sachet
Side effects/adverse reactions:
HAEM: Haemolytic anaemia in glucose-6-phosphate dehydrogenase deficiency
INTEG: Rash, urticaria, photosensitivity
RESP: Bronchospasm
CNS: Dizziness, headache, paraesthesia, convulsions, drowsiness, ataxia
EENT: Blurred vision
GI: Nausea, vomiting, anorexia,

diarrhoea, abdominal cramps
SYST: Fever, angioedema
MS: Muscle hypotonia, joint pain
Contraindications: Hypersensitivity, severe renal disease, hepatic disease, epilepsy
Precautions: Severe malnutrition, pregnancy, chronic disorders of central nervous system
Pharmacokinetics:
Readily absorbed, excreted in urine partly as metabolites, half-life variable
Interactions/incompatibilities:
• May increase extrapyramidal symptoms when used with phenothiazines
• Effects reduced by pyrantel pamoate
Treatment of overdose: Gastric lavage. Supportive treatment including anticonvulsants if necessary

NURSING CONSIDERATIONS

Assess:
• Stools during entire treatment, 1, 3, months after treatment; specimens must be sent to lab while still warm
Administer:
• Take in water or milk (Pripsen sachets)
• To be crushed or chewed
• Laxatives if constipated; not needed for drug to work
• Second course after 1 week off drug, if infection is severe
Evaluate:
• Nausea, vomiting
• Therapeutic response: expulsion of worms, 3 negative stool cultures after completion of treatment
• For allergic reaction: rash, itching, urticaria
• For infestation in other family members since transmission from person to person is common
Teach patient/family:
• Good hygiene: hand washing after bowel movement; avoid putting fingers in mouth; to take a daily bath or shower; to change bed linen daily
• That infested person should sleep alone
• To clean toilet daily with disinfectant
• Need for compliance with dosage schedule and duration of treatment
• That urine may turn orange or red
• To avoid hazardous activities since drowsiness occurs
• That seizures may recur in patient who is controlled on medication
Clinical assessment:
• Culture and sensitivity before drug therapy; drug may be given as soon as culture is taken
Lab. test interferences:
False positive: Urine glucose, tested with copper-reduction method (Clinitest)
Treatment of overdose: Supportive, drug may be removed by dialysis. Anticonvulsants such as diazepam or phenobarbitone may be appropriate

NURSING CONSIDERATIONS

Assess:
• Bowel pattern
• Fluid balance
• For penicillin sensitivity or previous allergy
Administer:
• After specimens sent for culture and sensitivity completed
• By slow bolus or, more usually, by infusion over ½ hr
• For IM use each g should be reconstituted with at least 2 ml water for injections or lignocaine 0.5–1% solution; IV injection should be reconstituted with at least 5 ml of water for injections per g and given over 3–5 min, or further diluted to at least 50 ml and infused over 20–40 min
Perform/provide:
• Resuscitation equipment if anaphylaxis should occur

• Adequate (2 litre) daily fluid intake

Evaluate:

• Therapeutic response: absence of fever, redness, inflammation, purulent drainage

• Fluid balance daily—bowel pattern daily for diarrhoea

• IV site for phlebitis or extravasation

• Urinalysis for haematuria

Teach patient/family:

• To notify nurse of diarrhoea/frequency of stools

• To report sore throat, fever, rashes

pipothiazine palmitate

Piportil Depot

Func. class.: Neuroleptic/antipsychotic

Chem. class.: Phenothiazine

Legal class.: POM

Action: Depresses cerebral cortex, hypothalamus, limbic system, which control activity; aggression; blocks neurotransmission produced by dopamine at synapse; exhibits antagonism of α-adrenergic, cholinergic effects

Uses: Maintenance in schizophrenia and related psychoses

Dosage and routes: Deep IM injection into gluteal muscle; test dose 25 mg, then further 25–50 mg after 4–7 days; then adjusted, according to response, in 25–50 mg increments every 4 weeks; usual maintenance range 50–100 mg every 4 weeks; maximum dose 200 mg every 4 weeks

Available forms include: Injection 50 mg/ml; 1-ml, 2-ml ampoules

Side effects/adverse reactions:

CVS: Hypotension, arrhythmias, atrioventricular block, ventricular tachycardia

HAEM: Agranulocytosis, leucopenia

INTEG: Pain, erythema, swelling, nodules at injection site, pallor, photosensitisation, contact sensitisation, rashes

CNS: Extrapyramidal symptoms, tardive dyskinesia, drowsiness, apathy, insomnia, depression, agitation, nightmares, blurred vision, tremor, rigidity, respiratory depression

GI: Dry mouth, constipation, obstructive jaundice

GU: Difficulty with micturition, impotence

EENT: Nasal congestion, ocular changes

MISC: Hypothermia, pyrexia, menstrual disturbances, galactorrhoea, gynaecomastia, weight gain, neuroleptic malignant syndrome

Contraindications: Coma, marked cerebral atherosclerosis, parkinsonism, bone marrow depression, phaechromocytoma, renal or liver failure, confusional states, severe cardiac insufficiency, hypersensitivity

Precautions: Cardiovascular disease, severe respiratory disease, renal or hepatic impairment, parkinsonism, epilepsy, acute infections, hypothyroidism, myasthenia gravis, leucopenia, history of jaundice, prostatic hypertrophy, elderly, alcohol withdrawal symptoms, brain damage, history of narrow angle glaucoma, thyrotoxicosis, pregnancy, lactation

Pharmacokinetics: Poorly understood

Interactions/incompatibilities:

• Increases CNS depression with: alcohol, barbiturates, other sedatives

• Increases the effects of: most antihypertensives, anticholinergic drugs including tricyclic antidepressants

- Decreased effects of: amphetamine, levodopa, bromocriptine, lysuride, pergolide, clonidine, guanethidine, adrenaline, hypoglycaemic drugs, anticonvulsants (lowered seizure threshold)
- Increased extrapyramidal effects with, and toxicity of, lithium

Clinical assessment:
- Administer small test dose to ensure patient does not experience undesirable side effects
- Adjust dosage and dosage interval to suit individual
- Adjust dosage of concurrently administered drugs if interaction occurs
- Immediate investigation of unexplained fever/infection

Treatment of overdose: Generalised vasodilation may occur, raising patient's legs may be sufficient, volume expanders may be required. Positive inotropic agents such as dopamine may be given for circulatory collapse if fluid replacement is insufficient. Anti-arrythmic agents (avoid lignocaine and long-acting types) may be required. Severe dystonic reactions respond to procyclidine (5–10 mg) or orphenadrine (20–40 mg) IM or IV. Convulsions treatment diazepam IV

NURSING CONSIDERATIONS

Assess:
- Baseline BP and pulse, weight

Administer:
- Deep IM in gluteal muscle
- Not more than 2–3 ml of oily injection at any one site

Evaluate:
- Pulse; arrhythmias and tachycardia may occur
- BP: hypotension may occur
- For development of jaundice—withhold drug if this develops

Teach patient/family:
- Not to drink alcohol whilst taking drug
- To avoid exposure to direct sunlight as skin may be sensitive
- To stand up slowly to avoid orthostatic hypotension
- That weight gain is possible whilst using this drug
- Seek medical advice before taking any medications

pirbuterol (inhaled)

Exirel

Func. class.: Bronchodilator

Chem. class.: Adrenergic B_2 stimulant

Legal class.: POM

Action: Causes bronchodilation by stimulating bronchial β-receptors

Uses: Asthma, bronchospasm associated with bronchitis and emphysema

Dosage and routes:
- *Adult and child over 12 yr:* Aerosol 1–2 puffs (0.2–0.4 mg) 3 or 4 times a day, may be increased to maximum 12 puffs a day. By mouth 10–15 mg 3 or 4 times a day

Available forms include: Capsules 10 mg, 15 mg; aerosol delivers 0.2 mg pirbuterol (as acetate) per actuation

Side effects/adverse reactions:

CNS: Tremors, anxiety, insomnia, headache

EENT: Irritation of nose, throat with inhaler

CV: Palpitations, tachycardia, hypertension, angina, hypotension, dysrhythmias

MS: Muscle cramps

RESP: Bronchospasm, dyspnoea, coughing especially after inhalation

MISC: Hypokalaemia

Contraindications: Hypersensitivity to sympathomimetics; concurrent use of non-selective β-blocker

Precautions: Lactation, pregnancy, coronary artery disease, dysrhythmias, hyperthyroidism, children under 12 yr

Pharmacokinetics:

By mouth: onset 1 hr, peak 1–2 hr, duration 6 hr. Half-life 2 hr, excreted in urine as sulphate conjugate

Inhalation: Onset 5–10 min, peak 15–30 min, duration 5 hr, plasma levels undetectable

Interactions/incompatibilities:

• Increased risk of hypokalaemia with: theophylline, aminophylline, choline theophyllinate, steroids, diuretics, long-term laxatives

• Decreased action of pirbuterol: β-blockers

Clinical assessment:

• Monitor serum potassium in patients at risk of hypokalaemia

Treatment of overdose: Symptomatic and supportive. Cardioselective β-blockers may be useful (caution in patients with history of bronchospasm)

NURSING CONSIDERATIONS

Assess:

• Respiratory function: vital capacity, forced expiratory volume, arterial blood gases

Administer:

• After shaking inhaler: instruct patient in correct inhaler technique

• Wait for 1 min between puffs

Perform/provide:

• Frequent mouthcare and drinks for dry mouth

Evaluate:

• Response to treatment: indicated by resolution of dyspnoea and wheezing during the hour following administration

• Improvement of peak expiratory flow rate

Teach patient/family:

• How to use inhaler. Ensure patient has read and understood the enclosed instructions

• To avoid getting aerosol in the eyes

• To wash and dry inhaler once daily

• Not to take non-prescription medicines as they may negate the effects of pirbuterol

• Provide information about all aspects of the drug and its administration: to avoid smoking and smokey atmospheres and exposure to respiratory infections

---

pirenzepine dihydrochloride

Gastrozepin

Func. class.: Selective antimuscarinic

Chem. class.: Dihydrobenzodiazepinone

Legal class.: POM

Action: Inhibits gastric acid and pepsin secretion

Uses: Gastric and duodenal ulceration

Dosage and routes:

• *Adult:* By mouth 50 mg twice daily 30 min before meals, increased if necessary to maximum of 150 mg daily in 3 divided doses for 4–6 weeks; in resistant cases for up to 3 months

Available forms include: Tablets 50 mg

Side effects/adverse reactions:

GI: Dry mouth

EENT: Visual disturbances

HAEM: Agranulocytosis, thrombocytopenia

Contraindications: Hypersensitivity; prostate enlargement; organic pyloric stenosis; paralytic ileus; closed-angle glaucoma or shallow anterior chamber; pregnancy

Precautions: Lactation, renal impairment

Pharmacokinetics: 25% absorbed orally (10–20% with food) mean half life of 12 hr, 90% excreted unchanged in faeces

Interactions/incompatibilities:

• Anticholinergic side effects may be enhanced by: atropine, antihistamines, butyrophenones, phenothiazines, tricyclic antidepressants

• Theoretical interaction with: MAOIs and sympathomimetics

Clinical assessment:

• Continue treatment for 4–6 weeks even when symptoms have subsided

Treatment of overdose: Symptomatic

NURSING CONSIDERATIONS

Administer:

• Give at least 30 min before meals, with liquid

Evaluate:

• For visual disturbances—patient may require assistance with activities

• Therapeutic response—lessening of symptoms

Teach patient/family:

• Consult clinician before taking non-prescribed medication

piroxicam

Feldene, Larapam, Pirozip

Func. class.: Non-steroidal anti-inflammatory drug

Chem. class.: Oxicam derivative

Legal class.: POM

Action: Inhibits prostaglandin synthesis by inhibiting an enzyme needed for biosynthesis; possesses analgesic, anti-inflammatory, antipyretic properties

Uses: Mild to moderate pain, osteoarthritis, rheumatoid arthritis

Dosage and routes:

• *Adult:* By mouth, per rectum in chronic conditions, normally 20 mg daily, occasionally 10 mg daily sufficient, maximum 30 mg daily. Acute gout: 40 mg daily for 5–7 days. Acute musculoskeletal disorders: 40 mg daily for 2 days, then 20 mg daily for 7–14 days. Daily doses may be divided

IM injection same as dose by mouth

• *Child over 6 yr:* By mouth in juvenile chronic arthritis, less than 15 kg, 5 mg daily; 16–25 kg, 10 mg daily; 26–45 kg, 15 mg daily; over 46 kg, 20 mg daily

Available forms include: Capsules 10 mg, 20 mg; dispersible tablets 10 mg, 20 mg; melt-in-mouth tablets 20 mg; suppositories 20 mg; injection 20 mg/ml

Side effects/adverse reactions:

GI: Nausea, anorexia, vomiting, diarrhoea, jaundice, cholestatic hepatitis, constipation, flatulence, cramps, peptic ulcer, gastrointestinal bleeding. Local pain; irritation, tenesmus with suppositories

CNS: Dizziness, drowsiness, fatigue, confusion, insomnia, anxiety, depression

CV: Peripheral oedema, palpitations

INTEG: Purpura, rash, pruritus, alopecia, epidermal necrolysis

GU: Nephrotoxicity: raised serum creatinine and blood urea nitrogen

HAEM: Blood dyscrasias

EENT: Tinnitus, hearing loss, blurred vision

SYST: Hypersensitivity reactions: anaphylaxis, angiodema, serum sickness

Contraindications: Hypersensitivity; hypersensitivity to aspirin or other NSAIDs; active, suspected or recurrent peptic ulceration; porphyria; last trimester of pregnancy; asthma. Suppositories only: inflammatory lesions of the rectum/anus, recent history of rectal/anal bleeding

Precautions: Pregnancy, lactation, children, bleeding disorders, upper GI disorders, cardiac disorders, hypersensitivity to other NSAIDs, renal disease, severe hepatic disease

Pharmacokinetics:

By mouth: Peak 2 hr, half-life 50 hr; metabolised in liver, excreted in urine (metabolites) excreted in breast milk, 99% protein bound

Interactions/incompatibilities:

- May increase action of oral anticoagulants, phenytoin, lithium, sulphonylurea hypoglycaemic agents, methotrexate

Clinical assessment:

- Monitor therapeutic response to, and blood levels of lithium, phenytoin during concurrent treatment
- Monitor therapeutic response to oral anticoagulants, sulphonylurea hypoglycaemics during concurrent therapy
- Opthalmic examination if visual problems develop
- Withdraw drug during methotrexate therapy

Treatment of overdose: Supportive and symptomatic. Activated charcoal may be useful

NURSING CONSIDERATIONS

Administer:

- With or after food
- Dissolve dispersible tablets in water
- Injection; deep I.M. injection into upper outer quadrant of buttock

Evaluate:

- Therapeutic response: decreased pain, stiffness, swelling in joints, ability to move more easily
- For eye, ear problems: blurred vision, tinnitus (may indicate toxicity)

Teach patient/family:

- To report blurred vision or ringing, roaring in ears (may indicate toxicity)
- To avoid driving or other hazardous activities if dizziness or drowsiness occurs
- To take with food or milk
- To report change in urine pattern, weight increase, oedema, pain increase in joints, fever, blood in urine (indicates nephrotoxicity)
- That therapeutic effects may take up to 1 month
- Report any persistent indigestion or black tar-like stools

---

piroxicam (topical)

Feldene Gel, Feldene Sports Gel

Func. class.: Nonsteroidal antiinflammatory

Chem. class.: Oxicam derivative

Legal class.: POM

Action: Inhibits prostaglandin synthesis by inhibiting an enzyme needed for biosynthesis; possesses analgesic, antiinflammatory properties

Uses: Topical application to superficial joints affected by osteoarthritis and musculoskeletal injuries

Dosage and routes:

- *Adult:* Massage approximately 1 g of Gel (3 cm strip) into the affected area 3–4 times a day

Side effects/adverse reactions:

INTEG: Erythema, rash, desquamation, pruritus

Contraindications: Hypersensitivity to piroxicam, aspirin or other NSAIDs; children

Precautions: Pregnancy, breast feeding, hypersensitivity to other non-steroidal antiinflammatories. Do not use on open wounds, mucosal surfances, infected lesions, dermatoses

Pharmacokinetics: Rapid equilibration by gel with tissue under site of application. In chronic use plasma levels rise to approximately one-twentieth dose found after 20 mg orally

Interactions/incompatibilities: Unlikely to occur at low plasma levels achieved

NURSING CONSIDERATIONS

Administer:

- Externally only
- Do not use occlusive dressings
- Massage into skin leaving no residual gel

Evaluate:

- Therapeutic response
- Side effects

Teach patient/family:

- How to use the gel
- Not to apply it to open or infected wounds
- To discontinue use and report any side effects

---

pivampicillin

Pondocillin

Func. class.: Broad spectrum antibiotic

Chem. class.: Pivaloyloxy methyl ester of ampicillin

Legal class.: POM

Action: Ampicillin derivative, which is rapidly broken down in GI tract to ampicillin to increase bioavailability from oral dose, bactericidal antibotic

Uses: Urinary tract infections, acute and chronic bronchitis, invasive salmonellosis, gonorrhoea, ear, nose and throat infection, gynaecological infections. Skin and soft tissue infections

Dosage and routes:

- *Adult:* By mouth 500 mg every 12 hr, doubled in severe infections
- *Child up to 1 yr:* By mouth 40–60 mg/kg daily in divided doses; *1–5 yr:* 350–525 mg daily; *6–10 yr:* 525–700 mg daily

Gonorrhoea

- *Adult:* By mouth 1.5–2 g as a single dose with 1 g of probenicid

Available forms include: Tablets, 500 mg; suspension, 175 mg/5 ml when reconstituted with water

Side effects/adverse reactions:

GI: Diarrhoea, nausea, vomiting, flatulence

INTEG: Rashes, urticaria

CV: Angioedema

MS: Joint pains

SYST: Fever, anaphylactic shock

CNS: Dizziness

Contraindications: Penicillin hypersensitivity, porphyria, glandular fever

Precautions: History of allergy, renal or hepatic impairment, cephalosporin hypersensitivity, pregnancy, lactation, lymphatic leukaemia

Pharmacokinetics: Rapidly hydrolysed to ampicillin by non-specific enzymes present in the serum, GI mucosa and other tissues. Plasma levels are 2–3 times higher than equimolar doses of ampicillin. Peak levels within 1 hr. Not affected by food, in GI tract

Interactions/incompatibilities: Reduced absorbtion with antacids

Treatment of overdose: Supportive measures

NURSING CONSIDERATIONS

Assess:

- Bowel pattern
- Fluid balance
- For penicillin hypersensitivity or allergy

Administer:

- To be taken with or after food
- After specimens have been sent for culture and sensitivity
- With food if needed for GI symptoms

Perform/provide:

- Resuscitation equipment if anaphylaxis occurs
- Adequate (2 litre) daily fluid intake

Evaluate:

- Therapeutic response: decreased fever, malaise, chills

• Daily fluid balance
• Bowel pattern daily; if severe diarrhoea occurs, report to clinician – may be discontinued

Teach patient/family:
• To complete antibiotic course as prescribed
• To report signs of rashes, joint pains, shortness of breath and other signs of sensitivity/ anaphylaxis immediately

pivmecillinam

Selexid
Func. class.: Antibiotic, broad spectrum
Chem. class.: Pivaloyloxymethyl ester of mecillinam
Legal class.: POM

Action: Hydrolysed to mecillinam *in vivo*, interferes with biosynthesis of bacterial cell wall

Uses: Acute uncomplicated cystitis, chronic or recurrent bacteriuria, salmonellosis, alternative antibiotic in treatment of acute typhoid fever. Highly active against most Enterobacteriaceae; less active against Gram positive organisms; *Ps. aeruginosa* and *Strep. faecalis* virtually resistant

Dosage and routes:

Cystitis
• *Adults:* By mouth 400 mg initially, then 200 mg 8 hrly for 3 days

Bacteriuria
• *Adults:* By mouth 400 mg every 6–8 hr
• *Child less than 40 kg:* 20–40 mg/ kg in 3 or 4 divided doses

Salmonellosis
• *Adults:* By mouth 1.2–2.4 g daily for 14 days; 14–28 days for carriers
• *Child less than 40 kg:* 30–60 mg/kg daily in 3 or 4 divided doses

Available forms include: Tablets, 200 mg; suspension, granules 100 mg/sachet

Side effects/adverse reactions:
GI: Diarrhoea, nausea, vomiting, indigestion
INTEG: Rashes, urticaria
SYST: Anaphylactic shock

Contraindications: Penicillin and cephalosporin hypersensitivity

Precautions: History of allergy, renal or hepatic impairment, pregnancy

Pharmacokinetics: Hydrolysed to mecillinam *in vivo*. Well absorbed from GI tract. Peak plasma concentrations of 5 mcg per ml have been achieved 1 to 2 hr after 400 mg dose. 50% of dose may be excreted as mecillinam in urine, mainly within 6 hr of a dose, serum half life is 1.2 hr

NURSING CONSIDERATIONS:

Assess:
• Baseline observations: temperature pulse and respiration
• Bacteriological screen: swabs, stool sample, etc.

Administer:
• To be taken with or after food, with plenty of water
• By mouth as directed, i.e. before or with food for better absorption
• With copious fluids
• Concurrent administration of probenecid delays oral excretion of mecillinam, producing sustained serum levels

Perform/provide:
• Secure container and storage at room temperature
• Fluid balance chart

Evaluate:
• Therapeutic response, decrease in fever and symptoms
• Signs of anaphylaxis: rash, etc.
• Side effects of GI disturbance

Teach patient/family:
• To finish course of prescribed antibiotics
• Health education issues to avoid

reoccurrence of symptoms
- Seek medical advice if symptoms/malaise reoccurs

pizotifen

Sanomigran
Func. class.: Antimigraine agent
Legal class.: POM

Action: Prevents abnormal dilation of cranial blood vessels and sensitisation of surrounding pain receptors

Uses: Prophylaxis of vascular headache, including classical migraine, common migraine, cluster headache

Dosage and routes:
- *Adult:* By mouth 1.5 mg at night or 500 mcg 3 times daily adjusted for response; usual range 0.5–3 mg daily; maximum single dose 3 mg, maximum daily dose 4.5 mg
- *Child:* By mouth up to 1.5 mg daily in divided doses; maximum single dose at night 1 mg

Available forms include: Tablets (as hydrogen maleate) 500 mcg, 1.5 mg; elixir (as hydrogen maleate) 250 mcg/5 ml

Side effects/adverse reactions:
CNS: Drowsiness, dizziness, stimulation in children
GI: Nausea
META: Weight gain
MS: Muscle pain

Precautions: Closed angle glaucoma, renal insufficiency, pregnancy, lactation, predisposition to urinary retention

Pharmacokinetics:
Readily absorbed from GI tract, metabolised with liver excreted as metabolites in urine

Interactions/incompatibilities:
- Increased sedation with: alcohol, antihistamines sedatives, hypnotics
- Decreased effect of: adrenergic neurone blocking antihypertensives

Treatment of overdose: Gastric lavage and diuresis. Severe hypotension should be corrected (caution: adrenaline may cause paradoxical effects). Convulsions managed with benzodiazepines or barbiturates

NURSING CONSIDERATIONS

Assess:
- Baseline weight

Administer:
- Give with or after food to avoid GI symptoms

Provide:
- Quiet, calm environment with decreased stimulation from noise, bright light or excessive talking

Evaluate:
- Weight daily, check for peripheral oedema in feet, legs
- For stress level, activity, recreation, coping mechanisms of patient
- Neurological status, level of consciousness, blurring vision, nausea, vomiting, tingling in extremities that occur preceding headache
- Ingestion of tyramine foods (pickled products, beer, red wine, mature cheese), food additives, preservatives, colourings, artificial sweeteners, chocolate, caffeine; all/any may precipitate these types of headache
- Therapeutic response: decrease in frequency, severity of headache

Teach patient/family:
- Not to use non-prescribed medications, serious drug interactions may occur
- To maintain dose at approved level, not to increase even if drug does not relieve headache
- To report side effects; increased vasoconstriction, starting with cold extremities, then paraesthesia, weakness
- That an increase in headaches

may occur when the drug is discontinued after long-term use
• Report at once: dyspnoea, paraesthesiae, urinary problems, pain in abdomen, chest, back, legs

plicamycin (mithramycin)

Mithracin
Func. class.: Antineoplastic, antibiotic
Chem. class.: Crystalline aglycone
Legal class.: POM

Action: Inhibits DNA, RNA, protein synthesis; may lower serum calcium levels by blocking osteoclast response to parathyroid hormone
Uses: Refractory hypercalcaemia associated with a variety of neoplasms, specifically where standard therapeutic methods have failed
Dosage and routes:
Doses are highly variable, and dependent on local treatment protocols, concomitant therapy and tumour type; the following dose schedules have been used
• *Adult:* IV 25 mcg/kg/day for 3–4 days, repeat at intervals of 1 week. Frequency may be reduced for maintenance
Available forms include: Injection 2.5 mg
Side effects/adverse reactions:
META: Decreased serum phosphorus, potassium
HAEM: Haemorrhage, thrombocytopenia, WBC count, increased clotting time
GI: Nausea, vomiting, anorexia, diarrhoea, stomatitis, increased liver enzymes
GU: Increased serum urea, creatinine, proteinuria
INTEG: Rash, cellulitis, local irritation at injection site flushing
CNS: Drowsiness, weakness, lethargy, headache, depression
SYST: Fever
Contraindications: Hypersensitivity, myelosuppression, bleeding disorders, pregnancy, breast-feeding
Precautions: Renal disease, hepatic disease, electrolyte imbalances
Pharmacokinetics: Crosses blood–brain barrier, excreted in urine; little known about pharmacokinetics
Interactions/incompatibilities:
• Increased toxicity: other antineoplastics or radiation
Clinical assessment:
• Full blood count, platelet count, prothrombin time, bleeding time before, regularly during and a few days after treatment
• Renal function: Monitor before, during treatment
• Liver function tests before, during therapy
Treatment of overdose: Supportive

NURSING CONSIDERATIONS

Administer:
• HANDLING: take safety precautions appropriate to antineoplastic agents; vesicant agent
• Following local antineoplastic (cytotoxic) policies
• After ensuring that clinician is aware of blood results
• IV; by IV infusion in 1 litre dextrose 5% or sodium chloride 0.9%, over 4–6 hours
• Other medications by mouth if possible. Avoid IV, IM, SC routes to prevent infection and bruising
• Anti-emetic 30–60 min before treatment
• All other medication as prescribed including analgesics, antibiotics, anti-emetics, antispasmodics
Perform/provide:
• Drug must not be handled by pregnant staff
• Staff to use protective garments/gloves/goggles
• Reconstitution in designated

aseptic area
• Usage immediately after mixing
• Strict medical asepsis, protective isolation if WBC levels are low
• Observe oral mucosa for ulceration/breakdown. Encourage oral hygiene 4 times a day
• Warm compresses at injection site for inflammation; check for extravasation

Evaluate:
• Observe for diarrhoea and administer anti-diarrhoea drugs as required
• Bleeding: haematuria, bruising or petechiae, mucosa or orifices 8 hrly
• For signs of thrombocytopenia and depression of clotting factors 10 days after administration
• Food preferences; list likes, dislikes
• Inflammation of mucosa, breaks in skin
• Yellowing of skin, sclera, dark urine, clay-coloured stools, itchy skin, abdominal pain, fever, diarrhoea
• Buccal cavity 8 hrly for dryness, sores, ulceration, white patches, oral pain, bleeding, dysphagia
• Local irritation, pain, burning at injection site (vesicant drug)
• Frequency of stools, characteristics, cramping
• Temperature if indicated

Teach patient/family:
• Why protective isolation precautions are necessary in same cases
• To report any complaints or side effects to nurse or clinician
• To avoid foods with citric acid, hot or rough texture
• To report to clinician any bleeding, white spots, ulcerations in the mouth; tell patient to examine mouth daily
• To avoid driving or activities requiring alertness, drowsiness may occur
• To report leg cramps, tingling of fingertips, weakness; may indicate hypokalaemia
• Can cause metallic taste in mouth: encourage bland diet

pneumococcal vaccine

Pneumovax II
Func. class.: Polyvalent pneumococcal vaccine
Chem. class.: Mixture of 23 purified polysaccharide capsular antigens from serotypes of *Streptococcus pneumoniae*
Legal class.: POM

Action: Promotes development of antibody-mediated immunity
Uses: Individuals at particular risk of contracting pneumococcal disease, e.g. those who have had a splenectomy
Dosage and routes: IM/subcutaneous injection 0.5 ml as single dose
Available forms include: 0.5 ml single-dose vial
Side effects/adverse reactions:
INTEG: Erythema, soreness, induration at injection site
SYSTEM: Fever, anaphylactic shock
HAEM: Relapse of idiopathic thrombocytopenic purpura
NEURO: Possibly paraesthesias, acute radiculopathy, Guillain-Barré syndrome
Contraindications: Children less than 2 yr, pregnancy, 10 days before and during immunosuppressive therapy, Hodgkin's disease suffers with history of extensive chemotherapy and/or nodal irradiation, breast feeding, hypersensitivity
Precautions: Cardiovascular or respiratory disease, previously immunised adult patients, children immunised within last 3 yr

Clinical assessment:
• Mark patient notes clearly to prevent revaccination

NURSING CONSIDERATIONS

Administer:
• After inspecting to ensure it is clear, colourless and free from suspended particles
• Undiluted
• IM or deep subcutaneous into deltoid muscle or lateral aspect of mid-thigh
• Do *not* inject intravascularly

Perform/provide:
• Refrigerated storage
• Adrenaline in case of anaphylaxis

Evaluate:
• For anaphylaxis

Teach patient/family:
• That local reaction (swelling, redness at injection site) is common for 48 hr and mild fever may occur
• No booster dose is required
• Protection will be afforded for up to 5 yr
• They may still contract pneumonia since protection is against only some of the serotypes

---

podophyllotoxin

Condyline, Warticon, Warticon Fem
Func. class.: Keratolytic
Chem. class.: Active constituent of podophyllum resin
Legal class.: POM

Action: Arrests mitosis of, and destroys the cells of, the hyperkeratotic layers and underlying epidermis of treated skin

Uses: Anogenital warts (condylomata acuminata)

Dosage and routes:
• *Adult:* Topically twice daily for 3 days, may be repeated after 7 days if necessary; maximum 5 treatment courses

Available forms include: Alcoholic solution 0.5%

Side effects/adverse reactions:
INTEG: Local irritation especially on second or third day of application

Contraindications: Hypersensitivity, open wounds

Precautions: Lesions larger than 4 cm^2 should be treated under the direct supervision of medical staff

Treatment of overdose: In topical overdose wash area thoroughly with soap and water. If ingested use gastric lavage, symptomatic and supportive treatment

NURSING CONSIDERATIONS

Assess:
• Local erythema
• Erosions, tenderness or inflammation

Administer:
• Patient receives 0.5% w/v podophyllotoxin solution, for 3 days, applied locally to warts. Four day treatment free interval. This cycle can be repeated for up to four weeks

Perform/provide:
• Leaflets provided with treatment
• Stop treatment if inflamata or itching ensues treatment

Evaluate:
• At intervals of four, six and ten weeks to assess presence/absence of warts
• Side effects, (inflammation or itching)

Teach patient/family:
• To return to clinic for assessment by physician after a 10 week period following treatment
• To return for assessment by clinician after a ten-week period following treatment
• Reasons for using solution regularly as instructed
• To stop treatment if side effects occur

podophyllum resin

Posalfilin, Podophyllin Paint Compound, BPC
Func. class.: Keratolytic
Chem. class.: Podophyllum derivative
Legal class.: POM

Action: Arrests mitosis by binding to tubulin, protein subunit of spindle microtubules; also interferes with movements of chromosomes
Uses: Venereal warts, keratoses, multiple superficial, epitheliomatoses
Dosage and routes:
Warts
• *Adult:* Topical, cover wart, cover with wax paper, bandage for 4–6 hr, wash, may be repeated weekly if needed
Keratoses/epitheliomatoses
• *Adult:* Topical, apply daily with applicator, let dry, remove tissue, may be reapplied if needed
Available forms include: Paint 15%
Side effects/adverse reactions:
HAEM: Thrombocytopenia, leucopenia
INTEG: Irritation of unaffected areas
CNS: Peripheral neuropathy, hallucination, confusion, dizziness, stupor, ataxia, hypotonin, convulsions, coma
GI: Nausea, vomiting, diarrhoea abdominal pain
Contraindications: Hypersensitivity, pregnancy, facial warts
Interactions/incompatibilities:
• Necrosis of skin: when used with other keratolytics
NURSING CONSIDERATIONS
Assess:
• Platelets, full blood count if systemic absorption occurs
Administer:
• Wear gloves to apply
• Only to affected area; protect surrounding normal skin
• Only to small areas or for short periods of time or absorption (systemic) may occur
• Avoid open wounds, face
• If a large number of warts are present, treat few at a time to minimise systemic absorption
Evaluate:
• Therapeutic response: decrease in size and amount of lesions
• Allergic reactions: irritation, redness, itching, stinging, burning; drug should be discontinued
• Blood dyscrasias if systemic absorption is suspected: decrease platelets
• Peripheral neuropathy; drug should be discontinued
Teach patient/family:
• That discomfort will begin after 12–24 hr, subside in 2–4 days
• Accurate and safe method of application

poliovirus vaccine, live, oral, trivalent

Func. class.: Vaccine
Legal class.: POM

Action: Produces specific antibodies for poliomyelitis
Uses: Prevention of polio
Dosage and routes: Consult manufacturer's data sheet
• *Adults:* (Unimmunised) one dose every 4 weeks for a total of three doses
• *Infants:* 1st dose at 2 months, 2nd and 3rd dose at intervals of 4 weeks
• *Reinforcement:* One dose at school entry, one further dose at school leaving
• Adult booster when exposure to the disease is likely, e.g. travel, health care workers at risk

Available forms include: Oral vaccine 1 dose or 10 dose
Side effects/adverse reactions:
SYST: Paralysis
Contraindications: Hypersensitivity, active infection, allergy to any component of the vaccine, efficacy impaired if subject has diarrhoea or vomiting, immunosuppression (an inactivated vaccine is available for the immunosuppressed patient)
Precautions: Pregnancy
Interactions/incompatibilities:
• Do not use TB skin test within 6 weeks of vaccine
• Do not use within 3 months of transfusion of whole blood, plasma, or use with immune serum globulin

NURSING CONSIDERATIONS

Assess:
• Active or suspected infection, diarrhoea or vomiting
• History of allergies, especially hypersensitivity to penicillin or streptomycin
Administer:
• Orally; after shaking well, dose is dropped onto sugar cube. Usually primary course 3 doses then reinforcing doses
• Give at same time as or with 3-week interval between other live vaccine
Perform/provide:
• Store vaccines at 0–4°C
Evaluate:
• For anaphylaxis; dyspnoea, bronchospasm, tachycardia, profuse sweating, collapse
• History of allergies, skin conditions reactions to vaccinations
Teach patient/family:
• That a reinforcing dose is needed by adults when exposure to disease is likely
• That there is a very slight risk of recipient paralysis from vaccination

polymyxin B sulphate

Func. class.: Antibiotic
Chem. class.: Polymyxin
Legal class.: POM

Action: Interferes with phospholipids, penetrates cell wall; changes occur immediately in bacterial membrane causing leakage of essential metabolites
Uses: Serious *PS. aeruginosa, E. aerogenes, K. pneumoniae, E. coli, H. influenzae* infections or when other antibiotics cannot be used
Dosage and routes:
• *Adult and child:* IV infusion 15,000–25,000 U/kg/day in divided doses every 12 hr, or as a continuous infusion. Total daily dosage must not exceed 2,000,000 units
• *Neonates:* A total of 15,000–45,000 U per kg bodyweight per day in low equally divided doses
Available forms include: Injection IV 500,000 U
Side effects/adverse reactions:
INTEG: Urticaria
CNS: Dizziness, weakness, paraesthesia
RESP: Paralysis
GU: Nephrotoxicity, azotemia, oliguria
SYST: Anaphylaxis
Contraindications: Hypersensitivity
Precautions: Pregnancy, renal impairment mysthenia gravis
Interactions/incompatibilities:
• Increased skeletal muscle relaxation: anesthetics, neuromuscular blockers (tubocurarine decamethonium, succinylcholine, gallamine)
• Increased nephrotoxicity, neurotoxicity: aminoglycosides, sodium citrate, parenteral quinine, parenteral quinidine, polypeptides, antibiotics with muscle relaxant properties
• Do not mix in solution or syringe

with cephalothin sodium, chloramphenicol sodium succinate, chlorothiazide, heparin, penicillins, tetracyclines, cobalt, magnesium, iron, amphotericin B, nitrofurantoin, prednisolone

Clinical assessment:

- Monitor serum urea, creatinine
- Renal studies: urinalysis, protein, blood
- Culture and sensitivity before drug therapy; drug may be taken as soon as culture is taken; culture and sensitivity may be done after completion of therapy

Treatment of overdose: Withdraw drug, maintain airway, administer, adrenaline, aminophylline, O_2, IV corticosteroids

NURSING CONSIDERATIONS

Assess:

- Any patient with compromised renal system; drug is excreted slowly in poor renal system function; toxicity may occur rapidly

Administer:

- IV after reconstituting with 300–500 ml Dextrose 5% given over 60–120 min
- After samples have been taken for culture and sensitivity

Perform/provide:

- Storage in dark area at room temperature
- Ensure resuscitation equipment and adrenaline nearby
- Adequate intake of fluids (2000 ml) during diarrhoea episodes

Evaluate:

- Fluid balance; report, oliguria
- Therapeutic response: absence of fever, purulent drainage, culture and sensitivity negative
- Skin eruptions, itching; drug should be discontinued
- Respiratory status: rate, character, dyspnoea, symptoms of neuromuscular blockade, tightness in chest; discontinue drug if these occur
- Allergies before initiation of treatment, reaction of each medication; note allergies on nursing care plan in bright red letters; notify all people giving drugs
- For flushing of face, dizziness, disorientation, weakness, paraesthesia, blurred vision, slurred speech, restlessness, irritability; indicate neurotoxicity

Teach patient/family:

- To report sore throat, fever, fatigue; could indicate superimposed infection

---

polynoxylin

Anaflex

Func. class.: Antibiotic/Antifungal

Chem. class.: Condensation product of formaldehyde and urea

Legal class.: P

Action: May act by the release of formaldehyde

Uses: Antibacterial and antifungal for use in mild skin, aural and nasal infections

Dosage and routes:

- *Topical:* Apply once or twice daily

Available forms include: Cream 10%

Side effects/adverse reactions:

INTEG: Local reaction to any constituents of topical preparation

Contraindications: None

NURSING CONSIDERATIONS

Administer:

- Cleanse skin before application

Perform/provide:

- Storage of cream below 25°C

Evaluate:

- Therapeutic response
- Lesions diminished

Teach patient/family:

- To seek medical advice if sign of infection worsening; may require systemic therapy

polythiazide

Nephril
Func. class.: Thiazide diuretic
Chem. class.: Sulphonamide derivative
Legal class.: POM

Action: Acts on distal tubule by increasing excretion of water, sodium, chloride, potassium
Uses: Oedema, hypertension
Dosage and routes:
• *Adult:* By mouth 1–4 mg/day
Available forms include: Tablets 1 mg
Side effects/adverse reactions:
GU: Frequency, polyuria, glucosuria
CNS: Paraesthesia, headache, dizziness, weakness
GI: Nausea, vomiting, anorexia, constipation, diarrhoea, cramps, pancreatitis, GI irritation, jaundice
EENT: Xanthopsia
INTEG: Rash, urticaria, purpura, photosensitivity, fever, necrotising angiitis
META: Hyperglycaemia, hyperuricaemia
HAEM: Aplastic anaemia, leucopenia, agranulocytosis, thrombocytopenia
CV: Orthostatic hypotension
ELECT: Hypokalaemia, hyponatraemia, hypochloraemia
Contraindications: Hypersensitivity to thiazides or sulphonamides, anuria
Precautions: Hypokalaemia, renal electrolyte imbalance disease, pregnancy, hepatic disease, gout, chronic obstructive airways disease, lupus erythematosus, diabetes mellitus, breast feeding
Pharmacokinetics:
By mouth: Onset 2 hr, peak 6 hr, duration 24–48 hr; excreted unchanged by kidneys, enters breast milk, half-life 26 hr
Interactions/incompatibilities:
• Increased toxicity of: lithium, non-depolarising skeletal muscle relaxants, cardiac glycosides
• Decreased effects of: antidiabetics
• Decreased absorption of: thiazides: cholestyramine, colestipol
• Decreased hypotensive response: indomethacin
• Increased action of: quinidine
Clinical assessment:
• BP lying, standing; postural hypotension may occur
• Electrolytes: potassium, sodium, chloride; include serum urea, blood sugar, full blood count, serum creatinine, blood pH, arterial blood gases
• Potassium replacement if potassium is less than 3.0 mmol/litre
Lab. test interferences:
Increase: Bromsulphthalein retention, calcium, amylase
Decrease: Protein bound iodine, phenolsulphthalein
Treatment of overdose: Lavage if taken orally, monitor electrolytes, supportive therapy

NURSING CONSIDERATIONS

Assess:
• Rate, depth, rhythm of respiration, effect of exertion
• Glucose in urine if patient is diabetic
Administer:
• In morning to avoid interference with sleep if using drug as a diuretic
• With food, if nausea occurs; absorption may be decreased slightly
Evaluate:
• Weight, fluid balance daily to determine fluid loss; effect of drug may be decreased if used daily
• Improvement in oedema of feet, legs, sacral area daily if medication is being used in congestive cardiac failure
• Signs of metabolic acidosis: drowsiness, restlessness
• Signs of hypokalaemia: postural

hypotension, malaise, fatigue, tachycardia, leg cramps, weakness
• Rashes, temperature elevation daily
• Confusion, especially in elderly; take safety precautions if needed
Teach patient/family:
• To increase fluid intake 2–3 litres/day unless contraindicated; to rise slowly from lying or sitting position
• To notify clinician of muscle weakness, cramps, nausea, dizziness
• Drug may be taken with food or milk
• That blood sugar may be increased in diabetics
• Take early in day to avoid nocturia

---

potassium bicarbonate/ potassium benzoate/ potassium chloride

Kay-Cee-L, Kloref, Kloref-S, Sando K, Leo-K, Slow-K, combination products
Func. class.: Electrolyte
Chem. class.: Potassium
Legal class.: P

Action: Necessary for adequate transmission of nerve impulses and cardiac contraction, renal function, intracellular ion maintenance
Uses: Prevention and treatment of hypokalaemia
Dosage and routes:
Potassium chloride
• *Adult:* Prevention of hypokalaemia: 25–50 mmols daily by mouth
• Treatment of hypokalaemia: 135–200 mmols daily by mouth
• *IV:* 20 mmols diluted to 500 ml, given over 2–3 hr. Repeat according to plasma levels
Available forms include: Many preparations; tablets, capsules, syrup, injections, infusion solutions
Side effects/adverse reactions:
CNS: Cardiac depression, arrhythmias, arrest, peaking T waves, lowered R and depressed RST, prolonged P-R interval, widened QRS complex
GI: Nausea, vomiting, cramps, pain, diarrhoea, oesophageal or small bowel ulceration
INTEG: Cold extremities
Contraindications: Renal disease, obstructions in digestive tract, (severe), severe haemolytic disease, Addison's disease, hyperkalaemia, acute dehydration, extensive tissue breakdown, e.g. severe burns, renal impairment, peptic ulcer or history of, concurrent treatment with anticholinergics, pregnancy
Precautions: Cardiac disease, potassium sparing diuretic therapy, systemic acidosis
Interactions/incompatibilities:
• Hyperkalaemia, potassium sparing, diuretic, or other potassium products
Pharmacokinetics:
By mouth: Excreted by kidneys and in faeces
Clinical assessment:
• ECG for peaking T waves, lowered R, depressed RST, prolonged P-R interval, widening QRS complex, hyperkalaemia; drug should be reduced or discontinued
• Potassium level during treatment (3.5–5.0 mmol/litre normal level)
• Cardiac status: rate, rhythm, CVP, if being monitored directly
NURSING CONSIDERATIONS
Assess:
• Baseline fluid balance
• Urea and electrolyte levels
• Digoxin toxicity if indicated
Administer:
• Orally—in tablet form; IV—dilute 20 mmols in 500 ml dextrose or sodium chloride solution

• IV infusion slowly over 2–3 hr
• Do not mix with other drugs
• Avoiding peripheral lines

Perform/provide:
• Storage at room temperature

Evaluate:
• Therapeutic response: absence of fatigue, muscle weakness
• Degree of cardiac arrhythmias, ST elevation or depression
• Fluid balance, urinary output

Teach patient/family:
• To add potassium-rich foods to diet: bananas, orange juice, avocados; whole grains, broccoli, carrots, prunes, cocoa after this medication is discontinued
• To avoid non-prescribed products: antacids, salt substitutes, analgesics, vitamin preparations
• To report symptoms of hyperkalaemia (lethargy, confusion, diarrhoea, nausea, vomiting, fainting, decreased output) or continued hypokalaemia (fatigue, weakness, polyuria, polydipsia, cardiac changes)

---

potassium canrenoate

Spiroctan-M
Func. class.: Diuretic
Chem. class.: Potassium salt of canrenone
Legal class.: POM

Action: Competitive inhibition of aldosterone

Uses: Oedema associated with secondary aldosteronism, liver failure, chronic decompensated heart disease, diagnosis and treatment of primary hyperaldosteronism

Dosage and routes: Slow IV injection/infusion 200–400 mg/day; up to 800 mg/day in exceptional cases

Available forms include: Injection 20 mg/ml, 10-ml ampoule

Side effects/adverse reactions:
META: Gynaecomastia (males), mastodynia
GI: Nausea, vomiting
CNS: Transient confusion syndrome (high doses)
INTEG: Pain, irritation at injection site
ELECT: Hyperkalaemia

Contraindications: Hyponatraemia, hyperkalaemia, renal failure, porphyria, Addison's disease, pregnancy, lactation

Precautions: Children

Pharmacokinetics: Diuresis normally commences within the first 24 hr, although long latent periods can be seen in refractory cases

Interactions/incompatibilities:
• Antagonism: anti-inflammatory analgesics, carbenoxolone, corticosteroids, corticotrophin
• Potentiation: Angiotension converting enzyme inhibitors
• Increased risk of renal failure: anti-inflammatory analgesics

Clinical assessment:
• Use only when treatment with other diuretic agents inadequate and when oral aldosterone antagonists cannot be used
• Adjust dosage to needs and response of individual
• Use for as short a time as possible
• Monitor electrolyte balance regularly in long-term use
• Prescribe anti-emetic for nausea and vomiting
• Full blood count, urine and electrolytes

Lab. test interferences:
Increase: Blood urea nitrogen

Treatment of overdose: Cease therapy, anti-emetics, potassium eliminating drug if hyperkalaemia

NURSING CONSIDERATIONS

Assess:
• Weight and fluid balance

Administer:

• Check visually for precipitation
• Do not add other drugs to injection solution
• Slowly over 2–3 mins to avoid pain and initiation at injection site
• Anti-emetics, as prescribed, for nausea and vomiting

Evaluate:
• Therapeutic response – fluid loss

potassium iodide

Aqueous Iodine Oral Solution (Lugol's solution)
Func. class.: Antithyroid agent
Chem. class.: Iodine compound
Legal class.: P

Action: Inhibits secretion of thyroid hormone, fosters colloid accumulation in thyroid follicles, decreases vascularity of gland
Uses: Preparation for thyroidectomy, adjunct in thyrotoxic crisis
Dosage and routes:
Thyrotoxic crisis
• *Adult and child:* By mouth 1 ml in water 3 times daily after meals
Preparation for thyroidectomy
• *Adult and child:* By mouth 0.1–0.3 ml three times a day (well diluted with milk or water)
Available forms include: Solution 10%
Side effects/adverse reactions:
ENDO: Hypothyroidism, hyperthyroid adenoma
INTEG: Rash, urticaria, angioneurotic oedema, acne, mucosal hemorrhage, fever
CNS: Headache
HAEM: Eosinophilia
GI: Nausea, diarrhoea, vomiting, small bowel lesions, upper gastric pain
MS: Arthralgia
EENT: Metallic taste, stomatitis, salivation, periorbital oedema
Contraindications: Hypersensitivity to iodine, hyperkalaemia, breast feeding
Precautions: Pregnancy, lactation, children, prolonged therapy
Pharmacokinetics:
By mouth: Onset 24–48 hr, peak 10–15 days after continuous therapy, uptake by thyroid gland or excreted in urine; crosses placenta
Interactions/incompatibilities:
• Lithium may add to hypothyroid effect
Lab. test interferences:
Interferes: Urinary 17-hydroxycorticosteroids

NURSING CONSIDERATIONS

Assess:
• Baseline pulse, BP, temperature daily
• Fluid balance
• Weight daily

Administer:
• Through straw to prevent tooth discolouration
• With milk or water
• At same time each day, to maintain drug level
• Lowest dose that relieves symptoms

Perform/provide:
• Fluids to 3–4 litres/day, unless contraindicated

Evaluate:
• Therapeutic effect: weight gain, decreased; pulse puffy hands, feet
• Overdose: peripheral oedema, heat intolerance, diaphoresis, palpitations, arrhythmias, severe tachycardia, increased temperature, delirium, CNS irritability
• Hypersensitivity: rash, enlarged cervical lymph nodes may indicate drug needs to be discontinued
• Hypoprothrombinaemia: bleeding, petechiae, ecchymosis
• Clinical response: after 3 weeks should include increased weight, pulse; decreased thyroxine

Teach patient/family:

• To abstain from breast feeding after delivery
• To take pulse daily
• To keep graph of weight, pulse, mood
• Avoid non-prescribed drugs that contain iodine
• That seafood, other iodine products may be restricted
• Not to discontinue this medication abruptly; thyroid crisis may occur
• That response may take several months if thyroid is large
• Discontinue drug, notify clinician if any of the following occur: fever, rash, metallic taste, swelling of throat, burning of mouth, throat, sore gums, teeth, severe GI distress, enlargement of thyroid, pinhead-sized spots or bruising

povidone-iodine

Betadine, Savlon Dry, Videne
Func. class.: Antiseptic
Chem. class.: Iodophore
Legal class.: P

Action: Destroys a wide variety of microorganisms after local irrigation by germicidal action due to the release of iodine
Uses: Cleansing wounds, disinfection, pre-operative skin preparation
Dosage and routes:
• *Adult and child:* Use as required for antisepsis
Available forms include: Paint 10%; spray 5%; solution 10%; scrub 7.5%; gargle 1%; powder spray 0.5–2.5%; pessaries 200 mg; vaginal gel 10%; vaginal cleansing kit 10%; scalp and skin cleanser solution 7.5%; skin cleanser solution 4%; dusting powder 5%; dressing 10%; ointment 10%
Side effects/adverse reactions:
INTEG: Irritation
Contraindications: Hypersensitivity to iodine; regular use during pregnancy, breast-feeding, in patients with thyroid disorders, renal impairment or on lithium therapy
Precautions: Extensive burns, broken skin

NURSING CONSIDERATIONS
(Refer to information provided by pharmacist)
• Do not apply to extensive burns or broken skin
• Surgical skin preparation—apply immediately before surgery for maximum germicidal action
Perform/provide:
• Consider patch testing for long term usage
Evaluate:
• Area of the body involved: irritation, rash, breaks, dryness, scales
Teach patient/family:
• To discontinue use if rash, irritation, or redness occurs and seek medical advice

pralidoxime mesylate

P25, 2 PAM Chloride
Func. class.: Antidote
Chem. class.: Quaternary ammonium oxide
Legal class.: POM

Action: Displaces enzymes at receptor site by reactivation of cholinesterase inhibited by phosphate esters
Uses: Organophosphate poisoning antidote as an adjunct to atropine
Dosage and routes:
Organophosphate poisoning
• *IM injection:* 1 g initially followed by 1–2 further doses if necessary
• *IV injection:* 1–2 g initially in 10–15 ml water for injections followed by a further 1–2 doses if necessary

• *IV infusion:* 1–2 g in 100 ml–0.9% saline over 15–30 mins. Usual maximum 12 g in 24 hr
• *Child:* 20–60 mg/kg as required
Available forms include: Injection IV 200 mg/ml (5 ml ampoule) from designated poison centres
Side effects/adverse reactions:
CNS: Dizziness, headache, drowsiness, visual disturbances
GI: Nausea
MS: Weakness, muscle rigidity
CV: Tachycardia
RESP: Hyperventilation, laryngospasm
Contraindications: Hypersensitivity, inorganic phosphates, carbonates, organophosphates with anticholinesterase activity
Precautions: Myasthenia gravis, pregnancy, renal insufficiency
Pharmacokinetics:
IV: Peak 5–15 min
IM: Peak 10–20 min
Half-life 1½ hr, metabolised in liver, excreted in urine (unchanged)

NURSING CONSIDERATIONS

Assess:
• Baseline vital signs and fluid balance

Administer:
• Only with resuscitation equipment available
• As soon as possible after poisoning; within 4 hr
• IM into deep muscle; IV slowly, diluted with water, over 5–10 minutes
• Concurrent dose of atropine

Evaluate:
• BP, pulse, fluid balance; observe for decreased urinary output for 48–72 hr after poisoning to determine atropine toxicity from poisoning effects
• Airway, need for assistance with respiration
• Respiratory status: rate, rhythm, characteristics

prazosin hydrochloride

Hypovase, Alphavase
Func. class.: Antihypertensive
Chem. class.: α-Blocker
Legal class.: POM

Action: Peripheral blood vessels are dilated, peripheral resistance lowered, reduction in blood pressure results from post-synaptic α-adrenergic receptors being blocked
Uses: Hypertension, refractory congestive heart failure, Raynaud's vasospasm. Benign prostatic hyperplasia
Dosage and routes:
Hypertension:
• *Adult:* By mouth initially 500 mcg 2–3 times a day for 3–7 days, increasing to 1 mg 2–3 times daily for further 3–7 days; dose may then be increased gradually according to response; maximum dose 20 mg daily in divided doses
Congestive heart failure
• *Adult:* By mouth 500 mcg 2–4 times daily increasing to 4 mg daily in divided doses; maintenance 4–20 mg daily in divided doses
Raynaud's syndrome
• *Adult:* By mouth 500 mcg twice daily for 3–7 days; adjust to response, maintenance 1–2 mg twice daily
Benign prostatic hypertrophy
• *Adult:* Initially 500 mcg twice daily for 3–7 days according to response, increasing to 2 mg twice daily
Available forms include: Tablets 0.5 mg, 1 mg, 2 mg, 5 mg
Side effects/adverse reactions:
CV: Palpitations, orthostatic hypotension, tachycardia, oedema
CNS: Dizziness, headache, drowsiness, anxiety, depression, vertigo, weakness, fatigue, hallucinations
GI: Nausea, vomiting, diarrhoea, constipation, abdominal pain,

pancreatitis, liver junction abnormalities
GU: Urinary frequency, incontinence, impotence, priapism
EENT: Blurred vision, epistaxis, tinnitus, dry mouth, red sclera
INTEG: Rash, pruritus, alopecia, lichen planus, fever
Contraindications: Hypersensitivity, congestive heart failure due to mechanical obstruction (e.g. aortic stenosis, mitral valve stenosis), pulmonary embolism, pericardial disease, children under 12 yr
Precautions: Pregnancy, children under 12 yr, aortic and mitral valve stenosis, lactation
Pharmacokinetics:
By mouth: Onset 2 hr, peak 1–3 hr, duration 6–12 hr; half-life 2–4 hr, metabolised in liver, excreted via bile, faeces (over 90%), in urine (under 10%)
Interactions/incompatibilities:
• Increased hypotensive effects: β-blockers, calcium channel antagonists
Clinical assessment:
• Jugular venous distension 4 hrly
• Blood urea, uric acid if on long-term therapy
Treatment of overdose: Administer volume expanders or vasopressors, discontinue drug, place in supine position

NURSING CONSIDERATIONS

Assess:
• Baseline BP, fluid balance, weight
Administer:
• Whole, do not chew or crush tablets
Evaluate:
• BP pulse 4 hrly
• Weight daily, fluid balance
• Oedema in feet, legs daily
• Skin turgor, dryness of mucous membranes for hydration status
• Rales, dyspnoea, orthopnoea
Teach patient/family:
• Fainting occasionally occurs after initial dose

prednisolone acetate/ prednisolone sodium phosphate (ophthalmic, otic)

Minims, Pred Forte, Predsol, combination product
Func. class.: Anti-inflammatory, Corticosteroid
Chem. class.: Glucocorticoid, immediate acting
Legal class.: POM

Action: Decreases inflammation, resulting in decreases in pain, photophobia, cellular infiltration
Uses: Inflammation of eye, lids, conjunctiva, cornea, uveitis, iridocyclitis, allergic condition, burns, foreign bodies, inflammatory conditions of the ear
Dosage and routes:
• *Adult and child:* Eyes: Instil 1–2 drops into conjunctival sac every 1–2 hr until controlled, then reduce frequency
• Ears: 2–3 drops every 2–3 hr until controlled, then reduce frequency
Available forms include: Suspension 1%; solution 0.5%
Side effects/adverse reactions:
EENT: Increased intra-ocular pressure, poor corneal wound healing, increased possibility of corneal infections, glaucoma exacerbation, cataracts, thinning of the cornea
Contraindications: Hypersensitivity, acute superficial herpes simplex, fungal/viral diseases of eye or conjunctiva, ocular tuberculosis infections of the eye
Precautions: Corneal abrasions, glaucoma, soft contact lenses, administration to 'red eyes'

NURSING CONSIDERATIONS

Administer:

• After shaking suspension instil into affected eye or ear

Evaluate:

• Allergic reactions: redness, itching, swelling, lacrimation

• Therapeutic response: absence of swelling, redness, exudate

Teach patient/family:

• Instillation method

• Wash hands thoroughly before administrations

• Not to share eye medications with others

• Discard eye-drops after 28 days of opening—discarding unused product

prednisolone/ prednisolone acetate/ prednisolone sodium phosphate/prednisolone sodium metasulphobenzoate

Deltacortril-Enteric, Deltastab, Precortisyl, Precortisyl-Forte, Prednesol, Sintisone, Predfoam, Predenema, Predsol

Func. class.: Corticosteroid

Chem. class.: Glucocorticoid, immediate acting

Legal class.: POM

Action: Decreases inflammation by suppression of migration of polymorphonuclear leucocytes, fibroblasts, reversal to increase capillary permeability and lysosomal stabilization

Uses: Severe inflammation, immunosuppression, neoplasms

Dosage and routes:

• *Adult:* By mouth 5–60 mg daily as a single dose. IM (acetate) 25–100 mg once or twice weekly. Intra-articular or soft tissue injection (acetate): 5–25 mg depending on size of joint (maximum 3 joints per day)

• *By rectum foam/retention enema:* 20 mg once or twice daily for 2–4 weeks

• Suppositories, 5 mg inserted at night and morning after a bowel movement

Available forms include: Tablets 1, 5, 25 mg; tablets EC 2.5, 5 mg; tablets soluble, 5 mg (sodium phosphate) injection, 25 mg/ml aqueous suspension (1 ml) acetate; enema (disodium phosphate) 20 mg, Foam Enema (metasulphobenzoate sodium) 20 mg

Side effects/adverse reactions:

INTEG: Acne, poor wound healing, ecchymosis, petechiae, hirsutism

CNS: Depression, headache, mood changes, insomnia

CV: Embolism, hypotension on rapid withdrawal

HAEM: Thrombocytopenia

MS: Fractures, osteoporosis, proximal myopathy, avascular osteonecrosis, tendon rupture

GI: Diarrhoea, nausea, abdominal distension, GI haemorrhage, increased appetite, pancreatitis, dyspepsia, peptic and esophageal ulceration, oesophageal candidiasis

EENT: Fungal infections, increased intraocular pressure, blurred vision

ELECT: Sodium and water retention, hypertension, hypokalaemic alkalosis

META: Suppression of hypothalamo-pituitary adrenal axis, growth retardation in children, menstrual irregularity, diabetogenic

Contraindications: Systemic injection, unless specific anti-injective therapy is employed

Precautions: Pregnancy, diabetes mellitus, glaucoma, osteoporosis, seizure disorders, ulcerative colitis, tuberculosis, hypertension, psychosis, peptic ulceration, previous steroid myopathy, children, ocular herpes simplex, family history of diabetes mellitus, family history of glaucoma

Pharmacokinetics:

By mouth: Peak 1–2 hr, duration 2 days

IM: Peak 3–45 hr

Interactions/incompatibilities:

• Decreased effects of: cholestyramine, colestipol, barbiturates, rifampicin, ephedrine, phenytoin, carbamazepine

• Decreased effects of: anticoagulants, anticonvulsants, antidiabetics, diuretics

• Increased side effects: alcohol, salicylates, amphotericin B, digitalis preparations, non-steroidal anti-inflammatory drugs, live vaccines

• Increased effect of: salicylates

• Diuretics: may cause excessive potassium loss

Clinical assessment:

• Potassium, blood sugar, urine glucose while on long-term therapy; hypokalaemia and hyperglycaemia

• Plasma cortisol levels during long-term therapy (normal level: 138–635 nmol/litre when drawn at 8 AM)

• Titrated dose, use lowest effective dose

• Radiography: bone density on long-term therapy

• Fluid balance, be alert for decreasing urinary output and increasing oedema

Lab. test interferences:

Increase: Cholesterol, sodium, blood glucose, uric acid, calcium, urine glucose

Decrease: Calcium, potassium, thyroxine, triiodothyronine, thyroid ^{131}I uptake test, urine 17-hydroxycorticosteroids, 17-ketosteroids, protein bound iodine

False negative: Skin allergy tests

NURSING CONSIDERATIONS

Assess:

• Baseline BP, pulse and weight

Administer:

• IM injection deeply in large mass, rotate sites, avoid deltoid

• In one dose in AM to prevent adrenal suppression. Avoid SC administration; damage may be done to tissue

• After shaking suspension (parenteral)

• With food or milk to decrease GI symptoms

Perform/provide:

• Assistance with movement in patient with bone tissue disease to prevent fractures

• Weight gain more than 2.5 kilo (to be reported)

• For chest pain

• Therapeutic response: ease of respirations, decreased inflammation

• Infection: increased temperature, WBC, even after withdrawal of medication; drug masks symptoms of infection

• Potassium depletion: paraesthesias, fatigue, nausea, vomiting, depression, polyuria, arrhythmias, weakness

• Oedema, hypotension, cardiac symptoms

• Mental status: affect, mood, behavioural changes, aggression

Teach patient/family:

• That warning card, as steroid user should be carried

• To notify clinician if therapeutic response decreases; dosage adjustment may be needed

• Not to discontinue this medication abruptly or adrenal crisis can result

• To avoid non-prescribed products: salicylates, alcohol in cough products, cold preparations unless directed by clinician

• Teach patient all aspects of drug use, including Cushingoid symptoms
• Symptoms of adrenal insufficiency; nausea, anorexia, fatigue, dizziness, dyspnoea, weakness, joint pain
• Supplement verbal information with instruction leaflet

prednisone

Decortisyl
Func. class.: Corticosteroid
Chem. class.: Glucocorticoid, immediate acting
Legal class.: POM

Action: Decreases inflammation by suppression of migration of polymorphonuclear leucocytes, fibroblasts, reversal to increase capillary permeability, and lysosomal stabilisation
Uses: Severe inflammation, immunosuppression, neoplasms, multiple sclerosis
Dosage and routes:
• *Adult:* By mouth 2.5–15 mg 2 to 4 times a day, then daily or alternate days maintenance
• *Child under 1 yr:* Not recommended; 1–7 yr: quarter to half adult dose; 7–12 yr: half to three quarters adult dose
Available forms include: Tablets 5 mg
Side effects/adverse reactions:
INTEG: Acne, poor wound healing, ecchymosis, petechiae, hirsuitism
CNS: Depression, headache, mood changes insomnia
CV: Hypotension on rapid withdrawal, embolism
HAEM: Thrombocytopenia
MS: Fractures, osteoporosis, proximal myopathy, avascular osteonecrosis, tendon rupture
GI: Diarrhoea, nausea, abdominal distention, GI haemorrhage, increased appetite, pancreatitis dyspepsia, peptic and oesophageal ulceration oesophageal candidiasis
EENT: Fungal infections, increased intraocular pressure, blurred vision
ELECT: Sodium and water retention, hypertension, hypokalaemic acidosis
META: Suppression of hypothalamo-pituitary adrenal axis, growth retardation in children, menstrual irregularities, diabetogenic
Contraindications: Systemic infection, unless specific anti-infective therapy is employed
Precautions: Pregnancy, diabetes mellitus, glaucoma, osteoporosis, seizure disorders, ulcerative colitis, tuberculosis, hypertension, psychosis, peptic ulceration, previous steroid myopathy children, ocular herpes simplex, family history of diabetes mellitus, family history of glaucoma
Pharmacokinetics:
By mouth: Peak 1–2 hr, duration 1–1½ days, half-life 3½–4 days
Interactions/incompatibilities:
• Decreased effects of: cholestyramine, colestipol, barbiturates, rifampicin, ephedrine, phenytoin, carbamazepine
• Decreased effects of: anticoagulants, anticonvulsants, antidiabetics, diuretics
• Increased side effects: alcohol, non-steroidal anti-inflammatory drugs, salicylates, amphotericin B, digitalis preparations, live vaccines
• Increased effects of: salicylates, oestrogens, indomethacin
• Diuretics may cause excessive potassium loss
Clinical assessment:
• Potassium, blood sugar, urine glucose while on long-term ther-

apy; hypokalaemia and hyperglycaemia
• Plasma cortisol levels during long-term therapy (normal level: 138–635 nmol/litre when drawn at 8 AM)

Lab. test interferences:
Increase: Cholesterol, sodium, blood glucose, uric acid, calcium, urine glucose
Decrease: Calcium, potassium, thyroxine, triiodothyronine, thyroid ^{131}I uptake test, urine 17-hydroxycorticosteroids, 17-ketosteroids, protein bound iodine
False negative: Skin allergy tests

NURSING CONSIDERATIONS

Assess:
• Baseline BP, pulse and weight
• With food or milk to decrease GI symptoms

Administer:
• Titrated dose, use lowest effective dose

Perform/provide:
• Assistance with movement in patient with bone tissue disease to prevent fractures

Evaluate:
• Weight weekly, notify clinician of weekly gain over 2 kg
• BP 4 hrly, pulse, notify clinician if chest pain occurs
• Fluid balance, be alert for decreasing urinary output and increasing oedema
• Avoid use of surgical tape
• Daily urinalysis when on high dosage
• Radiography: bone density on long-term therapy
• Infection: increased temperature, WBC, even after withdrawal of medication; drug masks symptoms of infection
• Potassium depletion: paraesthesias, fatigue, nausea, vomiting, depression, polyuria, arrhythmias, weakness
• Oedema, hypotension, cardiac symptoms
• Mental status: affect, mood, behavioural changes, aggression
• Therapeutic response: ease of respirations, decreased inflammation

Teach patient/family:
• That warning card as steroid user should be carried
• To notify clinician if therapeutic response decreases; dosage adjustment may be needed
• Not to discontinue this medication abruptly or adrenal crisis can result
• To avoid non-prescribed products: salicylates, alcohol in cough products, cold preparations unless directed by clinician
• Teach patient all aspects of drug use, including Cushingoid symptoms
• Symptoms of adrenal insufficiency: nausea, anorexia, fatigue, dizziness, dyspnoea, weakness, joint pain
• That wounds will take longer to heal
• To avoid use of surgical tape

---

prilocaine hydrochloride

Citanest, Citanest with Octapressin
Func. class.: Anaesthetic, local
Chem. class.: Aminoacylamide
Legal class.: POM

Action: Inhibits nerve impulses from sensory nerves, thereby producing anaesthesia

Uses: Infiltration, regional nerve block, spinal anaesthesia, regional IV analgesia, dental anaesthesia

Dosage and routes:
• Local injection, dose adjusted according to site of operation to maximum of 400 mg used alone or 600 mg if used with adrenaline or felypressin

Available forms include: Injection

1%, 10 mg/ml, 20 ml, 50 ml vials; injection 2%, 20 mg/ml, 10 ml; injection 0.5%, 5 mg/ml 20 ml, 50 ml vials; injection 4%, 40 mg/ml, 2-ml cartridge with octopressin; injection 3%, 30 mg/ml, 2-ml cartridge and self-aspirating cartridge

Side effects/adverse reactions:
CV: Cardiac arrest, bradycardia, hypotension, myocardial depression
CNS: Agitation, euphoria, convulsions, dizziness, tremors, unconsciousness
RESP: Respiratory depression
INTEG: Cutaneous, lesion, urticaria, oedema, anaphylactic reactions

Contraindications: Hypersensitivity, anaemia, methaemoglobinaemia

Precautions: Impaired cardiac conduction, renal or hepatic impairment, epilepsy, elderly or debilitated patients, impaired respiratory function

Pharmacokinetics: Rapidly metabolised mainly in the liver and also the kidneys. Principal metabolite excreted in urine is *o*-tomidine. Prilocaine crosses placenta during prolonged epidural anaesthesia producing methaemoglobinaemia in the foetus

Treatment of overdose: Maintain airway; administer O_2, vasopressor, IV fluids, anticonvulsants for seizures

NURSING CONSIDERATIONS

Assess:
- BP, pulse, respiration

Administer:
- With resuscitation equipment nearby
- Only drugs without preservatives for epidural or caudal anaesthesia

Perform/provide:
- Use new solution, discard part-used units

Evaluate:
- Therapeutic response, anaesthesia necessary for procedure
- Allergic reactions, rash, urticaria, itching
- Cardiac status, ECG for arrhythmias, pulse, BP during treatment
- Foetal heart tones if drug is used during labour

---

primaquine phosphate

Func. class.: Antimalarial
Chem. class.: Synthetic 8-aminoquinolone
Legal class.: P

Action: Action is unknown; thought to destroy exoerythrocytic forms by gametocidal action, and inhibition of mitochondrial respiration

Uses: Malaria caused by *Plasmodium vivax*, *Plasmodium ovale*

Dosage and routes:
- A blood schizonticide such as chloroquine should be given before primaquine to eliminate erythrocytic forms
- *Adult:* By mouth 15 mg primaquine base daily for 14–21 days
- *Child:* 0.2–0.3 mg primaquine base per kg body weight daily

Available forms include: Tablets 13.2 mg (7.5 mg base)

Side effects/adverse reactions:
GI: Nausea, vomiting, abdominal pain
HAEM: Haemolytic anemia, methaemoglobinaemia

Precautions: Hypersensitivity, lupus erythematosus, rheumatoid arthritis, methaemoglobulinaemia, G6PD deficiency, pregnancy, lactation, concurrent with drugs that induce haemolysis or bone marrow depression

Pharmacokinetics:
By mouth: Metabolised by liver

(metabolites), half-life 3.7–9.6 hr
Interactions/incompatibilities:
• Toxicity: mepacrine
Clinical assessment:
• Ophthalmic test if long-term treatment or drug dosage over 150 mg/day
• Liver studies every week: aspartate aminotransferase, alanine aminotransferase, bilirubin, if on long-term therapy
• Blood studies, full blood count, since blood dyscrasias occur
NURSING CONSIDERATIONS
Administer:
• Before or after meals at same time each day to maintain drug level
Evaluate:
• Therapeutic effect
Teach patient/family:
• To report any new symptoms

primidone

Mysoline
Func. class.: Anticonvulsant
Chem. class.: Barbiturate derivative
Legal class.: POM

Action: Raises seizure threshold is converted to active drug phenobarbitone
Uses: Management of grand mal and psychomotor (temporal lobe), epilepsy, focal or Jacksonian seizures, petit mal, myoclonic jerks and akinetic attacks. Management of essential tremor
Dosage and routes:
Epilepsy
• *Adult:* By mouth initially 125 mg at bedtime; increase according to response by 125 mg every 3 days to 500 mg daily in 2 divided doses; then increase according to response by 250 mg every 3 days to a maximum of 1.5 kg daily in divided doses
• *Child:* By mouth 20–30 mg/kg daily in 2 divided doses
Essential tremor
• *Adult:* By mouth initially 50 mg daily; increase over 2–3 weeks according to response to maximum 750 mg daily in divided doses
Available forms include: Tablets 250 mg; suspension 250 mg/5 ml
Side effects/adverse reactions:
HAEM: Thrombocytopenia, leucopenia, neutropenia, eosinophilia, megaloblastic anemia, lymphadenopathy, folic acid deficiency
CNS: Stimulation, drowsiness, dizziness, confusion, sedation, headache, flushing, hallucinations, coma, psychosis, ataxia
GI: Nausea, vomiting, anorexia
INTEG: Rash, oedema, lupus-like syndrome (rare)
EENT: Diplopia, nystagmus
GU: Impotence, polyuria
Contraindications: Severe respiratory depression, porphyria
Precautions: Chronic obstructive airways disease, hepatic disease, renal disease, hyperactive children, lactation, pregnancy
Pharmacokinetics:
By mouth: Peak 4 hr, excreted by kidneys, excreted in breast milk, half-life 3–24 hr. Metabolised to active metabolites including phenobarbitone
Interactions/incompatibilities:
• Decreased effects: Tricyclic antidepressants and antipsychotics (lower seizure threshold)
• Effects reduced (accelerated metabolism): disopyramide, quinidine, chloramphenicol, doxycycline, metronidazole, coumarin anticoagulants, tricyclic antidepressants, clonazepam, phenytoin, phenobarbitone, griseofulvin, felodipine, isradipine, corticosteroids, cyclosporin, sex hormones including oral contraceptives, theophylline, thyroxine

• Enhanced CNS side-effects with other CNS depressants including alcohol
Clinical assessment:
• Drug level: therapeutic level of derived phenobarbitone 15–40 mg/litre
Treatment of overdose: Aspiration of stomach contents if recently ingested, no specific antidote, give supportive treatment

NURSING CONSIDERATIONS

Administer:
• Total daily dose best given in two divided doses
• Oral suspension requires special diluent for low doses
Evaluate:
• Mental status: mood, alertness, effect, memory (long, short)
• Respiratory depression
• Blood dyscrasias: fever, sore throat, bruising, rash, jaundice
Teach patient/family:
• Emphasise necessity of taking drug at appropriate time and on a continuing basis
• All aspects of drug administration: action, route, dose, when to notify clinician
• About side effects

probenecid

Benemid
Func. class.: Uricosuric
Chem. class.: Sulphonamide derivative
Legal class.: POM

Action: Inhibits tubular reabsorption of urate, with increased excretion of uric acid, inhibits urinary excretion of β-lactam antibiotics
Uses: Treatment of hyperuricaemia in gout, gouty arthritis, adjunct to cephalosporin or penicillin treatment especially of gonorrhoea
Dosage and routes:
Gout/gouty arthritis
• *Adult:* By mouth 250 mg twice a day for 1 week, then 500 mg twice a day, increasing by 500 mg every 4 weeks if needed; not to exceed 2 g/day; maintenance: as long as patient is asymptomatic dosage may be reduced by 500 mg every 6 months to minimum effective dose
Adjunct in penicillin/cephalosporin treatment
• *Adult and child over 50 kg:* By mouth 500 mg four times a day
• *Child (over 2 yr) under 50 kg:* By mouth 25 mg/kg, then 10 mg/kg four times a day
Gonorrhoea
• *Adult:* By mouth 1 g with oral ampicillin or IM ½ hr before procaine penicillin or cefoxitin
Available forms include: Tablets 500 mg
Side effects/adverse reactions:
CNS: Drowsiness, headache, confusion, stimulation, dizziness, in overdose: EEG changes, convulsions
GU: Frequency, nephrotic syndrome. In gouty patients: haematuria, renal colic, urate stones
GI: Gastric irritation, nausea, vomiting, anorexia, hepatic necrosis, sore gums
INTEG: Rash, dermatitis, pruritus, flushing, alopecia
SYST: Fever, anaphylaxis
HAEM: Anaemia, haemolytic anaemia, leucopenia, aplastic anaemia
MISC: Exacerbation of gout
Contraindications: Acute gout, hypersensitivity, severe hepatic disease, history of blood dyscrasias, severe renal disease, child under 2 yr, renal urate stones, porphyria
Precautions: Pregnancy, lactation, peptic ulceration, low fluid intake
Pharmacokinetics:
By mouth: Peak 2–4 hr, duration

8 hr, half-life 8–10 hr; metabolised by liver, excreted in urine, 85–95% bound to plasma proteins
Interactions/incompatibilities:
• Increased blood levels of these drugs (significance uncertain): sulphonamides, dapsone, nalidixic acid, nitrofurantoin, acyclovir, PAS, indomethacin, ketoprofen, meclofamate, lorazepam rifampicin, naproxen, sodium iodothalamate and some other contrast media, β-lactam antibiotics, pantothenic acid
• Increased blood levels of these drugs, likely toxicity: methotrexate, sulphonylurea hypoglycaemics, zidovudine
• Decreased effect: salicylates, pyrazinamide
Clinical assessment:
• Uric acid levels within normal limits
Lab. test interferences:
False positive: Benedict's test
Decrease: Urinary 17-ketosteroids, phenolsulphthalein (PSP), sulphabromophthalein (BSP), *p*-aminohippuric acid (PAH)
Treatment of overdose: Induce emesis or gastric lavage. No specific antidote, treatment symptomatic including IV diazepam or short-acting barbiturate for CNS stimulation

NURSING CONSIDERATIONS

Assess:
• pH of urine
• Fluid balance
• Dietary intake
Administer:
• After food or with milk
• With a full glass of water
• With prophylactic colchicine or NSAID during initial therapy for gout (not aspirin or salicylate)
• With appropriate antibiotic for infections, after culture and sensitivity tests, including those for concurrent infections
Perform/provide:
• Low purine diet restricting: offal, anchovies, sardines, meat gravy, dried beans, meat extracts
Evaluate:
• Therapeutic response; resolution of infection
• Therapeutic result; dimunition of gout pain
• Recidivist tendencies
• Urinary pH and fluid balance regularly
Teach patient/family:
• To avoid non-prescribed preparations, particularly
• Necessity of taking entire course of medication as prescribed
• To drink at least 2 litres of fluid daily, avoiding alcohol
• To report side-effects, including GI pain, urinary symptoms
• That starting treatment may precipitate an acute attack
• Counselling about protection during sexual intercourse, contact tracing of partners if treating gonorrhoea

---

probucol

Lurselle
Func. class.: Hypolipidaemic
Chem. class.: Butylphenol derivative
Legal class.: POM

Action: Lowers elevated serum cholesterol, effect on triglycerides less consistent; underlying mechanisms unclear
Uses: Type IV hyperlipidaemia, Severe hypercholesterolemia dietary treatment unsuccessful
Dosage and routes:
• *Adult:* By mouth 500 mg twice daily with breakfast, supper
Available forms include: Tablets 250 mg
Side effects/adverse reactions:
GI: Nausea, vomiting, diarrhoea, constipation, anorexia, flatulence,

abdominal pain
INTEG: Flushing, alopecia, sweating, hyperthermia
CV: Palpitations, arrhythmias, prolonged QT interval
EENT: Visual disturbances
CNS: Palpitations, paraesthesias
SYST: Hypersensitivity reactions including angioedema
Contraindications: Hypersensitivity, breast-feeding
Precautions: Arrhythmias, myocardial damage, angina pectoris, pregnancy, children
Pharmacokinetics:
By mouth: Absorption low and variable, better with food; excreted in bile/faeces
Clinical assessment:
- ECG before treatment in patients with recent myocardial damage
- For signs of vitamin A, D, K deficiency

Evaluate:
- Therapeutic response: decreased triglycerides, cholesterol levels (hyperlipidaemia), diarrhoea, pruritus (excess bile area)

Lab. test interferences:
- *Increase:* Liver function studies, CPK, renal function studies, blood glucose

NURSING CONSIDERATIONS

Assess:
- Baseline BP and ECG
- Dietary habits and smoking status

Administer:
- Drug with meals
- Bowel pattern daily; increase fibre, fluid, in diet to prevent constipation occurring

Teach patient/family:
- That compliance is needed since toxicity may result if doses are missed
- That risk factors should be decreased: high fat diet, smoking, alcohol consumption, absence of exercise
- That non-prescribed preparations should be avoided unless directed by clinician
- About side effects; nausea: belching

procainamide hydrochloride

Procainamide Durules, Pronestyl
Func. class.: Anti-arrhythmic (Class Ia)
Chem. class.: Procaine analogue
Legal class.: POM

Action: Increases electrical stimulation threshold of ventricle, His Purkinje system, which stabilises cardiac membrane
Uses: Supraventricular tachyarrhythmias, ventricular arrhythmias, digitalis induced arrhythmias
Dosage and routes:
Ventricular arrhythmias
- *Adult:* By mouth 50 mg/kg daily in divided doses every 3–6 hr (control if possible using plasma concentration)
- *Adult:* By mouth, modified-release tablets, usual dose 2–3 tablets 3 times a day, adjust to plasma concentration
- *Adult:* Slow IV injection 100 mg at rate not exceeding 50 mg/min; maximum 1 g
- *Adult:* IV infusion, 500–600 mg; maintenance 2–6 mg/min; then oral treatment if necessary after 3–4 hr

Atrial fibrillation
- *Adult:* By mouth, higher doses than those used for ventricular arrhythmias may be required

Available forms include: Tablets 250 mg; modified-release tablets 500 mg; injection 100 mg/ml
Side effects/adverse reactions:
CNS: Headache, dizziness, confusion, psychosis, depression

GI: Nausea, vomiting, anorexia, diarrhoea, bitter taste, hepatitis
CV: Hypotension, cardiovascular collapse, arrest cardiac arrhythmias
HAEM: Lupus-like syndrome, agranulocytosis, neutropenia, thrombocytopenia, haemolytic anaemia
INTEG: Rash, urticaria, oedema, flushing
SYST: Chills, fever, allergic reactions
MS: Joint and muscle pain, muscle weakness

Contraindications: Hypersensitivity, heart block, heart failure, hypotension

Precautions: Pregnancy, lactation, renal disease, liver disease, congestive heart failure, respiratory depression, elderly, myasthenia gravis, asthma, SLE

Pharmacokinetics

By mouth: Peak 1–2 hr, duration 3 hr (8 hr extended)
Half-life 3 hr, metabolised in liver to active metabolites, excreted unchanged by kidneys (60%) effective concentration is 4–8 mcg/ml, toxicity rare below 12 mcg/ml

Interactions/incompatibilities:

• Increased effects of neuromuscular blockers neostigmine, pyridostigmine, propranolol, muscle relaxants, antihypertensives
• Increased myocardial depression with other anti-arrhythmics
• Increased procainamide serum levels with amiodarone, cimetidine
• Trimethoprim, propranolol
• Decreased effects of: sulphonamide antibiotics
• Risk of neutropenia/Stevens–Johnson syndrome with captopril

Clinical assessment:

• ECG continuously during acute therapy to determine increased P-R or QRS segments; if these develop, discontinue immediately; watch for increased ventricular ectopic beats
• Plasma concentrations
• Monthly serological tests for antinuclear factors suggestive of lupus-like syndrome; stop treatment if they occur
• Full blood count if symptoms suggest agranulocytosis

Treatment of overdose: Induce vomiting/use gastric lavage or administer activated charcoal if recent oral ingestion. No specific antidote. Monitor ECG. Removable by haemodialysis. General supportive measures include sympathomimetic agents and fluid expansion for cardiovascular symptoms. Temporary ventricular pacing may be needed

NURSING CONSIDERATIONS

Assess:

• Blood gases
• Baseline vital signs
• Fluid balance, electrolytes (potassium, sodium chloride)
• BP and ECG continuously for fluctuations during IV use

Evaluate:

• Therapeutic response: re-establish normal sinus rhythm
• Check site daily for infiltration or extravasation
• Malignant hyperthermia: tachypnoea, tachycardia, changes in BP, increased temperature
• Cardiac rate, respiration: rate, rhythm, character, continuously
• Respiratory status: rate, rhythm, lung fields, watch for respiratory depression
• CNS effects: dizziness, confusion, psychosis, paraesthesia, convulsions; drug should be discontinued
• Lung fields, bilateral rales may occur in congestive heart failure patient
• Increased respiration, increased pulse; drug should be discontinued

procaine HCl

Func. class.: Local anaesthetic
Chem. class.: Ester
Legal class.: POM

Action: Competes with calcium for sites in nerve membrane that control sodium transport across cell membrane; decreases rise of depolarisation phase of action potential
Uses: Local anaesthesia by infiltration and regional routes
Dosage and routes:
- Injection up to 1 g (200 ml of 0.5% solution or 100 ml of 1%) with adrenaline 1 in 200,000

Available forms include: Injection, 2%
Side effects/adverse reactions:
CNS: Anxiety, restlessness, convulsions, loss of consciousness, drowsiness, disorientation, tremors, shivering
CV: Myocardial depression, cardiac arrest, arrhythmias, bradycardia, hypotension, fetal bradycardia
GI: Nausea, vomiting
EENT: Blurred vision, tinnitus, pupil constriction
INTEG: Rash, urticaria, allergic reactions, oedema, burning, skin discolouration at injection site, pallor, sweating
RESP: Status asthmaticus, respiratory arrest, anaphylaxis
Contraindications: Hypersensitivity, severe liver disease, myasthenia gravis, complete heart block, solutions containing adrenaline should not be used in appendages
Precautions: Elderly
Pharmacokinetics:
Onset 2–5 min, duration 1 hr; metabolised by plasma cholinesterases, liver, excreted in urine (metabolites)
Interactions/incompatibilities:
- Arrhythmias: adrenaline, halothane, enflurane

Treatment of overdose: Airway, O_2, vasopressor, IV fluids, anticonvulsants for seizures

NURSING CONSIDERATIONS

Assess:
- Baseline BP, pulse, respiration before treatment

Administer:
- Only drugs that are not cloudy, do not contain precipitate
- Only with resuscitation equipment nearby
- Only drugs without preservatives for epidural or caudal anaesthesia

Evaluate:
- Therapeutic response: anaesthesia necessary for procedure
- Allergic reactions: rash, urticaria, itching
- Cardiac status: ECG for arrhythmias, pulse, BP during anaesthesia
- Fetal heart tones if drug is to be used during labour

Teach patient/family:
- Effect of injection

procarbazine

Natulan
Func. class.: Antineoplastic
Chem. class.: Methylhydrazine derivative
Legal class.: POM

Action: Inhibits DNA, RNA, protein synthesis; has multiple sites of action
Uses: Hodgkin's disease, cancers resistant to other therapy
Dosage and routes:
Doses are highly variable, and dependent on local treatment protocols, concomitant therapy and tumour type; the following dose schedules have been used

• *Adult:* By mouth usually in combination with other drugs at a dose of 100 mg/m^2 daily for 10–14 days repeated 4–6 weekly. As a single agent 50 mg daily increased over 6 days to 250–300 mg daily in divided doses, reducing once maximal response achieved to 50–150 mg daily in divided doses. Continue to cumulative total of at least 6 g
• *Child:* By mouth 50 mg daily for 7 days, then 100 mg/m^2 until desired response, leucopenia, or thrombocytopenia occurs

Available forms include: Capsules 50 mg (as hydrochloride)

Side effects/adverse reactions:
HAEM: Thrombocytopenia, anaemia, leucopenia, bleeding disorders
GI: Nausea, vomiting, anorexia, diarrhoea, constipation, dry mouth, stomatitis, impaired liver function
EENT: Retinal haemorrhage, papiloedema
INTEG: Rash, pruritus, alopecia, hyperpigmentation
CNS: Headache, insomnia, confusion, coma pain, chills, fever, sweating, paraesthesias, drowsiness, anxiety, tremor, convulsions
RESP: Cough, pneumonitis
CVS: Tachycardia, hypotension

Contraindications: Hypersensitivity, severe myelosuppression, severe hepatic/renal damage, pregnancy, breast-feeding

Precautions: Renal disease, hepatic disease, radiation therapy, phaeochromocytoma, epilepsy, elderly, cardiovascular disease

Pharmacokinetics: Half-life 1 hr; concentrates in liver, kidney, skin; metabolised in liver, excreted in urine; WBC nadir 2–3 weeks post-dose

Interactions/incompatibilities:
• Increased CNS depression given with: barbiturates, antihistamines, narcotics, phenothiazines
• Disulfiram-like reaction: ethyl alcohol
• Procarbazine is weak mono-MAOI; low risk of hypertension with: tricyclic antidepressants, narcotic analgesics; tyramine-rich foods, guanethidine, levodopa, reserpine, amphetamines and other sympathomimetics
• Hypertension: guanethidine, levodopa, methyldopa, reserpine

Clinical assessment:
• Full blood count, differential, platelet count weekly during treatment and until nadir blood counts have been passed; withhold drug if myelosuppression is excessive
• Renal function studies: before, during therapy
• Liver function tests before, during therapy

Treatment of overdose: Gastric lavage, supportive treatment, no specific antidotes, regular blood counts, blood products and/or filgrastim to treat myelosuppression

NURSING CONSIDERATIONS

Administer:
• HANDLING: take safety precautions appropriate to antineoplastic agents
• Following local antineoplastic (cytotoxic) policies
• After ensuring that clinician is aware of blood results
• By mouth; capsules should be swallowed whole, never opened
• Other medications by mouth if possible. Avoid IV, IM, SC routes to prevent infection and bruising
• Anti-emetic 30–60 min before treatment
• All other medication as prescribed including analgesics, antibiotics, anti-emetics, antispasmodics

Perform/provide:
• Strict medical asepsis and protection isolation if WBC levels are low

• Liquid diet: carbonated drinks, jelly; dry toast, plain biscuits may be added if patient is not nauseated or vomiting
• Storage in tight, light-resistant container in cool environment

Evaluate:
• Toxicity: facial flushing, epistaxis, thrombocytopenia; drug should be discontinued
• Bleeding: haematuria, bruising or petechiae, mucosa or orifices 8 hrly
• Skin rashes: drug should be discontinued
• Food preferences; list likes, dislikes
• Effects of alopecia on body image; discuss feelings about body changes
• Inflammation of mucosa, breaks in skin
• Yellowing of skin, sclera, dark urine, clay-coloured stools, itchy skin, abdominal pain, fever, diarrhoea
• Oral mucosa regularly for dryness, sores or ulceration, white patches, oral pain, dysphagia
• Local irritation, pain, burning at injection site
• GI symptoms: frequency of stools, cramping
• Acidosis, signs of dehydration: rapid respirations, poor skin turgor, decreased urine output, dry skin, restlessness, weakness

Teach patient/family:
• Why protective isolation precautions are necessary
• To report any complaints, side effects to nurse or clinician: cough, shortness of breath, fever, chills, sore throat, bleeding, bruising, vomiting blood, black tarry stools
• MAOI drug, avoid foods such as marmite, cheese, alcohol
• That hair may be lost during treatment and wig or hairpiece may be available in the NHS; tell patient that new hair may be different in colour, texture
• To avoid foods with citric acid, hot or rough texture
• To report any bleeding, white spots, ulcerations in mouth to physician; tell patient to examine mouth daily
• To avoid driving or activities requiring alertness; drowsiness may occur
• That contraceptive measures are recommended during therapy
• Avoid ingestion of alcohol, tyramine-containing foods; cold, hayfever, or weight-reducing products may cause serious drug interactions

---

prochlorperazine mesylate/ prochlorperazine maleate

Buccastem, Vertigon, Prozière, Stemetil, Stemetil Eff
Func. class.: Anti-emetic; neuroleptic/antipsychotic
Chem. class.: Phenothiazine
Legal class.: POM

Action: Acts centrally by blocking chemoreceptor trigger zone, which in turn acts on vomiting centre
Uses: Nausea, vomiting, Ménière's syndrome, psychoses
Dosage and routes:
Postoperative nausea/vomiting
• *Adult:* IM 12.5 mg 1–2 hr before anaesthesia; may repeat in 30 min; followed by oral medication after 6 hr as needed
Severe nausea/vomiting, Ménière's, labyrinthitis, anxiety
• *Adult:* By mouth 5–10 mg three or four times a day; modified release capsule 15 mg once or twice daily. Rectal 25 mg twice or three times a day; IM 12.5 mg followed by oral medication; buccal 3–6 mg twice a day

Schizophrenia, other psychoses
• *Adult:* IM 12.5–25 mg 2–3 times daily or rectal 25 mg 2–3 times daily until oral treatment possible. Oral starting dose 25 mg/day in divided doses increased at 4–7 day intervals until satisfactory to response obtained, usually 75–100 mg/day in divided doses
• *Child over 10 kg:* By mouth only, 250 mcg/kg two or three times a day

Available forms include: IM injection 12.5 mg/ml; tablets 5, 25 mg; modified release capsules 10, 15 mg; syrup 5 mg/5 ml, suppository 5 mg, 25 mg; buccal tablets 3 mg; effervescent granules 5 mg sachets

Side effects/adverse reactions:
CNS: Depression, restlessness, tremor, dystonia, dyskinesia, tardive dyskinesia, drowsiness, dizziness
GI: Nausea, vomiting, anorexia, dry mouth, diarrhoea, constipation, weight loss, metallic taste, cramps, jaundice
CV: Circulatory failure, hypotension, cardiac arrhythmias
RESP: Respiratory depression
HAEM: Leucopenia, agranulocytosis
EENT: Ocular changes, nasal congestion
INTEG: Skin rashes, photosensitivity, contact dermatitis greyish-mauve skin colouration
SYST: Neuroleptic malignant syndrome, hypothermia
ENDO: Gynaecomastia, galactorrhoea, amenorrhoea, impotence
GU: Urinary retention

Contraindications: Hypersensitivity to phenothiazines, coma, seizure, encephalopathy, bone marrow depression, pregnancy, breast-feeding, phaeochromocytoma

Precautions: Children under 2 yr, elderly, renal dysfunction, epilepsy, Parkinsonism, hypothyroidism, myasthenia gravis, prostate hypertrophy, narrow angle glaucoma, liver disease, phaechromocytoma, blood dyscrasias, bone marrow depression

Pharmacokinetics:
By mouth: Onset 30–40 min, duration 3–4 hr. Onset 30–40 min, duration 10–12 hr
Rectal: Onset 60 min, duration 3–4 hr
IM: Onset 10–20 min, duration 12 hr, metabolised by liver, excreted by kidneys, excreted in breast milk

Interactions/incompatibilities:
• Decreased effects: antacids, lithium, anti-cholinergic agents (antipsychotic effects)
• Increased anticholinergic action: anticholinergics, tricyclic antidepressants
• Do not mix with other drugs in syringe or solution
• Increased CNS depression given with: barbiturates, alcohol, other sedatives
• Increased hypotension with anaesthetics
• Risk of arrhythmias with anti-arrhythmics
• Effects increased: antihypertensives especially α-adrenoceptor blockers
• Effects reduced: amphetamine, levodopa, bromocriptine, lysuride, pergolide, clonidine, guanethidine, adrenaline, anticonvulsants
• Encephalopathy when administered with desferrioxamine

Clinical assessment:
• Carry out immediate haematological investigation if signs of unexplained infection/fever

Treatment of overdose: Gastric lavage and activated charcoal if within 6 hr of oral ingestion, no specific antidote, treatment supportive; volume expansion and inotropes in circulatory collapse, maintain normal body temperature, treat dystonias with anticholinergic

NURSING CONSIDERATIONS

Assess:

• Vital signs, BP; check patients with cardiac disease more often

Administer:

• IM deep injection in large muscle mass; withdraw to avoid IV administration

• Reduce dose to minimum and use for minimum time

• Stop treatment if jaundice develops

Evaluate:

• Therapeutic response: absence of nausea, vomiting

• Respiratory status before, during, after administration of emetic; check rate, rhythm, character; respiratory depression can occur rapidly with elderly or debilitated patients

Teach patient/family:

• Avoid hazardous activities, activities requiring alertness; dizziness may occur

---

procyclidine hydrochloride

Kemadrin, Arpicolin

Func. class.: Antimuscarinic

Chem. class.: Tertiary amine

Legal class.: POM

Action: Acts on acetylcholine receptors in CNS, which decrease involuntary movements

Uses: Parkinson symptoms, including those induced by antidopaminergic drugs

Dosage and routes:

• *Adult:* By mouth 2.5 mg three times a day after meals, titrated to patient response, not to exceed 60 mg/day; IV (in acute dystonia) IM 5–10 mg once repeated after 20 mins if necessary, maximum 20 mg daily

Available forms include: Tablets 5 mg, injection 5 mg/ml, syrup 2.5, 5 mg/5 ml

Side effects/adverse reactions:

CNS: Confusion, anxiety, restlessness, irritability, delusions, hallucinations, incoherence, dizziness

EENT: Blurred vision, photophobia, dilated pupils, difficulty swallowing

CV: Palpitations, tachycardia, postural hypotension

GI: Dryness of mouth, constipation, nausea, vomiting, abdominal distress, paralytic ileus

GU: Hesitancy, retention

INTEG: Flushing, dry skin

Contraindications: Tardive dyskinesia, closed-angle glaucoma, prostatic hypertrophy, urinary retention, gastrointestinal obstruction

Precautions: Pregnancy, elderly, lactation, prostatic hypertrophy, glaucoma, GI/GU obstruction, hepatic and renal impairment, cardiovascular disease. NB: Abuse potential

Pharmacokinetics:

By mouth: Onset 30–45 mins, duration 4–6 hr, plasma half-life 12 hr

Interactions/incompatibilities:

• Decreased action of: haloperidol, phenothiazines, buccal formulations (dry mouth), cisapride, ketoconazole

• Increased anticholinergic effect: antihistamines, MAOIs, phenothiazines, tricyclic antidepressants, other anticholinergic drugs

Treatment of overdose: Gastric lavage if recently ingested, supportive treatment including diazepam for convulsions

NURSING CONSIDERATIONS

Administer:

• With or after meals for GI problems, including a dry mouth; may be given with any fluid before for dry mouth; may be given with fluids other than water

Perform/provide:

• Mouthwashes, frequent drinks, to relieve dry mouth

Evaluate:

• Therapeutic response

• Parkinsonism: shuffling gait, muscle rigidity, involuntary movements

• Urinary hesitancy, retention

• Constipation; increase fluids, bulk, exercise if this occurs

• For tolerance over long-term therapy; dose may need to be increased or changed

• Mental status: affect, mood, CNS depression, worsening of mental symptoms during early therapy

Teach patient/family:

• Not to discontinue this drug abruptly; to taper off over 1 week

• To avoid non-prescribed medication: cough, cold preparations with alcohol, antihistamines unless directed by clinician

---

progesterone

Cyclogest, Gestone

Func. class.: Progestogen

Chem. class.: Steroid hormone

Legal class.: POM

Action: Prepares uterus to receive fertilised ovum, stimulates growth of mammary tissue, anti-neoplastic action against endometrial cancer

Uses: Amenorrhoea, premenstrual syndrome, abnormal uterine bleeding

Dosage and routes:

Amenorrhoea/uterine bleeding

• *Adult:* IM 5–10 mg daily for 5–10 days until 2 days before anticipated onset of menstruation

Pre-menstrual syndrome

• *Adult:* Rectal suppository/vaginal suppository 200–400 mg twice a day from day of symptom appearance to start of bleed

Embryo transfer

• Seek specialist advice

Available forms include: Injection IM 25, 50 mg/ml; rectal/vaginal suppository 200, 400 mg

Side effects/adverse reactions:

CNS: Dizziness, headache, migraines, depression, fatigue, insomnia

CV: Oedema

GI: Nausea, vomiting, anorexia, cramps, cholestatic jaundice; with rectal administration diarrhoea, flatulence

EENT: Diplopia, loss of vision, retinal lesions

GU: Amenorrhoea, cervical erosion, breakthrough bleeding, dysmenorrhoea, vaginal candidiasis, breast changes

INTEG: Rash, urticaria, acne, hirsutism, alopecia, oily skin, seborrhoea, pain at injection site

META: Weight gain, catabolism

Contraindications: Breast cancer, hypersensitivity, reproductive cancer, undiagnosed vaginal bleeding, high risk of arterial disease; rectal use in colitis; vaginal use in vaginal infection, immediately postpartum or with recurrent cystitis; thromboembolic disorder

Precautions: Pregnancy, lactation, hypertension, congestive cardiac failure, diabetes mellitus, bone disease, depression, migraine headache, convulsive disorders, hepatic disease, renal disease

Pharmacokinetics:

IM: Duration 24 hr

Excreted in urine, faeces, metabolised in liver

Interactions/incompatibilities:

• Vaginal preparation interferes with barrier contraceptives

• Raises plasma cyclosporin levels

Treatment of overdose: Unlikely

to be of significance, treatment symptomatic

NURSING CONSIDERATIONS

Assess:

• Baseline observations especially BP and weight

• Urinalysis to detect undiagnosed diabetes

Administer:

• IM injection given deep into buttock rather than thigh or deltoid

Evaluate:

• Therapeutic response: decrease abnormal uterine bleeding, absence of amenorrhoea

• BP and weight during therapy

• Mood changes

• For side effects

Teach patient/family:

• All aspects of drug usage, including Cushingoid symptoms

• About potential side effects including breast lumps, vaginal bleeding, oedema, jaundice, dark urine, clay-coloured stools, dyspnoea, headache, blurred vision, abdominal pain, numbness or stiffness in legs, chest pain; male to report impotence or gynaecomastia

• Oral preparation to be taken with food/milk

• To report suspected pregnancy promptly

---

promazine

Sparine

Func. class.: Antipsychotic, neuroleptic

Chem. class.: Phenothiazine

Legal class.: POM

Action: Depresses cerebral cortex, hypothalamus, limbic system, which control activity, aggression; blocks neurotransmission produced by dopamine at synapse; exhibits a strong α-adrenergic, cholinergic blocking action; as anti-emetic, inhibits medullary chemoreceptor trigger zone; mechanism for antipsychotic effects is unclear

Uses: Short-term management of psychomotor agitation; agitation, restlessness in elderly

Dosage and routes:

Psychomotor agitation

• *Adult:* By mouth 100–200 mg 4 times daily; IM 50 mg (25 mg elderly, debilitated, repeated after 6–8 hr if required

Agitation and restlessness

• *Elderly:* By mouth 25–50 mg up to 4 times daily

Available forms include: Syrup 50 mg (as embonate)/5 ml; injection IV, IM 50 mg/ml; tablets 25 mg, 50 mg, 100 mg

Side effects/adverse reactions:

RESP: Respiratory depression

CNS: Extrapyramidal symptoms: pseudoparkinsonism, akathisia, dystonia; tardive dyskinesia, drowsiness, headache, seizures, confusion, excitement, agitation, nightmares, insomnia

HAEM: Anaemia, leucopenia, leucocytosis, agranulocytosis

INTEG: Rash, photosensitivity, dermatitis, pallor, vascular spasm if injected IV undiluted

EENT: Blurred vision, nasal congestion, lens changes

GI: Dry mouth, nausea, vomiting, anorexia, constipation, jaundice

GU: Urinary retention, impotence

ENDO: Amenorrhoea, gynaecomastia

CV: Orthostatic hypotension, cardiac arrest, ECG changes, tachycardia

SYST: Neuroleptic malignant syndrome, hypothermia

Contraindications: Hypersensitivity, coma, child, brain damage, breast-feeding, bone marrow depression, pregnancy

Precautions: Seizure disorders,

blood dyscrasias, bone marrow depression, hepatic disease, cardiac disease, respiratory disease, renal failure, epilepsy, narrow angle glaucoma, hypothyroidism, myasthenia gravis, phaeochromocytoma, prostatic hypertrophy, parkinsonism

Pharmacokinetics:

By mouth: Onset erratic, peak 2–4 hr

IM: Onset 15 min, peak 1 hr, duration 4–6 hr

Metabolised by liver, excreted in urine, enters breast milk

Interactions/incompatibilities:

- Oversedation: other CNS depressants, alcohol, barbiturates
- Decreased absorption: aluminium hydroxide or magnesium hydroxide antacids
- Decreased effects of: lithium, levodopa, bromocriptine, lysuride, pergolide, anticonvulsants
- Increased effects of: antihypertensives
- Increased anticholinergic effects: anticholinergics, tricylic antidepressants
- Increased risk of arrhythmias with anti-arrhythmics
- Increased hypotension with anaesthetics
- Decreased absorption of tetracyclines with sparine suspension

Clinical assessment:

- Reduce dose to minimum and use for minimum time
- Stop treatment if jaundice develops
- Carry out immediate haematological investigation if signs of unexplained fever/infection

Treatment of overdose: Lavage if orally ingested, no specific antidote, supportive treatment of convulsions, hypotension, hypothermia

NURSING CONSIDERATIONS

Assess:

- Fluid balance
- Establish baseline BP, pulse and respiratory rate

Administer:

- With flavours to mask taste (citrus, chocolate)
- IM injection into large muscle mass

Perform/provide:

- Decreased noise input by dimming lights, avoiding loud noises
- Supervised ambulation until stabilised on medication; do not involve in strenuous exercise program because fainting is possible; patient should not stand still for long periods of time
- Increased fluids to prevent constipation
- Sips of water, mouthwashes for dry mouth

Evaluate:

- Therapeutic response: decrease in emotional excitement, hallucinations, delusions, paranoia, reorganization of patterns of thought, speech
- Swallowing of oral medication; check for hoarding or giving of medication to other patients
- Effect, orientation, level of consciousness, reflexes, gait, coordination, sleep pattern disturbances
- BP (standing and lying); pulse, respirations, 4 hrly during initial treatment; report drops of 30 mmHg
- Dizziness, faintness, palpitations, tachycardia on rising
- Uncoordinated movements including akathisia (inability to sit still, no pattern to movements), tardive dyskinesia (bizarre movements of jaw, mouth, tongue, extremities), pseudoparkinsonism (rigidity, tremors, pill rolling, shuffling gait)
- Constipation, urinary retention daily, if these occur increase bulk and water in diet

Teach patient/family:

• That postural hypotension occurs frequently, and to rise from sitting or lying position gradually
• To remain lying down after IM injection for at least 30 min
• To sit down in bathroom; avoid standing for long periods
• To avoid hot baths, hot showers, or stand up washes since hypotension may occur
• To avoid abrupt withdrawal of this drug or tremors may result; drugs should be withdrawn slowly
• To avoid non-prescribed preparations (cough, hayfever, cold) unless approved by clinician since serious drug interactions may occur; avoid use with alcohol or CNS depressants, increased drowsiness may occur
• To use a sunscreen during sun exposure to prevent burns
• Regarding compliance with drug regimen
• About possibility of uncoordinated movements and need to inform clinician immediately if these occur. Necessity for meticulous oral hygiene since oral candidiasis may occur
• To report sore throat, malaise, fever, bleeding, mouth sores; if these occur, full blood count should be taken and drug discontinued

promethazine

Avomine, Phenergan, Sominex
Func. class.: Antihistamine, antiemetic, sedative
Chem. class.: Phenothiazine
Legal class.: POM (injection), P (tablets, syrup)

Action: Acts on blood vessels, GI, respiratory system by competing with histamine for H_1-receptor site; decreases allergic response by blocking histamine

Uses: Motion sickness, rhinitis, allergy symptoms, sedation, nausea, pre-operative and post-operative sedation

Dosage and routes:

Nausea

• *Adult and child over 10 yr:* By mouth/IM 25 mg up to 4 times a day
• *Child:* By mouth every 6–8 hr, 2–5 yr 5 mg; 5–10 yr 10 mg or IM 6.25–12.5 mg

Motion sickness

• *Adult and child over 10 yr:* By mouth 25 mg once or twice a day, first dose the evening before travelling
• *Child:* By mouth, 5–10 yr 12.5–25 mg twice a day

Allergy/rhinitis

• *Adult and child over 10 yr:* By mouth 10–25 mg 3–4 times a day; slow IV, diluted, in emergency 25–50 mg
• *Child:* By mouth once or twice a day, 2–5 yr 5–15 mg; 5–10 yr 10–25 mg

Sedation

• *Adult and child over 10 yr:* By mouth/IM 25–50 mg at bedtime
• *Child:* By mouth at bedtime, 2–5 yr 15–20 mg; 5–10 yr 20–25 mg

Sedation (pre-operative/postoperative)

• *Adult:* By mouth/IM 25–50 mg
• *Child:* By mouth, 2–5 yr 15–20 mg; 5–10 yr 20–25 mg or IM 6.25–12.5 mg

Available forms include: Tablets 10, 20 mg (as hydrochloride); tablets 25 mg (as theoclate); syrup 5 mg/ml (as hydrochloride); injection 25 mg/ml (as hydrochloride)

Side effects/adverse reactions:

CNS: Dizziness, drowsiness, poor coordination, fatigue, confusion, neuritis, restlessness, headache, nightmares, hyperactivity in children, tremor, tics, dyskinesias

CV: Hypotension, palpitations, arrythmias
RESP: Increased thick secretions
HAEM: Thrombocytopenia, agranulocytosis, haemolytic anaemia
GI: Dry mouth, nausea, vomiting, anorexia, constipation, diarrhoea, jaundice
INTEG: Rash, urticaria, photosensitivity, pain at injection site
GU: Retention, dysuria, frequency
EENT: Blurred vision, dilated pupils, tinnitus, nasal stuffiness
SYST: Allergic reactions including anaphylaxis

Contraindications: Hypersensitivity to phenothiazines, lower respiratory tract disease, coma, CNS depression, neonates, porphyria, patients receiving MAOIs within 14 days

Precautions: Renal disease, cardiac disease, bronchial asthma, seizure disorder, hyperthyroidism, bronchitis, prostatic hypertrophy, bladder neck obstruction, pregnancy, lactation, narrow angle glaucoma

Pharmacokinetics:
By mouth: Onset 20 min, duration 4–6 hr, metabolised in liver, excreted by kidneys, GI tract (inactive metabolites)

Interactions/incompatibilities:
• Increased CNS depression: barbiturates, narcotics, hypnotics, tricyclic antidepressants, alcohol
• Increased anticholinergic effects with: anticholinergics, tricyclic antidepressants

Lab. test interferences:
False negative: Skin allergy tests
False positive/negative: Urine pregnancy test

Treatment of overdose: Administer ipecacuanha syrup or lavage, no specific antidote, provide symptomatic treatment, ensure adequate respiratory, circulatory status, diazepam for convulsions

NURSING CONSIDERATIONS

Assess:
• Fluid balance
• Urinalysis before treatment

Administer:
• IV only in an emergency, by slow intravenous injection after dilution with 10 times its volume with water for injection.
• Deep IM in large muscle; rotate site. IM injection painful, use oral route if possible
• Syrup is not suitable for diabetic patients
• Orally with meals if GI symptoms occur, absorption may slightly decrease

Perform/provide:
• Sips of water, mouthwashes for dryness
• Ensure oral medication is swallowed by elderly

Evaluate:
• When used as a sedative for elderly. Variations in dosage may be necessary if desired effect is to be obtained
• Therapeutic response: absence of running or congested nose or rashes, nausea and absence of motion sickness
• Respiratory status: rate, rhythm, increase in bronchial secretions, wheezing, chest tightness
• Cardiac status: palpitations, increased pulse, hypotension
• Be alert for retention, frequency or dysuria. Discontinue drugs if these occur

Teach patient/family:
• Avoid prolonged sunlight as photosensitive skin reaction may occur
• Ambulant patients when first using drug should not drive or operate machinery as drowsiness and disorientation may occur
• To notify clinician if confusion, over-sedation, hypotension occur

propafenone hydrochloride

Arythmol
Func. class.: Anti-arrhythmic (Class Ic)
Legal class.: POM

Action: Class 1C anti-arrhythmic with basic local anaesthetic activity and membrane-stabilising effects. Some beta-blocking activity has been reported
Uses: Prophylaxis and treatment of ventricular arrhythmias
Dosage and routes:
• *Adult:* By mouth initially 150 mg, three times a day, increasing at intervals of not less than 3 days to 300 mg twice daily, maximum 300 mg 3 times a day; reduce dose in patients under 70 kg
Available forms include: Tablets 150 mg, 300 mg
Side effects/adverse reactions:
GI: Nausea, vomiting, constipation, diarrhoea, dry mouth, cholestasis, bitter taste
CNS: Dizziness, fatigue, headache, blurred vision, seizures
HAEM: Blood dyscrasias
CV: Bradycardia, sinoatrial, atrioventricular or intraventricular blocks. Proarrhythmic effects. Postural hypotension
INTEG: Allergic skin reactions, lupus syndrome
Contraindications: Uncontrolled congestive heart failure, cardiogenic shock (except arrhythmia-induced), severe bradycardia, uncontrolled electrolyte disturbances, obstructive airways disease, marked hypotension, sinus node dysfunction, atrial conduction defects, second degree or greater atrioventricular block, bundle branch block or distal block unless patients are paced adequately, myasthenia gravis
Precautions: The weak negative inotropic effect of propafenone may assume importance in patients with cardiac failure. A reduction in dose is recommended in patients weighing less than 70 kg, and may also be necessary if liver or renal function is impaired. Elderly patients may respond to a lower dose
Pharmacokinetics: Peak levels after 2 to 3 hr
Interactions/incompatibilities:
• Propafenone potentiated by: other local anaesthetic type agent, cimetidine, quinidine. Reduced propafenone blood levels with: rifampicin
• Propafenone increases blood levels of: digoxin, warfarin, propranolol, metoprolol
Clinical assessment:
• Monitor concurrent therapy with oral anticoagulants closely; dose adjustment probably needed
• Halve dose of concurrent digoxin therapy and monitor levels

NURSING CONSIDERATIONS:
Assess:
• Baseline vital signs, ECG
Administer:
• Tablets should be swallowed whole with a drink after food
Perform/provide:
• Therapy should be initiated under hospital conditions with ECG monitoring and cardiovascular surveillance
Evaluate:
• Therapeutic effect
• BP continuously for fluctuations. Report changes to clinician
• For all side effects
Teach patient/family:
• That they should take special care if driving, operating machinery or performing any other hazardous task

• About potential side effects
• To report any change to clinician
• Rise slowly to sitting or standing position to minimise hypotension
• Not to stop medication without medical advice

propantheline bromide

Pro-Banthine
Func. class.: Gastrointestinal anticholinergic
Chem. class.: Synthetic quaternary ammonium compound
Legal class.: POM

Action: Inhibits muscarinic actions of acetylcholine at postganglionic parasympathetic neuroeffector sites
Uses: Treatment of peptic ulcer disease, irritable bowel syndrome, gastrointestinal conditions characterised by smooth muscle spasm, hyperhidrosis, enuresis
Dosage and routes:
• *Adult:* By mouth 15–30 mg up to four times a day before meals
Available forms include: Tablets 15 mg
Side effects/adverse reactions:
CNS: Confusion, stimulation in elderly, headache, insomnia, dizziness, drowsiness, anxiety, weakness, hallucinations, depression
GI: Dry mouth, constipation, paralytic ileus, heartburn, nausea, vomiting, dysphagia
GU: Hesitancy, retention, impotence
CV: Palpitations, tachycardia
EENT: Blurred vision, photophobia, mydriasis, cycloplegia, increased ocular tension
INTEG: Urticaria, rash, pruritus, anhidrosis, fever, flushing
SYST: Anaphylaxis, angioedema
Contraindications: Hypersensitivity to anticholinergics, narrow-angle glaucoma, GI obstruction, myasthenia gravis, paralytic ileus, GI atony, toxic megacolon, severe ulcerative colitis, obstruction of urinary tract, hiatus hernia with reflux oesophagitis, symptomatic reflux
Precautions: Hyperthyroidism, coronary artery disease, arrhythmias, congestive heart failure, ulcerative colitis, hypertension, hepatic disease, renal disease, elderly, prostatic hypertrophy, pregnancy, breast-feeding
Pharmacokinetics:
By mouth: Onset 30–45 min, duration 4–6 hr, plasma half-life 2–3 hr; metabolised by liver, GI system, excreted in urine, bile
Interactions/incompatibilities:
• Increased anticholinergic effect: amantadine, tricyclic anti-depressants, MAOIs, other anticholinergics, phenothiazines
• Decreased plasma levels of: phenothiazines
• Reduced GI effects of: domperidone, metoclopramide, cisapride
• Reduced effect of any concurent buccal tablets (dry mouth)
Treatment of overdose: Emesis/gastric lavage and activated charcoal, no specific antidote, treatment supportive, diazepam for CNS stimulation, consider physostigmine 500 mcg–2 mg IV in severe cases

NURSING CONSIDERATIONS

Assess:
• Baseline vital signs, cardiac status: checking for arrhythmias, increased rate, palpitations
Administer:
• 1 hr before meals for better absorption
Perform/provide:
• Frequent sips of water, mouthwashes for dryness of oral cavity
• Increased fluids, bulk, exercise to patient's lifestyle to decrease constipation

• Frequent mouth washes

Evaluate:

• Therapeutic response: absence of epigastric pain, bleeding, nausea, vomiting

• GI complaints: pain, bleeding (frank or occult), nausea, vomiting, anorexia

Teach patient/family:

• Avoid driving or other hazardous activities until stabilised on medication

• Avoid alcohol or other CNS depressants; will enhance sedating properties of this drug

propranolol hydrochloride

Angilol, Apsolol, Berkolol, Sloprolol, Inderal, Propanix, Cardinol, Half-Inderal LA, Inderal LA, Propanix SR, Beta-Prograne, Bedranol SR, Betadur CR

Func. class.: Antihypertensive, anti-anginal anti-arrhythmic, anti-migraine agent

Chem. class.: Non-selective β-blocker

Legal class.: POM

Action: Decreases preload, afterload, which is responsible for decreasing left ventricular end diastolic pressure, systemic vascular resistance

Uses: Hypertension, arrhythmias, migraine prophylaxis, thyrotoxic crisis, anxiety, anxiety-induced tachycardia, chronic stable angina pectoris, prophylaxis of angina pain, essential tremor

Dosage and routes:

Oral doses described below may be given once or twice daily using modified-release preparations

Hypertension

• *Adult:* By mouth 80 mg twice daily; maintenance usually 160–320 mg daily

Angina

• *Adult:* By mouth 40 mg 2–3 times daily; maintenance usually 120–240 mg daily

Myocardial infarction prophylaxis

• *Adult:* By mouth 40 mg 4 times daily for 2–3 days, then 80 mg twice daily, beginning 5–21 days after infarction

Portal hypertension

• *Adult:* By mouth initially 40 mg twice daily; increase to 80 mg twice daily according to heart rate; maximum 160 mg twice daily

Arrhythmias

• *Adult:* By mouth 10–40 mg 3–4 times daily

• *Adult:* IV injection 1 mg over 1 min; repeat at 2-min intervals; maximum 10 mg

• *Child:* By mouth (as a guide) 250–500 mcg/kg 3–4 times daily

• *Child:* Slow IV injection (as a guide) 25–50 mcg/kg; repeat 3–4 times a day if required

Hypertrophic obstructive cardiomyopathy

• *Adult:* By mouth 10–40 mg 3–4 times daily

Hyperthyroidism

• *Adult:* By mouth (adjunct) 10–40 mg 3–4 times daily

• *Adult:* IV injection (thyrotoxic crisis) 1 mg over 1 min; repeat at 2-min intervals if required; maximum 10 mg

• *Child:* By mouth (as a guide) 250–500 mcg/kg 3–4 times daily

• *Child:* Slow IV injection (as a guide) 25–50 mcg/kg; repeat 3–4 times a day if required

Phaeochromocytoma with alpha blocker

• *Adult:* By mouth 60 mg daily for 3 days before surgery; inoperable cases, 30 mg daily

• *Child:* By mouth (as a guide) 250–500 mcg/kg 3–4 times daily

Migraine prophylaxis

• *Adult:* By mouth 40 mg 2–3

times daily; maintenance 80–160 mg daily
• *Child:* By mouth (as a guide) 250–500 mcg/kg 3–4 times daily
Essential tremor
• *Adult:* By mouth 40 mg 2–3 times daily; maintenance 80–160 mg daily
Anxiety symptoms
• *Adult:* By mouth 40 mg twice daily; increase to 3 times daily if required
Available forms include: Capsules modified-release 80 mg, 160 mg; tablets 10 mg, 40 mg, 80 mg, 160 mg; injection 1 mg/ml; oral suspension 5 mg/5 ml, 50 mg/5 ml (both special order)
Side effects/adverse reactions:
RESP: Dyspnoea, bronchospasm
CV: Bradycardia, hypotension, congestive heart failure
HAEM: Agranulocytosis, thrombocytopenia
GI: Nausea, vomiting, diarrhoea, constipation, cramps, dry mouth
INTEG: Rash, pruritus, fever
CNS: Depression, hallucinations, dizziness, fatigue, lethargy, paraesthesias, nightmares
EENT: Dry eyes
MISC: Cold extremities
MS: Muscle fatigue
Contraindications: Bronchospasm, asthma, history of obstructive airways disease, metabolic acidosis, sinus bradycardia, partial heart block, uncontrolled congestive heart failure
Precautions: Diabetes mellitus, pregnancy, renal disease, lactation, congestive heart failure, hyperthyroidism, chronic obstructive airways disease, elderly
Pharmacokinetics:
By mouth: Onset 30 min, peak 1–1½ hr, duration 6 hr
IV: Onset 2 min, peak 15 min, duration 3–6 hr
Half-life 3–5 hr, metabolised by liver, crosses blood–brain barrier, excreted in breast milk
Interactions/incompatibilities:
• Risk of severe hypotension, asystole if verapamil is injected during propranolol therapy—avoid; risk less when given by mouth, but only if myocardium well preserved
• Severe hypertension with noradrenaline, adrenaline and if switched abruptly from clonidine
• Bradycardia, AV block with diltiazem, digoxin, amiodarone
• Severe hypotension, heart failure with nifedipine
• Enhanced effect of: hypoglycaemic agents (and masked hypoglycaemic symptoms), antihypertensives, chlorpromazine
• Increased toxicity with: lignocaine
• Hypotensive effects enhanced by: alcohol, anaesthetics, diuretics anxiolytics, hypnotics, fluvoxamine cimetidine
• Hypotensive effects reduced by: corticosteroids, oestrogens, rifampicin, thyroxine
• Reduced effects of: neostigmine, pyridostigmine
• Increased peripheral vasoconstriction with: ergotamine
Clinical assessment:
• Consider stopping treatment if skin rashes, dry eyes appear
Lab. test interferences:
• Determination of catecholamines by fluorescence, serum bilirubin by diazo method
Treatment of overdose: Gastric lavage; atropine 1–2 mg IV to counter bradycardia; glucagon 10 mg IV as cardiac stimulant repeated if needed; β-agonist if glucagon fails

NURSING CONSIDERATIONS

Assess:
• Baseline BP, pulse, respirations
• Weight
• Fluid balance
Administer:

• With full glass of water on empty stomach (oral tablet)
Evaluate:
• Pain: duration, time started, activity being performed, character
• Tolerance if taken over long period of time
• Therapeutic response; degree of palpitations, breathlessness and anxiety levels
• BP, heart and respiratory rates
• Observe for postural hypotension
Teach patient/family:
• That dose must be taken with a glass of water
• That drug may be taken before stressful activity: exercise, sexual activity
• That sublingual area may sting when drug comes in contact with mucous membranes
• To seek medical advice if dizziness, breathlessness or any other side effects are experienced
• To avoid hazardous activities if dizziness occurs
• Stress patient compliance with complete medical regimen
• To change position changes slowly to prevent fainting
• Decrease dosage over 2 weeks to prevent cardiac damage

---

propylthiouracil

Func. class.: Antithyroid agent
Chem. class.: Thioamide
Legal class.: POM

Action: Blocks synthesis of T_3, T_4 (triiodothyronine, thyroxine), inhibits organification of iodine
Uses: Hyperthyroidism
Dosage and routes:
• *Adult:* By mouth 300–600 mg daily in divided doses until euthyroid and then reduce to maintenance of 50–150 mg daily
Available forms include: Tablets 50 mg
Side effects/adverse reactions:
ENDO: Enlarged thyroid
INTEG: Rash, urticaria, pruritus, alopecia, hyperpigmentation,
GU: Irregular menses, nephritis
CNS: Drowsiness, headache, vertigo, fever
HAEM: Agranulocytosis, leucopenia, thrombocytopenia, hypothrombinaemia, lymphadenopathy
GI: Nausea, diarrhoea, vomiting, jaundice, hepatitis
MS: Myalgia, arthralgia
MISC: Lupus-like syndrome, fetal goitre
Contraindications: Hypersensitivity
Precautions: Bone marrow depression, hepatic disease, pregnancy, renal disease, lactation, large goitre
Pharmacokinetics:
By mouth: Rapidly absorbed, half-life 1–2 hr, excreted in urine, bile, breast milk, cross placenta
Clinicial assessment:
• Triiodothyronine, thyroxine, which is decreased; serum thyroid stimulating hormone, which is increased; free thyroxine index, which is increased if dosage is too low; discontinue drug 3–4 weeks before radioactive iodine uptake
• Blood for blood dyscrasias: leucopenia, thrombocytopenia, agranulocytosis
• Lowest dose that relieves symptoms
Treatment of overdose: No symptoms likely from single large dose, supportive

NURSING CONSIDERATIONS

Assess:
• Pulse, BP, temperature and night pulse
• Input and output of fluids
• Height, growth rate if given to children

• Weight daily prior to initial treatment at weekly intervals

Administer:

• Orally

• At same time daily in divided doses to maintain drug level

• Lowest dose that relieves symptoms

• With meals to decrease GI upset

Perform/provide:

• Fluids to 3–4 litres/day, unless contraindicated

• Removal of medication 4 weeks before radioactive iodine uptake test

Evaluate:

• Therapeutic effect: weight gain, decreased pulse, thyroxine and BP

• Overdose: peripheral oedema, heat intolerance, sweating, palpitations, arrhythmias, severe tachycardia, increased temperature, delirium, CNS irritability

• Hypersensitivity: rash, enlarged cervical lymph nodes, drug may need to be discontinued

• Hypoprothrombinaemia: bleeding, petechiae, ecchymosis

• Bone marrow depression: sore throat, fever, fatigue

Teach patient/family:

• To abstain from breast feeding after delivery

• Report redness, swelling, sore throat, mouth lesions, which indicate blood dyscrasias

• To keep graph of weight, pulse, mood

• That seafood, other iodine products may be restricted

• Not to discontinue this medication abruptly; thyroid crisis may occur; stress patient response

• That response may take several months if thyroid is large

• Symptoms/signs of overdose: periorbital oedema, cold intolerance, mental depression

• Symptoms of inadequate dose: tachycardia, diarrhoea, fever, irritability, weight loss

• That surgery may be necessary

• To only take other medication if directed by clinician

• That children show immediate behaviour personality changes

---

protamine sulphate

Prosulf

Func. class.: Heparin antagonist

Chem. class.: Low molecular weight protein

Legal class.: POM

Action: Produces stable complex when combined with heparin

Uses: Heparin overdose

Dosage and routes:

• *Adult:* IV 1 mg of protamine neutralises 100 U heparin (mucous) or 80 U heparin (lung) if given within 15 mins, administer slowly over 1–3 min; do not exceed 50 mg/10 min

• Reduce dose if given more than 15 mins after heparin as heparin is rapidly excreted

Available forms include: Injection IV 10 mg/ml

Side effects/adverse reactions:

CV: Hypotension, bradycardia

INTEG: Rash, dermatitis, urticaria, alopecia, flushing

HAEM: Bleeding (in overdose)

RESP: Dyspnoea

Contraindications: Hypersensitivity

Precautions: Pregnancy, breast feeding

Pharmacokinetics:

IV: Onset 5 min, duration 2 hr

Clinical assessment:

• Coagulation tests (activated partial thromboplastin time, ACT) 15 min after dose, then in several hours

NURSING CONSIDERATIONS

Assess:

• Vital signs

• Degree of bleeding

Administer:

- Dilution in sodium chloride 0.9% or 5% dextrose

Evaluate:
- Vital signs, BP every 30 min per first 3 hr
- Therapeutic response, diminution of bleeding
- Skin rash, urticaria, derma

protirelin

TRH, TRH-ROCHE
Func. class.: Thyrotrophin-releasing hormone
Chem. class.: Tripeptide
Legal class.: POM

Action: Stimulates secretion of thyroid stimulating hormone
Uses: Assessment of thyroid function and thyroid stimulating hormone reserve in hypopituitarism
Dosage and routes:
- *Adult:* IV injection 200 mcg
- *Child:* IV 1 mcg/kg

Available forms include: Injection 100 mcg/ml; 2-ml ampoule
Side effects/adverse reactions:
CNS: Dizziness
CV: Syncope, bronchospasm, tachycardia, hypertension
GI: Nausea, strange taste
GU: Desire to micturate
INTEG: Flushing
Precautions: Severe hypopituitarism, cardiac insufficiency, bronchial asthma, obstructive airways disease, pregnancy
Pharmacokinetics: IV: metabolised in plasma, possibly tissues, half-life 5–6 min
Interactions/incompatibilities: Not to be diluted
Clinical assessment:
- Take blood at 20, 60 min post-injection to detect peak/delayed TSH response

Treatment of overdose: Doses of up to 1 mg have not resulted in symptoms of overdose

NURSING CONSIDERATIONS

Assess:
- Pulse and BP; night pulse if possible
- Weight for children

Administer:
- After blood sample for control thyroid-stimulating hormone
- Intravenously, directly in vein as a single bolus injection
- Take a blood sample 20 min after injection for peak thyroid-stimulating hormone level
- 60 min after injection blood sample taken to detect a delayed thyroid-stimulating hormone level

Evaluate:
- Interpretation of results, by the response to protriptyline HCl from the basal values
- Effect of any other medication
- Side effects: usually mild and transient; nausea, desire to micturate, flushing, hypertension

Teach patient/family:
- Advise on result of test

protriptyline hydrochloride

Concordin
Func. class.: Antidepressant, tricyclic
Chem. class.: Dibenzocycloheptene—secondary amine
Legal class.: POM

Action: Blocks reuptake of noradrenaline, serotonin into nerve endings, increasing action of noradrenaline, serotonin in nerve cells
Uses: Depression
Dosage and routes:
- *Adult:* By mouth 15–40 mg daily in divided doses, may increase to 60 mg daily
- *Elderly:* By mouth, initially 5 mg 3 times a day, exceed 20 mg daily with caution

Available forms include: Tablets 5, 10 mg

Side effects/adverse reactions:

ENDO: Gynaecomastia, breast enlargement, galactorrhoea, changes in libido, changes in blood sugar

HAEM: Agranulocytosis, thrombocytopenia, eosinophilia, leucopenia

CNS: Dizziness, drowsiness, confusion, headache, anxiety, tremors, stimulation, weakness, insomnia, nightmares, extrapyramidal symptoms (elderly), increased psychiatric symptoms, paraesthesia, hallucinations, peripheral neuropathy, ataxia

GI: Diarrhoea, dry mouth, nausea, vomiting, paralytic ileus, decreased appetite, cramps, epigastric distress, jaundice, hepatitis, stomatitis, constipation, peculiar taste, black tongue

GU: Retention, impotence

INTEG: Rash, urticaria, sweating, pruritus, photosensitivity, flushing alopecia

CV: Orthostatic hypotension, ECG changes, tachycardia, hypertension, palpitations, myocardial infarction, stroke, heart block

EENT: Blurred vision, tinnitus, mydriasis

SYST: Hyperpyrexia, oedema, fever, weight gain/loss

Contraindications: Hypersensitivity to tricyclic antidepressants, recovery phase of myocardial infarction, heart block, severe liver disease, concurrent use of MAOIs, children under 16 yr, cardiac arrhythmias, mania, marked agitation, breast-feeding, porphyria

Precautions: Prostatic hypertrophy, suicidal patients, increased intra-ocular pressure, narrow-angle glaucoma, urinary retention, hepatic disease, hyperthyroidism, electroshock therapy, elective surgery, pregnancy, epilepsy, elderly, CV disorders

Pharmacokinetics:

By mouth: Peak plasma levels 8–12 hr, therapeutic effect 2–3 weeks; metabolised by liver, excreted by kidneys, half-life 54–198 hr

Interactions/incompatibilities:

- Decreased effects of: guanethidine, clonidine, debrisoquine, bethanidine, anticonvulsants, buccal medications (dry mouth)
- Increased effects of: alcohol, barbiturates, benzodiazepines, CNS depressants
- Hyperpyretic crisis, convulsions, hypertensive episode: MAOIs
- Inhalational anaesthetics increase risk of hypotension and arrhythmias
- Hypertension and/or arrhythmias with: sympathomimetic agents e.g. noradrenaline, adrenaline, ephedrine, phenylpropanolamine, isoprenaline
- Increased anticholinergic effects: anticholinergics, antihistamines, phenothiazines

Clinical assessment:

- ECG for flattening of T wave, bundle branch block, atrioventricular block, dysrhythmias in cardiac patients

Treatment of overdose: ECG monitoring, induce emesis, lavage, activated charcoal, administer anticonvulsant, dialysis ineffective

NURSING CONSIDERATIONS

Administer:

- Increased fluids, bulk in diet if constipation, urinary retention occur
- With food or milk for GI symptoms
- Dosage before bedtime if oversedation occurs during day; may take entire dose at bedtime; elderly may not tolerate once daily dosing
- Frequent mouthwashes, sips of water for dry mouth

Perform/provide:

- Assistance with movement during beginning therapy if drowsiness/dizziness occurs

Evaluate:

- Weight weekly, appetite may increase with drug
- Uncontrolled movements primarily in elderly: rigidity, dystonia, akathisia
- Mental status: mood, sensorium, affect, suicidal tendencies, increase in psychiatric symptoms: depression, panic
- Urinary retention, constipation
- Withdrawal symptoms: headache, nausea, vomiting, muscle pain, weakness; do not usually occur unless drug was discontinued abruptly

Teach patient/family:

- That therapeutic effects may take 2–3 weeks
- Use caution in driving or other activities requiring alertness because of drowsiness, dizziness, blurred vision
- To avoid alcohol ingestion, other CNS depressants unless prescribed
- Not to discontinue medication quickly after long-term use, may cause nausea, headache, malaise
- To wear sunscreen or large hat since photosensitivity may occur

proxymetacaine HCl (ophthalmic)

Ophthaine

Func. class.: Anaesthetic, ocular (short acting)

Chem. class.: Ester

Legal class.: POM

Action: Decreases ion permeability by stabilising neuronal membrane

Uses: Cataract extraction, tonometry, gonioscopy, removal of foreign bodies, suture removal, glaucoma surgery

Dosage and routes:

Glaucoma surgery and cataract extraction

- *Adult and child:* Instil 1 drop every 5–10 min for 5–7 doses

Tonometry/gonioscopy/suture removal

- *Adult and child:* Instil 1–2 drops 3 min before procedure

Available forms include: Solution 0.5%

Side effects/adverse reactions:

EENT: Blurred vision, stinging, burning, lacrimation, photophobia, conjunctival redness, iritis, stromal oedema, pupil dilation, corneal erosion (in chronic use), allergic keratitis

INTEG: Contact dermatitis

Contraindications: Hypersensitivity

Precautions: Abnormal levels of plasma esterases, allergies, hyperthyroidism, hypertension, cardiac disease

Pharmacokinetics:

Instil: Onset 13–30 seconds, duration 15–20 min

NURSING CONSIDERATIONS

Perform/provide:

- Protective covering for eye
- Storage in refrigerator

Teach patient/family:

- To report change in vision, with blurring or loss of sight, trouble breathing, sweating, flushing
- Not to touch or rub eye, which may further damage eye

pseudoephedrine HCl/ pseudoephedrine sulphate

Sudafed, Sudafed SA, Galpseud many combination products ~~NHS~~

Func. class.: Adrenergic agonist

Chem. class.: Substituted phenylethylamine, sympathomimetic

Legal class.: P (Sudafed-Co, Sudafed Expect, Actifed)

Action: Stimulates vascular adrenergic receptors causing vasoconstriction resulting in decongestant action particularly in nasal sinuses. May also stimulate heart and cause hypertension

Uses: Decongestant, nasal congestion

Dosage and routes:

• *Adult:* By mouth 60 mg 8 hrly, modified release capsules 120 mg 12 hrly

• *Child 6–12 yr:* By mouth 30 mg 8 hrly

• *Child 2–6 yr:* By mouth 15 mg 8 hrly

Available forms include: Capsules modified release 120 mg; syrup 30 mg/5 ml; tablets 60 mg

Side effects/adverse reactions:

CNS: Tremors, anxiety, insomnia, headache, dizziness, confusion, hallucinations, sleep disturbances

EENT: Dry nose, irritation of nose and throat

CV: Palpitations, tachycardia, hypertension

GI: Anorexia, nausea, vomiting

RESP: Depression

INTEG: Rashes

GU: Retention

Contraindications: Hypersensitivity to sympathomimetics, concurrent use of MAOIs, severe hypertension, coronary artery disease

Precautions: Pregnancy, cardiac disorders, hyperthyroidism, diabetes mellitus, prostatic hypertrophy, elevated intraocular pressure, breast feeding, hypertension

Pharmacokinetics:

By mouth: Onset 15–30 min, duration 4–6 hr, 8–12 hr (modified release), plasma half-life 5–8 hr metabolised in liver, excreted in breast milk

Interactions/incompatibilities:

• Do not use with MAOIs, β-blockers or tricyclic antidepressants, hypertensive crisis may occur

• Decreased effects of: hypotensive agents especially guanethidine, debrisoquine, bethanidine

Treatment of overdose: Gastric lavage and supportive measures, anticonvulsants and bladder catheterisation if necessary. Acid diuresis, dialysis speed elimination

NURSING CONSIDERATIONS

Assess:

• Respirations, pulse, BP

• Vital signs

Perform/provide:

• Refrigerated storage of reconstituted solution if refrigerated for no longer than 24 hr

• Do not use discoloured solutions

Evaluate:

• Paraesthesias and coldness of extremities, peripheral blood flow may decrease

• Insomnia, anxiety, dizziness, any urinary retention

• Therapeutic response: decreased nasal and sums congestion

Teach patient/family:

• Reason for drug administration

• To only take other medication if directed by clinician

---

pyrantel embonate

Combantrin

Func. class.: Anthelmintic

Chem. class.: Pyrimidine derivative

Legal class.: POM

Action: Causes paralysis in worm by neuroblockade, worms are expelled by normal peristalsis

Uses: Threadworm, hookworm, roundworms

Dosage and routes:

• *Adult and child over 6 months:* By mouth 10 mg/kg as a single dose, minimum 125 mg, maximum 1 g; repeat on 3 consecutive days for *Necator* (hookworm) if infection severe

Available forms include: Tablets 125 mg

Side effects/adverse reactions:
INTEG: Rash
CNS: Dizziness, headache, drowsiness, insomnia, weakness
GI: Nausea, vomiting, anorexia, diarrhoea, distension, elevations of liver enzymes
Contraindications: Hypersensitivity
Precautions: Hepatic disease, pregnancy
Pharmacokinetics:
By mouth: Poorly absorbed, metabolised in liver. More than 50% excreted in faeces, urine (unchanged/metabolites)
Interactions/incompatibilities:
- Antagonised by piperazine

Treatment of overdose: Gastric lavage supportive treatment

NURSING CONSIDERATIONS

Assess:
- Stools during entire treatment; specimens must be sent to lab while still warm; gloves must be worn whilst handling stools

Administer:
- Orally after meals to avoid GI symptoms

Perform/provide:
- Storage in tight, light-resistant containers in cool environment

Evaluate:
- For therapeutic response: expulsion of worms, 3 negative stool cultures after completion of treatment
- For allergic reaction: rash
- For diarrhoea during expulsion of worms
- Anorexia can result so observe diet and fluid intake

Teach patient/family:
- Proper hygiene after bowel movements including handwashing technique; wash hands before meals, tell patient to avoid putting fingers in mouth
- To take a bath or shower in the morning on rising, not to shake bed linen, change bed linen daily, wash in hot water
- To clean toilet daily with disinfectant
- Importance of compliance with dosage schedule, duration of treatment
- To drink fruit juice to help expel worms
- To wear shoes, wash all fruits, vegetables well before eating
- Wear gloves when handling stools
- Avoid hazardous activity if drowsiness occurs

---

pyrazinamide

Zinamide
Func. class.: Antitubercular
Chem. class.: Pyrazinoic acid amide
Legal class.: POM

Action: Bactericidal interference with lipid, nucleic acid biosynthesis
Uses: Tuberculosis, as an adjunctive to other drugs
Dosage and routes:
- *Adult:* By mouth 20–35 mg/kg/day in 3–4 divided doses, not to exceed 3 g/day

Available forms include: Tablets 500 mg
Side effects/adverse reactions:
INTEG: Photosensitivity, urticaria
CNS: Anorexia, malaise
GI: Hepatotoxicity, abnormal liver function tests, aggravation of peptic ulcer, nausea, vomiting
GU: Urinary difficulty, increased uric acid
HAEM: Sideroblastic anaemia
SYST: Fever
MS: Arthralgia, gout
Contraindications: Hypersensitivity, hepatic damage, lactation hyperuricaemia, gouty arthritis, porphyria
Precautions: Pregnancy, child, renal insufficiency, diabetes mellitus

Pharmacokinetics:
By mouth: Peak 2 hr, half-life 9–10 hr; metabolised in liver, excreted in urine (metabolites/unchanged drug)
Interactions/incompatibilities:
• Antagonises effects of probenicid, sulphinpyrazone as uricosurics
Clinical assessment:
• Liver function tests prior to therapy and every 2–4 weeks during therapy
• Renal status before, monthly, during therapy, including blood urate
Lab. test interferences:
• Certain urine dip-tests for ketones
Treatment of overdose: Gastric lavage, supportive treatment; high-carbohydrate, low-fat diet, probenecid for hyperuricaemia

NURSING CONSIDERATIONS

Assess:
• Temperature, baseline BP, pulse
• Culture and sensitivity prior to therapy
Administer:
• With meals to decrease GI symptoms
Evaluate:
• Hepatic status: decreased appetite, jaundice, dark urine, fatigue
Teach patient/family:
• The importance of compliance with regimen
• Inform about side effects. Patients must tell clinician immediately if these occur
• That scheduled appointments must be kept or relapse may occur
• Avoid alcohol while taking this drug

---

pyridostigmine bromide

Mestinon
Func. class.: Anticholinesterase, cholinergic
Chem. class.: Tertiary amine carbamate
Legal class.: POM

Action: Inhibits destruction of acetylcholine, which increases concentration at sites where acetylcholine is released; this facilitates transmission of impulses across myoneural junction
Uses: Myasthenia gravis, paralytic ileus, post-operative urinary retention
Dosage and routes:
Myasthenia gravis
• *Adult:* By mouth 30–120 mg given at intervals throughout the day, usually daily dose 300–1200 mg
• *Child over 6 yr:* Initially 60 mg, increased gradually usual dose 30–360 mg daily
• *Child under 6 yr:* Initially 30 mg, increased gradually usual dose range 30–360 mg daily
Other indications:
• *Adult:* By mouth 60–240 mg, frequency determined by patient needs
• *Child:* By mouth 15–60 mg, frequency determined by patient needs
Available forms include: Tablets 60 mg
Side effects/adverse reactions:
INTEG: Rash, urticaria, sweating
CNS: Confusion, weakness, convulsions, paralysis
GI: Nausea, diarrhoea, vomiting, cramps, involuntary defaecation
CV: Bradycardia, hypotension
GU: Frequency, incontinence
RESP: Bronchospasm, excessive secretions

EENT: Miosis, blurred vision, lacrimation, salivation

Note: Most effects described are dose-related and indicative of overdose

Contraindications: Gastrointestinal or urinary obstruction; hypersensitivity to drug or bromide

Precautions: Seizure disorders, bronchial asthma, coronary occlusion, hyperthyroidism, arrhythmias, peptic ulcer, pregnancy, lactation, parkinsonism, hypotension, vagotonia, bradycardia

Pharmacokinetics:

By mouth: Onset, 1–2 hr, duration 2½–4 hr, poorly absorbed, plasma half-life 3–4 hr

Metabolised in liver, excreted in urine largely unchanged

Interactions/incompatibilities:

- Decreased action of: gallamine, pancuronium, tubocurarine, atropine
- Increased action of: suxamethonium chloride
- Decreased action of aminoglycosides, anaesthetics, procainamide, quinidine, clindamycin, lincomycin, propranolol, lithium

NURSING CONSIDERATIONS

Assess:

- Vital signs, respiration 4 hrly
- Fluid balance, check for urinary retention or incontinence

Administer:

- Smaller doses required after thymectomy or when additional therapy (steroids, immunosuppressants) are given
- Larger doses after exercise or fatigue
- Dose titration needed to give best therapeutic response with minimum toxicity
- With food or milk to decrease GI symptoms
- On empty stomach for better absorption

Evaluate:

- Therapeutic response: increased muscle strength, hand grasp, improved gait, absence of laboured breathing (if severe)
- Bradycardia, hypotension, bronchospasm, headache, dizziness, convulsions, respiratory depression; drug should be discontinued if toxicity occurs

Teach patient/family:

- That drug is not a cure, it only relieves symptoms
- Emphasise importance of taking drug at time prescribed
- All aspects of drug: action, side effects, dose, symptoms of both over and under usage, when to notify clinician
- To wear ID specifying myasthenia gravis, drugs taken

---

pyridoxine HCl (vitamin B_6)

Benadon, Comploment Continus

Func. class.: Vitamin B_6, water soluble

Chem. class.: Methylpyridine derivative

Legal class.: Tablets: P. Injection: POM

Action: Necessary for fat, protein, carbohydrate metabolism; enhances glycogen release from liver and muscle tissue; needed as co-enzyme for metabolic transformations of a variety of amino acids

Uses: Vitamin B_6 deficiency associated with inborn errors of metabolism, seizures, isoniazid therapy, or oral contraceptives, premenstrual syndrome

Dosage and routes:

Deficiency states

• *Adult:* By mouth 25–50 mg up to three times a day
Isoniazid neuropathy
• *Prophylaxis:* By mouth 10 mg
• *Therapeutic:* By mouth 50 mg three times a day
Idiopathic sideroblastic anaemia
• *Adult:* By mouth 100–400 mg daily in divided doses
Premenstrual syndrome
• *Adult:* By mouth 50–100 mg daily
Available forms include: Tablets 10, 20, 50 mg; tablets modified release 100 mg; injection IM/IV 50 mg (with Vitamins B and C)
Side effects/adverse reactions:
SYST: Serious allergic reactions possible with Vitamins B and C injection
Contraindications:
Hypersensitivity
Pharmacokinetics:
By mouth/injection: Half-life 2–3 weeks, metabolised in liver, excreted in urine
Interactions/incompatibilities:
• Decreased effects of: levodopa

NURSING CONSIDERATIONS

Assess:
• Baseline vital signs
Evaluate:
• Therapeutic response: absence of nausea, vomiting, anorexia, skin lesions, glossitis, stomatitis, oedema, convulsions, restlessness
• Nutritional status:
• Pyridoxine levels during treatment
• Vital signs 4-hrly
• For hypersensitivity
Teach patient/family:
• Good dietary habits; foods such as brown bread, cereals, green vegetables, pulses, meat
• To avoid vitamin supplements unless directed by clinician

pyrimethamine

Daraprim, Fansidar (with sulfadoxine), Maloprim (with dapsone)
Func. class.: Antimalarial
Chem. class.: Folic acid antagonist
Legal class.: (Daraprim) P; combinations POM

Action: Inhibits folic acid metabolism in parasite, prevents transmission by stopping growth of fertilised gametes
Uses: Malaria, prophylaxis in conjunction with other agents
Dosage and routes:
Prophylaxis of malaria
Alone (not recommended by UK experts) or with dapsone (Maloprim)
• *Adults:* By mouth 1 tablet weekly
• *Child over 10 yr:* 1 tablet weekly
• *Child 5–10 yr:* ½ tablet weekly
With sulfadoxine (Fansidar) (not recommended by UK experts for prophylaxis)
• *Adults:* 1 tablet weekly
• *Child 9–14 yr:* ¾ tablet weekly
• *Child 4–8 yr:* ½ tablet weekly
• *Child under 4 yr:* ¼ tablet weekly
Acute attacks of malaria
With sulfadoxine (Fansidar)
• *Adult:* By mouth 2–3 tablets as a single dose alone or with quinine
• *Child 10–14 yr:* 2 tablets
• *Child 7–9 yr:* 1½ tablets
• *Child 4–6 yr:* 1 tablet
• *Child under 4 yr:* ½ tablet
Available forms include: Tablets 25 mg; 25 mg with 500 mg sulfadoxine (Fansidar); 12.5 mg with 100 mg dapsone (Maloprim)
Side effects/adverse reactions:
Pyrimethamine alone:
INTEG: Rash
HAEM: Megaloblastic anaemia
Additionally, with dapsone:
HAEM: Agranulocytosis, methaemoglobinaemia

Additionally, with sulfadoxine:
INTEG: Alopecia, Stevens–Johnson syndrome, Lyell's syndrome
GI: Nausea, vomiting, stomatitis, feeling of fullness, hepatitis
HAEM: Leucopenia, thrombocytopenia, agranulocytosis
RESP: Pulmonary infiltration
CNS: Fatigue, headache, polyneuritis
SYST: Fever

Contraindications: Hypersensitivity, allergy to sulphonamides (Fansidar, Maloprim), megaloblastic anaemia caused by folate deficiency. Fansidar only (sulfadoxine): prophylactic use in patients with severe renal/liver damage or blood dyscrasias, lactation. Dapsone only: G6PD deficiency

Precautions: Pregnancy

Pharmacokinetics:
By mouth: Peak 2 hr, half-life 111 hr; metabolised in liver, highly protein bound, excreted in urine (metabolites)

Interactions/incompatibilities:
- Increased antifolate effect when given with: cotrimoxazole, trimethoprim, phenytoin, methotrexate
- Theoretical risk of increased blood levels of oral anticoagulants, sulphonylurea, hypoglycaemics, phenytoin with Fansidar (sulfadoxine)

Treatment of overdose: Gastric lavage, anticonvulsant and respiratory support if needed

NURSING CONSIDERATIONS

Administer:
- Before or after meals at same time each day to maintain drug level and to decrease GI symptoms
- Stop treatment immediately if signs of muco-cutaneous toxicity seen with Fansidar
- Give folinic acid supplements during pregnancy

Teach patient/family:
- To report visual problems, fever, fatigue, bruising, bleeding; may indicate blood dyscrasias
- To take frequent rest periods when fatigued
- To take avoidance measures against mosquito bites, e.g. repellants, nets

quinalbarbitone sodium

Seconal Sodium, combination product
Func. class.: Sedative/hypnotic (short-acting)
Chem. class.: Barbiturate
Legal class.: CD (Sch 2) POM

Action: Depresses activity in brain cells primarily in reticular activating system in brainstem; selectively depresses neurones in posterior hypothalamus, limbic structures

Uses: Severe, intractable insomnia

Dosage and routes:
- *Adult:* By mouth 50–100 mg at bedtime

Available forms include: Capsules 50, 100 mg

Side effects/adverse reactions:
CNS: Lethargy, drowsiness, hangover, dizziness, confusion, agitation, anxiety, psychiatric disturbances, nightmares, hallucinations, headache, dependence, CNS depression, ataxia
GI: Nausea, vomiting, constipation
INTEG: Rash, urticaria, angioedema, exfoliative dermatitis
CV: Hypotension, bradycardia
RESP: Respiratory depression
HAEM: Megaloblastic anaemia (long-term treatment)

Contraindications: Hypersensitivity to barbiturates, history of drug/alcohol abuse, acute/chronic pain, debilitated patients, pregnancy, breast-feeding, dyspnoea or respiratory obstruction, severe liver impairment, porphyria, children/young adults, elderly, use for more than 14 days

Precautions: Mental depression, hepatic or renal dysfunction, shock, respiratory depression

Pharmacokinetics: Well absorbed by mouth. Metabolised by liver, excreted by kidneys (metabolites); half-life 15–40 hr

Interactions/incompatibilities:

• Increased CNS depression: alcohol, MAOIs, sedative, narcotics

• Decreased effect of these drugs: oral anticoagulants, calcium channel blockers, corticosteroids, disopyramide, griseofulvin, quinidine, oral contraceptives, phenytoin, tricyclic antidepressants, tetracyclines

Treatment of overdose: Supportive care; in severe poisoning consider haemodialysis or haemoperfusion

NURSING CONSIDERATIONS

Administer:

• ½–1 hr before bedtime for insomnia

Perform/provide:

• Assistance with mobility after receiving dose; drug causes drowsiness

Evaluate:

• Therapeutic response: ability to sleep at night, decreased amount of early morning awakening if taking drug for insomnia

• Unresolved pain, as drug may cause severe stimulation if pain is present

• Mental status: mood, memory (long, short)

• Physical dependency: more frequent requests for medication, shakes, anxiety

Teach patient/family:

• That hypersensitivity is common, particularly in elderly: headache, hangover, drowsiness, dizziness, excitement, occasionally confusion

• Best taken 30 min before retiring to bed

• That drug is indicated only for short-term treatment of insomnia and is probably ineffective after 2 weeks

• That physical dependency may result when used for extended periods of time (45–90 days depending on dose)

• To avoid driving or other activities requiring alertness

• To avoid alcohol ingestion or CNS depressants; serious CNS depression may result

• Not to discontinue medication quickly after long-term use; drug should be tapered over 1–2 weeks

• That withdrawal insomnia may occur after short-term use

• That effects may take 2 nights for benefits to be noticed

• Alternate measures to improve sleep (reading, warm bath, warm milk, TV, self-hypnosis, deep breathing)

---

quinapril

Accupro

Func. class.: Antihypertensive

Chem. class.: Angiotensin converting enzyme inhibitor, non-sulphydryl

Legal class.: POM

Action: Selectively suppresses renin-angiotensin-aldosterone system; the active metabolite quinaprilat inhibits angiotensin converting enzyme, prevents conversion of angiotensin I to angiotensin II

Uses: Adjunct to diuretics or cardiac glycosides in congestive heart failure; hypertension where standard therapy is ineffective or inappropriate

Dosage and routes:

Diuretics should be stopped if possible for 2−3 days before starting treatment to minimise the risk of a rapid fall in blood pressure and hypotension

Hypertension

• *Adult:* Initially 5 mg daily, adjusted according to response; maintenance usually 20−40 mg daily, in single or divided doses; up to 80 mg daily has been given; initial dose with concurrent diuretics, elderly, or in renal impairment, 2.5 mg daily

Congestive heart failure

• *Adult:* By mouth initially 2.5 mg daily under hospital supervision, adjusted according to response; usual maintenance, 10−20 mg daily in 2 divided doses; up to 40 mg daily may be given

Available forms include: Tablets 5 mg, 10 mg, 20 mg

Side effects/adverse reactions:

CNS: Headache, dizziness, insomnia, paraesthesia, nervousness, fatigue

RESP: Cough, upper respiratory tract infection, rhinitis

MS: Myalgia, weakness, back pain

GI: Nausea, vomiting, dyspepsia, abdominal pain

CV: Chest pain, hypotension

INTEG: Angioedema (discontinue immediately), rash

EENT: Sinusitis, pharyngitis, taste disturbances

GU: Renal impairment

Contraindications: Hypersensitivity, pregnancy, breast-feeding, aortic stenosis or outflow obstruction, renovascular disease, porphyria

Precautions: Severe heart failure, renal insufficiency, peripheral vascular disease, atherosclerosis, dehydration, low sodium diet

Interactions/incompatibilities:

• May decrease effect of: tetracyclines

• Possibly increased toxicity: lithium, potassium salts, potassium sparing diuretics, non-steroidal anti-inflammatory agents

• Increased effect of: alcohol, anaesthetics, other antihypotensives, β-blockers, diuretics, phenothiazines

• Decreased effect of: non-steroidal anti-inflammatory agents, corticosteroids, oestrogens, oral contraceptives

Clinical assessment:

• Monitor: renal function before or during therapy in renal insufficiency

• White cell count in collagen vascular disorders or with leucopenic drugs. Use relevant points as for captopril

NURSING CONSIDERATIONS

Assess:

• Baseline vital signs

• Apical/radial pulse before administration; notify physician of any significant changes

• Urinalysis for protein daily in first morning specimen, if protein is increased a 24 hr urinary protein should be collected

Administer:

• First dose under medical supervision in hospital

• IV infusion of 0.9% NaCl (as ordered) to expand fluid volume if severe hypotension occurs

Perform/provide:

• Supine or Trendelenburg position for severe hypotension, especially in early treatment

Evaluate:

• Therapeutic response

• BP, pulse every 4 hr; note rate, rhythm, quality during initial therapy

• Symptoms of congestive cardiac failure: oedema, dyspnoea

• Renal symptoms: polyuria, oliguria, frequency

Teach patient/family:

• Administer 1 hr before meals

• Not to discontinue drug abruptly

• Not to use non-prescribed (cough, cold, or allergy) products unless directed by clinician

• Stress patient compliance with dosage schedule, even if feeling better

• To rise slowly to sitting or standing position to minimise orthostatic hypotension

• Notify clinician of: persistant dry cough, sore throat, swelling of hands or feet, irregular heartbeat, chest pain, signs of angioedema

• May cause dizziness, fainting; light-headedness may occur during first few days of therapy

---

quinidine

Kiditard, Kinidin

Func. class.: Anti-arrhythmic (Class Ia)

Chem. class.: Quinine dextro isomer

Legal class.: POM

Action: Stabilises cardiac membrane and prolongs action potential duration

Uses: Atrial fibrillation, supraventricular and ventricular tachyarrhythmias

Dosage and routes:

Initial test dose to detect hypersensitivity reactions

• *Adult:* By mouth, quinidine sulphate, 200–400 mg 3–4 times a day

• *Adult:* By mouth, quinidine bisulphate, modified-release, 500 mg every 12 hr, adjusted as required

Available forms include: Quinine bisulphate: capsules modified-release 250 mg, tablets modified-release 250 mg; Quinine sulphate: tablets 200 mg

Side effects/adverse reactions:

CNS: Headache, dizziness, confusion, vertigo (signs of cinchonism)

EENT: Tinnitus, blurred vision, hearing loss (signs of cinchonism)

GI: Nausea, vomiting, abdominal pain, diarrhoea, granulomatous hepatitis

CV: Heart block, extrasystole, ventricular arrhythmias, widened QRS complex, cardiac arrest, hypotension

HAEM: Thrombocytopenia, haemolytic anaemia, aplastic anaemia

RESP: Asthma (hypersensitivity)

INTEG: Rash, urticaria, pruritus, purpura (signs of hypersensitivity); photosensitivity, lupus, flushing

SYST: Fever

Contraindications: Hypersensitivity, cardiac glycoside-induced arrhythmias, complete heart block

Precautions: Pregnancy, lactation, hypotension, liver disease, uncompensated cardiac failure, partial heart block, myocardial damage, conductive tissue disease, myasthenia gravis

Pharmacokinetics:

By mouth: Onset 2–3 hr, peak 1–3 hr, duration 6–8 hr; half-life 6–7 hr, metabolised in liver, excreted unchanged by kidneys

Interactions/incompatibilities:

• May increase effects of: neuromuscular blockers, digoxin, anticoagulants, β-blockers

• May increase effects of quinidine: cimetidine, verapamil, diuretics, antacids

• May decrease effects of: neostigmine, pyridostigmine

• May decrease effects of quinidine: rifampicin, antiepileptics, barbiturates

Clinical assessment
Assess:
• ECG continuously at high doses
• Blood levels at higher doses
Treatment of overdose: Symptomatic supportive care; monitor CV, respiratory, and renal function and blood electrolytes

NURSING CONSIDERATIONS

Assess:
• BP, TPR, ECG prior to therapy
Evaluate:
• Cardiac and respiratory rate, temperature, BP
• Observe for potential tachypnoea, tachycardia, pyrexia and changes in BP
• CNS effects: may cause dizziness, confusion, psychosis paraesthesias, convulsions
• Inform clinician if any of the above occur. Therapy may be discontinued

quinine bisulphate/ quinine dihydrochloride/ quinine hydrochloride/ quinine sulphate

Func. class.: Antimalarial
Chem. class.: Cinchona alkaloid
Legal class.: POM

Action: Inhibits parasite replications, transcription of DNA to RNA by forming complexes with DNA of parasite
Uses: *Plasmodium falciparum* malaria, nocturnal leg cramps
Dosage and routes:
Malaria
• *Adults:* By mouth 600 mg (dihydrochloride, hydrochloride, or sulphate) 8 hrly for 7 days (with pyrimethamine/sulfadoxine or tetracycline); IV infusion, loading dose of 20 mg/kg (of salts as above) over 4 hrs then 10 mg/kg (up to maximum 700 mg) over 4 hr every 8–12 hr, until course can be completed by mouth. Reduce maintenance to 5–7 mg/kg if given for more than 72 hr
• *Child:* By mouth 10 mg/kg of salts as above 8 hrly for 7 days (with pyrimethamine/sulfadoxine or tetracycline); IV infusion as for adult
Leg cramps
• *Adult:* By mouth 200 mg (sulphate) or 300 mg (bisulphate) at night
Available forms include: Tablets 300 mg (bisulphate, dihydrochloride, hydrochloride, sulphate) 125 mg (sulphate), 200 mg (sulphate); IV infusion (dihydrochloride) 300 mg/ml
Side effects/adverse reactions:
RESP: Asthma (hypersensitivity)
INTEG: Pruritus, rashes, purpura, angioedema (signs of hypersensitivity)
HAEM: Thrombocytopenia, agranulocytosis, hypothrombinaemia, haemolysis
CNS: Headache, confusion, vertigo, dizziness (signs of cinchonism)
EENT: Visual disturbances including temporary blindness, tinnitus, deafness (signs of cinchonism)
GI: Nausea, vomiting, diarrhoea, abdominal pain, hepatitis
CV: Heartblock, ventricular, arrhythmias, hypotension, circulatory failure
ENDO: Hypoglycaemia
GU: Renal failure
SYST: Fever
Contraindications: Hypersensitivity, haemolysis, optic neuritis, tinnitus, haemoglobinuria
Precautions: Pregnancy (avoid except in life threatening disease), atrial fibrillation, heart block or other cardiac disease, severe hepatic disease, myasthenia gravis, G6PD deficiency

Pharmacokinetics:
By mouth: Peak 1–3 hr, metabolised in liver, excreted in urine, half-life 4–5 hr

Interactions/incompatibilities:
• May increase effects of quinine: cimetidine
• May increase effects of: digoxin, neuromuscular blockers, anticoagulants

Treatment of overdose: Symptomatic supportive care; monitor CV, respiratory, and renal function

NURSING CONSIDERATIONS

Assess:
• BP, pulse

Administer:
• IV by slow infusion (injection is hazardous)
• Before/after meals at same time each day to maintain drug level
• At night if taking for leg cramps (nocturnal)

Perform/provide:
• Urinalysis for haemoglobin

Evaluate:
• Therapeutic effect: relief of symptoms
• If administered IV, watch for hypotension, tachycardia
• Signs of rhinitis, nausea, rashes, abdominal pain, visual disturbances

Teach patient/family:
• To avoid non-prescribed preparations: cold preparations, tonic water
• To inform prescribing clinician if already on anticoagulant therapy or digoxin
• To take regular exercise if experience night cramps

rabies vaccine

Merieux Inactivated Rabies Vaccine
Func. class.: Inactivated human diploid cell vaccine
Chem. class.: Inactivated Wistar Pm/Wl 38 1503–3M virus strain
Legal class.: POM

Action: Promotes development of rabies-specific antibodies

Uses: Active immunisation as prophylactic measure to personnel at risk of contracting rabies e.g. staff at animal quarantine stations, animal handlers, veterinary surgeons, field workers at risk of being bitten by wild animals, staff in attendance upon a patient suspected of or known to be suffering from rabies; post-exposure treatment of previously unvaccinated patients

Dosage and routes:
Prophylaxis
• Deep subcutaneous, IM injection initially 1 ml, then further 1 ml after 7 days, then further 1 ml after 28 days (Department of Health preferred schedule); reinforcing doses 1 ml every 1–3 yr depending on risk of infection

Staff in attendance on patients with rabies
• Intradermally, 4 doses of 0.1 ml injected at different sites on the same day
• For further advice contact Duty Medical Officer, Central Public Health Laboratory, Colindale Avenue, Colindale, London NW9 5HT, Tel 081–200 4400

Post-exposure treatment (no, or inadequate prophylaxis)
• Deep subcutaneous, IM injection 1 ml on day of exposure then 1 ml after 3, 7, 14, 30 and 90 days; rabies immunoglobulin should be given concurrently on day 0

Available forms include: Injection,

2.5 International Units single dose vial

Side effects/adverse reactions:

INTEG: Pain, erythema and induration of injection site pruritus, nausea

SYST: Fever, malaise or myalgia. Anaphylaxis

Interactions/incompatibilities:

• Reduced effect of vaccine: steroids, immunosuppressants

Clinical assessment:

• Do not wait for confirmation of rabies before administering first vaccination

• Cease injections if animal is found not to be rabid

• Use with care in allergy to neomycin (traces are present in vaccine)

• Prescribe protection against tetanus and infection for those with serious bites

• All contacts of a rabid subject should be vaccinated

NURSING CONSIDERATIONS

Administer:

• Use immediately after reconstitution

• Discard any vaccine unused within an hour of reconstitution

• Administer deep subcutaneous or IM into deltoid region—avoid the gluteal region

• Ensure adrenaline is readily available in case of anaphylactic reaction

• Ensure bite wounds are thoroughly cleansed with soapy water

Evaluate:

• For anaphylaxis

• For signs of local skin reactions and mild fever or malaise

Teach patient/family:

• That local and systemic side effects are common within 48 hr but are usually mild

• That all contacts will need vaccination if subject is rabid

• If vaccination is given prophylactically, further immunisation will be required if patient is exposed to rabies virus

---

ranitidine

Zantac

Func. class.: H_2 receptor antagonist

Chem. class.: Imidazole derivative

Legal class.: POM

Action: Inhibits histamine at H_2 receptor site in parietal cells, which inhibits gastric acid secretion

Uses: Duodenal ulcer, Zollinger-Ellison syndrome, benign gastric ulcer, reflux oesophagitis, prophylaxis for stress ulcer, Mendelson's syndrome

Dosage and routes:

Duodenal/Gastric ulceration

• *Adult:* By mouth 150 mg twice a day or 300 mg at bedtime for 4–8 weeks; may be increased to 300 mg twice a day in duodenal ulcer. Maintenance if required 150 mg at bedtime. IV Injection 50 mg diluted to 20 ml over 5 min every 6–8 hr. IV intermittent infusion 50 mg/100 ml over 2 hr every 6–8 hr, IM injection 50 mg 6–8 hrly. Continuous IV infusion in severely ill patients 0.125–0.25 mg/kg/hr

Oesophageal reflux

• *Adult:* By mouth 150 mg twice a day or 300 mg at night for up to 12 weeks, may be increased to 150 mg 4 times a day

Prevention of NSAID-associated duodenal ulcers

• *Adult:* By mouth 150 mg twice a day

Zollinger-Ellison syndrome

• *Adult:* By mouth 150 mg 3 times a day increasing if required to maximum 6 g daily

Mendelson's syndrome

• *Adult:* By mouth pre-operative: 150 mg 2 hr before induction and, preferably night before; IM or slow IV 50 mg, 45–60 min before anaesthesia
• *Obstetric*: By mouth 150 mg on commencement of labour then 150 mg 6 hrly; administer antacid (e.g. sodium citrate) prior to anaesthesia

Peptic ulcer in children
• By mouth 2–4 mg/kg twice a day to maximum 300 mg/day

Available forms include: Tablets 150 mg, 300 mg; injection 25 mg/ml IM, IV; syrup 75 mg in 5 ml; effervescent tablets 150 mg, 300 mg

Side effects/adverse reactions:
CNS: Headache, dizziness, confusion, hallucination
GI: Hepatotoxicity
CV: Bradycardia, atrioventricular block, asystole
HAEM: Leucopenia, thrombocytopenia, agranulocytosis
INTEG: Urticaria, rash, swelling/discomfort in breast (men)
SYST: Anaphylaxis, fever

Contraindications: Hypersensitivity

Precautions: Pregnancy, lactation, use in children is limited therefore caution is necessary, renal disease, may mask symptoms of undiagnosed gastric carcinoma

Pharmacokinetics:
By mouth: Peak 2–3 hr, metabolised by liver, excreted in urine largely unchanged, breast milk, half-life 2–3 hr

Interactions/incompatibilities:
• Decreased absorbtion of: itraconazole, ketoconazole

Treatment of overdose: No problem expected in overdose, supportive treatment only

NURSING CONSIDERATIONS

Assess:
• Establish baseline pulse then monitor pulse rate frequently
• Fluid balance

Administer:
• Effervescent tablets and granules should be dissolved in half a glass of water
• Dilute one ampoule to 20 ml and give slowly IV over at least 2 mins, preferably 5 mins
• Injection is compatible with 0.9% sodium chloride, 5% glucose, glucose 4%, sodium chloride 0.18% and compound sodium lactate

Teach patient/family:
• That gynaecomastia may occur but is reversible
• Avoid driving or other hazardous activities until patient is stabilised on this medication
• About appropriate diet
• To avoid black pepper, caffeine, alcohol, harsh spices, extremes in temperature of food
• To avoid non-prescribed preparations: aspirin, cough, cold preparations

remoxipride

Roxiam
Func. class.: Neuroleptic
Chem. class.: Substituted benzamide
Legal class.: POM

Action: Highly selective antagonism of the neurotransmitter dopamine of D_2 receptors in the brain; antagonism of dopamine in the cerebral cortex, hypothalamus and limbic system probably particularly important. Little sedative effect compared to older neuroleptics

Uses: Acute and chronic schizophrenic psychoses, and other psychoses where delusions, hallucinations and thought disorder are prominent symptoms, except those due to depressive illness

Dosage and routes:
• *Adult:* By mouth, initially 300 mg once daily adjusted according to individual response, effective dose usually in range 150–450 mg once daily; maximum 600 mg once daily; maintenance dose usually 150–300 mg once daily
• *Elderly:* By mouth, initially 150 mg once daily adjusted according to response
Renal or hepatic impairment: In severe renal (creatinine clearance less than 25 ml/min) or hepatic impairment a starting dose of 150 mg once daily is recommended
Available forms include: Capsules, modified release 150, 300 mg
Side effects/adverse reactions:
CNS: Tiredness, drowsiness, insomnia, concentration difficulties, restlessness, anxiety, agitation, aggressiveness, headache, dizziness, akathisia, hypokinesia, rigidity, tremor, acute dystonia, dyskinesia
CV: Hypotension
EENT: Dry mouth, salivation, blurred vision
ENDO: Menstrual disorders, gynaecomastia, galactorrhoea
GI: Nausea, constipation, elevated liver enzymes
GU: Micturition disorders
INTEG: Skin rash, urticaria
MISC: Changes in body weight
Precautions: Pregnancy; lactation; severe renal or hepatic impairment, Parkinson's disease; history of or current breast cancer
Interactions:
• Increased risk of extrapyramidal effects with: metoclopramide, tetrabenazine
• Antagonism of: bromocriptine, levodopa, lysuride, pergolide
Treatment of overdose: Careful observation; symptomatic and supportive treatment; IV antiparkinsonian therapy for extrapyramidal symptoms; benzodiazepines may be of value for agitation or excitation related to akathisia

NURSING CONSIDERATIONS

Assess:
• Baseline BP, body weight, urinary output, menstrual pattern
Administer:
• Without opening capsule
Evaluate:
• BP (for hypotension)
• Therapeutic effect
• For all side effects
Teach patient/family:
• Need for compliance with regime
• About side effects of drug
• Importance of reporting side effects to nurse or clinician
• Not to discontinue the drug suddenly

---

reproterol HCl (inhaled)

Bronchodil
Func. class.: Bronchodilator
Chem. class.: Adrenergic β-2 stimulant
Legal class.: POM

Action: Selective β-2 stimulation of receptors in respiratory smooth muscle producing bronchodilation
Uses: Reversible airways obstruction, bronchial asthma, chronic bronchitis and emphysema
Dosage and routes:
• *Adult:* Inhalation 0.5–1 mg (1–2 puffs), repeated after 3–6 hr if necessary; maintenance therapy 1 mg (2 puffs) 3 times daily
• *Child 6–12 yr:* Inhalation 0.5 mg (1 puff) every 3–6 hr; maintenance therapy 0.5 mg (1 puff) three times a day
Available forms include: Aerosol inhalation, 500 mcg metered dose inhaler
Side effects/adverse reactions:
CNS: Fine tremor, headache, nervous tension

CVS: Tachycardia
Contraindications: Hypersensitivity to the drug
Precautions: Hyperthyroidism, pregnancy, myocardial infarction, phaeochromocytoma
Interactions/incompatibilities:
• May inhibit action of this drug: other β-blockers
Clinical assessment:
• Monitor blood potassium levels before, during long-term therapy
Treatment of overdose:
Symptomatic relief only necessary

NURSING CONSIDERATIONS

Assess:
• Baseline pulserate; tachycardia may occur
Administer:
• Using correct inhaler technique
• Shake before use
• Wait for 1 min between puffs
Perform/provide:
• Store aerosol canister away from heat, do not puncture even when empty
• Replace nebuliser solutions daily
Evaluate:
• Patient technique with aerosol inhaler—poor technique may be mistaken for poor drug action
• For side effects of digital tremor, restlessness—children may need reassurance when these occur
• Therapeutic response—easier breathing
• Need for further measures if usual degree of relief not obtained
Teach patient/family:
• Correct technique—this should be re-assessed occasionally
• Not to exceed prescribed dose
• Children should always be supervised by responsible adult when using aerosol/nebuliser
• Check with clinician before taking unprescribed preparations
• Report to clinician at once if usual degree of relief is not obtained or if asthma is severe

---

rifampicin

Rifadin, Rimactane,
Func. class.: Anti-tubercular
Chem. class.: Rifamycin derivative
Legal class.: POM

Action: Inhibits DNA-dependent RNA polymerase, bactericidal
Uses: Pulmonary tuberculosis, leprosy, brucellosis, Legionnaires' Disease. Prophylaxis of meningococcal meningitis, *H. influenzae*
Dosage and routes:
Tuberculosis
• *Adult:* By mouth: 450–600 mg/day or 600–900 mg 3 times a week; IV infusion: 600 mg over 2–3 hr daily
• *Child:* By mouth 10–20 mg/kg/day not to exceed 600 mg/day or 15 mg/kg 3 times a week
Leprosy
• *Adult:* By mouth 600 mg once per month
Brucellosis, Legionnaires' disease, serious staphylococcal infection
• *Adult:* By mouth 600–1200 mg daily in 2–4 divided doses
Prophylaxis of meningococcal meningitis
• *Adult:* By mouth 600 mg twice daily for 2 days
• *Child (1–12 yr):* By mouth 10 mg/kg twice daily for 2 days
• *Child (3 months–1 yr):* By mouth 5 mg/kg twice daily for 2 days
Prophylaxis of H. influenzae
• *Adult and children in exposed household:* By mouth 20 mg/kg (maximum 600 mg) once daily for 4 days
Available forms include: Capsules 150, 300 mg; Syrup, 100 mg/5 ml; IV infusion, 300, 600 mg
Side effects/adverse reactions:
CV: Hypotension, shock
CNS: Headache, drowsiness, lethargy, confusion, peripheral

neuropathy, psychosis
GU: Acute renal failure
EENT: Blurred vision, optic neuritis, photophobia, conjunctivitis
HAEM: Haemolytic anaemia, thrombocytopenia, leucopenia, purpura, eosinophilia
GI: Anorexia, nausea, vomiting, diarrhoea, abdominal discomfort, pseudomembranous colitis, liver damage
INTEG: Rash, flushing
MISC: Flu-like syndrome, red colouration of body fluids
RESP: Wheezing, dyspnoea
MS: Myopathy

Contraindications: Hypersensitivity, jaundice

Precautions: Pregnancy, hepatic impairment, alcoholism, breast feeding, soft contact lenses (permanent red staining), for treatment should always be given in combination to prevent resistance occurring, porphyria

Pharmacokinetics:
By mouth: Peak 2–3 hr, duration greater than 24 hr, half-life 2–5 hr (dose dependent) metabolised in liver (active/inactive metabolites), excreted mostly in bile, also in urine as free drug excreted in breast milk

Interactions/incompatibilities:
• Decreased effect of: barbiturates, clofibrate, corticosteroids, dapsone, anticoagulants, oral antidiabetics, hormones, digoxin, PAS, oral contraceptives, digitalis, vitamin D, phenytoin, quinidine, mexiletine, methadone, theophylline, chloramphenicol, ketoconazole, cyclosporin A, azathioprine, β-blockers, verapamil, cimetidine

Clinical assessment:
• Liver function tests before treatment and at regular intervals
• Regular blood counts during prolonged therapy
• Do not restart therapy stopped because of serious toxicity
• Reduce dose to 8 mg/kg in hepatic impairment
• If restarting therapy after a break, start at dose of 75 mg/day and increase towards therapeutic dose by 75 mg/day. Side effects more likely upon restarting

Lab. test interferences:
Interference: Folate level, vitamin B_{12}, bromsulphthalein, radiographic gall bladder studies

Treatment of overdose: Gastric lavage, activated charcoal, consider forced diuresis, haemodialysis, general supportive measures

NURSING CONSIDERATIONS

Assess:
• Liver function test before and during treatment
• Signs of anaemia including regular blood count Hb
• Pulse, BP, respirations and temperature
• Input and output of fluids check for decrease in output, urinalysis
• Weight

Administer:
• To be given half to one hour before food; use with other agents for treatment of infections to limit development of resistance
• Orally before meals or 2 hr after
• IV by infusion only over 2–3 hr
• Anti-emetics if vomiting occurs
• With food if severe GI upset, but absorption of rifampicin decreased

Evaluate:
• Therapeutic effect containment and decreased infection. Prophylaxis use for contacts preventing diseases
• Hepatic status, decreased appetite, jaundice, dark urine, fatigue
• Hypotension, shock, confusion, psychosis
• Anaemia, purpura, thrombocytopenia
• Nausea, vomiting, rash, flushing, flu-like symptoms

• Effects of other drugs increased or decreased
• Culture and sensitivity to detect resistance

Teach patient/family:

• To report purpura and any signs of bleeding immediately
• To report signs of jaundice—yellowing skin, eyes, dark urine and faeces
• Women using oral contraception require another method of contraception
• That tests and treatment may take many months, but correct dosage will be scheduled and must be taken as directed
• That permanent red staining of soft contact lenses can occur during therapy
• That urine, faeces, saliva, sputum, sweat, tears may be coloured red-orange

---

rimiterol hydrobromide (inhaled)

Pulmadil, Pulmadil Auto
Func. class.: Bronchodilator
Chem. class.: Adrenergic β2 stimulant
Legal class.: POM

Action: Selective β_2 stimulation of receptors in respiratory smooth muscle producing bronchodilation
Uses: Reversible airways obstruction, especially when short action required
Dosage and routes:
• *Adult and child:* Inhalation (aerosol) 200–600 mcg (1–3 puffs) up to 8 times daily; do not repeat in less than 30 mins
Available forms include: Aerosol inhalation, 200 mcg metred dose inhaler
Side effects/adverse reactions:
CNS: Headache
INTEG: Rash
META: Hypokalaemia
RESP: Paradoxical bronchospasm
Contraindications: Hypersensitivity to the drug
Precautions: Pregnancy
Pharmacokinetics: Readily absorbed, subject to first pass metabolism and metabolism by catechol-*O*-methyltransferase. Very short half-life of less than 5 min
Interactions/incompatibilities:
• May inhibit effect β-blockers
Clinical assessment:
• Regular serum potassium monitoring
Treatment of overdose: Symptomatic relief only necessary

NURSING CONSIDERATIONS

Assess:
• Baseline pulse; Tachycardia may occur
Administer:
• Shake before use to disperse particles
• Using correct inhaler technique
• Wait for 1 min between puffs
Perform/provide:
• Do not puncture or burn container
Evaluate:
• Patient's technique to ensure correct
• Therapeutic response—improvement in respiratory status
Teach patient/family:
• Correct technique for administration—this should be checked periodically
• Administration of drug to children must always be supervised by a responsible adult
• Wait for 1 min between inhalations to allow assessment of response
• Not to administer more than eight treatments in any 24 hr
• Not to take any non-prescribed medication without consulting clinician

• Seek medical advice if the usual degree of symptomatic relief is not obtained

risperidone

Risperdal ▼
Func. class.: Antipsychotic
Chem. class.: Benzisoxazole-derivative
Legal class.: POM

Action: Potent antagonist of dopamine at D_2 receptors and serotonin at 5-HT_2 receptors. Also has antagonist properties at alpha$_2$-adrenergic receptors and, with lower potency, at alpha$_1$-adrenergic receptors and H_1-histaminergic receptors. Balanced central serotonin and dopamine antagonism may explain its efficacy against both positive and negative symptoms of psychosis, and its relatively low tendency to produce extrapyramidal side effects

Uses: Acute and chronic schizophrenic psychoses, and other psychotic conditions in which positive and/or negative symptoms are prominent

Dosage and routes:

• *Adult:* By mouth, initially 1 mg twice a day increased to 3 mg twice a day over 3 days; dosage may be maintained at this level or further adjusted. Usual optimum dosage is in the range 2–4 mg twice a day; doses above 5 mg twice a day should be used with caution; max. 8 mg twice a day

• *Elderly:* By mouth, initially 0.5 mg twice a day increased cautiously, if required, to 1–2 mg twice a day

• *Renal and hepatic impairment:* By mouth, initially 0.5 mg twice a day increased cautiously, if required, to 1–2 mg twice a day

Available forms include: Tablets 1, 2, 3, 4 mg

Side effects/adverse reactions:

CNS: Insomnia, agitation, anxiety, headache, somnolence, fatigue, dizziness, impaired concentration; extrapyramidal symptoms including tremor, rigidity, bradykinesia, akathisia, acute dystonia, seizures

CV: Orthostatic dizziness, orthostatic hypotension with reflex tachycardia

EENT: Rhinitis, hypersalivation

ELECT: Hyponatraemia

ENDO: Hyperprolactinaemia causing galactorrhoea and menstrual irregularities; inappropriate secretion of antidiuretic hormone causing hyponatraemia

GU: Erectile dysfunction, ejaculatory dysfunction, orgasmic dysfunction, menstrual disturbances

INTEG: Rash

MISC: Neuroleptic malignant syndrome, polydipsia

Contraindications: Hypersensitivity; breast-feeding

Precautions: Cardiovascular disease; Parkinson's disease; epilepsy; pregnancy

Pharmacokinetics: Completely absorbed following oral administration; peak plasma concentrations reached within 1–2 hr; metabolised to active metabolites, excreted in urine; elimination half-life of risperidone and its active metabolites 24 hr

Interactions: Antagonism of: amantidine, bromocriptine, levodopa, lysuride, pergolide

Treatment of overdose: Gastric lavage and administration of a laxative; cardiovascular monitoring including continuous electrocardiography; supportive treatment including IV fluids and/or sympathomimetic agents for hypotension and circulatory collapse

NURSING CONSIDERATIONS

Assess:

• Current psychotic status (including self-neglect) and medication; risk of hoarding or giving tablets to others
• BP, standing and lying
• Baseline weight

Administer:
• As prescribed and titrated gradually over first 3 days; thereafter dose individualised as necessary
• With or after food, but with a full glass of water

Perform/provide:
• Extra fluids and appropriate diet to help constipation

Evaluate:
• Therapeutic effect: reduction of symptoms (hallucinations, delusions, hostility, withdrawal, poverty of speech)
• Side effects: insomnia, agitation, orthostatic hypotension, extrapyramidal symptoms (distressing involuntary movements, particularly of the face and head)
• Weight; may be gained on Risperidone

Teach patient/family:
• To take medication as prescribed
• About side effects and to report these promptly to nurse or clinician
• To rise slowly from sitting or lying position if dizziness occurs
• Not to discontinue medication without seeking professional advice first

---

ritodrine HCl

Yutopar
Func. class.: Myometrial relaxant
Chem. class.: β_2-adrenergic agent
Legal class.: POM

Action: Reduces frequency, intensity of uterine contractions by stimulation of the β_2 receptors in uterine smooth muscle

Uses: Preterm labour, fetal asphyxia in labour where it is desired to obtain uterine relaxation

Dosage and routes:
• *Adult:* IV infusion 50 mcg/min, increased gradually by 50 mcg/min every 10 min until desired response or control maternal heart rate reaches 140 beats per minute, usually 150–350 mcg/min continue 12–48 hr after contractions have ceased. Then by mouth 10 mg given ½ hr before termination of IV, then 10 mg every 2 hr for 24 hr, then 10–20 mg every 4–6 hr, not to exceed 120 mg/day. IM 10 mg every 3–8 hrs continued 12–48 hr after contractions have ceased followed by oral therapy

Available forms include: Tablets 10 mg; IV/IM injection 10 mg/ml

Side effects/adverse reactions:
META: Hyperglycaemia in diabetics
CNS: Headache, anxiety, nervousness, tremor
GI: Nausea, vomiting, anorexia, malaise
CV: Tachycardia palpitation, hypotension
INTEG: Flushing, sweating

Contraindications: Hypersensitivity, antepartum haemorrhage which requires immediate delivery, eclampsia and severe pre-eclampsia, intra-uterine fetal death, chorioamnionitis, maternal cardiac disease, cord compression

Precautions: Heart disease, first 16 weeks of pregnancy, diabetes, hypertension, mild to moderate pre-eclampsia, hyperthyroidism

Pharmacokinetics:
Metabolised in liver, excreted in urine

Interactions/incompatibilities:
• Increased risk of hypokalaemia: potassium depleting diuretics, corticosteroids, theophylline
• Pulmonary oedema: corticosteroids

• Increased effects of: general anaesthetics

Clinical assessment:

• Maternal heart rate during infusion, maintain below 140 beats per minute

• Monitor blood glucose during IV infusion in diabetics

NURSING CONSIDERATIONS

Assess:

• Maternal, pulse rate

• For premature labour

• Intensity, length of uterine contractions

• Blood glucose in diabetics

Administer:

• By infusion pump, and monitor carefully

Perform/provide:

• Explanation of procedure

• Call bell

• Continuous CTG

Evaluate:

• Therapeutic response: decreased intensity, length of contraction, absence of preterm labour, decreased BP

• Maternal pulse rate

• Foetal heart rate

• Dilatation of cervix

Teach patient/family:

• To remain in bed during infusion

• Relevance of treatment

• Possible side effects

---

salbutamol (inhaled)

Aerolin Autohaler, Maxivent, Steri-Neb Salamol, Salbulin, Salbutamol Cyclocaps, Ventodisks, Ventolin

Func. class.: Bronchodilator

Chem. class.: Adrenergic β_2 stimulant

Legal class.: POM

Action: Selective β_2 stimulation of receptors in respiratory smooth muscle producing bronchodilation

Uses: Treatment of reversible obstructive airways disease

Dosage and routes:

Acute and intermittent asthma and wheezing

• *Adult:* By aerosol inhalation 100–200 mcg (1–2 puffs) as needed; by powder inhalation 200–400 mcg as needed

• *Child:* By aerosol inhalation 100 mcg (1 puff) as needed; by powder inhalation 200 mcg as needed

Prophylaxis of exercise-induced bronchospasm

• *Adult:* By aerosol inhalation 200 mcg (2 puffs); by powder inhalation 400 mcg

• *Child:* By aerosol inhalation 100 mcg (1 puff); by powder inhalation 200 mcg

Chronic maintenance therapy

• *Adult:* By aerosol inhalation 200 mcg (2 puffs) 3–4 times daily; by powder inhalation 400 mcg 3–4 times daily

• *Child:* By aerosol inhalation 100–200 mcg (1–2 puffs) 3–4 times daily; powder inhalation 200 mcg 3–4 times daily

Chronic bronchitis unresponsive to conventional therapy and severe acute asthma

• *Adult:* By nebulisation 2.5–5 mg repeated up to 4 times daily; may be increased to 10 mg in refractory, severe, acute asthma if side effects permit

• *Child:* By nebulisation 2.5–5 mg repeated up to 4 times daily

Available forms include: Metered-dose aerosol inhaler 100 mcg per actuation; breath-actuated aerosol inhalation 100 mcg per actuation; disks containing 8 powder blisters for use in Diskhaler device 200 mcg, 400 mcg per blister; capsules (Rotacaps, Cyclocap containing powder for inhalation via inhaler device (Rotahaler, Cyclohaler) 200, 400 mcg (as sulphate);

concentrated solution for use in nebuliser 5 mg/ml (as sulphate); isotonic solution for nebulisation, unit dose Nebules 2.5 mg, 5 mg (as sulphate) in 2.5 ml

Side effects/adverse reactions:
CV: Tachycardia, peripheral vasodilatation
CNS: Headache
ELEC: Hypokalaemia
INTEG: Urticaria
MS: Tremor, cramps
MISC: Hyperactivity in children, hypersensitivity reactions including anaphylaxis and angioedema
RESP: Paradoxical bronchospasm

Contraindications: Hypersensitivity

Precautions: Hyperthyroidism; pregnancy; breast feeding; hypokalaemic patients or those at risk of developing hypokalaemia because of concomitant therapy

Interactions:
• Increased risk of hypokalaemia with: aminophylline, corticosteroids, diuretics, theophylline
• Risk of acute angle closure glaucoma when nebulised with ipratroprium

Treatment of overdose: The preferred antidote is a cardio-selective β-blocker. However, such drugs must be used with extreme caution in patients with a history of bronchospasm

NURSING CONSIDERATIONS

Assess:
• Baseline vital signs, lung sounds, respiratory capacity

Administer:
• Using correct technique for each device, i.e.:
 – Diskhole blisters should only be pierced immediately before inhalation
 – nebuliser solution to be diluted with normal saline to a volume appropriate to the nebuliser
 – oxygen as the carrier gas when nebulising drug for patients with severe asthma attacks
 – air as the carrier gas for patients with chronic bronchitis and hypercapria
• After shaking aerosol, patient should exhale, place mouthpiece in mouth, press aerosol and inhale slowly, hold breath for 10 s and exhale slowly

Perform/provide:
• Storage: nebuliser solution protected from the light and used within one month of opening the bottle

Evaluate:
• Therapeutic effect, absence of dyspnoea, wheezing after 1 hr
• For side effects

Teach patient/family:
• Good technique in use of device
• How to store, use, clean and care for the inhaler and disks
• About the side effects of the drug, (shakiness, flushing, headache, dry mouth)
• To avoid getting solution in the eyes
• To avoid smoky atmospheres, people with respiratory infection
• Techniques for averting asthma attacks (use of space) and how to deal with attack if it occurs
• Not to exceed the prescribed dosage

salbutamol (oral, parenteral)

Ventolin, Ventolin CR, Volmax
Func. class.: Bronchodilator and uterine relaxant
Chem. class.: Adrenergic β_2 stimulant
Legal class.: POM

Action: Selective β_2 stimulation of receptors in respiratory smooth muscle producing bronchodilation and in uterus reducing frequency and intensity of uterine contractions

Uses: Treatment of reversible obstructive airways disease and the management of premature labour

Dosage and routes:

Obstructive airways disease

Severe bronchospasm and status asthmaticus

• *Adult:* By SC or IM injection 500 mcg repeated every 4 hr as required; IV 250 mcg injected slowly and repeated if necessary; IV infusion 5 mcg/min, adjusted according to response and heart rate usually in range 3–20 mcg/min, more if necessary

Routine management:

• *Adult:* By mouth 4 mg (occasionally up to 8 mg or as little as 2 mg) 3–4 times daily; modified release 8 mg twice daily

Elderly: By mouth 2 mg 3–4 times daily; modified release 8 mg twice daily

• *Child under 2 yr:* By mouth 100 mcg/kg body weight 4 times daily

• *Child 2–6 yr:* By mouth 1–2 mcg 3–4 times daily; modified release (in children over 3 yr) 4 mg twice daily

• *Child 6–12 yr:* By mouth 2 mg 3–4 times daily; modified release 4 mg twice daily

Prevention of premature labour:

• *Adult:* By IV infusion 10 mcg/min gradually increased to maximum 45 mcg/min until contractions have ceased, then gradually reduced; IV or IM injection 100–250 mcg repeated according to patient's response; subsequently by mouth 4 mg every 6–8 hr.

Available forms include: Injection 50, 500 mcg/ml (as sulphate); solution of IV infusion 1 mg/ml (as sulphate); syrup 2 mg/5ml; tablets 2, 4 mg; tablets, modified release 4, 8 mg

Side effects/adverse reactions:

CV: Tachycardia, peripheral vasodilatation, mild hypotension

CNS: Headache

ELECT: Hypokalaemia

GI: Nausea and vomiting when used for premature labour

INTEG: Urticaria, pain at IM injection site

MS: Tremor, cramps

MISC: Hyperactivity in children, hypersensitivity reactions including anaphylaxis and angio-oedema

RESP: Pulmonary oedema when used for premature labour

Contraindications: Hypersensitivity; management of threatened abortion or premature labour complicated by placenta praevia; antepartum haemorrhage; toxaemia of pregnancy; eclampsia; severe pre-eclampsia, intra-uterine infection

Precautions:

General: Hyperthyroidism; breast feeding; hypokalaemic patients or those at risk of developing hypokalaemia because of concomitant therapy; myocardial insufficiency; arrhythmias; hypertension; IV in diabetes mellitus

Obstructive airways disease: Pregnancy

Premature labour: Suspected cardiac disease; mild to moderate pre-eclampsia; overhydration

Interactions:

• Increased risk of hypokalaemia with: aminophylline, corticosteroids, diuretics, theophylline

• Antagonised by: β-blockers

Treatment of overdose: The preferred antidote is a cardio-selective β-blocker. However, such drugs must be used with extreme caution in patients with a history of bronchospasm

NURSING CONSIDERATIONS

Assess:

• Baseline vital signs, lung sounds and respiratory capacity in patients with obstructive airways disease

• Baseline vital signs and rate and strength of uterine contractions in premature labour patients
• Blood glucose if patient is diabetic

Administer:
• IV with appropriate technique and care of IV line, rate adjusted according to response. Salbutamol solution for IV infusion should be diluted to a concentration of not more than 500 mcg/ml before infusion. Parenteral preparation should be diluted with sodium chloride or dextrose or dextrose with sodium chloride
• By mouth – modified release tablets should be swallowed whole

Perform/provide:
Storage: protect from light. Store admixtures for not longer than 24 hr

Evaluate:
• Therapeutic effect, absence of dyspnoea (chest patients); cessation of contractions (pregnancy)
• For side effects including elevation of blood sugar in diabetics when given IV

Teach patient/family:
• About the function of the drug
• About the side effects of the drug, shakiness, flushing, headache, dry mouth
• That IM injection causes slight pain and stinging
• To avoid smoky atmospheres, people with respiratory infection
• Techniques for averting asthma attacks (use of space) and how to deal with attack if it occurs
• Not to exceed the prescribed dosage

salcatonin

Calsynar, Miacalcic
Func. class.: Thyroparathyroid agent (calcium regulator)
Chem. class.: Synthetic polypeptide hormone
Legal class.: POM

Action: Decreases: bone resorption, blood calcium levels; increases deposits of calcium in bones

Uses: Hypercalcaemia, postmenopausal osteoporosis of malignancy, Paget's Disease, pain associated with bone cancer

Dosage and routes:

Hypercalcaemia
• IM/Subcutaneous up to 8 units/kg 6–8 hrly adjusted as required; IV Infusion (Miacalcic) 5–10 units/kg over at least 6 hr in 500 ml physiological saline

Paget's disease
• IM/Subcutaneous initially 50–100 units 3 times weekly increased to daily if needed for 3–6 months

Bone pain (neoplastic disease)
• IM/Subcutaneous 200 units 6-hrly or 400 units 12-hrly for 24–48 hr

Post-menopausal osteoporosis
• IM/Subcutaneous 100 units/day plus calcium and vitamin D

Available forms include: Injectable subcutaneous/IM 50, 100, 200 units/ml; injectable IV 50, 100 units/ml

Side effects/adverse reactions:
INTEG: Rash, flushing, irritation at injection site
CNS: Dizziness
GU: Diuresis, calcitonin antibody formation
GI: Nausea, diarrhoea, vomiting, unpleasant taste
MS: Tingling of hands
SYST: Anaphylactic and other allergic reactions

Contraindications: Hypersensi-

tivity, pregnancy, breast-feeding
Precautions: Renal disease, pregnancy, children
Pharmacokinetics:
IM/Subcutaneous: Onset 15 min, peak 1 hr, elimination half-life 70–90 min, metabolised by kidneys, excreted as inactive metabolites
IV: Plasma half-life less than 15 min
Interactions/incompatibilities:
- Theoretically may enhance toxicity of cardiac glycosides by producing rapid change serum electrolytes
- Dilution for IV use results in potency loss of approximately 20%

Clinical assessment:
- Reductions in serum alkaline phosphatase, urinary hydroxyproline denote response in Paget's Disease; lowered serum calcium in hypercalcaemia. Check for response, continued response

Treatment of overdose: Not likely to be significant, treatment supportive.

NURSING CONSIDERATIONS

Assess:
- Nutritional status; diet for sources of vitamin D (milk, some seafood), calcium (dairy products, dark green vegetables), phosphates
- Systemic allergic reaction to drug: skin test before first dose

Administer:
- Do not give Miacalcic injection as bolus (contains phenol)
- With anti-emetic at night if GI symptoms

Perform/provide:
- Urinalysis
- Storage in refrigerator
- Restriction of sodium, potassium if required

Evaluate:
- Local reaction at injection site
- GI symptoms, polyuria, flushing, tingling, headache for sediment

Teach patient/family:
- Avoid non-prescribed medicines
- All aspects of drug: action, side effects, dose, when to notify clinician

salicylic acid

Func. class.: Keratolytic
Legal class.: GSL

Action: Corrects abnormal keratinization and causes peeling of skin
Uses: Dandruff, seborrhoeic dermatitis, psoriasis, multiple superficial epitheliomatoses, hyperkeratosis, tinea, removal of warts
Dosage and routes:
- *Adult and child:* Apply as required

Available forms include: Ointment 2%; collodion 12%; plaster 20%, 40%; lotion 2%. Also many combination products
Side effects/adverse reactions:
INTEG: Irritation, drying
CNS: Salicylism: hearing loss, tinnitus, dizziness
Contraindications:
Hypersensitivity
Treatment of overdose: Overdose not likely in normal use

NURSING CONSIDERATIONS

Administer:
- Only to intact skin; do not use on inflamed, broken skin
- Apply after wetting skin; wash thoroughly each morning after treatment

Evaluate:
- Therapeutic response: decrease in dandruff, size of lesions
- Salicylism: tinnitus, hearing loss, dizziness
- Allergic reactions: irritation, redness

Teach patient/family:
- To avoid contact with eyes, mucous membranes
- To apply lotion if drying occurs

salmeterol (inhaler) ▼

Serevent

Func. class.: Bronchodilator (long-acting)

Chem. class.: Adrenergic β_2 stimulant

Legal class.: POM

Action: Selective β_2 stimulation of receptors in respiratory smooth muscle producing bronchodilation; also has modulatory action on inflammatory processes in the lung, though the significance of these is currently unclear

Uses: Long-term treatment of reversible obstructive airways disease; not a replacement for oral or inhaled corticosteroids; unsuitable for the relief of acute asthmatic symptoms

Dosage and routes:

• *Adult:* By inhalation of powder (Diskhaler) or aerosol 50–100 mcg twice daily

Available forms include: Disks containing 4 powder blisters for use in Diskhaler device 50 mcg (as xinafoate) per blister; metered-dose aerosol inhaler 25 mcg (as xinafoate) per actuation

Side effects/adverse reactions:

CV: Palpitations

CNS: Headache

ELECT: Hypokalaemia

INTEG: Skin reactions, local irritation

MISC: Non-specific chest pain

MS: Tremor, cramps, arthralgia

RESP: Paradoxical bronchospasm

Contraindications: Hypersensitivity

Precautions: Hyperthyroidism; pregnancy; breast feeding; hypokalaemic patients or those at risk of developing hypokalaemia because of concomitant therapy

Interactions:

• Increased risk of hypokalaemia with: aminophylline, corticosteroids, diuretics, theophylline

Treatment of overdose: The preferred antidote is a cardio-selective β-blocker. However, such drugs must be used with extreme caution in patients with a history of bronchospasm

NURSING CONSIDERATIONS

Assess:

• Baseline vital signs, lung sounds, respiratory capacity

Administer:

• Using correct technique for device supplied, i.e.:

– Diskhole blisters should be pierced immediately before inhalation

– after shaking the aerosol, patient should exhale, place mouthpiece in mouth, press aerosol and inhale slowly, hold breath for 10 s and exhale slowly

Perform/provide:

• Storage protected from sunlight

Evaluate:

• Therapeutic response, absence of dyspnoea, wheezing

• For side effects

Teach patient/family:

• Good technique in use of device

• How to store disks, how to clean and care for the inhaler

• About side effects of the drug (shakiness, headache, cramps, dry mouth)

• To avoid smoky atmospheres, people with respiratory infection

• Techniques to avert asthma attack (use of space) and how to deal with attack if it occurs

• Not to exceed the prescribed dosage

selegiline

Eldepryl
Func. class.: Antiparkinsonian agent
Chem. class.: Monoamine-oxidase-*B* inhibitor
Legal class.: POM

Action: Prevents breakdown of dopamine in the brain, inhibits re-uptake of dopamine at the pre-synaptic dopamine receptor, thus prolonging the effect of endogenous dopamine and levodopa
Uses: Adjunctive treatment in Parkinson's disease
Dosage and routes:
• *By mouth:* 10 mg in morning or 5 mg at breakfast time and 5 mg at midday alone or as an adjunct to levodopa therapy
Available forms include: Tablets 5 mg
Side effects/adverse reactions:
CNS: Confusion, agitation, psychosis
CV: Hypotension
GI: Nausea, vomiting
Contraindications: Pregnancy
Precautions: Side effects of levodopa may be increased; concurrent levodopa dose may need to be reduced by 25–50%
Pharmacokinetics:
By mouth: Rapidly and completely absorbed, plasma half-life 39 hr, metabolised in liver, excreted in urine
Interactions/incompatibilities:
• Risk of hypertensive crises with: non-selective MAOIs
• Note: Selegiline does not require dietary restrictions of the type needed with non-specific MAOIs
Clinical assessment:
• Reduce concurrent levodopa dose if side-effects are increased with selegiline
Treatment of overdose: Low toxicity, observe 24–48 hr, symptomatic treatment
NURSING CONSIDERATIONS
Assess:
• Baseline BP—hypotension may occur
Administer:
• With breakfast and at midday or as single dose in the morning
Evaluate:
• Check to ensure patient has swallowed tablet
• Confusion: patient may need reassurance and careful explanations if confused
• Therapeutic response: reduction in parkinsonian symptoms

selenium sulphide

Selsun, Lenium
Func. class.: Antibiotic, topical
Legal class.: P

Action: Unknown
Uses: Dandruff, seborrhoea in scalp
Dosage and routes:
• *Adult and child:* Topical, wash hair with 1–2 tsp, leave on 2–3 min; rinse, repeat, use twice a week for 2 weeks then once a week or as needed
Available forms include: Shampoo 2.5%
Side effects/adverse reactions:
INTEG: Oiliness of hair/scalp, alopecia, discolouration of hair
Contraindications: Hypersensitivity, inflamed skin
Precautions: Child under 5 yr, pregnancy
Interactions/incompatibilities:
• Do not use within 2 days of dyeing, tinting, waving the hair
Treatment of overdose:
Unknown in normal use. If swallowed induce vomiting/gastric lavage, supportive treatment

NURSING CONSIDERATIONS

Perform/provide:

• Thorough hair rinsing after use

Evaluate:

• Toxicity: tremors, perspiration, pain in abdomen, weakness, anorexia

• Area of body involved, including time involved, what helps or aggravates condition

Teach patient/family:

• To avoid contact with eyes, genital area

• To discontinue use if rash or irritation occurs

• That drug may damage jewellery, remove before application

• That drug is not to be taken internally

• Should not be used within 48 hr of applying hair colouring or perm solution

senna

NHS Senokot

Func. class.: Laxative

Chem. class.: Anthraquinone glycoside

Legal class.: P/GSL (small packs)

Action: Stimulates peristalsis by action on Auerbach's plexus

Uses: Constipation, bowel preparation for surgery or examination, avoidance of straining after cerebral and cardiovascular disease

Dosage and routes:

• *Adult:* By mouth 2–4 tablets, 5–10 ml granules, 10–20 ml syrup at bedtime

• *Child (over 6 yr):* Half adult doses taken in the morning

• *Child (2–6 yr):* 2.5 ml–5 ml syrup in the morning

Available forms include: Tablets 7.5 mg; granules; 15 mg/5 ml; syrup 7.5 mg/5 ml, (as sennoside B)

Side effects/adverse reactions:

GI: Nausea, vomiting, anorexia, cramps, diarrhoea, loss of bowel tone

META: Hypokalaemia

Contraindications: Hypersensitivity; intestinal obstruction; abdominal pain (undiagnosed); acute surgical abdomen

Pharmacokinetics:

By mouth: Onset 6–24 hr; metabolised by liver, excreted in faeces

Interactions/incompatibilities: None known

Clinical assessment:

• Physical examination if 3 days of increasing dose fail to produce bowel motion

• Blood electrolytes if drug is used often by patient

Treatment of overdose: Supportive, plenty of fluid for diarrhoea

NURSING CONSIDERATIONS

Assess:

• Fluid balance

Administer:

• In morning or evening (oral dose)

• Tablets with a drink

• Granules may be stirred into hot milk, sprinkled in food or eaten as they are

Evaluate:

• Therapeutic response: return to normal bowel habit

• Cause of constipation; identify whether fluids, fibre, or exercise is missing from lifestyle

• Cramping, rectal bleeding, nausea, vomiting; seek medical advice if these occur

Teach patient/family:

• That normal bowel movements do not always occur daily

• That shortage of fluids, fibre, and lack of exercise contribute to constipation

• Not to use laxatives for long-term therapy; bowel tone will be lost

• Do not use in presence of

abdominal pain, nausea, vomiting
• Notify clinician if constipation unrelieved or if symptoms of electrolyte imbalance occur: muscle cramps, pain, weakness, dizziness

sermorelin ▼

Geref 50
Func. class.: Growth hormone releasing hormone (GHRH) analogue
Chem. class.: Peptide
Legal class.: POM

Action: Acts directly on the somatotrophs of the anterior pituitary, stimulating growth hormone (somatotrophin) release
Uses: Diagnostic agent used to test the functional capacity and response of growth hormone secreting cells of the anterior pituitary to stimulation
Dosage and routes:
• *Adult and Child:* By IV injection 1 mcg/kg body weight in the morning following an overnight fast
Available forms include: Injection 50 mcg
Side effects/adverse reactions:
INTEG: Facial heat, facial flushing, pain at injection site
Contraindications: Hypersensitivity; pregnancy; breast feeding
Precautions: Epilepsy; untreated hypothyroidism; obesity; hyperglycaemia; elevated plasma fatty acids
Interactions:
• Response to sermorelin influenced by drugs affecting growth hormone release including: growth hormone (discontinue 1–2 weeks before test), antithyroid drugs, NSAIDs, drugs affecting the release of somatostatin, insulin or glucocorticoids

NURSING CONSIDERATIONS
Assess:
• Fasting status
Administer:
• In the morning after overnight fast.
• Reconstituting injection with solvent immediately prior to use
Perform/provide:
• Storage of injection powder in refrigerator prior to reconstitution
Evaluate:
• For side effects
Teach patient/family:
• Reasons for administering drug

sertraline ▼

Lustral
Func. class.: Antidepressant
Chem. class.: Serotonin (5HT) reuptake inhibitor
Legal class.: POM

Action: Selectively inhibits reuptake of the central neurotransmitter serotonin with little effect on noradrenaline
Uses: Depressive illness
Dosage and routes:
• *Adult:* By mouth, starting dose 50 mg once a day, adjusted according to response; maximum daily dose 200 mg. Doses of 150 mg or more should not be used for periods exceeding 8 weeks
Available forms include: Tablets 50, 100 mg
Side effects/adverse reactions:
CNS: Tremor
EENT: Dry mouth
GI: Nausea, diarrhoea, dyspepsia, raised liver enzymes
GU: Ejaculatory delay
INTEG: Increased sweating
Contraindications: Hypersensitivity; unstable epilepsy; MAOIs within 14 days of starting treatment
Precautions: Pregnancy; breast

feeding; electroconvulsive therapy; epilepsy; hepatic and renal impairment
Interactions:
• Risk of toxicity with MAOIs—do not give sertraline with, or for 14 days after, MAOIs; do not give MAOIs for at least 7 days after stopping sertraline
• Risk of CNS toxicity with: lithium, sumatriptan, tryptophan
Treatment of overdose: Gastric lavage within 12 hr of ingestion; symptomatic and supportive treatment
NURSING CONSIDERATIONS
Assess:
• History of epilepsy, alcoholism
Administer:
• Tablets with food
Evaluate:
• Therapeutic response (dosage will be adjusted accordingly)
• For side effects
Teach patient/family:
• To take tablets with food
• Need for compliance with regime
• Not to take alcohol, or with MAOIs

silver nitrate

Func. class.: Keratolytic
Legal class.: P

Action: Possesses anti-infective, astringent, caustic properties
Uses: Cauterisation of lesions, warts, over-granulation of wounds
Dosage and routes:
• *Adult and child:* Apply as directed by clinician
Available forms include: Sticks
Side effects/adverse reactions:
INTEG: Skin discolouration
Contraindications: Hypersensitivity
NURSING CONSIDERATIONS
Administer:
• Apply to lesion only after protecting surrounding tissue with petroleum jelly
• After moistening stick with water
Evaluate:
• Therapeutic response: absence of lesions
Teach patient/family:
• To handle very carefully with dry hands or wearing surgical gloves
• To avoid contact with healthy tissue
• To avoid contact with clothing
• Not to moisten with saliva
• Keep away from children

silver sulphadiazine (topical)

Flamazine
Func. class.: Antibiotic
Chem. class.: Sulphonamide
Legal class.: POM

Action: Interferes with bacterial cell wall synthesis
Uses: Burns (2nd, 3rd degree), infected leg ulcers, pressure sores
Dosage and routes:
• *Adult and child:* Topical, apply to affected area usually daily; for leg ulcers apply at least 3 times a week
Available forms include: Cream 1%
Side effects/adverse reactions:
INTEG: Rash, urticaria, stinging, burning, itching
HAEM: Leucopenia
Contraindications: Hypersensitivity, premature infants and newborn
Precautions: Impaired renal function, pregnancy, impaired hepatic function, lactation
Pharmacokinetics: Up to 10% absorbed from large wounds, metabolism slow
Interactions/incompatibilities:
• Increased blood levels of: oral

hypoglycaemics, phenytoin

NURSING CONSIDERATIONS

Administer:

- Using aseptic technique
- After cleansing debris before each application
- Analgesic before application if needed
- Enough medication to cover burns completely, keep covered with medication at all times

Evaluate:

- Allergic reaction: burning, stinging, swelling, redness
- Therapeutic response: development of granulation tissue

Teach patient/family:

- That drug may be continued until graft can be done
- To move digits inside the plastic
- That grey coloured exudate is normal

---

simvastatin

Zocor

Func. class.: Hypolipidaemic agent
Chem. class.: HMG CoA reductase inhibitor
Legal class.: POM

Action: Competitive inhibitor of HMG CoA reductase

Uses: Primary hypercholesterolaemia unresponsive to other therapy, with a cholesterol level in excess of 7.8 mmol/l

Dosage and routes:

- *Adult:* By mouth initially 10 mg at night, adjusted at intervals of not less than 4 weeks; usual range 10–40 mg once daily at night

Available forms include: Tablets 10 mg, 20 mg

Side effects/adverse reactions:

CNS: Headache, fatigue
GI: Constipation, flatulence, nausea, dyspepsia, abdominal cramps, diarrhoea, raised liver enzymes
INTEG: Rash
MS: Myopathy

Contraindications: Active liver disease; pregnancy, women must be adequately protected by non-hormonal contraceptive methods; lactation

Precautions: Avoid conception for 1 month after treatment, history of liver disease/alcohol abuse

Pharmacokinetics: Simvastatin is activated by extensive first-pass metabolism to form active metabolites. Mainly excreted in the bile

Interactions/incompatibilities:

- Increased risk of myositis when given with: nicotinic acid, fibric acid derivatives, cyclosporin, other immunosuppressants
- Increased effects of: oral anticoagulants

Clinical assessment:

- Liver function tests before treatment then periodically
- Monitor serum creatine phosphokinase regularly in patients on drugs increasing risk of myositis

Treatment of overdose:
Supportive measures, monitor liver function

NURSING CONSIDERATIONS

Assess:

- For signs of vitamin A, D, K deficiency

Administer:

- Drug with meals if GI symptoms occur

Evaluate:

- Therapeutic response
- Bowel pattern daily; increase bulk, water in diet if constipation develops

Teach patient/family:

- To take tablet at night or with meals to reduce incidence of GI complications
- To have good fibre/fluid intake if prone to constipation
- To report any rash to clinician
- To remain on low fat diet to help the tablet work effectively

smallpox vaccine

Func. class.: Vaccine; live, attenuated
Legal class.: POM

Action: Stimulates production of specific antibodies against smallpox virus
Uses: Prevention of smallpox. Following global elimination of smallpox, vaccination is now only appropriate to those such as laboratory workers who are exposed to pox viruses such as vaccinia. Guidance for laboratory staff has been prepared by the Advisory Committee on Dangerous Pathogens and the Advisory Committee on Genetic Manipulation
Dosage and routes:
• *Adult:* Inoculate into the skin by scarification or pressure about 0.02 ml of reconstituted vaccine
• *Note:* Specialist advice should be sought on the need for primary immunisation and reinforcing doses
Available forms include: Injection ampoules with diluent
Side effects/adverse reactions:
CNS: Malaise, headache, post-vaccinal encephalitis
CV: Myocarditis, pericarditis
GI: Vomiting
GU: Glomerulonephritis, vaginitis
INTEG: Development of pustular lesion at site of application; urticaria; purpura; eczema vaccinatum
MISC: Regional lymphadenopathy
SYST: Fever; rigor; generalised vaccinia infection; secondary bacterial and viral infections
Contraindications: Eczema or history of eczema, acute illness, patients with compromised immunity including those suffering from malignant disease or receiving cytototoxic chemotherapy, immunosuppressive drugs, high doses of corticosteroids or radiotherapy
Note: Because of the lack of smallpox risk to the general population smallpox vaccination should be considered to be generally contraindicated unless recommended by an appropriate expert
Precautions: Pregnancy, breast-feeding
Interactions:
• Reduced effect and danger of systemic infections with: immunosuppressive agents including high-dose corticosteroids; cytotoxic chemotherapy; azathioprine
Incompatibilities:
• Alcohol—if skin is swabbed with alcohol prior to injection it must be allowed to dry completely before application
• Do not mix with any other vaccine or drug

NURSING CONSIDERATIONS

Assess:
• Vaccination status
Administer:
• After seeking specialist advice on technique of administration
• Using dilutent supplied
• On outer aspect of upper arm or mid thigh
• Covering the inoculation site with occlusive dressing
Perform/provide:
• Rubber or plastic gloves for administration (to be disposed of immediately after according to regulations related to disposal of dangerous pathogens)
• Wash hands thoroughly after handling vaccine
• NB Accidental infection of eyes by contaminated fingers may cause corneal scarring or blindness
• Equipment and facilities for dealing with anaphylactic reactions
Evaluate:
• For signs and symptoms of successful vaccination;
• For anaphylactic reaction

Teach patient/family:
• About side-effects of vaccination: sore, swollen area at site of injection, swollen glands, fever, malaise
• Not to wet the area of injection or to remove occlusive covering

sodium aurothiomalate

Myocrisin
Func. class.: Antirheumatic
Chem. class.: Gold complex
Legal class.: POM

Action: Anti-inflammatory action unknown; may decrease phagocytosis, lysosomal activity, prostaglandin synthesis
Uses: Active progressive, rheumatoid arthritis, juvenile chronic arthritis
Dosage and routes:
• *Adult:* Seek expert advice. Deep IM injection, 10 mg test dose in the first week followed by weekly doses of 50 mg until signs of remission. Benefit is not expected until 300 to 500 mg has been given. The dose of 50 mg is continued at 2-week intervals until full remission. The interval between injections is then gradually increased to 4 weeks, then after 18 months to 2 yrs to 6 weeks and then continued for 5 yr. If there is no remission after 1 g has been given and no signs of gold toxicity are present, 6 injections of 100 mg at weekly intervals may be given. If after this time no signs of remission occur alternative treatments should be considered
• *Child:* Progressive juvenile chronic arthritis, deep IM injection 1 mg/kg weekly to a maximum dose of 50 mg weekly. A test dose corresponding to one-tenth to one-fifth of calculated dose should be given for 2–3 weeks. The dosing interval should be gradually increased first to 2 weeks then to 4 weeks according to response and continued for 1–5 yr
Available forms include: IM injection 10, 20, 50 mg in 0.5 ml
Side effects/adverse reactions:
EENT: Gold deposits in the eye
HAEM: Thrombocytopenia, agranulocytosis, aplastic anaemia, leucopenia, eosinophilia
INTEG: Rash, pruritus, dermatitis, exfoliative dermatitis, angioneurotic oedema
GI: Stomatitis, nausea, vomiting, alopecia, diarrhoea, metallic taste, jaundice, hepatitis
GU: Proteinuria, haematuria, nephrosis
RESP: Pulmonary fibrosis
CNS: Weakness, flushing
CV: Palpitations
INTEG: Local irritation at injection site
Contraindications: Hypersensitivity to gold, systemic lupus erythematosus, exfoliative dermatitis, pregnancy, breast-feeding, severe renal disease, severe liver disease, blood disorders, porphyria
Precautions: Decreased tolerance in elderly, necrotising enterocolitis, pulmonary fibrosis, diabetes mellitus
Interactions/incompatibilities:
• Increased risk blood dyscrasias: when given in combination with other therapy, capable of inducing blood disorders; oxyphenbutazone, phenylbutazone
Clinical assessment:
• Before each injection, full blood count and test urine for albumin
• Annual chest X-ray should be carried out

NURSING CONSIDERATIONS

Assess:
• Urinalysis for protein before each injection
Administer:
• By deep IM injection followed by gentle massage of the area

Evaluate:
• Improvement in disease symptoms after 6–8 weeks
• Proteinuria
• Slow rashes or mouth ulcers

Teach patient/family:
• If appropriate to test own urine and record it
• Report any skin rashes or mouth ulcers
• Full effectiveness after approximately 2 months
• Importance of regular injections
• Gold card to be carried
• May experience change in taste
• May get itchy skin
• May get heavy periods
• May get easy bruising or bleeding gums or nose
• Must report symptoms to clinician

sodium bicarbonate

Func. class.: Alkalinizer
Chem. class.: $NaHCO_3$
Legal class.: GSL, Injection, POM

Action: Orally neutralises gastric acid, which forms water, NaCl, CO_2; increases plasma bicarbonate, which buffers hydrogen ion concentration; reverses acidosis

Uses: Acidosis (metabolic), cardiac arrest, alkalinisation (systemic/urinary) antacid

Dosage and routes:

Acidosis
• *Adult and child:* Slow IV injection, a strong solution (up to 8.4%) or by continuous IV infusion sodium bicarbonate (1.26%) may be infused with isotonic sodium chloride determined by blood gas values. Seek clinician's advice

Cardiac arrest
• *Adult and child:* IV bolus injection 50 ml of 8.4% or according to blood gas results. Seek clinician's advice
• *Infant:* Seek clinician's advice

Urinary alkalinisation
• *Adult:* 3 g in water every 2 hr until urinary pH exceeds 7, maintenance of alkaline urine 5–10 g daily

Antacid
• *Adult:* By mouth tablets: 2–6 tablets sucked when required; powder: 1–5 g in water when required

Available forms include: Tablets 300 mg; powder, ear drops
Injection: 8.4%, 4.2%
Infusion: 1.26%, 4.2%, 8.4%

Side effects/adverse reactions:
CNS: Irritability, headache, confusion, stimulation, tremors, twitching, tetany, weakness, convulsions, hypertonicity
CV: Irregular pulse, cardiac arrest
GI: Flatulence, belching, distension
META: Alkalosis
RESP: Shallow, slow respirations, cyanosis, apnoea
INTEG: Tissue necrosis at injection site

Contraindications: Hypertension, peptic ulcer, eclampsia, hypernatraemia, hypoventilation, hypocalcaemia, hypochlorudria, metabolic or respiratory alkalosis

Precautions: Congestive cardiac failure, hepatic and renal impairment

Pharmacokinetics:
By mouth: Onset 2 min, duration 10 min
IV: Onset 15 min, duration 1–2 hr, excreted in urine

Interactions/incompatibilities:
• Increases effects: salicylates, quinidine
• Reduces effects: 4-quindones; lithium, tetracyclines, penicillamine
• Do not mix solution with other drugs

Clinical assessment:
- Respiratory rate, rhythm, depth, notify clinician of abnormalities
- Electrolytes, blood pH, PO_2, bicarbonate, during treatment
- Alkalosis: irritability, confusion, twitching, hypertonicity, slow respirations, cyanosis, irregular pulse
- Milk-alkali syndrome: confusion, headache, nausea, vomiting, anorexia, urinary stones, hypercalcaemia

NURSING CONSIDERATIONS

Assess:
- Vital signs
- Blood gas analysis
- Acidotic balance

Evaluate:
- For side effects
- Vital signs, respiratory function
- Blood gas analysis
- Urinary output

Teach patient/family:
- To suck antacid tablets and drink with 200 ml water
- Not to take antacid with milk, or milk-alkali syndrome may result
- Not to use antacid for more than 2 weeks

---

sodium cellulose phosphate

Calcisorb
Func. class.: Antihypercalcaemic
Chem. class.: Phosphorylated cellulose
Legal class.: P

Action: Decreases hypercalcium by binding with calcium in lumen of stomach and intestine and facilitates excretion

Uses: Reduces calcium absorption from diet in treatment of hypercalciuria and recurrent formation of renal stones, and in osteopetrosis. Also used for idiopathic hypercalcaemia of infancy, hypercalcaemic sarcoidosis and treatment of vitamin D intoxication

Dosage and routes:
- *Adult:* By mouth 15 g/day divided as three 5 g doses with each meal
- *Child:* 10 g daily in divided doses with meals

Available forms include: Powder 5 g sachets

Side effects/adverse reactions:
GU: Hypomagnesuria
GI: Nausea, anorexia, diarrhoea, dyspepsia

Contraindications: Renal failure, congestive cardiac failure, pregnancy, lactation

Precautions: Children

Clinical assessment:
- Any associated increase in serum phosphate may be harmful

Interactions/incompatibilities:
- May decrease action of this drug: magnesium preparations
- Calcium and magnesium levels (serum, urinary) throughout treatment

NURSING CONSIDERATIONS

Administer:
- Powder may be dispersed in water, juice; taken with meals; sprinkled on food
- Stir powder into water or sprinkle on food

Perform/provide:
- Increase fluids to 3 litres/day; urinary output should be over 2 litres/day

Evaluate:
- Therapeutic response: absence of renal stone formation

Teach patient/family:
- To decrease calcium in diet; dairy products; decrease sodium, citrus fruits in diet; increased excretion of drug will occur; decrease oxalate (chocolate, tea, spinach) rhubarb, beetroot

sodium cromoglycate

Intal, Rynacrom
Func. class.: Antiasthmatic, antiallergic agent
Chem. class.: Mast cell stabiliser
Legal class.: Intal (POM) Rynacrom (P)

Action: Inhibits histamine, slow-reacting substance of anaphylaxis release from mast cells in respiratory tract; this decreases allergic response
Uses: Prophylaxis of asthma and allergic rhinitis
Dosage and routes:
Allergic rhinitis
- *Adults and children, insufflation:* 10 mg each nostril up to 4 times a day
- *Nasal drops:* Instil 2 drops each nostril 6 times a day
- *Nasal spray:* 1 spray into each nostril 2–4 times a day

Prophylaxis of asthma
- Regular use is necessary
- *Adults and children, aerosol inhalation:* 10 mg (2 puffs) 4 times daily increased up to 6–8 times daily. Additional dose may also be taken before exercise; maintenance 5 mg (1 puff) 4 times daily
- *Powder inhalation:* (Spincaps) 20 mg 4 times a day, increased to 6–8 times daily in severe cases
- *Nebuliser solution:* 20 mg inhaled 4 times a day up to 6 times daily

Available forms include: Rynacom: insufflation cartridge 10 mg, nasal drops 2%, nasal spray 4%, Intal: aerosol inhalation 5 mg, autohaler 5 mg, capsules for inhalation 20 mg, nebuliser solution 10 mg/ml
Side effects/adverse reactions:
EENT: Throat irritation, cough, nasal congestion, transient bronchospasm
Contraindications: Hypersensitivity to this drug or lactose; status asthmaticus
Precautions: Pregnancy, lactation
Pharmacokinetics:
Inhalation: Peak 15 min, duration 4–6 hr, excreted unchanged in faeces, half-life 80 min

NURSING CONSIDERATIONS

Administer:
- By inhalation/nebuliser/nasally only; not to be given by mouth
- Gargle, sips of water to decrease irritation in throat after use
- If nebuliser solution is mixed with other drugs, any unused solution should be discarded immediately and the nebuliser chamber thoroughly cleaned
- Where a concurrent aerosol bronchodilator is used give broncodilator first
- Give nebuliser solution with a power-operated nebuliser via a face mask or mouth piece; hand-operated nebulisers should not be used
- Mixed solutions must not be used if cloudy

Evaluate:
- Therapeutic response
- Respiratory status: respiratory rate, rhythm, characteristics, cough, wheezing, dyspnoea

Teach patient/family:
- To clear mucus before using
- Proper inhalation technique for each device
- That therapeutic effect may take up to 4 weeks
- Not to swallow capsule
- Not to use for asthma attack
- To continue regular usage

sodium cromoglycate (ophthalmic)

Opticrom
Func. class.: Anti-allergic drug
Chem. class.: Mast cell stabilizer
Legal class.: POM

Action: Inhibits degranulation of

mast cells after contact with antigens, which decreases release of histamine and slow-releasing-substance of anaphylaxis (SRS-A) from mast cell
Uses: Allergic and vernal conjunctivitis
Dosage and routes:
- *Adult:* Instil 1–2 drops in both eyes 4 times a day; ointment apply 2 or 3 times daily

Available forms include: Aqueous solution 2%, ointment 4%
Side effects/adverse reactions:
EENT: Stinging, transient blurring of vision with eye ointment
Contraindications: Hypersensitivity to benzalkonium chloride; soft contact lenses should not be worn during treatment with the eye drops; the eye ointment should not be used if contact lenses are worn

NURSING CONSIDERATIONS

Teach patient/family:
- Method of instillation, and not to touch dropper or take nozzle to eye
- Blurring of vision may occur following instillation of ointment
- To report stinging, burning, itching, lacrimation, puffiness
- Not to wear soft contact lens, use may be reinstituted 4–6 hr after therapy is discontinued

sodium fluoride

Fluor-A-Day, En-De-Kay, Fluorigord, Zymafluor oral-B Fluoride
Func. class.: Trace elements
Chem. class.: Fluoride ion
Legal class.: P

Action: Necessary for hard tooth enamel, and for resistance to periodontal disease; reduces acid production by dental bacteria
Uses: Prevention of dental caries
Dosage and routes:
- Dosage should be adjusted for fluoride content of the drinking water, diet and age

Child:
- Water content less than 300 mcg fluoride ions/l, up to 6 months, none; 6 months–2 years, 0.55 mcg daily (250 mcg fluoride ions)
- 2–4 yr, 1.1 mg daily (500 mcg fluoride ions)
- Over 4 yr, 2.2 mg daily (1 mg fluoride ions)
- Water content between 300 and 700 mcg fluoride ions/l up to 2 yr, none;
- 2–4 yr, 0.55 mg daily (250 mcg fluoride ions)
- Over 4 yr, 1.1 mg daily (500 mcg fluoride ions)
- Water content over 700 mcg fluoride ions/l

No supplementation recommended
Available forms include: Tablets: 0.55 mg (250 mcg fluoride ions), 1.1 mg (500 mcg fluoride ions), 2.2 mg (1 mg fluoride ions); Drops: 0.5 mg/0.15 ml (250 mcg fluoride ions), 0.275 mg/drop (125 mcg fluoride ions), 0.15% (250 mcg fluoride ions in 8 drops); Rinse: 2%, 0.05%, 0.2%
Side effects/adverse reactions:
Acute overdosage: Black tar-like stools, bloody vomit, diarrhoea, hypocalcaemia, other metabolic and electrolyte disturbances, tremors, hyperreflexia, paraesthesia, tetany, cardiac arrhythmias, shock, respiratory arrest, cardiac failure
Chronic overdosage: Gastric complaints, joint pain, stiffness, discolouration of teeth (white, yellowish-brown, black)
Contraindications: Hypersensitivity, areas where drinking water is fluoridated
Pharmacokinetics:
By mouth: Excreted in urine and faeces, breast milk
Interactions/incompatibilities:
- Avoid use with dairy products

Treatment of overdose: Gastric lavage, maintenance of high urine output and other symptomatic and supportive measures

NURSING CONSIDERATIONS

Assess:

• Use in children

Administer:

• Drops after meals with fluids or undiluted

Evaluate:

• Therapeutic response: absence of dental caries

• Nutritional status: increase fluoride content of water, decrease carbohydrate snacks, increase fish, tea, mineral water

Teach patient/family:

• Tablets should be sucked or dissolved in the mouth, do not swallow whole

• To monitor children using gel or rinse; not to be swallowed

• Not to drink, eat, or rinse mouth for at least ½ hr

• To apply after brushing and flossing at bedtime

• Store out of children's reach

---

sodium fusidate

Fucidin

Func. class.: Antibiotic, narrow-spectrum

Chem. class.: Fusidic acid salt

Legal class.: POM

Action: Inhibits bacterial protein synthesis and may be bacteriostatic or bactericidal

Uses: Staphylococcal infections, especially osteomyelitis, resistant to penicillins

Dosage and routes:

• *Adult:* By mouth 500 mg 8-hrly; doubled in severe infections or use appropriate combined therapy; suspension: 750 mg 8 hrly

• *Child:* By mouth 0–1 yr, 1 ml suspension/kg daily in 3 divided doses: 1–5 yr, 5 ml 3 times daily; 5–12 yr, 10 ml 3 times a day

• By slow IV infusion:

Adults greater than 50 kg: 580 mg diethanolamine fusidate (equivalent to 500 mg sodium fusidate) 3 times daily, infusion over 6 hr

Children and adult less than 50 kg: 6–7 mg of diethanolamine fusidate per kg 3 times a day, infusion over 6 hr

Staphylococcal skin infections

• Topical apply 2% cream ointment or gel 3 or 4 times daily

Bacterial conjunctivitis

• Instil 1% eye drops twice daily; continue for 48 hrs after healing

Available forms include: Tablets 250 mg (sodium fusidate); suspension 250 mg/5 ml (as fusidic acid); infusion powder for reconstitution 500 mg with buffer (as diethanolamine fusidate); gel 2%; cream 2%; ointment 2%; medicated dressing 2%; eye drops 1%

Side effects/adverse reactions:

GI: Nausea, vomiting

HAEM: Hypocalcaemia (high doses of I/V)

INTEG: Rashes, jaundice (reversible)

Contraindications: Hypersensitivity. Avoid IM or subcutaneous injections

Precautions: Hepatic impairment, pregnancy, lactation. Preterm infants, jaundice, acidotic infants

Pharmacokinetics: Mainly excreted in the bile. Suspension is fusidic acid and has only 70% bioavailability compared to the tablets which are the salt, sodium fusidate. Doses stated for suspension take this into account, and to avoid underdosing must be adhered to (e.g. 750 mg/15 ml fusidic acid is equivalent to 500 mg sodium fusidate)

Interactions/incompatibilities:

• Infusion should not be mixed

with amino-acid solutions or blood

Clinical assessment:

• Perform liver function tests periodically when high oral doses used over a long period and in patients with liver dysfunction

• Urea and electrolytes, liver function tests

• For severe or deep seated infections additional concurrent anti-staphylococcal antibiotic therapy may be necessary

Treatment of overdose: Symptomatic and supportive therapy

NURSING CONSIDERATIONS

Assess:

• Baseline fluid balance

Administer:

• If IV, reconstitute 580 mg of diethanolamine fusidate with 50 ml phosphate/citrate buffer, add to 500 ml infusion solution (for adults, children over 50 kg) and give by infusion over not less than 6 hrs

• By infusion into a large vein

• Over prescribed period

• Shake suspension before use

• Reconstitute powder for IV use with care and according to enclosed instructions

• Discard any unused IV solution once reconstituted

Evaluate:

• For local reaction at intravenous site

• For jaundice—if this persists (stop drug in consultation with medical staff)

• For other side effects

• For resistance (narrow spectrum antibiotic)

• Regular liver function tests

• Fluid balance

Venospasm, thromboplebilis and haemolysis (excessive doses)

sodium nitrite

Sodium Nitrite Injection (Special orders)

Func. class.: Antidote

Legal class.: POM

Action: Sodium nitrite converts haemaglobin to methaemaglobin; which competes with cytochrome oxidase for cyanide with the formation of cyanomethaemaglobin; thiosulphate aids the conversion or inactivation of cyanide to thiocyanate

Uses: In conjunction with sodium thiosulphate for emergency treatment of cyanide poisoning

Dosage and routes:

• IV injection 10 ml over 3 min, followed by 25 ml sodium thiosulphate injection 50% by IV injection 10 min

Available forms include: Injection 3% (30 mg/ml) in water for injections

Side effects/adverse reactions:

CV: Vasodilation

CNS: Headache

INTEG: Flushing

Clinical assessment:

• This drug is toxic if cyanides are not present

• Cyanide toxicity: blood screen

• Use only in conjunction with sodium thiosulphate

NURSING CONSIDERATIONS

Assess:

• Pulse, BP, respiration, check for apnoea

• ECG, blood gases, blood count

• Flushed face, red lips, cherry red mucous membranes

Administer:

• By IV injection, slowly over at least 3 min

• With resuscitation equipment available for assisted ventilation

Evaluate:

• For signs of vasodilation including flushing and headache
• Therapeutic response: normal blood gases, decreased carboxyhaemoglobin levels

sodium nitroprusside

Nipride
Func. class.: Antihypertensive
Chem. class.: Vasodilator, peripheral
Legal class.: POM

Action: Directly relaxes arteriolar, venous smooth muscle; resulting in reduction in cardiac preload, after-load
Uses: Hypertensive crisis, controlled hypotension in surgery, acute on chronic heart failure
Dosage and routes:
Hypertensive crisis
• *Adult:* Patients not on other antihypertensives, IV infusion, initial dose 0.3–1.0 mcg/kg/min, usual range 0.5–6.0 mcg/kg/min (20–400 mcg/min), maximum for short-term (several hours) treatment 8 mcg/kg/min; maximum total dose for longer periods but less than 14 days, 70 mg/kg for patients with normal renal function; lower doses for patients on other antihypertensives
Controlled hypotension in surgery
• *Adults:* IV infusion, maximum dose should not exceed 1.5 mcg/kg/min
Heart failure
• *Adults:* IV infusion, initially 10–15 mcg/min, increased every 5–10 min in 10–15 mcg/min increments as necessary; usual range 10–200 mcg/min; maximum 280 mcg/min (4 mcg/kg/min); infusion continued until patient stabilised on appropriate oral agents, normally up to 72 hours

Available forms include: Infusion 50 mg (hospital only)
Side effects/adverse reactions:
GI: Nausea, vomiting, abdominal pain retro-sternal discomfort
CNS: Dizziness, headache, agitation, twitching, restlessness, apprehension
EENT: Tinnitus, blurred vision
CVS: Palpitations
INTEG: Pain, irritation at injection site, sweating
METAB: Acidosis
Contraindications: Hypertension compensatory, vitamin B_{12} deficiency, liver disease, Leber's optic atrophy
Precautions: Pregnancy, lactation, children, fluid, electrolyte imbalances, hepatic disease, severe renal impairment, impaired cerebral circulation, hypothyroidism, elderly
Pharmacokinetics:
IV: Onset 1–2 min, duration 1–10 min after IV dose, half-life 4 days in patients with normal renal function; metabolised in liver, excreted in urine
Interactions/incompatibilities:
• Severe hypotension: anaesthetic agents, nitrates, other antihypertensives
• Do not mix with any drug in syringe or solution
Clinical assessment:
• Electrolytes: potassium, sodium, chloride, CO_2, bicarbonate, lactate
• Assess renal and hepatic function
• BP by direct means if possible, check ECG continuously
• Thiocyanate levels daily if on long-term treatment
• Monitor plasma-cyanide concentration
• Administer depending on BP reading every 15 min
Treatment of overdose: Cyanide intoxication; immediately
1. Stop infusion
2. Administer cyanide antidote

either IV administration of sodium thiosulphate or dicobalt edetate
3. Institute auxiliary treatment to support respiration

NURSING CONSIDERATIONS

Assess:
- Baseline vital signs, weight, renal function, electrolyte and bicarbonate levels

Administer:
- By infusion pump only

Perform/provide:
- Protect from direct sunlight with foil or brown paper, discard if gross colour changes in fluid
- Solution should not be used after a period of 24 hr from the time of preparation

Evaluate:
- Therapeutic response: decreased BP, absence of bleeding
- Nausea, vomiting, diarrhoea, abdominal pain
- Oedema in feet, legs daily
- Pain at infusion site
- Skin turgor, dryness of mucous membranes for hydration status

Teach patient/family:
- To report dizziness, headache, nausea or other side effects

---

sodium valproate

Epilim, Ortept
Func. class.: Anticonvulsant
Chem. class.: Carboxylic acid derivative
Legal class.: POM

Action: Increases levels of gamma-aminobutyric acid (GABA) in brain
Uses: All forms of epilepsy
Dosage and routes:
- *Adult:* By mouth, initially 600 mg daily in divided doses; increase according to response by 200 mg daily; usual range 1–2 g (20–30 mg/kg) daily in divided doses; maximum 2.5 g daily
- *Child:* By mouth, up to 20 kg (about 4 yr), initially 20 mg/kg in divided doses, increased according to plasma concentrations and response to 40 mg/kg daily; over 20 kg, initially 400 mg daily in divided doses, increased gradually according to response to 20–30 mg/kg, maximum 35 mg/kg daily
- *Adult:* Slow IV injection or IV infusion, when oral treatment is not possible; continuation of oral treatment, same as oral dose; initiation of treatment, slow IV injection 400–800 mg/kg (up to 10 mg/kg); then IV infusion up to 2.5 g daily; replace with oral treatment as soon as possible
- *Child:* Slow IV injection or infusion, as for adults, 20–30 mg/kg daily; increase according to plasma concentrations and response to 40 mg/kg

Available forms include: Tablets, enteric-coated, 200 mg, 500 mg; tablets, crushable, 100 mg; oral liquid 200 mg/5 ml; syrup 200 mg/5 ml
Side effects/adverse reactions:
HAEM: Thrombocytopenia, leucopenia, increased prothrombin time, inhibition of platelet aggregation, red cell hypoplasia
CNS: Sedation, incoordination, hallucinations, behavioural changes, tremors, lethargy, confusion
GI: Nausea, vomiting, gastric irritation, anorexia, cramps, hepatic failure, pancreatitis. Increased appetite and weight gain
INTEG: Rash, alopecia, bruising
GU: Amenorrhoea
METAB: Hyperammonaemia
CVS: Oedema
Contraindications: Active liver disease, porphyria
Precautions: Renal disease, pregnancy, lactation, children and patients with a history of liver dis-

ease, major surgery, diabetics, avoid sudden withdrawal

Pharmacokinetics:

By mouth: Onset 15–30 min, peak 1–4 hr, duration 4–6 hr

By mouth: Onset slow, duration 4–6 hr

Metabolised by liver, excreted by kidneys, faeces, excreted in breast milk, half-life 8–20 hr

Interactions/incompatibilities:

- Increased effects: MAOIs and other antidepressants
- Increased toxicity: salicylates, warfarin
- Dosage adjustment may be required in combination with other anticonvulsants

Clinical assessment:

- Full blood count and coagulation studies prior to undergoing surgery
- Liver function tests for first six months on therapy for patients most at risk or with prior history of liver disease
- Blood levels: therapeutic level 40–100 mg/litre (depending on time or sampling and presence of co-medication)

Lab. tests interferences: False positives in urine testing for possible diabetics

Treatment of overdose: Induced vomiting, gastric lavage assisted ventilation and other supportive measures may be necessary in massive overdose

NURSING CONSIDERATIONS

Administer:

- Tablets whole, not crushed or chewed
- Crushable tablets whole or crushed
- Oral formulations preferably after food
- IV injection reconstituted in solvent provided, slowly over 3–5 min
- IV infusion of reconstituted injection in glucose 5%, sodium chloride 0.9% or dextrose-saline

Evaluate:

- For signs of nausea, transient alopecia, false ketonuria, weight gain, purpuric rash/bruising
- Mental status: mood, alertness, affect, memory (long, short)
- Respiratory dysfunction: respiratory depression, character, rate, rhythm; hold drug if respirations are under 12/min or if pupils are dilated

Teach patient/family:

- That physical dependency may result when used for extended periods
- To avoid driving, other activities that require alertness
- Not to discontinue medication quickly after long-term use; convulsions may result
- To inform prescribing clinician if already taking anti-convulsants, especially phenobarbitone

---

sotalol hydrochloride

Beta-Cardone, Sotacor, combination products

Func. class.: Antihypertensive, anti-anginal, anti-arrhythmic

Chem. class.: Non-selective β-blocker

Legal class.: POM

Action: Decreases preload, afterload, which is responsible for decreasing left ventricular end diastolic pressure, systemic vascular resistance. Cardiac work and oxygen consumption are diminished

Uses: Hypertension, angina, arrhythmias, prophylaxis after infarction, thyrotoxicosis

Dosage and routes:

Hypertension

- *Adult:* By mouth initially 160 mg daily in 1–2 doses; maintenance 160 mg daily; maximum 600 mg daily

Angina
• *Adult:* By mouth initially 160 mg daily in 1–2 doses; maintenance 160 mg daily; maximum 600 mg daily
Arrhythmias
• *Adult:* By mouth 120–240 mg daily in single or divided doses
• *Adult:* Slow IV injection 20–60 mg over 2–3 min with ECG monitoring; repeat at 10-min intervals if necessary; maximum 100 mg over 3 min or longer
Myocardial infarction prophylaxis
• *Adult:* By mouth 320 mg daily starting 5–14 days after infarction
Hyperthyroidism (adjunct)
• *Adult:* By mouth 120–240 mg daily in single or divided doses
Available forms include: Tablets 40 mg, 80 mg, 160 mg, 200 mg; injection 10 mg/ml
Side effects/adverse reactions:
CV: Heart failure, bradycardia, peripheral vasoconstriction, atypical ventricular arrhythmias (torsade de pointes)
RESP: Bronchospasm
GI: Gastric disturbances, diarrhoea
INTEG: Rash
EENT: Dry eyes
Contraindications: Bronchospasm, asthma, history of obstructive airways disease, metabolic acidosis, sinus bradycardia, partial heart block, uncontrolled congestive heart failure
Precautions: Pregnancy (may cause fetal bradycardia), lactation, hepatic or renal impairment, avoid abrupt withdrawal in angina. In combined therapy clonidine should not be discontinued until several days after withdrawal of sotalol. Diabetes (may mask hypoglycaemic attack), anaesthesia, hypokalaemia, hypomagnesaemia
Pharmacokinetics: Completely absorbed from GI tract, peak plasma concentrations at 2–3 hr. Excreted unchanged in urine, not plasma protein bound. Plasma half-life 17 hr; low lipid solubility.
Interactions/incompatibilities:
• Increased effect: Adrenaline, amiodarone, amphetamines, antiarrhythmics, diltiazem, ergotamine, nifedipine, prenylamine, sympathomimetic amines, verapamil, diuretics
Clinical assessment:
• Creatinine clearance if kidney damage is diagnosed
• If given with thiazide or loop diuretic avoid hypokalaemia (note combination products)
• Stop therapy if severe or persistent diarrhoea; risk of hypokalaemia/hypomagnesaemia
Lab. test interferences:
Decrease: Blood glucose

NURSING CONSIDERATIONS

Assess:
• Baseline BP, pulse, respirations
• Fluid balance (for IV administration)
Administer:
• With 8 oz glass of water on empty stomach
Perform/provide:
• Peak flow if patient is chesty, wheezy or short of breath
Evaluate:
• For headache, lightheadedness, decreased BP; may indicate need for decreased dosage
• Pain: duration, time started, activity being performed
• Weight gain; report if less than 2.5 kg
• Tolerance, if taken over a long period of time
Teach patient/family:
• That drug should be taken before stressful activity or exercise
• That if taken sublingually, mucous membranes may sting
• To avoid potentially hazardous activities if dizziness occurs
• Stress patient compliance with complete medical regime and to

take medication as prescribed
• To make positional changes slowly to prevent fainting
• Decrease dosage over 2 weeks to prevent cardiac damage

spectinomycin hydrochloride

Trobicin
Func. class.: Antibiotic
Chem. class.: Aminoglycoside
Legal class.: POM

Action: Inhibits bacterial synthesis by binding to 30S subunit on ribosomes
Uses: Gonorrhoea
Dosage and routes:
• *Adult:* IM 2–4 g as single dose
• *Children over 2 yr:* 40 mg/kg, if no alternative treatment
Available forms include: Injection IM 2 g
Side effects/adverse reactions:
CNS: Dizziness, chills, fever, headache
HAEM: Anaemia
GI: Nausea, vomiting, increased blood urea nitrogen
GU: Decreased urine output
INTEG: Pain at injection site, urticaria, rash, pruritus, fever
SYST: Anaphylaxis
Contraindications: Hypersensitivity, syphilis
Precautions: Pregnancy
Pharmacokinetics:
IM: Peak 1–2 hr, duration up to 8 hr, half-life 1–3 hr, excreted in urine (active form)
Interactions/incompatibilities:
• Increases effect of lithium
Clinical assessment:
• Gonorrhoea culture after treatment
• Liver function tests; enzymes, aspartate aminotransferase, alanine aminotransferase, serum alkaline phosphatase following multiple doses
• Blood studies: haematocrit, Hb, blood creatinine if multiple diagnoses given
• Serologic test for syphilis 3 months after treatment

NURSING CONSIDERATIONS
Assess:
• Input and output of fluids, report decreased output
• Allergies before treatment, reaction of each medication
• Weight
• Gonorrhoea culture for sensitivity taken before initial dose
Administer:
• No more than 2 g per injection site
• After shaking vial vigorously. Add 3.2 ml water for injection to vial. Final volume is 5 ml
• IM upper outer quadrant of gluteal muscle
• With 20-gauge needle; no more than 5 ml per site
Perform/provide:
• Storage at room temperature; reconstituted solutions should be discarded after 24 hr
Evaluate:
• Therapeutic response, decreased dysuria, discharge
• Negative culture and sensitivity
• Side effects; dizziness, chills, fever, nausea, urticaria and mild discomfort at injection site
Teach patient/family:
• To avoid sexual contact with other people until negative culture is confirmed
• To treat sexual contacts simultaneously
• To practise safe sex
• That follow-up appointments are necessary to ensure syphilis has not been contacted and masked

spironolactone

Aldactone, Spirolone, Spiroctan, Lasitactone, Aldactide
Func. class.: Potassium-sparing diuretic
Chem. class.: Aldosterone antagonist
Legal class.: POM

Action: Competes with aldosterone at receptor sites in renal tubule, resulting in excretion of sodium chloride, water, retention of potassium, phosphate
Uses: Congestive cardiac failure, hepatic cirrhosis with ascites and oedema. Nephrotic syndrome, malignant ascites, primary aldosteronism (diagnosis and treatment)
Dosage and routes:
Congestive heart failure
• *Adults:* By mouth 100 mg daily increasing gradually if necessary up to 400 mg daily. Maintain 75–200 mg daily
Hepatic cirrhosis
• When with ascites and oedema urinary sodium/potassium ratio is greater than 1, 100 mg daily when ratio is less than 1 then 200–400 mg daily
Malignant ascites
• Initially 100–200 mg daily in severe cases up to 400 mg daily
Nephrotic syndrome
• 100–200 mg daily
Primary aldosteronism
• Long test: 400 mg daily for 3–4 weeks
• Short test: 400 mg daily for 4 days
• Pre-surgery: 100–400 mg daily prior to surgery
Available forms include: Tablets 25, 50, 100 mg; capsules 100 mg
Side effects/adverse reactions:
CNS: Headache, confusion, drowsiness, lethargy, ataxia
GI: Diarrhoea, cramps, hepatic cirrhosis
INTEG: Rash, pruritus, urticaria, fever
ENDO: Impotence, gynaecomastia, menstrual irregularities, breast soreness, mild androgenic effects e.g. hirsutism, deepening voice
ELECT: Hyperchloraemic metabolic acidosis, hyperkalaemia, increased blood urea
Contraindications: Hypersensitivity, anuria, severe renal disease, rapidly deteriorating renal function, hyperkalaemia, acute renal insufficiency, Addison's disease, porphyria
Precautions: Dehydration, hepatic disease, pregnancy, lactation, hyponatraemia, elderly
Pharmacokinetics:
By mouth: Onset 24–48 hr, peak 48–72 hr; metabolised in liver, excreted in urine
Interactions/incompatibilities:
• Diuretic effect antagonised by aspirin and indomethacin
• Increased action of: antihypertensives, digoxin
• Increased hyperkalaemia: potassium sparing diuretics, potassium products or angiotensin converting enzyme inhibitors
Lab. test interferences:
Interfere: certain serum digoxin assays
Treatment of overdose: Monitor electrolytes, administer IV fluids and electrolytes as necessary

NURSING CONSIDERATIONS

Assess:
• Baseline weight, fluid balance
Administer:
• In morning to avoid interference with sleep
• With food, if nausea occurs; absorption may be decreased slightly
Perform/provide:

• Fluid balance daily to determine fluid loss

Evaluate:

• Therapeutic effect

• Improvement in oedema of feet, legs, sacral area daily if medication is being used in congestive cardiac failure

• Improvement in CVP readings

• Signs of metabolic acidosis: drowsiness, restlessness

• Rashes, temperature elevation daily

• Confusion, especially in elderly, take safety precautions if needed

• Hydration: skin turgor, thirst, dry mucous membranes

Teach patient/family:

• That drowsiness, ataxia, mental confusion may occur; observe caution in driving (elderly patients should probably not drive at all)

• To notify clinician of cramps, diarrhoea, lethargy, thirst, headache, skin rash, menstrual abnormalities, deepening voice, breast enlargement

---

stanozolol

Stromba

Func. class.: Androgenic anabolic steroid

Chem. class.: Halogenated testosterone derivative

Legal class.: POM

Action: Anabolic agent with fibrinolytic properties. Alter the functional level of plasma C1 esterase inhibitor; enzyme which is depressed in hereditary angio-oedema. Protein building properties.

Uses: Prevention of hereditary angioedema, vascular manifestations of Behcet's disease

Dosage and routes:

Hereditary angio-oedema

• *Adult:* By mouth 2.5–10 mg daily to control attacks, reduced for maintenance (2.5 mg 3 times weekly may be sufficient)

• *Child 1–6 yr:* Initially 2.5 mg daily. 6–12 yr, initially 2.5–5 mg daily reduced for maintenance

Behcet's disease

• *Adult:* By mouth 10 mg daily

Available forms include: Tablets 5 mg

Side effects/adverse reactions:

INTEG: Rash, acneiform lesions, oily hair and skin, flushing, sweating, acne vulgaris, alopecia, hirsutism

CNS: Dizziness, headache, fatigue, tremors, paraesthesias, flushing, sweating, anxiety, lability, insomnia

MS: Cramps, spasms

CV: Increased BP

GU: Haematuria, amenorrhoea, vaginitis, decreased libido, decreased breast size, clitoral hypertrophy, testicular atrophy. In children prolonged use may lead to premature closure of the epiphyses

GI: Nausea, vomiting, constipation, weight gain, cholestatic jaundice, dyspepsia, peliosis hepatis, hepatic tumours

EENT: Voice change

Contraindications: Severe renal disease, severe cardiac disease, hepatic disease, hypersensitivity, pregnancy, lactation, prostate cancer, porphyria, premenopausal women except in life-threatening situations, male breast cancer

Precautions: Insulin dependent diabetes mellitus, cardiovascular disease

Pharmacokinetics: Metabolised in liver, excreted in faeces and urine. Highly protein bound

Interactions/incompatibilities:

• Increased effects of: oral anticoagulants and oral hypoglycaemic age

Clinical assessment:
• Electrolytes: potassium, sodium, chloride, calcium; cholesterol
• Liver function tests: enzymes, aspartate aminotransferase, alanine aminotransferase, bilirubin
• Thyroid function tests: Measure T_3 and T_4
Lab. test interferences:
Increase: Serum cholesterol, blood glucose, urine glucose
Decrease: Serum calcium, serum potassium, thyroxine, triiodothyranine, thyroid ^{131}I uptake test
Treatment of overdose: Observe and monitor liver function tests
NURSING CONSIDERATIONS
Assess:
• Weigh before initial treatment
• Input and output of fluids
Administer:
• Initial dose then reduce according to patient response. Lowest effective maintenance dose
• To children in short course with intervals between if possible
Perform/provide:
• Diet based on specific need of patient
• NB. This is a drug of abuse, particularly for athletes
Evaluate:
• Regular urinalysis
• Children in prolonged use for growth rate and premature closure of the epiphysis
• Weight gain greater than 2.5 kg a week
• Signs of masculinisation in female: increased libido, deepening of voice, breast tissue, enlarged clitoris, menstrual irregularities; male: gynaecomastia, impotence, testicular atrophy
• Therapeutic response, occurs in 4–6 weeks in osteoporosis, increased mobility. Control of angio-oedema
• Effect of any other drug therapy, e.g. anticoagulants increased
• Any adverse effects: report so increase, decrease or even discontinuing of the drug may occur especially if voice changes
Teach patient/family:
• Drug needs to be combined with complete health plan: diet, rest, exercise
• To notify clinician if therapeutic response decreases
• Not to discontinue this medication abruptly
• To notify clinician if any voice changes occur
• To understand body changes may occur including breast in men
• To test urine
• To weigh weekly and report changes greater than 2.5 kg a week
• About potential abuse

---

stilboestrol

Apstil
Func. class.: Oestrogen
Chem. class.: Non-steroidal synthetic oestrogen
Legal class.: POM

Action: Suppresses androgenic hormonal activity in the management of androgen-dependent carcinomas. Carcinogenic potential
Uses: Carcinoma of prostate, metastatic post-menopausal carcinoma of breast
Dosage and routes:
Prostatic cancer
• *Adult:* By mouth 1–3 mg daily
Breast cancer
• *Adult:* By mouth 10–20 mg daily
Available forms include: Tablets 1, 5 mg
Side effects/adverse reactions:
CNS: Dizziness, headache, migraines, depression, elation
CV: Hypotension, venous thrombosis, oedema, thromboembolism, stroke, pulmonary embolism, myocardial infarction

GI: Nausea, vomiting, diarrhoea, anorexia, pancreatitis, cramps, constipation, increased appetite, increased weight, cholestatic jaundice
EENT: Contact lens intolerance, increased myopia, astigmatism
GU: Amenorrhoea, cervical erosion, breakthrough bleeding, dysmenorrhoea, vaginal candidiasis, breast changes, gynaecomastia, testicular atrophy, impotence, increased risk of endometrial carcinoma
INTEG: Rash, urticaria, acne, hirsutism, alopecia, oily skin, seborrhoea, purpura, melasma
META: Folic acid deficiency, hypercalcaemia, hyperglycaemia
Contraindications: Premenopausal breast cancer, thromboembolic disorders, oestrogen-dependent neoplasms, genital bleeding (abnormal, undiagnosed), pregnancy, children, porphyria, hepatic disease, herpes gestationis, severe hypertension, thromboembolic disease, fibroids (uterine), hyperlipoproteinaemia
Precautions: Hypertension, asthma, blood dyscrasias, gallbladder disease, congestive cardiac failure, diabetes mellitus, migraine, epilepsy, depression, cardiac failure, contact lenses, cholestatic jaundice, renal dysfunction
Interactions/incompatibilities:
• Decreased action of: anticoagulants, oral hypoglycaemics, insulin
Clinical assessment:
• Liver function studies, including aspartate aminotransferase, alanine aminotransferase, bilirubin, alkaline phosphatase
• Monitor BP regularly, look for signs of thrombosis
Lab. test interferences:
Increase: Protein bound iodine retention test, T_4, thyroxine-binding globulin (TBG), prothrombin, factors VII, VIII, IX, X, triglycerides
Decrease: Glucose tolerance test
Treatment of overdose: Gastric lavage. Monitor plasma electrolytes, symptomatic support. Oestrogen-withdrawal bleeding may occur in female child

NURSING CONSIDERATIONS

Assess:
• Input and output of fluids, check for oedema and fluid retention
• Weigh before initial treatment and at weekly intervals
• Regular urinalysis
Administer:
• Titrated dose, use lowest effective dose
• Suitable analgesics and diuretics
• Orally with food or milk to decrease GI symptoms
Perform/provide:
• Store below 25°C in dry, light proof container
• Diet suitable to enhance each patients good health and aid any medical problems
Evaluate:
• Therapeutic response: decrease in tumour size in prostatic cancer and breast
• Oedema, hypertension, cardiac symptoms, jaundice, venous thrombosis
• Mental status: affect, mood, behavioural changes, aggression
• Signs of feminizing in men; impotence, testicular atrophy, enlarged breasts
• Females; withdrawal bleeding
• Effect of any other drug therapy e.g. decreased action of anticoagulants
Teach patient/family:
• To weigh weekly, report gain over 2 kg or weight losses more than 2 kg
• To report breast lumps, vaginal bleeding, oedema, jaundice, dark urine, clay coloured stools, dyspnoea, headache, blurred vision, abdominal pain, numbness or stiffness in legs, chest pain

- To avoid sunlight or wear sunscreen; photosensitivity can occur
- To understand body changes may occur
- To test urine for glucose
- That drug needs to be combined with complete health plan: diet, rest, exercise

---

streptokinase

Kabikinase, Streptase
Func. class.: Thrombolytic enzyme
Chem. class.: β-Haemolytic streptococcus filtrate (purified)
Legal class.: POM

Action: Activates conversion of plasminogen to plasmin (fibrinolysin): plasmin is able to dissolve clots (fibrin), fibrinogen, plasma proteins; induces dissolution of intravascular thrombi and emboli
Uses: Deep vein thrombosis, pulmonary embolism, arterial thromboembolism, arteriovenous cannula occlusion, lysis of coronary artery thrombi after myocardial infarction
Dosage and routes:
- *Adult:* IV infusion 250,000 units over 30 mins, then 100,000 units/hr or 24–72 hr depending on condition (seek specialist advice). Max. 3 days therapy
- Acute myocardial infarction, IV infusion 1,500,000 units over 60 min as a single dose
- Intracoronary administration, seek specialist advice
- Local application in blocked haemodialysis shunts, 10,000–25,000 units deposited in clotted section, seal on venous side. Repeat after 30–45 min if necessary
- *Child:* Reduce standard dose according to circulating volume (seek specialist advice)

Available forms include: Injection IV 100,000, 250,000, 600,000, 750,000, 1.5 million unit vials
Side effects/adverse reactions:
HAEM: Decreased haematocrit, bleeding
INTEG: Rash, urticaria, phlebitis at IV infusion site, itching, flushing, headache
CNS: Headache, fever, intracerebral haemorrhage
GI: Nausea, vomiting
RESP: Altered respirations, shortness of breath, bronchospasm
MS: Low back pain
CV: Hypertension, arrhythmias, hypotension
EENT: Periorbital oedema
Contraindications: Surgery or invasive procedure during proceeding 10 days, GI bleeding in previous 6 months. Thrombocytopenia, hepatic or renal disease, CVA, hypotension. Parturition (last 10 days). Ulcerative colitis, visceral carcinoma, menstrual bleeding, first 18 weeks of pregnancy (specialist advice). Subacute bacterial endocarditis, GU diseases associated with bleeding. Pulmonary disease with cavitation, acute pancreatitis, severe diabetes mellitus, severe hypertension (200 systolic or 100 diastolic)
Precautions: Arterial emboli from left side of heart, subsequent regimens may require test dose, elderly, pregnancy, mitral valve defects, atrial fibrillation, repeated therapy 5 days–12 months previously, recent streptococcal infections
Pharmacokinetics:
IV: Excreted in bile, urine, half-life under 20 min
Interactions/incompatibilities:
- Bleeding potential: Aspirin, indomethacin, phenylbutazone, anticoagulants, thyroid hormones, volatile oils, quinidine, allopurinol, sulphonamide, tetracyclines, valproic acid, dextrans

Clinical assessment:
• Blood studies (haematocrit, platelets, partial thromboplastin time, prothrombin time, thrombin time, activated partial thromboplastin time) before starting therapy; prothrombin time or activated partial thromboplastin time must be less than twice control before starting therapy. Measure thrombin time or prothrombin time every 3–4 hr during treatment
• Not effective if: deep vein thrombosis more than 14 days olds, occlusion of central retinal arteries more than 6–8 hr old, and thrombosis of central retinal vein more than 10 days old
• Anticoagulation with heparin or aspirin may be recommended after stop taking
• Streptokinase should not be given to same patient 5 days to 12 months since last dose
• Risk of allergic reaction, measure streptokinase serum antibody level
• Urokinase may be an alternative
Lab. test interferences:
Increase: Prothrombin time, activated partial thromboplastin time, thrombin time
Treatment of overdose: Haemorrhage controlled at site of injection as required. Serious life threatening haemorrhage controlled with aprotinin or IV tranexamic acid therapy (10 mg/kg slow IV injection)

NURSING CONSIDERATIONS

Assess:
• Vital baseline signs
Administer:
• By infusion over 1 hr in 100 mls NSaline, whilst observing for reperfusion arrhythmias [fairly common] for myocardial infarction
• By prescribed infusion intra-arterially, in specialist area, for arterial thrombosis
• Treatment with aspirin (150 mg daily) is recommended for prophylaxis for acute myocardial infarction for at least 4 weeks following thrombolysis
Perform/provide:
• Continuous electrocardiogram monitoring before, during and after infusion – particularly if post-myocardial infarction
• Resuscitation equipment as cardiac arrest/arrhythmias may occur
• Continuous observation of all puncture sites, IV sites for bleeding and general signs of bruising
• Daily urinanalysis
• Bed-rest during and after (under medical supervision) treatment
• Prescribed pain relief
Evaluate:
• BP, pulse; respirations, neurological signs, 4 hrly temperature
• 12 lead ECG and signs for cardiac history if post-myocardial infarction
• Therapeutic response. Avoidance of invasive procedures
• Pressure to bleeding sites – report immediately
• Allergy: fever, rash, loin pain, hypotension stop infusion, seek medical advice, may need anaphylaxis treatment before recommencement
Teach patient/family:
• Issue advice card: teach about further effects and health education issues relating to diagnosis

streptomycin sulphate

Func. class.: Antibiotic
Chem. class.: Aminoglycoside
Legal class.: POM

Action: Interferes with protein synthesis in bacterial cell by binding to ribosomal subunit, causing inaccurate peptide sequence to form in protein chain, causing bacterial death

Uses: Sensitive strains of *M. tuberculosis*; non-tuberculous infections such as septicaemia, bacterial endocarditis, chronic respiratory infections and pneumonia caused by sensitive strains of *K. pneumoniae*, and urinary tract infections due to *E. coli*

Dosage and routes:

Tuberculosis

- *Adult:* IM 1 g daily or 1 g 2–3 times a week depending on regimen, given with other antitubercular drugs usually for 2 months. Under 50 kg, over 40 yr age 500–750 mg IM daily or 750 mg 3 times a week
- *Child:* IM 15–20 mg/kg daily up to 1 g given with other antitubercular drugs

Tuberculous meningitis

- IM 30–40 mg/kg (maximum 1 g) daily; intrathecal 50 mg daily (adult) or 1 mg/kg daily (children)

Non-tuberculous infections

- *Adult:* IM 1 g daily for 3–7 days
- *Child:* IM 22–40 mg/kg daily (may use divided doses)

Available forms include: Injection vial 1 g

Side effects/adverse reactions:

GU: Oliguria, haematuria, renal damage, renal failure, nephrotoxicity

CNS: Confusion, depression, numbness, tremors, convulsions, neurotoxicity

EENT: Ototoxicity, deafness, visual disturbances, paraesthesia of mouth

GI: Nausea, vomiting, anorexia, increased alanine aminotransferase, aspartate aminotransferase, bilirubin, hepatomegaly, hepatic necrosis, splenomegaly

CV: Hypotension, myocarditis

INTEG: Rash, burning, urticaria, photosensitivity, dermatitis

Contraindications: Severe renal disease, hypersensitivity, suppurative otitis media, labyrinthine disturbances, pregnancy, myasthenia gravis

Precautions: Neonates, renal disease, lactation, hearing deficits, elderly

Pharmacokinetics:

IM: Onset rapid, peak 1–2 hr; plasma half-life 1–3 hr, not metabolised, excreted unchanged in urine

Interactions/incompatibilities:

- Increased ototoxicity, neurotoxicity, nephrotoxicity: other aminoglycosides, amphotericin B, polymyxin, vancomycin, ethacrynic acid, frusemide, mannitol, methoxyflurane, cisplatin, cephalosporins
- Decreased effects of: parenteral penicillins
- Increased effects: non-depolarising muscle relaxants

Clinical assessment:

- Serum peak, drawn at 60 min after IM injection, trough level drawn just before next dose
- For elderly, 24 hr serum level should not exceed 1 mcg/ml
- For renal impairment, initial dose 250–500 mg IM injection. No further dose given until serum level less than 20 mcg/ml. If 24 hr serum level greater than 3 mcg/ml reduce dose

Treatment of overdose: Haemodialysis, monitor serum levels of drug

NURSING CONSIDERATIONS

Assess:

- Fluid balance
- Weight before treatment; calculation of dosage is usually done based on ideal body weight, but may be calculated on actual body weight
- Hearing levels

Administer:

- After specimens have been taken for culture and sensitivity

• By deep IM injection in large muscle mass, rotate injection sites
• Drug in evenly spaced doses to maintain blood level
• Concentration of drug in injection must not exceed 5 mg/ml
• Intrathecally through spinal tap. After withdrawal of equal volume of cerebrospinal fluid, inject very slowly (at least 10 min) and observe vital signs. Watch for blood pressure and pulse changes
• Using gloves to avoid skin sensitisation to the powder when reconstituting
• By deep IM injection, changing the site for each injection, as a solution containing 1 g in 2–3 ml; intrathecally, as a solution containing no more than 5 mg/ml, over at least 10 min. Adjust dose according to renal function; 24-hour (trough) serum concentrations should not exceed 3 mg/l, or 1 mg/l in patients over 60 yrs

Perform/provide:
• Adequate fluids of 2–3 litres daily unless contraindicated to prevent irritation of tubules
• Supervise mobility, observe balance
• Dehydration: high specific gravity, decrease in skin turgor, dry mucous membranes, dark urine
• Overgrowth of infection: increased temperature, malaise, redness, pain, swelling, perineal itching, diarrhoea, stomatitis, change in cough, sputum
• Vestibular dysfunction: nausea, vomiting, dizziness, headache; drug should be discontinued if severe
• Storage in refrigerator

Evaluate:
• Therapeutic effect, absence of fever, draining wounds, clear sputum, painless micturition, negative culture and sensitivity after treatment
• Close attention to input and output of fluids
• Urinalysis daily for proteinuria, cells, casts; report sudden change in urine output
• Urine pH if drug is used for urinary tract infection; urine should be kept alkaline
• Renal impairment by securing urine for creatinine clearance testing, blood urea, serum creatinine; in renal impairment (creatinine clearance less than 80 ml/min) lower dosage should be given
• Deafness by audiometric testing, ringing, roaring in ears, vertigo. Assess hearing before, during, after treatment

Teach patient/family:
• To report headache, dizziness, symptoms of overgrowth of infection, renal impairment
• To report loss of hearing, ringing, roaring in ears, fullness in head
• To drink plenty of fluids for urinary infection. Water, milk, tea, etc.

---

sucralfate

Antepsin
Func. class.: Gastric protectant
Chem. class.: Aluminium hydroxide/sulphated sucrose complex
Legal class.: POM

Action: Forms a complex that adheres to ulcer site, inhibits pepsin, gastric juice, absorbs bile salts

Uses: Duodenal ulcer, gastric ulcer, chronic gastritis

Dosage and routes:
• *Adult:* By mouth 1 g 4 times a day 1 hr before meals and at bedtime or 2 g twice daily taken on

rising and at bedtime (maximum 8 g daily) for 4–6 weeks (12 weeks in resistant cases)

Prophylaxis of GI haemorrhage from stress ulceration:
- By mouth 1 g 6 times a day (maximum 8 g daily)

Available forms include: Tablets 1 g; suspension 1 g/5 ml

Side effects/adverse reactions:
CNS: Drowsiness, dizziness, sleeplessness, vertigo
GI: Dry mouth, constipation, nausea, vomiting, diarrhoea, indigestion
INTEG: Urticaria, rash, pruritus

Contraindications: Hypersensitivity, severe renal impairment

Precautions: Pregnancy, renal dysfunction, lactation, children

Pharmacokinetics:
By mouth: Minimal amounts absorbed from GI tract

Interactions/incompatibilities:
- Decreased effect: antacids
- Decreased action of: tetracyclines, cimetidine, phenytoin, digoxin

Clinical assessment:
- Severe renal impairment, measure serum aluminium
- Monitor blood urea, creatinine

NURSING CONSIDERATIONS

Assess:
- Pain levels
- Fluid balance

Administer:
- 1 hour before meals and at bedtime
- Antacid should not be taken half an hour before or after a dose
- Allow 2 hr separation between sucralfate and other drugs
- Tablets may be dispensed in 10–15 ml of water

Evaluate:
- Therapeutic response: absence of pain, nausea and vomiting
- Ability to tolerate normal diet

Teach patient/family:
- To reassess diet and avoid some foods and alcohol
- To take 1 hr before meals
- To complete full course
- To take other medications only if directed by clinician

sulconazole nitrate

Exelderm
Func. class.: Topical antifungal
Chem. class.: Imidazole
Legal class.: POM

Action: Alters the permeability of cell membranes of sensitive fungi

Uses: Fungal skin infections, tinea pedis, corporis, and cruris, pityriasis versicolor and candidiasis

Dosage and routes: Topical, apply 1–2 times daily continuing for 2–3 weeks after lesions have healed

Available forms include: Cream, 1%

Side effects/adverse reactions:
INTEG: Occasional skin irritation or sensitivity

Contraindications: Hypersensitivity

Precautions: Pregnancy

NURSING CONSIDERATIONS

Administer:
- After skin scrapings taken to confirm diagnosis
- Cleanse skin before application
- Massage gently into affected and surrounding skin areas
- Avoid contact with eyes

Evaluate:
- Sensitivity to drug—rashes, itching, discontinue drug

Teach patient/family:
- Correct method of application
- To avoid contact with eyes
- To inform clinician and stop using drug if sensitivity occurs
- To continue treatment for 2–3 weeks after improvement to prevent relapse

sulfametopyrazine

Kelfizine W
Func. class.: Antibiotic
Chem. class.: Sulphonamide
Legal class.: POM

Action: Long acting sulphonamide. Interferes with the synthesis of nucleic acids in sensitive organisms
Uses: Urinary tract infections, chronic bronchitis (including prophylaxis)
Dosage and routes:
• *Adult:* By mouth: 2 g as a single dose once per week
Available forms include: Tablets 2 g
Side effects/adverse reactions:
GI: Nausea, vomiting
HAEM: Eosinophilia, agranulocytosis, granulocytopenia, leucopenia, megaloblastic anaemia
INTEG: Erythema multiforme, rashes, epidermal necrolysis, purpura
Contraindications: Sulphonamide hypersensitivity, pregnancy, lactation
Precautions: Hepatic or renal impairment, photosensitivity, elderly, lactation
Pharmacokinetics: Readily absorbed from GI tract; 60% bound to plasma protein. High degree of renal tubular resorption and low hepatic metabolism gives half-life of 65 hr
Interactions/incompatibilities:
• Potentiation: pyrimethamine, coumarin derivatives, sulphonylureas, trimethoprim
• Antagonism: PABA
Clinical assessment:
• Avoid prescribing to those sensitive to other sulphonamides
• Regular blood picture for disorders
Treatment of overdose:
• Increase fluid intake for seven days to increase excretion of drug
• Give potassium citrate mixture or sodium bicarbonate to render urine alkaline and increase excretion of drug

NURSING CONSIDERATIONS
Assess:
• Fluid balance
Perform/provide:
• Regular mouthcare/mouthwashes if vomiting occurs
• Regular urinalysis if long-term therapy
Administer:
• By mouth, dissolved in water or orange squash
• After sample taken for culture and sensitivity
• Stir tablet into a half tumblerfull of water or orange squash
• At least 2 l daily fluid intake to avoid crystallisation in kidneys
• Anti-emetic for severe nausea and vomiting
Tests/investigations
Perform:
• Full blood count, urea and electrolytes, renal function
Evaluate:
• Urine – colour, fluid balance if drug given for urinary tract infection
• Signs of allergic reactions – rashes, erythema multiforme, dyspnoea
• Therapeutic response – absence of pain, fever, negative culture and sensitivity
• Blood dyscrasias – skin rash, fever, sore throat, bruising, bleeding, fatigue, joint pain
Teach patient/family:
• To dilute tablet in half tumblerful of fluid
• To take tablets only once per week
• To complete course of tablets even when symptoms improve or cease
• To avoid direct sunlight to skin – burning may occur
• To check with clinician before

taking non-prescribed medication
• To notify clinician at once of rash, fever, sore throat, bruising, bleeding, joint pain

sulindac

Clinoril
Func. class.: Non-steroidal anti-inflammatory drug
Chem. class.: Indeneacetic acid derivative
Legal class.: POM

Action: Inhibits prostaglandin synthesis by inhibiting an enzyme needed for biosynthesis; possesses analgesic, anti-inflammatory, anti-pyretic properties
Uses: Osteoarthritis, rheumatoid arthritis, ankylosing spondylitis, bursitis, tendinitis, tenosynovitis, acute gout
Dosage and routes:
• *Adult:* By mouth 200 mg twice a day, dose reduction may be possible in some patients; acute gout should respond within 7 days; limit treatment in peri-articular disorders to 7–10 days
Available forms include: Tablets 100 mg, 200 mg
Side effects/adverse reactions:
GI: Nausea, anorexia, vomiting, dyspepsia, convulsions, diarrhoea, jaundice, cholestatic hepatitis, constipation, flatulence, cramps, dry mouth, peptic ulcer, gastro-intestinal bleeding/perforation
CNS: Dizziness, drowsiness, fatigue, tremors, confusion, psychosis, insomnia, anxiety, depression, headache, vertigo, paraesthesia
CV: Peripheral oedema, palpitations, dysrhythmias, hypertension, congestive heart failure
INTEG: Purpura, rash, pruritus, sweating, alopecia, photosensitivity, toxic epidermal necrolysis
GU: Nephrotoxicity: dysuria, haematuria, oliguria, azotaemia, crystaluria, vaginal bleeding
HAEM: Blood dyscrasias
RESP: Bronchospasm, dyspnoea
EENT: Tinnitus, hearing loss, blurred vision, metallic taste, epistaxis
MISC: Allergic reactions including anaphylaxis
Contraindications: Hypersensitivity, hypersensitivity to aspirin or other NSAIDs, severe renal disease, severe hepatic disease, active or suspected GI bleeding or peptic ulcer, children, pregnancy, breast-feeding, asthma
Precautions: Elderly, cardiac disorders, hypersensitivity to other non-steroidal anti-inflammatory drugs, renal impairment, liver dysfunction, history of GI bleeding/peptic ulcer/kidney stones
Pharmacokinetics:
By mouth: Peak 2 hr, half-life 7–8 hr; activated by metabolism in liver (active sulphide metabolite half-life 16–17 hr, excreted in urine (metabolites), excreted in breast milk
Interactions/incompatibilities:
• May increase action of: oral anticoagulants, oral hypoglycaemics, lithium
• Decreased effect of sulindac, risk of peripheral neuropathy: dimethyl sulphoxide
• Increased risk of nephrotoxicity: cyclosporin, methotrexate, diuretics
• Decreased effect of sulindac: aspirin, diflunisal
Clinical assessment:
• Renal, liver function tests, before treatment, periodically thereafter if abnormality suspected
• Stop treatment permanently if patient develops unexplained fever, rash, liver changes, constitutional symptoms

Treatment of overdose: Empty stomach, activated charcoal, symptomatic treatment, no specific antidote

NURSING CONSIDERATIONS

Administer:
- With or after food
- With plenty of fluid if patient has history of renal stones

Evaluate:
- Therapeutic response: decreased pain, stiffness, swelling in joints, ability to move more easily
- For eye, ear problems: blurred vision, tinnitus (may indicate toxicity)
- Report any persistant indigestion and black tarry stools

Teach patient/family:
- To report blurred vision or ringing, roaring in ears (may indicate toxicity)
- To avoid driving or other hazardous activities if dizziness or drowsiness occurs
- To take with food or milk
- To report change in urine pattern, weight increase, oedema, pain increase in joints, fever, blood in urine (indicates nephrotoxicity)
- That therapeutic effects may take up to 1 month
- Report any persistant indigestion or black tarry stools

sulphacetamide sodium (ophthalmic)

Albucid, Minims, Sulphacetamide Sodium

Func. class.: Antibiotic
Chem. class.: Sulphonamide
Legal class.: POM

Action: Inhibits bacterial growth by preventing PABA conversion to folic acid

Uses: Conjunctivitis, superficial eye infections

Dosage and routes:
- *Adult and child:* Instil 2–4 drops 2–6 hrly

Available forms include: Sterile ophthalmic solution 10%

Side effects/adverse reactions:
EENT: Burning, stinging, swelling

Contraindications: Hypersensitivity to sulphonamides

NURSING CONSIDERATIONS

Administer:
- After washing hands, cleanse crusts or discharge from eye before application

Perform/provide:
- Storage at room temperature

Evaluate:
- Therapeutic response: absence of redness, inflammation, tearing
- Allergy: itching, lacrimation, redness, swelling

Teach patient/family:
- To use drug exactly as prescribed
- Not to rub eye
- Not to use eye makeup, towels, washcloths, eye medication of others; reinfection may occur
- That drug container tip should not be touched to eye
- To report itching, increased redness, burning, stinging; drug should be discontinued
- That blurred vision may occur when ointment is applied

sulphadiazine

Func. class.: Antibiotic
Chem. class.: Sulphonamide
Legal class.: POM

Action: Interferes with bacterial biosynthesis of proteins by competitive antagonism of para-aminobenzoic acid (PABA). Bacteriostatic antibiotic

Uses: Meningococcal meningitis and other gram-negative and -positive infections sensitive to sulphonamides

Dosage and routes:
• *Adult:* IM/IV 2 g initially, then 1 g 6-hrly for 2 days, then by mouth 1 g 6-hrly
• *Child over 2 months:* IM/IV 50 mg/kg once then 25 mg/kg 6-hrly for 2 days then by mouth 25 mg/kg 6-hrly
Available forms include: Tablets 500 mg, IM/IV injection 250 mg/ml (as sodium salt)
Side effects/adverse reactions:
SYST: Anaphylaxis, cyanosis
GI: Nausea, vomiting, abdominal pain, hepatitis, glossitis, diarrhoea, jaundice, anorexia
CNS: Headache, confusion, insomnia, hallucinations, depression, vertigo, fatigue, anxiety, drug fever, chills
HAEM: Leucopenia, thrombocytopenia, agranulocytosis, haemolytic anaemia, eosinophilia
INTEG: Rash, urticaria, Stevens-Johnson syndrome, erythema, photosensitivity, pain and inflammation at injection site
GU: Renal failure, toxic nephrosis, crystalluria, haematuria
CV: Vasculitis
Contraindications: Hypersensitivity to sulphonamides, premature/newborn babies under 6 weeks, renal or hepatic disease, porphyria
Precautions: Pregnancy, lactation, impaired hepatic or renal function, severe allergy, elderly
Pharmacokinetics:
By mouth: Rapidly absorbed, peak 3–6 hr; 30%–50% bound to plasma proteins, half-life 8–16 hr, excreted in urine, breast milk
Interactions/incompatibilities:
• Increased hypoglycemic response: sulphonylurea agents
• Increased anticoagulant effects: oral anticoagulants
• Decreased renal excretion of: methotrexate
• Increased renal toxicity of: cyclosporin
• Reduced effect of sulphadiazine: PABA, procaine and related local anaesthetics
Clinical assessment:
• Kidney function studies; blood urea, creatinine, urinalysis before and during treatment
• Monitor cotreatment with oral anticoagulants, sulphonylureas
• Discontinue if crystalluria followed by haematuria/oliguria occurs; increase fluid input, alkalinise urine with sodium bicarbonate
Treatment of overdose: Forced alkaline diuresis, symptomatic treatment

NURSING CONSIDERATIONS

Administer:
• After samples have been sent for culture and sensitivity
• With full glass of water to maintain adequate hydration; increase fluids to 2 l daily to decrease crystallisation in kidneys
• Do not administer subcutaneously or intrathecally
• Medication after culture and sensitivity; repeat culture and sensitivity after full course of medication completed
• Parenterally, diluted to not more than a 5% solution with water for injections, and given preferably by IV injection or in a suitable volume of infusion fluid by IV infusion; if necessary by deep IM injection. Oral therapy should commence after 2 days. Unsuitable for intrathecal or subcutaneous use due to high pH. By mouth, to be taken with plenty of water
Perform/provide:
• Resuscitation equipment; severe allergic reactions may occur
Evaluate:
• Therapeutic response: absence of pain, fever, culture and sensitivity negative
• Blood dyscrasias: skin rash,

fever, sore throat, bruising, bleeding, fatigue, joint pain

• Allergic reaction: rash, dermatitis, urticaria, pruritus, dyspnoea, bronchospasm

Teach patient/family:

• To take each oral dose with full glass of water to prevent crystalluria

• To complete full course of treatment to prevent superimposed infection

• To avoid sunlight or use sunscreen to prevent burns

• To avoid non-prescribed medicines (aspirin, vitamin C) unless directed by the clinician

• To use alternative contraceptive measures; decreased effectiveness of oral contraceptives may result

• To notify clinician if skin rash, sore throat, fever, mouth scores, unusual bruising, bleeding occur

sulphadimidine sodium

Sulphadimidine

Func. class.: Antibiotic

Chem. class.: Sulphonamide

Legal class.: POM

Action: Short acting, interferes with the synthesis of nucleic acids in sensitive microorganisms

Uses: Urinary tract infections, prophylaxis of meningococcal meningitis

Dosage and routes:

Urinary tract infections

• *Adult and child over 8 yr:* By mouth, initially 2 g then 0.5–1 g every 6–8 hr

Meningococcal prophylaxis (sensitive strains only)

• *Adult:* By mouth 1 g every 12 hr for 2 days

• *Child:* 3–12 months: By mouth 250 mg every 12 hr for 2 days over 1 yr: By mouth 500 mg every 12 hr for 2 days

Over 1 yr: By mouth 500 mg every 12 hr for 2 days

Available forms include: Tablets 500 mg

Side effects/adverse reactions:

SYST: Anaphylaxis, cyanosis

GI: Nausea, vomiting, abdominal pain, hepatitis, glossitis, diarrhoea, jaundice, anorexia

HAEM: Eosinophilia, agranulocytosis, leucopenia, thrombocytopenia, haemolytic anaemia

INTEG: Rashes, epidermal necrolysis, photosensitivity

CNS: Headache, confusion, insomnia, hallucinations depression, vertigo, fatigue, anxiety, drug fevers, chills

GU: Renal failure, toxic nephrosis, crystalluria, haematuria

CV: Vasculitis

Contraindications: Severe renal or hepatic disease, pregnancy at term, premature or newborn infants under 6 weeks, hypersensitivity to sulphonamides, porphyria

Precautions: Renal or hepatic impairment, elderly, lactation, pregnancy

Pharmacokinetics: Readily absorbed from GI tract, 50% bound to plasma protein. It penetrates into CSF, 40% of plasma concentration is as acetyl derivative. 50% of the dose will be excreted in the urine in 2 days

Interactions/incompatibilities:

• Potentiation of: oral anticoagulants, sulphonylureas

• Decreased renal excretion of: Methotrexate

• Increased renal toxicity of: cyclosporin

• Reduced effect of sulphadimidine: PABA, procaine and related local anaesthetics

Clinical assessment:

• Kidney function studies, before

and during treatment if impairment expected
• Blood counts at intervals during long-term treatment
• Discontinue if crystalluria develops; increase fluid input, alkanise urine with sodium bicarbonate
• Monitor cotreatment with oral anticoagulants, sulphonylureas

Treatment of overdose: Alkalinisation of the urine, with high fluid intake to produce at least 1.5 litres urine daily

NURSING CONSIDERATIONS

Assess:
• Fluid balance, urinalysis

Administer:
• By mouth, with plenty of water
• After sample taken for culture and sensitivity (repeat after full course completed)
• At least 2 l fluid/day to avoid crystallisation in kidneys
• Anti-emetic for severe nausea and vomiting

Evaluate:
• Fluid balance if drug given for urinary tract infection
• Urinalysis for crystals and blood
• Signs of allergic reactions—rashes, erythema multiforme, dyspnoea
• Therapeutic response—absence of pain, fever, negative culture and sensitivity
• Blood dyscrasias—skin rash, fever, sore throat, bruising, bleeding, fatigue, joint pain

Teach patient/family:
• Complete course of tablets even when symptoms improve or cease
• Drink plenty of fluids
• Avoid direct sunlight to skin—burning may occur
• Check with clinician before taking non-prescribed preparations
• Notify clinician at once of rash, fever, sore throat, bruising, bleeding, joint pain

sulphasalazine

Salazopyrin, Salazopyrin, EN-Tabs
Func. class.: Anti-inflammatory
Chem. class.: Aminosalicylate/sulphonamide complex
Legal class.: POM

Action: Metabolised by gut bacteria to release 5-aminosalicylate which has local anti-inflammatory action

Uses: Ulcerative colitis and Crohn's disease, active rheumatoid arthritis

Dosage and routes:

Ulcerative colitis, Crohn's disease
• *Adult:* By mouth, acute attack 1–2 g 4 times a day; maintenance 2 g daily in divided doses 6 hrly; suppositories 1 or 2 per rectum morning and at bedtime alone or with oral therapy; enema 1 daily at bedtime
• *Child over 2 years:* By mouth, acute attack. 40–60 mg/kg daily in divided doses; maintenance 20–30 mg/kg daily in 4 doses

Rheumatoid arthritis
• *Adult:* By mouth, 0.5 g as enteric-coated tablets daily increased by 0.5 g at weekly intervals to a maximum of 3 g daily in 2 divided doses

Available forms include: Tablets 500 mg; oral suspension 250 mg/5 ml; enteric-coated tablets 500 mg; suppository 500 mg; retention enema 3 g/100 ml single dose

Side effects/adverse reactions:

SYST: Anaphylaxis, lupus-like syndrome

GI: Nausea, vomiting, abdominal pain, stomatitis, hepatitis, glossitis, pancreatitis, diarrhoea, exacerbation of colitis, anorexia

CNS: Headache, confusion, insomnia, hallucinations, depression, vertigo, fatigue, anxiety, convulsions, drug fever, chills, neurotoxicity

HAEM: Leucopenia, neutropenia, thrombocytopenia, agranulocytosis, haemolytic anaemia, Heinz body anaemia, methaemoglobinaemia, hypoprothrombinaemia, folate deficiency anaemia

INTEG: Rash, urticaria, Stevens-Johnson syndrome, erythema, photosensitivity

GU: Renal failure, haematuria, nephrotic syndrome, crystalluria, azoospermia, orange urine

CV: Allergic myocarditis, allergic vasculitis

RESP: Pneumonitis

EENT: Staining of soft contact lenses, tinnitus

Contraindications: Hypersensitivity to sulphonamides or salicylates, children under 2 years, porphyria

Precautions: Impaired renal/hepatic function, severe allergy, G6PD deficiency, pregnancy

Pharmacokinetics:

By mouth: Partially absorbed, largely metabolised to 5-aminosalicylic acid and sulphapyridine by gut bacteria. Sulphapyridine mostly absorbed, excreted in urine; 5-aminosalicylic acid mostly excreted in faeces

Interactions/incompatibilities:

- Decreased absorption of: digoxin, folic acid
- Increased hypoglycaemic response: sulphonylurea agents
- Increased anticoagulant effects: oral anticoagulants
- Decreased renal excretion of: methotrexate
- Increased renal toxicity: cyclosporin

Clinical assessment:

- Liver function tests, full blood count monthly for first 3 months of treatment
- Renal function tests if impairment anticipated
- Monitor cotreatment with oral anticoagulants, sulphonylureas, digoxin

Treatment of overdose: Gastric lavage, supportive treatment, no specific antidote

NURSING CONSIDERATIONS

Assess:

- Fluid balance if acute attack ulceration colitis or Grohn's disease

Administer:

- Enteric coated tablets should be swallowed whole
- Give with food or milk
- With full glass of water to maintain adequate fluid intake; increase fluids to 2 l daily to decrease crystallisation in kidneys
- Total daily dose in evenly spaced doses to help minimise GI intolerance

Perform/provide:

- Resuscitation equipment; severe allergic reactions may occur

Evaluate:

- Therapeutic response
- Blood dyscrasias: skin rash, fever, sore throat, bruising, bleeding, fatigue, joint pain
- Allergic reaction: rash, dermatitis, urticaria, pruritus, dyspnoea, bronchospasm

Teach patient/family:

- To take with food or milk
- Take each oral dose with full glass of water to prevent crystalluria
- That drug may discolour urine orange−yellow
- That extended wear soft contact lenses may be permanently stained. Daily wear soft contacts and gas permeable lenses should respond to standard cleaning
- To complete full course of treatment to prevent superimposed infection
- To avoid sunlight or use sunscreen to prevent burns
- To notify clinician if skin rash, sore throat, fever, mouth sores,

unusual bruising, bleeding occur
• May cause temporary infertility in men reversible on discontinuance of drug
• Full effectiveness of drug reached in several weeks

sulphinpyrazone

Anturan
Func. class.: Uricosuric
Chem. class.: Pyrazolone
Legal class.: POM

Action: Inhibits tubular reabsorption of urates, with increased excretion of uric acid
Uses: Gout, hyperuricaemia
Dosage and routes:
Gout
• *Adult:* By mouth 100–200 mg then increased to 600 mg daily over 2–3 weeks, not to exceed 800 mg/day. Reduce dose once serum uric acid levels normal
Available forms include: Tablets 100, 200 mg
Side effects/adverse reactions:
GU: Renal calculi, renal colic, impaired renal function
GI: Gastric irritation, nausea, vomiting, hepatic necrosis, GI bleeding, jaundice
INTEG: Rash, pruritus, fever, photosensitivity
HAEM: Blood dyscrasias
RESP: Apnoea, irregular respirations
SYST: Sodium/water retention, precipitation of acute gout
Contraindications: Acute gout, blood dyscrasis, haemorrhagic diathesis, hypersensitivity to pyrazolone derivatives or NSAIDs (including aspirin), peptic or duodenal ulcers, porphyria, severe hepatic disease, severe renal disease
Precautions: Pregnancy, lactation, healed peptic ulcer, latent heart failure, impaired renal function
Pharmacokinetics:
By mouth: Peak 1–2 hr, half-life 3 hr, metabolized by liver, excreted in urine. 98% protein bound
Interactions/incompatibilities:
• Increased effect of: oral anticoagulants, sulphonylureas, phenytoin
• Decreased blood levels of: theophylline
• Effect reduced by: aspirin, pyrazinamide
Clinical assessment:
• Serum uric acid levels
• Full blood counts, renal function tests at regular intervals
Lab. test interferences:
Phenolsulphonphthalein, aminohippuric acid tests of renal function
Treatment of overdose: Empty stomach, gastric lavage, supportive treatment, no specific antidote

NURSING CONSIDERATIONS

Assess:
• Fluid balance; increase fluid intake to at least 2 L in 24 hours
• Urinalysis
Administer:
• With glass of water
• With food for GI symptoms
• With prophylactic colchicine or NSAID during initial therapy
Perform/provide:
• Ensure urine is alkaline
Evaluate:
• Therapeutic response: absence of pain, stiffness in joints
• Signs of renal impairment
Teach patient/family:
• To avoid high purine foods
• To avoid non-prescribed medicines, especially aspirin
• To report side-effects

sulpiride

Dolmatil, Sulpitil
Func. class.: Antipsychotic
Chem. class.: Substituted benzamide
Legal class.: POM

Action: Antagonist of central D_2 (dopamine 2) receptors
Uses: Treatment of acute and chronic schizophrenia
Dosage and routes:
Positive symptoms
• *Orally:* 400–800 mg daily in 2 divided doses increased up to 1200 mg–1800 mg daily
Negative symptoms
• 800 mg daily in 2 divided doses. Reducing dose to 200 mg daily will increase the alerting effect
Mixed +/− symptoms
• 400–600 mg twice daily
Nead not be administered on empty stomach
Available forms include: Tablets, 200 mg
Side effects/adverse reactions:
CNS: Extrapyramidal effects, tardive dyskinesia, akathisia, insommia, other sleep disturbances, aggravation of existing agitation
ENDO: Gynecomastia, galactorrhoea
Contraindications: Phaeochromocytoma; severe renal, hepatic or blood disease; alcoholic intoxication or other disorders with depressed CNS function
Precautions:
• Patients with extrapyramidal effects, hypertension, tumours
• Avoidance of alcohol
• Do not drive or operate machinery
• Reduce dose in mild-moderate renal impairment
• Pregnancy, especially first 16 weeks
• Breast-feeding – best avoided
Pharmacokinetics: Peak plasma levels after 2–4 hr, half-life 6–8 hr; excreted almost entirely as unchanged drug in the urine
Lab. test interferences: Serum glucose, serum cholesterol; sulpiride may interfere with these tests
Treatment of overdose: Alkaline osmotic diuresis. Anticholinergic treatment of extrapyramidal symptoms occur

NURSING CONSIDERATIONS

Assess:
• For hoarding or giving medicine to other patients
• Likelihood of compliance if self-medicating
• BP lying/standing
• For alcohol habit
Administer:
• By mouth, with or without food but with fluids
Perform/provide:
• Supervised ambulation until stabilised on medication
• Storage in a cool dry place
Evaluate:
• Therapeutic effect, reduction in schizophrenic symptoms
• Side effects, particularly extrapyramidal effects and aggravation of existing condition
• Effect of changes in body image (gynaecomastia, galactorrhoea) on patient
Teach patient/family:
• Dose may be taken with food and should be taken with full glass of water
• About side effects; to report any of these to nurse or clinician; that gynaecomastia, galactorrhoea are reversible when treatment is discontinued
• Not to take alcohol; not to drive or operate heavy machinery
• That medication should not be discontinued suddenly

sumatriptan

Imigran
Func. class.: Anti-migraine drug
Chem. class.: Serotonin antagonist
Legal class.: POM

Action: 5-hydroxytryptamine 1 (5-HT_1) receptor antagonist, centrally acting
Uses: Treatment of acute migraine attacks and cluster headache
Dosage and routes:
Migraine
• *Orally:* 100 mg single dose as early as possible after onset of attack, repeated if attack recurs; up to three doses in any 24 hr period. Food does not affect absorption
• *Subcutaneous injection:* 6 mg single dose as early as possible after onset of attack. May be repeated no earlier than 1 hr later if attack recurs; up to 2 doses in any 24 hr period
Drug is supplied in an autoinjector; instructions for use must be followed carefully
Cluster headache
• 6 mg by SC injection, repeated no earlier than 1 hr later; up to 2 doses in any 24 hr period
Available forms include: 6 mg auto-injector, 100 mg tablets
Side effects/adverse reactions:
CVS: Transient increases in blood pressure, chest pain, heaviness and tightness in chest or other parts of body
CNS: Drowsiness, dizziness
GI: Nausea and vomiting possible (relationship with sumatriptan not clear), altered liver function tests
INTEG: Flushing, transient pain at injection site
MS: Parasthesia, feeling of weakness
Contraindications: Hypersensitivity to drug; ischaemic heart disease; previous myocardial infarction or Prinzmetals angina; uncontrolled hypertension; patients taking ergotamine, monoamine oxidase inhibitors, 5-HT reuptake inhibitors or lithium
Precautions:
• Not to be used as prophylactic
• Conditions which predispose to heart disease
• Caution with driving or operating machinery if drowsiness is caused
• Impaired hepatic or renal function
• Pregnancy, breast-feeding
Pharmacokinetics:
• Maximum plasma concentrations occur after 25 min of SC administration and 0.5–5 hr of oral administration (although 70% of max. is attained after 45 min)
• Plasma half life is approx 2 hr. Sumatriptan is excreted in urine as metabolite and unchanged drug
Interactions:
• Must not be administered with mono-amine oxidase inhibitors (MAOIs), selective-serotonin re-uptake inhibitors (SSRI) or lithium
• Must not be administered within 24 hr after ergotamine has been administered, and ergotamine should not be administered within 6 hr of sumatriptan administration
Treatment of overdose: Monitor for at least 10 hr; standard supportive treatment supplied as required

NURSING CONSIDERATIONS

Assess:
• BP
• Other medication taken for migraine or other reasons
Administer:
• SC in auto-injector (supplied) as soon as attack starts
• By mouth as soon as attack

starts, with fluid (food does not affect absorption)

Perform/provide:

• Store: protect injection from light

Evaluate:

• Therapeutic effect; control of migraine and cluster headaches

• For side effects, changes in BP, pain, heaviness, tightness in chest

Teach patient/family:

• About the drug; that it must not be used prophylactically

• About side effects; to report any of these to nurse or clinician

• That driving and use of heavy machinery is inadvisable if drowsiness and dizziness occur

• How to use (and dispose of safely) the auto-injector

• That other medication (MAOIs) must not be taken and ergotamine not within 24 hr

---

suxamethonium chloride

Anectine, Scoline

Func. class.: Depolarising neuromuscular blocker

Legal class.: POM

Action: Inhibits transmission of nerve impulses by binding with cholinergic receptor sites, antagonising action of acetylcholine. Short acting depolarisation

Uses: Facilitation of endotracheal intubation, skeletal muscle relaxation during mechanical ventilation, surgery, or general anaesthesia

Dosage and routes:

• *Adult:* IV 20–100 mg repeated every 5–10 min as needed or followed by 2.5–4 mg/min by continuous IV infusion according to patient's need, not to exceed 500 mg/hr

• *Child:* IV 1–2 mg/kg initially then as for adult adjusted to body weight

Available forms include: Injection IV 50 mg/ml

Side effects/adverse reactions:

SYST: Anaphylaxis

CV: Bradycardia, tachycardia, increased, decreased BP, sinus arrest, arrhythmias

RESP: Prolonged apnoea, bronchospasm, cyanosis, respiratory depression

EENT: Increased secretions, increased intraocular pressure

GI: Increased secretions, increased bowel movement

MS: Weakness, muscle pain, fasciculations, prolonged relaxation

HAEM: Myoglobulinaemia

INTEG: Rash, flushing, pruritus, urticaria

ELECT: Transient hyperkalaemia

Contraindications: Hypersensitivity, family history of/current malignant hyperthermia, severe liver disease, decreased plasma pseudo/cholinesterase, myasthenia gravis, major muscle wasting, Duchenne muscular dystrophy, ophthalmic procedures when the anterior chamber of the eye is open, hyperkalaemia, patients with severe burns, recovering from major trauma, myotonia, acute narrow-angle glaucoma

Precautions: Pregnancy, cardiac disease, fractures—fasciculations may increase damage, dehydration, severe anaemia, malnutrition, neuromuscular disease, elderly, mothers within 6 weeks of giving birth, severe infection, phaeochromocytoma

Pharmacokinetics:

IV: Onset 1 min, peak 2–3 min, duration 6–10 min

IM: Onset 2–3 min

Hydrolysed in plasma, excreted in urine

Interactions/incompatibilities:

• Increased neuromuscular block-

ade: aminoglycosides, clindamycin, lincomycin, quinidine, local anaesthetics, polymyxin antibiotics, lithium, narcotic analgesics, oxytocin, procainamide, phenothiazines, phenelzine, alkylating agents, amphotericin, anticholinesterases (including organo-phosphorus pesticides and demecarium/ecothiopate eye drops), ketamine, quinine, verapamil
• Increased risk of cardiac arrhythmias given with: digoxin, other cardiac glycosides
• Reduced neuromuscular blockade: diazepam, propranolol

Clinical assessment:
• For electrolyte imbalances (potassium, magnesium); may lead to increased action of this drug

Treatment of overdose: Maintain airway, ventilate mechanically; consider anticholinesterase for secondary non-depolarising block

NURSING CONSIDERATIONS

Assess:
• History of malignant hyperthermia, myasthenia gravis or scolinic apnoea
• Vital signs (BP, pulse, respirations, airway)

Administer:
• Using nerve stimulator by anaesthetist to determine neuromuscular blockade
• By slow IV over 1–2 min (only by qualified person, usually an anaesthetist)

Perform/provide:
• Storage in light-resistant container at 4°C or less and do not resterilise
• Reassurance if communication is difficult during recovery from neuromuscular blockade

Evaluate:
• Vital signs, degree of respiratory function
• Check for urinary retention
• Therapeutic response: paralysis of jaw, eyelid, head, neck, rest of body
• Recovery: decreased paralysis of face, diaphragm, leg, arm, rest of body
• Allergic reactions: rash, fever, respiratory distress, pruritus; drug should be discontinued

Teach patient/family:
• That some muscular pain may occur during recovery

---

tamoxifen

Nolvadex, Tamofen, Noltam, Emblon, Oestrifen

Func. class.: Anti-neoplastic
Chem. class.: Hormone, anti-oestrogen
Legal class.: POM

Action: Inhibits cell division by binding to cytoplasmic oestrogen receptors

Uses: Breast cancer, anovulatory infertility

Dosage and routes:

Breast cancer
• *Adult:* By mouth 20–40 mg daily as a single dose or in two divided doses

Infertility
• *Adult:* By mouth 20 mg daily on days 2–5 of cycle, increasing if necessary to 40 mg and then 80 mg daily in subsequent cycles
If cycles irregular, start initial cause on any day, with subsequent cause starting 45 days later or on second day of cycle if menstruation occurs

Available forms include: Tablets 10, 20, 40 mg (as citrate)

Side effects/adverse reactions:
HAEM: Transient thrombocytopenia, deep vein thrombosis
GI: Gastrointestinal disturbances
GU: Vaginal bleeding, pruritus vulvae, cystic ovarian swelling (premenopausal women)

INTEG: Rash, dry skin
CNS: Headache, dizziness, depression, confusion
EENT: Ocular lesions, retinopathy, corneal opacity, blurred vision
ENDO: Hot flushes, amenorrhoea (in premenopausal women)
SYST: Fluid retention, tumour flare
Contraindications: Hypersensitivity, pregnancy, porphyria
Pharmacokinetics:
By mouth: Peak 4–7 hr, half-life 7–14 hr (1 week terminal), extensively metabolised, excreted in faeces, urine
Interactions/incompatibilities:
• Increased effect of: coumarin anticoagulants

NURSING CONSIDERATIONS

Administer:
• With food
Evaluate:
• Bleeding: haematuria, bruising, petechiae, mucosa or orifices daily if in acute condition
• Side effects especially if adding to patient's distress
• Symptoms indicating severe allergic reactions: rash, pruritus, urticaria, purpuric skin lesions, itching, flushing
Teach patient/family:
• To report any complaints, side effects to nurse or clinician
• That vaginal bleeding, pruritus, hot flashes, ocular lesions can occur, are reversible after discontinuing treatment

---

teicoplanin

Targocid
Func. class.: Antibiotic
Chem. class.: Glycopeptide
Legal class.: POM

Action: Bactericidal antibiotic which acts by binding to peptidoglycan units in the bacterial cell wall; with activity against both aerobic and anaerobic Gram-positive bacteria
Uses: Potentially serious Gram-positive infections including endocarditis, dialysis-associated peritonitis and serious infection due to multiply-resistant staphylococci
Dosage and routes:
Moderate infections
• *Adult:* IV injection (as a bolus or a 30-min infusion) 400 mg initially, maintenance IV or IM 200 mg/day
• *Children (under 14 yr):* IV 10 mg/kg every 12 hr for the first 3 doses followed by 6 mg/kg daily IV or IM
Severe infections
• *Adult:* IV injection every 12 hr for 3 doses initially, 400 mg, maintenance IV or IM 400 mg/day
• *Children under 14 yr:* IV injection 10 mg/kg every 12 hr for 3 doses initially, maintenance IV or IM 10 mg/kg/day
Available forms include: Injection 200 mg, 400 mg
Side effects/adverse reactions:
CNS: Dizziness, headache
EENT: Hearing loss, tinnitus, vestibular disturbances
INTEG: Erythema and local pain, thrombophlebitis, rash, pruritus
HAEM: Eosinophilia, leucopenia, neutropenia, thrombocytopenia, thrombocytosis
GU: Transient elevations of serum creatinine
GI: Nausea, vomiting, diarrhoea, raised liver enzyme values
RESP: Bronchospasm
SYST: Fever, anaphylaxis
Contraindications:
Hypersensitivity
Precautions: Hypersensitivity to vancomycin, pregnancy, lactation, renal insufficiency (renal and auditory function should be

monitored if therapy prolonged; dosage reduction required)
Pharmacokinetics: IV serum concentration exceeding typical MICs persist for 24 hr. 90 to 95% bound to serum albumin. Excreted unchanged by the kidney
Clinical assessment:
- Determination of teicoplanin serum concentrations may optimise therapy

NURSING CONSIDERATIONS:
Assess:
- Fluid balance
- Bowel pattern

Administer:
- Reconstitute with diluent provided; reconstituted solution may be given by direct IM, IV bolus injection or by IV infusion over 30 min. In severe infection trough (pre-dose) serum concentrations should not be below 10 mg/l. Adjust dose in renal insufficiency.
- After specimens have been sent for culture and sensitivity
- Prepare injection by slowly adding diluent to the drug vial, and rolling the vial gently until the powder is completely dissolved, taking care to avoid the formation of foam
- If the solution becomes foamy allow to stand for about 15 mins before use
- Reconstituted vials should be used immediately
- If this is not possible, keep at 4°C and discard within 24 hr
- Duration of therapy depends on infection; in endocarditis and osteomyelitis, treatment of 3 weeks or longer is recommended

Evaluate:
- For side effects
- Therapeutic response
- Observe injection site for signs of inflammation

Teach patient/family:
- To report side effects, tinnitus, etc.

temazepam

Func. class.: Sedative/hypnotic
Chem. class.: Benzodiazepine
Legal class.: CD (Sch 4) POM

Action: Produces CNS depression at limbic, thalamic, hypothalamic levels of the CNS; may be mediated by neurotransmitter gamma-aminobutyric acid (GABA); results are sedation, hypnosis, skeletal muscle relaxation, anticonvulsant activity, anxiolytic action
Uses: Insomnia (short term), premedication
Dosage and routes:
Insomnia
- *Adult:* By mouth 10–30 mg at bedtime increasing to 40–60 mg if needed; elderly patients may respond to 5–15 mg

Premedication
- *Adult:* By mouth 20–40 mg, 30–60 mins before surgical procedure

Available forms include: Capsules 10, 15, 20, 30 mg; Tablets 10, 20 mg; Oral solution 10 mg/5 ml
Side effects/adverse reactions:
CNS: Drowsiness, dizziness, confusion, depression, restless sleep, vivid dreams or nightmares, headache, dependence
GI: Gastro-intestinal disturbances
CV: Hypotension, palpitations
INTEG: Rash
EENT: Dry mouth
Contraindications: Hypersensitivity to benzodiazepines, children, acute pulmonary insufficiency; respiratory depression, obsessional or phobic states, chronic psychosis, porphyria
Precautions: Hepatic disease, renal disease, suicidal individuals, history of drug abuse, personality disorder, elderly, seizure disorders, pregnancy, lactation, arterio-

sclerosis; do not use for more than 2–4 weeks

Pharmacokinetics:

By mouth: Onset 30–45 min, duration 6–8 hr, half-life 8 hr; metabolised by liver, excreted by kidneys, excreted in breast milk

Interactions/incompatibilities:

- Increased sedative effects of alcohol, anaesthetics, antihistamines, antidepressants: cimetidine, disulfiram, narcotic analgesics
- Possibly reduced effect of: levodopa

NURSING CONSIDERATIONS

Administer:

- ½–1 hr before bedtime for sleeplessness

Evaluate:

- Therapeutic response: ability to sleep at night, decreased amount of early morning awakening if taking drug for insomnia
- Mental status: mood, alertness, affect, memory (long, short)

Teach patient/family:

- To avoid driving or other activities requiring alertness until drug is stabilized
- To avoid alcohol ingestion or CNS depressants; serious CNS depression may result
- That effects may take 2 nights for benefits to be noticed
- Alternative measures to improve sleep: reading, exercise several hours before bedtime, warm bath, warm milk, TV, self-hypnosis, deep breathing
- Hangover is common in elderly, but less common than with barbiturates

temocillin ▼

Temopen

Func. class.: Antibiotic

Chem. class.: Penicillinase-resistant penicillin

Legal class.: POM

Action: Interferes with biosynthesis of bacterial cell wall. It is active against many β-lactamase producing Gram-negative aerobes

Uses: Septicaemia, urinary tract infection, lower respiratory tract infections involving susceptible Gram-negative bacilli. Not active against Gram-positive bacteria

Dosage and routes:

- *Adult:* IM, IV injection, intermittent IV infusion, 1 to 2 g every 12 hr. In acute uncomplicated urinary tract infections 1 g daily, as single or divided doses

Available forms include: Injection 500 mg, 1 g (as sodium salt)

Side effects/adverse reactions:

INTEG: Pain at site of IM injection, rashes

GI: Diarrhoea

MS: Joint pains (hypersensitivity)

SYSTEM: Anaphylactic shock, fever (hypersensitivity)

Contraindications: Hypersensitivity to penicillin

Precautions: Pregnancy, breast feeding, renal insufficiency, history of allergy

Pharmacokinetics: Half-life 4 to 5 hr. 70% to 80% excreted in urine unchanged

Interactions/incompatibilities:

- Possibly decreased effect of: oral contraceptives
- Possibly decreased effect of temocillin: tetracyclines
- Increased antibacterial effect: aminoglycosides

NURSING CONSIDERATIONS:

- If a skin rash occurs treatment should be discontinued

• Solutions for IV injection should be prepared by dissolving 500 mg of powder in 10 ml of water for injections or 1–2 g of powder in 20 ml diluent
• The resulting solutions can be used for infusion by adding to an IV infusion solution
• Solutions for IM injection can be prepared by dissolving 500 mg of powder in 1.5 ml of water for injections or 1 g of powder in 2 ml of diluent
• If pain is experienced at the site of injection lignocaine hydrochloride 0.5 to 1% may be used in place of water for injections
• IV injection should be given by slow injection over 3–4 min and IV infusion over a period of 30–40 min
• Temocillin is compatible with water for injections, sodium chloride 0.9%, dextrose 5%
• Solutions should not be mixed with blood products or proteinaceous fluids or with intravenous lipid emulsions
• Powder should be stored in a dry place below 20°C
• Any part-used solutions should be discarded
• The solution should normally be administered within 30 mins of preparation; if this is not possible, it may be kept for up to 24 hr at 2 to 8°C
• Use relevant points in ticarcillin

NURSING CONSIDERATIONS

Assess:
• For known allergies to penicillin group
• Fluid balance
• Bowel pattern

Administer:
• After culture and sensitivity tests
• IV: By slow injection over 3–4 min or infusion over 30–40 min (drug is compatible with water, sodium chloride 0.9% or dextrose 5%)
• IM: By deep IM injection (may be mixed with lignocaine hydrochloride 0.5 to 1.0% if pain is experienced at site of injection)
• IM, as solution containing 1 g dissolved in 2 ml water for injections or lignocaine 0.5–1%; IV, as solution containing 1–2 g in 20 ml water for injections, by injection over 3–4 min or added to infusion and given over 30–40 min

Evaluate:
• Therapeutic response
• For allergic response, rashes, diarrhoea

---

tenoxicam

Mobiflex
Func. class.: Non-steroidal anti-inflammatory
Chem. class.: Oxicam
Legal class.: POM

Action: Inhibits prostaglandin synthesis; has marked anti-inflammatory and analgesic activity and some antipyretic activity
Uses: Osteoarthrosis, rheumatoid arthritis
Dosage and routes:
• *Adult:* By mouth, 20 mg daily in acute disorders usually 7 days, in severe cases maximum 14 days
Available forms include: Tablets 20 mg; milk granules 20 mg/sachet
Side effects/adverse reactions:
GI: Nausea, dyspepsia, abdominal pain, constipation, diarrhoea, flatulence, stomatitis, peptic ulcer, GI haemorrhage
HAEM: Blood dyscrasias
CNS: Headache, dizziness, depression, confusion, paraesthesia, vertigo, somnolence
INTEG: Rashes, erythema, pruritus, alopecia, photosensitivity
EENT: Swelling and irritation of eyes, blurred vision, tinnitus

CV: Palpitations
RESP: Dyspnoea
SYST: Weight changes, oedema
Contraindications: History of, active or suspected peptic ulcer, GI bleeding; gastritis; hypersensitivity to aspirin or other NSAIDS; hypersensitivity; pregnancy; breast feeding; children
Precautions: Renal or hepatic insufficiency, congestive heart failure, elderly
Pharmacokinetics:
By mouth: Rapidly and completely absorbed, extensively bound to plasma protein, elimination half life about 72 hr, extensively metabolised, excreted in urine and bile
Interactions/incompatibilities:
• Possibly increased toxicity: cyclosporin, diuretics, lithium, salicylates
• Possibly increased effects of: anticoagulants, anti-diabetic agents (sulphonylureas)

NURSING CONSIDERATIONS
Administer:
• With or after food
• With water
• Mix granules in water
Evaluate:
• Therapeutic response: decreased pain, stiffness, swelling in joints, ability to move more easily
• For eye, ear problems: blurred vision, tinnitus (may indicate toxicity)
Teach patient/family:
• To report blurred vision, ringing, roaring in ears (may indicate toxicity)
• To avoid driving or other hazardous activities if dizziness or drowsiness occurs
• To report change in urine pattern, weight increase, oedema, pain increase in joints, fever, blood in urine (indicates nephrotoxicity)
• That therapeutic effects may take up to 1 month

terbinafine (topical) ▼

Lamisil
Func. class.: Antifungal
Chem. class.: Allylamine
Legal class.: POM

Action: Interferes with fungal sterol biosynthesis leading to a deficiency of ergosterol and an accumulation of squalene resulting in fungal cell death
Uses: Yeast infections of the skin, principally those caused by *Candida* spp., also pityriasis
Dosage and routes:
• *Adult:* Topically to the affected area once or twice a day usually for 1–2 weeks
Available forms include: Cream 1%
Side effects/adverse reactions:
INTEG: Redness, itching or stinging at the site of application
Contraindications: Hypersensitivity
Precautions: Pregnancy; breast-feeding
Pharmacokinetics: Less than 5% terbinafine absorbed after topical application; metabolised in liver to inactive metabolites excreted in urine; elimination half-life 17 hr
Treatment of overdose: There is no experience of ingestion of terbinafine cream. If it occurs gastric emptying should be considered

NURSING CONSIDERATIONS
Assess:
• Skin condition
• Take swab for microbiological investigation before commencing treatment
Administer:
• After cleansing and drying affected area
• Rubbing in gently; wash hands thoroughly before and after application
Perform/provide:

• Affected areas in folds of skin may be covered with a gauze dressing

Evaluate:

• Absence of infection

Teach patient/family:

• To cleanse and dry skin thoroughly before application

• Not to stop treatment as soon as symptoms abate — regular application should continue for several more days to prevent recurrence

• To discontinue use and seek advice if side effects occur

---

terbutaline (inhaled)

Bricanyl (Turbohaler, Respules)

Func. class.: Bronchodilator

Chem. class.: Adrenergic β_2-stimulant

Legal class.: POM

Action: Causes bronchodilation by acting on β-receptors in bronchus and lung; has relatively little effect on cardiac receptors

Uses: Bronchospasm and the treatment of reversible obstructive airways disease

Dosage and routes:

By aerosol inhalation, acute and maintenance treatment

• *Adult and child:* 250–500 mcg (1–2 puffs) repeated after 6 hr if necessary; not more than 8 inhalations in 24 hr

By inhalation of powder (Turbohaler)

• *Adult and child:* 500 mcg (1 inhalation) as required: not more than 4 inhalations in any 24 hr

By inhalation of nebulised solution

• *Adult:* 5–10 mg 2–4 times daily; additional doses may be necessary in severe acute asthma

• *Child:* Up to 3 yr, 2 mg; 3–6 yr, 3 mg; 6–8 yr, 4 mg; over 8 yr, 5 mg; 2 to 4 times daily, respectively

Available forms include: Aerosol inhaler 250 mcg/metered inhalation. Powder inhaler 500 mcg/metered inhalation. Nebuliser solution 2.5 mg, 10 mg/ml

Side effects/adverse reactions:

CNS: Tremor, anxiety, headache

CV: Palpitations, tachycardia, arrhythmias

GI: Nausea

META: Hyperglycaemia

MS: Cramps

ELEC: Hypokalaemia

Contraindications: Hypersensitivity

Precautions: Pregnancy; cardiac disorders; hypothyroidism; diabetes mellitus; hypertension; elderly patients

Pharmacokinetics:

Onset: 5–30 min; duration 3–6 hr

Interactions:

• Decreased action: β-blockers

• Increased risk of hypokalaemia: corticosteroids, diuretics, xanthines

Treatment of overdose: Preferred antidote is cardioselective β-blocker, but use with extreme caution in patients with history of bronchospasm

NURSING CONSIDERATIONS

Assess:

• Baseline vital signs, lung sounds, respiratory capacity

Administer:

• Using correct technique for device

• Dilute nebuliser solution with sterile sodium chloride (0.9%) before use unless using Respules (2.5 mg/ml)

• After shaking aerosol, patient should exhale, place mouthpiece in mouth, press aerosol and inhale slowly tilting head back, hold breath for 10 seconds and exhale slowly

Perform/provide:

• Storage: nebuliser solution protected from the light and used within one month of opening bottle

• Discard Respules immediately after use

Evaluate:

• Therapeutic response: absence of dyspnoea and wheezing

• Tolerance over long-term therapy; dose may need to be increased or changed

Teach patient/family:

• Not to use non-prescribed medications; extra stimulation may occur

• Good technique in use of device

• How to store, use, clean and care for inhaler

• About side effects of drug: shakiness, flushing, headache, dry mouth

• To avoid getting solution in eyes

• Technique for averting asthma attacks (use of space) and how to deal with attacks if they occur

• Not to exceed prescribed dosage

• To avoid: smoking, smoke-filled rooms, persons with respiratory infections

terbutaline sulphate

Bricanyl, Bricanyl SA, Monovent

Func. class.: Bronchodilator

Chem. class.: Adrenergic β_2-stimulant

Legal class.: POM

Action: Causes bronchodilation by acting on β-receptors in bronchus and lung; has relatively little effect on cardiac receptors

Uses: Bronchospasm, premature labour

Dosage and routes:

Bronchospasm

• *Adult:* By mouth, 5 mg 2 or 3 times a day; subcutaneous/IM/slow IV injections 250–500 mg up to 4 times a day; IV infusion, solution of 3–5 mcg/ml at 1.5–5 mcg/min

• *Child: 3–7 yr:* By mouth; 0.75–1.5 mg three times a day

• *7–15 yr:* By mouth; 2.5 mg two or three times a day; subcutaneous slow IV/IM: 2–15 yr 10 mcg/kg (maximum 300 mcg)

Premature Labour

• *Adult:* IV infusion: 10 mcg/min for 1 hr, increased by 5 mcg every 10 min to maximum 20 mcg/min, until contractions stop; subsequently by subcutaneous injection, injection 250 mcg four times daily for 3 days and then by mouth 5 mg three times daily until 37th week of pregnancy

Available forms include: Tablets, 5 mg; tablets, modified release, 7.5 mg; aerosol, 0.25 mg/actuation; syrup, 0.3 mg/ml; injection, 0.5 mg/ml

Side effects/adverse reactions:

CNS: Tremors, anxiety, headache

CV: Palpitations, tachycardia, arrhythmias

GI: Nausea

META: Hypokalaemia, hyperglycaemia

MS: Cramp

Contraindications: Hypersensitivity to sympathomimetics

Precautions: Pregnancy, cardiac disorders, hyperthyroidism, diabetes mellitus, hypertension, elderly patients

Pharmacokinetics:

By mouth: Onset ½ hr, duration 4–8 hr

Subcutaneous: Onset 6–15 min, duration 1½–4 hr

Interactions/incompatibilities:

• Increased effects of both drugs: other sympathomimetics

• Decreased action: β-blockers

• Increased risk of hypokalaemia: corticosteroids, diuretics, xanthines

Treatment of overdose: Supportive symptomatic care; a cardioselective β-blocker may be helpful in arrhythmias, at the risk of inducing bronchoconstriction

NURSING CONSIDERATIONS

Evaluate:

• Therapeutic response: absence of dyspnoea and wheezing

• Tolerance over long-term therapy; dose may need to be increased or changed

Teach patient/family:

• Not to use non-prescribed medications; extra stimulation may occur

• On all aspects of drug; to avoid smoking, smoke-filled rooms, persons with respiratory infections

terfenadine

Triludan, Seldane

Func. class.: Antihistamine

Chem. class.: Butyrophenone derivative

Legal class.: P

Action: Acts peripherally on blood vessels, GI, respiratory system by competing with histamine for H_1-receptor site; decreases allergic response by blocking histamine

Uses: Allergic symptoms such as hayfever, rhinitis, and skin reactions

Dosage and routes:

• *Adult and child over 12 yr:* By mouth 60 mg twice a day or 120 mg in the morning

• *Child 6–12 yr:* By mouth 30 mg twice a day

• *Child 3–6 yr:* By mouth 15 mg twice a day

Available forms include: Tablets 60 mg, 120 mg; suspension 30 mg/5 ml

Side effects/adverse reactions:

CNS: Dizziness, headache, depression, convulsions, confusion, insomnia, nightmares, paraesthesia, tremor

CV: Palpitations, arrhythmias

RESP: Bronchospasm

GI: Abdominal pain, dyspepsia, jaundice, liver dysfunction

INTEG: Rash, alopecia photosensitivity, sweating, angioedema

GU: Menstrual disturbances

EENT: Visual disturbances

MS: Muscle pain

SYST: Anaphylaxis

Contraindications: Hypersensitivity; porphyria; hypokalaemia; prolonged QT interval; severe hepatic impairment

Precautions: Pregnancy, lactation, hepatic impairment

Pharmacokinetics:

By mouth: Peak 1–2 hr, 97% bound to plasma proteins, half-life is biphasic 3½ hr, 16–23 hr

Interactions/incompatibilities:

• Increased effect (reduced metabolism of terfenadine): ketoconazole, macrolide antibiotics

NURSING CONSIDERATIONS

Evaluate:

• Therapeutic response: absence of running or congested nose or rashes

Teach patient/family:

• All aspects of drug use; to notify clinician if confusion, sedation occurs

• To avoid driving or other hazardous activity if drowsiness occurs

testosterone

Func. class.: Androgenic anabolic steroid

Chem. class.: Steroid

Legal class.: POM

Action: Increases weight by building body tissue, increases potassium, phosphorus, chloride, nitrogen levels, increases bone development; controls development and maintenance of male sexual characteristics

Uses: Hypogonadism (male) menopausal disorders

Dosage and routes:

Hypogonadism

• *Adult:* By implantation 600 mg every 6 months

Menopausal disorders

• *Adult:* By implantation 50–100 mg every 4–8 months

Available forms include: Implant 100, 200 mg

Side effects/adverse reactions:

INTEG: Rash, acneiform lesions, oily hair, alopecia, hirsutism

MS: Closure of epiphyses in prepubertal males, increased bone growth

GU: Amenorrhoea, decreased female libido, decreased breast size, clitoral hypertrophy, prostatism in elderly men, testicular atrophy, suppression of spermatogenesis, priapism, precocious sexual development in prepubertal males

GI: Jaundice, hepatitis

META: Hypercalcaemia, sodium and fluid retention

Contraindications: Nephrosis, hypersensitivity, pregnancy, lactation, hypercalcaemia, breast cancer (men), prostatic carcinoma

Precautions: Ischaemic heart disease, cardiac, renal or hepatic impairment, epilepsy, migraine, skeletal metastases risk of exacerbating hypercalcaemia, hypertension, prepubertal males

Interactions/incompatibilities:

• Increased effects of: oral anticoagulants

NURSING CONSIDERATIONS

Assess:

• Baseline weight and BP

• Drug can be one of abuse, particularly by athletes

Perform/provide:

• Diet with increased calories and protein; decrease sodium if oedema occurs

Evaluate:

• Growth rate in children since growth rate may be uneven (linear/bone growth) when used for extended period

• Therapeutic response

• Cardiac symptoms, jaundice

• Observe for fluid retention

• Mental status: affect, mood, behavioural changes, aggression

• Signs of masculinisation in female: increased libido, deepening of voice, breast tissue, enlarged clitoris, menstrual irregularities; male: gynaecomastia, impotence, testicular atrophy

Teach patient/family:

• Drug needs to be combined with complete health plan: diet, rest, exercise

• To notify clinician if therapeutic response decreases

• Do not discontinue this medication abruptly

• Teach patient all aspects of drug usage, including changes in sex characteristics

• Women to report menstrual irregularities

• Drug can be abused

---

testosterone decanoate/ testosterone enanthate/ testosterone isocaproate/ testosterone phenylpropionate/ testosterone propionate/ testosterone undecanoate

Primoteston Depot, Restandol, Sustanon, Virormone

Func. class.: Androgenic anabolic steroid

Chem. class.: Steroid

Legal class.: POM

Action: Increases weight by building body tissue, increases potassium, phosphorus, chloride, nitrogen levels, increases bone development; controls development and maintenance of male sexual characteristics

Uses: Androgen deficiency, such as in hypogonadism (male), delayed puberty or cryptorchidism; breast cancer (female)

Dosage and routes:

Delayed puberty, cryptorchidism

• *Adult:* IM 50 mg (propionate) weekly

Breast cancer

• *Adult:* IM 100 mg (propionate) 2–3 times weekly; or 250 mg (enanthate) every 2–3 weeks

Hypogonadism

• *Adult:* IM 50 mg (propionate) 2–3 times weekly; or 250 mg (enanthate) every 2–3 weeks, reduced to every 3–6 weeks for maintenance; or 100 mg (isocaproate/phenylpropionate/propionate 2:2:1) every 2 weeks; or 250 mg (decanoate/isocaproate/phenylpropionate/propionate 10:6:6:3) every 3 weeks; By mouth 120–160 mg (undecanoate) daily for 2–3 weeks, then adjust in range 40–120 mg daily according to response

Available forms include: Capsules 40 mg (undecanoate); Injection 250 mg (enanthate)/ml, 50 mg (propionate)/ml, 100 mg (isocaproate 40 mg, phenylpropionate 40 mg, propionate 20 mg)/ml, 250 mg (decanoate 100 mg, isocaproate 60 mg, phenylpropionate 60 mg, propionate 30 mg)/ml

Side effects/adverse reactions:

INTEG: Rash, acneiform lesions, oily hair, skin, alopecia, hirsutism

MS: Closure of epiphyses in prepubertal males, increased bone growth

GU: Amenorrhoea, decreased female libido, decreased breast size, clitoral hypertrophy, prostatism in elderly man, testicular atrophy, suppression of spermatogenesis, priapism, precocious sexual development in prepubertal males

GI: Jaundice, hepatitis

META: Hypercalcaemia, sodium and fluid retention

Contraindications: Hypercalcaemia, nephrosis, breast cancer (men), prostatic carcinoma, hypersensitivity, pregnancy, lactation

Precautions: Ischaemic heart disease, cardiac, renal or hepatic impairment, hypertension, epilepsy, migraine, prepubertal males

Pharmacokinetics:

By mouth: Metabolised in liver, excreted in urine, breast milk

Interactions/incompatibilities:

• Increased effects of: oral anticoagulants

NURSING CONSIDERATIONS

Assess:

• Baseline weight and BP

• Growth rate in children since growth rate may be uneven (linear/bone growth) used for extended periods of time

Administer:

• Titrated dose; use lowest effective dose

• IM deep into large muscle mass

Perform/provide:

• Diet with increased calories, protein; decrease sodium if oedema occurs as medically directed

• Give iron in anaemia

Evaluate:

• Weight daily, notify clinician if weekly weight gain is over 2 kg

• BP 4 hrly

• Fluid balance; be alert for decreasing urinary output, increasing oedema

• Therapeutic response: occurs in 4–6 weeks in osteoporosis

• Oedema, hypertension, cardiac symptoms, jaundice

• Mental status: affect, mood, behavioural changes, aggression

- Signs of masculinisation in female: increased libido, deepening of voice, breast tissue, enlarged clitoris, menstrual irregularities; male: gynaecomastia, impotence, testicular atrophy
- Hypercalcaemia: lethargy, polyuria, polydipsia, nausea, vomiting, constipation; drug may need to be decreased
- Hypoglycaemia in diabetics, since oral anticoagulant action is decreased

Teach patient/family:

- Drug needs to be combined with complete health plan: Diet, rest, exercise
- To notify clinician if therapeutic response decreases
- Not to discontinue this medication abruptly
- Aspects of drug usage, including changes in sex characteristics
- Women to report menstrual irregularities
- That 1–3 month course is necessary for response in breast cancer
- That drug can be abused

---

tetanus vaccine; tetanus vaccine, adsorbed

Tet/Vac/FT, Tet/Vac/Ads, Clostet, Tetavax

Func. class.: Vaccine
Legal class.: POM

Action: Produces specific antibodies to tetanus

Uses: Prevention of tetanus (adsorbed vaccine preferred)

Dosage and routes:

- IM or deep subcutaneous injection 0.5 mls
- *Unimmunised adult and child over 10 yr:* Primary course 3 doses at 0, 4 and 8 weeks; 2 reinforcing doses given 10 yr after previous dose
- *Unimmunised child:* 3 doses (often given as triple vaccine) each four weeks apart with first booster at school entry (if 3 yrs elapsed since last dose), second booster between ages 15–19 yr
- *Immunised adult:* Boosters only required if sustaining a tetanus-prone wound

Side effects/adverse reactions:

INTEG: Local pain, redness and swelling at injection site
MS: Myalgia
SYST: Pyrexia, anaphylaxis
CNS: Headache, lethargy

Contraindications: Hypersensitivity, active infection, immunosuppression, patients who have received a booster in the preceding year

NURSING CONSIDERATIONS

Assess:

- Tetanus toxoid status
- History of reactions to vaccinations

Administer:

- Preferably by IM injection into deep muscle mass

Perform/provide:

- Record dose and lot number on notes
- Ensure patient has record card with dose, batch no and dates of next due injection or booster

Teach patient/family:

- Of importance of completing of primary course; second injection 6 weeks after first dose; booster
- That some local reaction may occur particularly if injection is given subcutaneously (swollen, red injection site)

tetrabenazine

Nitoman
Func. class.: Suppressor of choreiform movements
Chem. class.: Quinolizinone
Legal class.: POM

Action: Thought to deplete nerve endings of dopamine
Uses: Disorders of movement caused by Huntingdon's chorea, senile chorea, and related neurological conditions
Dosage and routes:
• *Adult:* By mouth; initially 12.5–25 mg 3 times daily, gradually increased by 12.5–25 mg/day every 3–4 days; maximum daily dose 200 mg
Available forms include: Tablets 25 mg
Side effects/adverse reactions:
CNS: Drowsiness, extrapyramidal symptoms, depression
CVS: Hypotension
GI: Disturbances
Contraindications: Lactation
Precautions: Pregnancy
Interactions/incompatibilities:
• CNS excitation, hypertension: MAOIs (within 14 days)
• Diminished effects of: reserpine, levodopa
Clinical assessment:
• Consider withdrawal of drug if patient becomes depressed
Treatment of overdose:
• Empty stomach; symptomatic treatment

NURSING CONSIDERATIONS
Assess:
• Baseline BP
Evaluate:
• Therapeutic response—improvement in movement disorders
• Onset of depression—drug may need to be withdrawn
• Side-effects, including hypotension
Teach patient/family:
• Rise slowly as fainting may occur
• Avoid potentially dangerous tasks requiring alertness (e.g. driving) as drowsiness may occur
• Check with clinician before taking non-prescribed preparations

tetracosactrin

Synacthen, Synacthen Depot
Func. class.: Corticotrophin analogue
Chem. class.: Synthetic polypeptide
Legal class.: POM

Action: Stimulates adrenal cortex to produce, secrete glucocorticoids, mineralocorticoids and, to a lesser extend, androgens
Uses: Testing adrenocortical function, short-term replacement of corticosteroids in Crohn's disease, rheumatoid arthritis
Dosage and routes:
Investigation of adrenocortical function
• *Adult:* IM/IV 250 mcg solution (short test) or 1 mg depot (long test)
• *Child:* IM/IV 250 mcg/1.73 m^2 body surface area solution (short test)
Depot injection for therapeutic purposes
• *Adult:* IM 1–2 mg daily reduced to 1 mg every 2–3 days then 1 mg weekly
• *Child:* IM 1 month–2 yr, initially 250 mcg daily reduced to 250 mcg every 2–8 days;
• *2–5 yr:* IM initially 250–500 mcg daily reduced to 250–500 mcg every 2–8 days
• *5–12 yr:* IM initially 0.25–1 mg daily reduced to 0.25–1 mg every 2–8 days

Available forms include: Injection 250 mcg/ml; depot injection 1 mg/ml (both as acetate)
Side effects/adverse reactions:
INTEG: Rash, urticaria, pruritus, flushing
CV: Sodium, water retention
SYST: Significant risk of anaphylaxis
Contraindications: Hypersensitivity, history of allergic disorders, e.g. asthma. Depot also contraindicated in: acute psychosis, infectious disease, Cushing's syndrome, peptic ulcer, refractory heart failure, adrenogenital syndrome, as therapy for adrenocortical insufficiency
Pharmacokinetics:
IV/IM: Onset 5 min, peak 1 hr, duration 2–4 hr
Depot preparations: Peak effect 8 hr, duration greater than 24 hr
Clinical assessment:
• When using diagnostically, take blood samples for cortisol levels 30 min after injection and also at hourly intervals up to 5 hr if depot preparation used
Treatment of overdose:
Symptomatic
NURSING CONSIDERATIONS
Assess:
• Weight
Administer:
• IV or IM with equipment/drugs in case of anaphylaxis
Perform/provide:
• Storage in a refrigerator at 2–8°C
• All equipment to deal with anaphylaxis
Evaluate:
• For all side effects including water retention
Teach patient/family:
• Of necessity to carry "Steroid ID" card at all times

tetracycline HCl

Achromycin, Panmycin, Sustamycin, Tetrabid-Organon, Tetrachel
Func. class.: Antibiotic, broad-spectrum
Chem. class.: Tetracycline
Legal class.: POM

Action: Inhibits protein synthesis in microorganisms
Uses: Early syphilis, chlamydial infections (trachoma, lymphogranuloma venereum, psittacosis, salpingitis, urethritis), *Mycoplasma* (respiratory and genital infections), exacerbations of chronic bronchitis, acne, refractory periodontal disease, brucellosis, rickettsia and other infections due to tetracycline-sensitive organisms. Malignant or cirrhotic pleural effusions
Dosage and routes:
• *Adult:* By mouth 250–500 mg every 6 hr or 250 mg modified release capsules 2 as one dose, then 1 every 12 hr; IM, 100 mg every 8–12 hr or 4–6 hr in severe infections; IV infusion 500 mg 12 hrly, maximum 2 g daily
Acne
• *Adult:* By mouth 250 mg three times a day for 3–4 weeks then 250 mg twice a day for 4 months or modified release capsules 250 mg once daily
Pleural effusions
• *Adult:* Via chest drain 500 mg IV preparation in 30–50 ml saline
Available forms include: Capsules 250 mg, modified release 250 mg; tablets 250 mg; powder for injection IM 100 mg; IV 250, 500 mg
Side effects/adverse reactions:
CNS: Headache, benign intracranial hypertension
HAEM: Eosinophilia, neutropenia, thrombocytopenia, haemolytic anaemia

EENT: Glossitis, decreased calcification and staining of deciduous teeth, oral candidiasis, visual disturbances
GI: Nausea, vomiting, diarrhoea, anorexia, enterocolitis, hepatotoxicity, flatulence, abdominal cramps, epigastric burning, pseudomembranous colitis, oesophageal ulceration
GU: Nephrotoxicity
INTEG: Rash, urticaria, photosensitivity, erythema, pruritus, pain and irritation of injection site

Contraindications: Hypersensitivity to tetracyclines, children under 12 yr, severe renal insufficiency, pregnancy, lactation, systemic lupus erythematosus

Precautions: Renal disease, hepatic disease

Pharmacokinetics:
By mouth: Peak 2–4 hr, only partially absorbed, half-life 6–10 hr; excreted in urine and faeces, excreted in breast milk, 20%–60% protein bound

Interactions/incompatibilities:
- Decreased absorption of tetracycline: antacids, dairy products, iron, quinapril, calcium salts, sucralfate, bismuth, zinc
- Increased effect of: oral anticoagulants
- Decreased effect: penicillins
- Nephrotoxicity enhanced by: methoxyflurane
- Reduced effect of: oral contraceptives

Clinical assessment:
- Monitor renal/hepatic function if pre-existing problems

Lab. test interferences:
False increase: Urinary catecholamines

Treatment of overdose: Gastric lavage, administer milk or antacid, supportive treatment

NURSING CONSIDERATIONS

Assess:
- Bowel pattern
- Fluid balance

Administer:
- By mouth, an hour before food or on an empty stomach; not to be taken with milk, iron preparations or antacids. By IM injection as a solution containing 100 mg dissolved in 2 ml water for injections injected deep into the gluteal region. IV, reconstituted with 5 ml water for injections per 250 mg and then diluted to at least 100 ml and up to 1000 ml with a suitable infusion fluid and infused at a rate not exceeding 100 ml in 5 min. Doses may need adjustment in renal impairment
- After specimens have been obtained and sent for culture and sensitivity
- 1 hr before or 2 hr after ferrous or milk products; 3 hr after antacid

Evaluate:
- Therapeutic response: decreased temperature, absence of lesions, negative culture and sensitivity
- Allergic reactions: rash, itching, pruritus, angioneurotic oedema
- Nausea, vomiting, diarrhoea; administer anti-emetic, antacids as ordered
- Overgrowth of infection: increased temperature, malaise, redness, pain, swelling, drainage, perineal itching, diarrhoea, changes in cough or sputum

Teach patient/family:
- Avoid sun exposure since burns may occur; sunscreen does not seem to decrease photosensitivity
- That all prescribed medication must be taken to prevent superimposed infection
- To avoid taking milk products at same time as tetracycline

tetracycline HCl (otic, ophthalmic)

Achromycin, Eye and Ear Ointment
Func. class.: Antibiotic
Chem. class.: Tetracycline
Legal class.: POM

Action: Inhibits bacterial cell-wall synthesis
Uses: Infection of eye, external otitis, trachoma
Dosage and routes:
• *Adult and child:* Ointment: apply up to 3 times daily, or more frequently if necessary
Trachoma
• *Adult and child:* Apply to eye 3 times daily for 6 weeks
Available forms include: Ointment 1%
Side effects/adverse reactions:
EENT: Poor corneal wound healing, overgrowth of non-susceptible organisms
Contraindications: Hypersensitivity
Precautions: Antibiotic hypersensitivity
Clinical assessment:
• Serious infections may require systemic treatment, especially trachoma
NURSING CONSIDERATIONS
Administer:
• After samples have been sent for culture and sensitivity
• After washing hands, cleanse crusts or discharge from eye before application
Evaluate:
• Therapeutic response: absence of redness, inflammation, tearing
• Allergy: itching, lacrimation, redness, swelling
Teach patient/family:
• To use drug exactly as prescribed
• Do not use eye make-up, towels, washclots, or eye medication of others, or reinfection may occur
• That drug container tip should not be touched to eye
• To report itching, increased redness, burning, stinging, swelling; drug should be discontinued
• That drug may cause blurred vision when ointment is applied
• Discard unused ointment 28 days after opening

tetracycline HCl (topical)

Topicycline, Achromycin
Func. class.: Antibiotic, topical
Chem. class.: Tetracycline
Legal class.: POM

Action: Interferes with microorganism phosphorylation, protein synthesis
Uses: Acne. Superficial pyogenic infections, prevention of wound infection caused by susceptible organisms
Dosage and routes:
Superficial infections
• *Adult and child:* Topical, apply ointment to affected area 1–3 times a day
Acne
• *Adult:* Apply solution twice a day
Available forms include: Ointment 3%; solution 0.22%
Side effects/adverse reactions:
INTEG: Rash, urticaria, stinging, burning, overgrowth of resistant organisms
Contraindications: Hypersensitivity
Precautions: Pregnancy, lactation
Clinical assessment:
• Systemic therapy may be required in serious infections
NURSING CONSIDERATIONS
Administer:
• After cleansing with soap, water before each application, dry well
• Enough medication to cover lesions completely
• Avoid eyes, nose and mouth

• Apply solution generously in acne, not just to individual lesions

Perform/provide:

• Storage in a cool place (8–15°C)

Evaluate:

• Allergic reaction: burning, stinging, swelling, redness

• Therapeutic response: decrease in size, number of lesions

Teach patient/family:

• Wash hands thoroughly before, after each application

• Apply with glove to prevent further infection

• Avoid use of non-prescribed creams, ointments, lotions unless directed by clinician

theophylline, theophylline sodium glycinate

Biophylline, Labophylline, Lasma, Nuelin, Nuelin SA, Slo-Phyllin, Theo-Dur, Uniphyllin-continus, combination products

Func. class.: Bronchodilator

Chem. class.: Xanthine

Legal class.: Oral formulations P; injectable POM

Action: Relaxes smooth muscle of respiratory system by blocking phosphodiesterase, which increases cyclic AMP

Uses: Asthma, bronchospasm associated with chronic bronchitis, reversible airway obstruction

Dosage and routes:

Note: The dosage of theophylline varies considerably with the formulation of the product. Once stabilized, patients should remain on the same brand. Doctors should not prescribe generically. Due to the potential toxicity of theophylline it is essential to maintain plasma concentrations at 10–20 mg/l; this may require adjustment of doses outside of ranges specified below. A night-time dose of a modified-release preparation is useful for nocturnal asthma or early morning wheezing. Dosage and route for each product are shown below:

Biophylline

Available forms: Syrup 125 mg theophylline hydrate (as sodium glycinate) per 5 ml; modified-release tablets 350 mg, 500 mg

Dosage:

• *Adult:* By mouth, syrup 125–250 mg 3 or 4 times a day; modified-release tablets, patient over 70 kg 500 mg every 12 hr, under 70 kg, 350 mg every 12 hr

• *Child 7–12 yr:* By mouth, syrup 62.5–125 mg 3 or 4 times a day

• *Child 2–6 yr:* By mouth 62.5 mg three or four times a day

Labophylline

Available forms: Injection 20 mg/ml with lysine

Dosage:

The initial doses that follow should be reduced by 50% in patients who have received oral xanthines in the previous 24 hr. Maintenance doses should be reduced in the elderly, heart failure

• *Adult:* Initial dose slow IV injection 200 mg over 15 min or IV infusion 4 mg/kg in 100 ml 0.9% sodium chloride or 5% glucose over 20–30 min. Maintenance: 0.5 mg/kg/hr for 12 hr then 0.4 mg/kg/hr in infusion of 0.9% sodium chloride or 5% glucose

• *Child:* Initial dose slow IV injection 4 mg/kg (over 15 min). Maintenance: over 6 yr 0.75 mg/kg/hr for 12 hr then 0.5 mg/kg/hr; 6 months–6 yr 1–0.8 mg/kg/hr for 12 hr then 0.6 mg/kg/hr

Lasma

Available forms: Modified-release tablets 300 mg

Dosage:

• *Adult:* 300 mg every 12 hr (or

600 mg at night in nocturnal asthma increased to 900 mg per day after 1 week in patients over 70 kg. Adjust dose in 150 mg increments

Nuelin

Available forms: Tablets 125 mg, liquid 60 mg theophylline hydrate (as sodium glycinate) per 5 ml

Dosage:

• *Adult:* By mouth, tablets 125 mg 3 or 4 times a day after meals increasing to 250 mg if required; liquid 120–240 mg 3 or 4 times a day after meals

• *Child 7–12 yr:* By mouth, tablets 62.5–125 mg 3 or 4 times a day after meals; liquid, 90–120 mg 3 or 4 times a day

• *Child 2–6 yr:* By mouth, liquid 60–90 mg 3 or 4 times a day

Nuelin SA

Available forms: modified-release tablets 175 mg, 250 mg (SA 250)

Dosage:

• *Adults:* By mouth 175–350 mg or 250–500 mg (SA 250) every 12 hr

• *Child over 6 yr:* By mouth 175 mg or 125–250 mg (SA 250) every 12 hr

Slo-Phyllin

Available forms: Capsules modified-release 60 mg, 125 mg, 250 mg

Dosage:

• *Adult:* By mouth 250–500 mg every 12 hr

• *Child 6–12 yr:* By mouth 125–250 mg every 12 hr

• *Child 2–6 yr:* By mouth 60–120 mg every 12 hr

Theo-Dur

Available forms: Modified-release tablets 200 mg, 300 mg

Dosage:

• *Adult:* By mouth 200–300 mg every 12 hr

• *Child over 35 kg:* By mouth 200 mg every 12 hr

• *Child under 35 kg:* By mouth 100 mg every 12 hr

Uniphyllin-continus

Available forms: Tablets, modified-release 200 mg, 300 mg, 400 mg

Dosage:

• *Adult:* By mouth, under 70 kg, 200 mg every 12 hr increasing to 300 mg 12 hrly after 1 week; over 70 kg, 300 mg every 12 hr increasing to 400 mg 12 hrly after 1 week

• *Child:* By mouth 9 mg/kg twice a day increasing if needed to maximum 16 mg/kg twice a day

Side effects/adverse reactions:

CNS: Anxiety, restlessness, insomnia, dizziness, convulsions, headache, light-headedness, delirium

CV: Palpitations, sinus tachycardia, other dysrhythmias

GI: Nausea, vomiting, anorexia, diarrhoea, dyspepsia, GI bleeding

RESP: Increased rate

Contraindications: Hypersensitivity to xanthines; concurrent use of other xanthines; porphyria; concommitant use of ephedrine in children

Precautions: Elderly, congestive cardiac failure, cor pulmonale, hepatic disease, active peptic ulcer disease, hyperthyroidism, hypertension, cardiac arrhythmias, alcoholism, epilepsy; lactation

Pharmacokinetics: By mouth, free drug rapidly and completely absorbed; kinetics dependent upon formulation, metabolised in liver, excreted in urine, breast milk

Interactions/incompatibilities:

• Increased theophylline plasma levels: allopurinol, disulfiram, frusemide, thiabendazole, oral contraceptives cimetidine, propranolol, erythromycin, viloxazine, mexiletine, ciprofloxacin, enoxacin, norfloxacin, diltiazem, verapamil

• Increased clearance of theophylline: barbiturates, carbamazepine, lithium, phenytoin, rifampicin, aminoglutethimide,

sulphinpyrazone, smoking, alcohol, primidone, interferon
• Increased risk of arrhythmias with: halothane
• Increased risk of hypokalaemia with: β-agonists
• Reduced plasma levels of: lithium
• Antagonism of adenosine

Clinical assessment:
• Theophylline blood levels (therapeutic level is 10–20 mg/l); toxicity may occur with small increase above 20 mg/l

NURSING CONSIDERATIONS

Assess:
• Baseline vital signs

Administer:
• By mouth; with or after meals to decrease GI symptoms
• Swallow modified-release tablets whole not chewed at prescribed regular intervals. Capsules may be opened and granules swallowed with soft food, e.g. yoghurt
• Same brand unless retitrate dose
• Infusion in 0.9% sodium chloride or 5% dextrose
• Injection slowly over 15–20 min

Evaluate:
• Heart rate; tachycardia can occur
• Monitor fluid balance; diuresis occurs, dehydration may result in elderly or children
• Respiratory rate, rhythm, depth
• Allergic reactions: rash, urticaria; if these occur, consult medical staff; drug may be discontinued

Teach patient/family:
• Avoid non-prescribed medications that contain theophylline or its derivatives
• To avoid hazardous activities; dizziness may occur
• Aspects of drug therapy: dosage, routes, side effects, when to notify the clinician
• If GI upset occurs, to take drug with water; seek advice if nausea/vomiting persists
• To swallow tablets whole

---

thiabendazole

Mintezol
Func. class.: Anthelmintic
Chem. class.: Benzimidazole derivative
Legal class.: POM

Action: Inhibits vital enzyme in worm

Uses: Strongyloidiasis, trichinosis, cutaneous and visceral larva migrans, dracontiasis; secondary treatment for threadworm when mixed with above infestations; adjunct in hookworm, whipworm, roundworm

Dosage and routes:
• *Adult and child:* By mouth 25 mg/kg (maximum 1.5 g) twice a day for variable number of days according to disease:

Strongyloidiasis, hookworm, roundworm, whipworm
• 2 days

Cutaneous larva migrans
• 2 days, repeated if necessary

Visceral larva migrans
• 7 days

Trichinosis
• 2–4 days

Dracontiasis
• 1 day (double dose in multiple infection)

Side effects/adverse reactions:
SYST: Anaphylaxis, collapse, angioneurotic oedema
GU: Haematuria, nephrotoxicity, crystalluria, enuresis, abnormal smell of urine
INTEG: Rash, pruritus, fever, flushing, perinal rash, dry mucous membranes, Stevens–Johnson syndrome

CNS: Dizziness, headache, drowsiness, weariness, irritability, convulsions, behavioural changes
EENT: Tinnitus, blurred vision, xanthopsia
GI: Nausea, vomiting, anorexia, diarrhoea, jaundice, liver damage, epigastric distress
CV: Hypotension
HAEM: Transient leucopenia
Contraindications: Hypersensitivity, pregnancy, lactation
Precautions: Severe malnutrition, hepatic disease, renal disease, anaemia, severe dehydration
Pharmacokinetics
By mouth: Well absorbed, peak 1–2 hr, metabolised completely by liver, excreted in faeces, urine
Interactions/incompatibilities:
- Increased plasma levels of: theophylline, other xanthines

Treatment of overdose: Induce emesis or gastric lavage, supportive treatment, no specific antidote

NURSING CONSIDERATIONS

Assess:
- Stools periodically during entire treatment; gloves must be worn when handling stools

Administer:
- By mouth with meals to avoid GI symptoms chewed before swallowing
- To be taken with food and chewed before swallowing

Teach patient/family:
- Proper hygiene after bowel movement including handwashing technique; tell patient to avoid putting fingers in mouth
- To observe diet and fluid intake
- That infected person should sleep alone and change bed linen daily
- Not to shake bed clothing
- To take a bath or shower with hot water each morning
- To clean toilet daily with disinfectant
- To wear gloves when handling stools
- Need for compliance with dosage schedule, duration of treatment
- To drink fruit juice to remove mucus that intestinal tapeworms burrow in; aids in expulsion of worms
- To avoid hazardous activities if drowsiness occurs
- To wash all fruit and vegetables
- To wear shoes

---

thiamine HCl (vitamin B_1)

Benerva, many combination products, (Pabrinex injection)
Func. class.: Vitamin B_1, water-soluble
Legal class.: Tablets P; Injection POM

Action: Used for pyruvate metabolism
Uses: Thiamine deficiency: beri-beri, Wernicke-Korsakoff syndrome; prophylactic in impaired absorption or where requirements are increased
Dosage and routes:
Prophylaxis
- *Adult:* By mouth 3–10 mg daily

Mild chronic deficiency
- By mouth 10–25 mg daily

Severe deficiency
- By mouth 200–300 mg daily

Check manufacturer's data sheet for dosage by injection
Available forms include: Tablets 25, 50, 100, 300 mg; injection IM, IV 250 mg (as part of vitamins B and C injection). Many combination products
Side effects/adverse reactions:
CNS: Weakness, restlessness
INTEG: Angioneurotic oedema, cyanosis, sweating, warmth (all primarily after injection)
SYST: Anaphylaxis (primarily after injection)
Contraindications: Hypersensitivity

Pharmacokinetics: Unused amounts excreted in urine (unchanged)

NURSING CONSIDERATIONS

Assess:

- Thiamine level
- Prophylactic or therapeutic treatment

Administer:

- Tablets orally with a drink or food
- Dilution with sodium chloride 0.9% or glucose 5% for IV infusion. Flush tubing before and after
- Intramuscular and intravenous preparation are combined vitamin preparations, and may not be interchangeable

NB: Do not give IM as an IV injection. IM rotate deep muscle sites.

- IV injections should be administered over at least 10 mins
- Facilities should be available for treating anaphylaxis when IV administered

Perform/provide:

- Storage of injections in light-resistant container and refrigerate
- Local treatment for any painful muscle sites after injection

Evaluate:

- Therapeutic response: absence of nausea, vomiting, anorexia, insomnia, tachycardia, paraesthesia, depression, muscle weakness
- After IM and IV treatment observe patient for anaphylaxis; cyanosis, sweating

Teach patient/family:

- To eat varied diet rich in vitamin B, includes yeast, pulses, whole wheat, vegetables
- To seek help for alcoholism
- Not to discontinue treatment without medical advice

thioguanine

Lanvis

Func. class.: Antineoplastic
Chem. class.: Purine analogue
Legal class.: POM

Action: Interferes with synthesis, utilization of purine nucleotides; effect is related to substitution of defective ribonucleotides into DNA

Uses: Acute myeloblastic, acute lymphoblastic and chronic granulocytic leukaemias

Dosage and routes:

Doses are highly variable, and dependent on local treatment protocols, concomitant therapy and tumour type; the following dose schedules have been used

- *Adult and child:* By mouth 2–2.5 mg/kg/day initially usually in combination with other antineoplastics

Available forms include: Tablets 40 mg

Side effects/adverse reactions:

HAEM: Thrombocytopenia, leucopenia, anaemia

GI: Nausea, vomiting, anorexia, diarrhoea, stomatitis, hepatotoxicity, gastritis

GU: Renal failure, hyperuricaemia, oliguria, haematuria, crystalluria

INTEG: Rash, dermatitis, dry skin

SYST: Fever

Contraindications: Prior drug resistance, pregnancy, breast-feeding

Precautions: Liver disease, bone marrow suppression, concurrent infections, pregnancy, potential carcinogen, teratogen

Pharmacokinetics: Oral form absorbed only 30%, metabolised in liver, excreted in urine as metabolites

Interactions/incompatibilities:

- Increased toxicity: radiation,

other anti-neoplastics

Clinical assessment:

- Full blood count, differential, platelet count at least weekly; withhold drug if excessive myelosuppression occurs
- Renal function tests, during therapy
- Liver function tests before, during therapy

Treatment of overdose: Gastric lavage, monitor blood picture. Supportive treatment including transfusion, filgrastim

NURSING CONSIDERATIONS

Monitor:

- Baseline vital signs, fluid balance

Administer:

- HANDLING: take safety precautions appropriate to antineoplastic agents
- Following local antineoplastic (cytotoxic) policies
- After ensuring that clinician is aware of blood results
- By mouth; give drug after evening meal and before bedtime. Tablets should not be crushed; take care not to inhale or ingest dust when breaking
- Other medications by mouth if possible. Avoid IV, IM, SC routes to prevent infection and bruising
- Anti-emetic 30–60 min before treatment
- Antacid immediately before thioguanine
- All other medication as prescribed including analgesics, antibiotics, anti-emetics, antispasmodics

Perform/provide:

- Strict medical asepsis, protective isolation if WBC levels are low
- Increase fluid intake to 2–3 litres/day to prevent urate deposits, calculi formation, unless contraindicated
- Strict oral hygiene with prescribed mouth washes
- Nutritious diet with iron, vitamin supplements as ordered

Evaluate:

- Fluid balance. Report fall in urine output to less than 30 ml/hr
- Temperature 4 hrly. Increase may indicate beginning of infection
- Bleeding: haematuria, bruising, petechiae, mucosa or orifices 8 hrly
- Hepatotoxicity: yellowing of skin, sclera, dark urine, clay-coloured stools, pruritus, abdominal pain, fever, diarrhoea
- Buccal cavity 8 hrly for dryness, sores, ulceration, white patches, oral pain, bleeding, dysphagia
- Symptoms indicating severe allergic reaction: rash, urticaria, itching, flushing

Teach patient/family:

- Why protective isolation precautions are needed
- To report any complaints, side effects to nurse or clinician: black tarry stools, chills, fever, sore throat, bleeding, bruising, cough, shortness of breath, dark, bloody urine
- To avoid foods with citric acid, hot or rough texture if stomatitis is present
- To report stomatitis: any bleeding, white spots, ulcerations in mouth; tell patient to examine mouth daily, report symptoms
- Contraceptive measures are recommended during therapy
- To drink 10–12 glasses of fluid/day
- To avoid vigorous brushing of teeth

thiopentone sodium

Intraval Sodium, Thiopentone Sodium (Non-proprietary)

Func. class.: Anaesthetic, general
Chem. class.: Barbiturate
Legal class.: POM

Action: Acts by depressing CNS to produce anaesthesia

Uses: Short general anaesthesia, induction anaesthesia before other anaesthetics
Dosage and routes:
• *Adult:* IV 100–150 mg (4–6 ml of 2.5% solution) over 10–15 secs repeated if necessary after 30 sec; *or* up to 4 mg/kg
• *Child:* Induction IV 2–7 mg/kg
Available forms include: Powder for injection IV 2.5 g/100 ml diluent (2.5%), 5.0 g/200 ml diluent (2.5%), 0.5 g/20 ml diluent (2.5%), 1 g/20 ml diluent (5%)
Side effects/adverse reactions:
RESP: Respiratory depression, bronchospasm
CNS: Retrograde amnesia, prolonged somnolence
CV: Tachycardia, hypotension, myocardial depression, arrhythmias
EENT: Sneezing, coughing, laryngeal spasm
INTEG: Chills, *shivering,* necrosis and pain at injection site, rash,
MS: Arthralgia
SYST: Fever, allergic reactions
Contraindications: Hypersensitivity, porphyria
Precautions: Drug addiction, elderly, adrenocortical insufficiency, cachexia and severe toxaemia, diabetes, raised plasma potassium or urea, severe cardiovascular disease, renal disease, hypotension, liver disease, myxoedema, dehydration, thyrotoxicosis, myasthenia gravis, asthma, increased intracranial pressure, muscular dystrophies, pregnancy, hypovolaemia, severe anaemia, status asthmaticus, severe haemorrhage, burns
Pharmacokinetics:
IV: Onset 30–40 sec; half-life 4–12 hr metabolised in liver
Interactions/incompatibilities:
• Increased action of thiopentone: CNS depressants, sulphonamides
• Do not mix with any other drug in solution or syringe
• Increased risk of arrhythmias with: tricyclic antidepressants, verapamil
• Increased hypotension with: antihypertensives, antipsychotics, β-blockers, verapamil
Treatment of overdose: Supportive

NURSING CONSIDERATIONS
Assess:
• Starvation status
• Vital signs and conciousness level before and 3–5 min after administration
Administer:
• Only with resuscitative equipment nearby
• IV slowly
• Discard unused solution within 24 hr
• Do not mix with any other drug in solution or syringe
Perform/provide:
• Sterile water to reconstitute powder
Evaluate:
• Therapeutic response to induction
• Arrhythmias or myocardial depression
• Signs of hypotension or bronchospasm in asthmatics
Teach patient/family:
• That patient will feel drowsy, disoriented before 'falling asleep'

thioridazine hydrochloride

Melleril
Func. class.: Antipsychotic, neuroleptic
Chem. class.: Phenothiazine, piperidine

Action: Depresses cerebral cortex, hypothalamus, limbic system, which control activity, aggression; blocks neurotransmission produced by dopamine at synapse; exhibits strong α-adrenergic, anticholinergic blocking action;

mechanism for antipsychotic effects is unclear. Less sedating; produces less extrapyramidal effects than other phenothiazines

Uses: Psychotic disorders, schizophrenia, severe behavioral problems in children, (alcohol withdrawal), agitation in elderly, short-term adjunct in anxiety

Dosage and routes:

Psychosis

• *Adult:* By mouth 150–600 mg daily in divided doses, maximum dose 800 mg a day in hospitalised patients (maximum 4 weeks) dose is gradually increased to desired response, then reduced to minimum maintenance

Severe mental/behavioural problems, non-psychotic emotional disturbances

• *Adult:* By mouth 75–200 mg daily

• *Child 1–5 yr:* By mouth 1 mg/kg daily

• *5–12 yr:* By mouth 75–150 mg daily (severe cases up to 300 mg daily)

Anxiety, agitation in elderly

• *Adult:* By mouth 30–100 mg daily

Available forms include: Tablets 10, 25, 50, 100 mg; suspension 25, 100 mg (thioridazine base)/5 ml; syrup 25 mg/5 ml

Side effects/adverse reactions:

CNS: Extrapyramidal symptoms (rare): pseudoparkinsonism, akathisia, dystonia, tardive dyskinesia; seizures, headache, sedation, mental dulling, dizziness, confusion, agitation, excitement

HAEM: Leucopenia, agranulocytosis

INTEG: Rash, photosensitivity, dermatitis

EENT: Blurred vision, glaucoma, nasal congestion decreased visual acuity, pigmentary retinopathy

GI: Dry mouth, nausea, vomiting, anorexia, constipation, diarrhoea, jaundice, weight gain, hepatitis

GU: Urinary retention, impotence, retrograde ejaculation

ENDO: Amenorrhoea, gynaecomastia, galactorrhoea

CV: Orthostatic hypotension, hypertension, cardiac arrest, ECG changes, tachycardia, arrythmias, oedema

Contraindications: Hypersensitivity, history of blood dyscrasias, coma, porphyria, CNS depression, children under 1 yr, breast-feeding, bone marrow depression

Precautions: Pregnancy, hepatic disease, cardiac disease, severe respiratory disease, renal failure, parkinsonism, narrow angle, glaucoma, prostatic hypertrophy, myasthenia gravis, epilepsy, phaeochromocytoma

Pharmacokinetics:

By mouth: Onset erratic, peak 2–4 hr; metabolised by liver, excreted in urine, enters breast milk, half-life 6–40 hr

Interactions/incompatibilities:

• Enhanced sedation with: alcohol, barbiturates other CNS depressants

• Decreased absorption of thioridazine: aluminium hydroxide or magnesium hydroxide antacids

• Decreased effects of: levodopa, antiepileptics (lowered seizure threshold), dopamine agonists

• Increased risk of extrapyramidal effects and neurotoxicity with: lithium

• Increased anticholinergic effects: anticholinergics, tricyclic antidepressants

• Increased hypotensive effect: anaesthetics, antihypertensives

• Increased risk of cardiac arrythmias with: antiarrythmias

Clinical assessment:

• Full blood counts monthly for first 3–4 months and if any unexplained infection, fever develops

• Liver function tests before,

during treatment if abnormality suspected
• Stop treatment if tardive dyskinesias develop
Lab. test interferences:
False positive: Pregnancy tests
False negative: Urinary 5-hydroxyindolocetic acid
Treatment of overdose: Lavage if orally injested, provide an airway, supportive treatment including plasma expanders for acute hypotension

NURSING CONSIDERATIONS

Assess:
• Establish baseline BP, pulse and respiratory rate
• Urinalysis is recommended before and during prolonged therapy
Administer:
• Antimuscarinic agent, if ordered; to be used if extrapyramidal symptoms occur
Perform/provide:
• Decreased noise input by dimming lights, avoiding loud noises
• Supervised ambulation until stabilised on medication; do not involve in strenuous exercise program because fainting is possible; patient should not stand still for long periods of time
• Increased fluids to prevent constipation
• Frequent sips of water for dry mouth
Evaluate:
• Swallowing of oral medication; check for hoarding or giving of medication to other patients
• Therapeutic response: decrease in emotional excitement, hallucinations, delusions, paranoia, reorganisation of patterns of thought, speech
• Affect, orientation, level of consciousness, reflexes, gait, coordination, sleep pattern disturbances
• BP (standing and lying) pulse and respirations 4 hrly during initial treatment; report drops of 30 mmHg
• Dizziness, faintness, palpitations, tachycardia on rising
• Extrapyramidal symptoms including akathisia (inability to sit still, no pattern to movements), tardive dyskinesia (bizarre movements of jaw, mouth, tongue, extremities), pseudoparkinsonism (rigidity, tremors, pill rolling, shuffling gait)
• Constipation, urinary retention daily; if these occur, increase bulk, water in diet
Teach patient/family:
• Postural hypotension occurs frequently; to rise from sitting or lying position gradually
• To avoid hot baths, hot showers, since hypotension may occur
• To avoid abrupt withdrawal of this drug or rapid relapse may result; drugs should be withdrawn slowly
• To avoid non-prescribed preparations (cough, hayfever, cold) unless approved by clinician since serious drug interactions may occur; avoid use with alcohol or CNS depressants, increased drowsiness may occur
• To use a sunscreen during sun exposure to prevent burns
• Compliance with drug regimen
• Necessity for meticulous oral hygiene since oral candidiasis may occur
• To report sore throat, malaise, fever, bleeding, mouth sores; if these occur, full blood count should be drawn and drug discontinued

thiotepa

Func. class.: Antineoplastic
Chem. class.: Alkylating agent
Legal class.: POM

Action: Alkylates DNA, RNA; inhibits enzymes that allow synthesis of amino acids in proteins; also responsible for cross-linking DNA strands

Uses: Breast, bladder, cancer, neoplastic effusions

Dosage and routes:
Doses are highly variable, and dependent on local treatment protocols, concomitant therapy and tumour type; the following dose schedules have been used

Breast cancer
- *Adult:* IM 15–30 mg 3 times a week for 2 weeks every 6–8 weeks or 15 mg daily for 4 days initially, followed in 3 weeks by 15 mg IM every 2–3 weeks

Neoplastic effusions
- *Adult:* Intracavity 10–65 mg in 20–60 ml sterile water repeated at weekly or 2 weekly intervals

Bladder cancer
- *Adult:* Instil up to 60 mg/60 ml water instilled in bladder once weekly for 4 weeks

Available forms include: Injection 15 mg

Side effects/adverse reactions:
CNS: Dizziness, headache
HAEM: Thrombocytopenia, leucopenia, pancytopenia
GI: Nausea, vomiting, anorexia
GU: Cystitis and rarely haemorrhagic cystitis
INTEG: Rash, pruritus, alopecia

Contraindications: Hypersensitivity, pregnancy, breast-feeding, WBC under 3000 and/or platelets under 100,000

Precautions: Radiation therapy, bone marrow suppression, pregnancy, lactation, children

Pharmacokinetics:
Onset slow, metabolised in liver, excreted in urine

Clinical assessment:
- Full blood count, differential, platelet count weekly; withhold drug if WBC is under 3000 or platelet count is under 100,000

Treatment of overdose: Gastric lavage, general supportive measures, blood transfusions if indicated

NURSING CONSIDERATIONS

Assess:
- Baseline TPR and fluid balance
- Nutritional status
- Reconstitution and administration by trained personnel. NB. Should not to be handled by pregnant staff

Administer:
- HANDLING: take safety precautions appropriate to antineoplastic agents
- Following local antineoplastic (cytotoxic) policies
- After ensuring that clinician is aware of blood results
- IV, IM, intrathecally
- Bladder instillation, after 8–12 hr dehydration. Dose must be retained for up to 2 hr with frequent repositioning of patient
- Intracavity into pleural or peritoneal cavity following drainage of effusion
- Other medications by mouth if possible. Avoid IV, IM, SC routes to prevent infection and bruising
- Anti-emetic 30–60 min before treatment
- All other medication as prescribed including analgesics, antibiotics, anti-emetics, antispasmodics

Perform/provide:
- Storage in light-resistant container, refrigerate
- Strict medical asepsis, protective isolation if WBC levels are low
- Special skin care

• Nutritious diet as tolerated
• Increased fluid intake to 2–3 litres/day to prevent urate deposits, calculi formation
• Scrupulous care of catheter
• Good mouth care
• Warm compresses at injection site for inflammation

Evaluate:
• Fluid balance and adequate fluid intake
• All side effects including GI disturbance
• Skin and mucosal condition

Teach patient/family:
• Of protective isolation precautions
• To report any complaints or side effects to nurse or clinician

---

thyroxine sodium

Eltroxin
Func. class.: Thyroid hormone
Legal class.: POM

Action: Increases metabolic rates, increases cardiac output, O_2 consumption, body temperature, blood volume, growth, development at cellular level

Uses: Hypothyroidism

Dosage and routes:
• *Adult:* By mouth 25–100 mcg daily, increased by 25–50 mcg every 1–4 weeks until desired response; maintenance dose 100–200 mcg daily as a single dose
• *Elderly:* Not advised to exceed maximum 50 mcg daily initially
• *Child:* By mouth 10 mcg/kg up to max. 50 mcg daily, may increase until desired response; reach 100 mcg daily at 5 yrs and adult doses by 12 yrs

Available forms include: Tablets 25, 50, 100 mcg

Side effects/adverse reactions:
INTEG: Sweating, flushing
CNS: Insomnia, headache, restlessness
CV: Tachycardia, palpitations, arrhythmas, angina
GI: Nausea, diarrhoea
MS: Muscular weakness, cramps in skeletal muscle

Contraindications: Hypersensitivity, thyrotoxicosis

Precautions: Elderly (reduced dose may be required), angina, pectoris, hypertension, ischaemia, myocardial insufficiency, diabetes mellitus/insipidus, cardiac disease, adrenal insufficiency

Pharmacokinetics:
Peak 12–48 hr, half-life 6–7 days; distributed throughout body tissues. 100 mcg thyroxine is equivalent in activity to 20–30 mcg liothyronine or 60 mg thyroid BP

Interactions/incompatibilities:
• Decreased absorption of this drug: cholestyramine
• Increased effects of: anticoagulants, sympathomimetics, tricyclic antidepressants, phenytoin
• Toxicity: digitalis preparations, catecholamines

Clinical assessment:
• Serum thyroxine and serum thyrotrophin levels in younger patients

Treatment of overdose: Gastric lavage or emesis if patient seen within several hours of taking dose. Treatment thereafter symptomatic. Thyroxine can recommence at lower dosage after a few days

NURSING CONSIDERATIONS

Assess:
• BP, pulse before each dose
• Weight
• Pretherapy ECG

Administer:
• Orally before breakfast as a single dose to decrease sleeplessness, and adjusted at 1–4 week intervals until normal metabolism maintained

• At same time daily to maintain drug level
• Lowest dose that relieves symptoms

Perform/provide:
• Store in childproof, light-resistant container
• Removal of medication 4 weeks before radio active iodine uptake test

Evaluate:
• Therapeutic response; increase in mental and physical ability, coursing increased weight loss, diuresis, appetite and absence of depression, constipation, peripheral oedema, cold intolerance, pale, cool, dry skin, brittle nails, alopecia, night blindness, paraesthesia, syncope, stupor, coarse hair, menorrhagia, coma, carotenaemia, skin, rosy cheeks
• Input and output of fluids to determine fluid loss
• Weigh before and during initial treatment
• Too rapid an increase in metabolism caused by excessive dosage/overdose; restlessness insomnia, sweating, flushing, headache cardiac arrhythmias, palpitation, tachycardia, diarrhoea, excessive weight loss, cramps in skeletal muscle and muscular weekness—stop treatment

Teach patient/family:
• Report nervousness, excitability, irritability, anxiety, may indicate too large a dose/overdose
• That children show immediate behaviour personality changes
• To read drug labels and avoid non-prescribed drugs containing iodine
• To avoid iodine food, salt iodinised, soy beans, tofu, turnips, some seafood, some bread

tiaprofenic acid

Surgam, Surgam SA
Func. class.: Non-steroidal anti-inflammatory drug
Chem. class.: Propionic acid derivative
Legal class.: POM

Action: Has both analgesic and anti-inflammatory effects
Uses: Pain and inflammation in rheumatic disease and other musculoskeletal disorders and soft tissue injury

Dosage and routes:
• By mouth 600 mg daily in 2–3 divided doses; modified-release 600 mg at night

Available forms include: Tablets 200 mg, 300 mg; capsules modified release 300 mg

Side effects/adverse reactions:
GI: Discomfort constipation, flatulence, bleeding, nausea, diarrhoea, dyspepsia, vomiting, anorexia, stomatitis
CV: Angioneurotic oedema
CNS: Headache, drowsiness
RESP: Asthma
INTEG: Rashes, photosensitivity, pruritus, alopecia
META: Fluid retention

Contraindications: Active or suspected peptic ulceration, children, hypersensitivity; hypersensitivity to aspirin or other NSAIDs; first and last trimester of pregnancy

Precautions: Elderly patients, history of peptic ulceration, allergic disorders, asthma, renal, cardiac, hepatic impairment (reduce dosage to 200 mg twice daily), pregnancy

Pharmacokinetics:
Readily absorbed from GI tract. Short half-life of 2 hr, highly bound to plasma protein. Excreted predominantly in the urine with smaller amounts in the bile

Interactions/incompatibilities: Anticoagulants, antihypertensives, cardiac glycosides, diuretics, hypoglycaemic agents, phenytoin, lithium

Clinical assessment:

- Renal and liver function tests, blood studies before treatment, periodically thereafter: blood urea, creatinine, aspartate aminotransferase, alanine aminotransferase, Hb

NURSING CONSIDERATIONS

Administer:

- With or after food or milk
- Modified-release capsule, swallow whole

Evaluate:

- Therapeutic response: decreased pain, stiffness, swelling in joints, ability to move more easily

Teach patient/family:

- To report change in urine pattern, weight increase, oedema, pain increase in joints, fever, blood in urine (indicates nephrotoxicity)
- Report any unresolved indigestion or black tar-like stools

---

tibolone ▼

Livial

Func. class.: Hormone replacement therapy

Legal class.: POM

Action: Oestrogenic, progestogenic and weak androgenic activity

Uses: Treatment of vasomotor symptoms (hot flushes, sweating), depressed mood and decreased libido resulting from natural or surgical menopause

Dosage and routes:

- *Orally:* 2.5 mg daily
- Should not be taken until 12 months after last menstrual bleed
- Need not be administered on empty stomach

Available forms include: Tablets, 2.5 mg

Side effects/adverse reactions:

CNS: Dizziness, headache

GI: Gastrointestinal upset

INTEG: Seborrhoeic dermatitis, increased facial hair growth

MISC: Change in body weight; vaginal bleeding; changes in liver function tests; ankle oedema

Contraindications: Pregnancy or lactation; known or suspected hormone-dependent tumours; cardiovascular, cerebrovascular disease, e.g. thrombophlebitis; thromboembolic disease; vaginal bleeding of unknown cause; severe liver disorders

Precautions: Renal impairment; epilepsy; migraine; diabetes mellitus; hypercholesterolaemia. Stop therapy if signs of thromboembolic disease, abnormal liver function or jaundice occur

Pharmacokinetics: Metabolised in the liver; metabolites excreted in urine and faeces

Interactions: Rifampicin, carbamazepine, phenobarbitone, phenytoin and primidone accelerate tibolone metabolism and may decrease its effectiveness

Treatment of overdose: Specific treatment is not required

NURSING CONSIDERATIONS

Assess:

- Menstrual history, including date of last menstrual bleed (must be 12 months or more)
- Eliminate any possibility of pregnancy
- BP, weight

Administer:

- By mouth, with or without food, but with fluids

Evaluate:

- Therapeutic effect; lessening of symptoms (hot flushes, sweats)
- Side effects: dizziness, headache, GI disturbance, ankle oedema

Teach patient/family:
• About side effects, including weight gain and increase in facial hair, and to report these to nurse or clinician
• To seek advice from clinician if unexpected vaginal bleeding occurs
• To check weight regularly

ticarcillin disodium

Ticar
Func. class.: Antibiotic, anti-pseudomonal
Chem. class.: Carboxypenicillin
Legal class.: POM

Action: Interferes with cell wall replication of susceptible organisms; osmotically unstable cell wall swells, bursts from osmotic pressure
Uses: Respiratory, soft tissue, urinary tract infections, bacterial septicaemia, general system infections, peritonitis, intra-abdominal sepsis, endocarditis effective for Gram-positive cocci (*S. aureus, S. faecalis, S. pneumoniae*), Gram-negative cocci (*N. gonorrhoeae*), Gram-positive bacilli (*C. perfringens, C. tetani*), Gram-negative bacilli (*Bacteroides* spp, *F. nucleatum, E. coli, P. mirabilis, Salmonella* spp, *M. morganii, P. rettgeri, Enterobacter* spp, *P. aeruginosa, Serratia* spp, *Peptococcus* spp, *Peptostreptococcus* spp, *Eubacterium* spp)
Dosage and routes:
• *Adult:* IV injection/infusion 15–20 g daily in divided doses every 4–8 hr. For the treatment of uncomplicated urinary tract infections IM/IV 3–4 g daily in divided doses every 4–8 hr
• *Child:* IV/IM 200–300 mg/kg daily in divided doses every 4–8 hr. For treatment of uncomplicated urinary tract infections 50–100 mg/kg daily in divided doses every 4–8 hr
Available forms include: Injection IM, IV 1, 5 g; IV infusion 5 g
Side effects/adverse reactions:
HAEM: Increased bleeding time, eosinophilia
GI: Nausea, vomiting, diarrhoea
META: Hypokalaemia
INTEG: Skin rashes
Contraindications: Hypersensitivity to penicillins
Precautions: Pregnancy, renal dysfunction (reduce dosage)
Pharmacokinetics:
IM: Peak 1 hr, duration 4–6 hr
IV: Peak 30–45 min, duration 4 hr, Half-life 70 min, small amount metabolised in liver, excreted in urine, breast milk
Interactions/incompatibilities:
• Increased antimicrobial effect of this drug: aminoglycosides, may be due to synergy
• Increased penicillin concentrations: probenecid
Clinical assessment:
• Blood studies: WBC, RBC, bleeding time
• Renal studies: urinalysis, protein, blood
• Culture and sensitivity before drug therapy
• Do not mix in some syringe with aminoglycosides
Treatment of overdose: Drug removed by haemodialysis, symptomatic support as required, increased risk of bleeding
NURSING CONSIDERATIONS
Assess:
• Baseline pattern
• Fluid balance
• Allergies before initiation of treatment, reaction of each medication; highlight allergies on patient's chart
Administer:
• For IM administration dissolve 1 g in 2 ml water for injections or

0.5% lignocaine hydrochloride; for IV use dissolved in 20 ml water for injections and give by injection over 3–4 min, or add to 100–150 ml infusion fluid and infuse over 30–40 min. Dosage may need adjustment in renal impairment
• By slow IV or infusion, lower doses

Perform/provide:
• Storage at 2 to 8°C; reconstituted solution for 24 hr at room temperature or 3 days refrigerated

Evaluate:
• Therapeutic response: absence of fever, purulent drainage, redness, inflammation
• Bowel pattern during treatment
• Fluid balance; report haematuria, oliguria since penicillin in high doses is nephrotoxic
• Skin eruptions after administration of penicillin to 1 week after discontinuing drug

Teach patient/family:
• To report sore throat, fever, fatigue: could indicate superimposed infection
• To wear or carry ID if allergic to penicillins

ticarcillin disodium/ clavulanate potassium

Timentin
Func. class.: Antibiotic, antipseudomonal
Chem. class.: Broad-spectrum penicillin
Legal class.: POM

Action: Interferes with cell wall replication of susceptible organisms; osmotically unstable cell wall swells, bursts from osmotic pressure

Uses: Respiratory, soft tissue, and urinary tract infections, bacterial septicaemia, general systemic infections, peritonitis, intra-abdominal sepsis, endocarditis, effective for gram-positive cocci (*S. aureus, S. faecalis, S. pneumoniae*), gram-negative cocci (*N. gonorrhoeae*), gram-positive bacilli (*C. perfringens, C. tetani*), gram-negative bacilli (*Bacteroides, F. nucleatum, E. coli, P. mirabilis, Salmonella, M. morganii, P. rettgeri, Enterobacter, P. aeruginosa, Serratia, Peptococcus, Peptostreptococcus, Eubacterium*)

Dosage and routes:
• *Adult:* IV infusion ticarcillin 3 g, clavulanate potassium 0.2 g every 4–8 hr
• *Child:* IV infusion ticarcillin 0.75 g, clavulanate 0.05 g/kg every 6–8 hr; in infants give every 12 hr during perinatal period

Available forms include: Injection IM, IV, 1.6 g and 3.2 g

Side effects/adverse reactions:
HAEM: Increased bleeding time, eosinophilia
GI: Nausea, vomiting, diarrhoea, hepatitis, cholestatic jaundice
INTEG: Skin rash
META: Hypokalaemia

Contraindications: Hypersensitivity to penicillins

Precautions: Neonates, severe hepatic dysfunction, renal impairment (reduce dosage)

Pharmacokinetics:
IV: Peak 30–45 min, duration 4 hr, half-life 64–68 min. Both components are well distributed in body fluids and tissue

Interactions/incompatibilities:
• Increased antimicrobial effect of this drug: aminoglycosides IV (mixed) due to synergy
• Increased penicillin concentrations: probenecid

Clinical assessment:
• Liver function tests
• Blood studies: WBC, RBC, hct, bleeding time
• Renal tests: urinalysis, protein, blood

• Culture and sensitivity before drug therapy

Treatment of overdose: Increased rate of bleeding, may be removed from circulation by dialysis

NURSING CONSIDERATIONS

Assess:

• Allergies before initiation of treatment, reaction of each medication; highlight allergies on chart, Kardex
• Fluid balance
• Bowel pattern
• Previous hypersensitivity to penicillins

Administer:

• After sample has been sent for culture and sensitivity
• By IV infusion in 50–150 ml of fluid over a period of 30–40 min. Dosage should be adjusted in renal impairment

Perform/provide:

• Storage at room temperature, reconstituted solution for up to 24 hr at room temperature in water for injections or 3 days refrigerated

Evaluate:

• Therapeutic response: absence of fever, purulent drainage, redness, inflammation
• Bowel pattern before, during treatment
• Fluid balance; report haematuria, oliguria since penicillin in high doses is nephrotoxic
• Any patient with compromised renal system, since drug is excreted slowly in poor renal system function; toxicity may occur rapidly
• Skin eruptions after administration of penicillin to 1 week after discontinuing drug
• Respiratory status: rate, character, wheezing, and tightness in chest

Teach patient/family:

• To report sore throat, fever, fatigue; could indicate superimposed infection
• To wear or carry ID if allergic to penicillins

---

timolol maleate (ophthalmic)

Timoptol

Func. class.: Antihypertensive, ocular

Chem. class.: Non-selective β-adrenergic blocker

Legal class.: POM

Action: Reduces production of aqueous humour

Uses: Elevated intra-ocular pressure, chronic open-angle glaucoma, secondary glaucoma, aphakic glaucoma, ocular hypertension

Dosage and routes:

• *Adult:* Instil 1 drop of 0.25% solution in affected eye twice a day; may increase to 1 drop of 0.5% solution twice a day if needed

Available forms include: Solution 0.25%, 0.5%

Side effects/adverse reactions:

CV: Bradycardia, arrhythmia, hypotension, syncope, heart block, CVA, cerebral ischaemia, congestive heart failure, palpitation, cardiac arrest

RESP: Bronchospasm, respiratory failure, dyspnoea

CNS: Weakness, fatigue, depression, anxiety, headache, confusion

EENT: Eye irritation, conjunctivitis, keratitis, visual disturbances

INTEG: Rash, urticaria

Contraindications: Hypersensitivity, asthma, 2nd/3rd degree heart block, severe obstructive pulmonary disease, sinus bradycardia, cardiac failure

Precautions: Pregnancy, soft contact lenses

Pharmacokinetics:

INSTIL: Onset 15–30 min, peak 1–2 hr, duration 24 hr

NURSING CONSIDERATIONS

Teach patient/family:

- To report change in vision, with blurring or loss of sight, trouble breathing, sweating, flushing
- Method of instillation, and not to touch dropper to eye
- That long-term therapy may be required
- That blurred vision will decrease with continued use of drug
- Discard remaining eye drops 28 days after opening

timolol maleate (systemic)

Blocadren, Betim, Combination products

Func. class.: Antihypertensive, antianginal, antimigraine agent

Chem. class.: Non-selective β-blocker

Legal class.: POM

Action: Competitively blocks stimulation of β-adrenergic receptor within vascular smooth muscle; produces chronotropic, inotropic activity (decreases rate of SA node discharge, increases recovery time), slows conduction of AV node, decreases heart rate, which decreases O_2 consumption in myocardium; also, decreases renin—aldosterone—angiotensin system, at high doses inhibits β2 receptors in bronchial system

Uses: Mild to moderate hypertension, prophylaxis after infarction, prophylaxis of angina pectoris, migraine

Dosage and routes:

Hypertension

- *Adult:* By mouth initially 5 mg twice a day, or 10 mg daily; maximum 60 mg daily

Angina

- *Adult:* By mouth initially 5 mg 2–3 times a day; maintenance 15–45 mg daily

Myocardial infarction prophylaxis

- *Adult:* Initially 5 mg twice a day then 10 mg twice a day after 2 days, 7–28 days after infarction (acute phase)

Migraine prophylaxis

- *Adult:* By mouth 10–20 mg daily

Available forms include: Tablets 10 mg

Side effects/adverse reactions:

CV: Hypotension, bradycardia, heart failure, heart block, coldness of limb extremities

CNS: Insomnia, dizziness, hallucinations, fatigue, insomnia, depression, paraesthesiae, disorientation, vertigo, nightmares

GI: Nausea, vomiting, *abdominal pain,* retroperitoneal fibrosis

INTEG: Rash, pruritus

RESP: Bronchospasm, dyspnoea

MS: Arthralgia

Contraindications: Bronchospasm, asthma, history of obstructive airways disease, metabolic acidosis, sinus bradycardia, partial heart block, uncontrolled congestive heart failure

Precautions: Pregnancy, lactation, diabetes mellitus, renal disease, cardiac failure/insufficiency, children

Pharmacokinetics:

By mouth: Peak 2–4 hr; half-life 3–4 hr, excreted 30%–45% unchanged, 60%–65% is metabolised by liver, excreted in breast milk

Interactions/incompatibilities:

- Increased hypotension, bradycardia: reserpine, hydralazine, methyldopa, prazosin, anticholinergics, alcohol, anaesthetics, anti-arrhythmics
- Decreased antihypertensive effects: indomethacin, NSAIDs
- Increased hypoglycaemic effects: insulin, anti-diabetics
- Decreased bronchodilation: theophyllines

Clinical assessment:

• Baselines in renal, liver function tests before therapy begins
• Reduced dosage in renal dysfunction

Treatment of overdose: Lavage, activated charcoal, IV atropine for bradycardia, IV β_2 stimulants for bronchospasm, administer vasopressor (noradrenaline), glucagon can reverse the effects of excessive beta blockade

NURSING CONSIDERATIONS

Assess:
• Baseline vital signs, weight and fluid balance
• Apex/radial pulse before administration; notify clinician of any significant changes

Administer:
• Orally, before meals, before bedtime

Perform/provide:
• Storage in dry area in a cool place, do not freeze

Evaluate:
• Therapeutic response: decreased BP after 1–2 weeks
• Oedema in feet, legs daily
• Fluid balance, weight daily if at risk of heart failure
• BP, pulse 4 hrly; note rate, rhythm, quality

Teach patient/family:
• Not to discontinue drug abruptly
• Not to use non-prescribed products containing α-adrenergic stimulants (nasal decongestants, cold preparations) unless directed by clinician/pharmacist
• To report bradycardia, dizziness, confusion, depression, fever, sore throat, shortness of breath to clinician
• To avoid alcohol, smoking, high sodium intake
• To avoid hazardous activities if dizziness is present
• To report symptoms of congestive heart failure: difficult breathing, especially on exertion or when lying down, night cough, swelling of extremities
• Take medication at bedtime to decrease effect of postural hypotension if it occurs

tinidazole

Fasigyn
Func. class.: Antibiotic/antiprotozoal
Chem. class.: Nitroimidazole derivative
Legal class.: POM

Action: Penetration of the drug into the cell of the micro-organism and subsequent damage of DNA strands or inhibition of their synthesis

Uses: Anaerobic bacterial and protozoal infections

Dosage and routes:

Anaerobic infections
• *Adult and child over 12 yr:* By mouth initially 2 g as single dose, then 1 g daily, as single or 2 equal doses, for 5–6 days

Non-specific vaginitis, trichomoniasis, giardiasis, acute ulcerative gingivitis
• *Adult:* By mouth 2 g as single dose; possible to repeat dose on day 2
• *Child:* By mouth 50–75 mg/kg as single dose may repeat dose

Intestinal amoebiasis
• *Adult:* By mouth 2 g/day for 2–3 days
• *Child:* By mouth 50–60 mg/kg/day for 3 days

Amoebic involvement of liver
• *Adult:* By mouth 1.5–2 g daily for 3–5 days
• *Child:* By mouth 50–60 mg/kg/day for 5 days

Prophylaxis of infection in abdominal surgery

• *Adult and children over 12 yr:* By mouth 2 g as single dose approx 12 hr before surgery
Available forms include: Tablets 500 mg
Side effects/adverse reactions:
CNS: Headache, drowsiness
HAEM: Leucopenia
GI: Nausea, vomiting, furry tongue, anorexia, metallic taste, diarrhoea
INTEG: Rashes, pruritus, urticaria, angioneurotic oedema
GU: Dark urine
Contraindications: Blood dyscrasias; organic neurological disorders, hypersensitivity; pregnancy, lactation
Precautions: Hepatic impairment
Pharmacokinetics: Completely absorbed through GI tract, peak plasma levels after 2 hr. Half-life is 12–14 hr. Plasma protein binding is approximately 12%
Interactions/incompatibilities:
• Reduced effect of: phenobarbitone
• Potentiation: nicoualone, phenytoin, warfarin, lithium
• Increased plasma concentrations: cimetidine
• Psychotic reactions: alcohol, disulfiram
Clinical assessment:
• Full blood count
Treatment of overdose:
• Gastric lavage if soon after ingestion
• Symptomatic and supportive treatment

NURSING CONSIDERATIONS
Administer:
• Tablets to be swallowed whole with or after food to minimise GI disturbances
Perform/provide:
• Mouthwashes to relieve furry tongue
Evaluate:
• Dizziness, lack of coordination, pruritus, joint pains. Discontinue drug
• Allergic reactions – fever, rigour, rash, itching. Discontinue drug
Teach patient/family:
• Take tablets with or after food
• Urine may turn dark red–brown
• Avoid alcohol – it may cause vomiting and abdominal cramps
• Proper hygiene and handwashing following bowel movements
• Report any side effects to clinician
• Check with clinician before taking non-prescribed preparations

---

tinzaparin

Innohep, Logiparin
Func. class.: Anticoagulant
Chem. class.: Low molecular weight heparin
Legal class.: POM

Action: Prevents conversion of fibrinogen to fibrin, with a longer duration of action than normal heparin
Uses: Prevention of deep vein thrombosis in patients undergoing surgery
Dosage and routes:
General surgery
• *Adult:* By SC injection 3500 IU 2 hr before surgery followed by 3,500 IU once daily for 7–10 days, post-operatively
Orthopaedic surgery
• *Adult:* By SC injection 50 IU/kg body weight 2 hr before surgery and then once daily for 7–10 days post-operatively; using prefilled syringes doses should be rounded off as follows: below 60 kg body weight 2500 IU once daily; 60–80 kg body weight 3500 IU once daily; above 80 kg body weight 4500 IU once daily

Available forms include: Prefilled syringes 2500, 3500, 4500 IU; injection ampoules 5000 IU
Side effects/adverse reactions:
GI: Raised liver enzymes
HAEM: Thrombocytopenia, haemorrhage
INTEG: Skin rashes and bruising at injection site
Contraindications: Hypersensitivity to heparin or sulphites; conditions where there is a risk of haemorrhage, e.g. generalised haemorrhage tendency, uncontrolled severe hypertension, active peptic ulcer, septic endocarditis, breast feeding
Precautions: Severe renal or hepatic impairment; history of asthma (associated with sulphite sensitivity), pregnancy
Pharmacokinetics: Around 90% absorbed after SC administration, absorption half-life 200 min, elimination half-life about 90 min; metabolised in liver, excreted in urine
Interactions:
• Increased risk of bleeding: aspirin, dipyridamole, NSAIDs, oral anticoagulants, dextran
Incompatibilities: Tinzaparin should not be mixed with other drugs or infusion solutions
Treatment of overdose: Withdraw tinzaparin therapy; in an emergency give protamine to neutralise tinzaparin

NURSING CONSIDERATIONS

Assess:
• Baseline vital signs including BP
Administer:
• Only by SC injection and not mixed with other drugs or solutions
Perform/provide:
• Disposal of syringes, including any remaining drug, after single use
• Regular monitoring for haemorrhage, including site of injection
Teach patient/family:
• About the drug and possible side effects
• To report any sign of bleeding, particularly at wound or injection sites
• Other techniques to avoid deep vein thrombosis (early mobilisation as appropriate, regular movement, deep breathing)

tobramycin (ophthalmic)

Tobralex
Func. class.: Antibiotic
Chem. class.: Aminoglycoside
Legal class.: POM

Action: Inhibits bacterial cell wall in organism by preventing amino acid and nucleotide incorporation into cell wall
Uses: Infection of eye
Dosage and routes:
• *Adult and child:* Instil 1–2 drops every 1–4 hr depending on infection
Available forms include: Solution 0.3%
Side effects/adverse reactions:
EENT: Lid itching, conjunctival erythema
Contraindications: Hypersensitivity
Precautions: Antibiotic hypersensitivity, prolonged use may result in antibiotic overgrowth of non-susceptible organisms including fungi

NURSING CONSIDERATIONS

Administer:
• After samples have been sent for culture and sensitivity
• After washing hands, cleanse crusts or discharge from eye before application
• Apply pressure on lacrimal sac for 1 min
Perform/provide:
• Storage of eye drops at 8–25°C,

discard 28 days after opening, sterile until opened

Evaluate:

• Therapeutic response: absence of redness, inflammation, tearing

• Allergy: itching, lacrimation, redness, swelling

Teach patient/family:

• To use drug exactly as prescribed

• Not to use eye make-up, towels, washcloths, and eye medication of others, or reinfection may occur

• That drug container tip should not be touched to eye

• To report itching, increased redness, burning, stinging; drug should be discontinued

• That drug may cause blurred vision when ointment is applied

• Discard 28 days after opening

---

tobramycin sulphate

Nebcin

Func. class.: Antibiotic
Chem. class.: Aminoglycoside
Legal class.: POM

Action: Interferes with protein synthesis in bacterial cell by binding to ribosomal subunit, causing inaccurate peptide sequence to form in protein chain, causing bacterial death

Uses: Severe systemic infections of CNS, respiratory, GI, urinary tract, bone, skin, soft tissues caused by susceptible organisms

Dosage and routes:

• *Adult:* IM/IV 3 mg/kg/day in divided doses every 8 hr; may give up to 5 mg/kg/day in divided doses every 6–8 hr

• *Child:* IM/IV 6–7.5 mg/kg/day in 3–4 equally divided doses

• *Neonates under 1 week:* IM/IV up to 4 mg/kg/day in divided doses every 12 hr

Available forms include: Injection IM, IV 10, 40 mg/ml

Side effects/adverse reactions:

GU: Oliguria, haematuria, renal damage, proteinuria, renal failure, nephrotoxicity

CNS: Confusion, vertigo, numbness, headache, fever

EENT: Ototoxicity, deafness, visual disturbances, tinnitis

HAEM: Agranulocytosis, thrombocytopenia, leucopenia, eosinophilia, anaemia

GI: Nausea, vomiting, diarrhoea, increased aspartate aminotransferase, alanine aminotransferase, bilirubin

INTEG: Rash, burning, urticaria

Contraindications: Intrathecal administration, hypersensitivity

Precautions: Neonates, renal disease (reduce dose) pregnancy, myasthenia gravis, lactation, hearing deficits parkinsonism, extensive burns

Pharmacokinetics:

IM: Onset rapid, peak 1–2 hr

IV: Onset immediate, peak 1–2 hr. Plasma half-life 1–3 hr, not metabolised, excreted unchanged in urine

Interactions/incompatibilities:

• Increased ototoxicity, neurotoxicity, nephrotoxicity: other aminoglycosides, amphotericin B, polymyxin, vancomycin, ethacrynic acid, frusemide, mannitol, cisplatin, cephalosporins

• Do not mix in solution or syringe: carbenicillin, ticarcillin, amphotericin B, cephalothin, erythromycin, heparin

• Increased effects: non-depolarising muscle relaxants

Clinical assessment:

• Serum peak, drawn at 30–60 min after IV infusion or 60 min after IM injection, trough level drawn just before next dose; blood level should not exceed 12 mg/l for prolonged periods; trough levels above 2 mg/l may indicate tissue accumulation

Treatment of overdose: Haemodialysis, monitor serum levels of drug

NURSING CONSIDERATIONS

Assess:

- Fluid balance
- Bowel pattern
- Weight before treatment; calculation of dosage is usually done based on ideal body weight, but may be calculated on actual body weight

Administer:

- After sample has been sent for culture and sensitivity
- If IV give diluted with 50–100 ml (adults) of 0.9% sodium chloride or dextrose 5% over a period of 20–60 min. Adjust dosage according to renal and auditory function; pre-dose (trough) concentrations should be less than 2 mg/l
- IM injection in large muscle mass, rotate injection sites
- Drug in evenly spaced doses to maintain blood level
- Bicarbonate to alkalinise urine if ordered in treating urinary tract infection, as drug is most active in an alkaline environment
- Culture and sensitivity before starting treatment to identify infecting organism

Perform/provide:

- Adequate fluids of 2–3 l/day unless contraindicated to prevent irritation of tubules
- Vital signs during infusion, watch for hypotension, change in pulse
- Flush IV line with or Dextrose 5% after infusion
- Supervised ambulation, other safety measures 0.9% sodium chloride if patient has vestibular dysfunction

Evaluate:

- IV site for thrombophlebitis including pain, redness, swelling ½-hrly, change site if needed; apply warm compresses to discontinued site
- Fluid balance, urinalysis daily for proteinuria, cells, casts; report sudden change in urine output
- Urine pH if drug is used for urinary tract infection; urine should be kept alkaline
- Therapeutic effect: absence of fever, draining wounds, negative culture and sensitivity after treatment
- Renal impairment (by securing urine for creatinine clearance testing), under
- Deafness by audiometric testing, ringing, roaring in ears, vertigo; assess hearing before, during, after treatment
- Dehydration: decrease in skin turgor, dry mucous membranes, dark urine
- Overgrowth of infection: increased temperature, malaise, redness, pain, swelling, perineal itching, diarrhoea, stomatitis, change in cough, sputum
- Culture and sensitivity before starting treatment to identify infecting organism
- Vestibular dysfunction: nausea, vomiting, dizziness, headache, drug should be discontinued if severe
- Injection and infusion sites for redness, swelling, abscesses; use warm compresses at site

Teach patient/family:

- To report headache, dizziness, symptoms of overgrowth of infection, renal impairment
- To report loss of hearing, ringing, roaring in ears, feeling of fullness in head

tocainide hydrochloride

Tonocard
Func. class.: Anti-arrhythmic (Class Ic)
Chem. class.: Lignocaine analogue
Legal class.: POM

Action: Increases electrical stimulation threshold of ventricale, His–Purkinje system, which stabilizes cardiac membrane
Uses: Ventricular tachycardia, arrhythmias, symptomatic and life threatening
Dosage and routes:
• *Adult:* By mouth 1.2 g daily in divided doses; maximum daily dose 2.5 g
Available forms include: Tablets 400 mg
Side effects/adverse reactions:
CNS: Headache, dizziness, involuntary movement, confusion, psychosis, restlessness, irritability, paraesthesias, tremor, convulsions
EENT: Tinnitus, blurred vision, hearing loss
GI: Nausea, vomiting, anorexia, diarrhoea
CV: Hypotension, bradycardia, angina, heart block, cardiovascular collapse (at high plasma concentrations), arrest, congestive heart failure
RESP: Dyspnoea, respiratory depression
HAEM: Agranulocytosis, aplastic anaemia, thrombocytopenia
INTEG: Rash, urticaria, oedema, swelling
Contraindications: Hypersensitivity to amides, 2nd or 3rd degree AV block (in the absence of a pacemaker)
Precautions: Pregnancy, lactation, children, renal disease, liver disease, respiratory depression, myasthenia gravis, uncompensated congestive heart failure, concurrent anti-arrhythmic agents, congestive heart failure
Pharmacokinetics:
By mouth: Peak 1 hr; half-life 10–17 hr, metabolised by liver, excreted in urine
Interactions/incompatibilities:
• May increase effects when used with: propranolol, quinidine
Clinical assessment:
• Chest X-ray, pulmonary function test during treatments
• Blood count weekly during first 12 wks of treatment
• Drug blood levels (therapeutic level 4–10 mcg/ml)
• Lung fields, bilateral rales may occur in congestive heart failure patient
Lab. test interferences:
Increase: Creatinine phosphokinase
Treatment of overdose: O_2, artificial ventilation, ECG, inotropic support

NURSING CONSIDERATIONS

Assess:
• Baseline BP and fluid balance
Administer:
• IV infusion under direction of anaesthetic with resuscitation facilities available
Evaluate:
• Toxicity: fine tremors, dizziness
• Fatigue, sore throat, fever, bruising, increased temperature
• Cardiac rate, respiration: rate, rhythm, character, ½ hrly
• Fluid balance ratio; check for decreasing output

tolazamide

Tolanase
Func. class.: Oral hypoglycaemic
Chem. class.: Sulphonylurea (1st generation)
Legal class.: POM

Action: Causes functioning β-cells

in pancreas to synthesise and release insulin, leading to drop in blood glucose levels; stimulation of insulin results in increased insulin binding; this drug not effective if patient lacks functioning β-cells

Uses: Maturity onset diabetes, mild to moderate severity

Dosage and routes:

• *Adult:* By mouth 100–250 mg daily adjusted according to patient response; maximum 1 g daily in divided doses if necessary

Available forms include: Tablets 100, 250 mg

Side effects/adverse reactions:

CNS: Headache, weakness, fatigue, lethargy, dizziness, vertigo

GI: Nausea, vomiting, diarrhoea, constipation, flatus, hepatotoxicity, jaundice, anorexia

HAEM: Leucopenia, thrombocytopenia, agranulocytosis, aplastic anaemia, pancytopenia, haemolytic anaemia

INTEG: Rash (rare) allergic reactions, pruritus, urticaria, eczema, photo-sensitivity), erythema

ENDO: Hypoglycaemia

Contraindications: Hypersensitivity to sulphonylureas; juvenile or brittle diabetes; renal or hepatic disease; pregnancy; surgery; trauma; diabetic ketoacidosis; coma; breast-feeding; porphyria

Precautions: Elderly, cardiac disease, thyroid disease, severe hypoglycaemic reactions

Pharmacokinetics:

By mouth: Completely absorbed by GI route; onset 1 hr, peak 4–8 hr, duration 20 hr; half-life 7 hr, metabolised in liver, excreted in urine (metabolites), breast milk, highly protein bound

Interactions/incompatibilities:

• May increase effects when taken with insulin, MAOIs, cimetidine, phenylbutazone and other NSAIDs, sulphonamides, chloramphenicol, probenecid, coumarin anticoagulants, β-blockers

• Decreased action of this drug: calcium channel blockers, corticosteroids, oral contraceptives, thiaide diuretics, thyroid preparations, oestrogens, phenothiazines, phenytoin, rifampicin, isoniazid

Treatment of overdose: Conscious patient, administer glucose or 3–4 lumps of table sugar with water. Repeat if necessary. Comatosed patient, administer IV glucose infusion or glucagon 1 mg by SC or IM injection to produce consciousness

NURSING CONSIDERATIONS

Administer:

• Drug 30 min before meals

Evaluate:

• Therapeutic response: decrease in polyuria, polydipsia, polyphagia, alertness, absence of dizziness, stable gait

• Hypoglycaemic/hyperglycaemic reaction that can occur soon after meals

Teach patient/family:

• To check for symptoms of cholestatic jaundice (dark urine, pruritus, yellow sclera); if these occur notify clinician

• To use a capillary blood glucose test while on this drug

• To avoid alcohol; disulfiram type reaction with alcohol

• To test urine glucose levels approximately 2 hr after each meal

• The symptoms of hypo/hyperglycaemia, what to do about each

• That this drug must be continued on 'a daily basis; explain consequence of discontinuing drug abruptly

• To take drug in morning to prevent hypoglycaemic reactions at night

• To avoid non-prescribed medications

• That diabetes is a life-long illness, drug will not cure disease

• That all food included in diet

plan must be eaten in order to prevent hypoglycaemia
• To carry medic alert ID as a diabetic

tolbutamide

Rastinon
Func. class.: Oral hypoglycaemic
Chem. class.: Sulphonylurea
Legal class.: POM

Action: Causes functioning β-cells in pancreas to synthesise and release insulin, leading to drop in blood glucose levels; stimulation of insulin results in increased insulin binding; this drug is not effective if patient lacks functioning β-cells
Uses: Maturity onset diabetes mild to moderate; NIDDM patients who have failed to be controlled by dietary means
Dosage and routes:
• *Adult:* By mouth 0.5–1.5 g (maximum 2 g) daily in divided doses, titrated to patient response
Available forms include: Tablets 500 mg
Side effects/adverse reactions:
CNS: Headache, weakness, paraesthesia
GI: Nausea, fullness, heartburn, hepatotoxicity, cholestatic jaundice
HAEM: Leucopenia, thrombocytopenia, agranulocytosis, aplastic anaemia, increased aspartate aminotransferase, alanine aminotransferase, alkaline phosphatase
INTEG: Rash, allergic reactions, pruritus, urticaria, eczema, photosensitivity, erythema
ENDO: Hypoglycaemia
MS: Joint pains
Contraindications: Hypersensitivity to sulphonylureas, juvenile or brittle diabetes, severe renal disease or hepatic disease, severe impairment of thyroid or adrenocortical function; breast-feeding; porphyria; surgery
Precautions: Pregnancy, elderly, cardiac disease, thyroid function, previous history of ketoacidosis, surgery, trauma, pregnancy, severe hypoglycaemic reactions
Pharmacokinetics:
By mouth: Completely absorbed by GI route; onset 30–60 min, peak 3–5 hr, duration 24 hr; half-life 7 hr, metabolised in liver, excreted in urine (metabolites), breast milk, 90%–95% is plasma protein bound
Interactions/incompatibilities:
• Increased effects of this drug: insulin, MAOIs, dicoumarol, salicylates, β-blockers, sulphonamides. NSAIDs, chloramphenicol
• Decreased action of this drug: calcium channel blockers, corticosteroids, oral contraceptives, thiazide diuretics, thyroid preparations, oestrogens, adrenaline, lithium, rifampicin, cyclophosphamide
Treatment of overdose: Conscious patient, administer glucose or 3–4 lumps of table sugar with water. Repeat if necessary. If comatosed patient, administer IV glucose infusion or glucagon 1 mg by subcutaneous or IM injection to produce consciousness

NURSING CONSIDERATIONS

Administer:
• Drug 30 min before meals
Perform/provide:
• Storage in tight container in cool environment, protected from light
Evaluate:
• Therapeutic response: decrease in polyuria, polydipsia, polyphagia, alertness, absence of dizziness, stable gait
• Hypoglycaemic/hyperglycaemic reaction that can occur soon after meals

Teach patient/family:

• To check for symptoms of cholestatic jaundice (dark urine, pruritus, yellow sclera); if these occur a clinician should be notified
• To use a capillary blood glucose test while on this drug
• To test urine glucose levels approximately 2 hr after each meal
• The symptoms of hypo/hyperglycaemia; what to do about each
• That this drug must be continued on a daily basis; explain consequence of discontinuing drug abruptly
• To take drug in morning to prevent hypoglycaemic reactions at night
• To avoid non-prescribed medications
• That diabetes is a life-long illness, drug will not cure disease
• That all food included in diet plan must be eaten in order to prevent hypoglycaemia (usually low fat, low carbohydrate diet)
• To carry a radioactive iodine uptake ID for emergency purposes
• Discuss with clinician if any of the following symptoms occur: dizziness, confusion, weakness, sweating, nausea, vomiting, skin rash

---

tolmetin sodium

Tolectin
Func. class.: Non-steroidal anti-inflammatory drug
Chem. class.: Pyrrole acetic acid derivative
Legal class.: POM

Action: Inhibits prostaglandin synthesis by decreasing an enzyme needed for biosynthesis; possesses analgesic, anti-inflammatory, antipyretic properties
Uses: Osteoarthritis, rheumatoid arthritis, ankylosing spondylitis, fibrositis, bursitis, juvenile arthritis
Dosage and routes:
• *Adult:* By mouth 600 mg–1800 mg daily in 2–4 divided doses, maximum 30 mg/kg daily, not to exceed 1.8 g/ day in 2–4 divided doses
Juvenile arthritis
• *Child:* By mouth 20–25 mg/kg daily in 3–4 divided doses; maximum 30 mg/kg daily up to 1.8 g/ day
• Not for use in children under 2 years
Available forms include: Capsules 200 mg, 400 mg
Side effects/adverse reactions:
GI: Nausea, anorexia, vomiting, diarrhoea, jaundice, cholestatic hepatitis, constipation, flatulence, cramps, dry mouth, peptic ulcer
CNS: Dizziness, drowsiness, fatigue, tremors, confusion, insomnia, anxiety, depression
INTEG: Purpura, rash, pruritus, sweating
GU: Nephrotoxicity
HAEM: Blood dyscrasias
EENT: Tinnitus, hearing loss, blurred vision
Contraindications: Hypersensitivity to this drug or other anti-inflammatory drugs, asthma, active or suspected peptic ulcer, last trimester of pregnancy, gastrointestinal bleeding. Avoid in patients currently receiving warfarin or oral anticoagulant drugs
Precautions: Pregnancy, lactation, bleeding disorders, GI disorders, cardiac disorders, elderly, renal/ hepatic disease
Interactions/incompatibilities:
• May increase action of coumarin, phenytoin, sulphonamides when used with this drug
Clinical assessment:
• Renal, liver tests, blood count: serum urea, creatinine, aspartate

aminotransferase, alanine aminotransferase, Hb before treatment, periodically thereafter
• Audiometric, ophthalmic examination before, during, after treatment

NURSING CONSIDERATIONS

Administer:
• With or after food or milk

Evaluate:
• Therapeutic response: decreased pain, stiffness, swelling in joints, ability to move more easily
• For eye, ear problems: blurred vision, tinnitus (may indicate toxicity)

Teach patient/family:
• To report blurred vision or ringing, roaring in ears (may indicate toxicity)
• To avoid driving or other hazardous activities if dizziness or drowsiness occurs
• To report change in urine pattern, weight increase, oedema, pain increase in joints, fever, blood in urine (indicates nephrotoxicity)
• That therapeutic effects may take up to 1 month to develop
• Avoid over-the-counter preparations; these may contain Aspirin

tranexamic acid

Cyklokapron
Func. class.: Haemostatic, antifibrinolytic
Legal class.: POM

Action: Competitively inhibits the activation of plasminogen to plasmin
Uses: Prophylaxis and treatment of haemorrhage following prostatectomy, conisation of the cervix, surgery in haemophiliacs, menorrhagia, traumatic hyphaema, management of dental extractions in haemophiliacs, hereditary angioneurotic, oedema, epistaxis, complications of thrombolysis, disseminated intravascular coagulation with predominant inactivation of the fibrinolytic system

Dosage and routes:
Seek specialist advice for treatment areas
• *Adult:* By mouth, 1–1.5 g 2–4 times daily depending on condition; slow IV injection, 1 g 3 times daily; by IV infusion 25–50 mg/kg body weight/day. Adjust dose in renal impairment

Available forms include: Tablets 500 mg, injection 100 mg/ml, syrup 500 mg/5 ml

Side effects/adverse reactions:
GI: Nausea, vomiting, abdominal cramps, diarrhoea
CV: Hypotension with too rapid injection

Contraindications: Hypersensitivity, history of thromboembolic disease
Precautions: Renal disease, pregnancy, lactation, upper urinary tract infection, haematuria

Clinical assessment:
• Fluid balance. If urinary output decreases the clinician must be informed and the drug discontinued
• Blood tests: clotting factors, platelets, signs and symptoms of thrombophlebitis
• Blood pressure and tachycardia
• Creatinine phosphokinase, urinalysis
• Liver function tests

NURSING CONSIDERATIONS

Assess:
• Baseline vital signs

Evaluate:
• Allergy, fever, rash, itching, jaundice
• Myopathy, weakness, fever, myoglobinaemia or oliguria, which indicate that drug should be discontinued
• Bleeding from mucous membranes, epistaxis, ecchymosis,

petechiae, haematuria, haematemesis

• Blood pressure and tachycardia

Teach patient/family:

• Any signs of bleeding must be reported, e.g. from gums, subcutaneously, in urine, stools or vomit

• To rise slowly when standing or sitting to avoid postural hypotension

tranylcypromine sulphate

Parnate

Func. class.: Antidepressant, (MAOI)

Chem. class.: Non-hydrazine MAOI

Legal class.: POM

Action: Increases concentrations of endogenous adrenaline, noradrenaline, serotonin, dopamine in storage sites in CNS by inhibition of monoamine oxidase; increased concentration reduces depression

Uses: Depressive illness, when uncontrolled by other means

Dosage and routes:

• *Adult:* By mouth 10 mg twice a day, may increase the second daily dose to 20 mg after 1 week. Usual maintenance dose: 10 mg daily

Available forms include: Tablets 10 mg

Side effects/adverse reactions:

HAEM: Dyscrasias

CNS: Dizziness, drowsiness, confusion, headache, anxiety, tremors, stimulation, weakness, hyperreflexia, mania, insomnia, restlessness, increased appetite, peripheral neuritis, dependence, fatigue

GI: Constipation, dry mouth, nausea, vomiting, diarrhoea, liver dysfunction

GU: Change in libido, frequency, difficulty in micturition

INTEG: Rash, flushing, increased perspiration

CV: Orthostatic hypotension, hypertension, dysrhythmias, hypertensive crisis (see Interactions below), palpitation

EENT: Blurred vision

SYST: Weight gain, oedema

Contraindications: Hypersensitivity to MAOIs, suspected cerebrovascular disease, blood dyscrasias, severe hepatic disease, phaeochromocytoma, porphyria, hyperthyroidism, within 1 week of other MAOIs or antidepressant drugs

Precautions: Convulsive disorders, hyperactivity, diabetes mellitus, pregnancy, lactation, elderly, surgery, alcohol/drug abuse, cardiovascular disease, concurrent electroconvulsive therapy

Pharmacokinetics:

Metabolised by liver, excreted by kidneys, elimination half-life 2–3 hr, excreted in breast milk. May take 3 weeks to start working, 5 weeks for maximal effect

Interactions/incompatibilities:

• CNS excitation or depression given with: pethidine and possibly other opiates, nefopam

• Serious CNS toxicity and/or hypertensive crisis given with, shortly before or after: other antidepressants including other MAOIs, rauwolfia alkaloids, oxypertine, sumatriptan, buspirone, tetrabenazine

• Hypertensive crisis with: levodopa, amphetamines, dexfenfluramine, diethylpropion, dopamine, dopexamine, ephedrine, fenfluramine, isometheptene, mazindol, pemoline, phentermine, phenylephrine, phenylpropanolamine, pseudoephedrine, other sympathomimetics, high tyramine foods (see below)

• Effect of oral hypoglycaemics, insulin reduced

Clinical assessment:

• Phentolamine for severe hypertension

• Check hepatic function if impairment suspected before, during treatment

Treatment of overdose: Lavage, activated charcoal, symptomatic and supportive treatment including phentolamine for severe hypertension

NURSING CONSIDERATIONS

Assess:

• Baseline vital signs

• BP (lying, standing), pulse

Administer:

• Increased fluids, bulk in diet if constipation, urinary retention occur

• With food or milk for GI symptoms

• Crushed if patient is unable to swallow medication whole

• Dosage at bedtime if oversedation occurs during day

• Mouthwashes, frequent sips of water for dry mouth

Perform/provide:

• Storage in tight container in cool environment

• Assistance with ambulation during beginning therapy since drowsiness/dizziness occurs

• Safety measures including cot sides

• Checking to see oral medication swallowed

Evaluate:

• Toxicity: increased headache, palpitation, discontinue drug immediately; prodromal signs of hypertensive crisis

• Mental status: mood, sensory, affect, memory (long, short), increase in psychiatric symptoms

• Urinary retention, constipation, oedema. Weight weekly

• Withdrawal symptoms: headache, nausea, vomiting, muscle pain, weakness

Teach patient/family:

• That therapeutic effects may take 1–4 weeks

• To avoid driving or other activities requiring alertness

• To avoid alcohol ingestion, CNS depressants or non-prescribed medications; particularly for colds, coughs, hay fever

• Not to discontinue medication quickly after long-term use

• To avoid high tyramine foods: mature cheese, sour cream, beer, wine, Marmite, Bovril, heavy red wines, broad beans, non-alcoholic beer, pickled products, liver, raisins, bananas, figs, avocados, meat tenderizers, chocolate, yogurt

• Report headache, palpitation, neck stiffness

---

trazodone HCl

Molipaxin

Func. class.: Antidepressant

Chem. class.: Triazolopyridine derivative

Legal class.: POM

Action: Unclear, may potentiate noradrenaline and antagonise serotonin in the brain

Uses: Depression, depression accompanied by anxiety

Dosage and routes:

• *Adult:* By mouth 150 mg/day in divided doses after meals, may be increased to 300 mg/day, or maximum 600 mg/day for hospitalised patients

Available forms include: Capsules 50, 100, tablets 150 mg, tablets modified release 150 mg, liquid 50 mg/5 ml

Side effects/adverse reactions:

CNS: Dizziness, drowsiness, con-

fusion, headache, tremor, stimulation, weakness, insomnia
GI: Diarrhoea, dry mouth, nausea, vomiting
GU: Priapism
INTEG: Rash
CV: Orthostatic hypotension, tachycardia, bradycardia
EENT: Blurred vision
SYST: Weight loss, oedema
Contraindications: Hypersensitivity, recent myocardial infarction, heart block, mania, porphyria
Precautions: Cardiovascular disease, hepatic disease, pregnancy, epilepsy, renal disease, lactation
Pharmacokinetics:
Metabolised by liver, excreted by kidneys, faeces; half-life 5–13 hr
Interactions/incompatibilities:
• Decreased effects of: guanethidine, clonidine
• Increased effects of: alcohol, barbiturates, benzodiazepines, and other CNS depressants
• Hyperpyretic crisis, convulsions, hypertensive episode given with or within 14 days of: MAOIs
Clinical assessment:
• Check hepatic and renal function if significant impairment considered likely
Treatment of overdose: Induce emesis, lavage, activated charcoal, symptomatic and supportive treatment

NURSING CONSIDERATIONS

Assess:
• BP (lying, standing), pulse
• Baseline weight
Administer:
• Increased fluids, fibre in diet if constipation, urinary retention occur
• After or with food
• In divided doses or entire daily dose may be given at night
• Mouthwashes, frequent sips of water for dry mouth
Perform/provide:
• Storage in tight, light-resistant container at room temperature
• Assistance with ambulation during beginning therapy since drowsiness/dizziness occurs
• Safety measures including siderails, primarily in elderly
• Checking to see oral medication swallowed
Evaluate:
• Weight weekly, appetite may increase with drug
• Uncoordinated movements primarily in elderly: rigidity, dystonia, akathisia
• Mental status: mood, sensory, affect, suicidal tendencies, increase in psychiatric symptoms: depression, panic
• Cardiovascular side-effects, particularly with high doses
• Urinary retention, constipation
• Withdrawal symptoms: headache, nausea, vomiting, muscle pain, weakness; do not usually occur unless drug was discontinued abruptly
Teach patient/family:
• That therapeutic effects may take 2–3 weeks
• Use caution in driving or other activities requiring alertness because of drowsiness, dizziness, blurred vision
• To avoid alcohol ingestion, other CNS depressants; drug enhances the effect of alcohol
• Not to discontinue medication quickly after long-term use, may cause nausea, headache, malaise

treosulfan

Treosulfan
Func. class.: Antineoplastic alkylating agent
Chem. class.: Busulphan derivative
Legal class.: POM

Action: Alkylates DNA, RNA; inhibits enzymes that allow synthesis of proteins; is also responsible for cross linking DNA strands

Uses: Ovarian carcinoma

Dosage and routes:

Doses are highly variable, and dependent on local treatment protocols, concomitant therapy and tumour type; the following dose schedules have been used

- *Adult:* By mouth 1–2 g daily in 3–4 divided doses to provide total dose of 21–28 g over initial 8 weeks, which includes treatment breaks
- *Adult:* IV 5–15 g every 1–3 weeks depending on blood count and concurrent chemotherapy

Available forms include: Capsules 250 mg; injection 5 g

Side effects/adverse reactions:

HAEM: Thrombocytopenia, leucopenia, pancytopenia, acute myeloid leukaemia

GI: Nausea, vomiting, diarrhoea, abdominal pain, weight loss

INTEG: Alopecia, dermatitis, skin pigmentation, local pain and necrosis following extravasation of IV infusion

Contraindications: Hypersensitivity, pregnancy, breast-feeding

Precautions: Radiotherapy, bone marrow depression, renal impairment, liver failure

Pharmacokinetics:

Activated *in vivo* by non-enzymic conversion to epoxide compounds

Clinical assessment:

- Prescribe anti-emetic to combat nausea and vomiting
- Monitor blood picture every 1–2 weeks
- Withdraw drug if white blood cell count is below 3×10^9/litre or platelet count below 100×10^9/litre

Treatment of overdose: Symptomatic and supportive treatment, including blood transfusion and filgrastim if appropriate

NURSING CONSIDERATIONS

Administer:

- HANDLING: take safety precautions appropriate to antineoplastic agents
- Following local antineoplastic (cytotoxic) policies
- After ensuring that clinician is aware of blood results
- IV; each 5 g vial of powder for injection should be dissolved in 100 ml water for injection
- Doses of up to 5 g as IV bolus injection
- Doses above 5 g as IV infusion at a rate of 5 g every 5–10 min
- By mouth; capsules must be swallowed whole and not opened or allowed to disintegrate in the mouth
- Other medications by mouth if possible. Avoid IV, IM, SC routes to prevent infection and bruising
- Anti-emetic 30–60 min before treatment
- All other medication as prescribed including analgesics, antibiotics, anti-emetics, antispasmodics

Perform/provide:

- Avoid extravasation into tissues as local pain and tissue damage will occur
- Analgesics as appropriate

Evaluate:

- IV site for signs of extravasation. Discontinue at once if this happens and use a different vein for remaining solution

Teach patient/family:

- To expect nausea and vomiting—take anti-emetics as prescribed
- Swallow capsules whole—do not allow to disintegrate in mouth
- About all side effects of drug and to report these immediately
- Reversible alopecia may occur

tretinoin

Retin-A, Retin-A Forte
Func. class.: Anti-acne agent, keratolytic
Chem. class.: Retinoid
Legal class.: POM

Action: Decreases cohesiveness of follicular epithelial cells, decreases microcomedone formation
Uses: Acne vulgaris in which comedones, papules and pustules predominate
Dosage and routes:
• *Adult and child:* Topical, cleanse area, apply to cover area lightly once or twice daily
Available forms include: Gel 0.01, 0.025%; lotion 0.025%; cream 0.025%, 0.05%
Side effects/adverse reactions:
INTEG: Rash, stinging, warmth, erythema, peeling, contact dermatitis, hypo/hyperpigmentation, photosensitivity
Contraindications: Hypersensitivity, family history of cutaneous epithelioma, pregnancy, sunburn
Precautions: Eczema, avoid application to broken skin
Pharmacokinetics:
Topical: Poor absorption, excreted in urine
Interactions/incompatibilities:
• Increased skin peeling when used with: medications containing agents such as sulphur, benzoyl peroxide, resorcinol, salicylic acid
Treatment of overdose: Gastric emptying if significant oral ingestion occurs

NURSING CONSIDERATIONS
Administer:
• Apply sparingly to cleansed skin; excessive application produces side effects without enhancing therapeutic effect
• Avoid oversaturation or contact with eyes, broken skin, accumulation in angles of the nose
• Do not apply at the same time as other skin medications
• Use the following with caution: medicated or abrasive soaps, cleansers that have a drying effect, products with high concentrations of alcohol astringent
• Wash hands after application
Perform/provide:
• Store in a cool place, protect lotion from light
Evaluate:
• Therapeutic response: decrease in size and number of lesions
• Area of body involved, including time involved, what helps or aggravates condition
Teach patient/family:
• To avoid application on normal skin or getting cream in eyes, nose, or other mucous membranes
• To avoid sunlight or sunlamps
• Treatment may cause warmth, stinging; dryness, peeling will occur
• Cosmetics may be used over drug, not to use shaving lotions
• That rash may occur during first 1–3 weeks of therapy
• That drug does not cure condition, only relieves symptoms

triamcinolone/ triamcinolone acetonide/ triamcinolone hexacetonide

Adcortyl, Kenalog Lederspan, Ledercort
Func. class.: Corticosteroid
Chem. class.: Synthetic fluorinated glucocorticoid
Legal class.: POM

Action: Decreases inflammation by suppression of migration of polymorphonuclear leucocytes, fibroblasts, reversal to increase capillary permeability and lysosomal stabilization. Immediate action

Uses: Severe inflammation, pain and stiffness associated with rheumatoid arthritis or osteoarthrosis, neoplasms, asthma (steroid dependent), bursitis, tendinitis, lichen planus, lichen simplex, collagen disorders, severe dermatitis and Stevens–Johnson syndrome, nephrotic syndrome, tenosynovitis, epicondylitis, hypertrophic scars, granuloma annulare, keloids, alopecia areata, seasonal or perennial allergic rhinitis, endocrine disorders, autoimmune haematological disorders, neoplastic disorders

Dosage and routes:

Bronchial asthma, rheumatoid arthritis, dermatoses

• *Adults and children over 34 kg:* By mouth 8–16 mg/day

• *Children less than 34 kg:* By mouth 4–12 mg/day

• *Adults and children over 6 yr:* By deep IM injection 40 mg (acetonide)

Rheumatic fever with severe carditis, nephrotic syndrome

• *Adult:* By mouth initially 16–20 mg/day

Collagen diseases, e.g. systemic lupus erythematosus

• *Adult:* By mouth, initially 20–30 mg/day

All doses should be adjusted according to individual requirements

Local joint inflammation or pain

• *Adult:* Intra-articular injection, small joint 2.5–10 mg (acetonide), large joint 5–40 mg (acetonide). A maximum of 80 mg over several sites can be given

• *Adult:* Intra-articular injection, small joint 2–6 mg (hexacetonide). Large joint 10–30 mg. Adjust dose and frequency according to individual requirements

Lichen simplex or planus, granuloma annulare, keloids, alopecia areata, hypertrophic scars

• *Adult:* Intradermal injections 2–3 mg (acetonide) depending on the size of the lesion. Maximum of 5 mg per site or total of 30 mg at several sites. Repeat if necessary at intervals of 1–2 weeks

• *Adult:* For intralesional or sublesional use 0.5 mg or less per square inch of affected skin (as hexacetonide)

Available forms include: Tablets 2, 4 mg; injection 10, 40 mg/ml acetonide; injection 5, 20 mg/ml hexacetonide

Side effects/adverse reactions:

INTEG: Acne, poor wound healing, bruising, striae, telangiectasia, ecchymosis, petechiae, weight gain, hirsutism, Cushingoid features

CNS: Depression, headache, mood changes intracranial hypertension, insomnia, aggravation of schizophrenia, dizziness

META: Sodium and water retention, hypokalaemic alkalosis, growth suppression in children, menstrual irregularity and amenorrhoea, impaired carbohydrate tolerance

CV: Hypertension, thrombophlebitis, thromboembolism, tachycardia

HAEM: Thrombocytopenia, leucocytosis

MS: Fractures, osteoporosis, sterile abscess, hyper- or hypopigmentation and subcutaneous and cutaneous atrophy at site of intradermal injection, weakness, proximal myopathy, avascular osteonecrosis, tendon rupture, local fat atrophy

GI: Diarrhoea, nausea, abdominal distension, peptic ulceration with perforation and haemorrhage, dyspepsia, GI haemorrhage, increased appetite, pancreatitis,

oesophageal candidiasis, oesophageal ulceration
EENT: Opportunistic infections, increased intraocular pressure, glaucoma, papilloedema, cataracts, blurred vision, corneal or scleral thinning, exacerbation of ophthalmic viral disease
Contraindications: Psychosis, hypersensitivity, exacerbation of viral disease, child less than 6 years, active tuberculosis, herpes simplex
Precautions: Pregnancy, diabetes mellitus, intestinal anastomoses, tuberculosis, viral, bacterial or fungal infection, hypertension, epilepsy, glaucoma, osteoporosis, ulcerative colitis, congestive heart disease, myasthenia gravis, acute glomerular nephritis, steroid myopathy, thrombophlebitis, peptic ulcer, epilepsy. Psychosis, elderly, chronic nephritis, metastatic carcinoma
Interactions/incompatibilities:
• Decreased effects of this drug: cholestyramine, colestipol, barbiturates, ripampicin, carbamazepine, phenytoin, theophylline
• Decreased effects of: anticoagulants, antidiabetics, antihypertensives, loop and thiazide diuretics, acetazolamide, vaccines
• Increased side effects: alcohol, salicylates, indomethacin
Clinical assessment:
• Serum potassium, blood sugar, urine glucose while on long-term therapy; hypokalaemia and hyperglycaemia
• Plasma cortisol levels during long-term therapy (normal level: 136–690 nmol/litre when drawn at 8 AM)

NURSING CONSIDERATIONS

Assess:
• Baseline weight, BP, pulse rate
• BP, pulse 4 hrly; notify clinician if chest pain occurs
• Fluid balance ratio, be alert for decreasing urinary output and increasing oedema

Administer:
• After shaking suspension (parenteral)
• Titrated dose, use lowest effective dose
• IM injection deeply in large muscle mass; rotate sites, avoid deltoid, use appropriate gauge needle
• In one dose in morning to prevent adrenal suppression. Avoid subcutaneous administration; damage may be done to tissue
• With food or milk to decrease GI symptoms

Perform/provide:
• Assistance with ambulation in patient with bone tissue disease to prevent fractures
• Weight daily, notify clinician if weekly gain is over 2–3 kg

Evaluate:
• Therapeutic response: ease of respirations, decreased inflammation
• Infection: increased temperature, WBC, even after withdrawal of medication. Drug masks infection symptoms
• Potassium depletion: paraesthesias, fatigue, nausea, vomiting, depression, polyuria, dysrhythmias, weakness
• Oedema, hypotension, cardiac symptoms
• Mental status: affect, mood, behavioural changes, aggression

Teach patient/family:
• That ID card as steroid user should be carried
• To notify clinician if therapeutic response decreases; dosage adjustment may be needed
• Not to discontinue this medication abruptly or adrenal crisis can result
• To avoid non-prescribed products: salicylates, alcohol in cough products, cold preparations unless directed by clinician
• Teach patient all aspects of

drug use, including Cushingoid symptoms
• Symptoms of adrenal insufficiency: nausea, anorexia, fatigue, dizziness, dyspnoea, weakness, joint pain

triamcinolone acetonide (oral cavity)

Adcortyl in Orabase
Func. class.: Corticosteroid
Chem. class.: Synthetic fluorinated glucocorticoid
Legal class.: POM

Action: Anti-inflammatory, anti-pruritic
Uses: Aphthous ulcers, ulcerative or denture stomatitis, desquamative gingivitis, erosive lichen planus, lesions of traumatic origin
Dosage and routes:
• *Adult and child:* Apply to the affected area two to four times a day. Do not rub in
Available forms include: Paste 0.1%
Side effects/adverse reactions:
INTEG: Irritation, sensitization
Contraindications: Hypersensitivity, to presence of fungal, viral, or bacterial infections of mouth or throat (unless treated), tuberculosis
Precautions: Child (maximum of 5 days), sepsis, pregnancy, prolonged usage

NURSING CONSIDERATIONS
Administer:
• After cleansing oral cavity
• Do not rub in
Evaluate:
• Allergy: rash, irritation, reddening, swelling
• Therapeutic response: absence of pain in affected area
• Infection: if affected area is infected, do not apply
Teach patient/family:
• To report rash, irritation, redness, swelling
• How to apply paste

triamcinolone acetonide (topical)

Adcortyl, Ledercort
Func. class.: Corticosteroid, topical
Chem. class.: Synthetic fluorinated glucocorticoid
Legal class.: POM

Action: Possesses anti-pruritic, anti-inflammatory actions
Uses: Psoriasis of the scalp, palms or soles only, eczema, contact dermatitis, pruritus, neurodermatitis
Dosage and routes:
• *Adult and child:* Apply sparingly to affected area two to four times a day, reducing frequency according to response
Available forms include: Ointment 0.1%; cream 0.1%
Side effects/adverse reactions:
INTEG: Burning, dryness, itching, increased sweating, lupus erythematosus like lesions, ecchymoses, irritation, hirsutism, atrophy, striae, secondary infection, impaired wound healing, facial erythema and telangiectasia, purpura, acneiform eruptions, petéchiae, thinning of the skin
Contraindications: Hypersensitivity to corticosteroids, fungal, viral or bacterial skin infections, tuberculosis, acne vulgaris, facial rosacea, perioral dermatitis or napkin eruptions
Precautions: Pregnancy, lactation, viral infections, bacterial infections, children (maximum of 5 days treatment)

NURSING CONSIDERATIONS

Administer:

• Only to affected areas; do not get in eyes

• Medication, then cover with occlusive dressing (only if prescribed), seal to normal skin, change 12 hrly; use occlusive dressing with extreme caution

• Only to dermatoses; do not use on weeping, denuded, or infected area

Perform/provide:

• Cleansing before application of drug

• Treatment for a few days after area has cleared

Evaluate:

• Therapeutic response: absence of severe itching, patches on skin, flaking

• Temperature; if fever develops, drug should be discontinued

Teach patient/family:

• To avoid sunlight on affected area; burns may occur

• That ointment is not a cure

• That rebound exacerbation may occur

---

triamterene

DYTAC

Func. class.: Potassium-sparing diuretic

Chem. class.: Diuretics

Legal class.: POM

Action: Acts on distal tubule to inhibit reabsorption of sodium, chloride

Uses: Oedema; in cardiac failure, cirrhosis of the liver, or nephrotic syndrome and that associated with corticosteroid treatment, may be used with other diuretics

Dosage and routes:

• *Adult:* By mouth 150–250 mg daily in divided doses after meals, reduce to alternate days after 1 week. Lower initial doses when given with other diuretics

Available forms include: Capsules 50 mg

Side effects/adverse reactions:

GI: Nausea, diarrhoea, vomiting, dry mouth, jaundice and elevated serum levels of liver enzymes

ELECT: Hyperkalaemia, hyponatraemia, metabolic acidosis

CNS: Weakness, headache

INTEG: Photosensitivity, rash

HAEM: Thrombocytopenia, megaloblastic anaemia

Contraindications: Hypersensitivity, anuria, severe renal disease, severe hepatic disease, hyperkalaemia, Addison's disease. Do not routinely administer with angiotensin converting enzyme (ACE) inhibitors

Precautions: Dehydration, pregnancy, hepatic disease, lactation, renal disease, cirrhosis, gout, other hypotensive agents as an additive effect may result

Pharmacokinetics:

By mouth: Onset 2 hr, peak 6–8 hr, duration 12–16 hr; half-life 3 hr; metabolised in liver, excreted in urine

Interactions/incompatibilities:

• Enhanced action of: antihypertensives

• Increased hyperkalaemia: other potassium sparing diuretics, potassium products, ACE inhibitors, NSAIDs, cyclosporin

Clinical assessment:

• Serum electrolytes: potassium, sodium, chloride; include serum urea, blood sugar, full blood count, serum creatinine, blood pH, arterial blood gases

Lab. test interferences:

Interfere: Bioassay of folic acid

Treatment of overdose: Lavage if taken orally, monitor electrolytes, administer IV fluids, dialysis

NURSING CONSIDERATIONS

Assess:
- Baseline weight
- Postural hypotension

Administer:
- With food

Perform/provide:
- Fluid balance daily to determine fluid loss; effect of drug may be diminished if taken daily

Evaluate:
- Improvement in oedema of feet, legs, sacral area daily if medication is being used in congestive heart failure
- Improvement in CVP and BP recordings
- Signs of metabolic acidosis: drowsiness, restlessness
- Rashes, temperature elevation daily
- Confusion, especially in elderly, take safety precautions if needed
- Hydration: skin turgor, thirst, dry mucous membranes

Teach patient/family:
- To take medication after meals
- To avoid prolonged exposure to sunlight since photosensitivity may occur
- Urine may appear blue in certain lights
- To notify clinician if weakness, headache, nausea, vomiting, dry mouth, fever, sore throat, mouth sores, unusual bleeding or bruising occurs
- Rise slowly from lying to sitting position

---

trientine dihydrochloride ▼

Func. class.: Heavy metal antagonist
Chem. class.: Chelating agent (thiol compound)
Legal class.: POM

Action: Binds with ions of lead, mercury, copper, iron, zinc to form a water-soluble complex excreted by kidneys

Uses: Wilson's disease (in patients intolerant of penicillamine)

Dosage and routes:
- *Adult:* By mouth 1.2–2.4 daily in 2–4 divided doses before food

Available forms include: Capsules 300 mg

Side effects/adverse reactions:
HAEM: Anaemia, iron deficiency
INTEG: Urticaria, fever
SYST: Hypersensitivity
GI: Nausea

Contraindications: Hypersensitivity

Precautions: Pregnancy

Pharmacokinetics:
By mouth: Peak 1 hr, metabolised in liver, excreted in urine

Interactions/incompatibilities:
- Decreased action: mineral supplements

Clinical assessment:
- Monitor hepatic renal studies: aspartate aminotransferase, alanine aminotransferase, alkaline phosphatase, blood urea, creatinine—CSM requests special records kept by pharmacist

NURSING CONSIDERATIONS

Assess:
NB. Special records must be kept by the pharmacist for this drug
- Fluid balance and urinalysis
- Baseline full blood count
- Dietary habits

Administer:
- On an empty stomach, ½–1 hr before meals
- Vitamin B_6 daily; depleted when this drug is used

Evaluate:
- Therapeutic response: improvement in neurologic, psychiatric symptoms
- Signs of anaemia
- Blood dyscrasias
- Side effects, nausea
- Urinalysis regularly

Teach patient/family:

• That therapeutic effect may take 1–3 months
• To avoid diet containing copper; this includes offal, shellfish, nuts, dried legumes, chocolate, wholegrain cereal
• That penicillamine-induced systemic lupus erythematosus may not resolve

trifluoperazine

Stelazine
Func. class.: Antipsychotic/ neuroleptic; anti-emetic
Chem. class.: Phenothiazine
Legal class.: POM

Action: Depresses cerebral cortex, hypothalamus, limbic system, which control activity, aggression; blocks neurotransmission produced by dopamine at synapse; exhibits strong α-adrenergic, anticholinergic blocking action; mechanism for antipsychotic effects is unclear
Uses: Psychotic disorders, non-psychotic anxiety, schizophrenia, symptomatic treatment of nausea and vomiting, severe psychomotor agitation
Dosage and routes:
Psychotic disorders
• *Adult:* By mouth 5 mg twice a day (high dosage) or 10 mg daily in modified-release form, increase by 5 mg after 1 week, then increasing at 5 mg intervals every 3 days. IM 1–3 mg in divided doses up to maximum 6 mg daily; child 50 mcg/kg daily in divided doses
• *Child:* By mouth initial dose not to exceed 5 mg in divided doses; IM *not recommended for children*, but 1 mg per 20 kg may be given daily in divided doses
Non-psychotic anxiety
• *Adult:* By mouth 1–2 mg twice a day (low dosage), or 2–4 mg modified-release, not to exceed 6 mg/day
• *Child 3–5 yr:* By mouth up to 1 mg daily in divided doses; 6–12 yr: By mouth maximum 4 mg daily in divided doses
Available forms include: All as hydrochloride. Tablets 1, 2, 5 mg; Spansule 2, 10, 15 mg; syrup concentrate 10 mg/ml for dilution prior to use, injection IM 1 mg/ml, Syrup 1 mg/5 ml
Side effects/adverse reactions:
RESP: Laryngospasm, dyspnoea, respiratory depression
CNS: Extrapyramidal symptoms: pseudoparkinsonism, akathisia, dystonia, tardive dyskinesia, seizures, headache, drowsiness, insomnia, restlesness, hyperpyrexia
HAEM: Leucopenia, pancytopenia; thrombocytopenia agranulocytosis
INTEG: Rash, photosensitivity, pigmentation
EENT: Blurred vision, glaucoma
GI: Dry mouth, nausea, vomiting, anorexia, constipation, diarrhoea, jaundice, weight gain
GU: Urinary retention, urinary frequency, enuresis, impotence, amenorrhoea, gynaecomastia
CV: Orthostatic hypotension, hypertension, cardiac arrest, ECG changes, tachycardia
MS: Muscular weakness
Contraindications: Hypersensitivity, coma, blood dyscrasias, severe hepatic disease, bone marrow depression, breast-feeding, pregnancy
Precautions: Breast cancer, epilepsy, Parkinson's disease, narrow angle glaucoma, pregnancy, lactation, children, elderly, cardiovascular disease, angina, prostatic hypertrophy, myasthenia gravis
Pharmacokinetics:

By mouth: Onset rapid, peak 2–3 hr, duration 12 hr, modified-release form. 60% released over 6–8 hr
IM: Onset immediate, peak 1 hr, duration 12 hr
Metabolised by liver, excreted in urine, enters breast milk

Interactions/incompatibilities:
• Oversedation: other CNS depressants, alcohol, barbiturate anaesthetics
• Decreased absorption: aluminium hydroxide or magnesium hydroxide antacids
• Decreased effects of: levodopa, anti-epileptics
• Increased effects of both drugs: antihypertensives, alcohol
• Increased anticholinergic effects: anticholinergics

Clinical assessment:
• Bilirubin, full blood count, liver function tests monthly
• Urinalysis is recommended before and during prolonged therapy

Treatment of overdose: Lavage if orally ingested, provide an airway; *do not induce vomiting*

NURSING CONSIDERATIONS

Assess:
• Swallowing of oral medication; check for hoarding or giving of medication to other patients
• Fluid balance
• Baseline vital signs including BP standing and lying

Perform/provide:
• Decreased noise input by dimming lights, avoiding loud noises
• Supervised ambulation until stabilised on medication; do not involve in strenuous exercise programme
• Increased fluids to prevent constipation
• Sips of water, mouthwashes for dry mouth

Evaluate:
• Therapeutic response: decrease in emotional excitement, hallucinations, delusions, paranoia, reorganization of patterns of thought, speech
• Affect, orientation, level of consciousness, reflexes, gait, coordination, sleep pattern disturbances
• BP standing and lying; also pulse, respirations 4 hrly during initial treatment; report drops of 30 mmHg
• Dizziness, faintness, palpitations, tachycardia on rising
• Extrapyramidal symptoms including akathisia (inability to sit still, no pattern to movements), tardive dyskinesia (bizarre movements of jaw, mouth, tongue, extremities), pseudoparkinsonism (rigidity, tremors, pill rolling, shuffling gait)
• Skin turgor daily
• Constipation, urinary retention daily

Teach patient/family:
• That orthostatic hypotension occurs frequently, and to rise from sitting or lying position gradually
• To remain lying down after IM injection for at least 30 min
• To avoid abrupt withdrawal of this drug or extrapyramidal symptoms may result; drugs should be withdrawn slowly
• To avoid non-prescribed preparations (cough, hayfever, cold) unless approved by clinician since serious drug interactions may occur; avoid use with alcohol or CNS depressants, increased drowsiness may occur
• To use a sunscreen during sun exposure to prevent burns
• Regarding compliance with drug regimen
• To report sore throat, malaise, fever, bleeding, mouth sores; if these occur, full blood count

should be drawn and drug discontinued
• In hot weather, heat stroke may occur; take extra precautions to stay cool
• To take additional fibre in diet and fluids if constipated
• Not to stand still for long periods of time

trifluperidol

Triperidol
Func. class.: Antipsychotic/neuroleptic
Chem. class.: Butyrophenone
Legal class.: POM

Action: Depresses cerebral cortex, hypothalamus, limbic system, which controls aggression; blocks neurotransmission produced by dopamine at synapse; exhibits strong α-adrenergic, anticholinergic blocking action
Uses: Schizophrenia and related psychoses, particularly mania
Dosage and routes:
• *Adult:* By mouth initially 500 mcg/day, adjusted by 500 mcg every 3–4 days according to response; maximum dose 6–8 mg/day
• *Child 5–12 yr:* By mouth initially 250 mcg/day adjusted according to response; maximum dose 2 mg/day
Available forms include: Tablets 500 mcg, 1 mg
Side effects/adverse reactions:
CNS: Extrapyramidal symptoms, tardive dyskinesia, sedation, drowsiness, apathy, nightmares, insomnia, depression, agitation, headache
CV: Hypotension
GU: Difficulty with micturition, menstrual disturbances, impotence
META: Galactorrhoea, gynaecomastia, changes in weight
INTEG: Photosensitization, contact sensitization, rashes, jaundice
GI: Nausea, loss of appetite, dyspepsia
Contraindications: Pregnancy, breast-feeding, comatose states, bone marrow depression, basal ganglia disease
Precautions: Parkinsonism, epilepsy, renal or hepatic impairment, elderly patients, closed-angle glaucoma
Interactions/incompatibilities:
• Oversedation: alcohol, other CNS depressants, barbiturates, anaesthetics
• Decreased absorption: antacids
• Decreased effects of: levodopa, anti-epileptics
• Increased effects of: antihypertensives
Clinical assessment:
• Bilirubin, full blood count, liver function tests monthly
Treatment of overdose: Supportive measures and anti-parkinsonian drugs as necessary

NURSING CONSIDERATIONS

Assess:
• Swallowing of oral medication, check for hoarding or giving medication to other patients
• Fluid balance
• Urinalysis, before and during therapy
Perform/provide:
• Decreased noise input by dimming lights, avoiding loud noises
• Supervised ambulation until stabilised on medication: do not involve in strenuous exercise programme because fainting is possible: patient should not stand still for long periods of time
• Increased fluids to prevent constipation
• Sips of water or mouthwashes for dry mouth
Evaluate:
• For extrapyramidal symptoms

• Orientation, level of consciousness, reflexes, coordination, sleep pattern; report any disturbances to clinician
• BP standing/lying; pulse and respirations 4-hrly during initial treatment; report drop in BP of 30 mmHg
• For constipation, urinary retention; if these occur, increase fibre and water in diet
• Therapeutic response: decrease in emotional excitement

Teach patient/family:
• That hypotension occurs; to rise from sitting or lying position gradually
• To avoid abrupt withdrawal of the drug—should be withdrawn slowly
• To avoid non-prescribed medication unless approved by clinician
• Avoid use with alcohol
• Keep to drug regime
• To report sore throat, malaise, fever, mouth sores

trimeprazine tartrate

Vallergan
Func. class.: Antihistamine
Chem. class.: Phenothiazine
Legal class.: POM

Action: Acts on blood vessels, GI, respiratory system by competing with histamine for H_1-receptor site; decreases allergic response by blocking histamine. Central sedative effect

Uses: Urticaria, pruritus, premedication for anaesthesia

Dosage and routes:
Urticaria/Pruritus
• *Adult:* By mouth 10 mg two or three times a day up to 100 mg (in intractable cases). Reduce dosage in elderly 10 mg once or twice a day
• *Children over 2 yrs:* By mouth 2.5–5 mg three or four times a day

Premedication
• *Children 2–7 yrs:* Maximum dosage 2 mg/kg

Available forms include: Tablets 10 mg; syrup 7.5 mg/5 ml, Forte syrup 30 mg/15 ml

Side effects/adverse reactions:
CNS: Drowsiness, insomnia, agitation, akathesia, Parkinsonism, tardive dyskinesia, dystonia
CV: Hypotension, tachycardia A-V block, atrial arrhythmia, ventricular fibrillation
RESP: Respiratory depression
HAEM: Agranulocytosis, leucopenia
GI: Dry mouth, jaundice
INTEG: Rash, urticaria, photosensitivity
ENDO: Hyperprolactinaemia, neuroleptic malignant syndrome
EENT: Nasal stuffiness, dry nose, throat, mouth

Contraindications: Hepatic or renal dysfunction, epilepsy, Parkinsonism, hypothyroidism, phaeochromocytoma, myasthenia gravis, prostatic hypertrophy, narrow-angle glaucoma, hypersensitivity to phenothiazines, breast-feeding; porphyria

Precautions: Children under 2 yr, pregnancy elderly

Interactions/incompatibilities:
• Increased CNS depression: barbiturates, hypnotics, tricyclic antidepressants, alcohol
• Decreased effect of: amphetamine, levodopa, clonidine, guanethidine, adrenaline, hypoglycaemic drugs
• Increased effect of this drug: MAOIs, anticholinergic drugs
• Increased effect of: antihypotensive drugs
• Decreased absorption of this drug: antacids, lithium

Clinical assessment:
• WBC during long-term therapy

Treatment of overdose: Administer lavage, activated charcoal, maintain airway

NURSING CONSIDERATIONS

Assess:

• Fluid balance

Administer:

• Preoperatively; 1–2 hrs before anaesthesia

• Syrup may be diluted with syrup (without preservative)

• With meals if GI symptoms occur; absorption may be slightly decreased

Perform/provide:

• Sips of water, frequent rinsing of mouth for dryness (except when used for premedication)

Evaluate:

• Therapeutic response: decreased itching associated with pruritus

Teach patient/family:

• All aspects of drug use; to notify clinician if side effects occur

• To avoid driving or other hazardous activity if drowsiness occurs

• To avoid concurrent use of alcohol or other CNS depressants

---

trimethoprim

Ipral, Monotrim, Syraprim, Trimogal, Trimopan

Func. class.: Antibiotic

Chem. class.: Pyrimidine derivative

Legal class.: POM

Action: Prevents bacterial synthesis by blocking enzyme reduction of dihydrofolic acid

Uses: Urinary tract infection, acute and chronic bronchitis, bronchopneumonia and lobar pneumonia

Dosage and routes:

• *Adult:* Acute infection by mouth, IV 200 mg every 12 hr; urinary tract infections, by mouth 300 mg daily or 200 mg twice a day. Chronic infections, and prophylaxis: By mouth, 100 mg at bedtime

• *Child:* By mouth 2–5 months, 25 mg twice a day; 6 months–5 yr 50 mg twice a day; 6 yr–12 yr 100 mg twice a day; IV 6–9 mg/kg daily in 2–3 divided doses

Available forms include: Tablets 100, 200, 300 mg; suspension 50 mg/5 ml; injection 20 mg (lactate)/ml

Side effects/adverse reactions:

INTEG: Pruritus, rash

HAEM: Depression of haemopoiesis

GI: Nausea, vomiting

Contraindications: Hypersensitivity, severe renal impairment, pregnancy, neonates, megaloblastic anaemia, lactation, blood dyscrasias

Precautions: Folate deficiency, mild or moderate renal disease

Pharmacokinetics:

By mouth: Peak 1–4 hr, half-life 8–11 hr, metabolised in liver, excreted in urine (unchanged 60%), breast milk

Interactions/incompatibilities:

• Increased concentration of procainamide

• Increased effect of anti-coagulants

• Elimination of digoxin and phenytoin may be enhanced

Clinical assessment:

• Nocturia; may indicate drug resistance

• Creatinine, urine cultures

Treatment of overdose: Gastric lavage and symptomatic treatment as necessary

NURSING CONSIDERATIONS

Administer:

• With full glass of water

• Culture and sensitivity before drug therapy; drug may be taken as soon as culture is taken

• Adjust dosage in renal impairment. IV by direct injection or

into a running IV infusion
Pharmaceutical precautions: Store below 25°C (suspension, injection) and protect from light. Oral suspension may be diluted with water or sorbitol solution; diluted suspension is stable for 14 days
Perform/provide:
• Adequate intake of fluids (2 litres) to decrease bacteria in bladder
Evaluate:
• Therapeutic response: absence of pain in bladder area, negative culture and sensitivity
• Skin eruptions
• Allergies before treatment, reaction of each medication; note allergies on chart, Kardex in bright red letters; notify all people giving drugs
Teach patient/family:
• Aspects of drug therapy: need to complete entire course of medication to ensure organism death (10–14 days); culture may be taken after completed course of medication
• To notify if nausea, vomiting

trimipramine maleate

Surmontil
Func. class.: Antidepressant, tricyclic
Chem. class.: Tertiary amine
Legal class.: POM

Action: Selectively inhibits serotonin uptake by brain; potentiates behavioural changes
Uses: Depression, particularly where sedation is required
Dosage and routes:
• *Adult:* By mouth 50–75 mg daily 2 hr prior to bedtime or 25 mg midday and 50 mg evening. Increased as necessary to maximum of 300 mg daily in divided doses
• *Elderly:* By mouth initially 10–25 mg three times a day, not recommended for use in children
Available forms include: Tablets 10, 25 mg; capsules 50 mg
Side effects/adverse reactions:
HAEM: Agranulocytosis, depression of bone marrow
CNS: Dizziness, drowsiness, tremors, peripheral neuropathy, increase in psychiatric symptoms convulsions
GI: Dry mouth, nausea, vomiting, jaundice, constipation
GU: Retention, interference with sexual function
INTEG: Rash, urticaria, sweating
CV: Orthostatic hypotension, tachycardia, palpitations
EENT: Blurred vision
Contraindications: Hypersensitivity to tricyclic antidepressants, recovery phase of myocardial infarction, concurrent use or within 2 weeks of monoamine oxidase inhibitor treatment. Lactation, mania, severe liver disease, any degree of heart block or other cardiac arrhythmia, porphyria
Precautions: Suicidal patients, severe depression, increased intraocular pressure, narrow-angle glaucoma, urinary retention, cardiac disease, hepatic disease, hyperthyroidism, elderly prostatic hypertrophy, epilepsy, pregnancy, concurrent use of anaesthetics (arrhythmias and hypotension)
Pharmacokinetics: Metabolised by liver, excreted by kidneys, steady state 2–6 days; half-life 7–30 hr
Interactions/incompatibilities:
• Decreased effects of: guanethidine, debrisoquine, bethanidine, clonidine, antiepileptics
• Increased effects of: sympathomimetics (adrenaline, noradrenaline, ephedrine, isoprenaline, phenylephrine, phenylpropanolamine), alcohol, barbiturates, benzodiazepines, CNS depressants, antihistamines

• Hyperpyretic crisis, convulsions, hypertensive episode: MAOIs
Clinical assessment:
• Blood studies: Full blood count, leucocytes, differential, cardiac enzymes if patient is receiving long-term therapy
• Hepatic studies: aspartate aminotransferase, alanine aminotransferase, bilirubin, creatinine
• ECG for flattening of T wave bundle branch block, AV block arrhythmias in cardiac patients
Treatment of overdose: ECG monitoring, induce emesis, lavage, activated charcoal, administer anticonvulsant, treat acidosis with 20 ml/kg sodium lactate

NURSING CONSIDERATIONS

Assess:
• BP lying, standing
• Baseline weight
Administer:
• Increased fluids, fibre in diet if constipation, urinary retention occur
• Frequent sips of water; mouthwashes for dry mouth
Perform/provide:
• Assistance with ambulation during beginning therapy since drowsiness/dizziness occurs
• Safety measures, including siderails primarily in elderly
• Checking to see oral medication swallowed
Evaluate:
• BP (lying, standing), pulse 4 hrly; if systolic BP drops 20 mmHg hold drug, notify clinician; take vital signs 4 hrly in patients with cardiovascular disease
• Weight weekly; appetite may increase with drug
• Mental status: mood, sensory affect, suicidal tendencies, increase in psychiatric symptoms: depression, panic
• Urinary retention, constipation
• Cardiovascular side effects, particularly with high doses
• Withdrawal symptoms: headache, nausea, vomiting, muscle pain, weakness; do not usually occur unless drug was discontinued abruptly
• Alcohol consumption; if alcohol is consumed, hold dose until morning (drug enhances effect of alcohol)
Teach patient/family:
• That therapeutic effects may take 2–3 weeks
• Use caution in driving or other activities requiring alertness because of drowsiness, dizziness, blurred vision
• To avoid alcohol ingestion, other CNS depressants and nonprescribed medications
• Not to discontinue medication quickly after long-term use, may cause nausea, headache, malaise

triprolidine hydrochloride

Pro Actidil, combination products
Func. class.: Antihistamine
Chem. class.: Alkylamine, H_1-receptor antagonist
Legal class.: P

Action: Acts on blood vessels, GI, respiratory system, by competing with histamine for H_1-receptor site; decreases allergic response by blocking histamine
Uses: Allergy, e.g. hay fever and urticaria
Dosage and routes:
• *Adult:* By mouth 10 mg early evening or 5–6 hr before retiring increased to 20 mg daily if symptoms severe
• *Child:* Not recommended
Available forms include: modified release tablets 10 mg
Side effects/adverse reactions:

CNS: Drowsiness
INTEG: Rash, urticaria, photosensitivity
Contraindications: Hypersensitivity to H_1-receptor antagonist; severe hepatic or renal dysfunction; porphyria
Precautions: Increased intraocular pressure, prostatic hypertrophy, pregnancy, lactation
Pharmacokinetics:
By mouth: Onset 20–60 min, duration 8–12 hr, detoxified in liver, excreted by kidneys (metabolites/free drug), half-life 20–24 hr
Interactions/incompatibilities:
• Increased CNS depressants: barbiturates, narcotics, hypnotics, tricyclic antidepressants, alcohol
• Decreased effect of: betahistine
Treatment of overdose: Gastric lavage, diazepam, vasopressors

NURSING CONSIDERATIONS

Administer:
• Swallowed whole
Perform/provide:
• Sips of water, frequent rinsing of mouth for dryness
• Storage in tight container at room temperature
Evaluate:
• Therapeutic response: decreased itching associated with urticaria
Teach patient/family:
• All aspects of drug use; to notify clinician if side effects occur
• To avoid driving or other hazardous activity if drowsiness occurs
• To avoid concurrent use of alcohol or other CNS depressants while taking this drug

tropicamide (ophthalmic)

Mydriacyl, Minims
Func. class.: Mydriatic, cycloplegic, anticholinergic
Chem. class.: Belladonna alkaloid
Legal class.: POM

Action: Paralysis of ciliary muscle, dilation of pupil
Uses: Fundus examination, cycloplegic refraction
Dosage and routes:
• *Adult and child:* Instil 1–2 drops of 1% solution, repeat in 5 min (refraction) or 1–2 drops of 0.5% solution 15–20 min before exam (fundus examination)
Available forms include: Solution 0.5%, 1%
Side effects/adverse reactions:
EENT: Raised intraocular pressure, stinging of eyes, photophobia, local hyperaemia, oedema
INTEG: Rash in children, dry skin, flushing
GI: Abdominal distension in infants, dry mouth, constipation, vomiting
CV: Bradycardia, tachycardia, palpitations, arrhythmias
GU: Urinary urgency, retention
CNS: Behavioural disturbances in children, giddiness, staggering
Contraindications: Hypersensitivity, narrow-angle glaucoma
Precautions: Infants, soft contact lenses, pregnancy, elderly, ocular hyperaemia
Pharmacokinetics:
INSTIL: Peak 15–20 min, (mydriasis), 20 min (cycloplegia), duration 2–6 hr (cycloplegia), 7 hr (mydriasis)
Interactions/incompatibilities:
Soft contact lenses (preparations with preservative)

NURSING CONSIDERATIONS

Evaluate:
• Eye pain, discontinue use

Teach patient/family:
- To report change in vision, with blurring or loss of sight, trouble breathing, sweating, flushing
- Method of instillation, including pressure on lacrimal sac for 1 min, and not to touch dropper to eye
- That blurred vision will decrease with repeated use of drug
- Not to engage in hazardous activities until able to see
- Wait 5 min to use other drops
- Contact lens wearers should seek advice from clinician before starting drops

tropisetron

Navoban ▼
Func. class.: Anti-emetic
Chem. class.: Serotonin 5-HT_3 antagonist
Legal class.: POM

Action: 5-HT_3 antagonists have complex actions antagonising serotonin at its receptor sites in both the CNS and the gut.
Uses: Prophylaxis of cancer chemotherapy-induced nausea and vomiting
Dosage and routes:
- *Adult:* By mouth or by IV injection/infusion, 5 mg once daily

Available forms include: Injection, 5 mg; tablets, 5 mg
Side effects/adverse reactions:
CNS: Headache, dizziness, fatigue
GI: Constipation, abdominal pain diarrhoea
Contraindications: Hypersensitivity, pregnancy, breast-feeding
Pharmacokinetics: Almost completely absorbed following oral administration; peak plasma concentrations reached within 3 hr; metabolised in the liver
Treatment of overdose: Syptomatic and supportive

NURSING CONSIDERATIONS

Assess:
- Vital signs (temperature, pulse, respiration, BP), fluid balance
- Full blood count, including platelets

Administer:
- By mouth each morning on rising, or at least one hr before food
- By injection given as slow IV bolus or into a running infusion, or as a short infusion in sodium chloride (0.9%), Ringer's solution or glucose (5%)

Perform/provide:
- All supportive measures for primary disease (care of skin, mouth; fluid balance; all other medication as prescribed)
- Storage: protect ampoules from direct sunlight

Evaluate:
- Therapeutic response: reduction or lessening of nausea and vomiting
- For side effects: headache, constipation

Teach patient/family:
- About the drug and its side effects
- To report any side effects to nurse or clinician

tubocurarine chloride

Jexin, Tubarine
Func. class.: Non-depolarising muscle relaxant
Chem. class.: Curare alkaloid
Legal class.: POM

Action: Inhibits transmission of nerve impulses by binding to cholinergic receptor sites, antagonising action of acetylcholine
Uses: Facilitation of endotracheal intubation, skeletal muscle relaxa-

tion during mechanical ventilation, surgery, or general anaesthesia, tetanus

Dosage and routes:

• *Adult:* IV bolus injection based upon initial dose of 15–30 mg (maximum 40 mg), supplementary doses of 5–10 mg as needed

• *Child:* IV bolus injection initial dose of 300–500 mcg/kg, then 60–100 mcg/kg as required. Add neonate IV 200–250 micrograms/kg, then 40–50 micrograms/kg as required

Available forms include: Injection IV 10 mg/ml

Side effects/adverse reactions:

CV: Bradycardia, tachycardia, decreased BP

RESP: Prolonged apnoea, bronchospasm, collapse, respiratory

INTEG: Rash, flushing, pruritus, urticaria, pain at injection site

Contraindications: Hypersensitivity, respiratory insufficiency, renal or hepatic impairment, asthma

Precautions: Pregnancy, lactation, respiratory disease, myasthenia gravis, gross obesity, myopathy, after poliomyelitis, repeat dose within 24 hr, family history of malignant hyperthermia

Pharmacokinetics:

IV: Onset 3–5 min, duration ½–hr; half-life 1–3 hr, degraded in liver, mainly excreted in urine unchanged

Interactions/incompatibilities:

• Increased hypotension: halothane

• Increased neuromuscular blockade: aminoglycosides, clindamycin, lincomycin, quinidine, volatile anaesthetics, polymyxin antibiotics, lithium, narcotic analgesics, thiazides, azlocillin, mezlocillin, nifedipine, verapamil, parenteral magnesium salts, β-blockers, tetracyclines

• Concurrent administration with depolarising relaxant may cause relaxation which is not reversible by neostigmine

• Neuromuscular blockade reduced by: azathioprine, mercaptopurine, lymphocytic antiglobulin

• Neuromuscular blockade reversed by: anticholinesterases

Clinical assessment:

• For electrolyte imbalances (potassium, magnesium); may lead to increased action of this drug

Treatment of overdose: Edrophonium or neostigmine, atropine, monitor, mechanical ventilation, monitor CV, electrolyte, respiratory status

NURSING CONSIDERATIONS

Assess:

• Vital signs (BP, pulse, respirations, airway)

• Anaesthetic history—NOT to be given to asthmatics, patients with renal or liver impairment

• Electrolyte levels

Administer:

Perform/provide:

• Storage in light-resistant area

Evaluate:

• Therapeutic response: level and degree of paralysis

• Vital signs, particularly respiratory rate

• Allergic reactions: rash, fever, respiratory distress, pruritus; drug should be discontinued

---

tulobuterol ▼

Brelomax, Respacal

Func. class.: Bronchodilator

Chem. class.: β_2-adrenergic agonist

Legal class.: POM

Action: Causes bronchodilatation by acting on β_2-receptors in bronchus and lung; has little effect on cardiac β_1-receptors

Uses: Prophylaxis and control of bronchospasm in reversible obstructive airways disease including asthma, chronic bronchitis and emphysema

Dosage and routes:

• *Adult:* By mouth; 2 mg twice−3 times daily

• *Child (over 10 yr):* By mouth; 1−2 mg twice daily

Available forms include: Tablets, 2 mg

Side effects/adverse reactions:

CNS: Tremor, stimulation, headache

CV: Palpitations, tachycardia

ELECT: Hypokalaemia

Contraindications: Hypersensitivity to sympathomimetic amines; moderate to severe renal failure; acute hepatic failure; chronic liver disease

Precautions: Pregnancy; breastfeeding; hyperthyroidism; diabetes mellitus; epilepsy; cardiovascular or coronary artery disease

Interactions:

• Increased risk of hypokalaemia: aminophylline, diuretics, corticosteroids, theophylline

• Reduced effects of both drugs: β-blockers

Treatment of overdose: The stomach should be emptied if this can be done within one hour of ingestion; symptomatic and supportive care; a cardioselective β-blocker may be helpful in arrhythmias, at the risk of inducing bronchoconstriction

NURSING CONSIDERATIONS

Assess:

• Baseline vital signs; lung sounds; respiratory capacity in patients with obstructive airways disease

• Blood glucose if patient is diabetic

Administer:

• By mouth as prescribed

Evaluate:

• Therapeutic effect: absence of dyspnoea; wheezing

• Side effects such as headache, palpitations

Teach patient/family:

• About the side effects of the drug: headache, palpitations

• To avoid smoky atmospheres, people with respiratory infections

• Techniques for avoiding asthma attacks (use of space) and how to deal with attack if it occurs

• Not to exceed the prescribed dose

---

typhoid vaccine (oral)

Vivotif

Func. class.: Oral vaccine

Chem. class.: Live attenuated organisms of *Salmonella typhi*

Legal class.: POM

Action: Promotes development of antibodies to *S. typhi*

Dosage and routes:

Primary immunization

• *Adult and child over 6 yr:* By mouth, 1 capsule, 1 hr before meals with a cold drink on alternate days × 3 doses

Reinforcement of immunity

• *Adult and child over 6 yr:* After a course of capsules protection exists for at least three years, though in typhoid endemic areas an annual booster is recommended. Booster courses consist of 3 doses, identical to primary immunization

Available forms include: Packs of 3 enteric coated capsules each containing at least 2,000 million viable organisms of attenuated *S. typhi* Ty 21a

Side effects/adverse reactions:

GI: Nausea, vomiting, diarrhoea, abdominal cramps

INTEG: Urticarial exanthema

Contraindications: Hypersensitivity, congenital or acquired immune deficiency including treatment with immunosuppressive drugs, acute febrile or gastrointestinal illness

Precautions: Pregnancy
Pharmacokinetics: Not applicable
Interactions/incompatibilities:
Vaccine inactivated by: Mefloquine (do not give within 12 hr), sulphonamides, antibiotics
Risk of systemic infection: Immunosuppressive drugs
Treatment of overdose: Not applicable

NURSING CONSIDERATIONS

Administer:
- Avoid administration during acute illness

Perform/provide:
- Record title, dose and batch no. of vaccine and date of administration

Teach patient/family:
- That side effects, including nausea, malaise and headache may be acute and require cessation of normal activities. These usually subside within 36 hr
- Report any neurological signs to clinician immediately

---

typhoid vaccines (injectable)

Typhoid Vaccine BP (whole, killed bacteria)
Typhim Vi (purified polysaccharide)
Func. class.: Monovalent vaccine
Legal class.: POM

Action: Promotes development of antibodies specific to *Salmonella typhi*
Uses: Active immunization against typhoid fever
Dosage and routes:
Typhoid Vaccine BP
Primary immunization
- *Adult:* Deep subcutaneous/IM injection, initially 0.5 ml; 2nd dose after 4–6 weeks 0.5 ml (or 0.1 ml intradermal)
- *Child 1–10 yr:* Deep subcutaneous/IM: unit 0.25 ml: 2nd dose 0.25 ml (or 0.1 ml intradermal)

Reinforcement of immunity
- Further doses every 3 yr approx on continued exposure

Typhim Vi
Primary immunization
- *Adult:* Deep subcutaneous/IM injection 0.5 ml single dose

Available forms include:
Typhoid Vaccine BP: Injection suspension, 1.5 ml vial containing more than 1,000 million organisms per ml *S. typhi*
Typhim Vi: Prefilled, single-dose syringe 25 mcg of *S. typhi*: Vi polysaccharide in 0.5 ml
Side effects/adverse reactions:
INTEG: Swelling, pain, tenderness at injection site
SYST: Malaise, fever, nausea, pyrexia
CNS: Headache. With Typhoid Vaccine BP: polyneuritis, myelitis
Contraindications: History of anaphylaxis, hypersensitivity, acute infection, children less than 1 yr, pregnancy
Precautions: Debilitated patients especially with previous history of typhoid vaccination

NURSING CONSIDERATIONS

Administer:
- Shake vial well before withdrawing dose
- Discard unused vaccine; at end of each vaccination review
- Record title, dose and batch no. of vaccine and date of administration
- Avoid administration during acute illness

Perform/provide:
- Ensure facilities available for management of prophylaxis

Teach patient/family:
- That side effects, including nausea, malaise and headache may be acute and require cessation of normal activities. These usually subside within 36 hr
- Report any neurological signs to clinician at once

urea hydrogen peroxide

Exterol

Func. class.: Cerulytic
Chem. class.: Urea compound
Legal class.: P

Action: Foaming action facilitates removal of impacted cerumen

Uses: Removal of impacted cerumen, urea soften cerumen

Dosage and routes:

• *Adult and child:* Instil 5–10 drops once or twice daily for 3–4 days

Available forms include: Solution 5%

Side effects/adverse reactions:

EENT: Itching, irritation in ear, redness

Contraindications: Hypersensitivity, ear surgery, perforated eardrum

Pharmacokinetics: Not known

Interactions/incompatibilities: None known

NURSING CONSIDERATIONS

Administer:

• With head tilted for 5–10 mins to retain drops
• By allowing drops to enter ear canal; do not touch dropper to ear
• Then irrigate ear if appropriate and necessary to remove wax

Evaluate:

• Therapeutic response: loosened cerumen, ability to hear better

Teach patient/family:

• Method of instillation, using aseptic technique
• Patients may experience effervescent feeling in ear after using drops

urofollitrophin

Metrodin

Func. class.: Gonadotrophin human follicle stimulating hormone
Chem. class.: Peptide hormone
Legal class.: POM

Action: Stimulates ovarian follicular growth

Uses: Induction of ovulation in infertile women with hypopituitarism or who have not responded to clomiphene and induction of multiple follicular growth in women undergoing assisted conception

Dosage and routes:

Hypothalamic-pituitary dysfunction

• IM initially 75–150 IU/day or 225–375 IU on alternate days increasing by 75 IU daily or 75–150 IU on alternate days until response optimal, then 10,000 IU human chorionic gonadotrophin 1–2 days after last dose. Reassess if unsuccessful after 6 ovulatory cycles

Assisted conception

• IM 150–225 IU, adjusted according to response, from day 5 of cycle until follicular development achieved in combination with clomiphene and human chorionic gonadotrophin. Other regimens are used

Available forms include: Powder for injection 75 IU/ampoule

Side effects/adverse reactions:

GI: Abdominal pain

INTEG: Rash, local reactions at injection site

GU: Multiple ovulation, ovarian hyperstimulation leading to ovarian rupture and peritoneal haemorrhage, multiple pregnancy

Contraindications: Hypersensitivity

Precautions: Ovarian cysts, adrenal or thyroid disease, hyperprolactinaemia, pituitary tumour

Pharmacokinetics: Metabolised in liver, excreted in faeces, stored in fat
Clinical assessment:
• Titrate dose to response assessed by measuring plasma/urinary oestrogen, or pelvic ultrasound scans
Treatment of overdose: Monitor degree of ovarian enlargement, give symptomatic relief, hospitalise if ovaries enlarged beyond 12 cm in diameter

NURSING CONSIDERATIONS

Assess:
• At the same time every day
Administer:
• By deep IM injection
Teach patient/family:
• Multiple births have been reported following treatment with this drug
• To inform clinician if low abdominal pain is experienced, as this may indicate the presence of an ovarian cyst, or rupture of a cyst
• Teach patient how to take and chart early morning temperature to determine if ovulation has occurred
• If pregnancy is suspected the clinician should be informed at once

urokinase

Ukidan
Func. class.: Thrombolytic enzyme
Chem. class.: Protein
Legal class.: POM

Action: Promotes thrombolysis by acting directly on endogenous fibrinolytic system to change plasminogen to plasmin
Uses: Vitreous haemorrhage, clotted AV shunts and IV cannulae, pulmonary embolism, deep vein thrombosis, peripheral vascular occlusion
Dosage and routes:
Pulmonary embolism
• *Adult:* IV infusion, initially 4400 IU/kg in 15 ml over 10 min, then 4400 IU/kg/hr for 12 hr
Deep vein thrombosis
• *Adult:* IV infusion, initially 4400 IU/kg in 15 ml over 10 min, then 4400 IU/kg/hr for 12–24 hr
Peripheral vascular occlusion
• Consult manufacturer's literature
AV shunts
• *Adult:* Instil 5000–37,500 IV in 2–3 ml 0.9% sodium chloride clamp off × 2–4 hr
Intraocular
• Intraocular injection: 5000–37,500 IV in 2 ml 0.9% sodium chloride
Available forms include: Powder for injection 5000, 25,000, 100,000 IU vials
Side effects/adverse reactions:
HAEM: Bleeding
INTEG: Local pain when injected into AV shunt
GI: Nausea, vomiting
GU: Haematuria
SYST: Elevated temperature following liberation of lysis products
Contraindications: Vitreous haemorrhage complicated by severe retinal disturbances, e.g. (retinal detachment), active bleeding, severe hypertension, recent surgery, pregnancy, severe hepatic or renal disease
Precautions: Known GI lesions prone to bleeding, multiple cardiac puncture as a consequence of cardio-pulmonary resuscitation, history of cerebro-vascular disease
Pharmacokinetics:
IV: Half-life 10–20 min, small amounts excreted in urine
Interactions/incompatibilities:
• Increased risk of bleeding given

with: Aspirin and other non-steroidal anti-inflammatories, anticoagulants
• Incompatible with: dextrose solutions when mixed
• Action prolonged by: dextrans
Clinical assessment:
• As soon as thrombi identified; not useful for thrombi over 1 week old
Treatment of overdose: Aprotinin, tranexamic acid or aminocaproic acid to antagonise. Clotting factors, red cells, whole blood for severe haemorrhage
NURSING CONSIDERATIONS
Assess:
• Baseline vital signs, BP, pulse, respiration, neurological signs, temperature, ECG
Administer:
• After reconstituting with 2 ml of 0.9% sodium chloride or water for injection; do not shake
Perform/provide:
• Bed rest during entire course of treatment
• Careful handling of patient to avoid bruising
• Avoidance of invasive procedures: injections, rectal temperature
• Treatment of fever with paracetamol or aspirin
• Pressure for 30 sec to minor bleeding sites; inform clinician if haemostasis not attained, apply pressure dressing
Evaluate:
• Vital signs, ECG and neurological observations
• Allergy: fever, rash, itching, chills, mild reaction may be treated with antihistamines
• Bleeding during first hr of treatment (most likely from site of injection but also haematuria, haematemesis, bleeding from mucous membranes, epistaxis, ecchymosis)
• Side effects: nausea, vomiting
Teach patient/family:
• About effects of drug
• To report any change indicating bleeding

---

ursodeoxycholic acid

Destolit, Ursofalk, combination products
Func. class.: Dissolution of gallstones
Chem. class.: 7β-epimer of chenodeoxycholic acid, bile acid
Legal class.: POM

Action: Dissolves cholesterol gallstones through desaturation of bile by cholesterol
Uses: Dissolution of radiolucent cholesterol gallstones
Dosage and routes:
• By mouth 8–12 mg/kg daily (up to 15 mg/kg daily in obese patients) in divided doses or as single dose at bedtime, for up to 2 yr; treatment should be continued for 3–4 months after stones dissolve
Available forms include: Tablets 150 mg; capsules 250 mg
Side effects/adverse reactions:
GI: Diarrhoea
INTEG: Pruritus
Contraindications: Radio-opaque stones; active gastric or duodenal ulcer; non-functioning gallbladder, liver disease; inflammatory diseases of small intestine or colon; pregnancy
Pharmacokinetics: Absorbed through GI-tract and undergoes enterohepatic recycling, excreted in faeces largely unchanged, some bacterial breakdown
Interactions/incompatibilities:
• Reduced effect of ursodeoxycholic acid: oestrogenic hormones, oral contraceptives, cholestyramine, colestipol

Treatment of overdose: Low toxicity, symptomatic relief only

NURSING CONSIDERATIONS

Assess:

• GI symptoms before commencing treatment

Administer:

• During meals for better absorption

• Whole—not to be crushed or chewed

• One dose always to be taken after the evening meal

Evaluate:

• GI symptoms, nausea, vomiting, abdominal pain, cramps, diarrhoea

Teach patient/family:

• Diarrhoea may occur initially; if persistent to consult clinician

• To take good, balanced diet, low in cholesterol

• That medication may need to be continued for up to 2 years

---

vaccine (measles, mumps and rubella vaccine, live, attenuated)

M-M-R$_{II}$

Func. class.: Vaccine, live, attenuated

Legal class.: POM

Action: Stimulates production of specific antibodies against viruses causing mumps, measles and rubella

Uses: Prevention of mumps, measles and rubella. In the UK, Health authorities have an obligation to ensure that children have received MMR vaccine by entry into primary school unless there is a valid contraindication, laboratory evidence of previous infection or parental refusal. MMR vaccine is unsuitable for prophylaxis following exposure to mumps or rubella since the antibody response is too slow

Dosage and routes:

• *Adult and child:* By SC or IM injection 0.5 ml

Note: Revaccination is not necessary except in children vaccinated in the first year of life

Available forms include: Injection, single dose vials with diluent

Side effects/adverse reactions:

CNS: Malaise, headache, polyneuropathy, dizziness, ataxia, febrile and afebrile convulsions, encephalitis

EENT: Sore throat, parotitis, nerve deafness, coryza, pharyngitis

GI: Nausea, vomiting

GU: Orchitis

HAEM: Thrombocytopenia, purpura

INTEG: Rash, injection site reactions including erythema, induration and tenderness; erythema multiforme

MISC: Regional lymphadenopathy

MS: Arthralgia, arthritis (usually transient)

RESP: Cough

SYST: Fever, anaphylaxis

Contraindications: Hypersensitivity (including history of anaphylactoid reactions to neomycin or chicken or eggs); pregnancy (should be avoided for 3 months after vaccination); children below 12 months unless at special risk (repeat at 15 months); untreated malignant disease; patients receiving high dose corticosteroids, other immunosuppressive drugs or radiotherapy; patients who have received other live virus vaccines within the previous month; ongoing acute febrile illness (defer vaccination)

Precautions: History of febrile convulsions, cerebral injury or other condition where stress due to fever should be avoided; within 3 months of blood or plasma transfusion or administration of human immunoglobulin (compromises immune response — test for success of vaccination); breast-feeding; family history of epilepsy; unsuitable for use with anti-Rh_0 (D) globulin in the immediate post-partum period when rubella vaccine alone should be used

Interactions:

• Less effective given within 3 months of previous: blood or plasma transfusion, human immunoglobulin

• Reduced effect and danger of systemic infections with: immunosuppressive agents including high-dose corticosteroids, cytotoxic chemotherapy, azathioprine

Incompatibilities:

• Alcohol — if skin is swabbed with alcohol prior to injection it must be allowed to dry completely before injecting

• Do not mix with any other vaccine or drug

Lab. test interferences: Depression of response to tuberculin skin test, if this test is to be done it should be done before or simultaneously with vaccination

Treatment of overdose: No cases reported; swallowing would inactivate virus; symptomatic and supportive treatment

NURSING CONSIDERATIONS

Assess:

• For contraindications (see Pharmacy section)

• Previous history of actual infection of MMR. This does not contraindicate vaccination

Administer:

• After checking expiry date

• Reconstituted only with dilutent provided by manufacturers; use within one hour of reconstitution

• If using alcohol to clean skin allow this to dry completely before injection

• By IM or SC injection into outer aspect of arm to adults and children

• Not mixed with other vaccines or drugs

• With adrenalin 1:1000 to hand in case of anaphylactic reaction

Perform/provide:

• Record name, date, dose, route, site batch number of vaccine in patient's notes

• Store in refrigerator (2°C–8°C) protected from light

• Patient with written record of name and date of vaccination

Evaluate:

• For anaphylactic reaction

• For local/systemic reactions; malaise, fever, rash are common

• By blood test after vaccination (for women of child-bearing age) to establish rubella immunity status

Teach patient/family:

• About possible side effects

• That women of child-bearing age should not become pregnant for 1–3 months after vaccination

• That MMR is not suitable for prophylaxis as antibody reaction is too slow to be of use

---

vancomycin HCl

Vancocin

Func. class.: Antibiotic
Chem. class.: Glycopeptide
Legal class.: POM

Action: Inhibits cell wall bacterial synthesis

Uses: Resistant staphylococcal infections, pseudomembranous colitis, staphylococcal enterocolitis, endocarditis, prophylaxis for dental procedures

Dosage and routes:

Serious staphylococcal infections

Doses should be adjusted according to plasma drug concentration

• *Adult:* IV infusion 500 mg every 6 hr or 1 g every 12 hr

• *Child:* IV infusion 40 mg/kg/day divided every 6 hr

• *Neonates:* IV 10 mg/kg every 12 hr

Pseudomembranous/staphylococcal enterocolitis

• *Adult:* By mouth 500 mg daily in divided doses for 7–10 days increased if necessary up to 2 g daily

• *Child:* By mouth 40 mg/kg/day in divided doses every 6–8 hr

Available forms include: Capsules 125, 250 mg; powder for injection IV 500 mg; injection may be given orally

Side effects/adverse reactions:
Serious side effects are unusual following oral dosing

CV: Cardiac arrest and vascular collapse after rapid infusion, vasculitis

EENT: Ototoxicity, permanent deafness, tinnitus

HAEM: Eosinophilia, neutropenia, thrombocytopenia

GI: Nausea

RESP: Wheezing, dyspnoea after rapid infusion

SYST: Anaphylaxis

GU: Nephrotoxicity: increased blood urea nitrogen, creatinine, albumin

INTEG: Chills, fever, rash, necrosis and thrombophlebitis at injection site, after rapid infusion: urticaria, pruritus

Contraindications:
Hypersensitivity

Precautions: Renal disease (adjust dose), pregnancy, lactation, elderly, neonates, decreased hearing

Pharmacokinetics:
Little oral absorption. After IV administration: peak 2 hr, half-life 3–13 hr, excreted in urine (active form). Therapeutic plasma levels: peak 18–26 mg/litre, trough 5–10 mg/litre

Interactions/incompatibilities:

• Ototoxicity or nephrotoxicity: aminoglycosides, cephalosporins notably cephalothin, colistin, polymyxin, bacitracin, cisplatin, amphotericin, loop diuretics

• Do not mix in solution or syringe with other drugs; check product information

• Exaggerated infusion reactions when given concomitantly with: anaesthetic agents

Clinical assessment:

• Blood levels at regular intervals

• Monitor renal function at regular intervals, adjust dose in renal impairment

• Signs of ototoxicity

• Blood studies: WBC

• Culture and sensitivity before drug therapy; drug may be taken as soon as culture is taken. Use less toxic agents where possible

Treatment of overdose: Supportive care with maintenance of glomerular filtration

NURSING CONSIDERATIONS

Assess:

• Fluid balance

• Bowel pattern

• Allergies before treatment, reaction of each medication; note allergies in nursing care plan in bright red letters; notify all people giving drugs

Administer:

• After samples have been sent for culture and sensitivity

• After reconstitution with 10 ml sterile water for injection 500 mg/100 ml; further dilution is needed for IV

• Infusion over 60 min; avoid extravasation

• Reconstitute with 5 ml water for injections per 250 mg; the resultant 50 mg/ml solution should be diluted with at least 50 ml of diluent per 250 mg for IV infusion over at least 60 mins; doses may also be given by continuous infusion, appropriately diluted. Adjust dosage in renal impairment (consult data sheet). Peak plasma concentrations should not exceed 30 mg/l; pre-dose (trough) concentrations should not exceed 10 mg/l

Perform/provide:

- Storage at 0–6°C – for up to 24 hr after reconstitution
- Adrenaline, resuscitation equipment on unit; anaphylaxis may occur
- Adequate intake of fluids (2 litres) to prevent nephrotoxicity
- Fluid balance ratio; report haematuria, oliguria since nephrotoxicity may occur
- BP during administration; sudden drop may indicate "red man" syndrome

Evaluate:

- Therapeutic response: absence of fever, sore throat
- Hearing loss, ringing, roaring in ears; drug should be discontinued
- Skin eruptions
- Respiratory status: rate, character, wheezing, tightness in chest

Teach patient/family:

- Aspects of drug therapy: need to complete entire course of medication to ensure organism death (7–10 days); culture may be taken after completed course of medication
- To report sore throat, fever, fatigue; could indicate superimposed infection
- That drug must be taken in equal intervals around clock to maintain blood levels

vasopressin (antidiuretic hormone)/(argipressin)

Pitressin

Func. class.: Pituitary hormone
Chem. class.: Lysine vasopressin
Legal class.: POM

Action: Promotes reabsorption of water by action on renal tubular epithelium, contracts smooth muscle

Uses: Pituitary diabetes insipidus, bleeding oesophageal varices

Dosage and routes:

Diabetes insipidus

- *Adult:* IM/subcutaneous 5–20 units every 4 hr as needed

Oesophageal varices

- IV 20 units in 100 ml dextrose 5% infused over 15 min

Available forms include: Injection IV, IM, subcutaneous 20 units/ml

Side effects/adverse reactions:

CNS: Drowsiness, headache, lethargy, tremor, vertigo
GU: Vulval pain, uterine cramp
GI: Nausea, cramps, belching, vomiting, urge to defecate
CV: Increased BP, anginal attack
INTEG: Sweating, pallor, urticaria
SYST: Anaphylaxis, water intoxication

Contraindications: Hypersensitivity, vascular disease (unless extreme caution), chronic nephritis

Precautions: Epilepsy, migraine asthma, congestive cardiac failure

Pharmacokinetics: Not absorbed orally, plasma half life 5–15 min

Interactions/incompatibilities:

- Increased antidiuretic effect: chlorpropamide, carbamazepine, clofibrate, tricyclic antidepressants
- Decreased antidiuretic effect: alcohol, lithium

Treatment of overdose: Monitor fluid balance carefully, hypertonic solutions for water intoxication, nitrates for angina pain

NURSING CONSIDERATIONS

Assess:

- Fluid balance
- Weight
- Pulse, BP, when giving drug IV or IM

Perform/provide:

- Storage injection between 2–8°C

Evaluate:

- Therapeutic response: absence of severe thirst, decreased urine output, osmolality
- Fluid balance ratio, weight daily, check for oedema in extremities, if water retention is severe, diuretic may be prescribed
- Water intoxication: lethargy, behavioural changes, disorientation, neuromuscular excitability

Teach patient/family:

- All aspects of drug: action, side effects, dose, when to notify clinician

vecuronium bromide

Norcuron

Func. class.: Non-depolarising neuromuscular relaxant

Chem. class.: Piperidinium derivative

Legal class.: POM

Action: Inhibits transmission of nerve impulses by binding with cholinergic receptor sites, antagonising action of acetylcholine

Uses: Facilitation of endotracheal intubation, skeletal muscle relaxation during mechanical ventilation, surgery, or general anaesthesia

Dosage and routes:

- *Adult and child:* IV bolus 0.08–0.10 mg/kg; incremental doses, 0.03–0.05 mg/kg, IV infusion 0.05–0.08 mg/kg/hr

Available forms include: Powder for IV use 10 mg vial and diluent (5 ml)

Side effects/adverse reactions:

RESP: Bronchospasm

EENT: Increased secretions

INTEG: Irritation at injection site

SYST: Anaphylaxis

Contraindications: Hypersensitivity

Precautions: Pregnancy, lactation, electrolyte imbalances, dehydration, neuromuscular disease, myasthenia gravis, obesity, after poliomyelitis

Pharmacokinetics:

IV: Onset 1–2 min, duration 20–30 mins; half-life 30–70 min, not metabolised, excreted in faeces

Interactions/incompatibilities:

- Increased neuromuscular blockade: aminoglycosides, clindamycin, lincomycin, quinidine, volatile anaesthetics, polymyxin antibiotics, lithium, narcotic analgesics, thiazides, azlocillin, mezlocillin, nifedipine, verapamil, parenteral magnesium salts, β-blockers, tetracyclines
- Neuromuscular blockade reduced by: chronic corticosteroids, azathioprine, mercaptopurine
- Neuromuscular blockade reversed by: anticholinesterases
- Concurrent administration with depolarising relaxant may cause relaxation which is not reversible by neostigmine

Clinical assessment:

- For electrolyte imbalances (potassium, magnesium); may lead to increased action of this drug

Treatment of overdose: Neostigmine, atropine, monitor vital signs; may require mechanical ventilation

NURSING CONSIDERATIONS

Assess:

- Baseline vital signs

Administer:
• Slowly over 1–2 min (by qualified anaesthetic personnel only)
• With resuscitation equipment nearby
Perform/provide:
• Storage in light-resistant area
• Nerve stimulator
Evaluate:
• Vital signs (BP, pulse, respirations, airway) until fully recovered; rate, depth, pattern of respirations, strength of hand grip
• Fluid balance; check for urinary retention, frequency, hesitancy
• Therapeutic response; degree of paralysis (jaw, neck, respiratory function)
• Heart rate for signs of distress
Administer:
• Using nerve stimulator by anaesthesiologist to determine neuromuscular blockade
• Anticholinesterase to reverse neuromuscular blockade
• By slow IV over 1–2 min (only by qualified person, usually an anaesthetist)
• Only slightly discoloured solution
Perform/provide:
• Reassurance if communication is difficult during recovery from neuromuscular blockade
Evaluate:
• Therapeutic response: paralysis of jaw, eyelid, head, neck, rest of body
• Recovery: decreased paralysis of face, diaphragm, leg, arm, rest of body
• Allergic reactions: rash, fever, respiratory distress, pruritus; drug should be discontinued

verapamil hydrochloride

Berkatens, Cordilox, Geangin, Half-Securon SR, Securon, Securon SR, Univer
Func. class.: Antihypertensive, anti-anguinal, anti-arrhythmic
Chem. class.: Calcium-channel
Legal class.: POM

Action: Inhibits calcium ion influx across cell membrane during cardiac depolarisation; produces relaxation of coronary vascular smooth muscle, dilates coronary arteries
Uses: Chronic stable angina pectoris, vasospastic angina, supraventricular arrhythmias, hypertension
Dosage and routes:
Hypertension
• *Adult:* By mouth, 240–480 mg daily in 2–3 divided doses; modified-release, initially 120 mg daily, up to 480 mg in divided doses if required
• *Child:* By mouth up to 10 mg/kg daily in divided doses according to severity
Angina
• *Adult:* By mouth, 80–120 mg 3 times daily; modified-release, 240 mg twice daily (in some cases once daily)
Supraventricular arrhythmias
• *Adult:* By mouth 40–120 mg 3 times daily; slow IV injection, 5–10 mg, further 5 mg after 5 min if required
• *Child:* By mouth, according to severity, up to 1 year, 20 mg 3 times a day; over 2 years, 40–120 mg 3 times a day; slow IV injection, up to 1 year, 0.1–0.2 mg/kg (usual range 0.75–2 mg), 1–15 years, 0.1–0.3 mg/kg (usual range 2–5 mg), repeat after 30 min if required
Available forms include: Tablets

80 mg, 120 mg, 160 mg; tablets, modified-release, 120 mg, 240 mg; capsules, modified-release, 120 mg, 180 mg, 240 mg; injection 2.5 mg/ml; oral suspension 40 mg/5 ml (special order)

Side effects/adverse reactions:
CV: Arrhythmias, oedema, worsening bradycardia, hypotension, heart block, asystole. Adverse CV effects much more likely after IV administration
GI: Nausea, vomiting, constipation, impaired liver function
INTEG: Rash, pruritus, flushing, photosensitivity
CNS: Headache, fatigue, dizziness
EENT: Gingival hyperplasia
ENDO: Gynaecomastia

Contraindications: Cardiogenic shock, sino-atrial block, history of heart failure or impaired left ventricular function

Precautions: Congestive heart failure, IV route in patients taking β-blockers, 1st degree heart block, atrial flutter or fibrillation complicating Wolff Parkinson White syndrome, myocardial infarction pregnancy

Pharmacokinetics:
IV: Onset 3 min, plasma half-life 2–8 hr
By mouth: Onset 1–2 hr, half-life (biphasic) 4–12 hr (terminal)
Metabolised by liver, excreted in urine (96% as metabolites), 90% protein bound

Interactions/incompatibilities:
- Increased hypotensive effects with: general anaesthetics, other antihypertensives, quinidine, antipsychotics
- Increased risk of bradycardia, heart block, myocardial depression with: amiodarone
- Increased effects of: carbamazepine, imipramine, non-depolarising muscle relaxants
- Severe hypotension, heart block, bradycardia, asystole with: β-blockers, especially if either agent given IV
- Increased blood levels of: digoxin, cyclosporin, theophylline
- Increased heart block and bradycardia with: cardiac glycosides
- Increased neurotoxicity with: lithium
- Cardiac status, ECG
- Blood levels of co-administered digoxin, theophylline

Treatment of overdose: Defibrillation, cardiac massage for asystole, atropine for AV block, vasopressor for hypotension

NURSING CONSIDERATIONS

Assess:
- Vital signs
- Baseline BP and respiratory rate

Perform/provide:
- Continuous ECG monitoring if given IV

Evaluate:
- Therapeutic response: decreased anginal pain
- BP, pulse, respiration

Teach patient/family:
- How to take pulse before taking drug; record or graph should be kept
- To avoid hazardous activities until dizziness is no longer a problem
- To limit caffeine consumption
- To avoid non-prescribed medicines unless approved by clinician
- Patient compliance P with all areas of medical regimen: diet, exercise, stress reduction, drug therapy
- To report any side effects, headache, dizziness or fatigue

vigabatrin

Sabril
Func. class.: Anticonvulsant
Chem. class.: GABA analogue
Legal class.: POM

Action: Selective irreversible inhibitor of GABA-transaminase, raises brain GABA levels
Uses: Treatment of epilepsy not satisfactorily controlled by other anti-epileptic drugs
Dosage and routes:
• *Adult:* By mouth, added to existing therapy, initially 2 g daily in single or 2 divided doses; adjust according to response by 0.5–1 g; maximum 4 g daily
• *Child:* By mouth, added to existing therapy, initially 40 mg/kg daily; increase according to response to 80–100 mg/kg daily; in terms of body weight: 10–15 kg, 0.5–1 g daily; 15–30 kg, 1–1.5 g daily; 30–50 kg, 1.3–3 g daily; over 50 kg 2–4 g daily
Available forms include: Tablets 500 mg; powder for oral solution 500 mg/sachet
Side effects/adverse reactions:
GI: Minor disturbances, changes in liver enzymes
CNS: Drowsiness, fatigue, dizziness, nervousness, irritability, depression, headache, confusion, aggression, psychosis, memory disturbance, paradoxical increase in seizure frequency. Excitation and agitation have been seen in children
HAEM: Slight decrease in haemoglobin
EENT: Diplopia
MISC: Weight gain
Contraindications: Pregnancy, breast-feeding
Precautions: Impaired renal function, elderly, history of psychosis, behavioural problems. Abrupt withdrawal may lead to rebound seizures. If treatment is to be discontinued it is recommended that the dose is reduced gradually over 2–4 weeks
Pharmacokinetics:
By mouth: Peak levels within 2 hr. Elimination half-life 5–8 hr via kidneys, not metabolised
Interactions/incompatibilities:
• Reduced blood levels of: phenytoin

NURSING CONSIDERATIONS

Assess:
• Baseline weight
• Renal function
Administer:
• Oral powder dissolved in water or soft drink
Evaluate:
• Weight gain
• GI disturbance
• Neurological function
Teach patient/family:
• That drug is to be taken in conjunction with other anti-epileptic drugs
• About side effects
• Not to discontinue drug suddenly; rebound stizates can occur
• Not to undertaken hazardous activity associated with machinery

vinblastine sulphate

Velbe
Func. class.: Antineoplastic
Chem. class.: *Vinca rosea* alkaloid
Legal class.: POM

Action: Inhibits mitotic activity, arrests cell cycle at metaphase; inhibits RNA synthesis
Uses: Breast, testicular cancer, leukaemias neuroblastoma, Hodgkin's and non-Hodgkin's lymphomas, mycosis fungoides, histiocytosis-X, renal cell carci-

noma, methotrexate–resistant choriocarcinoma and other sensitive tumours

Dosage and routes:

Doses are highly variable, and dependent on local treatment protocols, concomitant therapy and tumour type; the following dose schedules have been used

• *Adult and child:* IV 6 mg/m^2 usually no more frequently than every 7 days, for testicular tumours may increase dose to 0.2 mg/kg on each of two consecutive days every 3 weeks

Available forms include: Injection 1 mg/ml; injection 10 mg

Side effects/adverse reactions:

HAEM: Thrombocytopenia, leucopenia, anaemia

GI: Nausea, vomiting, anorexia, stomatitis, constipation, abdominal pain, haemorrhagic enterocolitis, rectal bleeding, diarrhoea, pharyngitis, adynamic ileus

INTEG: Rash, alopecia, pain and necrosis following extravasation

CV: Orthostatic hypotension, hypertension

CNS: Paraesthesias, peripheral neuropathy, depression, headache, convulsions, malaise, dizziness, weakness

ENDO: Inappropriate antidiuretic hormone secretion

MS: Myalgia, jaw pain, bone pain

Contraindications: Hypersensitivity, pregnancy, breast-feeding, bacterial infection, granulocytopenic patients; intrathecal administration, concurrent hepatic radiotherapy

Precautions: Hepatic disease

Pharmacokinetics: Terminal half-life in plasma 19 hr, metabolised in liver, excreted in urine, faeces, does not cross blood–brain barrier, 99% protein bound

Interactions/incompatibilities:

• Do not use with irradiation of liver

• Risk of bronchospasm, pulmonary infiltration and fibrosis with: mitomycin C

Clinical assessment:

• Liver function tests before, during therapy as needed or monthly

• Stop treatment if neurotoxicity develops

• Full blood count prior to each treatment, withhold if neutropenic

Treatment of overdose: Supportive treatment including anticonvulsants, transfusion products, filgrastim, cathartics

NURSING CONSIDERATIONS

Assess:

• Fluid balance, report fall in urine output of 30 ml/hr

• Monitor temperature 4 hrly may indicate beginning infection

Administer:

• HANDLING: take safety precautions appropriate to antineoplastic agents

• Following local antineoplastic (cytotoxic) policies

• After ensuring that clinician is aware of blood results

• IV; as bolus injection over 1 min or as IV injection over 1 min into tubing of fast-running sodium chloride 0.9% infusion

• Other medications by mouth if possible. Avoid IV, IM, SC routes to prevent infection and bruising if thrombocytopoenic

• Anti-emetic 30–60 min before treatment

• All other medication as prescribed including analgesics, antibiotics, anti-emetics, antispasmodics

Perform/provide:

• Trained personnel should reconstitute the drug in a designated area, adequate protective measures required. Avoid contact with eyes

• Not to be handled by pregnant personnel

• Strict medical asepsis, protective isolation if WBC levels are low
• Increase fluid intake to 2–3 litres/day to prevent urate deposits, calculi formation
• Strict oral hygiene with prescribed mouthwashes
• Brushing of teeth 2–3 times day with soft brush or cotton-tipped applicators for stomatitis; use unwaxed dental floss
• Warm compresses at injection site for inflammation
• Nutritious diet with iron, vitamin supplements
• Elevate head of bed to facilitate breathing

Evaluate:
• Bleeding: haematuria, guaiac, bruising or petechiae, mucosa of orifices 8 hrly
• Dyspnoea, rales, unproductive cough, chest pain, tachypnoea, fatigue, increased pulse, pallor, lethargy
• Effects of alopecia on body image; discuss feelings about changes in body image
• Oedema in feet, joint pain, stomach pain, shaking
• Inflammation of mucosa, breaks in skin
• Yellowing of skin and sclera, dark urine, clay-coloured stools, itchy skin, abdominal pain, fever, diarrhoea
• Buccal cavity 8 hrly for dryness, sores or ulceration, white patches, oral pain, bleeding, dysphagia
• Local irritation, pain, burning, discolouration at injection and infusion site
• Symptoms indicating severe allergic reaction: rash, pruritus, urticaria, purpuric skin lesions, itching, flushing
• Frequency of stools and characteristics: cramping, acidosis; signs of dehydration: rapid respirations, poor skin turgor, decreased urine output, dry skin, restlessness, weakness

Teach patient/family:
• Of protective isolation precautions
• To report any complaints or side effects to the nurse or clinician
• That impotence or amenorrhoea can occur, are reversible after discontinuing treatment
• To report any changes in breathing or coughing
• That hair may be lost during treatment, a wig or hairpiece may be available on the NHS; tell patient that new hair may be different in colour, texture
• To avoid foods with citric acid, hot or rough texture
• To report any bleeding, white spots or ulcerations in mouth to clinician; tell patient to examine mouth daily

---

vincristine sulphate

Oncovin
Func. class.: Antineoplastic
Chem. class.: Vinca alkaloid
Legal class.: POM

Action: Inhibits mitotic activity, arrests cell cycle at metaphase; inhibits RNA synthesis
Uses: Breast cancer, lung cancer, lymphomas, neuroblastoma, Hodgkin's and non-Hodgkin's lymphomas, acute lymphoblastic and other leukaemias, rhabdomyosarcoma, Wilms' tumour, osteogenic and other sarcomas, and other sensitive tumours
Dosage and routes:
Doses are highly variable, and dependent on local treatment protocols, concomitant therapy and tumour type; the following dose schedules have been used
• *Adult:* IV 1.4–1.5 mg/m^2 weekly not to exceed 2 mg a week

• *Child:* IV, under 10 kg, 0.05 mg/kg weekly

Available forms include: Injection 1 mg/ml; pre-filled syringes 1 mg, 2 mg; injection 1 mg, 2 mg, 5 mg

Side effects/adverse reactions:

HAEM: Granulocytopenia, rarely anaemia and thrombocytopenia

GI: Nausea, vomiting, anorexia, stomatitis, constipation, paralytic ileus, abdominal pain, diarrhoea

INTEG: Alopecia, rash, pain and necrosis following extravasation

SYST: Weight loss, fever, anaphylaxis

EENT: Optic atrophy

CV: Orthostatic hypotension, hypertension

CNS: Decreased reflexes, numbness, weakness, motor difficulties, CNS depression, cranial nerve palsies paralysis, neuritic pain, paraesthesia, difficulty walking, slapping gait, ataxia, foot drop, convulsions

MS: Muscle wasting, pain in limbs, bone, pharynx, jaw, myalgia

ENDO: Inappropriate secretion of antidiuretic hormone

GU: Polyuria, dysuria, retention, risk of uric acid nephropathy secondary to tumour lysis

Contraindications: Hypersensitivity, pregnancy; intrathecal administration, patients with demyelinating form of Charcot–Marie–Tooth syndrome, concurrent hepatic radiotherapy

Precautions: Hepatic disease, neuromuscular disease, infection, granulocytopenia

Pharmacokinetics: Terminal half-life 85 hr metabolised in liver, excreted in faeces, urine; does not cross blood–brain barrier, extensively protein bound

Interactions/incompatibilities:

• Do not use with irradiation of liver

• Risk of bronchospasm, pulmonary infiltration and fibrosis with: mitomycin

• Excretion slowed by: asparaginase (possibility of increased toxicity)

Clinical assessment:

• Liver function tests before, during therapy as needed or monthly

• Stop treatment if neurotoxicity develops

• Full blood count before each treatment, consider treatment carefully if neutropenic

Treatment of overdose: Supportive treatment including anticonvulsants, transfusion products, cathartics. Folinic acid may be protective in first 24 hr

NURSING CONSIDERATIONS

Assess:

• Baseline vital signs and fluid balance

Administer:

• HANDLING: take safety precautions appropriate to antineoplastic agents

• Following local antineoplastic (cytotoxic) policies

• After ensuring that clinician is aware of blood results

• IV: as an IV bolus injection into tubing of fast-running sodium chloride 0.9% infusion

• Other medications by mouth if possible. Avoid IV, IM, SC routes to prevent infection and bruising

• Anti-emetic 30–60 min before treatment

• All other medication as prescribed including analgesics, antibiotics, anti-emetics, antispasmodics

Perform/provide:

• Trained personnel, should reconstitute the drug in a designated area, adequate protective measures required. Avoid contact with the eyes

• Not to be handled by pregnant personnel

• Strict medical asepsis, protective

isolation if WBC levels are low
• Special skin care
• Strict oral hygiene with prescribed mouth washes
• Brushing of teeth 2–3 times day with soft brush or cotton-tipped applicators for stomatitis; use unwaxed dental floss
• Warm compresses at injection and infusion site for inflammation
• Nutritious diet with iron, vitamin supplements

Evaluate:
• Fluid balance, report fall in urine output of 30 ml/hr
• Monitor temperature 4 hrly may indicate beginning infection
• Bleeding: haematuria, bruising or petechiae, mucosa of orifices 8 hrly
• Dyspnoea, rales, unproductive cough, chest pain, tachypnoea, fatigue, increased pulse, pallor, lethargy
• Effects of alopecia on body image, allow patient to discuss feelings about changes in body image
• Oedema in feet, joint pain, stomach pain, shaking
• Inflammation of mucosa, breaks in skin
• Yellowing of skin and sclera, dark urine, clay-coloured stools, itchy skin, abdominal pain, fever, diarrhoea
• Buccal cavity 8 hrly for dryness, sores or ulceration, white patches, oral pain, bleeding, dysphagia
• Local irritation, pain, burning, discolouration at injection site
• Symptoms indicating severe allergic reaction: rash, pruritus, urticaria, purpuric skin lesions, itching, flushing
• Frequency of stools, characteristics: cramping, acidosis; signs of dehydration: rapid respirations, poor skin turgor, decreased urine output, dry skin, restlessness, weakness

Teach patient/family:
• About protective isolation precautions when indicated
• To report any complaints or side effects to nurse or clinician
• To report any bleeding, white spots or ulcerations in mouth to clinician; tell patient to examine mouth daily
• Good oral hygiene techniques; avoid vigorous brushing of teeth

---

vindesine sulphate

Eldisine
Func. class.: Antineoplastic
Chem. class.: Vinca alkaloid
Legal class.: POM

Action: Inhibits mitotic activity, arrests cell cycle at metaphase; inhibits RNA synthesis

Uses: Breast cancer, acute lymphoblastic, blastic crises of chronic myeloid leukaemia, malignant melanoma, and other sensitive tumours

Dosage and routes:
Doses are highly variable, and dependent on local treatment protocols, concomitant therapy and tumour type; the following dose schedules have been used
• *Adult:* IV 3 mg/m^2 every 7 days. Provided there is no granulocytopenia, dosage may be increased in 0.5 mg/m^2 steps at weekly intervals to maximum 4 mg/m^2
• *Child:* IV 4 mg/m^2 every 7 days

Available forms include: Injection 5 mg

Side effects/adverse reactions:
HAEM: Thrombocytopenia, leucopenia, anaemia, thrombocytosis
INTEG: Alopecia, pain and necrosis following extravasation
GI: Nausea, vomiting, anorexia, constipation, stomatitis, paralytic

ileus, abdominal pain, dysphagia, dyspepsia, diarrhoea
MS: Jaw pain, myalgia, bone and joint pain
CNS: Neuritis, paraesthesia, mental depression, loss of deep tendon reflexes, foot drop, headache, convulsions
Contraindications: Granulocytopenia, bacterial infection, demyelinating form of Charcot-Marie-Tooth syndrome, hypersensitivity, pregnancy, intrathecal administration, concurrent hepatic radiotherapy
Precautions: Renal disease, hepatic disease, neuromuscular disease
Pharmacokinetics: Terminal half-life greater than 20 hr, metabolised in liver, excreted in urine and bile, does not cross blood-brain barrier
Interactions/incompatibilities:
• Do not use with irradiation of liver
• Risk of bronchospasm, pulmonary infiltration and fibrosis with: mitomycin C
Clinical assessment:
• Liver function tests before, during therapy as needed or monthly
• Full blood count prior to each treatment, withhold if neutropenic
• Stop treatment if neurotoxicity develops

NURSING CONSIDERATIONS

Assess:
• Baseline fluid balance
Administer:
• HANDLING: take safety precautions appropriate to antineoplastic agents
• Following local antineoplastic (cytotoxic) policies
• After ensuring that clinician is aware of blood results
• IV: as an IV bolus or as injection into tubing of fast-running infusion
• Other medications by mouth if possible. Avoid IV, IM, SC routes to prevent infection and bruising
• Anti-emetic 30–60 min before treatment
• All other medication as prescribed including analgesics, antibiotics, anti-emetics, antispasmodics
Perform/provide:
• Should not be handled by pregnant staff
• Store at 2–8°C
• Reconstituted solutions stable for 30 days if refrigerated
• Strict medical asepsis, protective isolation if WBC levels are low
• All good supportive care including that of mouth and skin
• Warm compresses at injection and infusion site for inflammation
• Nutritious diet as tolerated
Evaluate:
• GI disturbances and abdominal bloating
• Signs of neuropathy
• Food preferences; list likes, dislikes
• Effects of alopecia on body image, discuss feelings about changes in body image
• All changes in condition
Teach patient/family:
• Of protective isolation precautions
• To report any complaints or side effects to nurse or clinician
• That hair may be lost during treatment, a wig or hairpiece may be available on the NHS; tell patient that new hair may be different in colour, texture
• That if neurological side effects occur they are usually reversible

vitamin A (retinol)

Ro-A-Vit, many combination products
Func. class.: Fat-soluble vitamin
Chem. class.: Retinol
Legal class.: Injection: POM, combination products: GSL

Action: Needed for epitheleal development, visual dark adaptation, skin and mucosal tissue repair
Uses: Vitamin A deficiency and prophylaxis
Dosage and routes:
Deficiency
• *Adults:* IM 100,000 units once monthly or in acute deficiency once weekly. Courses no longer than 6 weeks with 2-week interval. Liver disease, IM 100,000 units every 2–4 months (specialist use)
• *Child:* IM 50,000 units monthly
Children's Vitamin Drops
• *Child:* 1 month–5 yr, By mouth 5 drops daily
Available forms include: Injection 100,000 units (as palmitate) in 2 ml, oral combination products Children's Vitamin Drops (available under Welfare Food Scheme)
Side effects/adverse reactions:
Except for anaphylaxis to injection, described effects are symptoms of overdose
GI: Nausea, vomiting, anorexia, abdominal pain, jaundice, liver enlargement
CNS: Headache, increased intracranial pressure, lethargy, malaise
EENT: Gingivitis, papillaoedema, exophthalmos, inflammation of tongue and lips, tinnitus, visual disturbances
INTEG: Drying of skin and hair, pruritus, alopecia, erythema
MS: Arthraglia, retarded growth, bone pain and swelling
META: Hypercalcaemia
HAEM: Raised ESR
SYST: Anaphylaxis (after injection), weight loss
Contraindications: Hypersensitivity to vitamin A or injection vehicle, pregnancy
Precautions: Liver disease
Pharmacokinetics:
By mouth/injection: Stored in liver, fat; excreted (metabolites) in urine, faeces
Interactions/incompatibilities:
• Decreased absorption of this drug: liquid paraffin, cholestyramine, neomycin
Treatment of overdose: Discontinue drug

NURSING CONSIDERATIONS

Assess:
• Vitamin A deficiency: decreased growth, night blindness, dry, brittle nails, hair loss, urinary stones, increased infection
Administer:
• With food (orally) for better absorption
• Do not dilute or mix injection solution
Evaluate:
• Therapeutic response: increased growth rate, weight; absence of dry skin and mucuous membranes, night blindness
Teach patient/family:
• Not to use mineral oil while taking this drug
• To notify clinician of nausea, vomiting, lip cracking, loss of hair, headache
• Not to take more than the prescribed amount
• To take a Vitamin A-rich diet

vitamin D (cholecalciferol, vitamin D_3 or ergocalciferol, vitamin D_2)

Func. class.: Fat-soluble vitamin
Legal class.: Tablets P, Injection POM

Action: Needed for regulation of calcium, phosphate levels, normal bone development, parathyroid activity, neuromuscular functioning

Uses: Vitamin D deficiency, rickets, renal osteodystrophy, hypoparathyroidism

Dosage and routes:

Simple deficiency

- *Adult and children:* By mouth 400 units daily

Malabsorption/liver disease

- By mouth/IM up to 40,000 units daily

Hypoparathyroidism

- *Adult and child:* By mouth/IM up to 100,000 units daily

Available forms include: Tablets 400 (with 2.4 mmol calcium) 10,000 50,000 units; injection 300,000 units/ml

Side effects/adverse reactions: Described effects are symptoms of overdose

GI: Nausea, vomiting, anorexia, cramps, diarrhoea, constipation, metallic taste, dry mouth

CNS: Fatigue, weakness, drowsiness, convulsion, headache, vertigo

GU: Polyuria, nocturia, haematuria, albuminuria, renal failure

CV: Hypertension, dysrhythmias

MS: Decreased bone growth, bone pain, early muscle pain

INTEG: Pruritus, photophobia, sweating

MISC: Ectopic calcification

METAB: Raised serum and urine calcium and phosphate, thirst, weight loss

Contraindications: Hypersensitivity, hypercalcaemia

Precautions: Lactation, cardiovascular disease, renal calculi, renal dysfunction

Pharmacokinetics:

By mouth/injection: Well absorbed orally, stored in muscle, fat, liver, metabolised in liver and kidneys, excreted in bile (metabolites) and urine

Interactions/incompatibilities:

- Decreased effects of this drug: cholestyramine, colestipol, phenobarbitone, phenytoin, rifampicin

Clinical assessment:

- Blood calcium at regular intervals (initially weekly) and if nausea or vomiting present, also in patients receiving high dose therapy

Treatment of overdose: Empty stomach following recent bulk ingestion, monitor serum calcium, supportive treatments including IV fluids, calcitonin

NURSING CONSIDERATIONS

Assess:

- Nutritional status

Administer:

- IM injection in deep muscle mass, administer slowly

Evaluate:

- Therapeutic response: absence of rickets/osteomalacia, decrease in bone pain

Teach patient/family:

- Necessary foods to be included in diet: egg yolk, dairy products
- To avoid vitamin supplements unless directed by clinician
- To keep clinician's appointments to assess risk of toxicity/therapeutic benefit
- To report weakness, lethargy, headache, anorexia, loss of weight, nausea, vomiting, abdominal cramps, diarrhoea, constipation, excessive thirst, polyuria, muscle and bone pain

vitamin E (alpha tocapheryl acetate)

Ephynal, Vita-E, many combination products
Func. class.: Fat-soluble vitamin
Chem. class.: Tocopherols
Legal class.: GSL

Action: Anti-oxidant, co-factor for metabolic reactions
Uses: Vitamin E deficiency, in malabsorption syndrome. Need for supplementation in adults doubtful
Dosage and routes:
Cystic fibrosis
• *Adult:* By mouth 100–200 mg daily
• *Child (over 1 yr):* By mouth 100 mg daily
• *Child (under 1 yr):* By mouth 50 mg daily
Abetaliproteinaemia
• *Adult and child*: By mouth 50–100 mg/kg daily
Available forms include: Capsules 75, 200, 400 units. Chewable tablets 75 units; tablets (succinate) 50, 200 units; suspension 500 mg/5 ml
Side effects/adverse reactions:
CNS: Headache, fatigue
GI: Nausea, cramps, diarrhoea
Contraindications: Hypersensitivity
Pharmacokinetics:
By mouth: Metabolised in liver, excreted in bile
Interactions/incompatibilities:
• Increased action of: oral anticoagulants
Treatment of overdose: Supportive only, not likely to be significant
NURSING CONSIDERATIONS
Assess:
• Nutritional status
Evaluate:
• Clotting disturbances in patients previously stabilised on oral anticoagulants
• Therapeutic response: improvement in skin lesions, decreased oedema
Teach patient/family:
• Necessary foods to be included in diet: wheat germ, dark green leafy vegetables, nuts, eggs, liver, vegetable oils, dairy products, cereals
• To avoid vitamin supplements unless directed by clinician

warfarin sodium

Marevan
Func. class.: Anticoagulant
Chem. class.: Coumarin
Legal class.: POM

Action: Interferes with blood clotting by indirect means; depresses hepatic synthesis of vitamin K-dependent coagulation factors (II, VII, IX, X)
Uses: Prophylaxis is of embolisation in rheumatic heart disease and atrial fibrilation. Prophylaxis after insertion of prosthetic heart valve. Prophylaxis and treatment of venous thrombosis and pulmonary embolism. Transient ischaemic attacks
Dosage and routes:
• *Adult:* By mouth usual initial dose 10 mg daily, then titrated to International Normalised Ratio (INR) time daily; maintenance usualy 3–9 mg daily
Available forms include: Tablets 1 mg (Brown), 3 mg (Blue), 5 mg (Pink)
Side effects/adverse reactions:
GI: Diarrhoea, nausea, vomiting, pancreatitis
INTEG: Rash, alopecia
CNS: Fever
HAEM: Haemorrhage
EENT: Epistaxis

Contraindications: Severe hypertension, pericarditis, pericardial effusion, subacute endocarditis, severe hepatic or renal disease, increased fibrinolytic activity, following surgery on lung, prostate or uterus, peptic ulcer, pregnancy, hypersensitivity, haemorrhagic diathesis, blood dyscrasias, pre- and post-surgery on CNS or eyes, haemorrhage in GI, urogenital or respiratory tract and cardiovascular system

Precautions: Alcoholism, elderly, decreased dietary intake of Vitamin K, hepatic/renal dysfunction, concurrent administration of salicylates and other highly plasma protein-bound drugs

Pharmacokinetics:

By mouth: Onset 24 hr, peak 36–48 hr, duration 3–5 days, half-life ½–3 days; metabolised in liver, excreted in urine/faeces (active/inactive metabolites)

Interactions/incompatibilities:

• Increased action: allopurinol, chloramphenicol, clofibrate, amiodarone, diflunisal, heparin, steroids, cimetidine, disulfiram, thyroxine, glucagon, metronidazole, quinidine, sulindac, sulphinpyrazone, sulphonamides, tricyclic antidepressants, inhalation anaesthetics, salicylates, ethacrynic acid, indomethacin, mefenamic acid, oxyphenbutazone, phenylbutazone

• Decreased action: barbiturates, griseofulvin, haloperidol, carbamazepine, rifampicin, cholestyramine

• Increased or decreased action: chloral hydrate, glutethimide, sulphinpyrazone, triclofos sodium, alcohol

Clinical assessment:

• Blood counts (haematocrit, platelets, occult blood in stools) every 3 months

• International Normalised Ratio; use local laboratory guidelines to establish required ratio

Treatment of overdose: Administer Vitamin K and/or fresh frozen plasma

NURSING CONSIDERATIONS

Assess:

• Blood count, especially prothrombin time

• After prothrombin time

Administer:

• At same time each day to maintain steady blood levels

• Alone; NOT to be given with food

• Avoid all IM injections that may cause bleeding

Evaluate:

• Therapeutic response: decrease of deep vein thrombosis

• Signs of bleeding; gums, black tarry stools, haematuria epistaxis

• Fever, skin rash, urticaria

• Needed dosage change 1–2 wks

Teach patient/family:

• To avoid non-prescribed preparations that may cause serious drug interactions unless approved by clinician/pharmacist

• To carry an ID identifying drug taken

• Stress patient compliance

• On all aspects of: dosage, route, action, side effects, when to notify clinician

• To report any signs of bleeding: gums, under skin, urine, stools or epigastric pain

• To avoid hazardous activities (football, hockey, skiing) or dangerous work (driving)

xamoterol

Corwin
Func. class.: Inotropic agent
Chem. class.: β_1-adrenoceptor partial agonist
Legal class.: POM

Action: Acts on β_1-receptors; in mild heart failure it improves ventricular function with no increase in myocardial oxygen demand
Uses: Restricted by CSM to chronic mild heart failure in patients not breathless at rest but limited by symptoms on exertion
Dosage and routes: Treatment to be initiated in hospital after full assessment
• *Adult:* By mouth 200 mg for 1 week, then 200 mg twice daily
Available forms include: Tablets 200 mg (as fumarate)
Side effects/adverse reactions:
CNS: Headache, dizziness
CV: Chest pain, palpitations
GI: Disturbances
INTEG: Rashes
MS: Muscle cramp
Contraindications: Moderate to severe heart failure, breast-feeding, children (seek specialist advice)
Precautions: Cardiac outflow obstruction, arrhythmias, maintain concurrent digoxin in atrial fibrillation, chronic obstructive airways disease, bronchospasm, development of asthma, cardiac symptoms at rest, renal impairment, pregnancy, deterioration of heart failure (withdraw)
Interactions/incompatibilities:
• Beta-blockers – antagonism of effect of xamoterol and reduced beta-blockade
• Beta-agonists – competition for receptors
Clinical assessment:
• Fully assess severity of heart failure before starting treatment
• Monitor cardiac function
Treatment of overdose: Symptomatic conservative management
NURSING CONSIDERATIONS
Assess:
• Baseline vital signs
• Fluid balance
Administer:
• With meals to prevent GI symptoms
Evaluate:
• BP regularly
• Therapeutic response
• Exercise range – ease of breathing and respiration rate
• Coldness of extremities – peripheral blood flow may decrease
Teach patient/family:
• On all aspects of drug – avoid smoking and smoke-filled rooms
• Report any chest pain or palpitations, bronchospasm
• Not to drive as dizziness may occur

xipamide

Diurexan
Func. class.: Diuretic
Chem. class.: Thiazide related
Legal class.: POM

Action: Diuresis. Probably reduces peripheral vascular resistance. Reduces reabsorption of electrolytes from renal tubules increasing excretion of sodium and chloride ions and thereby water
Uses: Oedema, including congestive heart failure, hypertension
Dosage and routes: Adults by mouth
Oedema
• Initially 40 mg in morning increased to 80 mg if necessary; maintenance 20 mg in morning
Hypertension
• 20 mg in morning (may be in-

creased to 40 mg if necessary but if other anti-hypertensive therapy being given initial dose should not exceed 20 mg daily)

Available forms include: Tablets, scored 20 mg

Side effects/adverse reactions:

GU: Slight gastrointestinal disturbances

CNS: Mild dizziness

Contraindications: Hypercalcaemia, severe renal and hepatic impairment, Addison's disease, children, severe electrolyte deficiency, porphyria

Precautions: Pregnancy, diabetes, gout, renal or hepatic impairment, may cause hypokalaemia, prostatic hypertrophy, lactation

Pharmacokinetics: Absorption is rapid, peak plasma concentrations within 1–2 hr, 99% bound to plasma protein, plasma half-life 5–8 hr, excreted in urine, diuretic effect lasts up to 12 hr, antihypertensive effect lasts up to 24 hr or more

Interactions/incompatibilities:

- Increased toxicity of NSAIDs, calcium salts, cardiac glycosides, lithium
- If hypokalaemia increased toxicity and side effects of: amiodarone disopyramide, flecainide, quinidine, pimozide, sotalol, cardiac glycosides
- If hypokalaemia decreased effect of: lignocaine, mexiletine, tocainide
- Antagonise diuresis: NSAIDs, carbenoxolone, corticosteroids, oestrogens and combined oral contraceptives
- Reduced absorption caused by: cholestyramine, colestipol
- Decreased effect of: antidiabetics
- Enhanced hypotension: tricyclic antihypertensives (NB: α-blockers and ACE inhibitors)
- Increased risk of hypokalaemia: indapamide, corticosteroids, carbenoxolone, other diuretics

Clinical assessment:

- Lower or increase dose to achieve adequate control
- Monitor plasma electrolytes especially, potassium

Treatment of overdose: Maintain BP, restore blood volume, Correct electrolyte imbalance

NURSING CONSIDERATIONS

Assess:

- Baseline BP

Administer:

- In morning to avoid nocturia
- Ensure patient has ready access to toilet facilities
- With food if nausea occurs

Perform/provide:

- Weigh daily

Evaluate:

- Therapeutic effect: reduced oedema, lower blood pressure, reduction in weight
- For side effects – GI disturbance and mild dizziness
- Urine output for signs of acute urinary retention
- For signs of oedema

Teach patient/family:

- To take in morning to avoid nocturia
- To ensure toilet facilities readily available
- Not to perform tasks requiring alertness until sure they are not affected by dizziness
- To check with GP before taking other medications

xylometazoline HCl (nasal)

Otrivine

Func. class.: Nasal decongestant
Chem. class.: Sympathomimetic agent
Legal class.: GSL

Action: Marked α-adrenergic ac-

tivity. Vasoconstrictor with rapid and prolonged action—decreases congestion
Uses: Nasal congestion
Dosage and routes:
• *Adult and child over 12 yr:* Instil 2–3 drops or 1 spray in each nostril 2–3 times daily (0.1%) when required
• *Child:* 3 months–12 yr, instil 1–2 drops in each nostril once or twice a day (0.05%) when required
Available forms include: Nasal drops 0.1%, 0.05%; nasal spray 0.1%
Side effects/adverse reactions:
EENT: Irritation, sneezing, stinging, dryness, headache
CNS: In children—restlessness, sleep disturbance
After excessive use: tolerance and rebound congestion
Contraindications: Hypersensitivity to sympathomimetic amines, infants under 3 months, trans-sphenoidal hypophysectomy or surgery exposing the dura mater
Precautions: Avoid excessive use—do not use for more than 7 consecutive days, cardiovascular disease
Pharmacokinetics:
INSTIL: Onset 5–10 min, duration 5–6 hr; systemic absorption may occur
Treatment of overdose: No specific treatment—supportive measures

NURSING CONSIDERATIONS

Administer:
• Not more than 4 hrly
• For a maximum of 7 consecutive days unless otherwise prescribed
Perform/provide:
• Environmental humidification to decrease nasal congestion, dryness
Evaluate:
• Redness, swelling, pain in nasal passages
Teach patient/family:
• To avoid contamination of container
• Stinging may occur for a few applications; drying of mucosa may be decreased by environmental humidification
• To notify doctor if irregular pulse, insomnia, dizziness, or tremors occur
• Proper administration to avoid systemic absorption

yellow fever vaccine

Arilvax
Func. class.: Live attenuated vaccine 17D strain
Legal class.: POM

Action: Promotes development of antibodies specific to yellow fever virus
Uses: Active immunisation against yellow fever virus. Certificate of vaccination, in case of primary vaccination, is valid 10 yr from the 10th day after vaccination for re-vaccination within 10 yr, certificate is valid at once
Dosage and routes:
• *Adults and children over 9 months:* subcutaneous injection, 0.5 ml
Available forms include: Freeze-dried live vaccine 1-, 5-, 10-dose vial with diluent contains neomycin and polymyxin sulphates
Side effects/adverse reactions:
INTEG: Redness, swelling
CNS: Risk of encephalitis in infants under 9 months, headache
Contraindications: Presence of acute infection, impaired immune response, pregnancy, sensitivity to eggs or chick protein, neomycin or polymyxin. History of serious reaction to previous dose
Precautions: Infants under 9 months, within 6 weeks of administration of immune globulin. Al-

low minimum of 2 weeks after yellow fever vaccine before giving immune globulin. Interval of at least 3 wks between administration of other live vaccines. If not possible give simultaneously at different sites

Pharmacokinetics: Active immunity usually established within 10 days of primary vaccination and persists for many years

Interactions/incompatibilities:
• Not to be given while patient is being treated with nor within set time limit: corticosteroids, other immunosuppressive drugs
• Concurrent (within 3 wks) of other live vaccines

Clinical assessment:
• The decision to vaccinate during pregnancy or infants under 9 months must depend on the risk of exposure to the disease
• Do not prescribe for those sensitive to eggs or to neomycin or polymyxin
• Avoid vaccination within 6 weeks of immunoglobulin administration
• An interval of 3 weeks should lapse between administering any two live vaccines

NURSING CONSIDERATIONS

Assess:
• Active or suspected infection
• History of allergies, especially hypersensitivity to penicillin or eggs

Administer:
• Subcutaneously
• Ensure injection needle uncontaminated by spirit or disinfectant
• 5 ml for all ages
• With adrenaline 1:1000 and resuscitative equipment available
• Reconstitute with suitable sterile Arilvax solutions only
• After reconstitution keep cool and protect from light for up to one hr

Provide:
• Store at 2–3°C protected from light
• Dispose of remaining vaccine by incineration or disinfectant such as strong hydrochloride solution after one hr
• A record of injection, dose, lot number of vaccine, and date of administration

Evaluate:
• For anaphylaxis: dyspnoea, bronchospasm, tachycardia, profuse sweating, collapse
• History of allergies
• For local effects of soreness and redness at vaccination site

Teach patient/family:
• That there could be local effects of soreness and redness at vaccination site
• Immunity after primary injection commences after 10 days and lasts 10 yr reinforcing dose would then be required

---

zidovudine (formerly azidothymidine or AZT)

Retrovir
Func. class.: Antiviral
Chem. class.: Thymidine analogue
Legal class.: POM

Action: Inhibits replication of HIV virus by interfering with transcription of RNA and DNA

Uses: Management of advanced HIV disease such as AIDS or AIDS-related complex; early symptomatic or asymptomatic HIV infection with markers indicating risk of disease progression

Dosage and routes:

Asymptomatic
• *Adult:* Orally, 500 mg–1500 mg daily depending on the individual patient

Symptomatic

• *Adult:* Orally, 200 mg every 4 hr, decreasing to 100 mg every 4 hr in advanced disease, if not well tolerated. IV infusion 2.5 mg/kg every 4 hr for a maximum of 2 weeks
• *Children over 3 months:* Orally 180 mg/m^2 body surface area every 6 hr
• In haematological toxicity a brief interruption of therapy (2–4 weeks) or dose reduction may be necessary
• In hepatic impairment dosage reduction may be necessary, according to plasma levels

Available forms include: Capsules 100 mg, 250 mg, syrup 50 mg in 5 ml, injection (for dilution and infusion) 20 mg per ml (10 ml)

Side effects/adverse reactions:
HAEM: Neutropenia, leucopenia, anaemia
CNS: Fever, headache, malaise, asthenia, dizziness, insomnia, sweating, paraesthesia, somnolence, chills, anxiety, depression, loss of mental acuity
GI: Nausea, vomiting, diarrhoea, abdominal pain, anorexia, dyspepsia, flatulence
RESP: Dyspnoea, cough
EENT: Taste change
INTEG: Rash, pruritus, urticaria
MS: Myalgia
GU: Frequency
General: Chest pain, influenza-like syndrome, generalised pain

Contraindications: Hypersensitivity, neutrophils less than 0.75 × 10^9/litre or haemoglobin less than 7.5 g/decilitre; avoid in breast-feeding

Precautions: Pregnancy, children, renal and hepatic impairment, elderly, haematological toxicity, adjust dose if anaemia or myelosuppression. Pre-existing bone marrow compromise (lower dose)

Pharmacokinetics: In healthy adults
By mouth: Rapidly absorbed from GI tract, peak ½–1½ hr, metabolised in liver (inactive metabolites) and intracellularly, plasma half-life — 1 hr, excreted by kidneys (some tubular secretion). Plasma protein binding is relatively low

Interactions/incompatibilities:
• Limited experience — care with all combined regimes
• Increased risk of toxicity: amphotericin, doxorubicin, dapsone, flucytosine, ganciclovir (profound myelosuppression), interferon, vincristine, vinblastine, pentamidine, probenecid, and all nephrotoxic and myelosuppressive drugs
• Increased risk of: paracetamol, neutropenia
• Altered blood levels of: phenytoin
• Altered metabolism of zidovudine: aspirin, codeine, morphine, indomethacin, ketoprofen, naproxen, oxazepam, lorazepam, cimetidine, clofibrate, dapsone, isoprinosine, paracetamol
• Antagonise antiviral effect of zidovudine: nucleoside analogues
• Extreme lethargy: IV acyclovir
• Profound myelosuppression: ganciclovir

Clinical assessment:
• Full blood counts at least every 2 wks for first 3 months, thereafter at least monthly; if low, dose adjustments may be necessary or therapy may need to be discontinued and restarted after haematologic recovery; blood transfusions may be required
• Monitor plasma zidovudine (and its glucuronide) levels in renal and hepatic impairment
• Watch for signs of intolerance

Treatment of overdose: Observe closely for evidence of toxicity and give necessary supportive therapy. Haemodialysis enhances elimination of glucuronide metabolite but limited effect on zidovudine elimination

NURSING CONSIDERATIONS

Administer:

• By mouth, capsules should be swallowed whole

• Trimethoprim-sulfamethoxazole, pyrimethamine, or acyclovir as ordered to prevent opportunistic infections; if these drugs are given, watch for neurotoxicity

Perform/provide:

• Storage in cool environment, protect from light

Evaluate:

• Blood dyscrasias (anaemia, granulocytopenia): bruising, fatigue, bleeding, poor healing

Teach patient/family:

• Drug is not cure for AIDS, but will control symptoms

• To call clinician if sore throat, swollen lymph nodes, malaise, fever occur since other infections may occur

• That even with drug administration, patient is still infective and may pass AIDS virus on to others

• That follow-up visits must be continued since serious toxicity may occur, blood counts must be done every 2 weeks

• That drug must be taken every 4 hr around clock even during night

• That serious drug interactions may occur if non-prescribed products are ingested, check with clinician first

• That other drugs may be necessary to prevent other infections

zinc sulphate

Solvazinc, Zincomed, Z Span, many combination products

Func. class.: Trace element

Chem. class.: Zinc salt

Legal class.: P

Action: Needed for adequate healing, bone and joint development. Zinc is a constituent of many enzyme systems and an integral part of insulin

Uses: Demonstrated zinc deficiency

Dosage and routes:

• *Adult:* By mouth. Depends on individual formulation, 45–50 mg zinc 1–3 times daily

Available forms include: Effervescent tablets 200 mg (45 mg zinc); capsules 220 mg (50 mg zinc); modified-release capsules 61.8 mg (monohydrate) (22.5 mg zinc)

Side effects/adverse reactions:

GI: Abdominal pain, dyspepsia, GI irritation

Precautions: Renal failure

Pharmacokinetics: Partially absorbed from GI tract, excreted in faeces traces in urine

Interactions/incompatibilities:

• Reduced absorption of: ciprofloxacin tetracycline, oral iron, penicillamine

• Reduced absorption of zinc: tetracyclines, oral iron

Treatment of overdose: In gross overdose is corrosive; avoid gastric lavage or emesis; give demulcents (e.g. milk); chelating agents (e.g. dimercaprol, penicillamine, edetic acid) have been recommended. Absorption of zinc slowed by modified release. Give symptomatic and supportive therapy

NURSING CONSIDERATIONS

Administer:

• With meals to decrease gastric upset; avoid dairy products

Evaluate:

• Zinc levels during treatment

• Therapeutic response: absence of zinc deficiency

Teach patient/family:

• That element will need to be taken for 2 months to be effective

• To immediately report nausea, diarrhoea, rash, severe vomiting, restlessness

zinc sulphate (ophthalmic)

Sootheye

Func. class.: Astringent

Chem. class.: Zinc salt

Legal class.: P

Action: Vasoconstriction occurs by action on conjunctiva

Uses: Excessive lachrymation

Dosage and routes:

• *Adult and child over 2 yr:* Instil 1–2 drops two or three times a day

Available forms include: Solution—eye drops 0.25% 10 ml

Side effects/adverse reactions:

EENT: Eye irritation, burning

NURSING CONSIDERATION

Administer:

• Use aseptic technique and, for inpatient treatment, a separate bottle for each eye of each patient

Teach patient/family:

• To report change in vision, or irritation

• Method of instillation; tilt head backward, hold dropper over eye, drop medication inside lower lid, using pressure on inside corner of eye, hold 1 min, do not touch dropper to eye

zinc undecanoate and undecenoic acid (topical)

Mycota

Func. class.: Antibiotic, topical; antifungal

Legal class.: GSL

Uses: Skin infections, particularly tinea pedis

Dosage and routes:

• *Adult and child:* Topical apply to affected areas once or twice a day

Available forms include: Cream (undecanoate 20% undecenoic acid 5%), dusting powder (undecanoate 20%, undecenoic acid 2%), spray application (undecenoic acid 2.5%, dichlorophen 0.25%)

Side effects/adverse reactions:

None common

Contraindications:

Hypersensitivity

Precautions: Pregnancy, lactation

NURSING CONSIDERATIONS

Administer:

• Enough medication to cover lesions completely

• After cleansing with soap, water before each application, dry well

Evaluate for:

• Allergic reaction: burning, stinging, swelling, redness

• Therapeutic response: decrease in size, number of lesions

Teach patient/family:

• To apply with glove to prevent further infection

• To avoid use of non-prescribed creams, ointments, lotions unless approved by clinician

• To use medical asepsis (hand washing) before, after each application

• Not to walk barefoot

zopiclone

Zimovane
Func. class.: Hypnotic
Chem. class.: Cyclopyrrolone
Legal class.: POM

Action: Non-benzodiazepine hypnotic with high affinity for CNS binding sites of GABA macromolecular receptor complex
Uses: Short-term treatment of insomnia
Dosage and routes:
• *Adult:* By mouth 7.5 mg shortly before retiring, may be increased to 15 mg if patient does not respond
• *Elderly:* Initial dose of 3.75 mg nightly
Available forms include: Tablets 7.5 mg (scored)
Side effects/adverse reactions:
GI: A mild bitter or metallic aftertaste, nausea, vomiting
CNS: Irritability, confusion, anterograde amnesia, depressed mood, drowsiness on working, hallucinations, dizziness, lightheadedness, dependence, behavioural disturbances, incoordination
Contraindications: Avoid in pregnancy and breast-feeding, children
Precautions: Hepatic insufficiency, monitor withdrawal, elderly, history of drug abuse and psychiatric illness, avoid prolonged use (avoid abrupt withdrawal thereafter)
Pharmacokinetics: Short elimination half-life 3.5 to 6 hr
Interactions/incompatibilities:
• Enhanced sedative effect: CNS depressants, alcohol, anaesthetics, opioid analgesics, antidepressants, antihistamines, α-blockers, antipsychotics, baclofen, nabilone
• May decrease antidepressant activity of trimipramine
Clinical assessment:
• Monitor therapeutic effect and effect on alertness
• Monitor length of treatment—should be no longer than 4 weeks
Treatment of overdose: Supportive and in response to clinical signs and symptoms
NURSING CONSIDERATIONS:
Administer:
• At bedtime
Perform/provide:
• Mouthwash, drink to dispel bitter, metallic taste
Evaluate:
• Therapeutic effect
• GI disturbance including nausea, vomiting
Teach patient/family:
• Not to drive or operate machinery the day after treatment until established that performance is unimpaired
• Long-term continuous treatment is not recommended. A course of treatment should last no longer than 4 weeks
• Not to discontinue abruptly; rebound insomnia may occur

zuclopenthixol acetate

Clopixol, Acuphase
Func. class.: Antipsychotic, neuroleptic
Chem. class.: Thioxanthene
Legal class.: POM

Action: Believed to be related to dopamine receptor blocking effect
Uses: Short-term management of acute psychosis, mania or exacerbations of chronic psychosis
Dosage and routes:
• Treatment duration should not exceed 2 weeks

• *Adult:* By deep IM injection, 50–150 mg (elderly 50–100 mg), if necessary repeated after 2–3 days (1 additional dose may be needed 1–2 days after the first injection); maximum cumulative dose 400 mg per course and maximum 4 injections, if maintenance treatment necessary change to oral therapy 2–3 days after last injection or to a longer acting antipsychotic depot injection given concomitantly with last injection of zuclopenthixol acetate

Available forms include: Injection (oily) 50 mg per ml, 1 ml, 2 ml

Side effects/adverse reactions:

CNS: Extrapyramidal symptoms, sedation, confusional states, epileptic fits, drowsiness. Impaired temperature regulation

EENT: Dry mouth, nasal congestion, blurred vision

ENDO: Menstrual disturbances, gynaecomastia, galactorrhoea, amenorrhoea, hyperprolactinaemia, oligomenorrhoea

GI: Constipation

GU: Difficulty with micturition or retention

CV: Postural hypotension, tachycardia

INTEG: Pain, nodule formation at injection site

Contraindications: Children, Parkinsonism, coma, breast-feeding, bone marrow depression, porphyria. Acute alcohol, barbiturate or opiate poisoning

Precautions: Treatment should not exceed 2 weeks. Hepatic impairment, advanced renal disease, elderly, pregnancy, convulsive disorders, cardiovascular disease

Pharmacokinetics: Acetate is slowly released from oil depot and rapidly hydrolysed to release zuclopenthixol. Onset of sedation shortly after injection. Antipsychotic action persists 2–3 days. Metabolised in liver. Excreted in urine and faeces

Interactions/incompatibilities:

• Enhanced sedative effect: alcohol, anxiolytics and hypnotics, barbiturates and other CNS depressants

• Enhanced hypotensive effect: anaesthetics, antihypertensives (NB: ACE inhibitors), calcium-channel blockers

• Enhanced antimuscarinic effects: tricyclics, antimuscarinics

• Antagonism: anti-epileptics (convulsive threshold lowered), bromocriptine, levodopa, lysuride, pergolide, adrenergics

• Increased risk of extrapyramidal effects: methyldopa, metirosine, rauwolfia alkaloids, metoclopramide, lithium, tetrabenazine, piperazine

• Possible neurotoxicity: lithium

• Increased risk of ventricular arrhythmias: anti-arrhythmics which prolong QT interval

• Possible enhanced effect of zuclopenthixol: cimetidine

• Blocked antihypertensive effect of guanethidine and similarly acting compounds

• Mutual inhibition of metabolism: tricyclics antidepressants

• Reduced absorption of zuclopenthixol: antacids

• Do not mix in syringe with other injection fluids

Clinical assessment:

• Prescribe anticholinergic drugs only if Parkinsonian symptoms are a problem, and reassess requirements at regular intervals

• Monitor liver function

Treatment of overdose: No specific antidote. Symptomatic and supportive treatment. Support respiratory and cardiovascular systems. Adrenaline should not be given

NURSING CONSIDERATIONS

Assess:

• Baseline vital signs and fluid balance

Administer:

• With care; contact sensitisation can occur

• Do not mix with other injection fluids in syringe

• IM into gluteal muscle or lateral thigh

• Ensure, by aspiration before injecting, that drug not given intravascularly

• Not more than 2–3 ml only injection at any one site

• Do not stop drug abruptly—withdrawal must be slow

Evaluate:

• BP (lying and standing)—postural hypotension may occur

• Pulse—tachycardia and arrhythmias may present

• Temperature—hypothermia may occur

• Urine output and intake—urinary retention may occur

• Monitor therapeutic effect and side effects and adjust dose accordingly

• Monitor length of treatment—should not be more than 2 weeks

• Monitor accumulated dose given—should not exceed 400 mg and no more than 4 injections

• Monitor blood pressure (lying and standing)

• Check mouth to ensure patient swallowed tablets

• Patient may need help with walking and other tasks if blurred vision occurs

• For Parkinsonian symptoms—give anticholinergic drugs as prescribed

• Therapeutic response—improvement of schizophrenic state, reduction of aggression, agitation, hostility

---

NB: Stop drug and inform clinician at once if signs of neuroleptic malignant syndrome occur (hyperthermia, fluctuating consciousness, muscular rigidity, pallor, tachycardia, labile BP, sweating, urinary incontinence)

Teach patient/family:

• Rise slowly as fainting may occur

• Avoid alcohol

• Avoid driving and other activities requiring alertness until certain that drowsiness does not occur

• Check with clinician before taking non-prescribed preparation

• Side effects may include menstrual disturbances or impotence

• Not to stop taking drug suddenly

• Report any side effects to clinician

• That contact sensitisation can occur

zuclopenthixol decanoate

Clopixol, Clopixol Conc

Func. class.: Antipsychotic, neuroleptic

Chem. class.: Thioxanthene

Legal class.: POM

Action: Believed to be related to dopamine receptor blocking effect

Uses: Maintenance in schizophrenia and other psychoses, particularly with aggression and agitation, where compliance with oral medication is a problem

Dosage and routes:

• Deep IM into gluteal muscle

• *Adult:* Test dose initially 100 mg then after 7–28 days 100–200 mg or more, followed by 200–400 mg repeated at intervals of 2–4 weeks adjusted according to response; maximum 600 mg per week

Available forms include: Injection (oily) 200 mg per ml, 1 ml and 10 ml 500 mg per ml, 1 ml

Side effects/adverse reactions:

CNS: Tardive dyskinesia (carefully assess risk as may be irreversible). Extrapyramidal symptoms, sedation, confusional states, epileptic fits. Impaired temperature regulation

EENT: Dry mouth, nasal congestion, blurred vision

META: Alteration in weight, oedema

HAEM: Blood dyscrasias

ENDO: Menstrual disturbances, gynaecomastia, hyperprolactinaemia, oligomenorrhoea, galactorrhoea, amenorrhoea

INTEG: Erythema, swelling, pain, nodule formation at injection site

CV: Postural hypotension, tachycardia

GI: Constipation

GU: Difficulty with micturition or retention

Contraindications: Children, Parkinsonism, coma, breast-feeding, bone marrow depression, apathetic or withdrawn states—confusional states, porphyria. Acute alcohol, barbiturate or opiate poisoning

Precautions: Pregnancy, cardiovascular or severe respiratory disease, hepatic or renal disease, elderly, arrhythmias, convulsive disorders, arteriosclerosis, phaeochromocytoma, hypothyroidism, myasthenia gravis, prostatic hypertrophy, personal or family history of narrow-angle glaucoma, thyrotoxicosis, extrapyramidal disorders

Pharmacokinetics: Decanoic ester is slowly released from the oil depot and is rapidly hydrolysed to release zuclopenthixol which is relatively short-acting. Metabolised in liver. Excreted in urine and faeces

Interactions/incompatibilities:

- Enhanced sedative effect: alcohol, anxiolytics and hypnotics, barbiturates and other CNS depressants
- Enhanced hypotensive effect: anaesthetics, antihypertensives (NB: ACE inhibitors), calcium-channel blockers
- Enhanced antimuscarinic effects: tricyclics, antimuscarinics
- Antagonism: anti-epileptics (convulsive threshold lowered), bromocriptine, levodopa, lysuride, pergolide, adrenergics
- Increased risk of extrapyramidal effects: methyldopa, metirosine, rauwolfia alkaloids, metoclopramide, lithium, tetrabenazine, piperazine
- Possible neurotoxicity: lithium
- Increased risk of ventricular arrhythmias: anti-arrhythmics which prolong to QT interval
- Possible enhanced effect of zuclopenthixol: cimetidine
- Blocked antihypertensive effect of guanethidine and similarly acting compounds
- Mutual inhibition of metabolism: tricyclic antidepressants
- Reduced absorption of zuclopenthixol: antacids
- Do not mix in syringe with other injection fluids

Clinical assessment:

- Perform blood count
- Monitor liver function
- Prescribe anticholinergic drugs only if Parkinsonian symptoms are a problem, and reassess requirement at regular intervals

Treatment of overdose: Institute measures to support respiratory and cardiovascular systems. Adrenaline should not be given. There is no specific antidote

NURSING CONSIDERATIONS

Assess:
• Baseline vital signs and fluid balance
Administer:
• With care: contact sensitisation can occur
• Ensure, by aspiration before injecting, that drug not given intravascularly
• Not more than 2–3 ml only injection at any one site
• Do not stop drug abruptly—withdrawal must be slow
Evaluate:
• BP (lying and standing)—postural hypotension may occur
• Pulse—tachycardia and arrhythmias may present
• Temperature—hypothermia may occur
• Urine output and intake—urinary retention may occur
• Therapeutic effect and side effects and adjust dose accordingly
• Monitor accumulated dose given (see dose)
• Monitor blood pressure (lying and standing)
• Check mouth to ensure patient swallowed tablets
• Patient may need help with walking and other tasks if blurred vision occurs
• For Parkinsonian symptoms—give anticholinergic drugs as prescribed
• Therapeutic response—improvement of schizophrenic state, reduction of aggression, agitation, hostility

---

NB: Stop drug and inform clinician at once if signs of neuroleptic malignant syndrome occur (hyperthermia, fluctuating consciousness, muscular rigidity, pallor, tachycardia, labile BP, sweating, urinary incontinence)

Teach patient/family:
• Rise slowly as fainting may occur
• Avoid alcohol
• Avoid driving and other activities requiring alertness until certain that drowsiness does not occur
• Check with clinician before taking non-prescribed preparation
• Side effects may include menstrual disturbances or impotence
• Not to stop taking drug suddenly
• Report any side effects to clinician
• That contact sensitisation can occur

---

zuclopenthixol dihydrochloride

Clopixol
Func. class.: Antipsychotic, neuroleptic
Chem. class.: Thioxanthene
Legal class.: POM

Action: Believed to be related to dopamine receptor blocking effect
Uses: Schizophrenia and other psychoses, particularly when associated with agitated, aggressive or hostile behaviour
Dosage and routes:
• *Adult:* By mouth, initially 20–30 mg daily in divided doses increasing to maximum 150 mg daily if necessary; usual maintenance dose, 20–50 mg daily
Available forms include: Tablets, 2 mg, 10 mg, 25 mg (as dihydrochloride)
Side effects/adverse reactions:
GI: Constipation
GU: Difficulty with micturition or retention
META: Alteration in weight, oedema
HAEM: Blood dyscrasias
CNS: Tardive dyskinesia (carefully assess risk as may be irrever-

sible), extrapyramidal symptoms, sedation, confusional states, epileptic fits. Impaired temperature regulation
EENT: Dry mouth, nasal congestion, blurred vision
ENDO: Menstrual disturbances, gynaecomastia, hyperprolactinaemia, oligomenorrhoea, galactorrhoea, amenorrhoea
CV: Postural, hypotension, tachycardia

Contraindications: Children, Parkinsonism, coma, breast feeding, bone marrow depression, porphyria, apathetic or withdrawn states. Acute alcohol, barbiturate or opiate poisoning. Patients who cannot tolerate oral neuroleptic drugs

Precautions: Pregnancy, cardiovascular or severe respiratory disease, hepatic or renal disease, elderly, arrhythmias, convulsive disorders, arteriosclerosis, phaeochromocytoma, hypothyroidism, myasthenia gravis, prostatic hypertrophy, personal or family history of narrow angle glaucoma, thyrotoxicosis, extrapyramidal disorders

Pharmacokinetics: Metabolised in gut wall and in liver. Excreted in urine and faeces

Interactions/incompatibilities:
- Enhanced sedative effect: alcohol, anxiolytics and hypnotics, barbiturates and other CNS depressants
- Enhanced hypotensive effect: anaesthetics, antihypertensives (NB: ACE inhibitors), calcium-channel blockers
- Enhanced antimuscarinic effects: tricyclics, antimuscarinics
- Antagonism: anti-epileptics (convulsive threshold lowered), bromocriptine, levodopa, lysuride, pergolide, adrenergics
- Increased risk of extrapyramidal effects: methyldopa, metirosine, rauwolfia alkaloids, metoclopramide, lithium, tetrabenazine, piperazine
- Possible neurotoxicity: lithium
- Increased risk of ventricular arrhythmias: anti-arrhythmics which prolong a QT interval
- Blocked antihypertensive effect of guanethidine and similarly acting compounds
- Mutual inhibition of metabolism: tricyclic antidepressants
- Reduced absorption of zuclopenthixol: antacids
- Do not mix in syringe with other injection fluids

Clinical assessment:
- Perform blood count
- Monitor liver function
- Prescribe anticholinergic drugs only if Parkinsonian symptoms are a problem, and reassess requirement at regular intervals

Treatment of overdose: Measures to support the respiratory and cardiovascular systems should be instituted. Adrenaline should not be given. There is no specific antidote

NURSING CONSIDERATIONS

Assess:
- Baseline vital signs and weight before commencing medication

Administer:
- With care; contact sensitisation can occur
- Protect tablets from light and moisture
- Do not stop drug abruptly—withdrawal must be slow

Evaluate:
- BP (lying and standing)—postural hypotension may occur
- Pulse—tachycardia and arrhythmias may present
- Temperature—hypothermia may occur
- Urine output and intake—urinary retention may occur
- Therapeutic effect and side effects and adjust dose accordingly

- Monitor blood pressure (lying and standing)
- Check mouth to ensure patient has swallowed tablets
- Patient may need help with walking and other tasks if blurred vision occurs
- For Parkinsonian symptoms—give anticholinergic drugs as prescribed
- Therapeutic response—improvement of schizophrenic state, reduction of aggression, agitation, hostility
- For side effects

NB: Stop drug and inform clinician at once if signs of neuroleptic malignant syndrome occur (hyperthermia, fluctuating consciousness, muscular rigidity, pallor, tachycardia, labile BP, sweating, urinary incontinence

---

Teach patient/family:

- Rise slowly as fainting may occur
- Avoid alcohol
- Avoid driving and other activities requiring alertness until certain that drowsiness does not occur
- Check with clinician before taking non-prescribed preparation
- Side effects may include menstrual disturbances or impotence
- Not to stop taking drug suddenly
- Report any side effects to clinician
- That contact sensitisation can occur

Appendixes

Appendix 1: Exemptions from the Controls on Retail Sale: Midwives

There are certain exemptions from the restrictions that apply to General Sale List Medicines, Pharmacy Medicines or Prescription Only Medicines. The classes of persons and the bodies exempted, the medicinal products to which the exemptions apply, and the conditions (if any) which attach to the sale, supply or administration by these exempted persons [include midwives and the activities associated with their professional practice]...

Retail pharmacists may sell by wholesale to the exempted persons provided the sale constitutes no more than an inconsiderable part of the business, otherwise a wholesale dealers' licence is required.

Midwives: Sale or Supply

The restrictions do not apply to the supply or sale (but not offer for sale) of certain medicinal products by a certified midwife in the course of her professional practice.

The medicinal products to which this exemption applies are: (i) all medicinal products on a General Sale List and all Pharmacy Medicines; (ii) Prescription Only Medicines containing any of the following substances but no other Prescription Only Medicine: chloral hydrate, dichloralphenazone, ergometrine maleate (only when contained in a medicinal product which is not for parenteral administration), pentazocine hydrochloride, and triclofos sodium.

Midwives: Administration

Certified midwives may also administer parenterally in the course of their professional practice Prescription Only Medicines containing any of the following substances: ergometrine maleate, levallorphan tartrate, lignocaine, lignocaine hydrochloride, naloxone hydrochloride, oxytocins (natural and synthetic), pentazocine lactate, pethidine, pethidine hydrochloride, phytomenadione and promazine hydrochloride (in the case of lignocaine, lignocaine hydrochloride and promazine hydrochloride only while attending on a woman in childbirth).

***Medicines, Ethics and Practice. A Guide for Pharmacists* (1993), No. 11, October: Royal Pharmaceutical Society of Great Britain. Reproduced with the permission of the Controller of HMSO.**

Appendix 2: Guide to Therapeutic Drug Monitoring

<table>
<tr><th>Drug</th><th>Ideal sampling time</th><th>Plasma half-life (hrs)</th><th>Time to steady state</th><th>Comments on half-life</th><th>Accepted therapeutic range</th></tr>
<tr><td>Digoxin</td><td>At least 6–8 hrs after an IV or oral dose, or predose</td><td>36–51</td><td>7–14 days</td><td>Prolonged in renal failure and/or CCF</td><td>0.8–2.2 mcg/l</td></tr>
<tr><td>Carbamazepine</td><td rowspan="4">Immediately before an oral dose</td><td>5–27</td><td>Initiation of therapy 2–4 weeks, chronic therapy: 4 days</td><td>Start with low doses as high levels seen on initiating therapy prior to auto-induction of liver enzymes. Altered by other antiepileptics. (Reduced in children.)</td><td>Multiple antiepileptics
4–8 mg/l

Single drug
8–14 mg/l</td></tr>
<tr><td>Phenobarbitone</td><td>50–120</td><td>3 weeks</td><td>Altered by other antiepileptics. (Reduced in children.)</td><td>9–25 mg/l (paediatrics)
15–40 mg/l (adults)
greater than 15 mg/l (febrile convulsions)</td></tr>
<tr><td>Valproic acid</td><td>6–17</td><td>3 days</td><td>Altered by other antiepileptics. (Reduced in children.)</td><td>50–100 mg/l</td></tr>
<tr><td>Phenytoin</td><td>20–50</td><td>2–4 weeks</td><td>Dose dependent kinetics. Altered by other antiepileptics. (Reduced in children.)</td><td>7–16 mg/l</td></tr>
</table>

Theophylline	Aminophylline/ Theophylline 1 Slow release preparation 8 hrs after a dose or pre-dose 2 During a continuous IV infusion, preferably at 6 and 18 hrs	4–16	2 days	Prolonged in cardiac failure and/or cirrhosis. Reduced in smokers. (Reduced in children.)	10–20 mg/l (adults and paediatrics) 8–15 mg/l (neonates)
Lithium	12 hrs post dose	18–36	3–4 days	Prolonged by factors reducing GFR or renal function.	0.5–1.0 mmol/l minimum effective concentration mania prophylaxis potentially toxic concentration greater than 1.5 mmol/l

Note:
Ideal sampling time: This should be adhered to whenever possible. Drug levels taken at these times provide more meaningful information.
Time to steady state: This is the earliest time a drug level should be measured either following initiation of therapy or a change of dosage (unless therapeutic failure or toxicity is suspected).
Accepted therapeutic range: This is the range associated with optimal efficiency and minimal toxicity for the majority of patients. It is important to recognise that some patients will require levels outside of the quoted response.

**Department of Clinical Pharmacy,
Guy's Hospital**

Appendix 3: Drug and Poisons Information Services

The following regional and district drug information services will provide information and advice on drugs, and drug therapy by request:

England

Birmingham		021-311 1974
	or	021-378 2211 (extn 2296 /2297)
Bristol		0272 282867
Guildford		0483 504312
Ipswich		0473 704430
	or	0473 704431
Leeds		0532 430715
Leicester		0533 555779
Liverpool		051-236 4620 (extn 2126 /2127/2128)

London

Guy's Hospital		071-955 5000 (extn 3594/5892)
	or	071-378 0023
London Hospital		071-377 7487
	or	071-377 7488
Northwick Park		081-869 3973
Manchester		061-225 2063
	or	061-276 6270
Newcastle		091-232 1525
Oxford		0865 221808
	or	0865 221836
Southampton		0703 796908
	or	0703 796909

Northern Ireland

Belfast		0232 248095
Londonderry		0504 45171 (extn 3262)

Scotland

Aberdeen		0224 681818 (extn 52316)
Dundee		0382 60111 (extn 2351)
Edinburgh		031-229 2477 (extn 2094 /2416/2443)
	or	031-229 3901
Glasgow		041-552 4726
Inverness		0463 234151 (extn 288)
	or	0463 220157

Wales

Cardiff		0222 742979

For information on poisons and in some cases advice on laboratory analytical services, the following services are available:

Belfast		0232 240503
Birmingham		021-554 3801
Cardiff		0222 709901
Dublin		0001 379964
	or	0001 379966
Edinburgh		031-229 2477 031-228 2441 (Viewdata)
Leeds		0532 430715
	or	0532 432799
London		071-635 9191
	or	071-955 5095
Newcastle		091-232 5131

Appendix 4: Immunisation Against Infectious Diseases

The Department of Health, Welsh Office, Scottish Office and DHSS (Northern Ireland) publishes an informative and readable handbook, *Immunisation against Infectious Diseases*. The 1992 edition contains details of some important changes and additions of which the most noteworthy is probably the introduction of Haemophilus influenzae b vaccine. **Please refer to individual drug monographs for the most current vaccination schedules**. [Editor]

Immunisation for foreign travel

Introduction

Health advice for travellers is becoming increasingly complex as more people travel to more remote parts of the world and new, and sometimes, unfamiliar vaccines have to be considered. This [appendix] summarises those vaccines to be considered for foreign travel. Full details are contained in the individual chapters.

Advice to an individual traveller will depend on not only the country or countries to be visited, but also the area, the season, the type of holiday, the length of stay and the age and previous health of the traveller. It must also take into account entry regulations for each country if travelling to more than one, and must allow for last-minute excursions.

It is also important to remember that the commonest illnesses acquired abroad are preventable by measures other than vaccines:

(a) ***Diarrhoea*** occurs in up to 50% of travellers abroad. It and other diseases related to poor hygiene and sanitation, such as hepatitis A and typhoid, are largely preventable by keeping to simple rules regarding personal hygiene and the food and drink consumed.

(b) ***Malaria*** – about 2000 cases of malaria are reported in the UK each year in travellers. Most are due to failure to take, or poor compliance with, malarial chemoprophylaxis.

Vaccines

See table for summary of vaccines, doses and intervals.

Recommendations

(a) ***For all travellers***

This is an ideal opportunity to check that adults have completed tetanus and polio immunisations and that childhood immunisations are up to date.

(b) ***For areas where there is still indigenous poliomyelitis, such as Africa, Asia and Eastern Europe***

Poliomyelitis vaccine

(c) ***For areas of poor hygiene***

Typhoid

Hepatitis A

(d) ***For some countries, as a condition of entry***

Yellow fever

Meningococcal meningitis

(e) ***For visits to infected areas of a country***
Yellow fever
Meningococcal menigitis
(f) ***For infected areas, in some circumstances***
Cholera – to satisfy unofficial border demands
Rabies – remote travel out of reach of medical attention
Japanese encephalitis – stays of more than one month in rural areas in the months during and after rainfall, usually June–September.
Tick-borne encephalitis – camping/walking in warm forested areas of North Europe in late spring-summer.
BCG – stays over one month; close contact with local population

Whenever possible, the recommended intervals between doses and between vaccines should be followed. Most travellers' needs can be accommodated in two visits four to six weeks apart:

First visit
Yellow fever
Typhoid – 1st dose
Tetanus – booster
Hepatitis A – 1st dose if vaccine indicated (see below)

Second visit
Typhoid – 2nd dose
Polio – booster
Meningitis
Hepatitis A immunoglobulin – (or 2nd dose of vaccine)

For short-term travel and single holiday trips, one dose of immunoglobulin gives adequate protection against hepatitis A. Hepatitis A vaccine is an alternative for those who need longer-term protection or who travel frequently to endemic areas.

Where there is less than three weeks before departure, yellow fever and polio vaccines should be given on the same day.

If the polio and tetanus doses are the first, rather than boosters, the courses should be started earlier. If time does not allow this, the 2nd and 3rd doses can be completed after travel.

If rabies and/or Japanese encephalitis vaccines are required, at least one additional visit will be required.

For most vaccines, if time is short, a single dose will afford some useful protection.

Bibliography

International Travel and Health, Vaccination Requirements and Health Advice, WHO, Geneva, Switzerland. Published every year.
A guide on safe food for travellers, WHO, Geneva, Switzerland.

Useful telephone numbers

CDSC Travel Unit (for enquiries from the medical profession); Tel. 081-200 6868.
Malaria Reference Laboratory, pre-recorded message: 071-636 7921; (Egypt, Morocco, Turkey) 071-637 0248
For professional advice: 9.00–10.30am and 2.00–3.00pm 071-636 3924
Hospital for Tropical Diseases Travel Clinic (for enquiries from the medical profession): Tel. 071-637 9899.

Immunisation for foreign travel				
	Primary course	Interval between doses	Reinforcing doses	Comments
Diphtheria less than 10 years	3 doses usually as DTP	4 weeks	On exposure to a case	Adult: Immunity should be checked before vaccination using Schick test
greater than 10 years	Low dose vaccine 3 doses of 0.5ml SC or IM	4 weeks		
Tetanus less than 10 years	3 doses usually as DTP 0.5ml SC or IM	4 weeks	1 At school entry or 3 yrs after last dose 2 Before leaving school	
greater than 10 years	3 doses adsorbed vaccine of 0.5ml SC or IM	4 weeks	1 10 yrs after primary course 2 10 yrs later	
Poliomyelitis OPV	3 doses	4 weeks	1 At school entry 2 Before leaving school 3 Every 10 years if at continuing risk	Faecal excretion of vaccine virus up to 6/52; may be longer in immune suppressed
IPV	3 doses 0.5ml SC or IM	4 weeks	As above	
Hepatitis A (vaccine adults only)	2 doses 1.0ml IM	2–4 weeks	Single booster 6–12 months after primary course	
Immuno-globulin less than 10 yrs	2/12 protection: 125mg	3–5/12 protection 250mg IM		
greater than 10 yrs	2/12 protection: 250mg	3-5/12 protection 500mg IM		

Immunisation for foreign travel				
	Primary course	Interval between doses	Reinforcing doses	Comments
Typhoid Heat killed phenol preserved				
greater than 10 yrs	0.5ml SC or IM then 0.5ml SC or IM or 0.1 ml ID	4–6 weeks Valid greater than 10 days	0.5ml IM or SC or 0.1ml ID every 3 yrs	See monograph page 814 for details of oral vaccine
1–10 yrs Vi antigen	0.25ml SC or IM then 0.25 ml SC or IM or 0.1ml ID		0.25ml IM or SC or 0.1ml ID every 3 yrs or as required for travel	
Cholera greater than 10 yrs	1 dose 0.5ml SC or IM		1.0ml	
1–10 yrs	0.3ml SC or IM		0.5ml	
1–5 yrs	0.1 MC or IM		0.3ml every 6 months or as required for travel	
Yellow fever greater than 9/12	1 dose 0.5ml SC		Every 10 yrs	Given at designated centres only
Meningo-coccal A + C greater than 2/12	1 dose 0.5ml SC or IM		Every 3 yrs	May be less effective if less than 2 yrs of age

Immunisation for foreign travel				
	Primary course	**Interval between doses**	**Reinforcing doses**	**Comments**
Rabies greater than 1 yr	3 doses 1.0ml SC or IM or 0.1m ID	0, 7 and 28 days	Every 2–3 yrs	
Japanese Encephalitis children less than 3 yrs half dose	3 doses 1.0ml SC	0, 7–14 and 28 days	greater than 3 yrs × 1	Unlicensed vaccine — named patient only
	2 doses 1.0ml SC	4 weeks	greater than 1 yr × 1	Gives immunity for 1 yr
Tick-Borne Encephalitis	3 doses 0.5ml IM	0, 4–12 weeks then 9–12 months	Single dose × 1 up to 6 yrs greater than 10 course	Unlicensed vaccine — named patients only
	2 doses 0.5ml IM	4–12 weeks	Protection 1 year	
BCG	1 (greater than Heaf testing) 0.1ml ID		None	Valid after 2 months

Immunisation against Infectious Diseases **(1992), Department of Health Welsh Office, Scottish Office and Health Department DHSS (Northern Ireland): Reproduced with permission of the Controller of HMSO.**

Appendix 5
Wound Care Products Available on FP10 Prescription

The following products are commonly used for the treatment and dressing of various types of wounds. This information has been developed according to the most recent information available prior to publication of this book.[1,2] This appendix is intended only as a general reference to wound care products available on FP10 prescription of the 1993 Drug Tariff, and does not constitute an endorsement nor a criticism of any products listed. The following publications provide detailed information about individual products: manufacturer's product literature; *Formulary of Wound Management Products* by David A. Morgan, Media Medica Publications Ltd., Chichester; or *A Handbook of Surgical Dressings* by Stephen Thomas, The Surgical Materials Testing Laboratory, Bridgend.

Wound care product	Products allowed on FP10 prescription	Products not allowed on FP10 prescription
Absorbent Cottons BP		
Absorbent Cotton (Cotton Wool)	25g, 100g, 500g	Cotton wool balls, buds, pleats, unbleached (grey), non-absorbent.
Hospital Quality	Specification 1 100g, 500g	
Bandages		
Cotton Conforming Bandage BP	5cm, 7.5cm, 10cm, 15cm × 3.5m Type A, Type B	Bandage clips and fasteners.
Cotton Crepe Bandage BP	7.5cm, 10cm × 4.5m	

Crepe Bandage BP	5cm, 7.5cm, 10cm, 15cm	Stericrepe (Beacon & Janis).
Elastic Adhesive Bandage BP	5cm, 7.5cm, 10cm × 4.5m	
Elastic Diachylon Bandage, Ventilated BPC	7.5cm × 4.5m stretched	Plain, or non-ventilated Lestreflex.
Elastic Web Bandage BP	Blue line. 7.5cm, 10cm	Other sizes.
Elastic Web Bandage with Foot Loop DT	Specification 2a. Blue line with foot loop 7.5 cm	
Elastic Web Bandage without Foot Loop DT	Specification 2b. Red line. 7.5cm × 2.75cm, 7.5cm × 3.75m	
Heavy Cotton and Rubber Elastic Bandage BP	7.5cm	Elset and Elset S (Seton), Rayon and rubber elastic bandage.
High Compression Bandages (Extensible) i) PEC High Compression Bandage [Polyamide, Elastane & Cotton Compression (High) Extensible Bandage; "PECCHE" Bandage] ii) V.E.C. High Compression Bandage [Viscose, Elastane & Cotton Compression (High) Extensible Bandage; 'VECCHE' Bandage]	Specification 52. 7.5cm × 3m unstretched 10cm × 3m unstretched 7.5cm × 3m unstretched 10cm × 3m unstretched	

Wound care product	Products allowed on FP10 prescription	Products not allowed on FP10 prescription
Knitted Polyamide and Cellulose Contour Bandage BP	5cm, 7cm, 10cm, 15cm × 4m (stretched)	
Open Wove Type 1 BP (White Open Wove; WOW)	2.5cm, 5.0cm, 7.5cm, 10cm × 5m	
Plaster of Paris Bandage BP	7.5cm, 10cm × 2.7m	15cm × 2.7m Gypsona.
Polyamide and Cellulose Contour Bandage BP (Formerly: Nylon and Viscose Stretch Bandage)	5cm, 7.5cm, 10cm, 15cm × 4m (stretched)	
Porous Flexible Adhesive Bandage BP (Titanium Dioxide Elastic Adhesive Bandage)	Specification 3 7.5cm × 4.5m	
Suspensory Bandage Cotton DT (Scrotal Support)	Small, Medium, Large, Extra large **Type 1:** Cotton net bag with draw tapes and webbing waistband. **Type 2:** Cotton net bag with elastic edge and webbing waistband. **Type 3:** Cotton net bag with elastic edge and webbing waistband with insertion of elastic centre-front.	Athletic suspensory bandages, jockstraps, Litesome (Puma, distributed by Credenhill).

Triangular Calico Bandage BP (individually wrapped)	90cm side by 127 cm base	
Tubular Bandage (see Stockinette)		
		Zinc oxide self-adhesive bandage.
Zinc Paste Bandage BP	7.5cm × 6m	
Zinc Paste and Coal Tar Bandage BP	7.5cm × 6m	
Zinc Paste and Ichthammol Bandage BP	7.5cm × 6m	
Zinc Paste, Calamine and Clioquinol Bandage BP	7.5cm × 6m	
Zinc Paste and Calamine Bandage DT	Specification 5 (ii) 7.5cm × 6m	
Cellulose Wadding BP		
Cellulose Wadding	500g.	Robert Bailey Robinson.
Dressings (see also Wound Management Dressings)		
Boil Dressings	Pack containing two boil dressings and one healing dressing.	
Knitted Viscose Dressing BP (Formerly: Sterile Knitted Viscose Dressing)	Type 1: 9.5 cm × 9.5 cm Type 2: 9.5 cm × 9.5 cm	

Wound care product	Products allowed on FP10 prescription	Products not allowed on FP10 prescription
Multiple Dressing Pack No. 1	Carton containing: Absorbent cotton BP 25g, Absorbent cotton gauze BP 90cm × 1m, Open-wove bandage BP 3.5cm × 5m	
Multiple Dressing Pack No. 2	Carton containing: Absorbent cotton BP 100g, Absorbent cotton gauze BP 3 × 90cm × 1m, Open-wove bandage BP 2 × 5cm × 5m, 1 × 7.5cm × 5m	
Perforated Film Absorbent Dressing Sterile BP (PFA Dressing)	Type 1: 5cm × 5cm, 10cm × 10cm, 20cm × 10cm 1 box = 100 dressings 1 pack = 1 dressing Type 3: 5cm × 5cm, 10cm × 10cm, 20cm × 10cm. Type 4: 5cm × 5cm, 10cm × 10cm, 20cm × 10cm	Melolite, Mepore dressings.
Providone Iodine Fabric Dressing, Sterile	Specification 43 5cm × 5cm, 9.5cm × 9.5cm 1 pack = 1 dressing	
Semi-Permeable Adhesive Film Dressing (See: Vapour-Permeable Adhesive Film Dressing BP)		

Semi-Permeable Waterproof Plastic Wound Dressing BP Sterile (See: Vapour-Permeable Waterproof Plastic Wound Dressing BP Sterile)		
Standard Dressing No. 4	Medium elastic adhesive wound dressing BPC 1963. Pack of 3.	Standard Dressing Nos. 1–3, 5–15.
Standard Dressing No. 16	Eye pad with bandage BPC, sterile	Eye pads without bandage, Opticlude eye patch.
Sterile Dressing Pack DT	Specification 10 Pack contains: Gauze and cotton tissue pad 8.5 cm × 20cm, Gauze swabs 12 ply, 4 × 10cm × 10cm, Absorbent cotton balls 4 × 0.9g, Absorbent paper towel 45cm × 50cm, Water-repellent inner wrapper 50cm × 50cm. 1 box = 12 packs	
Sterile Dressing Pack with Non-Woven Pads	Specification 35 Pack contains: Non-woven fabric covered dressing pad (Surgipad) 10cm × 20cm, Non-woven fabric swabs (Topper 8) 4 × 10cm × 10cm, Absorbent cotton wool balls 4 × 0.8g, Absorbent paper towel 45cm × 51cm, Water-repellent inner wrapper 50cm × 50cm	Surgipad when ordered alone.

Wound care product	Products allowed on FP10 prescription	Products not allowed on FP10 prescription
Vapour-Permeable Adhesive Film Dressing BP (Formerly: Semi-permeable Adhesive Film Dressing)	Type 1: 10cm × 12cm Type 2: 10cm × 12cm Type 3: 10.2cm × 12.7cm Type 4: 10cm × 14cm 1 box = 10 dressings	Tegadem Plus, Tegadem Pouch, other sizes of Opsite, Spyrosorb, Spyroflex.
Vapour-Permeable Waterproof Plastic Wound Dressing BP Sterile (Formerly: Semi-permeable Waterproof Plastic Wound Dressing)	8.5 × 6cm	
Gauzes		
Absorbent Cotton Gauze Type 13 Light BP (Absorbent Gauze) Sterile	 1m, 3m, 5m, 10m, × 90cm	 X-ray detectable, soluble, muslin.
Non-sterile	25m roll.	50m, 100m rolls.
Gauze Dressings		
(Impregnated) Chlorhexidine Gauze Dressing BP, Sterile (Chlorhexidine Tulle Gras)	5cm × 5cm, 10cm × 10cm.	M & M Tulle, cod liver oil and honey tulle.

Framycetin Gauze Dressing BP, Sterile (Framycetin Tulle Gras)	10cm × 10cm.	
Paraffin Gauze Dressing BP, Sterile (Tulle Gras Dressing) Sodium Fusidate Gauze Dressing, Sterile BP	10cm × 10cm one-piece pack or 10-piece pack. 1 box = 10 piece pack 10cm × 10cm.	Vaseline sterile gauze.
Gauze Tissues		
Gauze and Cellulose Wadding Tissue BP (Formerly Cellulose Tissue)	500g.	
Gauze and Cotton Tissue (Gamgee Tissue) (Formerly Absorbent Gauze Tissue, Gauze Tissue) (i) Gauze and Cotton Tissue BP (ii) Gauze and Cotton Tissue DT (Hospital quality)	 500g – blue label. 500g – pink label.	Yellow label gamgee.

Wound care product	Products allowed on FP10 prescription	Products not allowed on FP10 prescription
Lint		
Absorbent Lint BP (White Lint, Plain Lint, Cotton Lint; Absorbent Cotton Lint)	25g, 100g, 500g.	
Boric Acid Lint BPC '63 (Pink Lint, Boric Acid Lint, Boric Lint)	100g.	25g boric acid lint.
Plasters		
Belladonna Adhesive Plaster BP	Medium 19cm × 12.5cm. Large 28cm × 17.5cm.	Allcocks plaster, mustard plaster, belladonna plaster with red felt backing, Salonpas plasters.
Salicylic Acid Adhesive Plaster (See Chiropody Appliances)		
Spool Plasters (See Surgical Adhesive Tapes)		
Stockinette		
Cotton Stockinette, Bleached BP Heavyweight (Cotton Stockinette) (Formerly Cotton Surgical Tubular Stockinette, Plain Cotton Stockinette)	2.5cm × 1m. 5cm × 1m. 7.5cm ×1m. 10cm × 6m. **N.B.** 1m for use as a base for Plaster of Paris or other bandages. 6m length for use as a compression bandage.	Tubegauz, Tubegauz applicators, Scholl finger bandage, Tubiton, Tubinette.

Elasticated Surgical Tubular Bandage BP (Formerly Elasticated Surgical Tubular Stockinette, ESTS, Elasticated Stockinette)	6.25cm × 0.5m, Size B. 6.25cm × 1m, Size G4 (Tubigrip only) 6.75cm × 0.5m, Size C. 6.75cm × 1m Size G4RT (Tubigrip only) 7.5cm × 0.5m, Size D. 7.5cm × 1m Size G4X (Tubigrip only) 8.75cm × 0.5m, Size E. 8.75 × 1m, Size E 10cm × 0.5m, Size F. 10cm × 1m Size G5 (Tubigrip only) 12cm × 0.5m, Size G. 12cm × 1m Size G6 (Tubigrip only)	Other sizes, 10m rolls, flesh colour rolls; all sizes, Tubigrip SSB (shaped support bandage), Tubigrip lumbar/abdominal support bandage, back support, hip spica, Tenoshape.
Elasticated Surgical Tubular Stockinette, Foam Padded a) Heel, elbow or knee b) Sacral	Specification 25. Small 'P4' 6.5cm × 60cm. Medium 'P4X' 7.5cm × 60cm. Large 'P5' 10cm × 60cm. Small 'P9' 22cm × 27cm. Medium 'P9' 28cm × 27cm. Large 'P9' 35cm × 27cm.	Tubifoam, Tubipad 4m rolls.
Elasticated Viscose Stockinette (Lightweight Elasticated Viscose Tubular Bandage)	Specification 46. Green line: Medium limb 5cm × 1m Blue line: Large limb: 7.5cm × 1m Yellow line: OS limb, heads, trunks (child) 10.75cm × 1m Beige line: Trunks (adult) 17.5cm × 1m	Tubifast applicator, Tubifast red line, Tubifast starter pack.

Wound care product	Products allowed on FP10 prescription	Products not allowed on FP10 prescription
Elasticated Net Surgical Tubular Stockinette DT	Specification 26.	
Type A	Size C. Arm/leg 1.8cm × 40cm. Size E. Thigh/head 2.5cm × 60cm. Size F. Trunk (adult) 4.5cm × 60cm. Size G. Trunk (OS adult) 5.4cm × 60cm.	
Type B	Now withdrawn	Setonet
Type C	Now withdrawn	Macrofix
Ribbed Cotton and Viscose Surgical Tubular Stockinette BP	For use as a protective dressing with tar-based and other non-steroidal ointments.	
Type A	Lightweight	
Type B	Heavyweight	
	Sizing for types A and B: Arm/leg (child), arm (adult) 5cm × 5m. Arm (OS adult), leg (adult) 7.5cm × 5m. Leg (OS adult) 10cm × 5m. Trunk (child) 15cm × 5m. Trunk (adult) 20cm × 5m. Trunk (OS adult) 25cm × 5m.	

Surgical Adhesive Tapes (Plasters)		
Elastic Adhesive Tape BP Elastic Surgical Adhesive Tape) (Formerly Zinc Oxide Elastic Adhesive Plaster; Elastic Adhesive Plaster; Zinc Oxide Elastic Self-Adhesive Plaster)	2.5cm × 1.5m. 2.5cm × 4.5m. 5cm × 4.5m (See Elastic Adhesive Bandage).	Haelan tape, Hypafix tape.
Impermeable Plastic Adhesive Tape BP (Impermeable Plastic surgical Adhesive Tape) (Formerly Plastic Adhesive Strapping; Waterproof Strapping; Waterproof Plastic Surgical Adhesive Tape; Waterproof Plastic Self-Adhesive Plaster)	2.5cm × 3m. 2.5cm × 5m. 5cm × 5m 7.5cm × 5m	Other sizes, X-ray detectable plasters. Bandaid, Ultraplast, Airstrip.
Impermeable Plastic Synthetic Adhesive Tape BP (Impermeable Plastic Surgical Synthetic Adhesive Tape) (Formerly Waterproof Plastic Surgical Synthetic Adhesive Tape)	2.5cm × 5m. 5cm × 5m.	Dermiclear, Durapore, Transpore.
Permeable Woven Synthetic Adhesive Tape BP (Permeable Woven Surgical Synthetic Adhesive Tape)	1.25 × 5m. 2.5cm × 5m. 5cm × 5m.	
Permeable Non-Woven Synthetic Adhesive Tape BP (Permeable Non-Woven Surgical Synthetic Adhesive Tape)	1.25cm × 5m. 2.5cm × 5m. 5cm × 5m.	MeFix tape, Scanpor ostomy tape.

Wood care product	Products allowed on FP10 prescription	Products not allowed on FP10 prescription
Zinc Oxide Adhesive Tape BP (Zinc Oxide Surgical Adhesive Tape) (Formerly Zinc Oxide Self-Adhesive Plaster, Zinc Oxide Plaster, Adhesive Plaster)	1.25cm × 3m, 5m. 2.5cm × 1m, 3m, 5m. 5cm × 5m. 7.5cm × 5m. If no size specified, supply 2.5cm × 1m.	
Swabs		
Gauze swabs		X-ray detachable swabs, eye squares.
Gauze Swab, Type 13 Light BP, Non-Sterile	8 ply, 10cm × 10cm. 100 pads per packet.	Other thicknesses (plies), sizes and quantities, Nu-Gauze (J&J).
Gauze Swab, Type 13 Light BP, Sterile	8 ply, 7.5cm × 7.5cm. 5 pads per packet.	Other thicknesses (plies), sizes and quantities. Telfa pads (Kendall), Nu-Gauze, (J&J).
Filmated Gauze Swab BP Non-Sterile	8 ply, 10cm × 10cm. 100 pads per packet.	
Non-Woven Fabric Swabs		
Non-Woven Fabric Swab DT Non-Sterile	Specification 28. 4 ply, 10cm × 10cm. 100 pads per packet.	Sof-wick (J&J), Topper 12 (J&J)

Sterile	4 ply, 7.5cm × 7.5cm. 5 pads per packet. Alternative to gauze swabs, sterile.	Sof-Wick (J&J), Topper 12 (J&J)
Filmated Non-Woven Fabric Swab DT	Specification 29. 8 ply, 10cm × 10cm. 100 pads per packet. Alternative to Filmated Gauze Swabs, BP.	
Wound Management Dressings		
Calcium Alginate Dressing, Sterile	Specification 41 Type 1: 5cm × 5cm, 10cm × 10cm 1 box = 10 dressings Type 2: 5cm × 5cm, 7.5cm × 12cm 1 box = 10 dressings	Sorbsan 10cm × 20cm, Sorbsan ribbon, Sorbsan packing, Sorbsan SA2000, Sorbsan +. Kaltostat other sizes, Kaltostat Fortex, Kaltostat cavity dressing, Kaltocarb, Kaltoclude.
Dextranomer Paste Pad Dressing, Sterile	Specification 49 Each pad 4cm × 6 containing a past of Dextranomer 90% 1 sachet = 3g 1 box = 7 dressings	

Wound care product	Products allowed on FP10 prescription	Products not allowed on FP10 prescription
Hydrocolloidal Semi-Permeable Dressing, Sterile	Specification 42 Type 1b: 10cm × 10cm (S150), 1 box = 10 dressings 15cm × 15cm (S151), 1 box = 10 dressings 15cm × 20cm (S153), 1 box = 10 dressings 20cm × 20cm (S152), 1 box = 5 dressings	Granuflex original dressings, compression bandage, granules, paste, transparent, ulcer pack, bordered.
	Type 2: 10cm × 10cm (3213) 1 box = 10 dressings 15cm × 15cm (3218) 1 box = 5 dressings 20cm × 20cm (3223) 1 box = 5 dressings	Comfeel pressure relieving dressing, transparent sheets, wound management powder, paste.
	Type 3 10cm × 12cm (Hydrocolloidal area 7cm × 9cm) 1 box = 10 dressings 13cm × 15cm (Hydrocolloidal area 10cm × 12cm) 1 box = 5 dressings	Tegasorb 17cm × 20cm.

Hydrogel Dressing-Starch Co-Polymer, Sterile	Specification 50 15g sachet 1 box = 10 sachets	25 g sachet.
Polyurethane Foam Dressing BP, Sterile	7.5cm × 7.5cm 1 box = 5 dressings 10cm × 10cm 1 box = 5 dressings 17.5cm × 10cm 1 box = 25 dressings 20 cm × 15 cm 1 box = 20 dressings	Lyofoam 'A', 'C', or 'T'; Synthadem, Dalzofoam.

References

1. *British National Formulary (BNF)* (1993), No 25, March: British Medical Association and the Royal Pharmaceutical Society of Great Britain.
2. *The NPA Guide to the Drug Tariff and NHS Dispensing for England and Wales* (July, 1993): The National Pharmaceutical Association.

Appendix 6: Standards for the Administration of Medicines United Kingdom Central Council for Nursing, Midwifery and Health Visiting October 1992

Introduction

1. This standards paper replaces the Council's advisory paper 'Administration of Medicines' (issued in 1986) (1), and the supplementary circular 'The Administration of Medicines' (PC 88/05) (2). The Council has prepared this paper to assist practitioners to fulfil the expectations which it has of them, to serve more effectively the interests of patients and clients, and to maintain and enhance standards of practice.
2. The administration of medicines is an important aspect of the professional practice of persons whose names are on the Council's register. It is not solely a mechanistic task to be performed in

strict compliance with the written prescription of a medical practitioner. It requires thought and the exercise of professional judgement which is directed to:

2.1 confirming the correctness of the prescription;

2.2 judging the suitability of administration at the scheduled time of administration;

2.3 reinforcing the positive effect of the treatment;

2.4 enhancing the understanding of patients in respect of their prescribed medication and the avoidance of misuse of these and other medicines and

2.5 assisting in assessing the efficiency of medicines and the identification of side effects and interactions

3. To meet the standards set out in this paper is to honour, in this aspect of practice, the Council's expectation (set out in the Council's 'Code of Professional Conduct') (3) that:

> **"As a registered nurse, midwife or health visitor you are personally accountable for your practice and, in the exercise of your professional accountability must:**
>
> 1. act always in such a manner as to promote and safeguard the interests and well-being of patients and clients;
> 2. ensure that no action or omission on your part, or within your sphere of responsibility, is detrimental to the interests, condition or safety of patients and clients;
> 3. maintain and improve your professional knowledge and competence;
> 4. acknowledge any limitations in your knowledge and competence and decline any duties or responsibilities unless able to perform them in a safe and skilled manner."

4. This extract from the 'Code of Professional Conduct' applies to all persons on the Council's register irrespective of the part of the register on which their name appears. Although the content of pre-registration education programmes varies, dependent on the part and level of the register involved, the Council expects that, in this area of practice as in all others, all practitioners will have taken steps to develop their knowledge and competence and will have been assisted to this end. The word 'practitioner' is, therefore, used in the remainder of this paper to refer to all registered nurses, midwives and health visitors, each of whom must recognise the personal professional accountability which they bear for their actions. The Council therefore imposes no arbitrary boundaries between the role of the first level and second level registered practitioner in this respect.

Treatment with medicines

5. The treatment of a patient with medicines for therapeutic, diagnostic or preventative purposes is a process which involves prescribing, dispensing, administering, receiving and recording. The word 'patient' is used for convenience, but implies not only a patient in a hospital or nursing home, but also a resident of a residential home, a client in her or his own home or in a community

home, a person attending a clinic or a general practitioner's surgery and an employee attending a workplace occupational health department. 'Patient' refers to the person receiving a prescribed medicine. Each medicine has a product licence, which means that authority has been given to a manufacturer to market a particular product for administration in a particular dosage range and by specified routes.

Prescription

6. The practitioner administering a medicine against a prescription written by a registered medical practitioner, like the pharmacist responsible for dispensing it, can reasonably expect that the prescription satisfies the following criteria:
   - 6.1 that it is based, whenever possible, on the patient's awareness of the purpose of the treatment and consent (commonly implicit);
   - 6.2 that the prescription is either clearly written, typed or computer-generated, and that the entry is indelible and dated;
   - 6.3 that, where the new prescription replaces an earlier prescription, the latter has been cancelled clearly and the cancellation signed and dated by an authorised medical practitioner;
   - 6.4 that, where a prescribed substance (which replaces an earlier prescription) has been provided for a person residing at home or in a residential care home and who is dependent on others to assist with the administration, information about the change has been properly communicated;
   - 6.5 that the prescription provides clear and unequivocal identification of the patient for whom the medicine is intended;
   - 6.6 that the substance to be administered is clearly specified and, where appropriate, its form (for example tablet, capsule, suppository) stated, together with the strength, dosage, timing and frequency of administration and route of administration;
   - 6.7 that, where the prescription is provided in an out-patients or community setting, it states the duration of the course before review;
   - 6.8 that, in the case of controlled drugs, the dosage is written, together with the number of dosage units or total course if in an out-patient or community setting, the whole being in the prescriber's own handwriting;
   - 6.9 that all other prescriptions will, as a minimum, have been signed by the prescribing doctor and dated;
   - 6.10 that the registered medical practitioner understands that the administration of medicines on verbal instructions, whether she or he is present or absent, other than in exceptional circumstances, is not acceptable unless covered by the protocol method referred to in paragraph 6.11;
   - 6.11 that it is understood that, unless provided for in a specific protocol, instruction by telephone to a practitioner to administer a previously unprescribed substance is not acceptable,

the use of facsimile transmission (fax) being the preferred method in exceptional circumstances or isolated locations and

6.12 that, where it is the wish of the professional staff concerned that practitioners in a particular setting be authorised to administer, on their own authority, certain medicines, a local protocol has been agreed between medical practitioners, nurses and midwives and the pharmacist.

Dispensing

7. The practitioner administering a medicine dispensed by a pharmacist in response to a medical prescription can reasonably expect that:

7.1 the pharmacist has checked that the prescription is written correctly so as to avoid misunderstanding or error and is signed by an authorised prescriber;

7.2 the pharmacist is satisfied that any newly prescribed medicines will not dangerously interact with or nullify each other;

7.3 the pharmacist has provided the medicine in a form relevant for administration to the particular patient, provided it in an appropriate container giving the relevant information and advised appropriately on storage and security conditions;

7.4 where the substance is prescribed in a dose or to be administered by a route which falls outside its product licence, unless to be administered from a stock supply, the pharmacist will have taken steps to ensure that the prescriber is aware and has chosen to exceed that licence;

7.5 where the prescription for a specific item falls outside the terms of the product licence, whether as to its route of administration, the dosage or some other key factor, the pharmacist will have ensured that the prescriber is aware of this fact and, mindful of her or his accountability in the matter, has made a record on the prescription to this effect and has agreed to dispense the medicine ordered;

7.6 if the prescription bears any written amendments made and signed by the pharmacist, the prescriber has been consulted and advised and the amendments have been accepted and

7.7 the pharmacist, in pursuit of her or his role in monitoring the adverse side effects of medicines, wishes to be sent any information that the administering practitioner deems relevant.

Standards for the administration of medicines

8. Notwithstanding the expected adherence by registered medical practitioners and pharmacists to the criteria set out in paragraphs 6 and 7 of this paper, the nurse, midwife or health visitor must, in administering any medicines, in assisting with administration or overseeing any self-administration of medicines, exercise professional judgement and apply knowledge and skill to the situation that pertains at the time.

9. This means that, as a matter of basic principal, whether adminis-

tering a medicine, assisting in its administration or overseeing self-administration, the practitioner will be satisfied that she or he:

9.1 has an understanding of substances used for therapeutic purposes;
9.2 is able to justify any actions taken and
9.3 is prepared to be accountable for the action taken

10. Against this background, the practitioner, acting in the interests of the patients, will:
10.1 be certain of the identity of the patient to whom the medicine is to be administered;
10.2 ensure that she or he is aware of the patient's current assessment and planned programme of care;
10.3 pay due regard to the environment in which that care is being given;
10.4 scrutinise carefully, in the interests of safety, the prescription, where available, and the information provided on the relevant containers;
10.5 question the medical practitioner or pharmacist, as appropriate, if the prescription or container information is illegible, unclear, ambiguous or incomplete or where it is believed that the dosage or route of administration falls outside the product licence for the particular substance and, where believed necessary, refuse to administer the prescribed substance;
10.6 refuse to prepare substances for injection in advance of their immediate use and refuse to administer a medicine not placed in a container or drawn into a syringe by her or him, in her or his presence, or prepared by a pharmacist, except in the specific circumstances described in paragraph 40 of this paper and others where similar issues arise and
10.7 draw the attention of patients, as appropriate, to patient information leaflets concerning their prescribed medicines.

11. In addition, acting in the interests of the patient, the practitioner will:
11.1 check the expiry date of any medicine, if on the container;
11.2 carefully consider the dosage, method of administration, route and timing of administration in the context of the condition of the specific patient at the operative time;
11.3 carefully consider whether any of the prescribed medicines will or may dangerously interact with each other;
11.4 determine whether it is necessary or advisable to withhold the medicine pending consultation with the prescribing medical practitioner, the pharmacist or a fellow professional colleague;
11.5 contact the prescriber without delay where contra-indications to the administration of any prescribed medicine are observed, first taking the advice of the pharmacist where considered appropriate;
11.6 make clear, accurate and contemporaneous record of the administration of all medicines administered or deliberately

withheld, ensuring that any written entries and the signature are clear and legible;

11.7 where a medicine is refused by the patient, or the parent refuses to administer or allow administration of that medicine, make a clear, accurate record of the fact without delay, consider whether the refusal of that medicine compromises the patient's condition or the effect of other medicines, assess the situation and contact the prescriber;

11.8 use the opportunity which administration of a medicine provides for emphasising, to patients and their carers, the importance and implications of the prescribed treatment and for enhancing their understanding of its effects and side effects;

11.9 record the positive and negative effects of the medicine and make them known to the prescribing medical practitioner and the pharmacist and

11.10 take all possible steps to ensure that replaced prescription entries are correctly deleted to avoid duplication of medicines.

Applying the standards in a range of settings

Who can administer medicines?

12. There is a wide spectrum of situation in which medicines are administered ranging, at one extreme, from the patient in an intensive therapy unit who is totally dependent of registered professional staff for her or his care to, at the other extreme, the person in her or his own home administering her or his own medicines or being assisted in this respect by a relative or another person. The answer to the question of who can administer a medicine must largely depend on where within that spectrum the recipient of the medicines lies.

Administration in the hospital setting

13. It is the Council's position that, at or near the first stated end of that spectrum, assessment of response to treatment and speedy recognition of contra-indications and side effects are of great importance. Therefore, prescribed medicines should only be administered by registered practitioners who are competent for the purpose and aware of their personal accountability.

14. In this context it is the Council's position that, in the majority of circumstances, a first-level registered nurse, a midwife, or a second-level nurse, each of whom has demonstrated the necessary knowledge and competence, should be able to administer medicines without involving a second person. Exceptions to this might be:

14.1 where the practitioner is instructing a student;

14.2 where the patient's condition makes it necessary and

14.3 where local circumstances make the involvement of two persons desirable in the interests of the patients (for example, in areas of specialist care, such as a paediatric unit without sufficient specialist paediatric nurses or in other acute units dependent on temporary agency or other locum staff).

15. In respect of the administration of intravenous drugs by practitioners, it is the Council's position that this is acceptable, provided that, as in all other aspects of practice, the practitioner is satisfied with her or his competence and mindful or her or his personal accountability.
16. The Council is opposed to the involvement of persons who are not registered practitioners in the administration of medicines in acute care settings and with ill or dependent patients, since the requirements of paragraphs 8 to 11 inclusive of this paper cannot then be satisfied. It accepts, however, that the professional judgement of an individual practitioner should be used to identify those situations in which informal carers might be instructed and prepared to accept a delegated responsibility in this respect.

Administration in the domestic or quasi-domestic setting

17. It is evident that in this setting, on the majority of occasions, there is no involvement of registered practitioners. Where a practitioner engaged in community practice dose become involved in assisting with or overseeing administration, then she or he must observe paragraphs 8 to 11 of this paper and apply them to the required degree. She or he must also recognise that, even if not employed in posts requiring registration with the Council, she or he remains accountable to the Council.
18. The same principles apply where prescribed medicines are being administered to residents in small community homes or in residential care homes. To the maximum degree possible, though related to their ability to manage the care and administration of their prescribed medicines and comprehend their significance, the residents should be regarded as if in their own home. Where assistance is required, the person providing it fills the role of an informal carer, family member or friend. However, as with the situation described in paragraph 17, where a professional practitioner is involved, a personal accountability is borne. The advice of a community pharmacist should be sought when necessary.

Self-administration of medicines in hospitals or registered nursing homes

19. The Council welcomes and supports the development of self-administration of medicines and administration by parents to children wherever it is appropriate and the necessary security and storage arrangements are available.
20. For the hospital patient approaching discharge, but who will continue on a prescribed medicines regimen following the return home, there are obvious benefits in adjusting to the responsibility of self-administration while still having access to professional support. It is accepted that, to facilitate this transition, practitioners may assist patients to administer their medicines safely by preparing a form of medication card containing information transcribed from other sources.

21. For the long-stay patient, whether in hospital or a nursing home, self-administration can help foster a feeling of independence and control in one aspect of life.
22. It is essential, however, that where self-administration is introduced for all or some patients, arrangements must be in place for the appropriate, safe and secure storage of the medicines, access to which is limited to the specific patient.

The use of monitored dosage systems

23. Monitored dosage systems, for the purpose of this paper, are systems which involve a community pharmacist, in response to the full prescription of medicines for a specific person, dispensing those medicines into a special container with sections for days of the week and times within those days and delivering the container, or supplying the medicines in a special container or blister packs, with appropriate additional information, to the nursing home, residential care home or domestic residence. The Council is aware of the development of such monitored dosage systems and accepts, provided they are able to satisfy strict criteria established by the Royal Pharmaceutical Society of Great Britain and other official pharmaceutical organisations, that substances which react to each other are not supplied in this way, and that they are suitable for the intended purpose as judged by the nursing profession and have a valuable place in the administration of medicines.
24. While, to the present, their use has been primarily in registered nursing homes and some community or residential care homes, there seems no reason why, provided the systems can satisfy the standards referred to in paragraph 25, their use should not be extended.
25. In order to be acceptable for use in hospitals or registered nursing homes, the containers for the medicines must:
    25.1 satisfy the requirements of the Royal Pharmaceutical Society of Great Britain for an original container;
    25.2 be filled by a pharmacist and sealed by her or him or under her or his control and delivered complete to the user;
    25.3 be accompanied by clear and comprehensive documentation which forms the medical practitioner's prescription;
    25.4 bear the means of identifying tablets of similar appearance so that, should it be necessary to withhold one tablet (for example Digoxin), it can be identified from those in the container space for the particular time and day;
    25.5 be able to be stored in a secure place and
    25.6 make it apparent if the containers (be they blister packs or spaces within a container) have been tampered with between the closure and sealing by the pharmacist and the time of administration.
26. While the introduction of a monitored dosage system transfers to the pharmacist the responsibility for being satisfied that the container is filled and sealed correctly so as to comply with the prescription, it does not alter the fact that the practitioner administering the medicines must still consider the appropriateness of each medicine as the time of administration falls due. It is not the

case, therefore, that the use of a monitored dosage system allows the administration of medicines to be undertaken by unqualified personnel.

27. It is not acceptable, in lieu of a pharmacist-filled monitored dosage system container, for a practitioner to transfer medicines from their original containers into an unsealed container for administration at a later stage by another person, whether or not that person is a registered practitioner. This is an unsafe practice, which carries risks for both practitioner and patient. Similarly, it is not acceptable to interfere with a sealed section at any time between its closure by the pharmacist and the scheduled time of administration.

The role of nurses, midwives and health visitors in community practice in the administration of medicines

28. Any practitioner who, whether as a planned intervention or incidentally, becomes involved in administering a medicine or assisting with or overseeing such administration, must apply paragraphs 8 to 11 of this paper to the degree to which they are relevant.
29. Where a practitioner working in the community becomes involved in obtaining prescribed medicines for patients, she or he must recognise her or his responsibility for safe transit and correct delivery.
30. Community psychiatric nurses whose practice involves them in providing assistance to patients to reduce and eliminate their dependence on addictive drugs should ensure that they are aware of the potential value of short-term prescriptions and encourage their use where appropriate in the long-term interests of their clients. They must not resort to holding or carrying prescribed controlled drugs to avoid their misuse by those clients.
31. Special arrangements and certain exemptions apply to occupational health nurses. These are described in Information Document 11 and the Appendixes of 'A Guide to an Occupational Health Nursing Service: A Handbook for Employers and Nurses', published by the Royal College of Nursing (4).
32. Some practitioners employed in the community, including in particular community nurses, practice nurses and health visitors, in order to enhance disease prevention, will receive requests to participate in vaccination and immunisation programmes. Normally these requests will be accompanied by specific named prescriptions or be covered by a protocol setting out the arrangements within which substances can be administered to certain categories of persons who meet the stated criteria. The facility provided by the 'Medicines Act 1968' (5) for substances to be administered to a number of people in response to an advanced 'direction' is valuable in this respect. Where it has not been possible to anticipate the possible need for preventive treatment and there is no relevant protocol or advance direction, particularly in respect of patients about to travel abroad and requiring preven-

tive treatment, a telephone conversation with a registered medical practitioner will suffice as authorisation for a single administration. It is not, however, sufficient as a basis for supplying a quantity of medicines.

Midwives and midwifery practice

33. Midwives should refer to the current editions of both the Council's 'Midwives Rules' (6) and 'A Midwife's Code of Practice' (7), and specifically to the sections concerning administration of medicines. At the time of publication of this paper, 'Midwives' Rules' sets out the practising midwife's responsibility in respect of the administration of medicines and other forms of pain relief. 'A Midwife's Code of Practice' refers to the authority provided by the 'Medicines Act 1968' and the 'Misuse of Drugs Act 1971' (8), and regulations made as a result, for midwives to obtain and administer certain substances.

What if the Council's standards in paragraphs 8 to 11 cannot be applied?

34. There are certain situations in which practitioners are involved in the administration of medicines where some of the criteria stated above either cannot be applied or, if applied, would introduce dangerous delay with consequent risk to patients. These will include occupational health settings in some industries, small hospitals with no resident medical staff and possibly some specialist units within larger hospitals and some community settings.

35. With the exception of the administration of substances for the purpose of vaccination or immunisation described in paragraph 32 above, in any situation to which a practitioner may be expected or required to administer 'prescription-only medicines' which have not been directly prescribed for a named patient by a registered medical practitioner who has examined the patient and made a diagnosis, it is essential that a clear local policy be determined and made known to all practitioners involved with prescribing and administration. This will make it possible for action to be taken in patients' interests while protecting practitioners from the risk of complaint which might otherwise jeopardise their position.

36. Therefore, where such a situation will or may apply, a local policy should be agreed and documented which:
    - 36.1 states the circumstances in which particular 'prescription-only medicines' may be administered in advance of examination by a doctor;
    - 36.2 ensures the relevant knowledge and skill of those to be involved in administration;
    - 36.3 describes the form, route and dosage range of the medicines so authorised and
    - 36.4 wherever possible, satisfies the requirements of Section 58 of the 'Medicines Act 1968' as a 'direction'.

Substances for topical application

37. The standards set out in this paper apply, to the degree to which they are relevant, to substances used for wound dressing and other topical applications. Where a practitioner uses a substance or product which has not been prescribed, she or he must have considered the matter sufficiently to be able to justify its use in the particular circumstances.

The administration of homeopathic or herbal substances

38. Homeopathic and herbal medicines are subject to the licensing provisions of the 'Medicines Act 1968', although those on the market when that Act became operative (which means most of those now available) received product licenses without any evaluation of their efficacy, safety or quality. Practitioners should, therefore, make themselves generally aware of common substances used in their particular area of practice. It is necessary to respect the right of individuals to administer to themselves, or to request a practitioner to assist in the administration or substances in these categories. If, when faced with a patient or client whose desire to receive medicines of this kind appears to create potential difficulties, or if it is felt that the substances might either be an inappropriate response to the presenting symptoms or likely to negate or enhance the effect of prescribed medicines, the practitioner, acting in the interests of the patient or client, should consider contacting the relevant registered medical practitioner, but must also be mindful of the need not to override the patient's rights.

Complementary and alternative therapies

39. Some registered nurses, midwives and health visitors, having first undertaken successfully a training in complementary or alternative therapy which involves the use of substances such as essential oils, apply their specialist knowledge and skill in their practice. It is essential that practice in these respects, as in all others, is based upon sound principles, available knowledge and skill. The importance of consent to the use of such treatment must be recognised. So, too, must the practitioner's personal accountability for her or his professional practice.

Practitioners assuming responsibility for care which includes medicines being administered which were previously checked by other practitioners

40. Paragraph 10.6 of this paper referred to the unacceptability of a practitioner administering a substance drawn into a syringe or container by another practitioner when the practitioner taking over responsibility for the patient was not present. An exception

to this is an already established intravenous infusion, the use of a syringe pump or some other kind of continuous or intermittent infusion or injection apparatus, where a valid prescription exists, a responsible practitioner has signed for the container of fluid and any additives being administered and the container are clearly and indelibly labelled. The label must clearly show the contents and be signed and dated. The same measures must apply equally to other means of administration of such substances through, for example, central venous, arterial or epidural lines. Strict discipline must be applied to the recording of any substances being administered by any of the methods referred to in this paragraph and to reporting procedures between staff as they change and transfer responsibility for care.

Management of errors or incidents in the administration of medicines

41. In a number of its Annual Reports, the Council has recorded its concern that practitioners who have made mistakes under pressure of work, and have been honest and open about those mistakes to their senior staff, appear often to have been made the subject of disciplinary action in a way which seems likely to discourage the reporting of incidents and therefore be to the potential detriment of patients and of standards.
42. When considering allegations of misconduct arising out of errors in the administration of medicines, the Council's Professional Conduct Committee takes great care to distinguish between those cases where the error was the result of reckless practice and was concealed and those which resulted from serious pressure of work and where there was immediate, honest disclosure in the patient's interest. The Council recognises the prerogative of managers to take local disciplinary action where it is considered to be appropriate but urges that they also consider each incident in its particular context and similarly discriminate between the two categories described.
43. The Council's position is that all errors and incidents require a thorough and careful investigation which takes full account of the circumstances and context of the event and the position of the practitioner involved. Events of this kind call equally for sensitive management and a comprehensive assessment of all the circumstances before a professional and managerial decision is reached on the appropriate way to proceed.

Future arrangements for prescribing by nurses

44. In March 1992 the Act of Parliament entitled the 'Medicinal Products: Prescription by Nurses etc. Act 1992' (9) became law. This legislation came into operation in October 1993. The legislation will permit nurses with a district nursing or health visiting qualification to prescribe certain products from a Nurse Prescribers' Formulary. The statutory rules, yet to be completed, will specify the categories of nurses who can prescribe under this

limited legislation. The Council will issue further information concerning this important new legislation prior to it becoming operative.

45. Enquiries in respect of this Council paper should be directed to the:

Registrar and Chief Executive
United Kingdom Central Council
for Nursing, Midwifery and
Health Visiting
23 Portland Place
London WC1 3AF

References

1. United Kingdom Central Council for Nursing, Midwifery and Health Visiting, 'Administration of Medicines; A UKCC Advisory Paper; A framework to assist individual professional judgement and the development of local policies and guidelines', April 1986.
2. United Kingdom Central Council for Nursing, Midwifery and Health Visiting, 'The Administration of Medicines', PC 88/05, September 1988.
3. United Kingdom Central Council for Nursing, Midwifery and Health Visiting, 'Code of Professional Conduct for the Nurse, Midwife and Health Visitor', Third Edition, June 1992.
4. Royal College of Nursing, 'A Guide to an Occupational Health Nursing Service; A Handbook for Employers and Nurses', Second Edition 1991.
5. 'Medicines Act 1968', Her Majesty's Stationary Office, London, Reprinted 1986.
6. United Kingdom Central Council for Nursing, Midwifery and Health Visiting, 'Midwives' Rules', March 1991.
7. United Kingdom Central Council for Nursing, Midwifery and Health Visiting, 'A Midwife's Code of Practice', March 1991.
8. 'Misuse of Drugs Act 1971', Her Majesty's Stationary Office, London, Reprinted 1985.
9. 'Medicinal Products: Prescription by Nurses, etc. Act 1992', Her Majesty's Stationary Office, London, 1992.

Bibliography

ABPI Data Sheet Compendium (1993–1994): Datapharm Publications Ltd.

American Hospital Formulary Service. Drug Information 93 (1993): American Society of Hospital Pharmacists.

British National Formulary (BNF) (1993), No. 25, March: British Medical Association and the Royal Pharmaceutical Society of Great Britain.

Dollery, Professor, Sir C.T. (ed.) *Therapeutic Drugs* (1991), Vols 1 and 2: Churchill Livingstone.

Goodman Gilman, A., Rall, T.W., Nies, A.S., Taylor, P. (eds) *The Pharmacological Basis of Therapeutics* (1990): Pergamon Press, Inc.

Immunisation against Infectious Diseases (1992), Department of Health Welsh Office, Scottish Office and Health Department DHSS (Northern Ireland).

Martindale, The Extra Pharmacopoeia (1993), 30th edn: Pharmaceutical Press.

Medicines, Ethics and Practice. A Guide for Pharmacists (1993), No. 11, October: Royal Pharmaceutical Society of Great Britain.

Stockley, I.H. *Drug Interactions* (1991), 2nd edn: Blackwell Scientific Publications.

index of generic drugs and trade names

Index of generic drugs by functional classes

Central nervous system disorders

Ear, nose and throat disorders

Endocrine system disorders

Eye disorders

Gastrointestinal system disorders

Infection

Obstetrics, gynaecology and urinary tract disorders

Respiratory system disorders

Skin disorders

Vaccines and immunological agents